## SUPRATENTORIAL COMPARTMENT ( ____ )

**Table of Illustrated Differential Diagnoses is continued on inside back cover.**

# MAGNETIC RESONANCE IMAGING OF CNS DISEASE

*A Teaching File*

Second Edition

# MAGNETIC RESONANCE IMAGING OF CNS DISEASE

*A Teaching File*

## DOUGLAS H. YOCK, JR., MD

Departments of Neuroscience and Radiology
Abbott Northwestern Hospital
Minneapolis, Minnesota

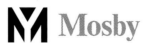 Mosby

St. Louis   London   Philadelphia   Sydney   Toronto

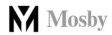

*Editor:* Janice Gaillard
*Developmental Editor:* Danielle Burke
*Project Manager:* Pat Joiner
*Designer:* Mark Oberkrom

Mosby, Inc.
11830 Westline Industrial Drive
St. Louis, Missouri 63146

Printed in the United States of America

**International Standard Book Number 0-323-01172-1**

01  02  03  04  05  TG/MVY  9  8  7  6  5  4  3  2  1

# FOREWORD

When Doug Yock asked me if I would write the Foreword to the second edition of *Magnetic Resonance Imaging of CNS Disease: A Teaching File,* I was immediately flattered, then humbled. My thoughts went back to 25 years ago, when I had the happy privilege to work with Doug at the Stanford University Medical Center. He was a resident, and I was a junior faculty member just finishing a neuroradiology fellowship. I think he taught me more than I did him; we had a wonderful time. Hans Newton said to me later, after Doug had spent some time with him at the University of California–San Francisco, "How do you get these stars at Stanford?" He was envious of our good fortune and rightfully so.

We tried hard to get Doug to stay in California, but Minnesota beckoned. For 25 years we have hoped that he would return! However, he did take a little of us with him; the nidus of his first Teaching File CT book came from cases he painstakingly collected at Stanford. When that book came out, it quickly became a favorite of mine and my residents; it was comprehensive, meticulously prepared, transparently organized, and useful far beyond the mere atlas.

It was no surprise when Dr. Yock followed this achievement with the publication of his MRI CNS Teaching File, and it was even better than his first book. Over 1000 cases, all arranged in a logical, didactic style, served simultaneously as a textbook of neuroradiology, a review atlas, and a reference. This is my favorite neuroradiology book (and I have them all). I use it primarily as a reference whenever I have a difficult case. I loan it to my residents and fellows. The pictorial index at the back of the book is especially valuable, an inspired appendix to an already overflowing cornucopia of delights.

This second edition miraculously surpasses the first. Over half the images are new; techniques such as diffusion-weighted imaging are included; differential diagnoses are brilliantly illustrated. Even a casual perusal impresses the reader with the quality of the illustrations, the selection of images, and the concise discussions. Everything in it reflects the thoughtfulness that is the hallmark of Dr. Yock's works.

It is truly a pleasure and an honor to introduce this book. Congratulations to the author for what is destined to be a most successful and popular edition. I know it will be the next book on my shelf.

**Barton Lane, MD**
Professor of Radiology and Neurosurgery
Stanford University Medical Center
Chief of Radiology
Palo Alto Veterans Administration Medical Center
Palo Alto, California

# PREFACE

This edition has been largely rewritten to incorporate technical advances and growing clinical experience. About half of the cases in the previous collection have been replaced with better examples, and many additional pathologies are newly presented. Several chapters have been expanded and divided, including those covering tumors of the posterior fossa, inflammatory and metabolic disorders, infarction and anoxia, hemorrhage and vascular lesions, and spinal tumors. The pictorial index has also been enlarged.

The structure of the teaching file is unchanged. Each page centers on a pair of scans demonstrating typical or unusual appearances of a particular disorder. Facing pages usually form a group of four images illustrating the MR spectrum of one condition or the potential resemblance of different processes.

Cases have been sequenced to build an expanding fund of knowledge. Cross-references connect the cases to point out similarities or distinctions.

The text concentrates on the interpretation of MR scans. Common diagnostic problems are stressed, and useful clues are suggested, with 150 illustrated "Differential Diagnoses." Discussions often include clinical correlation and pathophysiology.

Images and text have been edited to provide an overview that is thorough but reasonably concise. An effort has been made to balance scope and focus.

The organization and emphasis of the book are intended to support learning, review, and reference. Each chapter can be read from beginning to end as a series of miniconferences, scanned as a survey of pathology, or explored as a library of images for comparison to a specific case.

However this collection is used, I hope that it will be a helpful catalogue of CNS disease as viewed through the window of magnetic resonance imaging.

**Douglas H. Yock, Jr., MD**

# ACKNOWLEDGMENTS

Most of the MR studies in this collection were performed at Abbott Northwestern Hospital in Minneapolis by an outstanding group of skilled technologists. Several scans from Centennial Lakes/Edina Imaging Center and the Minnesota Diagnostic Center have also been included. Additional cases were generously contributed by Drs. Lanning Houston, Brian Larkin, Daniel Loes, Eduard Michel, Hugh Neeson, Mary Jo Nelson, Charles Truwit, and Clarke Tungseth of Minneapolis; John Huston of Rochester; Mory Jahangir of New Prague; David Kispert of St. Paul; Robert McGeachie of Duluth; Matthew Stone of Bismarck, North Dakota; and W. Michael Hensley of Parkersburg, West Virginia.

Drs. Anthony Cook, William Ford, Stephen Fry, David Larson, Mark Myers, John Steely, and David Tubman shared in the daily supervision of MR procedures and in the selection of teaching material. Dr. Larson and Dr. Steely reviewed the manuscript; I thank them for their willingness to undertake this time-consuming task.

Karla Fredrick, Patti Gutbrod, and Marilyn Miller processed the text with a remarkable combination of diligence and cheerfulness.

Gordon Sprenger, Robert Spinner, and Mark Dixon of Abbott Northwestern Hospital encouraged this project and have supported the development of a strong neuroscience program, from which the following cases are drawn. The neurologists and neurosurgeons at Abbott Northwestern have contributed directly and indirectly to the book through active practices and collegial exchange.

Janice Gaillard and her associates at Elsevier Health Sciences in Philadelphia and St. Louis provided editorial guidance for this edition. Carol Weis and her colleagues at Top Graphics in St. Louis were thorough, responsive, and efficient as they worked carefully on a tight schedule to manage the many details of production.

I remain grateful to the outstanding neuroradiologists who introduced me to their field: William Marshall, William Scott, and Barton Lane at Stanford University and T. Hans Newton and David Norman at the University of California in San Francisco.

My family deserves recognition for supporting yet another writing project with continued patience and understanding.

Finally, I thank the readers of the previous Teaching File books who have offered encouragement. Your comments are sincerely appreciated as motivation and reward.

DHY

# CONTENTS

# NOTES TO READERS

1. Axial and coronal scans are displayed with the patient's right on the reader's left.

2. All scans were performed at 1.0 T or 1.5 T.

3. Scan parameters (TR/TE) are specified only for sequences with intermediate weighting. Images with contrast predominantly determined by T1 or T2 relaxation are simply labeled as either *T1-weighted* or *T2-weighted*.

4. Abbreviations used for scan techniques are as follows:

      SE = spin echo (conventional spin echo)
     FSE = fast spin echo (rapid spin echo, turbo spin echo)
     GRE = gradient echo (gradient recalled echo, gradient refocused echo)
   FLAIR = fluid-attenuated inversion recovery
     MTS = magnetization transfer suppression/saturation

# MAGNETIC RESONANCE IMAGING OF CNS DISEASE

*A Teaching File*

# CHAPTER 1

# Metastases

### Case 1

39-year-old man complaining of headaches.
(sagittal, noncontrast T1-weighted SE scan)

### Case 2

69-year-old woman presenting with confusion.
(sagittal, noncontrast T1-weighted SE scan)

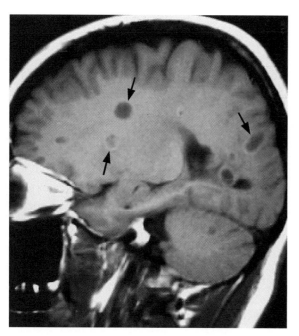

**Metastatic Adenocarcinoma of Unknown Origin**

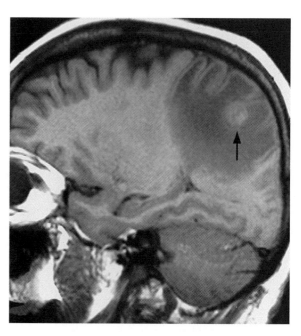

**Metastatic Carcinoma of the Breast**

Metastases are the most common adult intracranial neoplasms. Carcinomas of the breast and lung cause the greatest number of these lesions, although melanoma and hypernephroma metastasize to the brain with higher frequency. An intracranial mass accounts for the initial presentation of carcinoma in up to 10% of cases.

Nonhemorrhagic cerebral metastases are usually seen on T1-weighted MR scans as lesions of low signal intensity. The metastases themselves are typically well defined, as in Case 1 *(arrows)*. There is often surprisingly little reactive edema to obscure the interface between metastatic tissue and adjacent cerebral parenchyma. The appearance of multiple, sharply demarcated or "punched out" metastases may mimic multifocal inflammatory lesions.

Alternatively, extensive cerebral edema may surround and obscure an inciting metastatic nodule. In Case 2, the central metastasis is only faintly visible *(arrow)* within a large zone of T1 prolongation due to edema. As a result, the overall appearance in this case mimics that of a larger neoplasm, such as a primary glioma (compare to Case 71). Contrast enhancement is useful in this situation to (1) clearly define the enhancing metastasis within the larger area of abnormal signal and (2) disclose additional lesions to confirm multiplicity and favor a metastatic process.

### Case 3

58-year-old woman with no cerebral symptoms.
(axial, noncontrast T2-weighted SE scan)

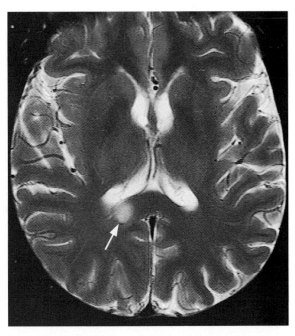

**Metastatic Carcinoma of the Breast**

### Case 4

41-year-old woman presenting with seizures.
(axial, noncontrast T2-weighted SE scan)

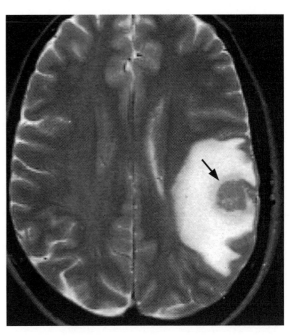

**Metastatic Carcinoma of the Breast**

The detection of nonhemorrhagic cerebral metastases on T2-weighted images depends on the presence of abnormal signal intensity within the lesion and/or the occurrence of surrounding edema. A small metastatic nodule with little edema is present in the major forceps on the right in Case 3 *(arrow)*. Multiple small metastases should be included in the differential diagnosis of focal lesions of high signal intensity on T2-weighted scans (see Cases 495 and 496). The lesion in Case 3 demonstrated enhancement after contrast was administered (see Case 17).

Case 4 represents the T2-weighted equivalent of Case 2. A central metastasis is largely isointense but is clearly outlined by a surrounding sea of edema. In other cases, a metastasis with long T2 values may be completely obscured by the increase in water content within adjacent white matter. The edema provoked by a cerebral metastasis is often more responsible for symptoms than the mass effect of the underlying neoplasm.

Some small metastases are themselves invisible on noncontrast scans but are localized by the focal edema that they incite. When one or more such lesions are found in subcortical white matter, the pattern may resemble inflammatory or demyelinating pathologies, such as progressive multifocal leukoencephalopathy (see Cases 398-401). Postcontrast scans usually narrow the differential diagnosis.

### Case 5

41-year-old man presenting with ataxia.
(axial, noncontrast T2-weighted SE scan)

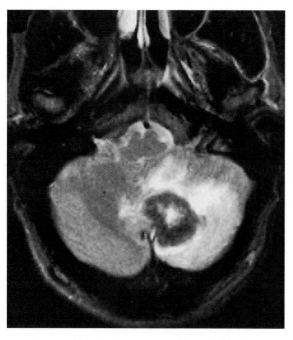

**Metastatic Adenocarcinoma of the Colon**

### Case 6

50-year-old woman presenting with a seizure.
(axial, noncontrast T2-weighted FSE scan)

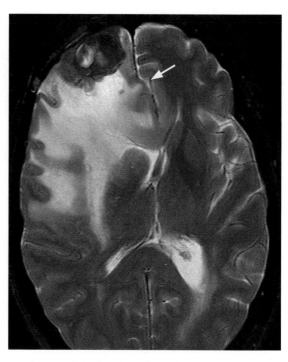

**Metastatic Adenocarcinoma of the Colon**
(recurrent)

Most cerebral metastases demonstrate high signal intensity or isointensity on T2-weighted scans, as seen in Cases 3 and 4. A minority of metastatic lesions are associated with T2-shortening, causing low signal intensity on long TR, long TE spin echo images.

Such T2-shortening may be due to hemorrhage within the metastasis (see Cases 9 and 10) or to the presence of paramagnetic material (e.g., melanin; see Case 8). Other metastases demonstrate low signal intensity on T2-weighted scans in the absence of blood products or paramagnetic molecules.

Metastases from adenocarcinoma of the colon are particularly likely to present this appearance. Short T2 values in such cases reflect some intrinsic property of the tumor tissue, possibly the presence of thickly proteinaceous material within the cells. This characteristic MR finding often correlates with increased attenuation values of the lesions on precontrast CT scans.

The cerebellum is a favorite site for intracranial metastases, as in Case 5. In fact, metastatic disease is the most common cause of a cerebellar mass in an adult (see Cases 10 and 22 for other examples).

Like the tumor in Case 5, the recurrent superficial mass in Case 6 demonstrates a small zone of central necrosis surrounded by tissue of low signal intensity. Extensive edema spreads throughout white matter of the right frontal lobe and continues posteriorly into the external capsule. The right caudate and lentiform nuclei are medially displaced, and there is prominent subfalcial herniation *(arrow)*.

Cerebral metastases are often found near the junction of gray and white matter. The superficial location reflects the high perfusion of cerebral cortex and is similar to the distribution of hematogenous cerebral infection.

### Case 7

49-year-old man presenting with a seizure.
(axial, noncontrast T1-weighted SE scan)

### Case 8

41-year-old woman being evaluated for
metastases from a known melanoma.
(axial, noncontrast T2-weighted SE scan)

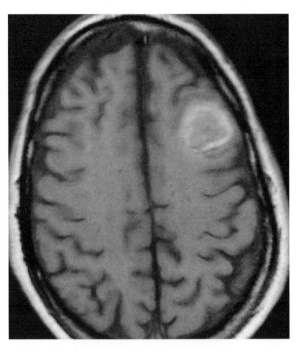

**Metastatic Melanoma**

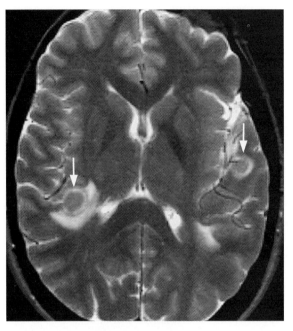

**Metastatic Melanoma**

Melanoma is among the primary tumors associated with hemorrhagic cerebral metastases (see Cases 9-12). However, even in the absence of hemorrhage, cerebral metastases from melanoma often demonstrate T1-shortening and mild T2-shortening.

The presence of the melanin molecule with its unpaired electrons is believed to account for the observed paramagnetic effects on signal intensity, although metallic ions (especially ferric iron) bound to melanin may contribute. Amelanotic metastases from primary melanomas are not associated with shortening of T1 or T2 values in the absence of hemorrhage.

The left frontal mass in Case 7 demonstrates a rim of short T1 values that resembles the margin of a benign intracerebral hematoma in the early subacute phase (see Case 675). The multiple lesions in Case 8 *(arrows)* are nearly isointense to brain but are defined by a surrounding collar of edema.

Melanoma ranks as the third most common cause of cerebral metastases, after carcinomas of the breast and lung.

### Case 9

63-year-old man presenting with right leg paresis.
(sagittal, noncontrast T1-weighted SE scan)

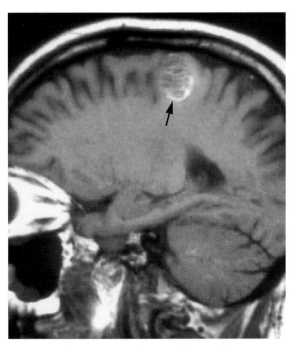

**Metastatic Carcinoma of the Lung**

### Case 10

61-year-old woman presenting with ataxia that
became acutely worse ten days prior to admission.
(coronal, noncontrast T1-weighted SE scan)

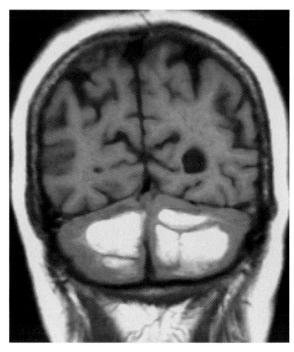

**Metastatic Carcinoma of the Colon**

---

The subcortical location and sharply defined margins of the lesion in Case 9 raise the possibility of metastatic disease. The high signal intensity on the T1-weighted image further suggests the presence of subacute or chronic hemorrhage within the lesion. (See Cases 673-676 for discussion of alterations in signal intensity caused by blood products of various ages.)

This feature narrows the likely diagnoses to those primary tumors that cause vascular metastases: melanoma, choriocarcinoma, hypernephroma, bronchogenic carcinoma, and occasionally breast carcinoma. Although hemorrhage into a cerebral metastasis is often the presenting event in metastatic melanoma, a renal or pulmonary neoplasm would be more common in a 63-year-old man.

Hemorrhagic metastases, such as the mass in Case 9, may simulate the appearance or cavernous angiomas or other "occult" vascular malformations (see Cases 761-764).

Occasionally a hemorrhagic glioma presents in a similar manner.

In Case 10, large areas of T1-shortening suggesting subacute hemorrhage are present in both cerebellar hemispheres. Spontaneous cerebellar hemorrhage is rarely bilateral. The presence of hemorrhagic masses on both sides of midline should raise the possibility of underlying structural lesions. This case is another example of the spectrum of presentations of cerebellar metastases in adults.

Hemorrhage into a cerebral or cerebellar neoplasm is one mechanism by which such subacute or chronic lesions may cause acute symptoms. Other mechanisms include the sudden triggering of reactive cerebral edema, ventricular obstruction causing acute hydrocephalus, and critical vascular compression by an enlarging mass. Between 1% and 5% of "strokes" are found to be the result of an underlying neoplasm.

### Case 11

66-year-old woman presenting with confusion.
(axial, noncontrast T2-weighted FSE scan)

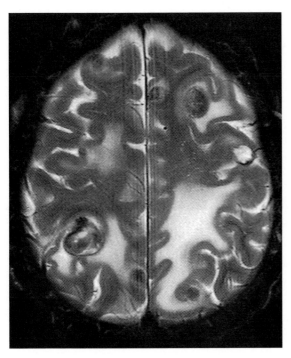

**Metastatic Hypernephroma**

### Case 12

66-year-old man presenting with personality
changes and right hemiparesis.
(axial, noncontrast scan; SE 2700/45)

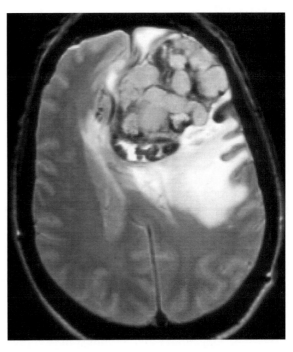

**Metastatic Carcinoma of the Lung**

---

Zones of low signal intensity within a cerebral mass on T2-weighted scans may be due to blood products, calcification, tissue that is densely fibrous or thickly proteinaceous, or flow voids in large vessels.

The multiple superficial nodules in Case 11 demonstrated areas of high signal intensity comparable to Case 9 on T1-weighted images. This combination of short T1 and T2 values suggests hemorrhagic lesions. The differential diagnosis includes multiple cavernous angiomas (see Cases 761-765), coagulopathy, trauma (see Cases 687 and 690), arteritis, and dural sinus thrombosis (see Case 650). However, the subcortical location and nodular morphology of these hemorrhagic masses and the prominent associated edema are most compatible with metastatic disease.

Case 12 illustrates the large size and complex architecture of some cerebral metastases. The combination of these features in a solitary lesion may mimic a primary glial neoplasm. A multinodular or "botryoid" configuration is somewhat unusual for metastatic disease (see Case 22 for similar morphology). Further complexity is caused by the areas of T2-shortening scattered throughout the tumor, which were pathologically proved to represent subacute hemorrhage. A giant cavernous angioma or thrombosed AVM is occasionally encountered with morphology resembling Case 12 (see Case 749).

Case 766 presents an additional example of smaller hemorrhagic cerebral metastases on long TR spin echo scans. MR detection of such lesions can be enhanced by the use of gradient echo sequences that are sensitive to the local field inhomogeneities associated with blood products.

Subfalcial herniation is present in Case 12. The combination of the metastasis and surrounding edema causes prominent frontal mass effect with a large midline shift.

## Case 13

84-year-old man presenting with confusion
and mild hemiparesis.
(sagittal, noncontrast T1-weighted SE scan)

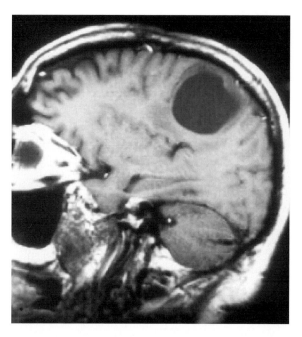

**Metastatic Squamous Cell Carcinoma of the Lung**

## Case 14

61-year-old woman presenting with
right homonymous hemianopsia.
(axial, noncontrast T2-weighted FSE scan)

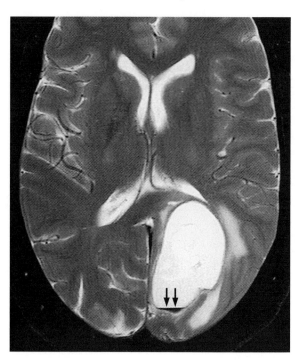

**Metastatic Adenocarcinoma of the Colon**

Large metastases may contain cystic or necrotic areas that are apparent even on noncontrast scans. The rim of tumor tissue surrounding the cyst may be surprisingly thin and uniform, as in Cases 13 and 14. In such instances, the alternative diagnosis of benign cyst or abscess may be considered. Solitary cystic metastases may also resemble malignant gliomas (see Cases 100 and 101), and the two tumors should be grouped together in the differential diagnosis.

A cystic appearance is often associated with metastatic squamous cell carcinoma, as in Case 13. Up to 50% of cerebral metastases from pulmonary squamous cell tumors are solitary, compared with about 30% of all intracranial metastases.

Case 14 demonstrates that metastatic adenocarcinomas can present similarly. A small sedimentation level of blood products is present at the posterior margin of the mass *(arrows)*, confirming the presence of a cystic cavity.

Moderate edema surrounds both of these tumors. Associated mass effect depresses the sylvian fissure and deforms adjacent sulci in Case 13. In Case 14, the trigone of the left lateral ventricle is displaced and compressed.

### Case 15

50-year-old woman presenting with seizures.
(axial, postcontrast T1-weighted SE scan)

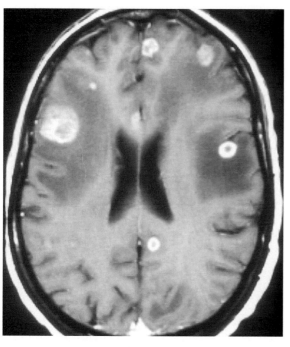

**Metastatic Carcinoma of the Breast**

### Case 16

84-year-old man presenting with confusion.
(coronal, postcontrast T1-weighted SE scan)

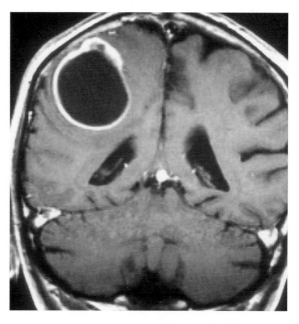

**Metastatic Squamous Cell Carcinoma of the Lung**
(same patient as Case 13)

---

Multiplicity is a hallmark of metastatic disease. The size, shape, enhancement pattern, and edema of individual lesions may vary substantially, as demonstrated in Case 15.

Small cerebral metastases are often inapparent on noncontrast scans because they are nearly isointense and have not incited reactive edema. Contrast enhancement may be the only clue to the presence of such lesions. The detection of small metastases can be of clinical importance in determining the nature of an accompanying larger mass and/or judging the appropriateness of surgery for a "solitary" lesion. Postcontrast scans using magnetization transfer suppression techniques are currently the most sensitive method to demonstrate enhancing metastases.

Large cerebral metastases may retain the well-defined, homogeneously enhancing character of small lesions. When such masses are located near a dural surface, the appearance can mimic a meningioma (see Case 198).

Other metastases demonstrate peripheral enhancement surrounding a central nonenhancing zone. The central area of little or no enhancement may represent a cyst, necrosis, or a slowly equilibrating compartment that accumulates contrast on later scans. Several lesions in Case 15 illustrate central areas of nonenhancement, while the mass in Case 16 appears to contain a large cyst. The enhancing margin of a metastatic lesion may be quite smooth and regular as in Case 16, but an irregular appearance of variable thickness is more characteristic (see Case 101).

## Case 17

58-year-old woman with no cerebral symptoms.
(axial, postcontrast T1-weighted SE scan)

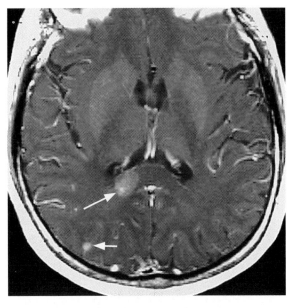

**Metastatic Carcinoma of the Breast**
(same patient as Case 3)

## Case 18

58-year-old man presenting with seizures.
(axial, postcontrast T1-weighted SE scan)

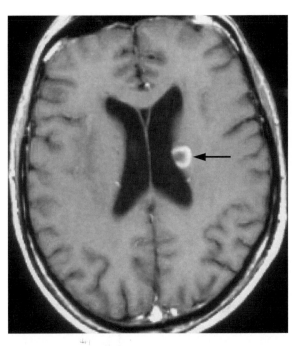

**Metastatic Carcinoma of the Lung**

---

Although superficial location is characteristic of hematogenous metastases, deep lesions are also encountered. The periventricular region is a common location for metastatic involvement by systemic lymphomas and carcinomas. Tumor cells can arrive at this site hematogenously, through CSF seeding from a metastasis near the cerebral surface, or as a result of hematogenous seeding of the highly vascular choroid plexus.

Case 17 presents a postcontrast scan of the small lesion illustrated in Case 3 *(long arrow)*. The junction of the splenium of the corpus callosum and the major forceps is a frequent site of deep hemispheric metastasis. Larger lesions in this location may resemble malignant gliomas or primary cerebral lymphomas (see Case 70).

Metastases along the ventricular margin may be focal, multifocal, or diffuse. The small, rim-enhancing mass within the corona radiata in Case 18 mimics an inflammatory lesion (e.g., active multiple sclerosis or toxoplasmosis; compare to Cases 382 and 477). The differential diagnosis of larger subependymal masses includes primary CNS neoplasms such as glioma or ependymoma, lymphoma, and giant cell astrocytoma associated with tuberous sclerosis.

Uniform enhancement of metastatic disease lining the ventricular margins may be seen with systemic lymphoma, metastatic melanoma, and metastatic carcinomas of the breast and lung (especially small cell). The differential diagnosis of enhancing ventricular margins also includes ependymal seeding or subependymal spread of gliomas and other primary CNS tumors (see Cases 110 and 111), primary CNS lymphoma, and inflammatory ventriculitis (see Case 432).

A tiny superficial metastasis is present at the posterior margin of the right cerebral hemisphere in Case 17 *(short arrow)*.

## Case 19

53-year-old man with a three-day history
of confusion.
(axial, noncontrast scan; SE 3500/34)

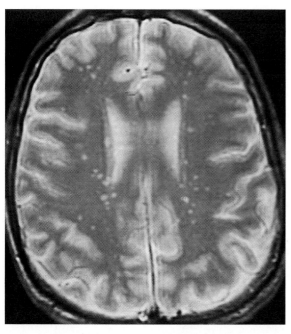

**Metastatic Carcinoma of the Lung**

## Case 20

35-year-old woman presenting with headaches.
(axial, postcontrast T1-weighted SE scan)

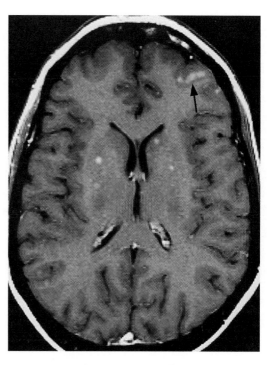

**Metastatic Carcinoma of the Breast**

Small cerebral metastases are sometimes remarkably numerous and uniform in size and morphology. The multiple foci of T2 prolongation in Case 19 demonstrated equivocal contrast enhancement and were subsequently discovered to represent metastases from a pulmonary carcinoma.

Tiny hematogenous metastases may be even more diffuse, with no abnormal enhancement to increase definition. Such "miliary" lesions may be appreciated only as a finely granular texture of increased signal intensity on T2-weighted scans, particularly within cortex and the basal ganglia.

Alternatively, multiple tiny enhancing metastases may be found within deep nuclei (as in Case 20) and/or within the cortical mantle. This appearance may resemble disseminated infection, noninfectious inflammatory processes, primary CNS lymphoma, subacute multifocal infarction, or vasculitis.

Leptomeningeal metastasis (or "carcinomatous meningitis") is present in the left frontal region in Case 20 (*arrow;* see Cases 29-31).

### Case 21

71-year-old man presenting with
a left sixth nerve palsy.
(axial, noncontrast T2-weighted SE scan)

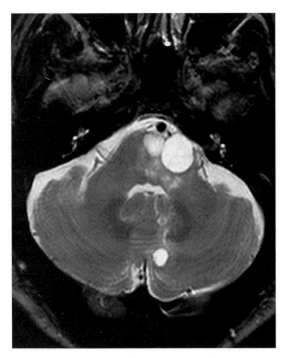

**Metastatic Adenocarcinoma of the Lung**

### Case 22

58-year-old woman presenting with abnormal gait.
(axial, postcontrast T1-weighted SE scan)

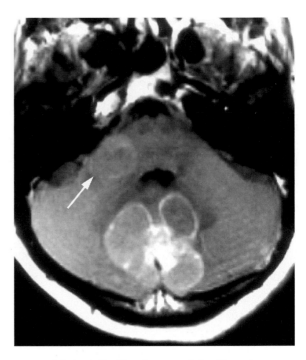

**Metastatic Carcinoma of the Breast**

The posterior fossa is a frequent site of intraaxial and extraaxial metastatic disease. Experience with CT scanning has previously established a high incidence of cerebellar metastases. More recently, MR has documented frequent intramedullary metastases involving the brainstem (and spinal cord).

The region of the mid pons and brachium pontis is a common location for metastases, as illustrated in Case 21. A large intraaxial metastasis at this site can bulge exophytically into the cerebellopontine angle cistern, potentially affecting multiple cranial nerves and mimicking an extraaxial mass (see Case 198).

The strikingly lobulated morphology of the cerebellar mass in Case 22 is unusual but within the spectrum of metastatic disease (compare to Case 12). The correct diagnosis is supported by the presence of a second lesion in the right brachium pontis *(arrow)*.

In younger adults, metastases with a "punched out" appearance as illustrated in Case 21 may resemble inflammatory disease of parasitic or demyelinating origin. (Case 1 is a good example.)

## Case 23

59-year-old woman scanned to
exclude cerebral metastases.
(sagittal, noncontrast T1-weighted SE scan)

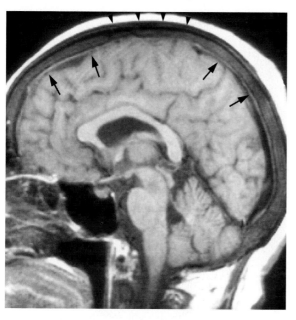

**Metastatic Carcinoma of the Breast**

## Case 24

25-year-old man presenting with
an enlarging scalp mass.
(sagittal, noncontrast T1-weighted SE scan)

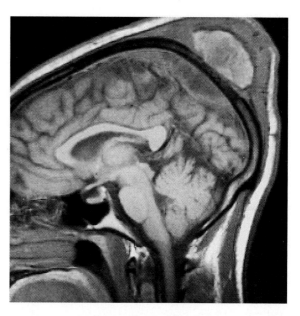

**Systemic Lymphoma**

---

Calvarial involvement by metastatic disease may be confined to bone or associated with adjacent soft tissue masses. In Case 23, the normal high signal intensity of fatty marrow in the diploic space of the skull on T1-weighted images has been uniformly replaced. This abnormally low signal intensity of the calvarium predominantly represents metastatic cellular infiltration, although reactive sclerosis may contribute in some cases (especially in metastatic carcinoma of the prostate). Only mild thickening of the underlying dura *(arrows)* and overlying scalp soft tissue *(arrowheads)* is present.

By contrast, Case 24 demonstrates large intracranial and extracranial soft tissue masses accompanying calvarial involvement by lymphoma. Dural-based metastases may also occur without overlying calvarial lesions, as seen in Cases 25, 26, and 28.

Occasional meningiomas present as transcranial masses similar to Case 24 (see Case 44). Such tumors may involve the skull base (e.g., with extension into the infratemporal fossa), as well as the convexity.

## Case 25

68-year-old man presenting with headaches
and facial weakness.
(axial, postcontrast T1-weighted SE scan)

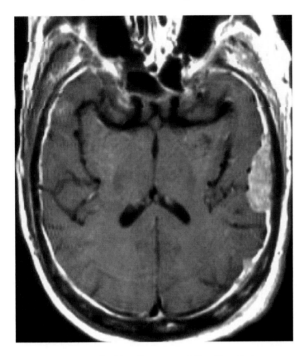

**Metastatic Carcinoma of the Prostate**

## Case 26

50-year-old woman presenting with
mediastinal adenopathy.
(coronal, postcontrast T1-weighted SE scan)

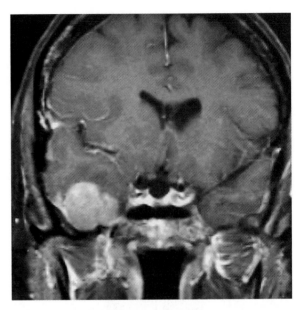

**Systemic Lymphoma**

Metastatic involvement of the dura may be an isolated primary process or reflect extension from either calvarial or cerebral lesions. The morphology of dural metastases may be mass-like, as in the above cases, or plaque-like, as illustrated on the next page.

In Case 25, thickened dural enhancement surrounds both cerebral hemispheres. Superimposed mass-like nodularity is present on the left. The nodules represent neoplastic tissue, while the more uniform surrounding enhancement is likely reactive. A separate dural-based mass was present in the cerebellopontine angle cistern, correlating with the patient's facial palsy.

Dural thickening and enhancement are commonly found adjacent to intracranial meningiomas (see Cases 50 and 52) or as a diffuse reactive process after lumbar puncture, cranial surgery, or in circumstances of intracranial hypotension (see Case 540).

Inflammatory disease can also result in meningeal thickening and enhancement. Granulomatous disorders such as tuberculosis, sarcoidosis, and meningovascular syphilis may present an appearance similar to Case 25, with uniform and/or nodular dural thickening. Other rare causes of diffuse dural thickening include Wegener's granulomatosis, rheumatoid arthritis, granulomatous angiitis, Erdheim Chester disease (lipid granulomatosis), and idiopathic hypertrophic pachymeningitis.

The extraaxial mass at the floor of the right middle cranial fossa in Case 26 proved to be due to primary involvement of the dura by systemic lymphoma. A similar lesion in the same location is occasionally seen in children with leukemia.

### Case 27

2-year-old boy presenting with irritability
and tremor.
(axial, noncontrast T2-weighted SE scan)

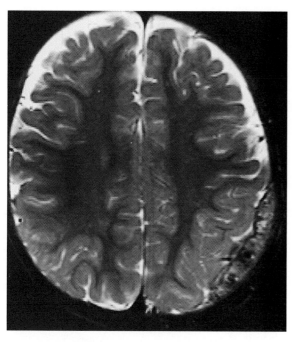

**Metastatic Neuroblastoma**
(containing hemorrhage)

### Case 28

53-year-old man presenting with headaches.
(axial, postcontrast T1-weighted SE scan)

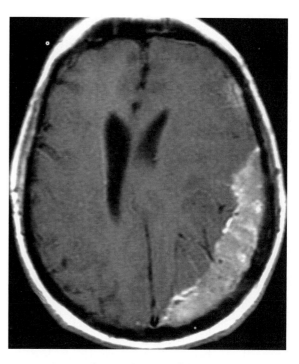

**Metastatic Carcinoma of the Prostate**

---

Dural-based metastases are often plaque-like, resembling the morphology of subdural collections. Cases 27 and 28 illustrate that this appearance may be encountered in both pediatric and adult patients.

Neuroblastoma should be a leading consideration (along with leukemia, lymphoma, and other "small blue cell" tumors) when epidural disease is discovered in a young child. Adjacent bone involvement may be present or inapparent. Physical examination of the patient in Case 27 demonstrated a large abdominal mass.

The dural-based metastasis in Case 28 is sharply demarcated from underlying cerebral tissue. This feature, together with homogeneous contrast enhancement, resembles a plaque-like meningioma. Like meningiomas, dural-based metastases may be associated with reactive changes in adjacent bone and vascular supply from dural arteries. The most common primary tumors to present in this matter are carcinomas of the prostate and breast.

Dural metastatic disease is occasionally associated with subdural hemorrhage. This condition, termed *pachymeningitis interna hemorrhagica,* is particularly frequent in patients with metastatic carcinoma of the breast. The heterogeneous areas of T2-shortening noted in the mass in Case 27 probably represent hemorrhage within the tumor tissue itself.

Case 701 presents a noncontrast scan of the patient in Case 28.

### Case 29

50-year-old woman presenting with
mediastinal adenopathy.
(coronal, postcontrast T1-weighted SE scan)

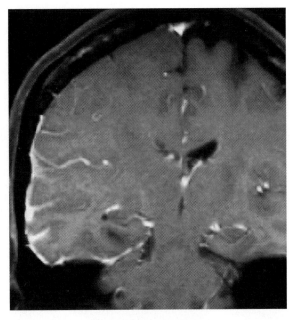

**Systemic Lymphoma**
(same patient as Case 26)

### Case 30

35-year-old woman presenting with a seizure.
(axial, postcontrast T1-weighted SE scan)

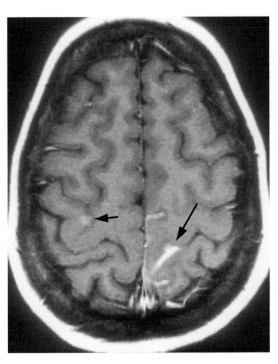

**Metastatic Carcinoma of the Breast**

Metastatic disease can involve the leptomeninges together with or separate from dural invasion. Neoplastic cells probably reach this location via seeding from superficial cerebral metastases rather than from direct hematogenous dissemination in most cases. Enhancing meningeal tumor may occupy sulci diffusely or focally with nodular or linear patterns.

In Case 29, enhancing tumor coats the surface of the right posterior temporal and inferior parietal lobes. The thin layer of abnormal tissue adjacent to the inner table extends medially into sulci and the sylvian fissure, distinguishing this pial process from dural metastases as illustrated previously.

Case 30 demonstrates more focal leptomeningeal metastases. A small nodule is present within a sulcus in the posterior right frontal region *(short arrow)*. A linear pattern of enhancing tumor fills sulci at the medial left hemisphere vertex *(long arrow)*.

On noncontrast scans, leptomeningeal carcinomatosis displaces CSF from the affected subarachnoid spaces, causing reduced visualization of sulci and cisterns. Tumor tissue within the subarachnoid space can be demonstrated directly on FLAIR images (see Case 720).

FLAIR scans after contrast administration have been reported to be the most sensitive single technique for detecting subtle leptomeningeal metastases.

Communicating hydrocephalus may develop in association with meningeal carcinomatosis, as with other meningeal pathologies. Conversely, benign leptomeningeal enhancement has been reported in cases of chronic or severe obstructive hydrocephalus, possibly reflecting vascular stasis due to increased intracranial pressure.

**Case 31**

34-year-old woman presenting with headaches.
(axial, postcontrast T1-weighted SE scan)

**Case 32**

29-year-old man presenting with seizures.
(axial, postcontrast T1-weighted SE scan)

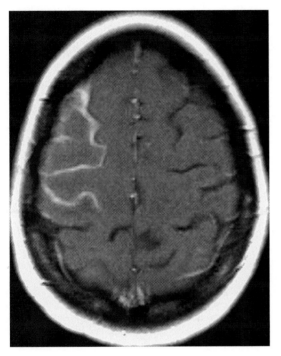

**Metastatic Carcinoma of the Breast**

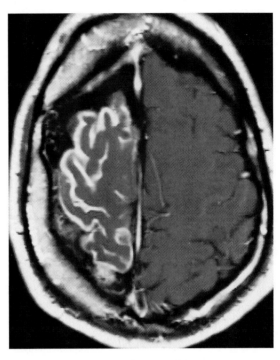

**Sturge-Weber Syndrome**

---

Leptomeningeal carcinomatosis is one of many pathologies that can present as abnormal enhancement within sulci and cisterns. Case 31 is a typical example, demonstrating metastatic tumor in the right superior frontal sulcus, as well as the superior portion of the precentral and central sulci. (See Case 720 for a precontrast scan of this patient.) Even in young adults, metastatic disease must unfortunately be included in the differential diagnosis of parenchymal and meningeal pathology.

The enhancement of the cerebral surface in Case 32 is due to the extensive meningeal angioma that characterizes

Sturge-Weber syndrome (see Cases 908-911). The typical clinical association with a facial angioma and accompanying hemicranial abnormalities (underlying cerebral atrophy and cortical calcification with thickening of the overlying calvarium) usually establish the diagnosis.

Other potential causes of sulcal enhancement include meningitis (see Cases 428-430), superficial enhancement in acute/subacute infarction (see Cases 578 and 579), meningeal congestion secondary to dural sinus thrombosis, and contrast enhancement occurring after subarachnoid hemorrhage.

# REFERENCES

Ahmadi H, Hilton DR, Segall HD, et al: Dural invasion by craniofacial and calvarial neoplasm: MR imaging and histopathologic evaluation. *Radiology* 188:747-750,1993.

Ahmadi H, Hilton DR, Segall HD, et al:Surgical implications of magnetic resonance-enhanced dura. *Neurosurgery* 35:370-88, 1994.

Atlas SW, Grossman TI, Gomori JM, et al: Hemorrhagic intracranial malignant neoplasms: spin echo MR imaging. *Radiology* 164:71-78, 1987.

Atlas SW, Grossman TI, Gomori JM, et al: MR imaging of intracranial metastatic melanoma. *J Comput Assist Tomogr* 11:577-582, 1987.

Bentson JR, Steckel RJ, Kagan AR: Diagnostic imaging in clinical cancer management: brain metastases. *Invest Radiol* 23:335-341, 1988.

Boorstein JM, Wong KT, Grossman RI, et al: Metastatic lesions of the brain: imaging with magnetization transfer. *Radiology* 191:799-806,1994.

Carrier DA, Mawad ME, Kirkpatrick JB, Schmid MF: Metastatic adenocarcinoma to the brain: MR with pathologic correlation. *AJNR* 15:155-160,1994.

Claussen C, Laniado M, Schorner W, et al: Gadolinium-DTPA in MR imaging of glioblastomas and intracranial metastases. *AJNR* 6:669-674, 1985.

Davis PC, Friedman NC, Fry SM, et al: Leptomeningeal metastasis: MR imaging. *Radiology* 163:449-454, 1987.

Davis PC, Hudgins PA, Peterman SB, Hoffman JC Jr: Diagnosis of cerebral metastases: double-dose delayed CT vs contrast-enhanced MR imaging. *AJNR* 12:293-300, 1991.

Destian S, Sze G, Krol G, et al: MR imaging of hemorrhagic intracranial neoplasms. *AJNR* 9:1115-1122, 1988.

Egelhoff JC, Ross JS, Modic MT, et al: MR imaging of metastatic GI adenocarcinoma in brain. *AJNR* 13:1221-1224, 1992.

Elster AD, MYM Chen: Can nonenhancing white matter lesions in cancer patients be disregarded? *AJNR* 13:1309-1315, 1992.

Escott EJ: A variety of appearances of malignant melanoma in the head: a review. *Radiographics* 21:625-639, 2001.

Essig M, Knopp MV, Schoenberg SO, et al: Assessment with contrast-enhanced fast fluid-attenuated inversion-recovery MR imaging. *Radiology* 210:551-557, 1999.

Gebarski SS, Blaivas MA: Imaging of normal leptomeningeal melanin. *AJNR* 17:55-60, 1996.

Healy ME, Hesselink JR, Press GA, Middleton MS: Increased detection of intracranial metastases with intravenous Gd-DTPA. *Radiology* 165:619-624, 1987

Kallmes DF, Gray L, Glass JP: High-dose gadolinium-enhanced MRI for diagnosis of meningeal metastases. *Neuroradiology* 40:23-26, 1998.

Krol D, Sze G, Malkin M, Walker R: MR of cranial and spinal meningeal carcinomatosis: compassion with CT and myelography. *AJNR* 9:709-714, 1988.

Laine FJ, Braun IF, Jensen ME, et al: Perineural tumor extension through the foramen ovale: evaluation with MR imaging. *Radiology* 174:65-72, 1990.

Lee JH, Lee BH, Choe DH, et al: Magnetic resonance imaging of brain metastases: Is T2-hypointensity a valid sign for adenocarcinoma? *Int J Neurorad* 4:263-265, 1998.

Lee Y-Y, Tien RD, Bruner JM, et al: Locualted intracranial leptomeningeal metastases: CT and MR characteristics. *AJNR* 10:1171-1180, 1989

Maki DD, Grossman RI: Patterns of disease spread in metastatic breast carcinoma: influence of estrogen and progesterone receptor status. *AJNR* 21:1064-1066, 2000.

Matthews VP, Caldemeyer KS, Ulmer JL, et al: Effects of contrast dose, delayed imaging, and magnetization transfer saturation on gadolinium-enhanced MR imaging of brain lesions. *JMRI* 7:14-22, 1997.

Mayr NA, Yuh WTC, Muhonen MG, et al: Cost-effectiveness of high-dose MR contrast studies in the evaluation of brain metastases. *AJNR* 15:1053-1061, 1994.

McKenzie CR, Rengachary SS, McGregor DH, et al: Subdural hematoma associated with metastatic neoplasms. *Neurosurgery* 27:619-625, 1990.

Nemzek W, Poirier V, Salamat MS, Yu T: Carcinomatous encephalitis (miliary metastases): lack of contrast enhancement. *AJNR* 14:540-542, 1993.

Olsen WI, Winkler MI, Ross DA: Carcinomatous encephalitis: CT and MR findings. *AJNR* 8:553-554, 1987.

Ortiz O, Schochet S, Bastug D: Imaging evaluation and clinicopathologic correlation of mass lesions involving the calvaria. II. Tumoral and inflammatory lesions. *Int J Neurorad* 5:151-165, 1999.

Paako E, Patronas NJ, Schellinger D: Meningeal Gd-DTPA enhancement is patients with malignancies. *J Comput Assist Tomogr* 14:542-546, 1990.

Peretti-Viton P, Taieb D, Viton JM, et al: Contrast-enhanced magnetisation transfer MRI in metastatic lesions of the brain. *Neuroradiology* 40:783-787, 1998.

Peterson AM, Meltzer CC, Evanson EJ, et al: MR imaging response of brain metastases after gamma knife stereotactic radiosurgery. *Radiology* 211:807-814, 1999.

Phillips ME, Ryals TJ, Kambhu SA, et al: Neoplastic vs. inflammatory meningeal enhancement with Gd-DTPA. *J Comput Assist Tomogr* 14:536-541, 1990.

Rippe DJ, Boyko OB, Friedman HS, et al: Gd-DTPA enhanced MR imaging of leptomeningeal spread of intracranial CNS tumor in children. *AJNR* 11:329, 1990.

Rodesch G, Van Bogaret P, Mavroudakis N, et al: Neuroradiologic findings in leptomeningeal carcinomatiosis: the value interest of gadolinium-enhanced MRI. *Neuroradiology* 32:26-32, 1990.

Russell EJ, Geremia GK, Johnson CE, et al: Multiple cerebral metastased: detectability with Gd-DTPA-enhanced MR imaging. *Radiology* 165:609-618, 1987.

Schubiger O, Haller D: Metastases to the pituitary-hypothalamic axis. *Neuroradiology* 34:131-134, 1992.

Shirai H, Imai S, Kajihara Y, et al: MRI in carcinomatosis encephalitis. *Neuroradiology* 39:437-440, 1997.

Singh SK, Agris JM, Leeds NE, Ginsberg LE: Intracranial leptomeningeal metastases: comparison of depiction at FLAIR and contrast-enhanced MR imaging. *Radiology* 217:50-53, 2000.

Sze G, Johnson C, Kawamura Y, et al: Comparison of single- and triple-dose contrast material in the MR screening of brain metastases. *AJNR* 19:821-828, 1998.

Sze G, Milano E, Johnson C, et al: Detection of brain metastases comparison of contrast-enhanced MR with unenhanced MR and enhanced CT. *AJNR* 11:785-792, 1990.

Sze G, Shin J, Krol G, et al: Intraparenchymal brain metastases: MR imaging versus contrast-enhanced CT. *Radiology* 168:187-194, 1988.

Sze G, Soletsky S, Bronen R, Krol G: MR imaging of the cranial meninges with emphasis on contrast enhancement and meningeal carcinomatosis. *AJNR* 10:965-975, 1989.

Tsuchiya K, Katase S, Yoshino A, Hachiya J: Use of contrast-enhanced fluid attenuated inversion recovery magnetic resonance imaging in the diagnosis of metastatic brain tumors. *Int J Neurorad* 5:9-15, 1999.

Turner DM, Graf CJ: Nontraumatic subdural hematoma secondary to dural metastasis: case report and review of the literature. *Neurosurgery* 11:678-680, 1982.

Tyrrell RI, Bundschuh CV, Modic MT: Dural carcinomatosis: MR demonstration. *J Comput Assist Tomogr* 11:329-332, 1987.

van de Pol M, van Oosterhout AGM, Wilmink JT, et al: MRI in detection of brain metastases at initial staging of small-cell lung cancer. *Neuroradiology* 38:207-210, 1996.

Watanabe M, Tanaka, R, Takeda N: Correlation of MRI and clinical features in meningeal carcinomatiosis. *Neuroradiology* 35:521-515, 1993.

West MS, Russell EJ, Berit R, et al : Calvarial and skull based metastases: comparison of nonenhanced and Gd-DTPA-enhanced MR images. *Radiology* 174: 85-92, 1990.

Woodruff WW Jr, Djang WT, Mc Lendon RE, et al: Intracerebral malignant melanoma: high-field MR imaging. *Radiology* 165:209-213, 1987.

Yousem DM, Patrone PM, Grossman RI: Leptomeningeal metastasis: MR evaluation. *J Comput Assist Tomogr* 14: 255-261, 1990.

Yuh WTC, Engelken JD, Muhonin MG, et al: Experience with high dose gadolinium MR imaging in the evaluation of brain metastases. *AJNR* 13:335-345, 1992.

Yuh WTC, Fisher DJ, Runge VM, et al: Phase III multicenter trial of high-dose gadoteridol in MR evaluation of brain metastases. *AJNR* 15:1037-1052, 1994.

Yuh WTC, Mayr-Yuh NA, Koci TM, et al: Metastatic lesions involving the cerebellopontine angle, *AJNR* 14:99-106, 1993.

Yuh WTC, Tali ET, Nguyen HD, et al: The effect of contrast dose, imaging time, and lesion size in the MR detection of intracerebral metastasis. *AJNR* 16:373-380, 1995.

# CHAPTER 2

# Meningiomas

## Case 33

55-year-old man presenting with headaches.
(sagittal, noncontrast T1-weighted SE scan)

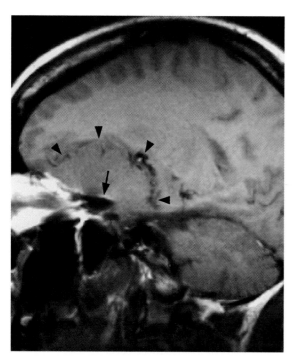

**Sphenoid Wing Meningioma**

## Case 34

51-year-old woman presenting with
homonymous hemianopsia.
(sagittal, noncontrast T1-weighted SE scan)

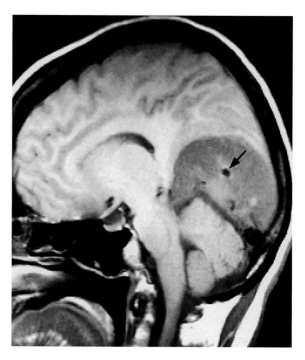

**Tentorial Meningioma**

Meningiomas arise from arachnoidal "cap" cells, presenting as extraaxial masses with a dural base. Even large tumors may cause relatively little edema and mass effect. This quiescent appearance implies slow growth, with gradual invagination into adjacent parenchyma.

The signal intensity of meningiomas is usually homogeneous on all pulse sequences, analogous to their characteristically uniform CT attenuation. Margins of the tumor may be very smooth, as in Case 34, or distinctly lobulated, as in Case 33.

Many meningiomas are nearly isointense with adjacent cerebral cortex on T1-weighted images. Small tumors may be inapparent on scans performed without contrast material. Larger isointense meningiomas are defined by distortions of anatomy. In Case 33, the tumor disrupts the normal pattern of cortical convolutions in the affected area.

Other meningiomas demonstrate lower signal intensity than cerebral parenchyma on T1-weighted scans, as in Case 34. Dense calcifications may cause focal areas of very low intensity *(arrow)*.

The margin of a meningioma on T1-weighted images is often highlighted by a rim of low signal intensity. Flow voids within vessels (usually veins) at the perimeter of the tumor may contribute to this definition, as in Case 33 *(arrowheads)*. More commonly, the "pseudocapsule" demarcating an otherwise isointense meningioma is due to a collar of displaced subarachnoid space (see Cases 35 and 36).

Meningiomas account for 15% to 20% of intracranial tumors, with a peak age incidence at 45 years and a moderate predominance in women. Less than 10% of intracranial meningiomas cause specific symptoms.

Hyperostosis and exaggerated pneumatization of the anterior clinoid process are present at the base of the meningioma in Case 33 *(arrow)*.

### Case 35

81-year-old man presenting with confusion.
(axial, noncontrast T2-weighted FSE scan)

### Case 36

71-year-old man presenting with headaches.
(axial, noncontrast T2-weighted SE scan)

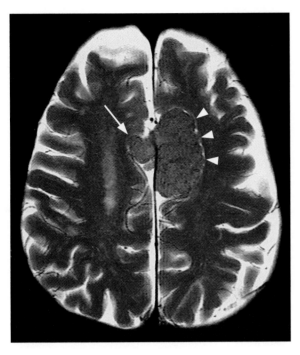

**Falx Meningioma**

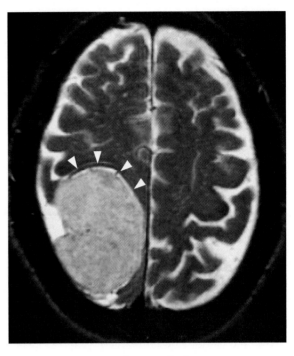

**Convexity Meningioma**

Many meningiomas are nearly isointense with cerebral cortex on T2-weighted images. This isointensity may obscure small lesions on noncontrast scans.

A collar of edema and/or a ring of prominent CSF surrounding a meningioma may help to define it, as seen laterally in Case 35 *(arrowheads)*. The tumor in this case is typically homogeneous, with a lobulation crossing the interhemispheric fissure beneath the free margin of the falx *(arrow)*.

Meningiomas may alternatively demonstrate high signal intensity on T2-weighted scans, as illustrated in Case 36. This appearance often correlates with syncytial or angioblastic histology. Tumors that are more nearly isointense on T2-weighted images tend to represent fibroblastic or transitional varieties.

The meningioma in Case 36 demonstrates the size that can be attained by a slowly growing intracranial mass. The surrounding brain gradually accommodates the expanding tumor, with symptoms remaining mild and nonspecific until the lesion is very large. The absence of reactive edema also attests to slow growth, while a rim of displaced subarachnoid space *(arrowheads)* outlines the margin of the tumor.

Occasional meningiomas have lower signal intensity than gray matter on T2-weighted images (see Case 67). This appearance may reflect unusual calcification, blood products, and/or a densely fibrous stroma with little water content. The psammomatous calcification of meningiomas characteristically demonstrated on CT scans is rarely detected on MR studies.

23

### Case 37

74-year-old woman presenting with blurred vision.
(axial, noncontrast T2-weighted FSE scan)

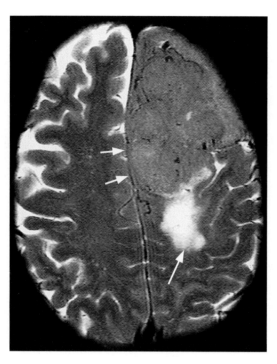

**Convexity Meningioma**

### Case 38

24-year-old man presenting with lightheadedness
and slurred speech.
(coronal, noncontrast T1-weighted SE scan)

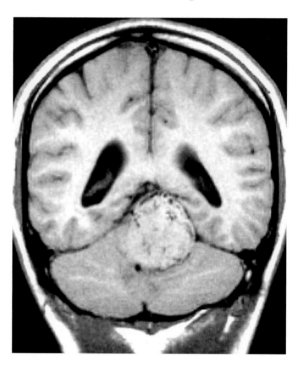

**Tentorial Meningioma**

Large vessels surrounding or within a meningioma may be a prominent feature of the CT or MR presentation. Scattered focal and tubular zones of low signal intensity throughout the left frontal mass in Case 37 represent multiple flow voids. The tumor is otherwise characteristically homogeneous. Localized edema is present in the centrum semiovale posterior to the lesion *(long arrow)*. Slow growth of the mass has caused contralateral bowing of the falx *(short arrows)*.

The impressive vascularity of some meningiomas may lead to diagnostic confusion. In Case 38, the posterior fossa mass containing multiple vascular channels in a young adult could be assumed to represent a hemangioblastoma (see Cases 183-186). The tumor proved to be a meningioma arising from the tentorium.

Case 93 presents an additional example of large vessels within a meningioma.

## Case 39

70-year-old woman presenting with diplopia.
(axial, noncontrast scan; SE 2500/28)

## Case 40

57-year-old woman presenting with
bilateral leg weakness.
(coronal, noncontrast scan; SE 2500/30)

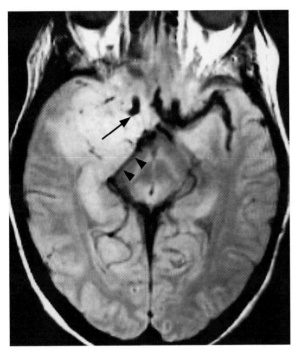

**Spenoid Wing Meningioma**

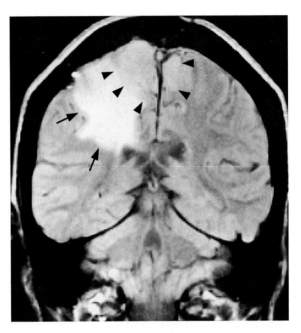

**Falx Meningioma**
(recurrent)

---

The absence of signal ("flow void") within cerebral arteries on routine spin echo MR sequences helps to define the status of vessels adjacent to tumors. In Case 39, a parasellar meningioma surrounds the supraclinoid internal carotid artery *(arrow)*. The mass crosses the tentorial margin to flatten the right side of the midbrain *(arrowheads)*.

Encasement of adjacent arteries is a characteristic feature of meningiomas in the sphenoid region. However, this finding is not histologically specific; pituitary adenomas may present a similar appearance (see Cases 232, 233, and 236).

Case 40 demonstrates that the coronal plane is useful for evaluating lesions involving the falx or tentorium. In this instance, the relatively isointense signal of meningioma tissue is seen on both sides of the falx *(arrowheads)*. In addition, the expected flow void within the lumen of the superior sagittal sinus has been replaced by tissue with signal intensity matching the adjacent meningioma. Tumor invasion and/or occlusion of a dural sinus can be confirmed by venographic MR techniques.

The meningioma in Case 40 has triggered marked edema on one side of the falx *(arrows)*, with no edema contralaterally. The mechanisms by which meningiomas incite reactive edema are unclear. Relevant factors probably include the thickness of cortex separating a tumor from underlying white matter and the presence or absence of venous compression. Edema is often a major cause of mass effect and symptomatology.

Paresis of the lower extremities may lead to initial clinical suspicion of spinal cord dysfunction in patients like Case 40. It is important to remember that parasagittal lesions near the cerebral vertex can also produce bilateral leg symptoms (through compression or invasion of the motor and sensory tracts from the medial portion of the precentral and postcentral gyri).

### Case 41

43-year-old woman presenting with impaired vision.
(sagittal, noncontrast T1-weighted SE scan)

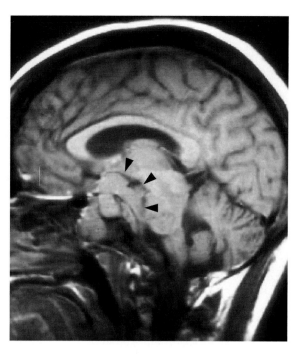

**Parasellar Meningioma**

### Case 42

72-year-old woman presenting with
right–sided proptosis.
(axial, noncontrast scan; SE 2700/45)

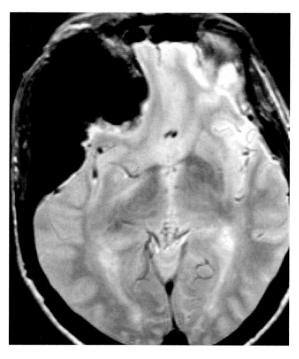

**Spenoid Wing Meningioma**

---

Hyperostosis frequently develops at the base of intracranial meningiomas. The sclerosis may accompany calvarial invasion or be an independent reaction to adjacent tumor.

In Case 41, isointense meningioma tissue fills the sella turcica. Tumor components occupy the suprasellar cistern and sphenoid sinus. The basisphenoid bone and clivus demonstrate very low signal intensity, reflecting dense reactive hyperostosis.

A similar appearance is occasionally caused by an inflammatory lesion at the skull base. For example, aspergillosis originating in the sphenoid sinus (typically in a diabetic patient) may provoke a sclerotic bone reaction (and encase parasellar vessels) to closely resemble a basal meningioma.

Case 42 illustrates marked thickening of bone due to a meningioma permeating the sphenoid wing ("intraosseous

meningioma"). Sphenoid involvement by sclerosing meningiomas may have both cerebral and orbital consequences, with proptosis resulting from bone deformity. Associated soft tissue components of tumor may be found in the middle cranial fossa, the orbit, and extracranially in the infratemporal fossa.

Fibrous dysplasia may also cause prominent thickening of bone of the skull base or face. However, fibrous dysplasia usually demonstrates homogeneous, intermediate signal intensity on MR scans (correlating with the characteristic "ground-glass" texture on x-rays and CT scans), rather than the markedly low signal of hyperostotic meningioma bone. Furthermore, fibrous dysphasia usually presents in the first decade of life, although the disorder is occasionally discovered in older adults.

## Case 43

49-year-old woman presenting with
decreased vision.
(sagittal, noncontrast T1-weighted SE scan)

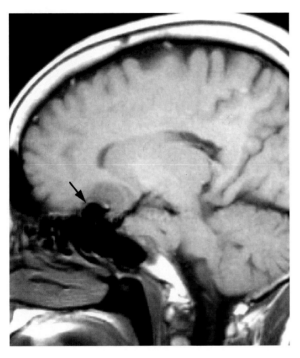

**Planum Sphenoidale and Parasellar Meningioma**

## Case 44

74-year-old man presenting with a scalp mass.
(sagittal, noncontrast T1-weighted SE scan)

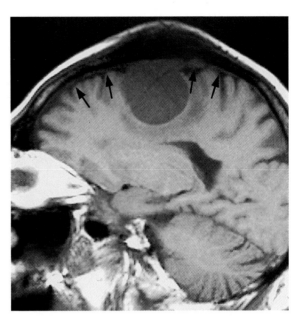

**Transcranial Convexity Meningioma**

---

Meningiomas arising from the anterior skull base may be associated with characteristic bone changes. The planum sphenoidale often becomes thickened in association with subfrontal tumors. Such dense hyperostosis of the planum causes low signal intensity comparable to Cases 41 and 42.

A more unique and highly typical change is tumor-induced remodelling of the planum sphenoidale, so that the sphenoid sinus is expanded along the base of the overlying meningioma. Case 43 demonstrates this "blistering" or elevation of the roof of the sinus toward the meningioma

*(arrow).* This seemingly paradoxical expansion of a sinus in the direction of an overlying mass is analogous to excessive pneumatization of the sphenoid wing occasionally seen adjacent to an arachnoid cyst.

The convexity meningioma in Case 44 has grown through the skull to present as a scalp mass at the vertex. The involved bone is both permeated and sclerotic. The spherical intracranial portion of the tumor is bordered by dural thickening *(arrows)* and surrounded by edema. Compare Case 44 to the transcranial metastasis in Case 24.

### Case 45

45-year-old man presenting with a seizure.
(axial, postcontrast T1-weighted SE scan)

### Case 46

31-year-old woman presenting with headaches.
(sagittal, postcontrast T1-weighted SE scan)

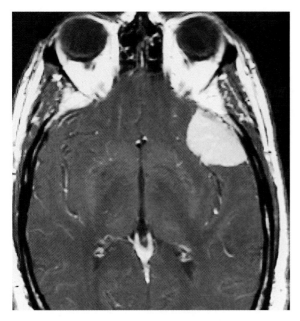

**Sphenoid Wing Meningioma**

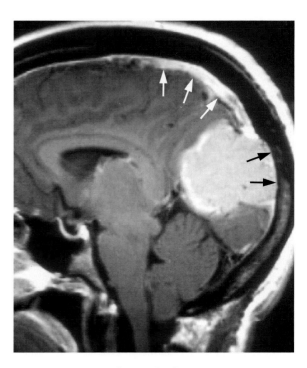

**Falx Meningioma**

Contrast enhancement within meningiomas is usually intense and uniform, regardless of tumor size. The sharply defined enhancement of the mass in Case 45 is typical. A faint fan-like pattern of linear striation radiates through the tumor from a central point at its base. This occasional but characteristic feature of meningiomas probably reflects the pattern of dural vascular supply (see Case 54A for another example).

The meningioma in Case 46 is larger but still demonstrates homogeneous enhancement. In this case, axial CT scans had suggested a tentorial origin for the tumor. Coronal and sagittal MR scans corrected this impression by demonstrating a broad base against the occipital inner table *(black arrows)*.

Contrast enhancement extending superiorly from the mass in Case 46 *(white arrows)* represents stasis in the superior sagittal sinus, which is compressed and/or invaded by the meningioma. Waves or ripples of compressed gray and white matter are seen in the cerebral hemisphere anterior to the tumor. This accordion-like morphology (including a band of displaced cortex between the superficial mass and underlying white matter) helps to establish the lesion as extraaxial.

Meningiomas of the sphenoid wing are often associated with extensive edema in the adjacent temporal lobe. Noncontrast scans in such cases may erroneously suggest an intraaxial neoplasm if the inciting meningioma is small and/or isointense. Postcontrast images resembling Case 45 establish the correct diagnosis.

### Case 47

61-year-old man with an abnormal CT scan
after trauma.
(coronal, postcontrast T1-weighted SE scan)

### Case 48

18-year-old woman presenting with a seizure.
(axial, postcontrast T1-weighted SE scan)

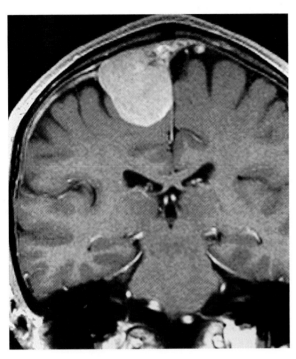

**Meningioma**

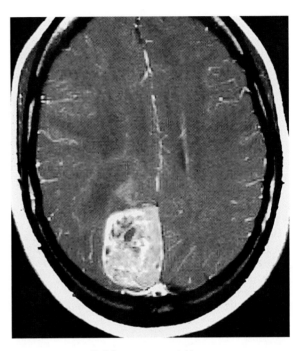

**Glioblastoma Multiforme**
(with invasion of the falx)

A mass at the surface of the brain may represent extraaxial or intraaxial pathology. The multiplanar display of MR usually helps to make this distinction, although occasional cases are indeterminate.

The meningioma in Case 47 demonstrates characteristically intense and homogeneous enhancement. The tumor probably arises from dura of the parasagittal convexity, although it may also be adherent to the falx. Mass effect from the lesion displaces underlying cortex with compression of the cingulate sulcus and mild inferior displacement of the right lateral ventricle.

As discussed in Chapter 1, metastases should be considered along with meningiomas in the differential diagnosis of dural-based tumors. Both pathologies are characteristically well defined with uniform contrast enhancement. Both may be associated with adjacent dural thickening, reactive bone changes, and angiographic supply by dural arteries.

Case 48 illustrates that superficial intraaxial tumors may (1) be well defined and (2) invade dura, mimicking the appearance of meningiomas or other extraaxial masses. The moderate heterogeneity of enhancement in this case does not exclude the diagnosis of meningioma (see Case 53), while the tumor's sharp margins and broad interface with the falx resemble a dural-based lesion.

### Case 49

72-year-old woman presenting with
right-sided proptosis.
(axial, postcontrast T1-weighted SE scan)

### Case 50

66-year-old man presenting with
transient expressive aphasia.
(axial, postcontrast T1-weighted SE scan)

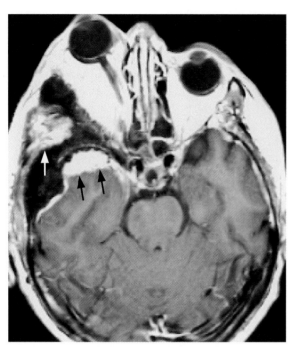

**Sphenoid Wing Meningioma**
(same patient as Case 42)

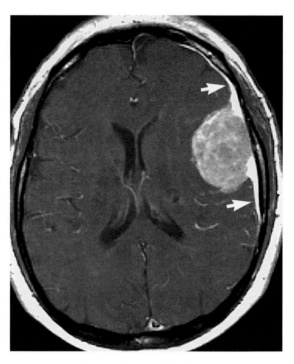

**Convexity Meningioma**

Some meningiomas spread along the inner table as relatively flat sheets of tissue. This "en plaque" morphology may be seen alone or in association with spherical or osseous components. The superficial location, homogeneous signal intensity, and marked contrast enhancement of such tumors remain characteristic.

Case 49 presents a postcontrast scan of the meningioma illustrated in Case 42. A plaque-like layer of enhancing tumor tissue is well defined along the anterior margin of the middle cranial fossa *(black arrows)*. Enhancing meningioma is also present within the infratemporal fossa *(white arrow)* and within the orbit (where it is difficult to distinguish from retrobulbar fat without fat suppression). Note the marked thickening of the right sphenoid bone and the prominent right-sided proptosis.

A layer of thickened dural enhancement extending away from the base of a meningioma is a common MR feature, as seen in Case 50 *(arrows)*. In some cases, such thickening correlates with either en plaque extension of tumor or the presence of meningiomatous islands surrounding the main lesion. In many cases, the "tail" of dural enhancement near the base of a meningioma represents reactive thickening, without tumor involvement.

Although an enhancing dural tail is commonly seen at the base of meningiomas, the finding is not specific. Metastases, acoustic schwannomas, and other superficial masses may be associated with adjacent dural thickening.

Case 53 illustrates another meningioma with an en plaque component. An additional example of a dural tail adjacent to meningiomas is seen in Case 52.

### Case 51A

1-year-old boy presenting with a one-month
history of staring and lip smacking.
(sagittal, noncontrast T1-weighted SE scan)

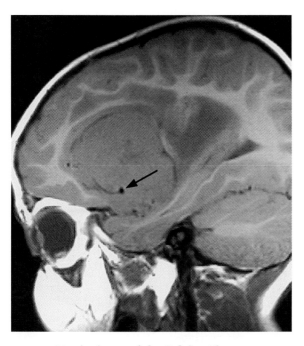

**Meningioma of the Sylvian Fissure**

### Case 51B

Same patient.
(axial, postcontrast T1-weighted SE scan with MTS)

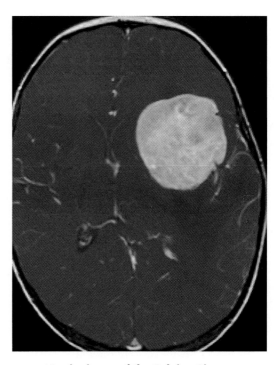

**Meningioma of the Sylvian Fissure**

As illustrated in the preceding cases of this chapter, a dural base is a characteristic diagnostic feature of extraventricular meningiomas. However, occasional intracranial meningiomas have no dural attachment, presumably arising from rests of meningeal cells. One recognized location for such tumors is the sylvian fissure, particularly in the pediatric age group.

The large mass in Case 51 is a typical example. The appearance of the lesion is characteristic of a meningioma: homogeneous, well-defined tissue with intense, uniform enhancement. A thin "CSF cleft" at the superior and posterior margins of the tumor in Case 51A favors extraaxial origin, while the relatively modest mass effect of the lesion suggests a slowly growing tumor. However, the mass has no connection with dura of the skull base or convexity.

The sagittal scan demonstrates tumor surrounding the flow void of the horizontal or "M1" segment of the middle cerebral artery *(arrow)*. Such encasement of adjacent vessels is a well-recognized property of meningiomas, as discussed in Case 39. The edema posterior to the tumor may be either reactive or ischemic secondary to compression of arterial branches.

Pediatric meningiomas arising from a dural base may have unusual appearances, tending to be larger and more aggressive than adult tumors.

Rare intracranial schwannomas or fibromas are also included in the differential diagnosis of round, uniformly enhancing intradural masses in children.

## Case 52

44-year-woman presenting with signs
of increased intracranial pressure.
(sagittal, postcontrast T1-weighted SE scan)

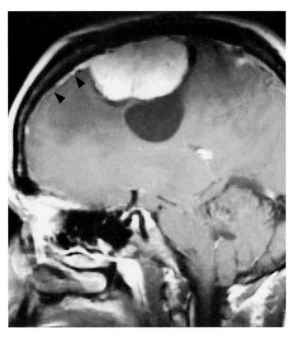

**Convexity Meningioma**

## Case 53

51-year-old woman presenting with right
homonymous hemianopsia.
(coronal, postcontrast T1-weighted GRE scan)

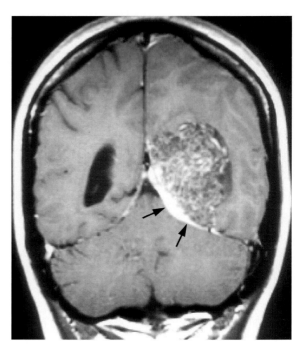

**Tentorial Meningioma**

---

Because the typical appearance of meningiomas is one of the most reliable stereotypes on CT and MR scans, atypical appearances can be confusing. A small number of meningiomas contain or are associated with nonenhancing areas. These may be due to necrosis, old hemorrhage, cyst formation, or fat within the meningioma tissue or reflect loculation of adjacent CSF.

In Case 52, a large cyst is present deep to the enhancing tumor. A more laminar halo of CSF-like intensity values is seen along the remainder of the tissue margin. This finding and the eccentric morphology of the cyst suggest that it represents a loculation of fluid adjacent to the meningioma, rather than an intratumoral cavity. A small, enhancing dural tail extends anteriorly from the main mass (*arrowheads;* see Cases 49 and 50).

Case 53 demonstrates heterogeneous, nonenhancing areas that are clearly within the substance of the tumor. The correct diagnosis depends on the typical dural-based morphology, including localized thickening of the tentorium *(arrows).* Compare Care 53 to the homogeneously enhancing tentorial meningiomas in Cases 59 and 60.

In some cases, inhomogeneous enhancement of a meningioma may combine with irregular margins and prominent edema to mimic a malignant glioma or metastasis. Coronal scans can help to correctly identify such tumors by demonstration that the mass arises from a dural base. However, superficial gliomas may invade the dura (see Case 48), and dural-based metastases must also be considered.

There is little correlation between atypical MR features and aggressive growth or recurrence of meningiomas (discussed in Case 54). Most inhomogeneous tumors have benign courses, and most "malignant" meningiomas originally demonstrate conventional homogeneity.

### Case 54A

72-year-old woman presenting with headaches
and personality change.
(sagittal, postcontrast T1-weighted
SE scan with MTS)

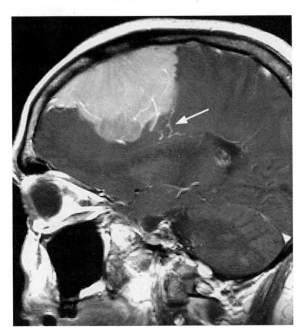

**Convexity Meningioma**

### Case 54B

Same patient.
(axial, postcontrast T1-weighted SE scan with MTS)

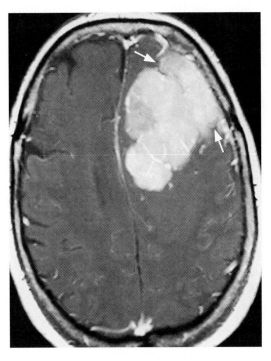

**Convexity Meningioma**

As noted on the preceding page, it is difficult to relate the imaging features of meningiomas to their subsequent biological behavior. Seemingly simple tumors recur after surgery, and complex-appearing meningiomas may follow a benign clinical course.

However, several morphological characteristics have been associated with parenchymal invasion and recurrence of meningiomas. These include a "mushrooming," plaque-like component or "pannus" extending over the cerebral surface from the major mass, abnormally prominent deep venous drainage from the tumor region (suggesting cortical invasion), and frond-like margins invaginating into underlying cerebral parenchyma.

Case 54 illustrates a plaque-like component (*arrows*, Case 54B) and prominent deep venous drainage (*arrow*, Case 54A). These findings combine with the lobulation and deep invagination of the mass to suggest an aggressive tumor with an increased risk of recurrence after resection.

A pattern of linear striations radiating into the tumor from the center of its base can be faintly appreciated in Case 54A. This morphology often correlates with a fan-like distribution of the tumor's dural arterial supply (see Case 45 for another example).

Dural-based hemangiopericytomas can resemble aggressive meningiomas and should be considered in the differential diagnosis of such masses. These highly vascular tumors arise from "pericytes," contractile cells surrounding capillaries. Their frequent meningeal origin and intense contrast enhancement mimic meningiomas, but they are more likely to recur locally and/or metastasize. Imaging clues to the diagnosis of hemangiopericytoma include more lobulation, a narrower base, more prominent and tortuous internal vessels, and more destruction of adjacent bone than expected for a meningioma.

## Case 55

54-year-old woman presenting with
decreased vision in the right eye.
(sagittal, noncontrast T1-weighted SE scan)

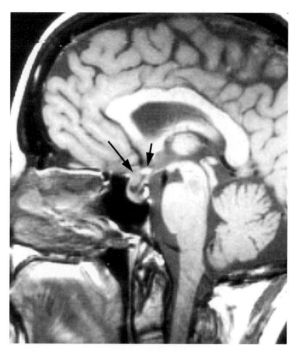

**Tuberculum Meningioma**

## Case 56

55-year-old man presenting with headaches.
(coronal, postcontrast T1-weighted SE scan)

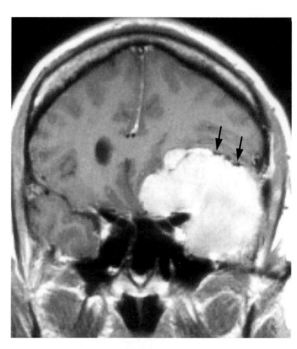

**Sphenoid Wing Meningioma**
(same patient as Case 33)

Along with the typical dural base, tissue homogeneity, sharp demarcation, and intense contrast enhancement of meningiomas, several characteristic locations of these tumors can help support the diagnosis. One common area of origin is the sphenoid ridge, either in the midline (i.e., tuberculum sella region) or laterally (along the sphenoid wing).

Sagittal MR scans provide excellent definition of even small lesions affecting the optic chiasm or pituitary infundibulum. In Case 55, a focal mound of homogeneous soft tissue *(long arrow)* is perched on the tuberculum sella, immediately anterior to the optic chiasm *(short arrow)*. This tiny meningioma was symptomatic by virtue of

is critical location. (Contrast this early presentation with the late manifestation of the large convexity meningioma in Case 36.)

Case 56 illustrates a typical meningioma of the sphenoid wing. The large mass crosses the sphenoid ridge to involve both the middle cranial fossa and the anterior cranial fossa. Prominent vessels at its superior margin *(arrows)* may include displaced branches of the middle cerebral artery, as well as large veins on the surface of the tumor. Contrast enhancement is characteristically intense and uniform. A hint of radial striation is present within the tumor (compare to Cases 45 and 54).

# DIFFERENTIAL DIAGNOSIS:
## DURAL-BASED, ENHANCING MASS ALONG THE SPHENOID WING

### Case 57

24-year-old man studied in follow-up
of prior acoustic schwannoma.
(axial, postcontrast T1-weighted SE scan)

### Case 58

84-year-old man presenting with confusion.
(axial, postcontrast T1-weighted SE scan)

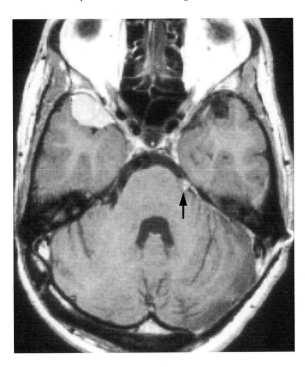

**Meningioma**
(in type 2 neurofibromatosis)

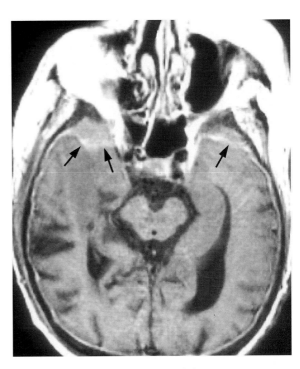

**Metastatic Carcinoma of the Prostate**
(dural-based)

---

As discussed in Chapter 1, metastases to the skull or dura may produce focal extraaxial masses. Such lesions may closely resemble meningiomas in location, definition, and contrast enhancement. The two types of epidural masses may also be indistinguishable at angiography, with similar dural arterial supply and tumor stains.

The most common tumor to mimic meningioma in this manner is metastatic prostate carcinoma, particularly along the sphenoid wing, as in Case 58. Melanoma, breast carcinoma, and renal carcinoma can cause similar appearances.

Superficial gliomas may invade the dura and occasionally mimic meningiomas in other respects as well (see Case 48). Intracranial lymphoma is often dural-based (see Case 26) and should be included in the differential diagnosis of meningioma-like lesions.

Neurofibromatosis type 2 is discussed in Cases 207 and 208. In Case 57, an area of enhancement along the cisternal segment of the trigeminal nerve on the left *(arrow)* suggests a small schwannoma at this site.

### Case 59

46-year-old woman presenting with right facial pain.
(axial, postcontrast T1-weighted SE scan with MTS)

### Case 60

78-year-old woman presenting with ataxia.
(coronal, postcontrast T1-weighted SE scan)

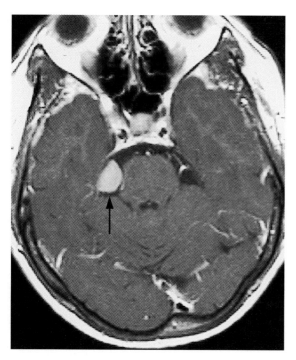

**Tentorial Meningioma**

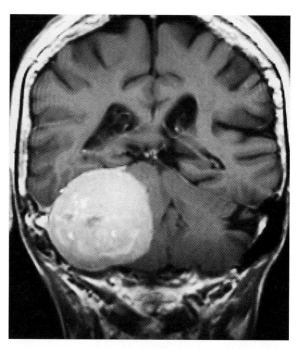

**Tentorial Meningioma**

Meningiomas arising from the tentorium may be plaque-like lesions mimicking pachymeningitis or spherical masses projecting inferiorly or superiorly.

The small tumor in Case 59 *(arrow)* is based along the inferior margin of the tentorium near the petrous apex. The lesion extends medially and inferiorly to involve the expected location of the cisternal segment of the trigeminal nerve, correlating with the patient's facial pain. The differential diagnosis in Case 59 would include a mass originating from the trigeminal nerve itself (e.g., schwannoma, lymphoma, or metastasis), but the flat lateral margin of the tumor favors a dural-based process.

Case 60 presents a much larger meningioma, occupying most of the posterior fossa on the right. It is difficult to specify the origin of the tumor, since it abuts the dura superiorly, laterally, and inferiorly. At surgery, the mass was found to arise from the inferior surface of the tentorium. There is relatively little mass effect for the size of the lesion, suggesting a slowly expanding process.

Intraaxial cerebellar tumors arising near the superior pial surface (e.g., hemangioblastoma or lateral medulloblastoma) may resemble the tentorial base of an inferiorly growing meningioma (see Cases 180 and 187), but other features usually enable differential diagnosis.

Cases 34 and 53 present examples of superiorly projecting tentorial meningiomas.

## Case 61

45-year-woman presenting with diplopia.
(axial, postcontrast T1-weighted SE scan)

## Case 62

68-year-old man.
(sagittal, postcontrast T1-weighted SE scan)

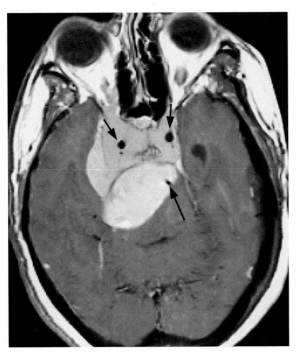

**Prepontine and Parasellar Meningioma**

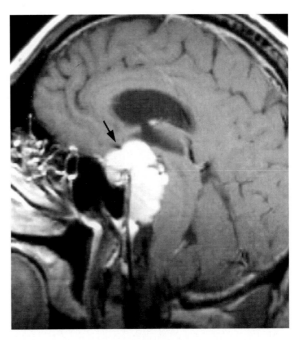

**Clivus Meningioma**

Meningiomas commonly extend across the tentorial hiatus from origins in either the parasellar region or the cerebellopontine angle. The morphology of transtentorial meningiomas may be plaque-like or lobular. The posterior fossa components of such tumors may occupy the prepontine or cerebellopontine angle cisterns, or both. The middle fossa components of transtentorial meningiomas commonly involve the cavernous sinus and may grow further laterally to displace the temporal lobe.

The meningioma in Case 61 expands the cavernous sinus bilaterally. The parasellar portions of the internal carotid arteries are encased on both sides *(short arrows)*. The prepontine component of the mass displaces and surrounds the basiler artery *(long arrow; see Case 220 for a sagittal view of this lesion.)*

In Case 62, a mildly lobulated meningioma is based against the clivus, dorsum sella, and diaphragm sella. The suprasellar component of such a lesion may cause visual or endocrine symptoms, while the interpeduncular and prepontine components may cause cranial neuropathies. Major arterial channels *(arrow)* are seen at the rostral pole of the tumor, partially restraining its growth and contributing to a lobulated morphology.

Trigeminal schwannomas can closely mimic the appearance of parasellar or transtentorial meningiomas. The contrast enhancement pattern of large trigeminal schwannomas is often more patchy or inhomogeneous than that of meningiomas (see Case 203), resembling the typical tumor stain at angiography. The differential diagnosis of an enhancing, extraaxial mass spanning the petrous apex in an adult also includes metastasis and lymphoma.

Some meningiomas are transtentorial by virtue of tentorial origin or invasion (see Case 53). Such tumors may extend along the superior and/or inferior surface of the tentorium and are not confined by the tentorial hiatus.

### Case 63

86-year-old man presenting with dizziness.
(axial, noncontrast T2-weighted SE scan)

### Case 64

48-year-old woman presenting with neck pain,
bilateral hand numbness, and right leg weakness.
(sagittal, postcontrast T1-weighted SE scan)

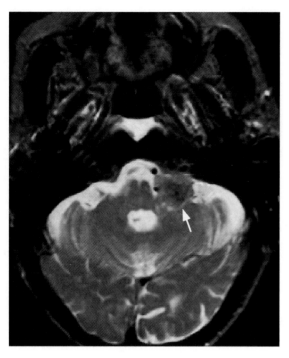

**Meningioma Near the Jugular Foramen**

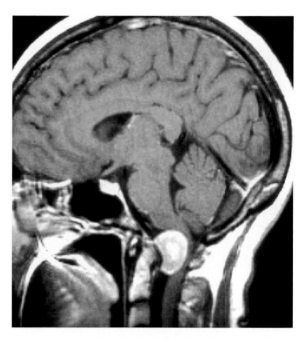

**Foramen Magnum Meningioma**

Meningiomas may occur at all levels within the cerebellopontine angle. Superiorly located tumors frequently cross the tentorial hiatus to involve the parasellar region, as seen in Case 61. Meningiomas occupying the midportion of the cerebellopontine angle cistern may mimic acoustic schwannomas (see Case 197). Finally, meningiomas may be found at the inferior margin of the cerebellopontine angle, as in Case 63. Such tumors may distort lower cranial nerves and/or compromise the foramen magnum.

Schwannomas and glomus jugulare tumors (see Cases 209 and 211) would be included in the differential diagnosis of a mass near the jugular foramen. The low signal in-

tensity of the lesion in Case 63 and the lack of associated expansion of the jugular foramen on adjacent scans make these alternative diagnoses unlikely.

The meningioma in Case 64 occupies a strategic location *within* the foramen magnum. Slow growth of this tumor has caused gradual thinning of the cervicomedullary junction, which can become remarkably attenuated before symptoms are manifest. (Compare to long-standing bony compromise of the craniocervical junction, as in Cases 990 and 1168). A concentric circular texture or architecture can be appreciated within the homogeneous enhancement of the tumor, an occasional finding in meningiomas.

### Case 65

35-year-old woman presenting with headaches
and tinnitus.
(axial, postcontrast T1-weighted SE scan)

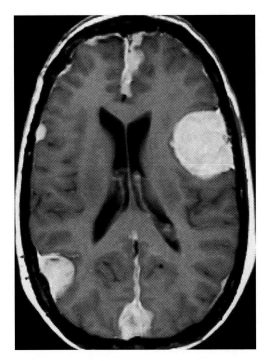

**Multiple Convexity and Falx Meningiomas**
(in neurofibromatosis type 2)

### Case 66

41-year-old man presenting with hearing loss.
(axial, postcontrast T1-weighted SE scan)

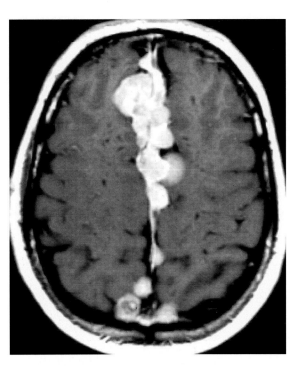

**Meningiomatosis of the Falx**
(in neurofibromatosis type 2)

Multiple intracranial meningiomas may be seen sporadically, but they are more commonly encountered in association with type 2 neurofibromatosis ("bilateral acoustic neurofibromatosis"). This syndrome, previously identified as "central" neurofibromatosis, is caused by a mutation on chromosome 22 and is genetically distinct from neurofibromatosis type 1 (see Cases 904-907).

Apart from their multiplicity, the meningiomas in the above scans are typical in appearance. The homogeneous, intense enhancement of the dural-based masses is characteristic.

Multifocal recurrence of aggressive meningiomas may be encountered after resection of an initially solitary lesion.

Sarcomatous transformation can occur in originally benign tumors. Some histological varieties (e.g., papillary and angioblastic meningiomas) are themselves associated with tendency toward recurrence and parenchymal invasion.

Induction of meningiomas has been reported after both high and low doses of radiation. The latency period in such cases may be as long as 20 years, correlating inversely with radiation dose and directly with patient age at the time of exposure. Radiation-induced meningiomas are typically rapidly growing and aggressive tumors with frequent multiplicity.

### Case 67

43-year-old woman presenting with
right homonymous hemianopsia.
(axial, noncontrast T2-weighted FSE scan)

### Case 68

76-year-old woman presenting with dementia.
(axial, postcontrast T1-weighted SE scan)

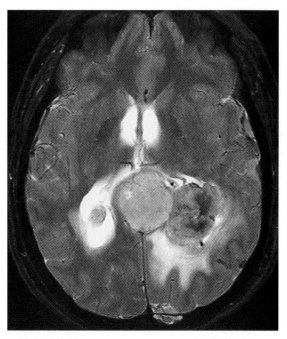

**Trigone and Subsplenial Meningiomas**
(in neurofibromatosis type 2)

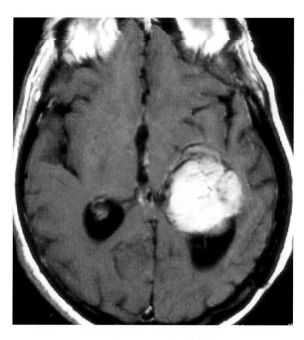

**Trigone Meningioma**

Intraventricular tumors account for about 2% of intracranial meningiomas. They most commonly occur within the atrium of the lateral ventricle, with greater frequency on the left side.

The left trigone meningioma in Case 67 is more heterogeneous than the adjacent midline tumor occupying the pineal region. Zones of low signal intensity within the mass may represent calcification, blood products, or densely fibrous stroma. Prominent vessels are seen at the margin of the lesion, and reactive edema is present within white matter of the occipital lobe. The small mass within the atrium of the right lateral ventricle may represent an additional small meningioma or unrelated enlargement of the choroid plexus.

Intraventricular tumors may displace CSF as they grow, causing relatively little parenchymal mass effect. However, trigone lesions frequently "trap" the ipsilateral temporal horn, which enlarges due to continuing CSF production by choroid plexus within the obstructed segment (see Case 791). The meningioma in Case 68 was associated with mild dilatation of the left temporal horn, probably not related to the patient's symptoms.

Meningiomas within the lateral ventricles are relatively more common in neurofibromatosis type 2 than in sporadic cases.

**Case 69**

67-year-old woman presenting with headaches
and dizziness.
(axial, postcontrast T1-weighted SE scan)

**Case 70**

53-year-old woman presenting with a seizure.
(axial, postcontrast T1-weighted SE scan with MTS)

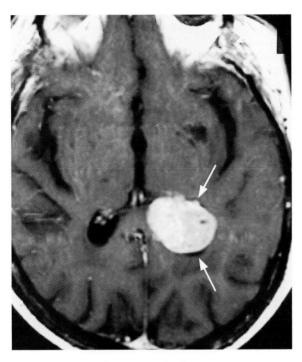

**Trigone Meningioma**
(intraventricular)

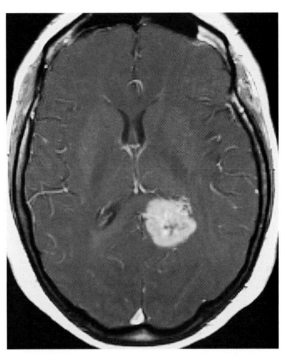

**Metastatic Carcinoma of the Lung**
(periventricular)

---

The distinction between intraventricular and periventricular lesions can be difficult, as illustrated above. Careful examination of multiple imaging planes may help to localize the tumor. When standard MR images are indeterminate, angiographic demonstration of tumor supply by choroidal arteries favors intraventricular origin of a mass.

Small rims of CSF both anterior and posterior to the tumor in Case 69 *(arrows)* suggest that it has originated and expanded within the ventricular trigone. In contrast, the metastasis in Case 70 has arisen within the left major forceps, with growth compressing the adjacent atrium of the lateral ventricle. As discussed in Chapter 1, the junction of

the splenium of the corpus callosum and the major forceps is a common location for intracerebral metastases.

Systemic tumors can also cause intraventricular metastases via hematogenous seeding of the choroid plexus (see Case 353).

The differential diagnosis of a uniformly enhancing mass in the trigone of the lateral ventricle includes choroid plexus papilloma (more commonly seen in children; see Cases 328-330), ependymoma (see Case 124), and vascular malformation (including an angioma in Sturge-Weber syndrome; see Case 911).

# REFERENCES

Ahmadi J, Hinton DR, Segall HD, Couldwell WT, et al: Dural invasion by craniofacial and calvarial neoplasms: MR imaging and histopathologic evaluation. *Radiology* 188:747-749, 1993.

Ahmadi J, Hinton DR, Segall HD, et al: Surgical implications of magnetic resonance-enhanced dura. *Neurosurgery* 35:370-377, 1994.

Aoki S, Barkovich AJ, Nishimura K, et al: Neurofibromatosis types 1 and 2: cranial MR findings. *Radiology* 172:527-534, 1989.

Aoki S, Sasaki Y, Machida T, Tanioka H: Contrast enhanced MR images in patients with meningiomas: importance of enhancements of the dura adjacent to the tumor. *AJNR* 11:935-938, 1990.

Berry I, Brant-Zawadzki M, Osaki L, et al: Gadolinium-DTPA in clinical MR of the brain: 2. Extraaxial lesion and normal structures. *AJNR* 7:789-793, 1986.

Bourekas EC, Wildenhain P, Lewin JS, et al: The dural tail sign revisited. *AJNR* 16:1514-1516, 1995.

Bradac GB, Schorner W, et al: Cavernous sinus meningiomas: an MRI study. *Neuroradiology* 29:758-581, 1987.

Breger RK, Papke RA, Pojunas KW, et al: Benign extraaxial tumors: contrast enhancement with Gd-DTPA. *Radiology* 163:427-430, 1987.

Buetow MP, Burton PC, Smirniotopoulos JG: Typical, atypical, and misleading features in meningioma. *Radiographics* 11:1087-1100, 1991.

Bydder GM, Kingsley DPE, Brown J, et al: MR imaging of meningiomas including studies with and without gadolinium-DTPA. *J Comput Assist Tomogr* 9:690-697, 1985.

Carpeggiani P, Crisi G, Trevisan C: MRI of intracranial meningiomas: Correlations with histology and physical consistency. *Neuroradiology* 35:532-536, 1993.

Carvalho GA, Matthies C, Tatagiba M, et al: Impact of computed tomographic and magnetic resonance imaging findings on surgical outcome in petroclival meningioma. *Neurosurgery* 47:1287-1295, 2000.

Castillo M, Davis PC, Ross WK, Hoffman JC Jr: Meningioma of the chiasm and optic nerves: CT and MR findings. *J Comput Assist Tomogr* 13:679-681, 1989.

Chen TC, Zee CS, Miller CA, et al: Magnetic resonance imaging and pathological correlates of meningiomas. *Neurosurgery* 31:1015-1022, 1992.

Chiechi MV, Smirniotopoulos JR, Mena H: Intracranial hemangiopericytomas: MR and CT features: *AJNR* 17:1365-1371, 1996.

Croutch KL, Wong WHM, Coufal F, et al: En plaque meningioma of the basilar meninges and Meckel's cave: MR appearance. *AJNR* 16:949-951, 1995.

Curnes JT: MR imaging of peripheral intracranial neoplasms: extra-axial versus intra-axial masses. *J Comput Assist Tomogr* 11:932-934, 1987.

Daemerel P, William G, Lammeus M, et al: Inracranial meningiomas: correlation between MR imaging and histology in fifty patients. *J Comput Assist Tomogr* 15:45-51, 1991.

Darling CF, Byrd SE, Reyes-Mugica M, et al: MR of pediatric intracranial meningiomas. *AJNR* 15:435-444, 1994.

Dolinskas CA, Simeone FA: Surgical site after resection of a meningioma. *AJNR* 19:419-426, 1998.

Elster AD, Challa VE, Gilbert TH, et al: Meningiomas: MR and histopathologic features. *Radiology* 170:857-862, 1089

Feliciani M, Ruscalleda J, Rovira A, et al: Cystic meningiomas in adults: computed tomographic and magnetic resonance imaging features in 15 cases. *Int J Neurorad* 4:21-32, 1998.

Fujii K, Fujita N, Hirabuki N, et al: Neuromas and meningiomas evaluation of early enhancement with dynamic MR imaging. *AJNR* 13:1215-1220, 1992.

George AE, Russell EJ, Kricheff II: White matter buckling: CT sign of extraaxial mass. *AJNR* 1:425-460, 1980.

Germano IM, Edwards MSB, Davis RI, Schiffer D: Intracranial meningiomas of the fist two decade of life. *J Neurosurg* 80:447-453, 1994.

Glasier CM, Husain MM, Chadduck W, Boop FA: Meningiomas in children: MR and histopathologic findings, *AJNR* 14:237-241, 1993.

Goldsher D, Litt AW, Pinto RS, et al: Dural "tail" associated with meningiomas on Gd-DTPA-enhanced MR images: characteristics, differential diagnostic value, and possible implications of treatment. *Radiology* 176:447-450, 1990.

Guidetti B, Delfini R, Gagliardi FM, Vagnozzi R: Meningiomas of the lateral ventricles: clinical, neuroradiologic, and surgical considerations in 19 cases. *Surg Neurol* 24:364-370, 1985.

Gupta S, Gupta RK, Banerjee D, Gujral RB: Problems with the "dural tail" sign. *Neuroradiology* 35:541-542, 1993.

Haughton VM, Rimm AA, Czervionke LF, et al: Sensitivity of Gd-DTPA-enhanced MR imaging of benign extraaxial tumors. *Radiology* 166:829-834, 1988.

Hirsch VM, Sekar LN, Lanzino G, et al: Meningiomas involving the cavernous sinus: value of imaging for predicting surgical complications. *Am J Roentgenol* 160:1083-1088, 1993.

Hope JKA, Armstrong DA, Babyn PS, et al: Primary meningeal tumors in children: correlation of clinical and CT findings with histologic type and prognosis. *AJNR* 13:1355-1364, 1992.

Ikushima I, Korogi Y, Kuratsu J, et al: Dynamic MRI of meningiomas and schwannomas: is differential diagnosis possible? *Neuroradiology* 39:633-638, 1997.

Jaaskelainen J, Haltia M, Servo A: Atypical and anaplastic meningiomas: radiology, surgery, radiotherapy and outcome. *Surg Neurol* 25: 233-242, 1986.

Kaplan RD, Coon S, Drayer BP, et al: MR characteristics of meningioma subtypes at 1.5 Tesla. *J Comput Assist Tomogr* 16: 366-371, 1992.

Katayama Y, Tsubokawa T, Tanaka A, Koshinaga M, et al: Magnetic resonance imaging of xanthomatous meningioma. *Neruoradiology* 35:187-189, 1992.

Kulali A, Ilcayto R, Fiskeci C: Cystic meningiomas. *Acta Neurochir (Wein)* 111:108-113, 1991.

Kuratsu J, Kochi M, Ushio Y: Incidence and clinical features of asymptomatic meningiomas. *J Neurosurg* 92:766-770, 2000.

Larson TL, Talbot JM, Wong ML: Geniculate ganglion meningiomas: CT and MR appearance. *AJNR* 16:1144-1146, 1995.

Lee A, Wallace C, Rewcastle B, Sutherland G: Metastases to meningioma. *AJNR* 19:1120-1122, 1998.

Mack EE, Wilson CB: Meningiomas induced by high-dose cranial irradiation. *J Neurosurg* 79:28-31, 1993.

Mahmood A, Caccamo DV, Tomecek FJ, Malik GM: Atypical and malignant meningiomas: a clinicopathological review. *Neurosurgery* 33:955-963, 1993.

Majos C, Cucurella G, Aguilera C, et al: Intraventricular meningiomas: MR imaging and MR spectroscopic finding in two cases. *AJNR* 20:882-885, 1999.

Mamourian AC, Lewandowski AE, Towfighi J: Cystic intraparenchymal meningioma in a chills: case report. *AJNR* 12:366-367, 1991.

Mawhinney RR, Buckley JH, Holloand IM, Worthington BS: The value of magnetic resonance imaging in the diagnosis of intracranial meningiomas. *Clin Radiol* 37:429-439, 1986.

Meltzer CC, Smirniotopoulos JG, Fukui MB: The dural tail. *Int J Neurorad* 4:33-40, 1998.

Moss R, Roskwald G, Chou S, et al: Radiation-induced meningiomas in pediatric patients. *Neurosurgery* 22:758, 1988.

Nagele I, Petersen D, Klose U, et al: The "dural tail" adjacent to meningiomas studied by dynamic contrast-enhanced MRI: a comparison with histopathology. *Neuroradiology* 36:303-307, 1994.

Naul LG, Hise JH, Bauserman SC, Todd FD: CT and MR of meningeal melanocytoma. *AJNR* 12:315-316, 1991.

Odake G: Cystic meningiomas report of three patients. *Neurosurgery* 30:935-940, 1992.

Perry RD, Parker GD, Hallinan JH: CT and MR imaging of fourth ventricular meningiomas. *J Comput Assist Tomogr* 14:276-280, 1990.

Roda JM, Bencosme JA, Perez-Higuelias A, Frail M: Simultaneous multiple intracranial and spinal meningiomas. *Neurochirugie* 35:92-94, 1992.

Rohringer M, Sutherland G, Louw DF, Sima AAF: Incidence and clinicopathological features of meningioma. *J Neurosurg* 71:665-672, 1989.

Ruscalleda J, Feliciani M, Avila A, et al: Neuroradiological features of intracranial and intraorbital meningeal haemangiopericytomas. *Neuroradiology* 36:440-445, 1994.

Salibi SS, Nauta HJW, Brem H et al: Lipomeningioma: report of three cases and review of the literature. *Neurosurgery* 25: 122-125, 1989.

Sheporaitis L, Osborn AG, Smirniotopoulos JG, Clunie DA, et al: Radiologic-pathologic correlation: intracranial meningioma. *AJNR* 13: 29-37, 1992.

Siegelman ES, Mishkin MM, Taveras JT: Past, present, and future of radiology of meningioma. *Radiographics* 11: 899-910, 1991.

Sklar EML, Schatz NJ, Glaser JS, et al: Optic tract edema in a meningioma of the tuberculum sellae. *AJNR* 21:1661-1663, 2000.

Spagnoli MV, Goldberg HI, Grossman RI, et al: Intracranial meningiomas high-field MR imaging. *Radiology* 161:369-375, 1986.

Sze G, Soletsky S, Bronen R, et al: MR imaging of the cranial meninges. *AJNR* 10: 965, 1989.

Taylor SI, Barakos JA, Harsh GR IV, Wilson CB: Magnetic resonance imaging of tuberculum sellae meningiomas: preventing preoperative misdiagnosis as pituitary adenoma. *Neurosurgery* 31:621-627, 1992.

Terasaki KK, Zee CS.: Evolution of central necrosis is a meningioma: CT and MR features. *J Comput Assist Tomogr* 14: 464-466, 1990.

Terstegge K, Schörner W, Henkes H, Heye N, et al: Hyperostosis in meningiomas: MR findings in patients with recurrent meningioma of the sphenoid wings, *AJNR* 15:55-560, 1994.

Tokumaru A, O'uchi T, Eguchi T, et al: Prominent meningeal enhancement adjacent to meningioma on Gd-DTPA-enhanced MR images: histopathologic correlation. *Radiology* 175:431-433, 1990.

Wagle VG, Villemure JG, Melanson D, et al: Diagnostic potential of magnetic resonance in cases of foramen magnum meningiomas. *Neurosurgery* 21:622-626, 1987.

Wasenko JJ, Hochhauser L, Stopa EG, Winfield JA: Cystic meningiomas: MR characteristics and surgical considerations. *AJNR* 15:1959-1965, 1999.

Watabe T, Azuma T: T1 and T2 measurements of meningiomas and neuromas before and after Gd-DTPA. *AJNR* 10:463-470, 1989.

Wilms G, Lammens M, Marchal G, et al: Prominent dural enhancement adjacent to nonmeneingiomatous malignant lesions on contrast-enhanced MR images. *AJNR* 12: 761-764, 1991.

Wilms G, Lammens M, Marchal G, et al: Thickening of dura surrounding meningiomas: MR features. *J Comput Assist Tomogr* 13:763-768, 1989.

Yeakley JW, Kulkarni M, McArdle CB, et al: High-resolution MR imaging of juxtasellar meningiomas with CT and angiographic correlation. *AJNR* 9:279-285, 1988.

Yoon HK, Na DG, Byun HS, et al: MRI of primary meningeal tumors in children. *Neuroradiology* 41:512-516, 1999.

Young SC, Grossman RI, Goldberg HI, et al: MR of vascular encasement in parasellar masses: comparison with angiography and CT. *AJNR* 9:35-38, 1988.

Zagzag D, Gomori JN, Rappaport ZH, Shalet MN: Cystic meningiomas presenting as a ring lesion. *AJNR* 7:911-912, 1986.

Zee CS, Chin T, Segall HD, et al: Magnetic resonance imaging of meningiomas. *Semin US CT MR* 13: 154-169, 1992.

Zimmerman RD, Fleming CA, Saint-Louis LA, et al: Magnetic resonance imaging of meningiomas. *AJNR* 6:149-157, 1985.

# CHAPTER 3

# Gliomas

### Case 71

30-year-old woman presenting with seizures, beginning with lip twitching and mouth opening. (sagittal, noncontrast T1-weighted SE scan)

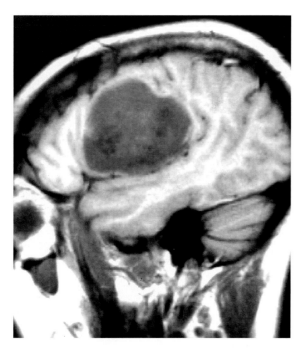

**Grade II Astrocytoma**

### Case 72

4-year-old boy presenting with seizures. (coronal, postcontrast T1-weighted SE scan)

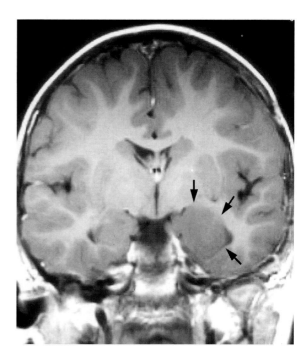

**Grade II Astrocytoma**

---

The current classification of gliomas by the World Health Organization recognizes three "special," "circumscribed," or "grade I" histologies: pilocytic astrocytoma, subependymal giant cell astrocytoma, and pleomorphic xanthoastrocytoma. The remaining "diffuse" or "infiltrating" gliomas are divided into grades II, III, and IV. Grade II tumors are often referred to as "low grade" lesions, while grade III and grade IV tumors are considered to be "high grade" gliomas (see Cases 86-89).

In the absence of hemorrhage or dense calcification, the signal intensity of low grade gliomas on T1-weighted images is usually homogeneous and comparable to or lower than that of gray matter. Cases 71 and 72 are typical examples.

The margin of gliomas such as Case 71 may be surprisingly distinct and smooth on MR scans as compared to their poor definition on CT studies. This sharp demarcation belies the biological potential of the tumors: most are infiltrating neoplasms that tend to increase in grade over time.

In other patients, low grade glial neoplasms present as amorphous thickening of cortical gray matter, as illustrated in Case 72 (*arrow*; see also Case 77). The deep temporal lobe is a common location for low grade tumors in children and young adults, and the history of seizures is typical for these patients (see Case 526 for an additional example). The absence of abnormal contrast enhancement in Case 72 is frequent in low grade astrocytomas.

An appearance comparable to Case 72 in an adult could be caused by herpes encephalitis or limbic encephalitis, an unusual paraneoplastic disorder most commonly associated with oat cell carcinoma of the lung (see Cases 443-447).

### Case 73

26-year-old woman presenting with seizures.
(coronal, noncontrast T2-weighted SE scan)

### Case 74

7-year-old girl presenting with seizures.
(axial, noncontrast T2-weighted SE scan)

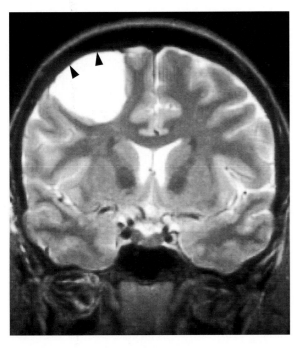

**Grade II Astrocytoma**

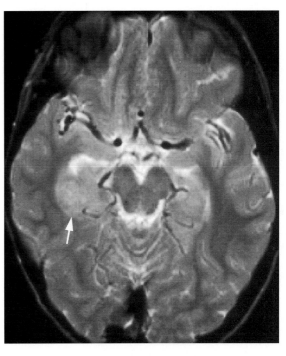

**Grade II Astrocytoma**

---

The signal intensity of low grade gliomas on long TR spin echo images may range from isointensity to very high values. High intensity (as in Case 73) is more common, reflecting high water content in the tumor region.

The glioma in Case 73 demonstrates little mass effect for its size, suggesting a long-standing, slow-growing lesion. The absence of reactive cerebral edema also supports a chronic, low grade process. Subtle erosion of the overlying calvarium is equivocally present *(arrowheads)*, again favoring a long history of gradual evolution (compare to Cases 116, 338, 340, and 809).

The peripheral base and sharply defined margins of a superficial glioma can resemble a localized cerebral infarct. Clues to the correct diagnosis include rounded rather than linear borders and the absence of an acute neurological deficit. MR scans typically demonstrate a characteristic gyriform morphology within subacute infarcts, illustrated in Cases 554, 559, and 565.

Occasional gliomas (both low and high grade) remain nearly isointense to gray matter on T2-weighted scans. This appearance, seen in the medial right temporal lobe of Case 74 *(arrow)*, often correlates with precontrast high attenuation on CT scans. Both features suggest dense cellularity with little cytoplasmic or extracellular water. Other tumors that can present a similar appearance are germinomas (see Case 294) and primary cerebral lymphomas (see Cases 348 and 349).

### Case 75

6-year-old boy presenting with seizures.
(axial, postcontrast T1-weighted SE scan)

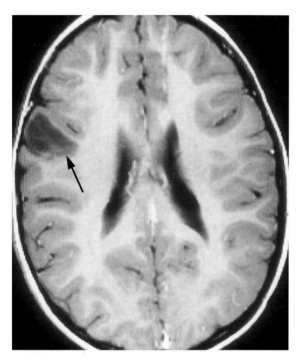

**Grade II Astrocytoma**

### Case 76

2-year-old girl presenting with seizures.
(axial, noncontrast T2-weighted SE scan)

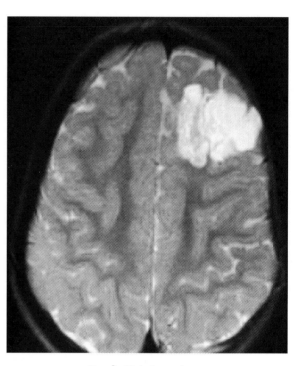

**Grade II Astrocytoma**

Many low grade gliomas are superficial lesions, involving cerebral cortex and commonly presenting with seizures. Such lesions are frequently encountered in children. The tumors are typically well defined and can often be resected with good long-term survival.

As illustrated in Cases 75 and 76, these cortical gliomas of childhood usually demonstrate long T1 and T2 values. Contrast enhancement is typically minimal or absent. The slow growth of the tumors may cause erosion of the adjacent inner table.

If the lesion is small, as in Case 75, a cortical/subcortical hamartoma of tuberous sclerosis might be considered in the differential diagnosis (see Cases 893 and 900). A search

for associated lesions, particularly subependymal nodules, is important is assessing this possibility.

The moderate lobulation of the superficial glioma in Case 76 is intermediate between the smoothly rounded margins of Case 73 and the gyriform infiltration in Case 78.

Dysembryoplastic neuroepithelial tumors (DNET) may similarly present as superficial lesions causing cortical thickening in young patients. These masses most commonly occur in the temporal or frontal lobes, often demonstrating a "mega-gyric" and/or multinodular morphology (see Cases 338-341). A history of seizures, associated calvarial erosion, and a lack of contrast enhancement may closely resemble the presentation of a low grade glioma.

### Case 77

41-year-old man presenting with seizures.
(coronal, postcontrast T1-weighted SE scan)

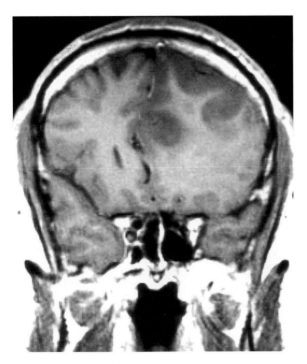

**Grade II Astrocytoma**

### Case 78

37-year-old man presenting with
sudden onset of disorientation.
(axial, noncontrast T2-weighted SE scan)

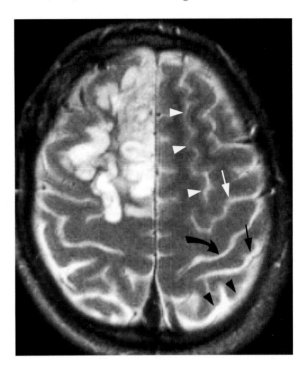

**Grade II Astrocytoma**
(recurrent)

Low grade gliomas sometimes infiltrate cortex rather than developing into a centralized mass. The resulting gyriform pattern of signal abnormality (with long T1 and T2 values) may resemble cortical edema from other etiologies, such as subacute infarction or meningitis. The clinical setting usually distinguishes among these diagnostic possibilities, but occasional gliomas present with stroke-like suddenness in the reported onset of symptoms.

The glioma in Case 77 has thickened cortex of the left frontal lobe both medially and laterally. There is no evidence of laminar T1-shortening within the involved gyri, a common finding in subacute infarcts (see Cases 572 and 573). Furthermore, the zone of abnormality affects two major vascular distributions (the anterior and middle cerebral arteries), an unusual occurrence in cerebral infarction.

In Case 78, the possibility of cortical infarction could be considered. However, this lesion also crosses the watershed between the anterior and middle cerebral artery distributions. This fact, together with the observation that the lateral involvement is mainly *sub*cortical, favors a diagnosis of infiltrating neoplasm rather than infarction.

As discussed on the preceding page, dysembryoplastic neuroepithelial tumors should be considered in the differential diagnosis of a gyriform mass involving cortex of the frontal and temporal lobes.

The normal sulcal anatomy in the rolandic region is well seen on the left side in Case 78. The superior frontal sulcus *(white arrowheads)* follows a parasagittal course before intersecting posteriorly (at a right angle) with the precentral sulcus *(white arrow)*. The intraparietal sulcus *(black arrowheads)* angles obliquely across the posterior parietal vertex before merging anteriorly with the postcentral sulcus *(black arrow)*. The central sulcus *(large curved arrow)* lies between the precentral and the postcentral sulci as the middle member of the three major laterally directed sulci.

## Case 79

3-year-old girl presenting with left hemiparesis.
(axial, noncontrast FLAIR scan)

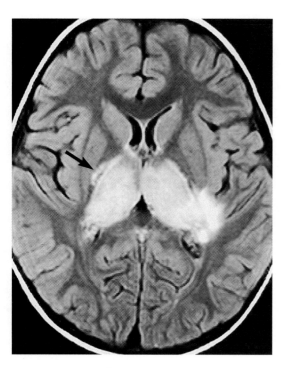

**Grade II Astrocytoma**

## Case 80

4-year-old girl presenting with headaches.
(axial, noncontrast T2-weighted FSE scan)

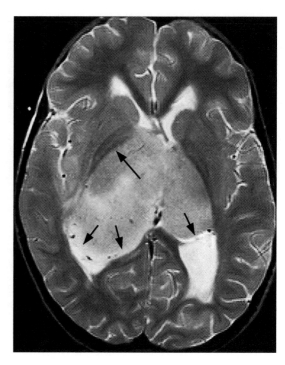

**Grade III Astrocytoma**

Gliomas may involve the thalamus bilaterally, crossing through and expanding the massa intermedia. This morphology is most commonly encountered in children but occasionally occurs in adults. The extent of thalamic infiltration may be remarkably symmetrical, as in Case 79, or variably asymmetrical, as in Case 80.

Signal intensity of the tumor is usually homogeneous, with mildly to moderately prolonged T2 values. Case 80 illustrates that thalamic gliomas with dense cellularity may demonstrate only mild hyperintensity on long TR images.

Reactive edema is present lateral to the tumor in Case 79. The involvement of the globus pallidus and posterior limb of the internal capsule on the right *(arrow)* correlates with the patient's hemiparesis.

The slow-growing glioma in Case 80 has caused marked displacement of the right lentiform nucleus *(long arrow).* Expansion of the pulvinar of the thalamus *(short arrows)* is associated with compression of the lateral ventricular trigones, right greater than left.

The differential diagnosis of bithalamic lesions includes inflammatory and vascular etiologies, such as acute disseminated encephalomyelitis (see Cases 394 and 396), viral encephalitis (see Case 656), infarction secondary to compromise of the rostral basilar artery (see Case 655), anoxia (see Case 666), and edema due to deep venous thrombosis (see Case 654).

### Case 81

18-year-old man presenting with seizures.
(coronal, noncontrast T1-weighted GRE scan)

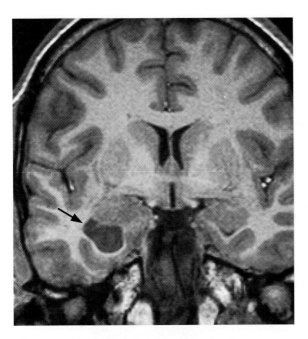

**Grade II Astrocytoma**

### Case 82

18-month-old girl presenting with a seizure.
(coronal, noncontrast T2-weighted FSE scan)

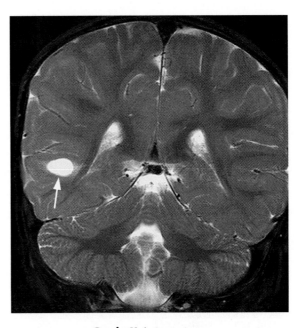

**Grade II Astrocytoma**

---

The usually well-defined margins of low grade gliomas on MR scans may result in the demonstration of very small tumors. The masses in Cases 81 and 82 *(arrows)* are only about 1 cm in diameter, but their long T1 and T2 values clearly demarcate them as foci of abnormal tissue. The appearance of these lesions is not specific, but focal glioma should be considered in the differential diagnosis, particularly in these clinical contexts.

Lesions in or near the hippocampal formation (as in Case 81) commonly cause seizures because of the low excitation threshold of neurons in this region. The medial temporal lobe can be difficult to assess on CT scans, and coronal MR studies are appropriate as an initial examination or following a negative CT study in such patients. (See Cases 467, 526, and 763 for other examples of small structural lesions within the temporal lobes of patients with seizures.) Compare the definition of the lesion in Case 81 with that in Case 72.

The very focal glioma in Case 82 resembles a cyst because of high water content and discrete margins. Such as-

trocytomas may contain cells with large amounts of cytoplasm, extensive extracellular fluid, and/or microcystic areas. MR documentation that a "watery" lesion is truly cystic requires a sedimentation level (see Case 95) or demonstration of facilitated diffusion characteristics.

The onset of seizures in an adult is a worrisome event. Cerebral masses are detected in approximately 20% of such cases. Seizures are a particularly common symptom of low grade neoplasms; up to 50% of oligodendrogliomas present in this manner.

Possible nonneoplastic causes of a localized subcortical zone of prolonged T2 values in a child with seizures include tuberous sclerosis (see Cases 900-902) and focal cortical dysplasia (see Case 879).

Calcification within a focal glioma may cause localized signal loss due to physical replacement of protons and/or susceptibility effects that accelerate proton relaxation. The lesion may then resemble a cavernous hemangioma (see Cases 761-764).

## Case 83A

47-year-old man presenting with
an episode of confusion.
(axial, noncontrast FLAIR scan)

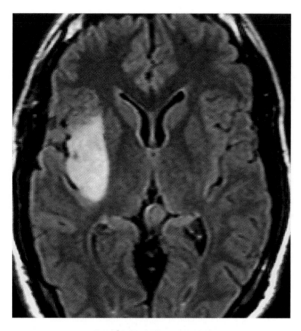

**Grade II Astrocytoma**

## Case 83B

Same patient.
(single voxel proton spectroscopy,
PRESS technique, SE 1500/135)

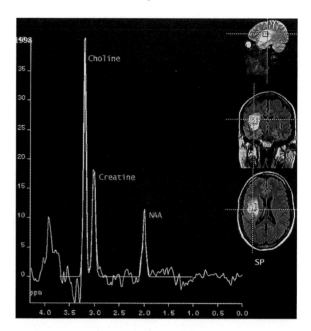

**Grade II Astrocytoma**

The clinical presentation and MR appearance of low grade gliomas may overlap those of other pathologies, such as cerebral infarction or encephalitis. MR spectroscopy can help to establish the diagnosis when the imaging characteristics of a lesion are ambiguous.

A zone of T2 prolongation and mild mass effect involves the insula and subinsular region in Case 83A. The morphology and location of the process are nonspecific; possible etiologies include nonneoplastic lesions (e.g., recent infarction), as well as a primary tumor.

Three key metabolites are labelled in the proton spectrum of the lesion in Case 83B. *N*-Acetyl aspartate (NAA), located at 2.0 ppm, is an amino acid found within nerve cells; its abundance correlates with the presence of healthy neurons and/or axons, with reduction of NAA suggesting damage to and/or replacement of the normal neuronal population. Creatine (and phosphocreatine), located at 3.0 ppm, is a component of cellular energy metabolism. Choline, positioned at 3.2 ppm, is incorporated in the metabolism of cell membranes; elevation of this peak is believed to reflect increased turnover of membranes or myelin and can be seen in neoplastic, demyelinating, or reparative states.

The metabolic profile in Case 83B indicates an abnormally low amount of NAA together with an elevation of choline. This combination suggests destruction or replacement of normal neurons by a process with increased turnover of membranes. Although nonspecific (an unusual demyelinating lesion could have similar characteristics), the pattern is most compatible with neoplasm.

The proton spectrum of recent cerebral infarction would be expected to show an elevated lactate peak at 1.3 ppm with little initial alteration of the NAA and choline levels. (NAA is observed to decrease a few days after cerebral infarction.)

Proton spectroscopy can also be useful in following the course of treated gliomas. The typical spectrum of residual or recurrent tumor (with a high choline peak) is distinct from the typical spectrum of radiation necrosis (lack of NAA, creatine, and choline peaks; elevated lactic acid). Mixtures of residual/recurrent tumor and post-therapeutic necrosis are present in most cases; three-dimensional techniques (e.g., chemical shift imaging or "CSI") are helpful for accurately sampling these heterogeneous lesions.

Spectra similar to Case 83B often can be demonstrated within tissue 1 or 2 centimeters beyond the margins of T2-prolongation or contrast enhancement in glial tumors. Lactate and/or lipid peaks, both occurring at 1.3 ppm, have been correlated with necrosis, high grade, and poor prognosis in gliomas.

## Case 84

30-year-old woman presenting with
right hemiparesis and aphasia.
(axial, postcontrast T1-weighted SE scan with MTS)

## Case 85

63-year-old man presenting with confusion.
(coronal, postcontrast T1-weighted SE scan)

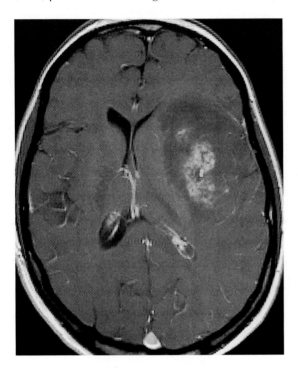

**Grade II Astrocytoma**

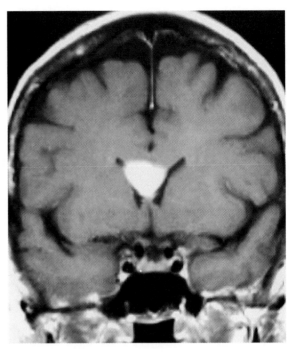

**Grade II Astrocytoma**

Many low grade gliomas demonstrate little or no contrast enhancement (see Case 72 for an example).

When present, enhancement of low grade astrocytomas is often partial or patchy, as illustrated in Case 84. Postcontrast MR scans have proved to be more sensitive than CT studies to mild abnormality of the blood-brain barrier. Enhancement of low grade lesions may be correspondingly more apparent or impressive on MR images than on CT scans.

Other low grade glial neoplasms enhance intensely, as in Case 85. The morphology of such enhancement is often solid and smoothly marginated, contrasting with the more irregular patterns characteristic of malignant gliomas. (See Cases 98 and 99, and compare Case 85 to Case 107.)

The presence of prominent contrast enhancement does not necessarily imply high grade malignancy of a glial tumor. For example, low grade pilocytic astrocytomas in children typically enhance intensely. Conversely, the absence of contrast enhancement does not exclude malignant histology; see Cases 102 and 103.

### Case 86

4-year-old boy presenting with headaches
and hemiparesis.
(sagittal, noncontrast T1-weighted SE scan)

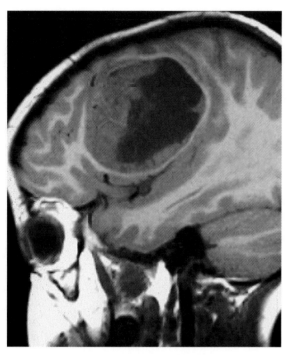

**Glioblastoma Multiforme**

### Case 87

38-year-old woman presenting with
auditory disturbance.
(coronal, noncontrast T1-weighted SE scan)

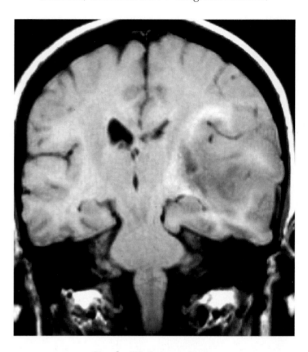

**Grade III Astrocytoma**

Anaplastic astrocytoma (grade III astrocytoma) and glioblastoma multiforme (grade IV astrocytoma) are often described together as "malignant" or "high grade" gliomas.

The MR spectrum of malignant gliomas overlaps that of low grade neoplasms, and occasional tumors have intermediate characteristics. However, the features of most high grade tumors are different from those of the lower grade lesions illustrated on the previous pages.

High grade gliomas typically demonstrate heterogeneous tissue texture and signal intensity on T1-weighted images. This complex architecture reflects variable cellularity, as well as the common presence of necrosis, hemorrhage, and cysts.

The posterior half of the large frontal mass in Case 86 is grossly cystic, traversed by septations leading to scattered mural nodules. The solid anterior portion demonstrates mixed tissue components and several low intensity foci, which may represent large vessels or dense calcifications.

Case 87 illustrates a more infiltrating morphology of a high grade glioma. The size of the mass and the variable tissue components suggest malignant histology.

### Case 88

38-year-old woman presenting with
auditory disturbance.
(axial, noncontrast scan; SE 3000/30)

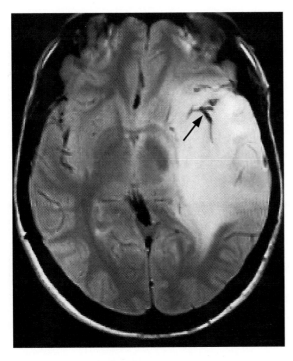

**Grade III Astrocytoma**
(same patient as Case 87)

### Case 89

61-year-old woman presenting with
severe headaches.
(axial, noncontrast T2-weighted SE scan)

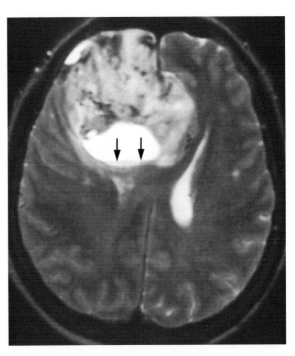

**Glioblastoma Multiforme**

---

On long TR spin echo scans, the appearance of malignant gliomas is usually dominated by high signal intensity. This prolongation of T2 values (and increased proton density) is attributable to both the tumor tissue and reactive "edema." Pathological studies have shown that tumor cells are actually present within (and beyond) the "edema" surrounding even well-defined masses.

The tumor in Case 88 is homogeneous, extending throughout an area that approximates the distribution of the middle cerebral artery. (Note the displaced flow void of the patent middle cerebral artery near its genu; *arrow*.) Many gliomas are found in the perisylvian region, where they may mimic recent infarction. The clinical context, confluent (rather than gyriform) edema, and predominant white matter involvement of a glioma usually allow distinction from ischemic lesions.

In Case 89, a much more heterogeneous glioma has grown to and around the dural margin of the anterior falx. The area of greatest signal intensity within the lesion is a fluid-filled cyst, which demonstrates a sedimentation level posteriorly *(arrows)*. Small, dark areas within the remainder of the mass represent hemorrhagic foci, which were seen as high intensity zones on a T1-weighted scan. (Compare to the appearance of hemorrhage and calcification within oligodendrogliomas in Cases 113-116.)

An aggressive meningioma or meningeal sarcoma arising from the falx and invading cerebral parenchyma could be considered in the differential diagnosis of Case 89. A postcontrast scan may help to distinguish between these possibilities.

**Case 90**

56-year-old man presenting with a seizure.
(axial, noncontrast T2-weighted FSE scan)

**Case 91**

68-year-old woman presenting with left hemiparesis.
(axial, noncontrast T2-weighted FSE scan)

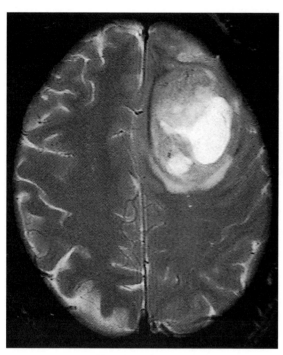

**Glioblastoma Multiforme**

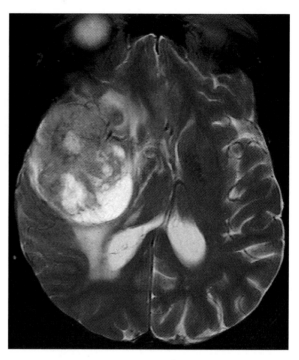

**Metastatic Carcinoma of the Lung**

---

The typical heterogeneity of malignant gliomas immediately suggests this diagnosis when a complex cerebral tumor is discovered in an adult. Case 90 is representative of such lesions.

Case 91 demonstrates that parenchymal metastases can present a very similar appearance of mixed signal abnormality. When a heterogeneous metastasis is large and solitary, the mass can be indistinguishable from a high grade glioma (see Cases 12 and 16 for other examples).

The high intensity zones within each of the above masses indicate water-like regions that may be necrotic,

cystic, or microcystic. More isointense areas likely represent cellular tissue. A small amount of edema is present near the margins of the tumor in each case.

Perfusion-weighted images may help to distinguish malignant primary tumors from metastatic lesions. High grade gliomas typically demonstrate increased relative cerebral blood volume in the zone of edema outside of the central mass, implying infiltrating tumor. Relative cerebral blood volume is usually not increased (and may be reduced due to capillary compression) in the region of edema surrounding a metastatic tumor.

### Case 92

70-year-old man presenting with left hemiparesis.
(axial, noncontrast scan; SE 3000/45)

### Case 93

55-year-old man presenting with headaches.
(axial, noncontrast scan; SE 2500/45)

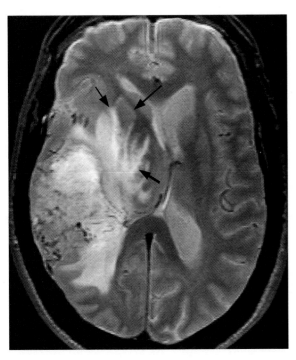

**Glioblastoma Multiforme**

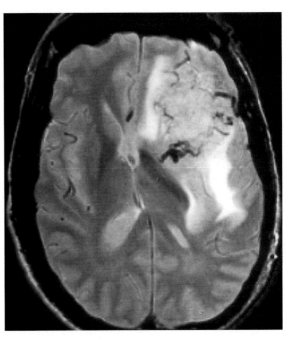

**Sphenoid Wing Meningioma**
(same patient as Case 33)

---

Large, bizarre vessels within a glial neoplasm are a strong indication of malignant histology. The irregular caliber, course, and branching pattern of the flow voids in Case 92 represent the MRI equivalent of tumor vascularity as previously defined by cerebral angiography.

The tumor vessels in Case 93 are equally large, but they are less irregular than in Case 92. Compare this appearance to the meningioma in Case 38.

Both of these tumors demonstrate moderately high signal intensity with surrounding edema. The edema in Case 92

tracks anteriorly to involve the internal *(short thick arrow)* and external *(short thin arrow)* capsules, surrounding the displaced lentiform nucleus *(long arrow)*. Both cases illustrate subfalcial herniation, with contralateral shift of the pericallosal arteries.

As discussed in Case 45, meningiomas of the sphenoid wing may incite extensive edema within the temporal lobe and adjacent hemisphere. The edema may be more impressive than the tumor itself, which can be overlooked on noncontrast scans.

### Case 94

6-year-old boy with a history of seizures.
(sagittal, noncontrast T1-weighted SE scan)

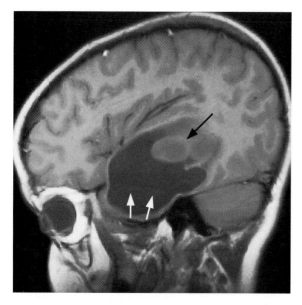

**Grade III Astrocytoma**

### Case 95

56-year-old woman presenting with hemiparesis.
(axial, noncontrast T2-weighted SE scan)

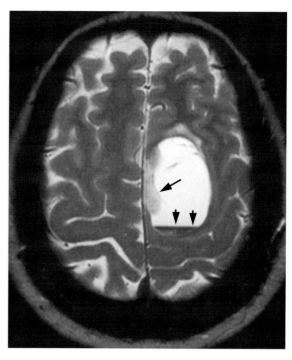

**Glioblastoma Multiforme**

Many low and high grade gliomas contain one or more cysts. When a tumor cyst is large and unilocular, palliative drainage may provide symptomatic improvement by reducing mass effect. Repeated aspiration or continuous drainage may be necessary due to rapid reaccumulation of fluid.

A reliable MR (or CT) indication of a truly cystic tumor is a sedimentation level within the lesion, as demonstrated in Case 95 *(short arrows)*. The dense material settling in the dependent portion of a cyst may be cellular debris, hemorrhage, or accumulated contrast material. The very low signal intensity of the sedimentation layer in Case 95 suggests blood products, as discussed in Chapter 13.

In the absence of a sedimentation level, a cyst can be suspected when the content of the lesion remains completely homogeneous on all pulse sequences. Some solid tumors (particularly astrocytomas with gelatinous consistency) are remarkably uniform (see Cases 131 and 138), so care must be taken before a mass can be labeled as "cystic." Diffusion-weighted imaging is useful to establish the cystic nature of an indeterminate lesion.

In Case 94, a complex mural nodule of tumor tissue is found along the posterior wall of the cyst *(black arrow)*. A thin septum is faintly visible within the cyst *(white arrows)*. Such partitions are better seen on MR scans than on CT studies but are difficult to resolve and can be missed entirely.

The malignant glioma in Case 95 demonstrates an elongated mural nodule medially *(long arrow)*. Septations cross the anterior portion of the cyst, and a small amount of edema is present anterior to the mass. Since the medial margin of the tumor is adjacent to the falx, the possibility of an atypical extraaxial lesion (e.g., meningioma) might be considered. Angiography demonstrated pial rather than dural arterial supply, and a cystic glioblastoma was confirmed at surgery.

### Case 96

13-year-old boy presenting with a seizure.
(sagittal, noncontrast T1-weighted SE scan)

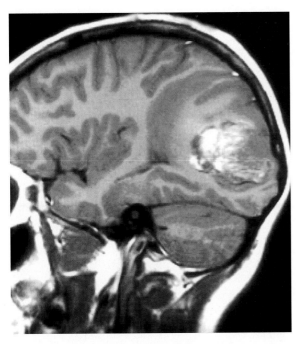

**Glioblastoma Multiforme**

### Case 97

17-year-old man with sudden loss of consciousness.
(axial, noncontrast T2-weighted FSE scan)

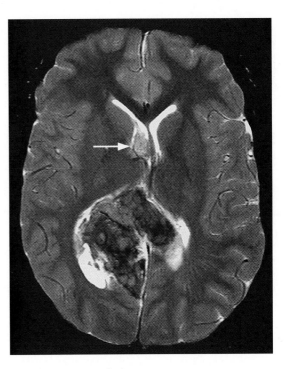

**Grade II Astrocytoma**

Macroscopic hemorrhage is relatively uncommon in gliomas, occurring in about 5%. Among low grade gliomas, oligodendrogliomas make up a disproportionate share of lesions presenting with gross hemorrhage. Malignant gliomas are characterized angiographically by neovascularity, which represents a likely source of bleeding (see Case 92).

Patchy T1-shortening is present throughout the occipital mass in Case 96, reflecting the presence of methemoglobin and implying subacute hemorrhage (see discussion of Cases 673-676). The texture or architecture of the lesion is more complex than the usual laminated morphology of a benign hematoma (compare to Case 675). This feature combines with the prominent surrounding edema to suggest that the hemorrhage is superimposed on an underlying structural lesion.

Recent hemorrhage demonstrates low signal intensity on T2-weighted images, as seen throughout the large mass in Case 97. The tumor expands the posterior body and splenium of the corpus callosum and extends into the major forceps on the right (compare to Cases 104 and 105). The trigones of the lateral ventricles are displaced anterolaterally and compressed. Associated intraventricular hemorrhage is present in the right frontal horn *(arrow)*.

Rupture of an arteriovenous malformation is the most common cause of sudden intracerebral hemorrhage in a child or adolescent (see Case 752) and was suspected after an initial CT scan in Case 97. However, the MR demonstration of lobulated architecture within the lesion and extension across the corpus callosum raised the likelihood of a hemorrhagic neoplasm, which was confirmed at surgery. Together, Cases 96 and 97 illustrate that both low and high grade gliomas can present with gross hemorrhage.

It is sometimes difficult to determine on initial studies whether a focal hemorrhage is benign or malignant. Clues to the latter etiology on subsequent scans include (1) unusually slow evolution/degradation of blood products; (2) discontinuity or irregularity of the hemosiderin ring formed at the perimeter of the lesion; and (3) persistent or increasing perilesional edema.

**Case 98**

50-year-old woman presenting with apathy.
(coronal, postcontrast T1-weighted SE scan)

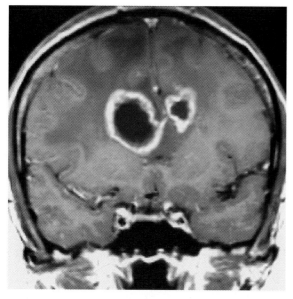

**Glioblastoma Multiforme**
(of the corpus callosum)

**Case 99**

4-year-old boy presenting with headaches.
(axial, postcontrast T1-weighted SE scan)

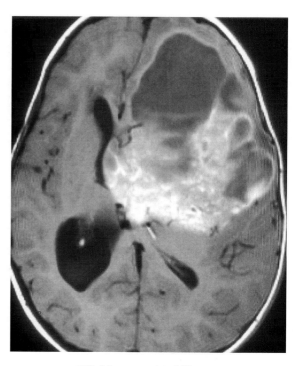

**Glioblastoma Multiforme**
(same patient as Case 86)

Most malignant gliomas demonstrate definite contrast enhancement. However, the pattern of abnormal enhancement can be quite variable.

In some anaplastic astrocytomas, contrast enhancement is surprisingly circumscribed and homogeneous. A nodular morphology may predominate, resembling Case 85.

More characteristic of malignant gliomas is the irregular, thick-walled peripheral enhancement illustrated in Case 98. The nonenhancing center of the tumor may gradually fill in with contrast material on delayed scans.

Complex mixed cystic and solid patterns are also common, as in Case 99 (see also Case 107). Areas of intense nodular enhancement are often combined with rim-enhancing zones to give a coarsely heterogeneous appearance.

A contrast-enhanced scan performed within days after surgery for a malignant glioma is useful (1) to assess completeness of resection and (2) as a baseline to evaluate subsequent tumor recurrence. Benign, reactive enhancement at the margins of resection may be seen even on early postoperative scans; however, such enhancement is usually laminar in morphology and relatively mild in degree. Prominent nodules of abnormal enhancement on initial postoperative scans suggest residual tumor (which in turn correlates with early local recurrence and poor prognosis). Benign enhancement at the borders of tumor resection can normally persist for several months.

Tissue changes may become apparent on proton spectroscopic studies (showing increasing choline levels) or perfusion-weighted scans (demonstrating increasing cerebral blood volume) before abnormal contrast enhancement develops in an area of extending or recurring glioma.

### Case 100

80-year-old woman being evaluated
for a possible stroke.
(axial, postcontrast T1-weighted SE scan)

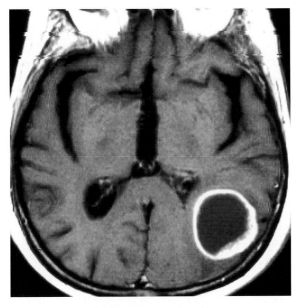

**Glioblastoma Multiforme**

### Case 101

37-year-old woman presenting with a seizure.
(axial, postcontrast T1-weighted SE scan)

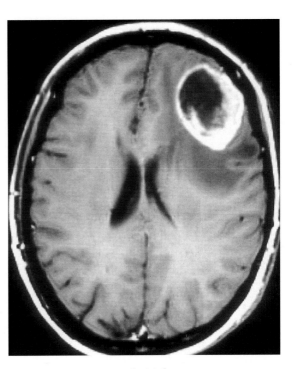

**Metastatic Melanoma**

The enhancing rim of the mass in Case 100 is relatively uniform in thickness and contour. While this appearance falls within the spectrum of malignant tumors, inflammatory lesions (e.g., pyogenic abscess or toxoplasmosis) should be considered in the differential diagnosis (see Cases 463-466).

Within the tumor category, a thick rim of contrast enhancement is not specific for high grade gliomas. Metastases, as in Case 101, and primary CNS lymphoma (especially in immunocompromised patients; see Case 357) may present a similar appearance.

Perfusion-weighted images can contribute to the MR distinction between primary and metastatic tumors by demonstrating increased cerebral blood volume outside of the enhancing mass in the former case and not in the latter. Similarly, proton spectroscopy of tissue surrounding the "margins" of a central mass may show elevated choline levels implying infiltrating tumor in cases of glioma, whereas the spectrum of tissue bordering a metastasis is unremarkable.

Both frontal lobe lesions and posterior parietal masses may become quite large without causing specific neurological deficits. A gradual change in alertness or orientation of an elderly patient may reach a threshold of detection that mimics the clinical presentation of a cerebrovascular accident.

### Case 102

4-year-old girl presenting with headaches.
(axial, postcontrast T1-weighted SE scan)

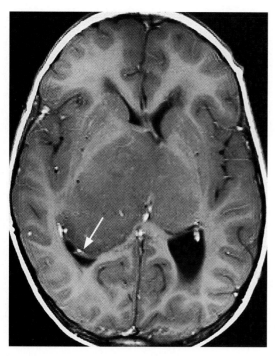

**Grade III Astrocytoma**
(same patient as Case 80)

### Case 103

36-year-old man presenting with transient confusion.
(axial, postcontrast T1-weighted SE scan with MTS)

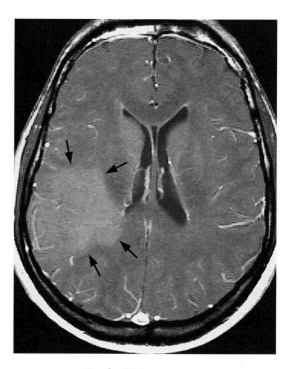

**Grade III Astrocytoma**

---

Occasional high grade gliomas do not demonstrate significant contrast enhancement. This behavior is most frequently associated with deep hemispheric lesions of dense cellularity. Specific locations where poorly enhancing malignant gliomas may be seen include the thalamus (as in Case 102) and the medial temporal lobe.

The bithalamic mass in Case 102 is asymmetrically larger on the right, where tumor extends from the foramen of Monro to the displaced choroid plexus within the trigone of the lateral ventricle *(arrow).* The lesion effaces the third ventricle, causing moderate hydrocephalus. (See Case 80 for a T2-weighted precontrast scan of this patient.)

Case 103 illustrates the need for caution in assessing contrast enhancement on scans performed with magnetization transfer suppression (MTS) techniques. MTS often increases the conspicuity of enhancement by decreasing the signal intensity of nonenhancing tissues. However, the technique may simultaneously create unrelated image contrast due to the different (usually reduced) magnetization transfer behavior of pathological tissue as compared to normal parenchyma. That is, a zone of mildly "increased" signal intensity on an MTS scan may reflect the intrinsic tissue characteristics of a pathological process rather than enhancement. In Case 103, a follow-up MTS scan without contrast enhancement was identical to the postcontrast image above.

The homogeneous mass in Case 103 has infiltrated an extensive region but causes relatively little mass effect. Although this combination and the lack of contrast enhancement might suggest a low grade process, occasional malignant gliomas present similarly. (See discussion of gliomatosis cerebri in Case 112.)

Elevated cerebral blood volume on perfusion-weighted scans and high choline levels on proton spectroscopy are clues to the high grade of a glial neoplasm even in the absence of abnormal enhancement.

## Case 104

33-year-old woman presenting with headaches.
(axial, noncontrast scan; SE 2500/28)

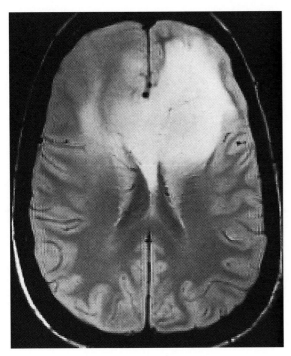

**Glioblastoma Multiforme**

## Case 105

62-year-old woman presenting with
rapidly worsening vision.
(axial, noncontrast T2-weighted SE scan)

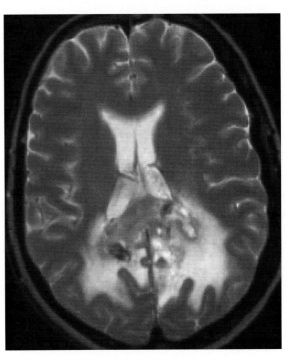

**Glioblastoma Multiforme**

---

The corpus callosum is commonly involved by glial tumors, which may arise within it or grow medially from hemispheric origins.

Callosal gliomas often have "wings" extending symmetrically or asymmetrically into both cerebral hemispheres. The resulting "butterfly" morphology is well demonstrated on axial or coronal views.

The glioma in Case 104 crosses the genu of the corpus collosum and thickens the minor forceps. The tumor in Case 105 traverses the splenium of the corpus callosum and infiltrates the major forceps. The signal intensity of the tumor in Case 104 is uniformly high, while Case 105 demonstrates heterogeneous isointesity suggesting dense cellularity with a high nuclear to cytoplasmic ratio. Pri-mary CNS lymphoma frequently involves the corpus callosum (see cases 350 and 354) and would be a diagnostic consideration in Case 105.

A number of nonneoplastic disorders can cause abnormal signal intensity and expansion of the corpus callosum resembling a tumor. Among these are multiple sclerosis, acute disseminated encephalomyelitis, and progressive multifocal leukoencephalopathy. HIV encephalitis may extend into the corpus callosum. Machiafava Bignami syndrome is a rare demyelinating disorder associated with alcohol consumption that frequently involves the corpus callosum.

Both of the above tumors infiltrate the septum pellucidum. Septal involvement is often a clue to the glial origin of smaller tumors near the foramen of Monro.

**Case 106**

5-year-old boy.
(coronal, noncontrast T1-weighted SE scan)

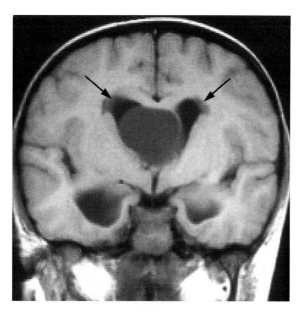

**Grade II Astrocytoma**
(cystic)

**Case 107**

66-year-old man.
(coronal, postcontrast T1-weighted SE scan)

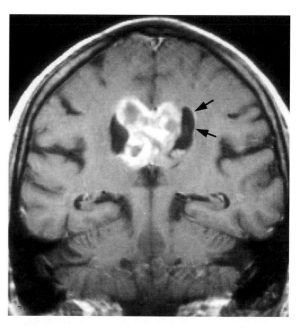

**Glioblastoma Multiforme**

As illustrated in Cases 104 and 105, gliomas of the corpus callosum frequently extend into the septum pellucidum. Less commonly, gliomas arise from or are centered in this structure.

The midline cystic glioma in Case 106 could be confused with a number of other lesions. Benign cysts occur in the septum pellucidum (see Case 845) but usually demonstrate intensity values comparable to CSF. Colloid cysts of the third ventricle may reach this size and have long T1 values (see Case 283), but the mass in Case 106 is centered above the roof of the third ventricle. Similarly, the location of the lesion as demonstrated by the coronal MR plane is superior to the normal range of craniopharyngiomas (which are occasionally found within the third ventricle but not above it).

Functionally, the cystic septal glioma in Case 106 has acted like a colloid cyst, obstructing the foramina of Monro to cause bilateral hydrocephalus. A small amount of periventricular edema caps the frontal horns bilaterally *(arrows)*.

In Case 107, a solid glioma expands the posterior portion of the septum pellucidum. The pattern of thick, heterogeneous contrast enhancement is typical for a malignant glial neoplasm. (Compare to the homogeneous enhancement of the low grade callosal/septal astrocytoma in Case 85.) The tumor invades the corpus callosum, and there is subtle evidence of subependymal extension on the left *(arrows)*.

Central neurocytomas (see Cases 342 and 343) are commonly attached to the septum pellucidum and should be considered in the differential diagnosis of a septal mass.

An additional septal glioma is presented in Case 345.

### Case 108

4-day-old girl with hydrocephalus diagnosed
on an intrauterine ultrasound.
(axial, noncontrast T2-weighted FSE scan)

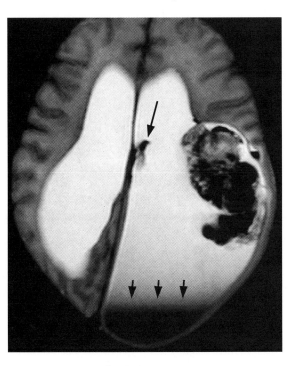

**Grade III Astrocytoma**
(with hemorrhage)

### Case 109

34-year-old woman presenting with headaches.
(axial, postcontrast T1-weighted SE scan)

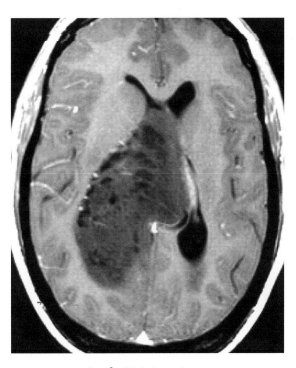

**Grade III Astrocytoma**

Partially or completely intraventricular astrocytomas may occur in children and adults.

Prominent T2-shortening within the tumor in Case 108 is attributable to extensive hemorrhage. A sedimentation level of blood products is present in the dilated left occipital horn *(short arrows),* and a thin layer of siderosis is suggested along the ependymal margins of the lateral ventricles more anteriorly (see discussion of Cases 721 and 722). At surgery, the large hemorrhagic tumor mass was found to be attached to the lateral wall of the lateral ventricle. The smaller, low intensity mass along the medial margin of the left lateral ventricle *(long arrow)* proved to be simple thrombus rather than a tumor implant.

The intraventricular mass in Case 109 is another example of a minimally enhancing high grade glioma. Multiple small cysts within the tumor were confirmed in the surgical specimen.

Oligodendrogliomas and ependymomas can also arise within or in proximity to the ventricular system (see Cases 123, 124, and 344). The differential diagnosis of intraventricular tumors should additionally include giant cell astro-

cytomas (see Cases 896 and 897) and central neurocytomas (see Cases 342 and 343). A choroid plexus papilloma could be considered in Case 108, although the location of the mass is lateral and superior to the expected position of such tumors within the trigone. Intraventricular meningiomas are usually homogeneous and enhancing masses (see Cases 68 and 69).

An intraventricular location allows a tumor to enlarge by displacing CSF, with relatively little mass effect on adjacent parenchyma. However, eventual ventricular obstruction can lead to rapidly increasing intracranial pressure. The marked hydrocephalus in Case 108 was due to intraventricular hemorrhage (with secondary clogging of the aqueduct and arachnoid granulations) rather than to compression of CSF pathways by the tumor itself.

Case 108 demonstrates that astrocytomas are among the intracranial tumors that can originate in utero and present at birth or during infancy. Other potential congenital neoplasms include teratomas, primitive neuroectodermal tumors, and choroid plexus papillomas or carcinomas.

## Case 110

39-year-old man presenting with confusion.
(axial, postcontrast T1-weighted SE scan with MTS)

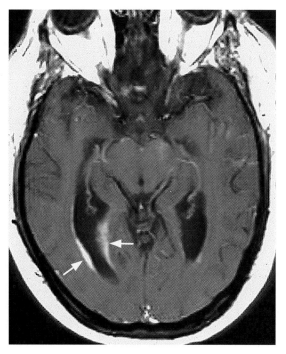

**Ependymal Seeding**
(from grade III astrocytoma adjacent
to the left frontal horn)

## Case 111

13-year-old boy being followed
after surgery for a brain tumor.
(axial, noncontrast FLAIR scan)

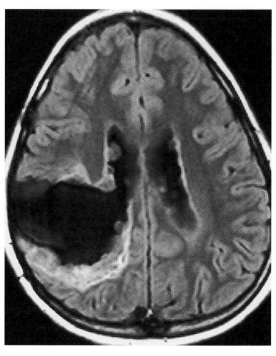

**Ependymal Seeding**
(by recurrent grade III astrocytoma)

---

Malignant gliomas frequently involve the ependymal surface or subependymal region of the ventricular system. Tumor spread along ventricular margins may represent direct extension from a primary mass or CSF "seeding" leading to distant implantation of tumor cells.

The above cases illustrate the variable morphology of ependymal involvement due to CSF dissemination of high grade gliomas. Smooth, relatively uniform thickening and enhancement along the margins of the occipital horn in Case 110 *(arrows)* was due to CSF-borne spread of a left frontal glioma.

A similar periventricular cast of tumor could be caused by CSF seeding from other CNS neoplasms (e.g., germinoma or primitive neuroectodermal tumor) or hematogenous metastases from systemic tumors (e.g., melanoma, oat cell carcinoma of the lung, and carcinoma of the breast). Primary CNS lymphoma (see Cases 352 and 434) or sec-

ondary brain involvement by systemic lymphoma (see Case 433) may present a comparable appearance. Inflammatory ventriculitis would also be included in the differential diagnosis of Case 110 (see Case 432).

Multinodular involvement of the ventricular surface in Case 111 matches the morphology along the margins of the large resection cavity. Although the small masses studding the ependymal surface of the right lateral ventricle could represent direct subependymal extension of tumor from the original resection site, the lesions within the contralateral ventricle suggest that CSF seeding has occurred.

Equivocal contrast enhancement at the anterior margin of the midbrain in Case 110 may represent leptomeningeal involvement by CSF-borne tumor. Faint ependymal enhancement is present at the borders of the left occipital horn.

### Case 112A

86-year-old woman presenting with dementia.
(axial, noncontrast T2-weighted FSE scan)

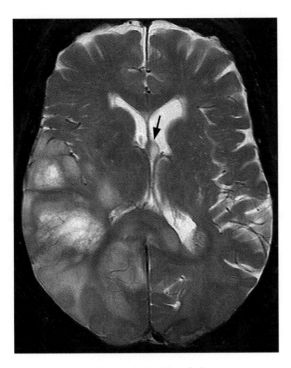

**Gliomatosis Cerebri**

### Case 112B

Same patient.
(coronal, postcontrast T1-weighted
SE scan with MTS)

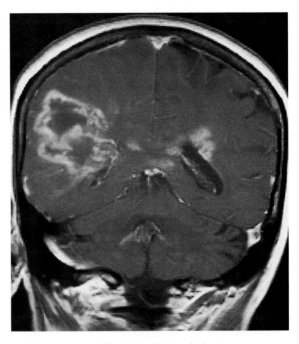

**Gliomatosis Cerebri**

---

Occasional patients present with extensive, bihemispheral involvement by gliomatous infiltration. In most of these cases, there is microscopic continuity of tumor linking the affected areas, and the widespread process may be called *gliomatosis cerebri.* In other instances, the multiple sites of tumor involvement appear to be radiographically and pathologically distinct. Cases of such "multicentric glioma" are probably rare, reflecting a generalized neoplastic susceptibility rather than extensive infiltration from a single source.

Patients with gliomatosis cerebri are often clinically problematic, with vague and generalized symptoms. In this uncertain context the widespread involvement apparent on imaging studies such as Case 112A may raise consideration of encephalitis or other inflammatory or metabolic disorders (compare to Cases 427, 442, 483, 485, and 486). The lesions of gliomatosis cerebri often enhance minimally if at all, compounding the diagnostic confusion.

Infiltration and expansion of white matter tracts is a characteristic feature of gliomatosis cerebri and can help to sug-

gest the diagnosis. The tumor in Case 112 has crossed through the splenium of the corpus callosum to extend along the margins of the left lateral ventricle. Involvement of the fornix on the left (*arrow;* Case 112A) confirms the impression of infiltrating neoplasm following axonal pathways.

The irregular contrast enhancement in Case 112B is typical of solitary malignant gliomas but more intense than usual in gliomatosis cerebri. When a few isolated islands of enhancement occur in such cases, they are commonly found to be connected by sheets of nonenhancing neoplasm.

Multivoxel proton spectroscopy can be helpful in defining the extent of tumor in gliomatosis cerebri.

Primary CNS lymphoma should be considered in the differential diagnosis of bihemispheral infiltrating disease (see Cases 346, 351, and 354).

Another example of gliomatosis cerebri is presented as Case 484.

## Case 113

54-year-old man presenting with seizures.
(sagittal, noncontrast T1-weighted SE scan)

## Case 114

41-year-old woman presenting with
headaches and blackouts.
(sagittal, noncontrast T1-weighted SE scan)

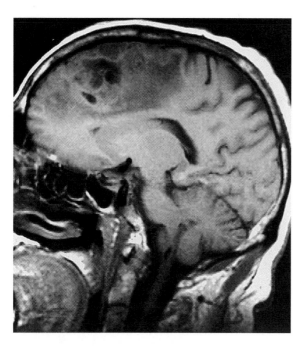

**Oligodendroglioma**

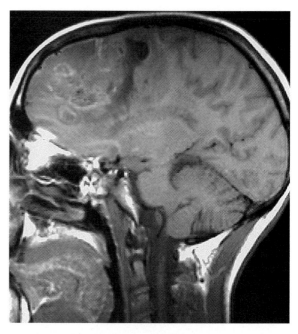

**Oligodendroglioma**
(anaplastic)

---

Oligodendrogliomas are much less common than astrocytomas, accounting for about 5% of primary gliomas. The frontal lobe is a characteristic location for these lesions, and cortical involvement is frequent. Fifty to seventy percent of patients with oligodendrogliomas present with seizures.

The typical MRI appearance of oligodendrogliomas is coarsely heterogeneous, as illustrated above. Both calcification and hemorrhage are more common in oligodendrogliomas than in astrocytomas, often accompanied by focal necrosis and cyst formation.

Areas of low signal intensity within the tumors in Cases 113 and 114 may represent either dense calcification or fluid-filled cysts.

The arcs and rims of T1-shortening in the anterior portion of the mass in Case 114 could reflect subacute hemorrhage and/or mineralization. A CT scan demonstrated fine and coarse calcification.

## Case 115

41-year-old woman presenting with headaches.
(axial, noncontrast T2-weighted FSE scan)

## Case 116

40-year-old man presenting with confusion.
(axial, noncontrast FLAIR scan)

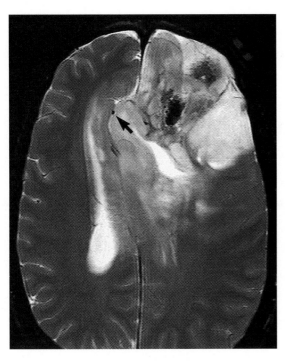

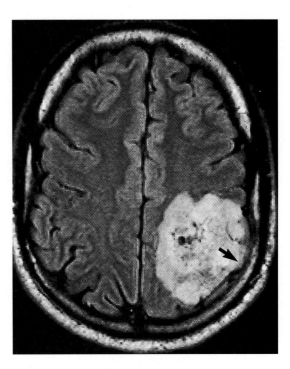

**Oligodendroglioma**
(anaplastic; same patient as Case 114)

**Oligodendroglioma**

Case 115 presents a T2-weighted scan of the patient in Case 114. Characteristic heterogeneity and nodularity of the oligodendroglioma are again apparent. Zones of relatively isointense tumor suggesting dense cellularity are interspersed with more watery tissue, areas of marked T2 prolongation (likely reflecting cysts or necrosis), and regions of low signal intensity (compatible with hemorrhage and/or calcification). The large tumor has infiltrated the corpus callosum and causes subfalcial herniation of the frontal lobe with displacement of the pericallosal artery *(arrow)*.

Although some oligodendrogliomas are anaplastic, many are slow-growing, low grade lesions. Such tumors are usually well defined with little surrounding edema, as illustrated in Case 116. Chronicity of the mass in this case is also suggested by erosion of the inner table *(arrow;* compare to Cases 73, 338, 340, and 809). Again the tumor is multinodular and heterogeneous. The central areas of low signal intensity correlated with dense calcification on a preceding CT scan.

Compare Case 115 to the hemorrhagic metastasis in Case 12 and the glioblastoma in Case 89.

### Case 117

7-year-old girl presenting with seizures.
(axial, noncontrast scan; SE 2500/28)

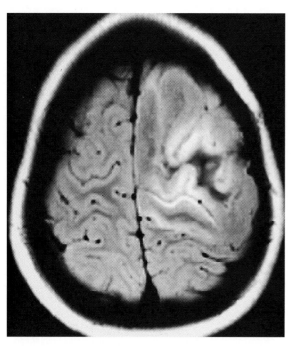

**Grade II Astrocytoma**

### Case 118

54-year-old man presenting with seizures.
(axial, noncontrast FLAIR scan)

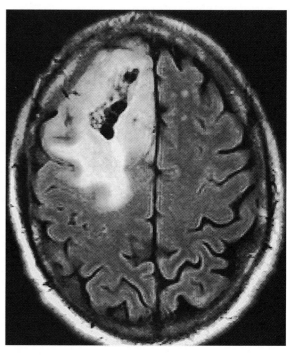

**Oligodendroglioma**
(same patient as Case 113)

---

The prominent zones of low signal intensity in each of the above tumors matched the morphology of dense calcifications on accompanying CT scans. T2-shortening due to intratumoral hemorrhage could otherwise be considered as a cause of these hypointense regions.

The homogeneous signal intensity of most low grade gliomas (see Cases 71 through 74) may be altered by calcification and/or hemorrhage. Hemorrhage is unusual in low grade astrocytomas, while calcification is demonstrated by CT scans in 10% to 20%.

Oligodendrogliomas are more frequently calcified than any other glial tumors, with a large majority demonstrating this finding. Despite a lower incidence of calcification in as-trocytomas, the much greater frequency of this histology makes astrocytoma the most commonly calcified glial neoplasm.

Small amounts of intratumoral calcification are usually inapparent on spin echo studies. Gradient echo scans emphasizing susceptibility effects are more sensitive in detecting parenchymal mineralization.

Dense calcifications usually result in zones of low signal intensity on all pulse sequences due to the associated low concentration of imageable protons. The morphology of intratumoral calcification may be stellate, as in Case 117, or nodular, as seen in Case 118.

## Case 119

53-year-old man presenting with a seizure.
(axial, postcontrast T1-weighted SE scan)

## Case 120

40-year-old man presenting with confusion.
(axial, postcontrast T1-weighted SE scan with MTS)

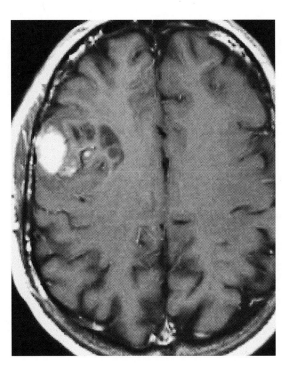

**Oligodendroglioma**

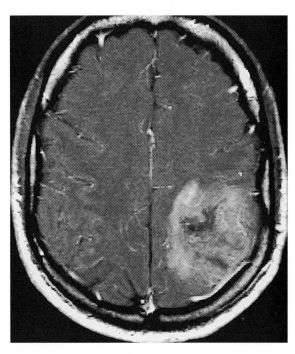

**Oligodendroglioma**
(same patient as Case 116)

---

Contrast enhancement within oligodendrogliomas is highly variable. Some tumors are largely nonenhancing. Others, such as Case 119, demonstrate intense patchy or nodular enhancement within portions of the lesion, contributing to the characteristic heterogeneity of these masses. Relatively uniform enhancement (surrounding areas of calcification, hemorrhage, or necrosis), as in Case 120, is less common.

Prominent enhancing vessels are seen within the tumor in Case 120. This feature is unusual in low grade oligodendrogliomas and raises the possibility of malignant transformation.

## Case 121A

16-year-old boy presenting with seizures.
(axial, noncontrast T2-weighted SE scan)

## Case 121B

Same patient.
(sagittal, postcontrast T1-weighted SE scan)

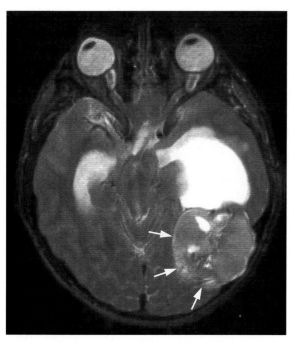

**Pleomorphic Xanthoastrocytoma**

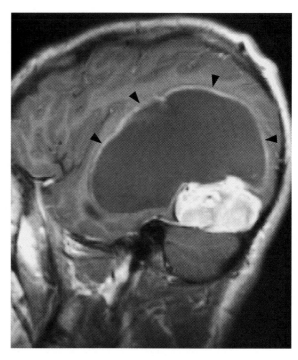

**Pleomorphic Xanthoastrocytoma**

Pleomorphic xanthoastrocytoma is a glioma subtype that occurs in young patients and is usually associated with a good prognosis. The clinical picture is typically one of seizures in an adolescent or young adult. Characteristic imaging features include a superficial location in the temporal lobe, calcification, and cyst formation. Histological examination demonstrates lipid-laden cytoplasm within tumor cells.

Case 121 is a good example of a cystic tumor with a mural nodule. Note that both the nodule and the perimeter of the cyst (*arrowheads*, Case 121B) demonstrate contrast enhancement. The midbrain in Case 121A is severely compressed by the combination of left temporal mass effect (with herniation of the uncus and parahippocampal gyrus) and hydrocephalus. Papilledema due to increased intracranial pressure distends the optic nerve sheaths and causes mild but definite flattening at the posterior margin of the globe bilaterally.

Several other primary tumors may present similar clinical and imaging features. Gangliogliomas can occur in any location above or below the tentorium (see Cases 128 and 149) but are most commonly encountered in the temporal lobes of young adults. Cyst formation and calcification are common.

Supratentorial pilocytic astrocytomas in children can also resemble the morphology of Case 121, with a mural nodule at the margin of a large cyst.

Dysembryoplastic neuroepithelial tumors (DNET) have recently been recognized as another neoplasm often affecting the temporal lobe in young patients with seizures (see Cases 338-341). However, DNETs rarely contain cysts as large as illustrated in this case.

Pleomorphic xanthoastrocytoma is one of three gliomas classified as "circumscribed" (i.e., not diffuse or infiltrating) and "grade I" by the World Health Organization. (The others are pilocytic astrocytoma and subependymal giant cell astrocytoma.)

# DESMOPLASTIC INFANTILE GANGLIOGLIOMAS

### Case 122A

8-month-old boy presenting with seizures.
(coronal, noncontrast T2-weighted FSE scan)

### Case 122B

Same patient.
(coronal, postcontrast T1-weighted SE scan)

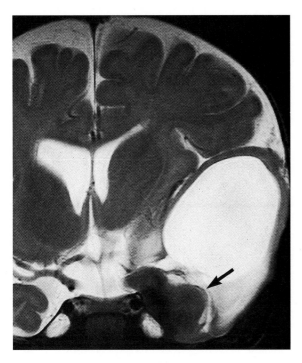

**Desmoplastic Infantile Ganglioglioma**

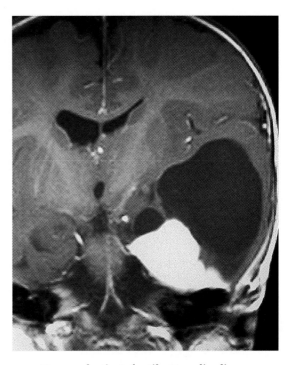

**Desmoplastic Infantile Ganglioglioma**

Gangliogliomas are tumors containing neoplastic cells of both neuronal and glial origin. The name *ganglioglioma* is applied to mixed tumors when the glial element is dominant; a mixed tumor that is largely neuronal is termed a *ganglioneuroma* or *gangliocytoma*. Pathologists use a variety of criteria and immunohistochemical stains to distinguish a true ganglioglioma from an astrocytoma containing normal neurons that have been engulfed by infiltrating tumor.

Gangliogliomas are most common in children and young adults, representing about 5% of pediatric brain tumors. They are usually slow-growing, often presenting with seizures. Temporal lobe location, calcification, and cyst formation are common characteristics of these lesions (see Cases 128 and 149). Contrast enhancement may be absent or focally intense. The combination of these features results in a more heterogeneous appearance than most low grade astrocytomas.

Desmoplastic infantile gangliogliomas are an unusual but stereotypical variant of this pathology. The tumors have been reported only in infants. They are often bulky intraaxial masses involving the surface of the brain. Large cysts are characteristically present adjacent to enhancing, meningeal-based tissue, at least part of which is densely fibrous.

Case 122A illustrates characteristic imaging features. The large intraaxial cyst expanding the left temporal lobe abuts a superficial mass of very low signal intensity *(arrow)*. There was no evidence of calcification or hemorrhage within the lesion on a CT scan, so that the hypointensity of the mass probably reflects desmoplasia.

Intense, homogeneous enhancement at the medial and inferior surfaces of the temporal lobe in Case 122B resembles a dural-based tumor. There is no enhancement at the margins of the cyst, which may be reactive rather than neoplastic.

Resection of desmoplastic infantile gangliogliomas is usually curative.

## Case 123

21-year-old man presenting with headaches.
(axial, postcontrast T1-weighted SE scan)

## Case 124

2-year-old girl presenting with nausea and vomiting.
(axial, noncontrast scan; SE 2500/25)

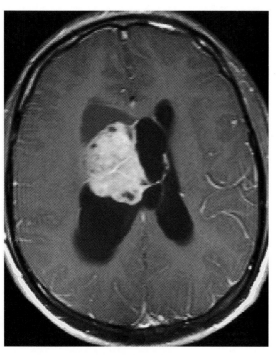

**Ependymoma**

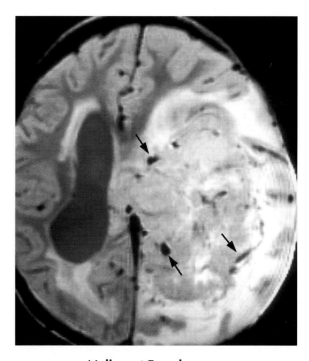

**Malignant Ependymoma**

About one-third of intracranial ependymomas occur in the supratentorial compartment. Supratentorial ependymomas can be found in children or adults, adjacent to the ventricular system or within cerebral parenchyma. (See Cases 157-162 for examples of the more common fourth ventricular ependymomas in children.)

The mass in Case 123 expands the body and frontal horn of the right lateral ventricle. The tumor is heterogeneous, with mixed solid and cystic components. Calcification is also common within intraventricular ependymomas. The typically complex morphology of these tumors may mimic the appearance of oligodendrogliomas or central neurocytomas (see Cases 342 and 343). (Also compare Case 123 to the pineoblastoma in Case 306.)

In Case 124, an aggressive-looking mass fills and expands the left lateral ventricle. Extensive hemispheric edema suggests parenchymal invasion. Large flow voids within the tumor *(arrows)* imply that it is highly vascular. The combination of these features favors a malignant lesion, with the differential diagnosis in a 2-year-old child including a choroid plexus neoplasm (carcinoma or papilloma; see Cases 328-333) as well as an aggressive ependymoma.

Contrast enhancement within ependymomas is variable. Some tumors demonstrate considerably less extensive and intense enhancement than Case 123.

Subependymomas may also present as masses within the lateral ventricles (sees Cases 129 and 344). Although some subependymomas are homogeneous, others closely resemble the more complex appearance of ependymomas.

The portion of the ventricle anterior to the tumor in Case 123 is obstructed, with higher signal intensity than normal CSF due to increased content of cells and/or protein. Periventricular edema is present along the margins of the hydrocephalic right lateral ventricle in Case 124.

### Case 125

4-year-old girl presenting with headaches,
nausea, and vomiting.
(axial, noncontrast T2-weighted SE scan)

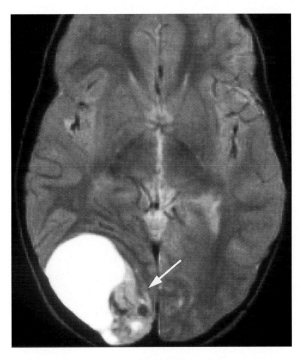

**Ependymoma**

### Case 126

12-year-old girl presenting with headaches
and left hemiparesis.
(axial, noncontrast T2-weighted FSE scan)

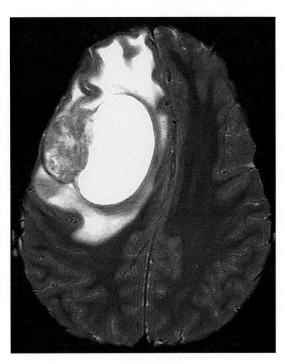

**Ependymoma**

---

Unlike posterior fossa ependymomas, supratentorial ependymomas are often parenchymal (i.e., not related to the ventricular system). They occur most commonly in the frontal and occipital lobes. Many such tumors are associated with large cysts.

Case 125 is a typical example. A mural nodule *(arrow)* is present at the posterior margin of the tumor cyst. Tissue within the nodule is heterogeneous, with areas of low signal intensity suggesting hemorrhage or calcification. The lesion is not adjacent to the ventricular system, having presumably arisen from an ependymal rest within the hemisphere.

The ependymoma in Case 126 is also extraventricular, heterogeneous, and partially cystic. Extensive surrounding edema suggests an aggressive tumor. Contrast enhancement was present within the mural nodule and at the margin of the cyst (see Case 127).

The differential diagnosis of a malignant-appearing cerebral neoplasm in a child includes ependymoma, glioblastoma multiforme, primitive neuroectodermal tumor (see Case 336), teratoma (see Case 309), and rhabdoid tumors (see discussion of Case 309).

### Case 127

12-year-old girl presenting with headaches
and left hemiparesis.
(coronal, postcontrast T1-weighted
SE scan with MTS)

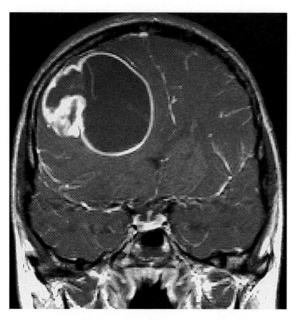

**Ependymoma**
(same patient as Case 126)

### Case 128

16-year-old girl presenting with seizures.
(coronal, postcontrast T1-weighted
SE scan with MTS)

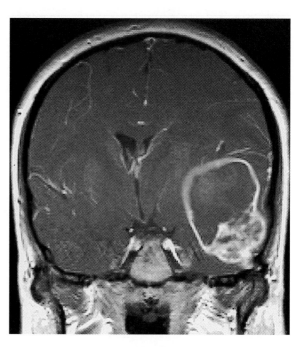

**Ganglioglioma**

Several tumors can present as a grossly cystic mass within the cerebral hemisphere of a child. The large cyst and mural nodule in Case 127 are typical of extraventricular supratentorial ependymomas. Pleomorphic xanthoastrocytomas may cause a similar appearance (see Case 121), as can hemispheric pilocytic astrocytomas.

Small cysts are often found in gangliogliomas. A grossly cystic tumor, as in Case 128, is less common (but see Case 122).

The temporal lobe location of the mass and the presentation with seizures in Case 128 are typical of gangliogliomas. Dysembryoplastic neuroepithelial tumors (DNETs) share these features and often contain small cyst-like regions (see Cases 338-341), but DNETs rarely form large cysts with mural nodules.

Cysts associated with astrocytomas and primitive neuroectodermal tumors are typically more irregular than the above lesions (but see Case 94).

Gangliogliomas carry a good prognosis after resection. Rare malignant transformation arises from the glial component of the tumor in most cases.

## Case 129A

42-year-old woman presenting with headaches.
(sagittal, noncontrast T1-weighted SE scan)

## Case 129B

Same patient.
(axial, noncontrast scan; SE 2600/45)

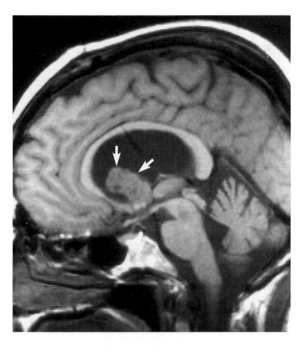

**Subependymoma**

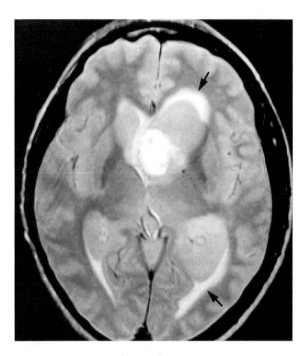

**Subependymoma**

Subependymomas are low grade glial neoplasms arising along the ventricular margins. Histological examination often demonstrates a mixture of ependymal and astrocytic cell types. Most subependymomas are incidental masses found by imaging or autopsy. They most commonly involve the fourth ventricle in older patients, with a male predominance. Supratentorial subependymomas are typically found in the frontal horn of the lateral ventricle, often attached to the septum pellucidum.

The tumors are rarely symptomatic unless they grow to obstruct CSF pathways. In this case, the mass has blocked the foramen of Monro, presenting like a colloid cyst (compare to Cases 282-285). Periventricular edema is present (*arrows,* Case 129B) due to hydrocephalus.

The mildly lobulated contour of the mass in Case 129A is typical of subependymomas, but choroid plexus papillomas or subependymal giant cell astrocytomas can have a similar appearance (compare to Cases 334 and 896). Relatively homogeneous high signal intensity is common on long TR images. Occasional subependymomas contain cysts and calcification causing more heterogeneity. Such tumors may resemble ependymomas or central neurocytomas (see Case 344 for an example).

Contrast enhancement within subependymomas is usually mild or absent, distinguishing them from subependymal giant cell astrocytomas which may occur in a similar location (see Case 897).

# REFERENCES

Albery FK, Forsting M, Sartor, K, et al: Early postoperative magnetic resonance imaging after resection of malignant glioma: objective evaluation of residual tumor and its influence on regrowth and prognosis. *Neurosurgery* 34:45-61, 1994.

Altman NR: MR and CT characteristics of gangliocytoma: a rare cause of epilepsy in children. *AJNR* 9:917-921, 1998.

Asari S, Makabe T, Katayama S, et al: Assessment of the pathological grade of astrocytic gliomas using an MRI score. *Neuroradiology* 36:308-310, 1994.

Atlas SW: Adult supratentorial tumors. *Semin Roentgenol* 25:130-154, 1990.

Atlas SW, Grossman RI, Gomori JM, et al: Hemorrhagic intracranial malignant neoplasms: spin-echo MR imaging. *Radiology* 164:71-77, 1987.

Bagley LJ, Grossman RI, Judy KD, et al: Gliomas: correlation of magnetic susceptibility artifact with histologic grade. *Radiology* 202:511-516, 1997.

Barnard RO, Geddes JF: The incidence of multifocal gliomas: a histologic study of large hemispere sections. *Cancer* 60:1519-1531, 1987.

Bendszus M, Warmuth-Metz M, Klein R, et al: MR spectroscopy in gliomatosis cerebri. *AJNR* 21:375-380, 2000.

Benitez WI, Glasier CM, Husain M, et al: MR findings in childhood gangliogliomas. *J Comput Assist Tomogr* 14:712-716, 1990.

Bird C, Drayer B, Medina M, et al: Gd-DTPA enhanced MR inaging in pediatric patients after brain tumor resection. *Radiology* 169: 123, 1988.

Burnette WC, Nesbit GM, Hall FW: Radiologic-pathologic correlation in oligodendroglioma. *Int J Neurorad* 3:503-510, 1997.

Burtscher IM, Skagerberg G, Geijer B, et al: Proton MR spectroscopy and preoperative diagnostic accuracy: an evaluation of intracranial mass lesions characterized by stereotactic biopsy findings. *AJNR* 21:84-93, 2000.

Butzen J, Prost R, Chetty V, et al: Discrimination between neoplastic and nonneoplastic brain lesions by use of proton MR spectroscopy: the limits of accuracy with a logistic regression model. *AJNR* 21:1213-1219, 2000.

Bynevelt M, Britton J, Seymour H, et al: FLAIR imaging in the follow-up of low-grade gliomas: time to dispense with the dual-echo? *Neuroradiology* 43:129-133, 2001.

Castillo C, Davis PC, Takei Y, Hoffman JC Jr.: Intracaranial gangliomas: MR, CT, and clinical findings in 18 patients. *AJNR* 11:4109-114, 1990.

Castillo M, Scatliff JH, Bouldin TW, Sowki K: Radiologic-pathologic correlation: intracranial astrocytoma. *AJNR* 13:1609-1616, 1992.

Centeno LS, Lee AA, Winter J, Barba D: Supratentorial ependymomas: neuroimaging and pathological correlation. *J Neurosurg* 64:209-215,1986.

Chiechi MV, Smirniotopoulos JG, Jones RV: Intracranial subependymomas: CT and MR imaging features in 24 cases. *Am J Roentgenol* 165:1245-1250, 1995.

Claussen C, Laniado M, Schorner W, et al: Gadolinium-DTPA in MR imaging of glioblastoma and intracranial metastases. *AJNR* 6:669-674, 1985.

Dean BL, Drauer BP, Bird CR, et al: Gliomas: classification with MR imaging. *Radiology* 174:411-415, 1990.

del Carpio-O'Donovan R, Korah I, Salazar A, Melancon D: Gliomatous cerebri. *Radiology* 198:831-835, 1996.

Destian S, Sze G, Krol G, et al: MR imaging of hemorrhagic intracranial neoplasms. *AJNR* 9:1115-1122, 1988.

Earnest F IV, Kelly PI, Scheithauer BW, et al: Cerebral astrocytomas: histopathologic correlation of MR and CT contrast enhancement with stereotatic biopsy. *Radiology* 166:823-827, 1988.

Elster AD, DiPersio DA, Cranial postoperative site: assessment with contrast-enhanced MR imaging. *Radiology* 174:93-98, 1990.

Faerber EN, Roman NV: Central nervous system tumors of childhood. *Radiol Clin North Am* 35:1301-1328, 1997.

Felsberg GJ, Silver SA, Brown MT, Tien RD: Radiologic-pathologic correlation. Gliosis cerebri. *AJNR* 15:1745-1754, 1994.

Forsting M, Albert FK, Kunze S, et al: Extirpation of glioblastomas: MR and CT follow-up of residual tumor and regrowth patterns. *AJNR* 14:77-78, 1993.

Furie DM, Provenzale JM: Supratentorial ependymomas and subependymomas: CT and MR appearance. *J Comput Assist Tomog* 19:518-525, 1995.

Galanis E, Buckner JC, Novotny P, et al: Efficacy of neuroradiological imaging, neurological examination, and symptom status in follow-up assessment of patients with high-grade gliomas. *J Neurosurg* 93:201-207, 2000.

Graff PA, Albright AL, Pang D: Dissemination of supratentorial malignant gliomas via the cerebrospinal fluid in children. *Neurosurgery* 30:64-71, 1992.

Graif M, Bydder GM, Steiner RE, et al: Contrast-enhanced MR imaging of malignant brain tumors. *AJNR* 6: 855-862, 1985.

Hashimoto M, Fujimoto K, Shioda S, Masuzawa T: Magnetic resonance imaging of glanglion cell tumors. *Neuroradiology* 35:181-184, 1993.

Haustain J, Laniado M, Niendorf H-P, et al: Administration of Gadopentetate Dimeglumine in MR imaging of intracranial tumors: dosage and field strength. *AJNR* 13:1199-1206, 1992.

Henry RG, Vigneron DB, Fischbein NJ, et al: Comparison of relative cerebral blood volume and proton spectroscopy in patients with treated gliomas. *AJNR* 21:357-366, 2000.

Hirai T, Korogi Y, Sugahara T, et al: Evaluation of infiltrative intraaxial brain tumors with turbo fluid attenuated inversion recovery sequences. *Int J Neurorad* 5:1-8, 1999.

Hoeffel C, Boukobza M, Polivka M, et al: MR manifestations of subependymomas. *AJNR* 16:2121-2129, 1995.

Hwang J-H, Egnaczyk GF, Ballard E, et al: Proton MR spectroscopic characteristics of pediatric pilocytic astrocytomas. *AJNR* 19:535-540, 1998.

Jelinek J, Smirniotopoulus JG, Parisi JE, Kanzer M: Lateral ventricular neoplasms of the brain. *AJNR* 11:567-574, 1990.

Johnson PC, Hunt SJ, Drayer BP: Human cerebral gliomas: correlation of postmortem MR imaging and neuropathologic findings. *Radiology* 170:211-218.

Kepes JJ: Pleomorphic xanthoastrocytoma: the birth of a diagnosis and a concept. *Brain Pathol* 3:269-274, 1993.

Kim DG, Han MH, Lee SH, et al:MRI of intracranial subependymoma: report of a case. *Neuroradiology* 35:185-186, 1993.

Knopp EA, Cha S, Johnson G, et al: Glial neoplasms: dynamic contrast-enhanced T2*-weighted MR imaging. *Radiology* 211:791-798, 1999.

Kondziolka D, Lunsford LD, Martinez AJ: Unreliability of contemporary neurodiagnostic imaging in evaluating suspected adult supratentorial (low-grade) astrocytoma. *J Neurosurg* 79:533-536, 1993.

Koslow SA, Claassen D, Hirsch WL, Jungreis CA: Gliomatosis cerebri: a case report with autopsy correlation. *Neuroradiology* 34:331-333, 1992.

Kumar AJ, Leeds NE, Fuller GN, et al: Malignant gliomas: MR imaging spectrum of radiation therapy-and chemotherapy-induced necrosis of the brain after treatment. *Radiology* 217:377-384, 2000.

Lee BCP, Kneeland JB, Cahill PT, Deck MDF: MR recognition of supratentorial tumors. *AJNR* 6: 871-878, 1985.

Lee Y-Y, Van Tassel P: Intracranial oligodendrogliomas: imaging findings in 35 untreated cases. *AJNR* 10:119-127, 1989.

Lee Y-Y, Van Tassel P: Intracranial oligodendrogliomas: imaging findings in 35 untreated cases. *Am J Roentgenol* 152:361-369, 1989.

Lee Y-Y, Van Tassel P, Bruner JM, et al: Juvenile pilocytic astrocytomas: CT and MR characteristics. *AJNR* 10:363-370, 1989.

Leite CC, Jinkins JR, Bazan III C, et al: MR of subarachnoid seeding from CNS glial tumors. *Int J Neurorad* 2:561-569, 1996.

Lunsford LD, Martinez AJ, Latchaw RE: Magnetic resonance imaging does not define tumor boundaries. *Acta Radiol [Suppl]* 369:154-156, 1986.

MacKay IM, Budder GM, Young IR: MR imaging of central nervous system tumors that do not display increase in T1 of T2. *J Comput Assist Tomogr* 9:1055-1061, 1985.

Madison MT, Hall WA, Latchaw RE, Loes DJ: Radiologic diagnosis staging, and follow-up of adult central nervous system primary malignant glioma. *Radiol Clin North Am* 32:183-196, 1994.

Margetts JC, Kalyan-Raman VP: Giant-celled glioblastomas of brain: a clinical pathological and radiological study of ten cases (including immunohistochemistry and ultrastructure). *Cancer* 63:524-531, 1989.

Nelson, SJ: Imaging of brain tumors after therapy. *Neuroimaging Clin North Am* 9:801-820, 1999.

Norfray JF, Tomita T, Byrd SE, et al: Clinical impact of MR spectroscopy when MR imaging is indeterminate for pediatric brain tumors. *Am J Roentgenol* 173:119-126, 1999.

Oser AB, Moran CJ, Kaufman BA, Park TS: Intracranial tumor in children: MR imaging findings within 24 hours of craniotomy. *Radiology* 205:807-812, 1997.

Palma I, Guidetti B: Cystic pilocytic of the cerebral hemispheres. *J Neurosurg* 62:811-815, 1985.

Palma I, Celli P, Cantore G: Supratentorial ependymomas of the first two decades of life: long-term follow-up of 20 cases (including two subependymomas). *Neurosurgery* 32:169-175, 1993

Partlow GD, del Carpio-O'Donovan R, Melanson D, Peters TM: Bilateral thalamic glioma: review of eight cases with personality change and mental deterioration. *AJNR* 13:1225-1230, 1992.

Pierallini A, Bonamini M, Osti MF, et al: Supratentorial glioblastoma: neuroradiologic findings and survival after surgery and radiotherapy. *Neuroradiology* 38:S26-S30, 1996.

Pierallini A, Bonamini M, Pantano P, et al: Radiological assessment of necrosis in glioblastoma: variability and prognostic value. *Neuroradiology* 40:150-153, 1998.

Poptani H, Gupta RK, Roy R, et al: Characterization of intracranial mass lesions with in vivo proton MR spectroscopy. *AJNR* 16:1593-1604, 1995.

Pronin IN, Holodny AI, Petraikin AV: MRI of high-grade glial tumors: correlation between the degree of contrast enhancement and the volume of surrounding edema. *Neuroradiology* 39:348-350, 1997.

Provenzale JM, Ali U, Barboriak DP, et al: Comparison of patient age with MR imaging features of gangliogliomas. *Am J Roentgenol* 174:859-862, 2000.

Rand SD, Prost R, Haughton V, et al: Accuracy of single-voxel proton MR spectroscopy in distinguishing neoplastic from non-neoplastic brain lesions. *AJNR* 18:1695-1704, 1997.

Rees JH, Smirniotopoulos JG, Jones RV, Wong K: Glioblastoma multiforme: radiologic-pathologic correlation. *Radiographics* 16:1413-1438, 1996.

Ricci PE: Imaging of adult brain tumors. *Neuroimaging Clin North Am* 9:651-670, 1999.

Rippe DJ, Boyko OB, Fuller GN, et al: Gadopentetate-dimeglumine enhanced MR imaging of gliomatosis cerebri: appearance mimicking leptomeningeal tumor dissemination. *AJNR* 11:800-801, 1990.

Roberts HC, Roberts TPL, Brasch RC, Dillon WP: Quantitative measurement of microvascular permeability in human brain tumors achieved using dynamic contrast-enhanced MR imaging: correlation with histologic grade. *AJNR* 21:891-898, 2000.

Rogers LR, Weinstein MA, Estes ML, et al: Diffuse bilateral cerebral astrocytomas with atypical neuroimaging studies. *J Neurosurg* 81:817-821, 1994.

Ross IB, Robitaille Y, Villemure J-G, Tampieri D: Diagnosis and management of gliomatosis cerebri: recent trends. *Surg Neurol* 36:431-440, 1991.

Russo CP, Frederickson K, Smoker WRK, et al: Pleomorphic xanthoastrocytoma: report of two cases and review of the literature. *Int J Neurorad* 2:570-578, 1996.

Rutherfoord GS, Hewlett RH, Truter R: Contrast enhanced imaging is critical to glioma nosology and grading. *Int J Neurorad* 1:28-38, 1995.

Sartoretti-Schefer S, Aguzzi A, Wichmann W, Valavanis A: Gangliogliomas: correlation between appearance on magnetic resonance imaging and tumor histology. *Int J Neurorad* 4:357-365, 1998.

Sato N, Bronen RA, Sze G, et al: Postoperative changes in the brain: MR imaging findings in patients without neoplasms. *Radiology* 204:839-846, 1997.

Serra A, Strain J, Ruyle S: Desmoplastic cerebral astrocytoma of infancy: report and review of the imaging characteristics. *Am J Roentgenol* 166:1459-1461, 1996.

Schimizu H, Kumabe T, Shirane R, Yoshimoto T: Correlation between proton MR spectroscopy and Ki-67 labeling index in gliomas. *AJNR* 21:659-665, 2000.

Shaw EG, Scheithauer BW, O'Fallon JR, et al: Oligodendrogliomas: the mayo clinic experience. *J Neurosurg* 76:428-434, 1992.

Shin YM, Chang KH, Han MH, Myung NH, et al: Glionatosis cerebri: comparison of MR and CT features. *Am J Roentgenol* 161:859-862, 1993.

Smirniotopoulos JG: The new WHO classification of brain tumors. *Neuroimaging Clin North Am* 9:595-614, 1999.

Spagnoli MV, Grossman RI, Packer RJ, et al: Magnetic resonance determination of gliomatosis cerebri. *Neuroradiology* 29:15-18, 1987.

Spoto GP, Press GA, Hesselink JR, Solomon M: Intracranial ependymoma and subependymoma: MR manifestations. *AJNR* 11: 83-91, 1990.

Strong JA, Hatten HP Jr, Brown MT, et al: Pilocytic astrocytoma: correlation between the initial imaging features and clinical aggressiveness. *Am J Roentgenol* 161:369-372, 1993.

Tampieri D, Moumdijian R, Melanson D, Ethier R: Intracerebral gangliogliomas in patients with partial complex seizures, CT and MR findings. *AJNR* 12: 49-755, 1991.

Tenreiro-Picon OR, Kamath SV, Knorr JR, et al: Desmoplastic infantile ganglioglioma: CT and MRI features. *Pediatr Radiol* 25:540-543, 1995.

Tervonen O, Forbes G, Scheithauer BW, Dietz MJ: Diffuse "fibrillary" astrocytomas: correlation of MRI features with histopathologic parameters and tumor grade. *Neuroradiology* 34:173-178, 1992.

Tien RD, Cardenas CA, Rajagopalan S: pleomorphic xanthoastrocytoma of the brain: MR findings in six patients. *Am J Roentgenol* 159:1287-1290, 1992.

Tien RD, Felsberg GJ, Friedman H et al: MR imaging of high grade cerebral gliomas: value of diffusion-weighted echoplanar pulse sequences, *Am J Roentgenol* 162:671-677, 1994.

Tshuciya K, Makita K, Furui S, Mitta K: MRI appearance of calcified regions within intracranial tumors, *Neuroradiology* 35:341-344, 1993.

Wtanabe M, Tanka R, Takeda N: Magnetic resonance imaging and histopathology of cerebral gliomas. *Neuroradiology* 35:463-469, 1992.

Yanaka K, Kamozaki T, Kobayashi E, et al: MR imaging of diffuse glioma. *AJNR* 13:349-351, 1992.

Yoshino MT, Lusio R: Pleomorphic xanthoastrocytoma. *AJNR* 13:1330-1332, 1992.

Yuh WTC, Nguyen HD, Tali ET, et al: Delineation of gliomas with various doses of MR contrast material. *AJNR* 15:983-989, 1994.

# CHAPTER 4

# Tumors of the Posterior Fossa and Skull Base in Children

### Case 130

9-year-old boy presenting with diplopia.
(sagittal, noncontrast T1-weighted SE scan)

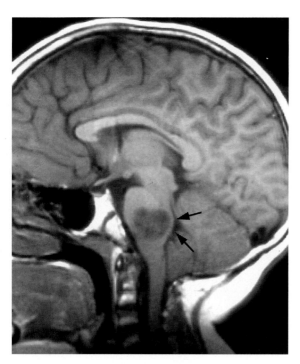

**Brainstem Glioma**

### Case 131

2-year-old girl presenting with ataxia.
(sagittal, noncontrast T1-weighted SE scan)

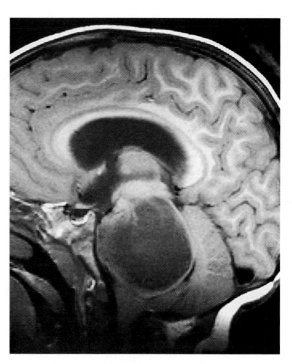

**Brainstem Glioma**

Gliomas cause the great majority of brainstem masses in children. Metastases, vascular malformations, and inflammatory disorders are more common in adults.

Brainstem gliomas in children are heterogeneous clinically and radiographically. The margins of the tumors may be well defined, as in these cases, or indistinct (see Case 132). In Case 130, the pons is expanded in anteroposterior diameter by a sharply demarcated mass of low signal intensity. The normal linear floor of the fourth ventricle is convex posteriorly *(arrows)*.

The larger mass in Case 131 compresses and displaces the fourth ventricle. In addition, exophytic tumor extends ventrally into the prepontine cistern. Bilateral anterior exophytic extension of pontine gliomas may surround and encase the basilar artery (see Case 133).

Although many brainstem gliomas demonstrate prolongation of T1 as seen above, other tumors may be isointense on short TR images. High signal intensity within the brainstem on noncontrast T1-weighted scans suggests hemorrhage within a tumor or the alternative diagnosis of a vascular malformation (especially cavernous hemangioma; see Case 767).

The location of childhood gliomas within the brainstem correlates with prognosis. Focal tumors of the midbrain and medulla are associated with longer average survival than pontine or diffuse gliomas.

Most pontine gliomas are classified histologically as fibrillary astrocytomas. These tumors carry a worse prognosis than the less common pilocytic astrocytomas, which are typically better defined and often exophytic.

## Case 132

14-year-old girl presenting with gait abnormality.
(axial, noncontrast T2-weighted FSE scan)

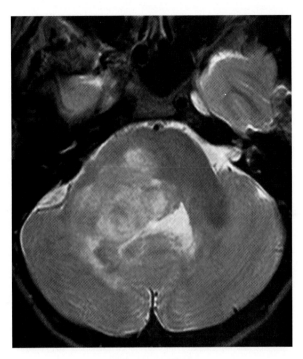

**Brainstem Glioma**

## Case 133

15-year-old girl presenting with diplopia, facial
weakness, nausea, and vomiting.
(axial, noncontrast T2-weighted SE scan)

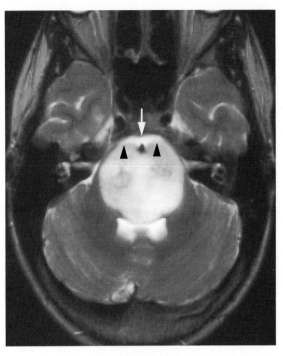

**Brainstem Glioma**

Most brainstem gliomas are readily detected on long TR spin echo images due to prominent high signal intensity. The pattern may be patchy and poorly defined, as in Case 132, or confluent and well marginated, as in Case 133.

The tumor in Case 132 is markedly asymmetrical (compare the width of the right middle cerebellar peduncle to that on the left), while the mass in Case 133 is centered in the midline. Case 133 illustrates bilateral anterior, exophytic extension of the glioma into the prepontine cistern *(arrowheads);* the basilar artery *(arrow)* is partially surrounded by tumor (compare to Case 134).

Occasionally a demyelinating process involves the brainstem in young adults, causing multifocal or diffuse edema that can mimic a glioma. Multiple sclerosis and acute disseminated encephalomyelitis may both present in this manner. Relatively rapid onset of symptoms, accompanying cerebral lesions, and an inflammatory CSF profile help distinguish such cases from brainstem neoplasms.

Neurofibromatosis type 1 may be associated with patchy areas of high signal intensity within the brainstem and cerebellar peduncles on T2-weighted images (see Cases 906-907). These lesions usually represent immature or disorganized tissue rather than true neoplasms. They generally do not demonstrate mass effect or abnormal contrast enhancement.

## Case 134

2-year-old girl presenting with ataxia.
(axial, postcontrast T1-weighted SE scan)

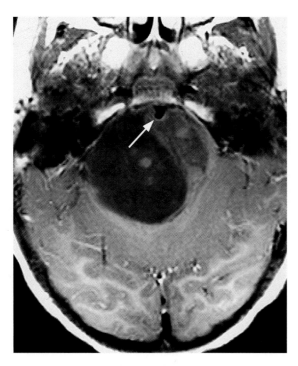

**Brainstem Glioma**
(same patient as Case 131)

## Case 135

13-year-old boy presenting with headaches
and diplopia.
(axial, postcontrast T1-weighted SE scan with MTS)

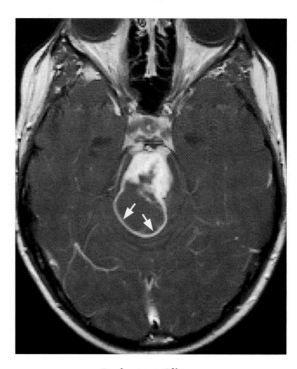

**Brainstem Glioma**

---

Contrast enhancement of brainstem gliomas is variable in extent and morphology. Even large and heterogeneous tumors may demonstrate little or no enhancement, as in Case 134.

Alternatively, both focal and diffuse gliomas of the brainstem may enhance intensely, with solid and/or peripheral components as illustrated by Case 135. (See Cases 140 and 141 for additional examples of heterogeneous enhancement within brainstem tumors.) As in the case of optic/hypothalamic tumors, pilocytic astrocytomas of the brainstem usually demonstrate impressive enhancement despite their low grade

histology. Enhancement within a brainstem glioma may develop or increase during the course of radiation therapy.

The above cases illustrate two common patterns of expansion in brainstem tumors. *Ventral* growth of the glioma in Case 134 has nearly surrounded the basilar artery *(arrow)*. In Case 135, the tumor is *dorsally* exophytic *(arrows)*, with posterior lobulation displacing and compressing the cerebellar vermis. A third potential growth pattern is anterolateral extension into the cerebellopontine angle, usually observed with originally eccentric lesions (see Case 141).

### Case 136

10-year-old boy shunted for hydrocephalus,
previously attributed to benign aqueductal stenosis.
(sagittal, noncontrast T1-weighted SE scan)

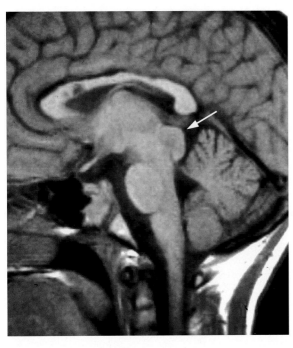

**Midbrain Glioma**

### Case 137

13-year-old girl presenting with headaches.
(axial, noncontrast T2-weighted FSE scan)

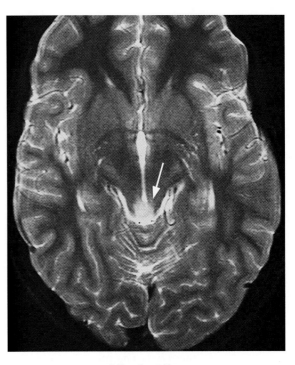

**Midbrain Glioma**

Some brainstem gliomas are focal, low grade lesions. Many of these tumors are relatively isodense on CT scans and isointense on T1-weighted MR images. Their detection is based on distortion of anatomy and/or abnormal signal intensity on T2-weighted scans.

In Case 136, a small glioma expands the midbrain tectum *(arrow)*, bulging into the quadrigeminal cistern. (Compare the diameter and morphology of the dorsal midbrain to Case 138.) The localized mass effect of the tumor effaces the aqueduct and accounts for the history of hydrocephalus. Benign aqueductal stenosis (see Cases 800-803) should be a diagnosis of exclusion after careful examination of the midbrain, best performed by MR.

Case 137 illustrates another focal glioma involving the midbrain tectum, a common location for these low grade tumors. The dorsal midbrain is mildly expanded, with mass effect obstructing the junction of the aqueduct and third ventricle.

Other pathologies may present as focal brainstem lesions, particularly in adults. Cavernous hemangiomas usually demonstrate complex signal intensity with components of short T1 and short T2 (see Cases 767 and 768), distinguishing them from most brainstem gliomas. Metastases to the brainstem are often accompanied by edema and typically enhance more intensely than brainstem gliomas (see Case 189). Demyelinating disease most frequently involves the pons or middle cerebellar peduncles (see Cases 378, 379, 381, and 405), and is often multifocal with a suggestive clinical context. Pineal lesions occupying the quadrigeminal cistern may resemble a dorsal midbrain mass (see Cases 294 and 295).

A small area of low signal intensity within the anterior body of the corpus callosum in Case 136 is related to prior shunting.

## Case 138

2-year-old girl whose parents reported
a stumbling gait.
(sagittal, noncontrast T1-weighted SE scan)

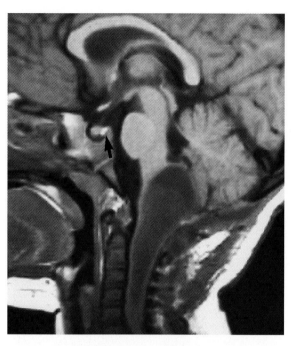

**Medullary Glioma**

## Case 139

40-year-old woman presenting with dysphagia
and asymmetrical reflexes.
(axial, noncontrast T2-weighted FSE scan)

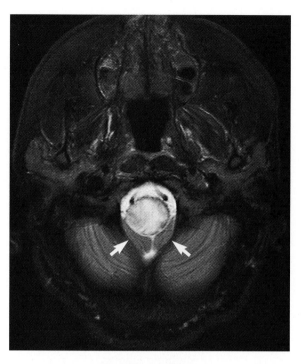

**Medullary Glioma**

---

Gliomas may involve the medulla with sparing of the more rostral brainstem. Such tumors are often dorsally exophytic, as illustrated in Case 138. The decussation of fiber tracks at the pontomedullary junction is a relative barrier to the superior growth of a low grade tumor, which may instead bulge posteriorly into the vallecula, deforming the caudal fourth ventricle. The mass in Case 138 extends well into the cervical spinal cord, a common feature of medullary gliomas.

Despite the homogeneously low signal intensity of the tumor in Case 138, it was found to be solid at surgery. Many astrocytomas of the posterior fossa and cerebral hemispheres demonstrate uniform regions of long T1 and long T2 values that represent homogeneously hydrated tissue rather than true cysts. The diagnosis of a cystic neoplasm can be made when a sedimentation level is observed but should not be otherwise presumed.

Case 139 is an example of a brainstem glioma in an adult. The medulla is diffusely expanded, causing mild posterior compression of the cerebellar tonsils *(arrows)*. The tumor demonstrates uniformly prolonged T2 values, resembling Case 133. (See Case 137 for discussion of the differential diagnosis of a brainstem mass in an adult.)

Case 138 illustrates the normal "bright spot" in the posterior portion of the sella turcica representing the neurohypophysis *(arrow;* see Cases 246 and 247).

## Case 140

6-year-old girl presenting with right hemiparesis.
(axial, postcontrast T1-weighted SE scan with MTS)

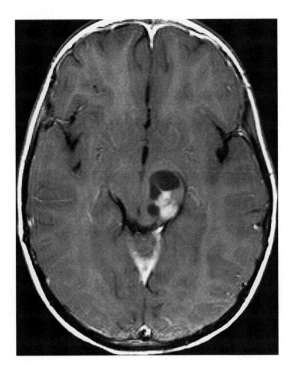

**Midbrain Glioma**

## Case 141

7-year-old girl presenting with a right
sixth nerve palsy.
(axial, postcontrast T1-weighted SE scan)

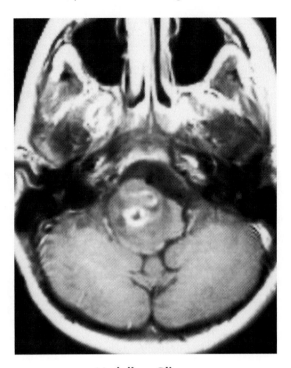

**Medullary Glioma**

---

Although many brainstem gliomas are centrally located and symmetrical, eccentric tumors occur at all levels.

The mass expanding the left cerebral peduncle in Case 140 is heterogeneous, with lobular morphology and both enhancing and nonenhancing components. Eccentric gliomas of the midbrain frequently extend superiorly to involve the thalamus. The asymmetry of such lesions can be a clue to their brainstem origin in the differential diagnosis of pineal region masses.

Case 141 illustrates an eccentric glioma of the medulla that extends exophytically into the inferior portion of the cerebellopontine angle cistern. Exophytic growth of brainstem or cerebellar gliomas must be considered along with extraaxial lesions when a cisternal mass is found in the posterior fossa. See Case 132 for an illustration of an eccentric pontine glioma and Case 163 for an example of eccentric posterolateral extension of a medullary glioma.

### Case 142

4-year-old girl presenting with clumsiness
and headaches.
(sagittal, noncontrast T1-weighted SE scan)

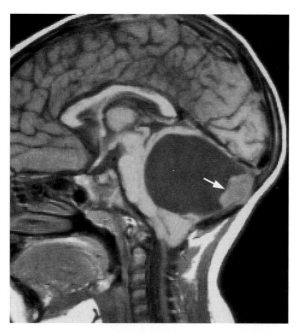

**Cystic Cerebellar Astrocytoma**

### Case 143

16-month-old boy presenting with vomiting
and impaired crawling/walking.
(sagittal, noncontrast T1-weighted SE scan)

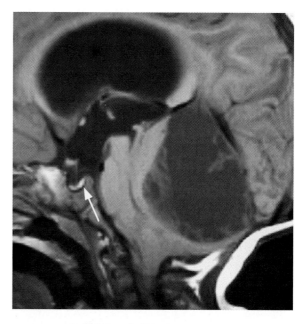

**Solid Cerebellar Astrocytoma**

Gliomas of the cerebellum are among the most common posterior fossa tumors in children. Most of these "juvenile cerebellar astrocytomas" are histologically pilocytic and noninfiltrating, correlating with benign behavior and a relatively good prognosis. (See Case 181 for discussion of the more aggressive "diffuse" category of cerebellar astrocytomas.)

The majority of juvenile cerebellar astrocytomas are cystic. A discreet mural nodule of tumor tissue is often present at the margin of the cyst, as seen posteriorly in Case 142 *(arrow)*. In other cases, the entire perimeter of the cyst is lined by a layer of tumor (see Case 147). Mural nodules at the margin of cystic cerebellar astrocytomas typically enhance, sometimes mimicking the appearance of hemangioblastomas (see Cases 183-186).

Solid cerebellar astrocytomas may be encountered in children and adults. The solid nature of some of these tumors is suggested by intermediate signal intensity, heterogeneity, and/or diffuse contrast enhancement. In other instances, homogeneous zones of long T1 and long T2 values (as in Case 143) or well-defined nonenhancing areas may falsely suggest the presence of cysts. The tumor in Case

143 was solid at surgery, demonstrating gelatinous tissue with microcystic histology that accounted for the pseudocystic MR appearance. As discussed in Case 138, the diagnosis of a cyst cannot be based on homogeneity of nonenhancing tissue.

The tumor cyst in Case 142 was centered in the midline and was mistaken for an enlarged fourth ventricle on an outside CT scan. When hydrocephalus is found on CT studies, it is important to carefully examine the third and fourth ventricles to distinguish possible enlargement from an obstructing, low attenuation lesion. (See Case 806 for another example.)

In both of the above cases the large cerebellar masses have caused anterior displacement and compression of the brainstem. (Compare the brainstem diameter in these scans to Case 136.) Both cases demonstrate kinking and occlusion of the aqueduct and herniation of the cerebellar tonsils.

A ventriculostomy had been performed prior to the MRI scan in Case 142. The normal "bright spot" of the neurohypophysis is seen in Case 143 *(arrow)*.

### Case 144

9-year-old boy presenting with headaches
and ataxia.
(axial, noncontrast T2-weighted FSE scan)

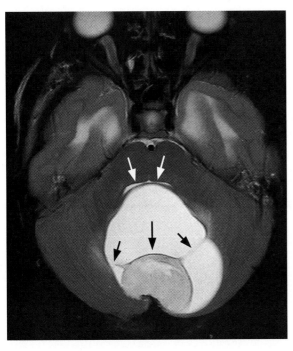

**Cystic Cerebellar Astrocytoma**

### Case 145

8-year-old girl presenting with headaches.
(axial, noncontrast T2-weighted FSE scan)

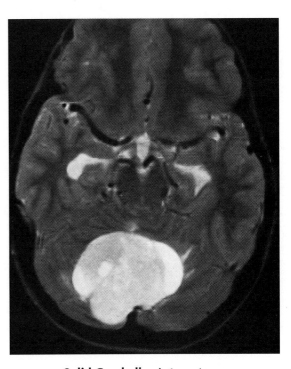

**Solid Cerebellar Astrocytoma**

The cystic components of cerebellar astrocytomas are well demonstrated on T2-weighted scans as zones of homogeneous high signal intensity. These fluid collections sharply define the less intense tissue components of the tumor.

In Case 144, a mural nodule at the posterior margin of the astrocytoma *(long arrow)* resembles Case 142. Septations extend from the nodule to the wall of the cyst *(short arrows)*.

Relatively isointense solid tissue predominates within the center of the cerebellar astrocytoma in Case 145. Small cysts are present at the periphery of the tumor. The overall morphology of the lesion overlaps the spectrum of medulloblastomas (compare to Case 153), although the mass is superior and posterior to the fourth ventricular location typical of most medulloblastomas in children.

A small amount of patchy edema surrounds each of the above lesions. Both have compressed the fourth ventricle *(arrows* in Case 144), causing obstructive dilatation of the temporal horns (with periventricular edema in Case 144). Hydrocephalus is usually present at the time of presentation in patients with cerebellar astrocytomas. Children with brainstem gliomas often present with neurological dysfunction prior to the development of ventricular obstruction.

## Case 146

14-year-old boy presenting with headaches
and blurred vision.
(coronal, postcontrast T1-weighted SE scan)

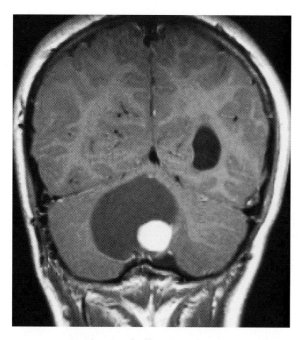

**Cystic Cerebellar Astrocytoma**

## Case 147

5-year-old boy presenting with ataxia.
(coronal, postcontrast T1-weighted SE scan)

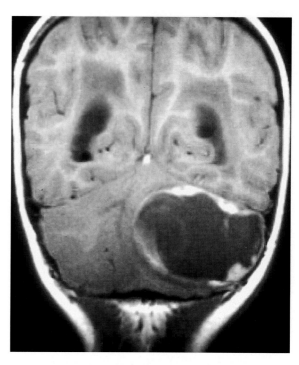

**Cystic Cerebellar Astrocytoma**

The mural nodules of cystic cerebellar astrocytomas typically enhance intensely and uniformly, as in Case 146. The remainder of the cyst wall may enhance completely, partially, or not at all.

Other cerebellar astrocytomas demonstrate more irregular peripheral enhancement of variable thickness, illustrated by Case 147. The presence of complex marginal enhancement in such cases does not imply high grade malignancy or poor prognosis, as is more generally true in supratentorial gliomas (see Cases 98 and 99).

Postcontrast scans may also demonstrate otherwise inapparent septations or bands of tumor tissue traversing a large cyst. Case 147 illustrates a multilocular cyst, in contrast to the unilocular lesion in Case 146.

Cerebellar astrocytomas that are histologically "diffuse" are commonly solid and often demonstrate patchy enhancement (see Case 181).

Hemangioblastomas can present an appearance very similar to Case 146 in young adults.

# DIFFERENTIAL DIAGNOSIS:
## HETEROGENEOUSLY ENHANCING MASS EFFACING THE FOURTH VENTRICLE

**Case 148**

30-year-old man presenting with headaches
and ataxia.
(coronal, postcontrast T1-weighted SE scan)

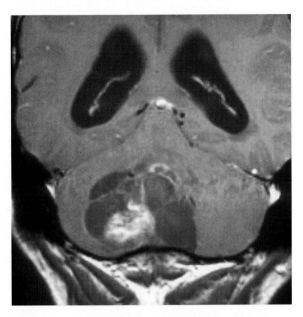

**Cerebellar Astrocytoma**

**Case 149**

15-year-old girl presenting with blurred vision
and found to have papilledema.
(coronal, postcontrast T1-weighted SE scan)

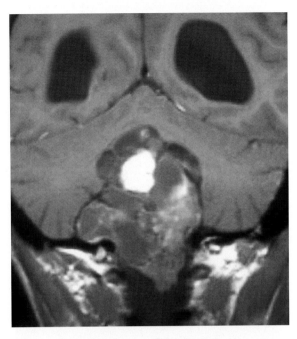

**Ganglioglioma of the Brainstem**

---

In both of these cases, a large mass near the midline of the posterior fossa has compressed the fourth ventricle, causing obstructive hydrocephalus. In each case the mass is lobulated and heterogeneous, with enhancing rims and nodules mixed with nonenhancing regions.

Although this appearance is well within the spectrum of cerebellar astrocytomas, it is not specific. The ganglioglioma in Case 149 extends dorsally from the brainstem to occupy and expand the vallecula.

Ganglioglioma is an unusual tumor in the differential diagnosis, but one which characteristically demonstrates this complex, multinodular morphology (see Cases 122 and 128). Other masses that could present a similar appearance in an adolescent or young adult would include hemangio-

blastomas of the cerebellum or brainstem and fourth ventricular masses such as ependymomas (see Cases 158 and 161).

Gangliogliomas contain a mixture of neuronal cells, which are usually mature, and glial cells of variable differentiation and aggressiveness. Most of these tumors occur before age 30, with the large majority located in the temporal lobe and presenting with seizures. Calcification and cysts are common; contrast enhancement is variable.

Note the caudal extension of the tumor in Case 149 through the foramen magnum to involve the cervical spinal canal. As illustrated here, the coronal and sagittal planes of MR are ideal for demonstrating lesions that span the craniocervical junction.

### Case 150

9-year-old girl presenting with a two-week history
of headaches and new onset of diplopia.
(sagittal, noncontrast T1-weighted SE scan)

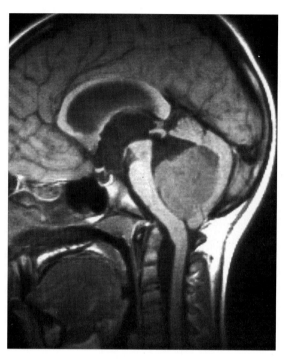

**Medulloblastoma**

### Case 151

10-year-old girl presenting with headaches.
(sagittal, noncontrast T1-weighted SE scan)

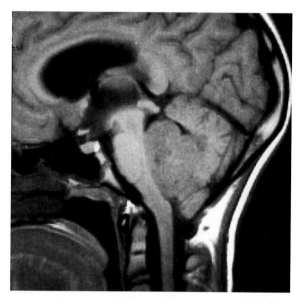

**Medulloblastoma**

Medulloblastomas rank with cerebellar astrocytomas as the most common posterior fossa tumors in children. Medulloblastomas are highly cellular masses arising from primitive cells in the neuroepithelial roof of the fourth ventricle (external granular layer of the inferior medullary velum). Many pathologists classify these neoplasms as "primitive neuroectodermal tumors."

Medulloblastomas usually present as midline masses filling, expanding, and obstructing the fourth ventricle. The sagittal MR plane clearly demonstrates the fourth ventricular location of these tumors, as in the above examples.

In Case 150, both the brainstem and the cerebellum are displaced and compressed. Hydrocephalus has caused bowing of the corpus callosum and prominent inferior ballooning of the floor of the third ventricle. The rostral fourth ventricle and aqueduct are distended due to the more caudal ventricular obstruction. The aqueduct has been shortened or "assimilated" into the superior expansion of the fourth ventricle.

Case 151 demonstrates the same features, which are slightly less severe. Note that in both cases the inferiorly displaced cerebellar tonsils enclose the caudal margin of the tumor, in contrast to Cases 157 and 158.

Medulloblastomas are often relatively homogeneous on MR scans, correlating with their usually uniform attenuation on CT studies. Calcification and cysts occur but are rarely prominent. Overall signal intensity is usually less that that of the surrounding brainstem and cerebellum.

The typical appearance of a medulloblastoma as in the above cases can occasionally be mimicked by a midline astrocytoma arising near the margins of the fourth ventricle. It is important to remember that (1) many solid astrocytomas present as homogeneous masses on noncontrast scans and (2) cystic or solid astrocytomas may occupy the midline.

### Case 152

9-year-old boy presenting with headaches.
(axial, noncontrast T2-weighted SE scan)

### Case 153

4-year-old boy presenting with nausea and vomiting.
(axial, noncontrast T2-weighted SE scan)

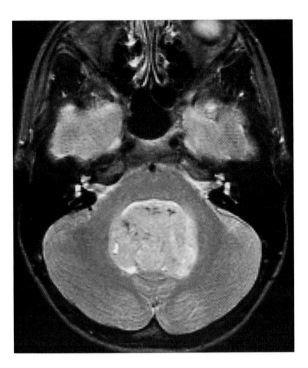

**Medulloblastoma**

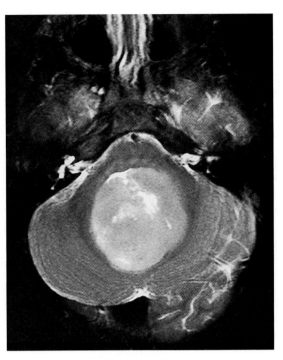

**Medulloblastoma**

Axial views demonstrate the midline location of most medulloblastomas in the pediatric age group. In the above cases the tumor has filled and enlarged the fourth ventricle, forming an expanded cast of this chamber.

The uniform cellularity of most medulloblastomas creates an overall impression of relatively homogeneous tissue. Mild heterogeneity is common due to the presence of small cysts (illustrated in the above cases by foci of high signal intensity) and/or calcification (illustrated by the punctate areas of low intensity in Case 152). Intratumoral hemorrhage is rare.

The masses in Cases 152 and 153 demonstrate that the background signal intensity of medulloblastomas on T2-weighted images is characteristically lower than other tumor types, reflecting dense packing of cells and a high nuclear to cytoplasmic ratio. (Compare to germinomas, as in Case 294, and CNS lymphoma, as in Cases 348 and 349.)

Nearly half of the children who develop medulloblastomas come to attention by age 5, with about 75% presenting by age 10.

### Case 154

4-year-old boy presenting with nausea and vomiting.
(axial, postcontrast T1-weighted SE scan)

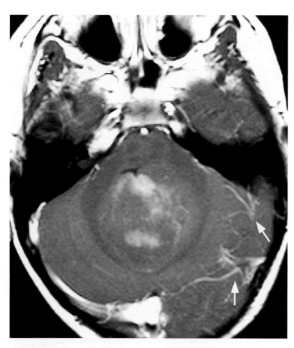

**Medulloblastoma**
(same patient as Case 153)

### Case 155

9-year-old boy presenting with headaches.
(axial, postcontrast T1-weighted SE scan)

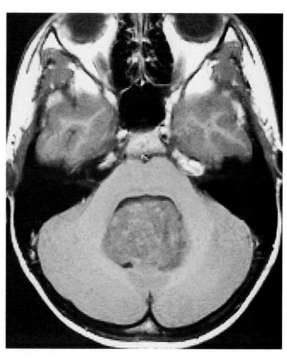

**Medulloblastoma**
(same patient as Case 152)

---

Contrast enhancement in medulloblastomas is surprisingly variable in extent and morphology. Many tumors enhance uniformly and intensely (see Case 180). However, heterogeneous or patchy enhancement, as in Case 154, or relative lack of enhancement, as in Case 155, is frequently encountered.

Medulloblastomas are among the primary CNS neoplasms commonly associated with seeding of the cerebrospinal fluid. (Others include ependymomas, germinomas, pineal cell tumors, and malignant gliomas.) About 20% of cases demonstrate CSF dissemination at the time of diagnosis. For this reason, a search for enhancing subarachnoid spaces is appropriate on initial and follow-up scans in

these patients. The most common sites of subarachnoid dissemination from medulloblastomas are sulci over the superior surface of the cerebellar hemispheres and vermis (see Case 165) and CSF spaces at the inferior margin of the frontal lobes. Occasional CSF-borne metastases from primitive neuroectodermal tumors are nonenhancing.

Note the prominent veins near the tentorium on the left in Case 154 *(arrows)*. These normal vessels drain the inferior surfaces of the temporal and occipital lobes, passing through or near the tentorial dura to reach the transverse sinus. Their location adjacent to the tentorium distinguishes them from components of a vascular malformation. (See Case 273 for another example.)

### Case 156A

17-year-old boy presenting with a two-week history of nausea, vomiting, and headaches.
(axial, noncontrast T2-weighted FSE scan)

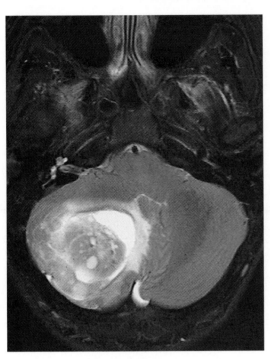

**Medulloblastoma**

### Case 156B

Same patient.
(sagittal, postcontrast T1-weighted SE scan)

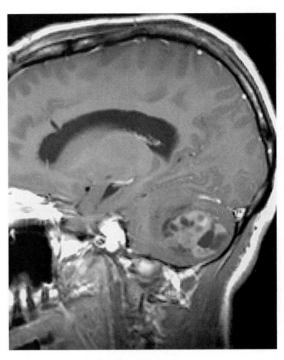

**Medulloblastoma**

Medulloblastomas may arise in the cerebellar hemispheres of older children and young adults (see Cases 177 and 180 for additional examples). Such lateral tumors are frequently associated with prominent fibrosis and have been called *desmoplastic medulloblastomas* or *cerebellar sarcomas.*

The MR characteristics of hemispheric medulloblastomas usually resemble those of vermian tumors and suggest the correct diagnosis. The solid component of the tumor in Case 156A illustrates modest heterogeneity superimposed on a background of uniform isointensity implying dense cellularity. The overall appearance is comparable to Cases 152 and 153.

However, the cystic portion of the mass combines with its hemispheric location to mimic a cerebellar astrocytoma (compare to Case 145). The enhancement pattern in Case 156B falls within the spectrum of medulloblastomas but also overlaps that of astrocytomas. These two histologies must often be considered together in the differential diagnosis of a mass within the cerebellar hemisphere of an adolescent or adult.

Hemispheric medulloblastomas can also resemble other neoplasms. They frequently reach the cerebellar surface, a feature shared by hemangioblastomas (see Cases 183-187). Infiltration of the overlying meninges can occur, potentially mimicking a meningioma. Exophytic enlargement can resemble extraaxial masses in the cerebellopontine angle (see Case 178). Alternatively, an infiltrating pattern of growth may suggest the appearance of Lhermitte-Duclos disease (see Case 182).

A ventriculostomy catheter enters the frontal horn of the lateral ventricle in Case 156B.

### Case 157

23-year-old woman presenting with nausea,
dizziness, and headaches.
(sagittal, noncontrast T1-weighted SE scan)

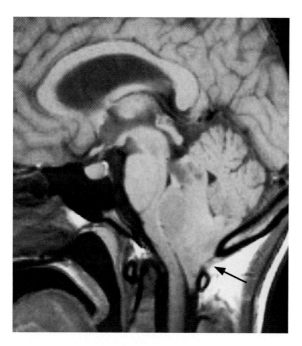

**Ependymoma**

### Case 158

22-month-old girl presenting with vomiting
and ataxia.
(sagittal, noncontrast T1-weighted SE scan)

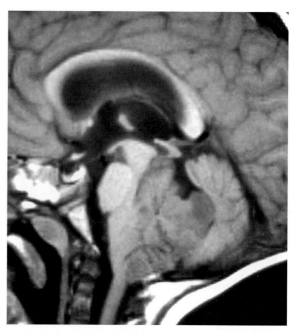

**Ependymoma**

Ependymomas arising from the fourth ventricle may be encountered in children and adults. Their location mimics the more common medulloblastomas, but other MR features usually suggest the correct diagnosis. Ependymomas are frequently calcified, and they often contain cysts. Together with occasional hemorrhage, these components result in a more heterogeneous mixture of signal intensities than is usually seen in medulloblastomas. The areas of low signal intensity near the superior margin of the tumor in Case 157 correlated with large calcifications on the patient's CT scan.

Another important feature of ependymomas illustrated above is the common dorsal expansion through the foramen of Magendie into the vallecula. Further caudal extension through the foramen magnum is seen in both cases (*arrow*, Case 157). This appearance of tumor flowing out of the fourth ventricle contrasts with the usually contained morphology of medulloblastomas, as seen in Cases 150 and

151. Ependymomas with extraventricular extension molding to the confines of the vallecula and subarachnoid space have been referred to as "plastic" ependymomas.

A third potential distinction between the typical MR appearances of ependymomas and medulloblastomas is their site of origin or attachment. Medulloblastomas are often more easily demarcated from the brainstem than from the vermis, where these tumors usually arise at the inferior medullary velum (see Case 150). By contrast, fourth ventricular ependymomas, as in Case 158, are often better separated from the vermis than from the dorsal brainstem, where they are frequently attached at surgery.

Like medulloblastomas, ependymomas typically fill and obstruct the fourth ventricle, causing hydrocephalus. Symptoms of nausea and vomiting may precede the development of overt hydrocephalus due to early tumor involvement of the dorsal medulla.

### Case 159

13-year-old boy presenting with a stumbling gait.
(axial, noncontrast T2-weighted SE scan)

### Case 160

18-month-old boy presenting with irritability
and vomiting.
(coronal, postcontrast T1-weighted SE scan)

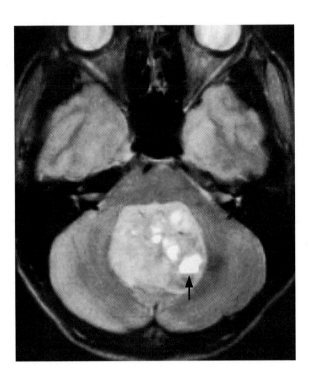

**Ependymoma**

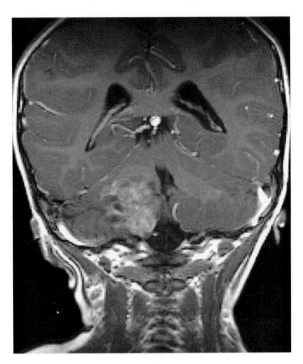

**Ependymoma**

T2-weighted scans of ependymomas often demonstrate multiple small areas of high signal intensity that potentially represent cysts. A sedimentation level is present in at least one of the cystic areas in Case 159 *(arrow)*, confirming a small fluid collection. While occasional medulloblastomas demonstrate comparable heterogeneity (see Cases 153 and 156), this complex internal architecture is more characteristic of ependymomas. The background signal intensity of ependymomas on T2-weighted scans is usually intermediate, similar to medulloblastomas (compare to Case 153 and see Case 161 for another example).

Enhancement within ependymomas is often less homogeneous and intense than seen in typical medulloblastomas. Tumor margins may be irregular and poorly de-

fined, and lobulation is frequent. Case 160 illustrates these features and the fact that ependymomas may arise eccentrically from the anterolateral recess of the fourth ventricle (as in this case) or within the cerebellopontine angle cistern (see Case 162).

Leptomeningial dissemination of tumor (see Cases 165-167) may be present at the time of diagnosis of ependymomas, but this finding is less common on initial scans than in cases of medulloblastoma.

Ependymomas of the fourth ventricle carry a poorer prognosis than medulloblastomas arising in the same location. Like medulloblastomas, infratentorial ependymomas are twice as common in boys as in girls.

## Case 161

22-month-old girl presenting with vomiting.
(axial, noncontrast T2-weighted SE scan)

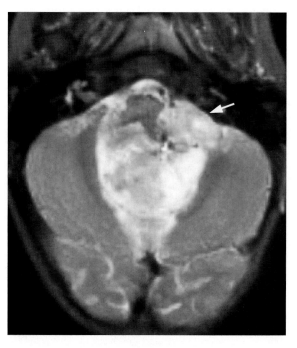

**Ependymoma**
(same patient as Case 158)

## Case 162

5-year-old boy presenting with headaches
and diplopia.
(coronal, noncontrast T1-weighted SE scan)

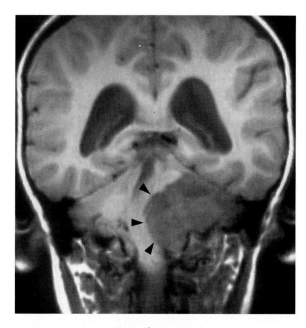

**Ependymoma**

---

In addition to the caudal extension illustrated in Cases 157 and 158, fourth ventricular ependymomas may grow laterally through the foramina of Luschka to accumulate in the cerebellopontine angle. In some cases the bulk of the tumor occupies this secondary location. In extreme cases the brainstem may be surrounded by cisternal neoplasm.

Case 161 illustrates a significant component of tumor within the left cerebellopontine angle *(arrow)*. This portion of the mass is causing displacement and rotation of the brainstem, with probable distortion of the ipsilateral cranial nerves.

Prominent asymmetrical extension of a fourth ventricular tumor into the cerebellopontine angle favors the diagnosis of ependymoma. Medulloblastomas may grow anteriorly into the anterolateral recesses of the fourth ventricle, but such extension is usually more symmetrical and less bulky than that seen with ependymomas.

Case 162 demonstrates that ependymoma should be considered in the differential diagnosis of a cerebellopontine angle mass in a child. Choroid plexus papilloma, meningioma, schwannoma, histiocytosis, rhadomyosarcoma, and metastasis (e.g., neuroblastoma or lymphoma) are other possibilities, although all are rare.

### Case 163

12-year-old girl with neurofibromatosis type 1,
presenting with dysarthria and ataxia.
(axial, noncontrast T2-weighted FSE scan)

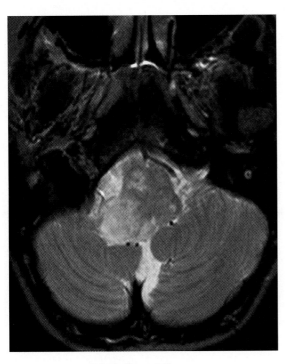

**Medullary Glioma**

### Case 164

18-month-old boy presenting with irritability
and vomiting.
(axial, noncontrast T2-weighted FSE scan)

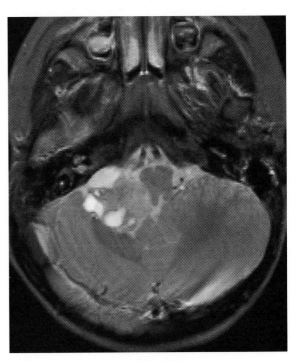

**Ependymoma**
(same patient as Case 160)

---

Several types of infratentorial tumors in children can arise or extend laterally to involve the region of the foramen of Luschka and the cerebellopontine angle cistern.

Exophytic growth of brainstem gliomas has been discussed in Cases 132-135. Case 163 presents another example. The medulla is grossly expanded (compare the diameter of the brainstem to Case 164), with greatest bulk in the region of the right inferior cerebellar peduncle. The right lateral recess of the fourth ventricle is posteriorly displaced and compressed by the mass effect of the tumor. (Compare to the anterolateral exophytic growth of the medullary glioma in Case 141.)

By contrast, the heterogeneous mass in Case 164 widens the lateral recess of the fourth ventricle, displacing both the medulla and the cerebellum. The tumor appears to be extraaxial with respect to these structures, having arisen in the plane between them. Comparison of Case 164 with Case 161 indicates that ependymomas may either extend through or arise within the lateral recess of the fourth ventricle.

Medulloblastomas and cerebellar astrocytomas can also grow exophytically into cisterns lateral to the brainstem (see Case 178). Intraaxial neoplasms are a primary consideration when a mass is encountered in the cerebellopontine angle of a child.

### Case 165A

8-year-old boy, six months after resection
of a fourth ventricular medulloblastoma.
(axial, noncontrast scan; SE 2500/45)

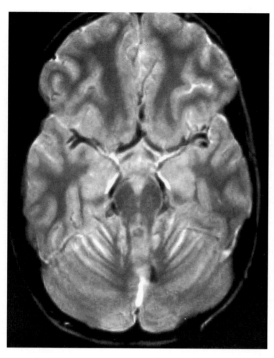

**Meningeal Recurrence of Medulloblastoma**

### Case 165B

Same patient.
(coronal, postcontrast T1-weighted SE scan)

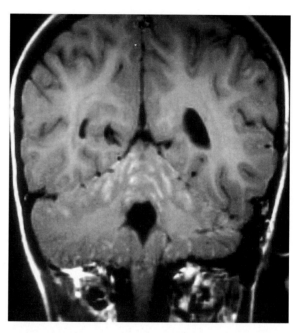

**Meningeal Recurrence of Medulloblastoma**

In addition to the caudal or lateral extension of fourth ventricular tumors discussed previously, medulloblastomas and aggressive ependymomas can spread by seeding of CSF spaces. Evidence of such fluid-borne leptomeningeal metastases may be present at the time of diagnosis or develop subsequently, as in this case. Involvement of the spinal canal is common.

Leptomeningeal tumor can be detected on noncontrast T1-weighted scans by subtle lack of sulcal definition in one or more areas. As CSF within sulci is replaced by tissue, the surface of the cerebellum or cerebral hemispheres becomes abnormally smooth and indistinct.

FLAIR or long TR/short TE spin echo images are often the most sensitive noncontrast scans for detection of meningeal disease (see Case 720). In Case 165A, the presence of leptomeningeal tumor is suggested by superficial areas of high signal intensity following the cortical contour of the cere-

bellum. These linear or curvilinear zones of long T2 may represent tumor within sulci and/or reactive edema in adjacent cerebellar folia. The overall pattern of high water content with a cortical or gyriform morphology may resemble subacute infarction (see Cases 626 and 627).

In Case 165B, the multiple foci of contrast enhancement apparently within cerebellar parenchyma represent cross-sections of subarachnoid tumor filling the sulci between folia. Meningeal tumor frequently takes the form of a uniform coating or "frosting" on the surface of the brain or spinal cord (see also Cases 29 and 1048). Large nodular components may develop at any location within sulci or cisterns.

Meningeal involvement by medulloblastomas, ependymomas, and metastases from other primary CNS or systemic tumors is often most apparent over the superior surface of the cerebellum. Coronal postcontrast scans are especially useful in demonstrating such pathology.

# DIFFERENTIAL DIAGNOSIS:
## ENHANCING LEPTOMENINGEAL TUMOR

### Case 166

1-year-old boy presenting with hydrocephalus.
(axial, postcontrast T1-weighted SE scan)

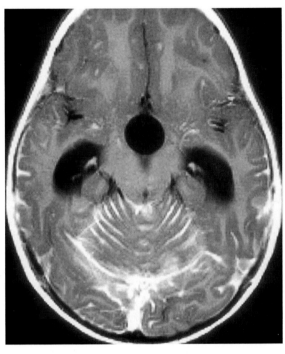

**CSF Seeding from a Pineoblastoma**

### Case 167

58-year-old woman presenting with bilateral
hearing loss.
(axial, postcontrast T1-weighted SE scan)

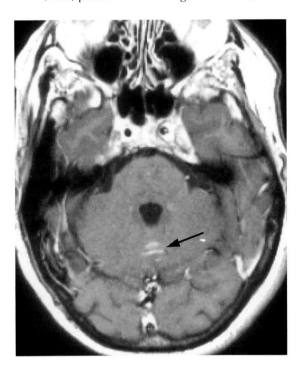

**Metastatic Carcinoma of the Breast**

---

Leptomeningeal involvement by tumor may represent CSF seeding from intracerebral neoplasms or metastatic spread of extracranial masses. Case 166 illustrates the former mechanism. Enhancing tumor fills sulci between cerebellar folia, comparable to the appearance in Case 165. Supratentorial subarachnoid spaces are also occupied by enhancing neoplasm. Primary brain tumors with a propensity for CSF spread include medulloblastomas, ependymomas, germinomas, pineal cell tumors, malignant gliomas, and choroid plexus tumors.

The patient in Case 167 presented with hearing loss and contrast enhancement in the internal auditory canals (see Case 202). The focal but definite enhancement within su-

perior vermian sulci *(arrow)* suggested that the auditory canal lesions might reflect meningeal disease. As a result, CSF cytology was obtained and metastatic adenocarcinoma was discovered. The systemic tumors that most commonly cause leptomeningeal metastases are melanoma, carcinoma of the breast, and carcinoma of the lung.

Abnormal meningeal enhancement may be seen in a number of nonneoplastic conditions. Among these are various forms of meningitis (see Case 430), the acute phase of cerebral infarction (see Cases 578 and 579), dural sinus thrombosis, and Sturge-Weber syndrome (see Case 910).

## Case 168

5-year-old girl presenting with right arm weakness.
(sagittal, noncontrast T1-weighted SE scan)

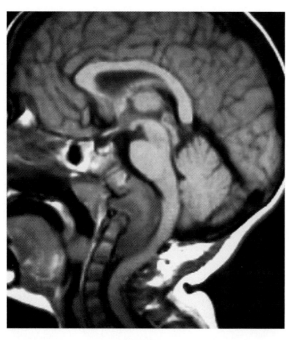

**Chordoma**

## Case 169

19-year-old woman presenting with weakness
of the tongue.
(sagittal, noncontrast T1-weighted SE scan)

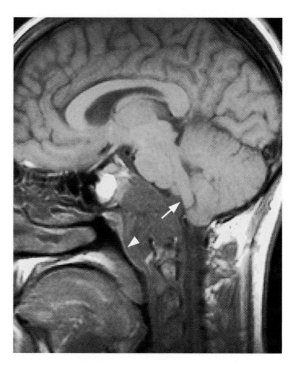

**Chordoma**

Chordomas arise from remnants of the primitive notochord, most frequently involving the clivus (35%) or sacrum (50%). Chordomas may also originate in the petrous or parasellar regions (see Case 219), mimicking other petrous tumors or parasellar meningiomas.

In Case 168, a large soft tissue mass expands from the caudal aspect of the clivus. The tumor has grown inferiorly to occupy the ventral two-thirds of the foramen magnum and cervical spinal canal. There is marked posterior displacement and distortion of the cervicomedullary junction. Prominent nasopharyngeal soft tissue is present, which can be a normal variant in children due to adenoid hypertrophy.

Case 169 demonstrates a lobulated chordoma replacing the entire clivus and extending into the nasopharynx (*arrowhead*) and the posterior fossa (*arrow*). The tumor is intermediate in signal intensity and quite homogeneous. (The zone of high signal intensity within the posterior portion of the sphenoid sinus probably represents inflammatory disease or hemorrhage rather than neoplasm.)

Calcification occurs within chordomas but is less well appreciated on MR scans than on CT images. Occasional chordomas demonstrate short T1 components (see Case 219), reflecting hemorrhage, mucinous content, or the effects of matrix calcification.

Rare clival chordomas project intracranially from an intact skull base, mimicking a meningioma of the clivus. Chordomas may also occur in the prepontine region with no attachment to the clivus, arising from notochordal remnants in this location.

## Case 170A

19-year-old woman presenting with weakness
of the tongue.
(axial, noncontrast T2-weighted FSE scan)

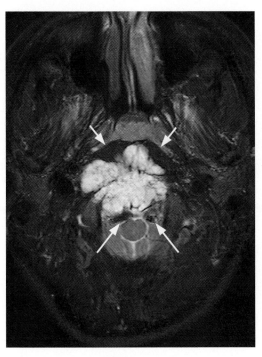

**Chordoma**
(same patient as Case 169)

## Case 170B

Same patient.
(coronal, postcontrast T1-weighted
SE scan with MTS)

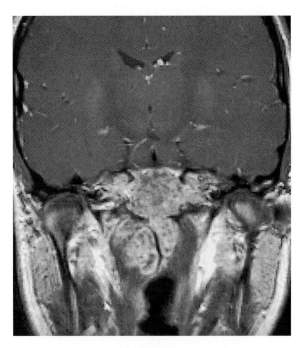

**Chordoma**

The very high signal intensity and lobulated contour of the mass in Case 170A are characteristic features of chordomas on T2-weighted scans. Long T2 values reflect the largely aqueous matrix of these tumors. Occasional chordomas demonstrate greater heterogeneity, with components of T1 and T2 shortening due to hemorrhage.

The tumor in Case 170A is centered in the midline, completely replacing the clivus. Anterior growth of the mass has displaced prevertebral musculature *(short arrows)* and nasopharyngeal mucosa. The posterior fossa components of the lesion cause dorsal displacement of the distal vertebral arteries *(long arrows)* and medulla.

Contrast enhancement within chordomas may be minimal, mottled, or quite homogeneous. Case 170B presents a typical pattern of moderate heterogeneity. Enhancing tumor occupies the entire mid portion of the skull base, including the petrous apices bilaterally. See Case 219 for another example of enhancement within a chordoma.

A large schwannoma traversing a neural foramen at the skull base can closely resemble the long T2 values and contrast enhancement of a clival chordoma. (See Case 204 for an example.)

### Case 171A

10-year-old girl presenting with retarded
growth and headaches.
(axial, noncontrast T2-weighted SE scan)

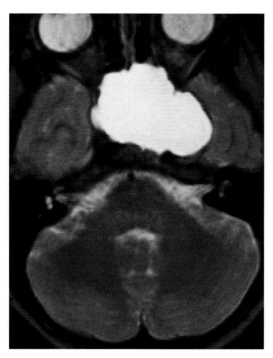

**Craniopharyngioma**

### Case 171B

Same patient.
(coronal, postcontrast T1-weighted SE scan)

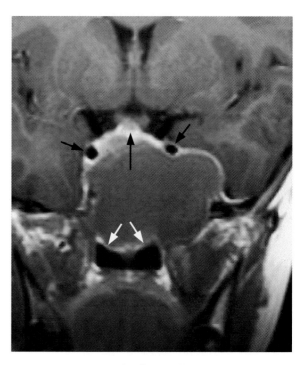

**Craniopharyngioma**

Although the majority of craniopharyngiomas are suprasellar and/or intrasellar in location, infrasellar lesions may occur along the course of Rathke's pouch. Such masses can fill and expand the basisphenoid bone and/or sphenoid sinus, as in this patient.

Uniformly high signal intensity is seen throughout the lesion in Case 171A, suggesting homogeneous fluid content. This appearance combines with lobulated lateral extensions of the mass to resemble a chordoma such as Case 170. However, the postcontrast scan in Case 171B demonstrates that enhancement is limited to the margins of the lesion, a pattern that would be unusual for a chordoma (compare to Case 170B) and that favors the diagnosis of a cystic craniopharyngioma. The center of the mass within the sphenoid bone is also more anterior than the usual clival origin of midline chordomas, as illustrated in Case 170.

Note the marked elevation of the pituitary gland *(long black arrow)* nearly reaching the optic chiasm in Case 171B. The parasellar segments of the internal carotid arteries *(short black arrows)* are also superiorly displaced, and the inferior margin of the tumor bulges into the nasopharynx *(white arrows)*.

A mucocele of the sphenoid sinus should be considered in the differential diagnosis when a lesion like Case 171 is encountered in an adult. The sphenoid sinus is rarely pneumatized in children, and mucoceles of any sinus are uncommon in the pediatric population.

### Case 172A

14-year-old boy presenting with diplopia.
(coronal, noncontrast T1-weighted SE scan)

### Case 172B

Same patient.
(coronal, postcontrast T1-weighted SE scan)

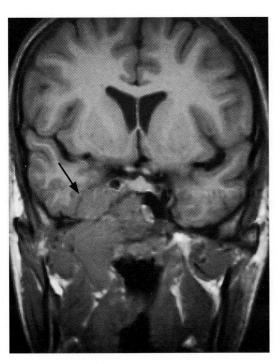

**Rhabdomyosarcoma**

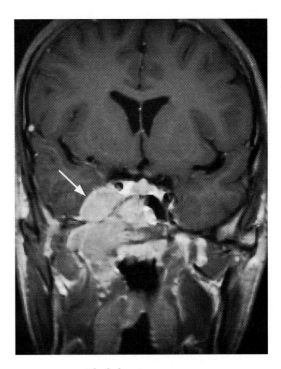

**Rhabdomyosarcoma**

A number of pathologies can cause aggressive destruction of the skull base in children. Rhabdomyosarcoma is the most common of these, frequently extending intracranially by traversing foramina and fissures or by direct erosion through bone.

Case 172 demonstrates an extradural intracranial component of the tumor within the middle cranial fossa on the right *(arrows)*, superiorly displacing the right cavernous sinus. The bulk of the tumor replaces the right sphenoid and pterygoid bones, obliterating fat planes beneath the skull base.

Rhabdomyosarcomas are typically isointense to muscle on T1-weighted scans and variably heterogeneous with increased signal intensity (compared to muscle) on T2-weighted images. Contrast enhancement is usually intense and uniform, as in Case 172B. Fat saturation sequences are useful to distinguish enhancing tumor from normal fat planes beneath the skull base.

Lymphoma, neuroblastoma, granulocytic sarcoma (leukemia), and Langerhans cell histiocytosis would be included in the differential diagnosis of a destructive lesion involving the base of the skull in a child.

### Case 173

10-year-old boy presenting with headaches.
(coronal, noncontrast T1-weighted SE scan)

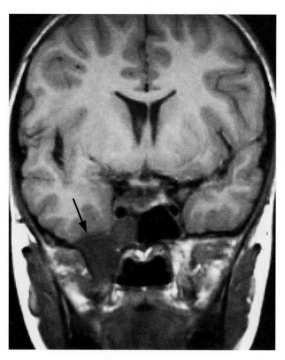

**Fibrous Dysplasia**

### Case 174

21-year-old woman presenting with decreased
visual acuity.
(axial, noncontrast T2-weighted FSE scan)

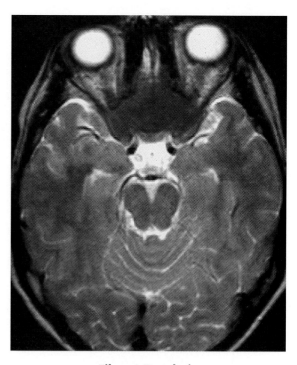

**Fibrous Dysplasia**

Fibrous dysplasia may involve the skull base in children or adults and should be considered in the differential diagnosis of osseous pathology. Location within the basisphenoid or basiocciput is common. The lesions are frequently discovered incidentally, as in Case 173.

On noncontrast scans, fibrous dysplasia typically demonstrates homogeneous, finely granular low-to-intermediate signal intensity, corresponding to the characteristic "ground glass" pattern on radiographs and CT scans. This smooth, uniform texture is apparent within the right sphenoid sinus and pterygoid plates in Case 173 and within the planum sphenoidale and anterior clinoid processes in Case 174.

Fibrous dysplasia commonly causes expansion of bone, with notable preservation of cortical margins. Associated compromise of neural foramina may lead to symptoms, as with other bone dysplasias (e.g., osteopetrosis). In Case 174, the optic canals are narrowed by thickening of the osseous margins.

In adults, metastatic carcinoma of the prostate can involve the skull base with low signal intensity on T2-weighted scans and a uniform, granular texture resembling fibrous dysplasia. Hyperostosis associated with a meningioma of the skull base would also be included in the differential diagnosis of Case 174 (compare to Cases 41 and 42).

### Case 175

38-year-old woman presenting with headaches.
(axial, postcontrast T1-weighted SE scan)

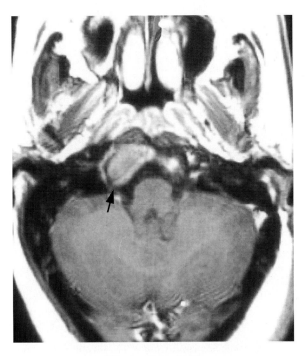

**Fibrous Dysplasia**

### Case 176

21-year-old woman presenting with decreased
visual acuity.
(coronal, postcontrast T1-weighted SE scan)

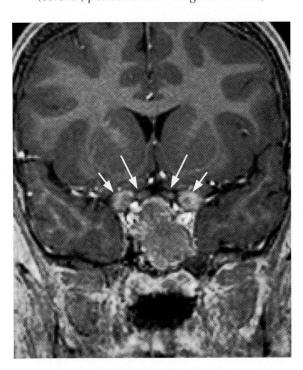

**Fibrous Dysplasia**
(same patient as Case 174)

Contrast enhancement within bone involved by fibrous dysplasia is usually intense and uniform, matching the degree of homogeneity on precontrast scans.

In Case 175, the right side of the clivus is expanded *(arrow)* and demonstrates diffuse enhancement. (This would be more convincingly shown by a pulse sequence with fat saturation.)

Homogeneous enhancement in Case 176 involves the body of the sphenoid bone and the anterior clinoid processes *(short arrows)*, which are moderately expanded. (Compare to the mottled enhancement of the chordoma in Case 170B.) The intracranial segments of the optic nerves *(long arrows)* are visible medial to the processes. There is no evidence of an intracranial or suprasellar mass to suggest meningioma arising from the planum or tuberculum sella.

# REFERENCES

Albright AL, Packer RJ, Zimmerman R, Rorke LB, et al: Magnetic resonance scans should replace biopsies for the diagnosis of diffuse brain stem gliomas: a report from the children's cancer group, *Neurosurgery* 33:1026-1030, 1993.

Bilaniuk LT, Molloy PT, Zimmerman RA, et al: Neurofibromatosis type 1: brain stem tumours. *Neuroradiology* 39:642-653, 1997.

Bosley TM, Cohen DA, Schatz MJ, Zimmerman Ra, et al: Comparison of metrizamide computed tomography and magnetic resonance imaging in evaluation of lesions at the cervicomedullary junction. *Neurology* 35:485-492, 1985.

Brown RV, Sage MR, Brophy BP: CT and Mr findings in patients with chordomas of the petrous apex. *AJNR* 11:121-124, 1990.

Byrne JV, Kendall BE, Kingsley DPE, et al: Lesions of the brain stem: assessment by magnetic resonance imaging. *Neuroradiology* 31:129, 1989.

Cassleman JW, Dejonge I, Neyt L, et al: MRI in craniofacial fibrous dysplasia. *Neuroradiology* 35:234-237, 1993.

Chaljub G, Van fleet R, Guinto FC Jr, et al: MR imaging of clival and paraclival lesions. *Am J Roentgenol* 159:1069-1074, 1992.

Chang T, Teng MMH, Ling JF: Posterior cranial fossa tumors in childhood. *Neuroradiology* 35:274-278, 1993.

David R, Lamki N, Fan S, et al: The many faces of neuroblastoma. *Radiographics* 9:859-882, 1989.

Donna J, Halperin EC, Friedman HS, Boyko OB: Subfrontal recurrence of medulloblastoma. *AJNR* 13:1617-1618, 1992.

Doucet V, Peretti-Viton P, Figarella-Branger D, et al: MRI of intracranial chordomas. Extent of tumour and contrast enhancement: criteria for differential diagnosis. *Neuroradiology* 39: 571-576, 1997.

Epstein FJ, Farmer J-P: Brain stem glioma growth patterns. *J Neurosurgery* 78:408-412, 1993.

Faerber EN, Roman NV: Central nervous system tumors of childhood. *Radiol Clin North Am* 35:1301-1328, 1997.

Fernandez-Latorre F, Menor-Serrano F, Alonso-Charterina S, Arenas-Jimenez J: Langerhans' cell histiocytosis of the temporal bone in pediatric patients: imaging and follow-up. *Am J Roentgenol* 174:217-222, 2000.

Fischbein NJ, Kaplan MJ, Holliday RA, Dillon WP: Recurrence of clival chordoma along the surgical pathway. *AJNR* 21:578-583, 2000.

Fischbein NJ, Prados MD, Wara W, et al: Radiologic classification of brain stem tumors: correlation of magnetic resonance imaging appearance with clinical outcome. *Pediatr Neurosurg* 24:9-23, 1996.

Fukui MB, Hogg JP, Martinez AJ: Extraaxial ependymoma of the posterior fossa. *AJNR* 18:1179-1181, 1997.

Good CD, Wade AM, Hayward RD, et al: Surveillance neuroimaging in childhood intracranial ependymoma: how effective, how often, and for how long? *J Neurosurg* 94:27-32, 2001.

Gusnard DA: Cerebellar neoplasms in children. *Semin Roentgenol* 25: 263-278, 1990.

Hudgins PA, Davis PC, Hoffman JC Jr: Gadopentetate Dimeglumine-enhanced MR imaging in children following surgery for brain tumor: spectrum of meningeal findings. *AJNR* 12:301-308, 1991.

Hueftle M, Han J, Kaufman B, et al: MR imaging of brainstem gliomas. *J Comput Assist Tomogr* 9:263, 1985.

Jan M, Dweik A, Destrieux C, Djebbari Y: Fronto-orbital sphenoidal fibrous dysplasia. *Neurosurgery* 34:544-547, 1994.

Kane AG, Robles HA, Smirniotopolous JG, et al: Diffuse pontine astrocytoma. *AJNR* 14:941-945, 1993.

Kimura F, Kim KS, Friedman HS, et al: MR imaging of the normal and abnormal clivus. *AJNR* 11:1015-1021, 1990.

Kochi M, Mihara Y, Takada A, et al: MRI of subarachnoid dissemination of medulloblastoma. *Neuroradiology* 33:264-268, 1991.

Laine FL, Nadel L, Brain IF: CT and MR imaging of the central skull base: 2. Pathologic spectrum. *Radiographics* 10:797, 1990.

Lee BCP, Deck MDF, Kneeland JB, Cahill PT: MR imaging of the craniocervical junction. *AJNR* 6:209-213, 1985.

Lee BCP, Kneeland JB, Walker RW, et al: MR imaging of brain stem tumors. *AJNR* 6:159-164, 1985.

Lee Y-Y, Van Tassel P, Bruner JM, et al: Juvenile pilocytic astrocytomas: CT and MR characteristics. *AJNR* 10:363-370, 1989.

Leproux F, De Toffel B, Aesch B, Cotty P: MRI of cranial chordomas: the value of gadolinium. *Neuroradiology* 35:543-545, 1991.

Lizak PF, Woodruff WW: Posterior fossa neoplasms: multiplanar imaging. *Semin US CT MR* 13:182-206, 1992.

Luh GY, Bird CR: Imaging of brain tumors in the pediatric population. *Neuroimaging Clin North Am* 9:691-716, 1999.

Lyons MK, Kelly PJ: Posterior fossa ependymoma: report of 30 cases and review of the literature. *Neurosurgery* 28:659-661, 1991.

Maleci A, Cervoni L, Delfini R: Medulloblastoma in children and in adults: a comparative study. *Acta Neurochir (Wien)* 19:62-67, 1992.

May PL, Blaser SI, Hoffman HJ, et al: Benign intrinsic tectal "tumors" in children. *J Neurosurg* 74:867-871, 1991.

Meyers SP, Hirsch WL Jr, Curtin HD, et al: Chordomas of the skull base: MR features. *AJNR* 13:1627-1636, 1992.

Meyers SP, Hirsch WL, Curtin HD, Barnes L, et al: Chondrosarcomas of the skull base: MR imaging features. *Radiology* 184: 103-108, 1992.

Meyers SP, Kemp SS, Tarr RW: MR imaging features of medulloblastoma. *Am J Roentgenol* 158:865-895, 1992.

Meyers SP, Wildenhain S, Chess MA, Tarr RW: Postoperative evaluation for intracranial recurrence of medulloblastoma: MR findings with gadopentetate dimeglumine. *AJNR* 15:1425-1434, 1994.

Mueller DP, Moore SA, Sato RY, Yuh WTC: MR spectrum of medulloblastoma. *Clin Imaging* 16:250-255, 1992.

Okada Y, Aoki S, Barkovich AJ, et al: Cranial bone marrow in children: assessment of normal development with MR imaging. *Radiology* 171:161-164, 1989.

Oot RF, Melville GE, New PFJ, et al: the role of MR and CT in evaluating clival chondroma and chondrosarcomas. *AJNR* 9:715-723, 1988.

Peterman SB, Steiner RE, Bydder GM, et al: Nuclear magnetic resonance imaging (NMR) of brain stem tumors. *Neuroradiology* 27:202-207, 1985.

Poussaint TY, Kowal JR, Barnes PD, et al: Tectal tumors of childhood: clinical and imaging follow-up. *AJNR* 19:977-983, 1998.

Rippe DJ, Boyko OB, Friedman HS, et al: Gd-DTPA-enhanced MR imaging of leptomeningeal spread of primary intracranial CNS tumors in children. *AJNR* 11:329-332, 1990.

Robles HA, Smirniotopoulos JG, figueroa RE: Understanding the radiology of intracranial primitive neuroectodermal tumors from a pathological perspective: a review. *Semin US CT MR* 13:170-181, 1992.

Rollins N, Mendelsohn D, Mulne A, et al: Recurrent medulloblastoma: frequency of tumor enhancement on Gd-DPTA MR imaging. *AJNR* 11:583-587, 1990.

Rollins NK, Nisen P, Shapiro KN: The use of early postoperative MR in detecting residual juvenile cerebellar pilocytic astrocytoma. *AJNR* 19:151-156, 1998.

Sen CN, Sekhar LN, Schramm VL, et al: Chordoma and chondrosarcoma of the cranial base: an 8-year experience. *Neurosurgery* 25:921-941, 1989.

Sherman J, Citrin C, Barkovich A, et al: MR imaging of the tectum. *AJNR* 8:59, 1987.

Shigeki A, Dillon WP, Barkovich AJ, Normal D: Marrow conversion before pneumatization of the sphenoid sinus: assessment with MR imaging. *Radiology* 172:373-375, 1989.

Spoto GP, Press GA, Hesselink JR, Solomon M: Intracranial ependymomas and subependymoma: MR manifestations. *AJNR* 11:83-91, 1990.

Stroink AR, Hoffman HJ, Hendrick EB, Humphreys RP: Diagnosis and management of pediatric brain stem gliomas. *J Neurosurg* 65:745-750, 1986.

Strong JA, Hatten HP Jr, Brown MT, et al: Pilocytic astrocytoma: correlation between the initial imaging features and clinical aggressiveness. *Am J Roentgenol* 161:369-372, 1993.

Sun B, Wang CC, Wang J: MRI characteristics of midbrain tumours. *Neuroradiology* 41:158-162, 1999.

Sze G, Vichanco LS, Brant-Zawadzki M, et al: Chordomas: MR imaging. *Radiology* 166:187-191, 1993.

Tortori-Donati P, Fondelli MP, Cama A, et al: Ependymomas of the posterior cranial fossa: CT and MRI findings. *Neuroradiology* 37:238-243, 1995.

Tortori-Donati P, Fondelli MP, Rossi A, et all: Medulloblastoma in children: CT and MRI findings. *Neuroradiology* 38:352-359, 1996.

Vandertop WP, Hoffman HJ, Drake JM, et al: Focal midbrain tumors in children. *Neurosurgery* 31:186-194, 1992.

Weber AL, Liebsch NJ, Sanchez R. Sweriduc ST: Chordomas of the skull base: radiologic and clinical evaluation. *Neuroimaging Clin North Am* 4:515-527, 1994.

Yano M, Tajima S, Tanaka, Y, et al: Magnetic resonance imaging of craniofacial fibrous dysplasia. *Ann Plast Surg* 30:371-374, 1993.

# CHAPTER 5

# Tumors of the Posterior Fossa and Skull Base in Adults

## Case 177

26-year-old man presenting with
headaches and ataxia.
(axial, noncontrast T2-weighted FSE scan)

## Case 178

32-year-old man presenting with
left-sided hearing loss.
(axial, noncontrast FLAIR scan)

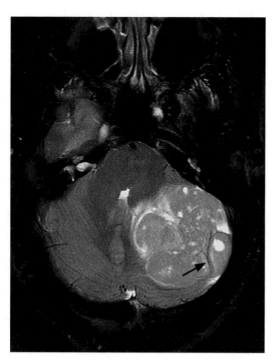

**Medulloblastoma**

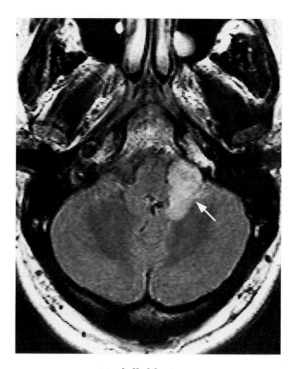

**Medulloblastoma**

Medulloblastomas in adolescents and adults are often eccentric, arising from the cerebellar hemisphere rather than the vermis. Lateral medulloblastomas may remain intraaxial, as in Case 177, and should be considered along with astrocytomas and hemangioblastomas in the differential diagnosis of a mass within the cerebellar hemisphere of a young adult. (See Case 156 for an additional example.)

The small cysts and otherwise homogeneously isointense tissue of the tumor in Case 177 are comparable to the typical appearance of midline medulloblastomas in children, as discussed in Chapter 4. This dense cellularity and the usually uniform contrast enhancement (see Case 180) offer clues to the correct diagnosis.

Occasional hemispheric medulloblastomas grow exophytically into the cerebellopontine angle and can cause symptoms suggesting an extraaxial process. Case 178 illustrates this pattern. The majority of the tumor occupies a cisternal location, presumably distorting the eighth cranial nerve as it approaches the cochlear nuclei (which lie in the dorsal lateral medulla, immediately anterior to the lateral recess of the fourth ventricle).

An exophytic astrocytoma arising from the brachium pontis or cerebellum could present an appearance similar to Case 178. The morphology of the tumor is comparable to many pediatric ependymomas (see Cases 160-162), but adult infratentorial ependymomas are rarely eccentric (see Case 179).

Case 177 demonstrates relatively little edema and mass effect for the size of the tumor. The pial base and prominent vessel *(arrow)* at the margin of the mass are features that are typical of hemangioblastomas (see Cases 183-187), but the predominantly solid and uniform appearance of the tumor would be unusual for a hemangioblastoma of this size.

Adult medulloblastomas are frequently associated with prominent fibrosis and described as "desmoplastic." This histological feature does not have prognostic significance.

Late relapse is more common in adult medulloblastomas than in pediatric cases, and prolonged postoperative surveillance is warranted.

## Case 179A

34-year-old man presenting with headaches.
(axial, noncontrast T2-weighted FSE scan)

## Case 179B

Same patient.
(coronal, postcontrast T1-weighted
SE scan with MTS)

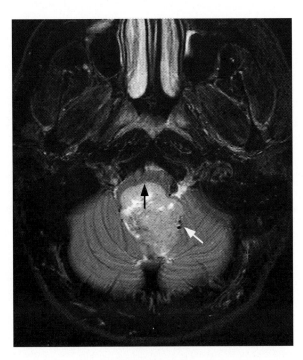

**Ependymoma**

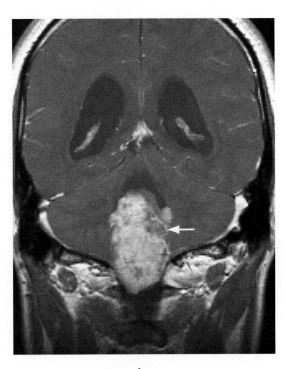

**Ependymoma**

The age distribution of infratentorial ependymomas includes a peak among young adults (ages 25-35), as well as one in early childhood (ages 1-5). The adult tumors share the imaging characteristics of the pediatric lesions discussed in Chapter 4.

Most adult ependymomas of the posterior fossa are slow-growing masses arising within the fourth ventricle. Lateral extension into the cerebellopontine angle is less frequently observed than in children (see Cases 161, 162, and 164), in distinction to the more common eccentricity of adult medulloblastomas as discussed on the previous page.

Case 179A demonstrates a mildly heterogenous mass growing inferiorly from the fourth ventricle to extend within the vallecula, anteriorly displacing and compressing the medulla *(black arrow)*. The coronal scan in Case 179B shows that the caudal extension of tumor passes through the foramen magnum into the cervical spinal

canal, a feature characteristic of pediatric ependymomas (see Cases 157 and 158 and compare to Cases 186 and 335). The mildly lobulated tumor obstructs the fourth ventricle, causing moderate hydrocephalus.

The differential diagnosis in Case 179 includes a solid hemangioblastoma, given the prominent vessels at the margins of the mass *(white arrows;* compare to Case 184). However, the lesion seems very well demarcated from the dorsal medulla, which would be the expected site of origin for a hemangioblastoma in this location. Furthermore, the low signal intensity in Case 179A suggests denser cellularity than is usually seen in hemangioblastomas. An exophytic glioma of the cerebellum or brainstem, a choroid plexus papilloma of the fourth ventricle (see Case 335), or a subependymoma could also be considered among diagnostic possibilities.

### Case 180

26-year-old man presenting with
headaches and ataxia.
(coronal, postcontrast T1-weighted
SE scan with MTS)

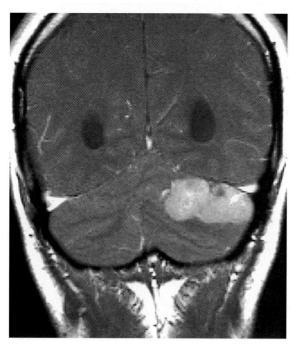

**Medulloblastoma**
(same patient as Case 177)

### Case 181

23-year-old woman presenting with ataxia.
(coronal, postcontrast T1-weighted SE scan)

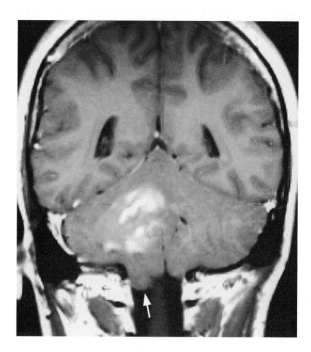

**Astrocytoma**

Metastases and hemangioblastomas are the most frequently encountered cerebellar masses in adults. However, the cerebellar tumors of childhood may also occur in older patients, as illustrated above.

Case 180 presents a postcontrast scan of the hemispheric medulloblastoma in Case 177. The uniform enhancement of this tumor is a common characteristic of midline pediatric medulloblastomas. This homogeneous appearance combines with the superficial base of the mass to mimic a tentorial meningioma (compare to Cases 60 and 188). A solid hemangioblastoma, which typically arises at the pial surface, would be included in the differential diagnosis (see Case 187).

Enhancement within the astrocytoma in Case 181 is intense but patchy and poorly defined. This pattern is more amorphous than would be expected for a hemangioblastoma, medulloblastoma, or metastasis. The tumor proved to be a diffuse astrocytoma, a histological variant that is more infiltrating and carries a poorer prognosis than the juvenile pilocytic tumors discussed in Chapter 4. Mass effect from lesion in Case 181 has caused ipsilateral tonsillar herniation *(arrow)*.

Primary or metastatic lymphoma should also be considered in the differential diagnosis of cerebellar masses in adults (see Case 348).

# LHERMITTE-DUCLOS DISEASE
## (DYSPLASTIC GANGLIOCYTOMA OF THE CEREBELLUM)

### Case 182A

36-year-old man presenting with ataxia.
(axial, noncontrast T1-weighted SE scan)

### Case 182B

Same patient.
(axial, noncontrast T2-weighted SE scan)

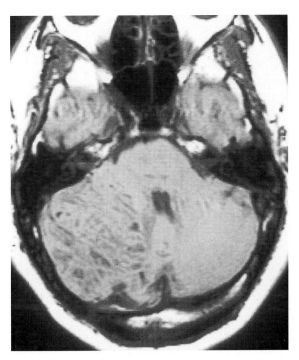

**Lhermitte-Duclos Disease**

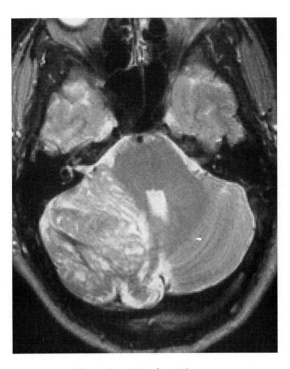

**Lhermitte-Duclos Disease**

Lhermitte-Duclos disease is an unusual cause of a cerebellar mass in an adult. This lesion is viewed by some pathologists as a hypertrophic malformation or hamartoma. However, the associated masses have been demonstrated to enlarge over time and to recur after resection, acting much like low grade neoplasms.

The entitiy is now commonly referred to as "dysplastic gangliocytoma of the cerebellum." It most frequently affects young men. Gross pathology demonstrates localized thickening of cerebellar folia. Microscopic examination shows large, dysplastic neurons within the granular layer of cerebellar cortex and excessive myelination of axons in the molecular layer.

The usual pattern of corrugated, thickened folia seen in this case is characteristic of the disorder and correlates with the hypertrophic folia seen pathologically. Relatively isointense cerebellar cortex is surrounded by an overall background of prolonged T1 and T2 values in the above images. Other reported cases have demonstrated more extensive high intensity abnormality on T2-weighted scans.

This patient had undergone prior resection of a right cerebellar mass. Follow-up studies over a period of years documented recurrence of the lesion.

Lhermitte-Duclos disease may be found in association with Cowden disease, a neurocutaneous syndrome of multiple hamartomas and neoplasms involving mucous membranes and skin, as well as solid organs (breast, colon, thyroid gland, and ovaries).

115

### Case 183

48-year-old woman presenting with
headaches and ataxia.
(coronal, noncontrast T1-weighted SE scan)

### Case 184

48-year-old man presenting with
neck pain and abnormal gait.
(axial, noncontrast T2-weighted FSE scan)

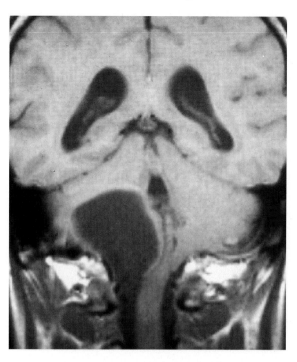

**Cerebellar Hemangioblastoma**

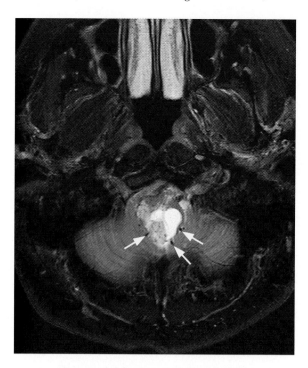

**Hemangioblastoma of the Medulla**

Hemangioblastomas are relatively uncommon tumors of the posterior fossa and spinal cord, usually discovered in adults ages 25 to 50. The masses are often cystic and highly vascular. An intensely enhancing mural nodule is characteristic.

Clues to the diagnosis on noncontrast scans include the suspicion of a cystic tumor and the presence of prominent vessels within or surrounding the lesion. Case 183 demonstrates a rounded zone of homogeneously long T1 values involving the inferior right cerebellar hemisphere. An enhancing mural nodule was demonstrated on postcontrast scans, and the tumor proved to be grossly cystic at surgery.

In Case 184, foci of low signal intensity *(arrows)* are present at the margin of a small mass containing cystic and solid components. These signal voids suggest flow within enlarged arteries and favor a highly vascular neoplasm. (Compare to the discussion of glomus tumors in Cases 209 and 210.)

Another useful diagnostic feature is the usual superficial location of hemangioblastomas. These tumors characteristically arise at the pial surface of the cerebellum or brain-

stem. (See Case 621 for an additional example.) Multiplanar MR display is helpful in establishing this relationship.

Hemangioblastomas are an important component of von Hippel-Lindau (VHL) syndrome, a multisystem disorder that may also include retinal angiomas, hypernephroma, pheochromocytoma, and cysts of the pancreas and kidney. This syndrome is inherited with a pattern of autosomal dominance (chromosome 3); sporadic mutations are rare. Hemangioblastomas occur in 40% to 80% of VHL syndrome patients, with three-fourths of these tumors involving the cerebellum. Multiple hemangioblastomas and spinal hemangioblastomas (see Cases 1099 and 1100) are much more common in VHL syndrome than in spontaneous cases. Screening and surveillance for additional lesions are appropriate when a hemangioblastoma is diagnosed.

Hemangioblastomas are among the tumors that may span the craniocervical junction, crowding the foramen magnum and causing occipital or cervical pain, as in Case 184. The foramen magnum should be carefully examined on all MR scans of the neck.

### Case 185

38-year-old woman presenting with
headaches and ataxia.
(axial, postcontrast T1-weighted SE scan with MTS)

### Case 186

16-year-old boy presenting with
nausea and vomiting.
(coronal, postcontrast T1-weighted SE scan)

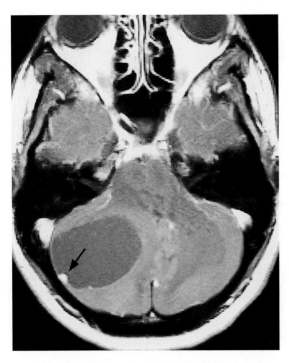

**Cerebellar Hemangioblastoma**

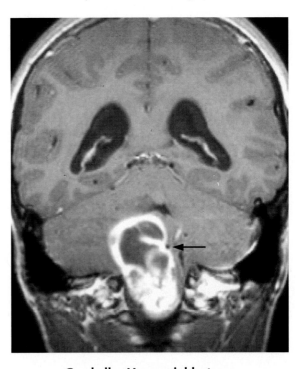

**Cerebellar Hemangioblastoma**

Intense contrast enhancement is characteristic of hemangioblastomas. The absence of this feature should suggest an alternative diagnosis. Enhancement may be seen throughout a solid hemangioblastoma (see Case 187) or at the margin of cystic lesions. Marginal enhancement may occur only within a mural nodule or along the entire perimeter of a cyst.

In Case 185, a tiny nodule of enhancement *(arrow)* is demonstrated at the posterolateral margin of the large, smooth cyst. Faint linear enhancement continues medially along the posterior border of the lesion.

The CT and MR appearance of hemangioblastomas and cystic cerebellar astrocytomas can be indistinguishable. Both tumors may have a prominently enhancing mural nodule with little or no enhancement along the remainder of the cyst wall (compare Case 185 to Case 146). Prominent vascular channels and contact with the pial surface are features regularly seen in hemangioblastomas and less commonly associated with astrocytomas. Angiography can be

diagnostic in the evaluation of a cystic cerebellar tumor: the mural nodule of a hemangioblastoma is intensely vascular, while the mural nodule of a cystic astrocytoma is often hypovascular.

Case 186 presents a more complex hemangioblastoma, with solid tissue and rims of enhancement surrounding and separating several cystic loculations. Flow voids due to large vessels *(arrow)* can be identified at the perimeter of the tumor. The mass expands the cerebellar tonsil, which herniates caudally through the foramen magnum.

Isolated cerebellar hemangioblastomas are a manifestation of von Hippel-Lindau disease in about 20% of cases. Funduscopic examination and evaluation of the kidneys are warranted when a possible cerebellar hemangioblastoma is discovered.

Hemangioblastomas are often not encapsulated or well-circumscribed at surgery or histologically. Postoperative recurrence has been reported in up to 20% of these tumors.

### Case 187

28-year-old man presenting with ataxia.
(coronal, postcontrast T1-weighted SE scan)

### Case 188

79-year-old woman presenting with
headaches and dizziness.
(coronal, postcontrast T1-weighted SE scan)

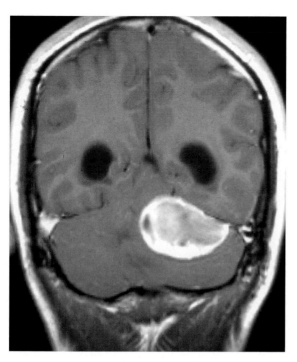

**Cerebellar Hemangioblastoma**

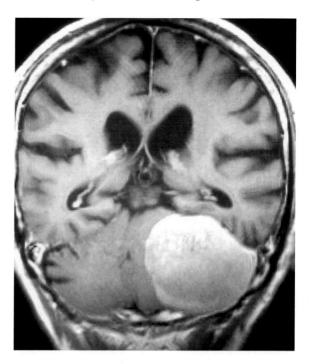

**Tentorial Meningioma**

The typical pial base of a hemangioblastoma may occasionally resemble the dural base of a meningioma. Since some meningiomas may demonstrate large vessels (see Cases 37 and 38) like hemangioblastomas, the two tumors can be confusingly similar in appearance. Contrast enhancement within meningiomas is usually more homogeneous than that of hemangioblastomas, as seen in the above cases. However, some hemangioblastomas are solidly enhancing, while some meningiomas are not (see Case 53).

The presence of relatively little mass effect for the size of the tumor, as in Case 188, favors a slow-growing mass such as a meningioma. By contrast, prominent edema and tonsillar herniation were demonstrated on other scans in association with the smaller but more rapidly enlarging hemangioblastoma in Case 187.

Angiography will usually distinguish between the above tumors, demonstrating pial supply to a hemangioblastoma and dural supply to a meningioma. A search for small additional lesions elsewhere in the cerebellum or brainstem is warranted to support the diagnosis of hemangioblastoma.

Medulloblastomas involving the cerebellar hemispheres of adults (so-called *cerebellar sarcomas*) often reach the pial surface and should be included in this differential diagnosis (see Case 180). Metastases should also be considered whenever a cerebellar mass is encountered in an adult.

# DIFFERENTIAL DIAGNOSIS:
## BRAINSTEM MASS IN AN ADULT

### Case 189

54-year-old woman presenting with left facial pain.
(axial, postcontrast T1-weighted SE scan)

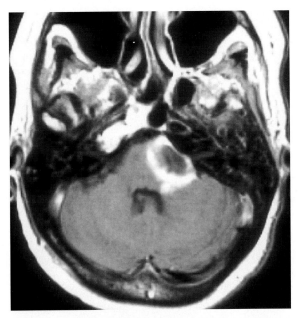

**Metastatic Carcinoma of the Breast**

### Case 190

45-year-old man who collapsed at work.
(axial, noncontrast T2-weighted FSE scan)

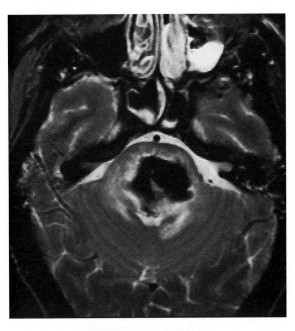

**Pontine Hemorrhage**

---

Although gliomas are the most frequent causes of brainstem masses in children, they are less common in adults. Other neoplasms, inflammatory processes, and vascular lesions must be included in the differential diagnosis of brainstem lesions in adulthood.

The region of the mid pons and brachium pontis is a common location for brain metastases, illustrated in Case 189. A large, intraaxial metastasis at this site can bulge exophytically into the cerebellopontine angle cistern, mimicking an extraaxial mass (see Case 198).

A number of inflammatory pathologies can cause swelling and signal abnormality within the brainstem. Among them are multiple sclerosis, acute disseminated encephalomyelitis, central pontine myelinolysis, tuberculosis, and *Listeria* rhombencephalitis; these are discussed in Chapters 8 and 9.

Case 190 illustrates that brainstem masses may be vascular rather than neoplastic. The large, irregular zone of low signal intensity within the pons represents a subacute hematoma, with deoxyhemoglobin and intracellular methemoglobin causing marked shortening of T2 values. A rim of surrounding edema is present. The brainstem is expanded, with posterior displacement of the fourth ventricle (compare to Case 133).

The patient in Case 190 was hypertensive, and the pontine hemorrhage was believed to be spontaneous. Rupture of a vascular malformation could present identically. The pons is a common location for cavernous angiomas, which can themselves be mass-like (see Cases 767 and 768) or cause recurrent hemorrhages, usually in association with a venous malformation (see Case 770). Capillary telangiectasias are also common in the brainstem (see Case 774) but rarely present with hemorrhage.

A retention cyst is seen in the left maxillary sinus in Case 190, and mucosal thickening lines the margins of the sphenoid sinus.

### Case 191

43-year-old woman presenting with
right-sided hearing loss.
(coronal, noncontrast T1-weighted SE scan)

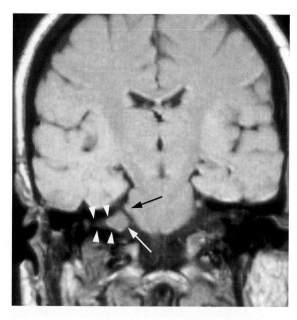

**Acoustic Schwannoma**

### Case 192

60-year-old woman with right facial numbness and
a ten-year history of right-sided hearing loss.
(coronal, noncontrast T1-weighted SE scan)

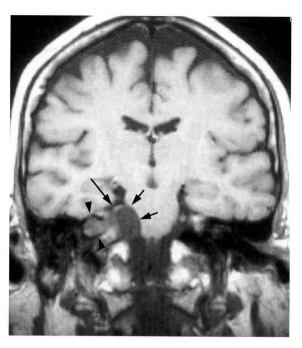

**Acoustic Schwannoma**

Acoustic schwannomas represent about 10% of primary intracranial tumors and account for the majority of masses in the cerebellopontine angle. They are typically well-defined lesions with smoothly rounded margins, centered at the internal auditory meatus.

In Case 191, the small schwannoma *(white arrow)* extends from the medial aspect of the internal auditory canal (IAC; *arrowheads*) into the cerebellopontine angle cistern, without contacting the adjacent fifth cranial nerve *(black arrow)*. The uniform, intermediate intensity of this mass is typical of small schwannomas.

Case 192 illustrates a larger, more complex schwannoma. The solid component of this tumor expands the IAC *(arrowheads;* compare to Case 191) and extends through the porus acusticus. A large cyst is present more medially, deforming the pons *(short arrows)* and elevating the fifth cranial nerve *(long arrow;* compare to the normal fifth nerve on the left side).

Cysts are commonly found in association with acoustic schwannomas. Many such "cysts" represent loculations of CSF surrounded by thickened arachnoid membranes adjacent to a tumor. Cystic degeneration within schwannomas is also common. When a partially cystic schwannoma invaginates into adjacent parenchyma, the appearance may resemble a hemangioblastoma arising at the pial surface.

Almost all patients who present with acoustic schwannomas have hearing loss, the presence or absence of which can be valuable in the differential diagnosis. Facial numbness due to distortion of the fifth nerve (as in Case 192) is a common secondary symptom of large eighth nerve tumors. The seventh cranial nerve is resistant to compressive dysfunction, and facial paresis rarely accompanies acoustic schwannomas preoperatively.

Because most schwannomas arise from the vestibular portion of the eighth nerve, these tumors are most accurately termed *vestibular schwannomas*. However, long-standing usage and the predominance of auditory symptoms explain the common "acoustic" nomenclature.

### Case 193

69-year-old man presenting with
left-sided hearing loss.
(axial, noncontrast T2-weighted SE scan)

### Case 194

39-year-old man presenting with right-sided hearing
loss and impaired rapid alternating movements.
(axial, noncontrast T2-weighted FSE scan)

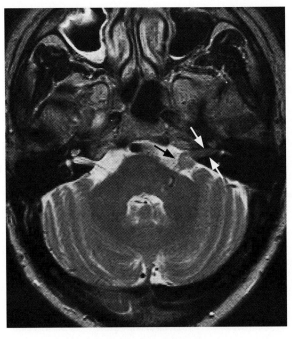

**Acoustic Schwannoma**

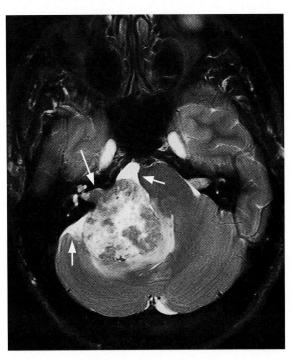

**Acoustic Schwannoma**

Small acoustic schwannomas may be isointense or hyperintense as compared to the brainstem on T2-weighted scans. In Case 193, a small isointense mass projects into the cerebellopontine angle cistern from the left internal auditory meatus *(black arrow)*. The internal auditory canal (IAC) is filled with tissue of low signal intensity *(white arrows)*, displacing the normal content of CSF (compare to the contralateral IAC). The combination of tumor filling the IAC and bulging medially into the adjacent cistern causes a "club" or "ice cream cone" morphology that is typical of small acoustic schwannomas.

Larger schwannomas may remain homogeneous, but a heterogeneous pattern of mixed tissue components is more common in tumors exceeding 2 cm in diameter. Case 194 is a good example, demonstrating irregular necrotic or cystic zones interspersed with more cellular tissue. Note the small intracanalicular portion of the tumor, which causes flaring of the IAC *(long arrow)*.

The cisternal component of the slowly growing schwannoma in Case 194 has gradually invaginated far into the adjacent parenchyma. Only a thin band of compressed tissue separates the tumor from the fourth ventricle. Proximity to the ventricular system is not a reliable criterion for distinguishing between intraaxial and extraaxial lesions.

The extraaxial origin of a cerebellopontine angle mass is usually indicated by contralateral brainstem displacement, causing widening of the cisterns at the margins of the tumor. Cisternal widening is seen anterior and posterior to the mass in Case 194 *(short arrows; also see Case 195)*.

Compare Case 194 to Case 182B.

### Case 195

38-year-old woman presenting with
right-sided hearing loss.
(axial, postcontrast T1-weighted SE scan)

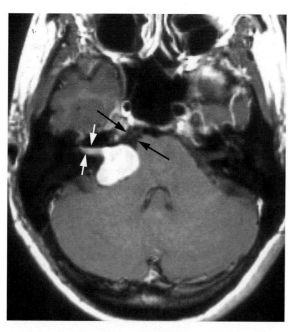

**Acoustic Schwannoma**

### Case 196

73-year-old woman after transmastoid resection
of a left-sided acoustic schwannoma.
(axial, postcontrast T1-weighted SE scan)

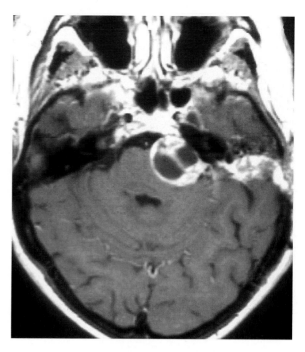

**Acoustic Schwannoma**

Contrast enhancement in schwannomas is usually intense. This characteristic allows detection of even very small eighth nerve lesions (see Case 200).

Uniformly enhancing schwannomas like Case 195 must often be considered in the differential diagnosis of meningiomas, particularly in the posterior fossa and parasellar regions. However, nonenhancing zones are common within large schwannomas, as illustrated by the recurrent tumor in Case 196. Occasional schwannomas are almost entirely cystic, with only a thin rim of enhancement distinguishing them from other extraaxial pathologies (such as an epidermoid cyst).

Case 195 is a good example of ipsilateral cisternal widening *(black arrows)* in association with an extraaxial mass.

This case also demonstrates the common appearance of a bulbous cisternal schwannoma in continuity with a stem or pedicle of enhancement occupying the mildly expanded IAC *(white arrows)*. The degree of IAC erosion is not necessarily related to the overall size of an acoustic schwannoma, which may expand exophytically in the adjacent cistern (see Case 194).

High signal intensity within the left mastoid region in Case 196 is mainly due to a fat graft placed at the time of previous surgery. Contrast-enhanced scans performed with fat saturation techniques are useful to eliminate potential confusion between fat packing and enhancing tumor in cases with a history of transmastoid surgery.

# DIFFERENTIAL DIAGNOSIS:
## ENHANCING MASS WITHIN THE CEREBELLOPONTINE ANGLE

### Case 197

38-year-old woman presenting with left facial pain.
(coronal, postcontrast T1-weighted SE scan)

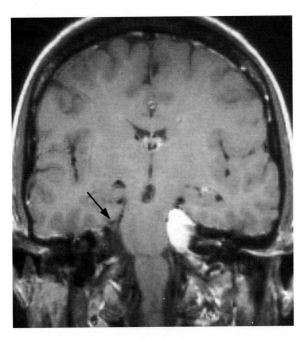

**Meningioma**

### Case 198

38-year-old woman presenting with
mild ataxia and tinnitus.
(axial, postcontrast T1-weighted SE scan)

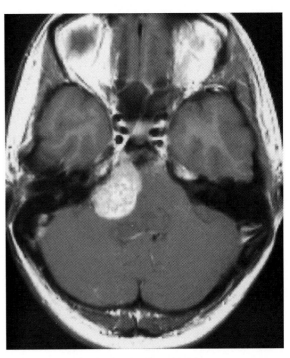

**Metastatic Adenocarcinoma**
(intraaxial; unknown origin)

---

A number of pathologies can present as enhancing extraaxial masses with the cerebellopontine angle cistern. Meningioma is the most common benign tumor to mimic an acoustic schwannoma in this location, as in Case 197.

The CT and MR appearance of meningiomas and acoustic schwannomas may be very similar. However, several potential discriminating features can be noted. Relatively low signal intensity on T2-weighted images is more common in meningiomas than schwannomas (but see Case 193). Most posterior fossa meningiomas are centered above or below the IAC, rather than at the internal auditory meatus. Cerebellopontine angle meningiomas can extend into the IAC, but few are associated with significant widening of the canal or with hearing loss. Finally, cerebellopontine angle meningiomas typically have a broader base against the petrous bone than schwannomas.

Other benign lesions in the CT differential diagnosis often have characteristic MR appearances (e.g., aneurysms and glomus jugulare tumors).

Malignant neoplasms can also present in the cerebellopontine angle. Extraaxial, dural-based metastases in this location may occur with carcinomas of the prostate, breast, and lung. Lymphoma should also be considered in this differential diagnosis.

Case 198 demonstrates that superficial parenchymal lesions may grow exophytically to mimic an extraaxial mass. The apparent dural base, intense enhancement, and sharp definition of this mass closely resemble the expected characteristics of a meningioma. The only disconcerting feature is the unusual texture within the lesion. As discussed in Chapter 2, meningiomas are usually quite homogenous or demonstrate radial or circular tissue patterns.

The meningioma in Case 197 distorts the left fifth cranial nerve near its entrance to the pons (compare to the normal trigeminal nerve on the right; *arrow*), causing the patient's facial pain. See Case 189 for an example of an intraaxial metastasis presenting similarly while resembling Case 198.

Compare the above scans to Cases 211-213.

## Case 199

49-year-old woman presenting with tinnitus and
reduced speech discrimination in the left ear.
(axial, noncontrast T2-weighted FSE scan)

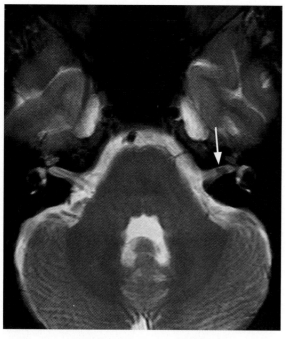

**Acoustic Schwannoma**

## Case 200

46-year-old man presenting with right-sided
hearing loss and vertigo.
(axial, postcontrast T1-weighted SE scan)

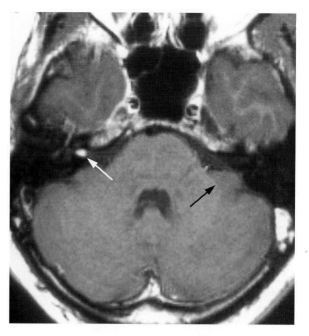

**Acoustic Schwannoma**

Symptoms of hearing loss or impaired discrimination can be caused by very small acoustic schwannomas compressing the cochlear nerve within the IAC. Tumors arising within the confines of the IAC typically cause symptoms at an earlier stage than masses that predominantly involve the cisternal portion of the nerve.

Intracanalicular acoustic schwannomas may be identified as soft tissue masses within the IAC on noncontrast MR images. Definition of small intracanalicular lesions is favored by strongly T2-weighted scans with high spatial resolution (e.g., rapid spin echo sequences using a 512 matrix, as in Case 199, or three-dimensional gradient echo sequences such as *constructive interference in a steady state* or *CISS*).

Contrast-enhanced MR scans reliably demonstrate intracanalicular schwannomas measuring only a few millimeters in diameter. The tumor in Case 200 *(white arrow)* is a tiny mass, entirely within the confines of the IAC.

Scans through the IAC often display soft tissue nodules near the posterior margin of the cerebellopontine angle cistern *(black arrow,* Case 200), which represent the normal flocculus of the cerebellum. These rounded structures are occasionally misinterpreted as extraaxial masses, especially if head tilt causes assymetrical visualization. However, the normal flocculus is located posterior to the IAC and does not enhance appreciably.

# DIFFERENTIAL DIAGNOSIS:
## FOCAL CONTRAST ENHANCEMENT IN THE REGION OF THE INTERNAL AUDITORY CANAL

### Case 201

55-year-old man presenting with vertigo.
(coronal, postcontrast T1-weighted SE scan)

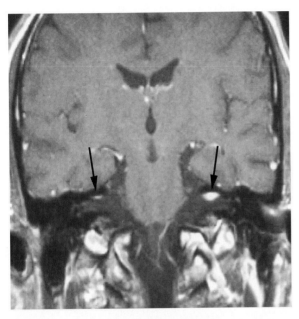

**Normal Petrosal Veins**

### Case 202

58-year-old woman presenting with
bilateral hearing loss.
(axial, postcontrast T1-weighted SE scan)

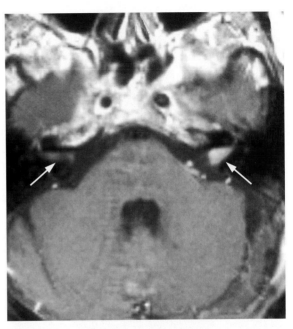

**Leptomeningeal Metastases**
(from carcinoma of the breast)

---

Normal vascular structures can cause contrast enhancement near or within the IAC, mimicking a small acoustic schwannoma. The petrosal venous system is typically located slightly superior to the internal auditory meatus. Considerable right/left symmetry in the size of these veins is common, as illustrated in Case 201 *(arrows)*. Attention to the margins of the IAC and comparison with the contralateral side will usually establish the nature of an enhancing vascular pseudotumor.

Areas of fatty marrow within the petrous apex are common and are frequently asymmetrical (see Case 215). These focal zones of high signal intensity can be mistaken for enhancing masses on T1-weighted postcontrast images. Attention to the precise location of the high signal region with respect to the IAC usually resolves confusion. A fat saturation scan can be performed in ambiguous cases. Precontrast T1-weighted images or fat saturation sequences will also distinguish rare lipomas of the IAC from enhancing schwannomas.

Abnormal contrast enhancement within the IAC on MR studies is not specific for acoustic schwannomas. Hemangiomas or inflammation of the facial nerve can present a similar appearance. Meningeal disease (e.g., carcinomatosis as in Case 202, sarcoidosis or lymphoma as in Case 492) can extend into the IAC with associated abnormal enhancement. Finally, reactive meningeal changes after surgery to remove a schwannoma can lead to intracanalicular enhancement, so postoperative scans must be interpreted cautiously.

In Case 202, the patient's bilateral hearing loss was the presenting symptom of metastatic breast carcinoma. The presence of abnormal meningeal enhancement involving the superior vermis (see Case 167), as well as the IACs, led to CSF cytology, which in turn established the diagnosis.

Enhancement of the membranous labyrinth may be noted on IAC studies performed to "rule out acoustic schwannoma." This evidence of labyrinthitis may correlate with the patient's symptoms and should be sought on otherwise negative scans of the petrous bones.

### Case 203A

39-year-old woman presenting with right facial pain.
(axial, noncontrast T1-weighted SE scan)

### Case 203B

Same patient.
(axial, postcontrast T1-weighted SE scan)

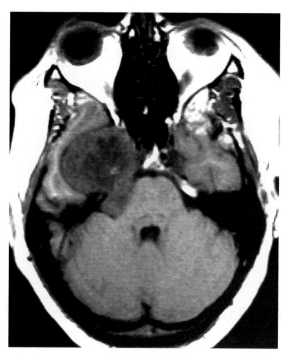

**Trigeminal Schwannoma**

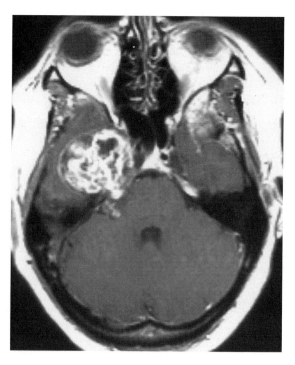

**Trigeminal Schwannoma**

Trigeminal schwannomas commonly arise near the gasserian ganglion, which is located within Meckel's cave in the posterior portion of the cavernous sinus.

Small trigeminal schwannomas may cause local widening of the cavernous sinus and should be included in the differential diagnosis discussed in Cases 278 and 279. Care must be taken not to overread apparent symmetry in the morphology of normal Meckel's caves caused by rotation or tilt of the head (see Case 405).

Larger tumors often acquire a dumbbell shape with components in the middle and posterior fossa. The middle fossa expansion of trigeminal schwannomas is characteristically extradural, while extension posteriorly along the cisternal course of the fifth nerve represents an intradural mass.

The precontrast appearance of the schwannoma in Case 203A is nonspecific and cannot be distinguished from a parasellar meningioma. (A T2-weighted scan demonstrated a granular texture and high signal intensity.) However, the irregular enhancement pattern in Case 203B is characteris-

tic of large schwannomas and would be distinctly unusual for a meningioma (compare to Cases 61 and 204B).

Lymphoma and metastasis should be considered in the differential diagnosis of enhancing masses spanning the petrous apex. Parasagittal chordomas or chondrosarcomas may also cross the petrous apex and can demonstrate speckled or "swiss cheese" patterns of enhancement (see Cases 218 and 219).

Trigeminal schwannomas are among the lesions to be sought in patients with tic douloureux. A more classic finding in such cases is looping of a vessel near the "entry zone" of the fifth cranial nerve as it joins the pons (see discussion of Cases 778 and 779). In most cases of trigeminal neuralgia, scans are unremarkable and symptoms are attributed to "microvascular compression" of the fifth nerve.

Neuritis (e.g., due to herpes) and meningeal neoplasm should be considered in the differential diagnosis of thickening and/or enhancement of the cisternal segment of the trigeminal nerve (see Cases 206 and 497).

## Case 204A

37-year-old woman, two years after partial resection of a hypoglossal schwannoma.
(axial, noncontrast T2-weighted FSE scan)

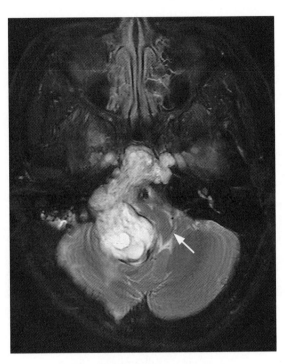

**Hypoglossal Schwannoma**

## Case 204B

Same patient.
(axial, postcontrast T1-weighted SE scan)

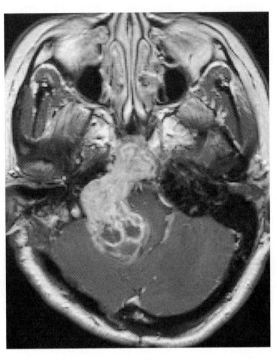

**Hypoglossal Schwannoma**

Schwannomas of other cranial nerves usually have MR characteristics comparable to acoustic and trigeminal tumors. High signal intensity on T2-weighted images and intense contrast enhancement are typical, as illustrated above.

The large tumor in Case 204 has grossly expanded the hypoglossal canal, eroding bone of the petrous apex and clivus. The intracranial component of the schwannoma displaces and compresses the medulla (*arrow,* Case 204A), while the extracranial component bulges into the nasopharynx. Such dumbbell morphology following the course of the cranial nerve through a foramen is highly suggestive of a schwannoma. The well-defined, smoothly rounded margins of the lesion are characteristic, as is the mixed solid and peripheral pattern of contrast enhancement.

The differential diagnosis in this case would include schwannomas arising from other cranial nerves (most commonly the ninth) near the jugular foramen. There is no evidence of prominent vascular channels, which would be expected in a glomus tumor of this size (compare to Cases 209 and 210). The transcranial extent, lobulated morphology, and long T2 values of the mass resemble a chordoma (compare to Cases 168-170), but the centering of the lesion at the hypoglossal canal and the intense enhancement favor the correct diagnosis.

Chondrosarcomas of the skull base (see Case 218) can present as lobulated masses in the cerebellopontine angle with prolonged T2 values and intense contrast enhancement resembling a schwannoma.

# DIFFERENTIAL DIAGNOSIS:
## ENHANCING MASS INVOLVING A CRANIAL NERVE

### Case 205

53-year-old man presenting with diplopia
due to a left oculomotor palsy.
(coronal, postcontrast T1-weighted SE scan)

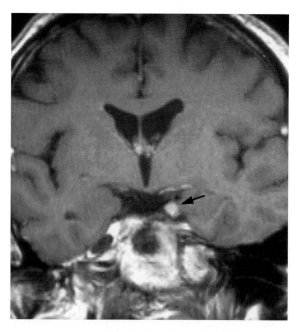

**Third Nerve Schwannoma**

### Case 206

13-year-old girl presenting with headaches.
(coronal, postcontrast T1-weighted SE scan)

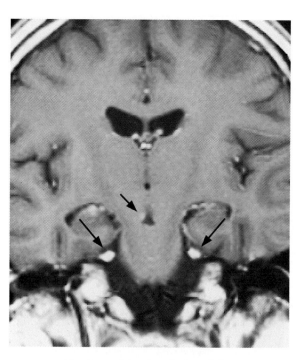

**Meningeal Leukemia Involving
the Fifth Cranial Nerves**

---

Abnormal enlargement and/or enhancement of a cranial nerve may reflect a mass arising from the nerve itself (e.g., schwannoma or hemangioma) or meningeal disease adherent to its surface. Case 205 illustrates the intense contrast enhancement typical of small schwannomas. The left third nerve *(arrow)* is involved between the interpeduncular fossa and the cavernous sinus.

Case 206 demonstrates abnormal enhancement of the cisternal segments of the trigeminal nerves bilaterally *(long arrows;* compare to the normal nonenhancing fifth nerves in Case 201). There is also faint enhancement of the proximal right third nerve *(short arrow)*. These findings reflect

leukemic infiltration of the meninges covering the nerves. A similar appearance can be caused by meningeal carcinomatosis from solid systemic neoplasms (e.g., melanoma and breast carcinoma; see Case 202). CSF seeding from primary intracranial tumors may also result in tumor deposits affecting one or more cranial nerves.

Inflammatory meningeal disease (e.g., tuberculosis, sarcoidosis, and meningovascular syphilis) and neuritis (e.g., Lyme disease and herpes zoster oticus and ophthalmicus) should be included in the differential diagnosis of abnormally enhancing cranial nerves (see Cases 497 and 498).

### Case 207

20-year-old man presenting with right-sided
hearing loss and facial numbness.
(axial, noncontrast scan; SE 2800/30)

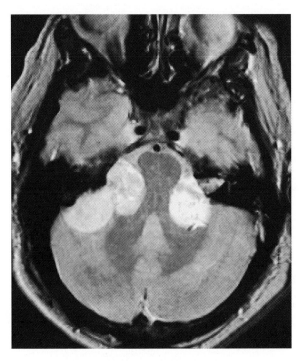

**Bilateral Acoustic Schwannomas**

### Case 208

37-year-old woman being followed
with type 2 neurofibromatosis.
(coronal, postcontrast T1-weighted
SE scan with MTS)

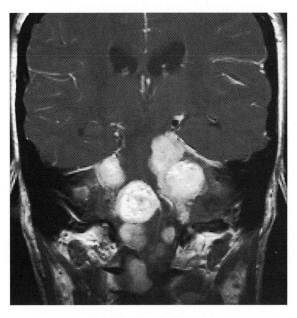

**Multiple Schwannomas**
(and meningiomas)

---

Bilateral acoustic schwannomas, as in Case 207, strongly suggest the diagnosis of neurofibromatosis. *Bilateral acoustic neurofibromatosis* (BANF) has now been designated *type 2* neurofibromatosis and is clinically and genetically distinct from the more common *type 1* neurofibromatosis or von Recklinghausen's disease (which is discussed in Cases 904-907).

The tumors in Case 207 are unusually homogeneous for their size. Many schwannomas develop cystic or necrotic regions as they enlarge (see Cases 194, 196, and 204). The high signal intensity of the masses is a typical feature of schwannomas on long TR images, although isointense tumors are also common.

In addition to acoustic schwannomas at early ages, patients with type 2 neurofibromatosis may present with schwannomas of other cranial nerves and/or with one or more cranial meningiomas. The multiple infratentorial masses in Case 208 probably include both schwannomas and meningiomas. Cases 65 and 66 illustrate multiple supratentorial meningiomas in patients with type 2 neurofibromatosis.

The bilateral acoustic schwannomas in type 2 neurofibromatosis are often very asymmetrical in size. When an eighth nerve tumor is detected in a young adult, a careful search should be made for a smaller contralateral lesion.

## Case 209A

70-year-old woman presenting with dysphagia.
(sagittal, noncontrast T1-weighted SE scan)

## Case 209B

Same patient.
(axial, noncontrast T2-weighted SE scan)

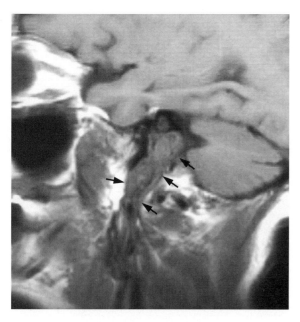

**Glomus Jugulare Tumor**

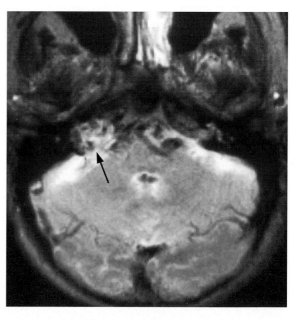

**Glomus Jugulare Tumor**

Glomus tumors (chemodectomas, paragangliomas) originate from paraganglionic cells in numerous locations, including the carotid sinus (carotid body tumor), jugular bulb (glomus jugulare), and middle ear (glomus tympanicum). Glomus tumors are multiple in about 3% of spontaneous cases and about 25% of familial cases. Although most of these neoplasms are histologically benign, they may be locally invasive. Associated bone erosion is often irregular and poorly defined, suggesting malignancy.

Glomus jugulare tumors typically enlarge the jugular foramen and span the skull base, as seen in this case. The sagittal view (Case 209A) demonstrates that the region of the jugular foramen is expanded and filled with the intensity of soft tissue rather than the signal void of flowing blood *(arrows)*. The tumor is seen to extend below the skull base, involving the cervical portion of the internal jugular vein.

A useful feature in distinguishing glomus tumors from a normal jugular bulb (or from other masses such as schwannomas) is the typical granular texture of glomus lesions due to flow voids within the highly vascular tissue. On spin echo images these small circular and tubular areas of low signal intensity cause a characteristic "salt and pepper" pattern. Compare this appearance in Case 209B to the more homogeneous texture of the jugular foramen in Case 214A.

The zones of low signal intensity within the left cerebellopontine angle cistern in Case 209B were due to tortuous looping of the distal left vertebral artery.

## Case 210

60-year-old woman found to
have a middle ear mass.
(axial partition, noncontrast three-dimensional
time-of-flight GRE sequence)

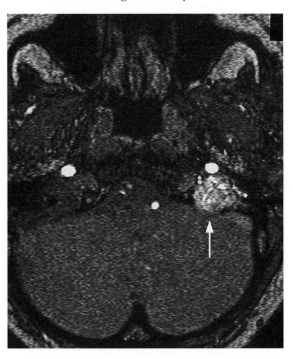

**Glomus Jugulare Tumor**

## Case 211

63-year-old man presenting with dysfunction
of cranial nerves IX to XII on the left.
(axial, postcontrast T1-weighted SE scan)

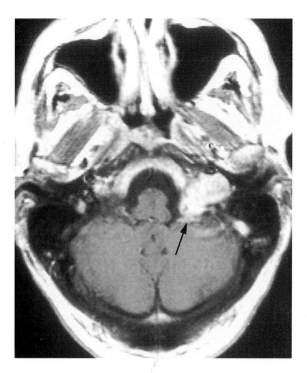

**Glomus Jugulare Tumor**

---

Glomus tumors are characteristically highly vascular. The source image from a time-of-flight MR angiographic sequence in Case 210 demonstrates multiple small arteries containing flow-related enhancement within the mass filling the left jugular foramen. (Flow-related enhancement is also seen in the internal carotid arteries and in the distal left vertebral artery.) This appearance confirms the abundant blood supply to the tumor and correlates with the typical "salt and pepper" texture of the tissue on nonangiographic scans such as Case 209.

Intense contrast enhancement is a usual feature of glomus tumors, as illustrated in Case 211. The uniformly enhancing mass has expanded the jugular foramen and extends medially into the cerebellopontine angle cistern. The cisternal component of the tumor continued superiorly to reach the level of the internal auditory canal, where it mimicked an acoustic schwannoma. Care must be taken to establish the rostral and caudal limits of cisternal masses.

Glomus jugulare tumors occur more frequently in women than in men, with female/male incidence ratios as high as 5 to 1 in some series.

# DIFFERENTIAL DIAGNOSIS:
## ENHANCING EXTRAAXIAL MASS NEAR THE JUGULAR FORAMEN

### Case 212

37-year-old woman presenting with dysfunction of cranial nerves IX to XII on the right.
(coronal, postcontrast T1-weighted SE scan with MTS)

### Case 213

86-year-old man presenting with dysfunction of cranial nerves IX to XI on the left.
(coronal, postcontrast T1-weighted SE scan)

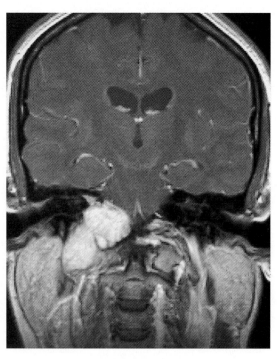

**Schwannoma**

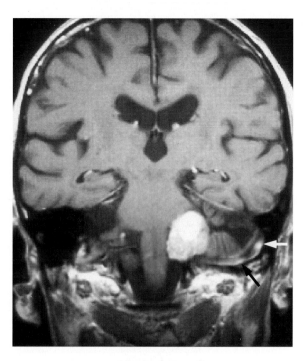

**Meningioma**

A number of enhancing masses can arise within or extend to the jugular foramen. As seen in Case 212, schwannomas of cranial nerves IX through XII may expand and transverse the jugular foramen, closely resembling a glomus tumor. The margins of the jugular foramen are usually smoother and better defined when enlarged by a schwannoma than when eroded by a glomus tumor. A more reliable distinguishing feature is the usual absence of prominent vessels within a schwannoma on routine or angiographic images, while appreciable internal vascularity is a hallmark of glomus tumors.

The extraaxial tumor in Case 213 is located slightly posterior to the junction of the sigmoid sinus *(arrows)* and jugular vein. It was not associated with prominent vessels or erosion of the jugular foramen, making a glomus tumor unlikely. However, a schwannoma of one of the lower cranial nerves could present a very similar appearance. Perfusion-weighted scans may assist in distinguishing between these two extraaxial masses: meningiomas contain high blood volume, while schwannomas usually do not.

Dural-based metastases and lymphoma should be included in the differential diagnosis of solidly enhancing extraaxial masses near the jugular bulb.

**Case 214A**

66-year-old man presenting with
bilateral hearing loss.
(axial, noncontrast scan; SE 3600/22)

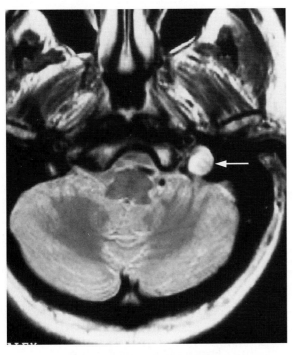

Large (Normal) Jugular Foramen

**Case 214B**

Same patient.
(axial source image from a noncontrast
two-dimensional time-of-flight GRE sequence)

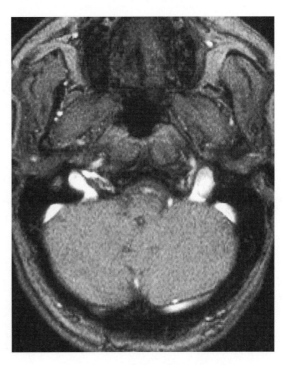

Large (Normal) Jugular Foramen

High signal intensity fills the large left jugular foramen in Case 214A *(arrow)*. This appearance could suggest a mass, such as a glomus jugulare tumor or a schwannoma. Instead, the finding represents normal slow flow within a large jugular vein.

MR scans performed with motion-refocusing pulse sequences, after contrast injection, and/or in circumstances of slow jugular flow, may normally demonstrate isointense or high signal within the jugular vein. The combination of a large jugular foramen and prominent intraluminal signal may falsely mimic a neoplasm.

Several clues help differentiate a normal jugular bulb from a foraminal tumor on MR scans. First, the bony margins of normally large foramina are more smoothly rounded and better defined than the erosive appearance usually

seen with glomus tumors. (This quality may be better appreciated on CT examinations.)

Second, as illustrated in Cases 209 and 210, glomus tumors of medium or large size usually contain multiple flow voids, which give the lesion a characteristically coarse texture. This pattern is distinct from the more amorphous appearance of slow flow within a large vessel.

Finally, MR venography or single slice gradient echo images in the axial plane may be used to establish flow-related enhancement within a patent jugular vein. In Case 214B, flow-related enhancement produces high signal intensity within both jugular foramina. Although the intensity within the large left foramen is slightly heterogenous (reflecting different flow velocities and phases), no filling defect displaces flow from any segment of the foramen.

## Case 215A

47-year-old man presenting with
a right sixth nerve palsy.
(axial, postcontrast T1-weighted SE scan)

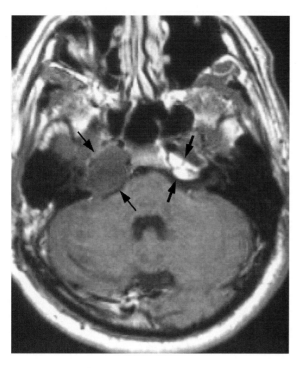

**Primary Epidermoid Tumor**

## Case 215B

Same patient.
(axial, noncontrast T2-weighted SE scan)

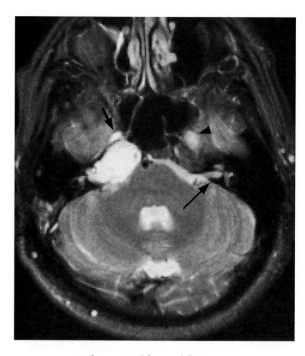

**Primary Epidermoid Tumor**

---

The petrous apex can be involved by a number of benign and malignant neoplasms. Among the former are primary epidermoid tumors. These gradually enlarging masses result from accumulation of squamous debris within a rest of keratinizing epithelium enclosed during formation of the skull. They are distinct from the secondary cholesteotomas that may develop as a complication of inflammatory disease in the middle ear and mastoid region.

Epidermoid tumors of the petrous apex are characteristically expansile lesions, with thinning rather than destruction of bony margins. Like intracranial epidermoid tumors, these masses usually demonstrate long T1 and long T2 values, as seen in this case. Minimal contrast enhancement may be present at the perimeter of the lesion, but the center is nonenhancing. This combination of features (long T1, expansion of bone, and lack of enhancement) is highly suggestive of the correct diagnosis.

An unusual mucocele or abscess within an apical petrous air cell could be considered in the differential diagnosis.

An eccentric skull base chordoma (see Case 219) or chondrosarcoma (see Case 218), or a schwannoma might resemble the appearance of Case 215B but would be expected to enhance.

Case 215A demonstrates fatty marrow within the left petrous apex *(thick arrows)*, a common normal variant that is often asymmetrical. On non–fat-suppressed coronal postcontrast scans, similar areas can be mistaken for enhancement in a mass involving the cerebellopontine angle (e.g., acoustic schwannoma). Note that the signal intensity of this region is substantially decreased on the T2-weighted scan (Case 215B).

Conversely, CSF within the IACs is much more apparent on T2-weighted images *(long arrow,* Case 215B) than on T1-weighted scans. Comparing the right and left sides in this image, it is clear that the petrous apex tumor has extended posteriorly to involve the right IAC. The anterior margin of the mass displaces and compresses Meckel's cave *(short arrow;* compare to the normal left side indicated by the *arrowhead).*

### Case 216

42-year-old man with a history
of chronic otitis media.
(sagittal, noncontrast T1-weighted SE scan)

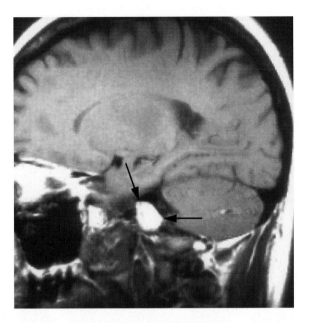

**Cholesterol Granuloma**

### Case 217

51-year-old man presenting with headaches.
(axial, noncontrast T2*-weighted GRE scan)

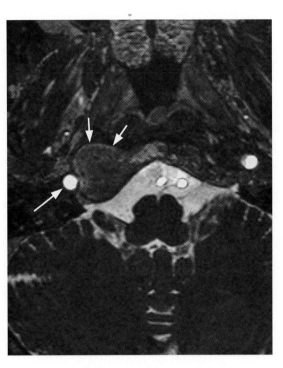

**Cholesterol Granuloma**

Cholesterol granulomas (also called "cholesterol cysts") are among the benign pathologies that may involve the petrous apex. These lesions represent obstructed air cells that have become filled with old blood products from recurrent small hemorrhages.

Like primary epidermoid tumors, cholesterol granulomas are expansile, slow-growing masses. However, these two pathologies follow nearly opposite patterns of signal intensity. The presence of methemoglobin causes cholesterol granulomas to characteristically demonstrate high signal intensity on noncontrast T1-weighted images, as shown in Case 216 *(arrows)*. The presence of deoxyhemoglobin and/or hemosiderin often results in low signal intensity on T2- or T2*-weighted scans, as seen in Case 217 *(short arrows)*. Cholesterol granulomas may alternatively contain high signal regions on long TR images, or a mixture of high and low signal intensity, depending on the proportion and nature of blood products within the cyst fluid.

Note that the well-defined, smoothly marginated lesion in Case 217 is immediately adjacent to the flow-related enhancement within the internal carotid artery *(long arrow)*. Large cholesterol granulomas can surround the petrous segment of this vessel and/or extend into the middle ear. An aneurysm of the internal carotid artery is a rare alternative cause of a slowly expanding mass within the petrous bone, usually demonstrating distinctive lamellar thrombus and/or an expanded zone of flow-related signal changes.

The list of benign expansile bone tumors of the skull base also includes osteoblastomas and aneurysmal bone cysts. Like cholesterol granulomas, aneurysmal bone cysts contain blood products, usually evident as sedimentation levels within a multiloculated architecture.

Fatty marrow within the petrous apex is characterized by short T1 and T2 values (see Case 215). The lack of bone expansion should distinguish this normal variation from a cholesterol granuloma. In equivocal cases, a scan using fat-suppression technique can establish the nature of T1-shortening within the petrous apex.

### Case 218A

48-year-old woman presenting with
a left sixth nerve palsy.
(axial, noncontrast T2-weighted FSE scan)

### Case 218B

Same patient.
(axial, postcontrast T1-weighted SE scan with MTS)

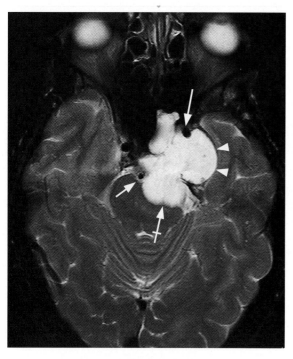

**Chondrosarcoma**

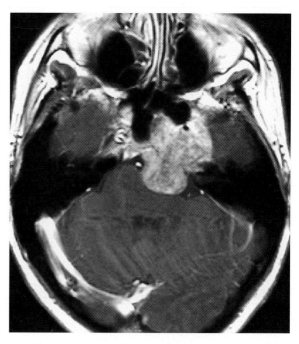

**Chondrosarcoma**

Chondrosarcomas of the skull base are slow-growing tumors that most frequently arise in the region of the petro-occipital synchondrosis. From this parasagittal origin, the lesions expand to erode the lateral aspect of the clivus and/or sphenoid bone and the petrous apex. Further growth leads to masses in the parasellar region and/or posterior fossa.

The tumor in Case 218A has replaced the sphenoid bone on the left, extending into and enlarging the left cavernous sinus *(arrowheads)*. The anterior margin of the mass partially surrounds the internal carotid artery *(long arrow)*. Posteriorly, the lesion crosses the tentorial hiatus to border the basilar artery *(short arrow)* and deform the cerebral peduncle *(crossed arrow)*.

The long T2 values within the tumor are typical of neoplasms with a chondroid matrix. This characteristic and the lobulated morphology of the mass resemble the MR features of chordomas involving the skull base (see Case 170A as well as Case 219). The usual parasagittal location of chondrosarcomas can help distinguish them from chordomas, which more commonly arise near the midline. (However, chordomas can also originate parasagittally; see Case 219.) Matrix calcification is a more common and prominent feature of chondrosarcomas than of chordomas, but mineralization is often not apparent on MR images.

Chondrosarcomas usually enhance intensely with variable heterogeneity. The pattern demonstrated in Case 218B is typical but nonspecific (compare to the chordoma in Case 170B).

A large schwannoma could present an appearance similar to the above scans (see Case 204). A meningioma of the skull base could also be included in the differential diagnosis of Case 218B, but the homogeneous T2 prolongation of Case 218A would be very atypical.

## Case 219A

58-year-old man presenting with right-sided
hearing loss and sixth nerve palsy.
(coronal, noncontrast T1-weighted SE scan)

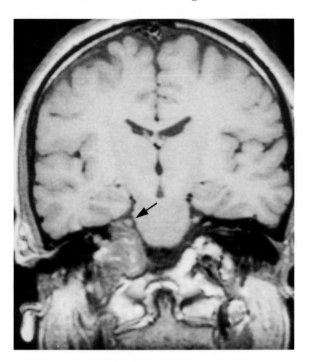

**Chordoma**

## Case 219B

Same patient.
(axial, postcontrast T1-weighted SE scan)

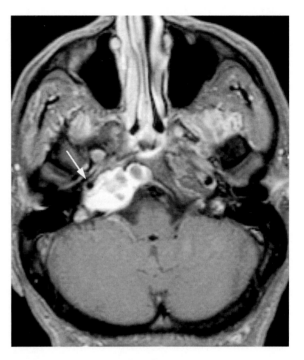

**Chordoma**

Chordomas often involve the center of the skull base, as illustrated in Cases 168-170. However, chordomas may also arise several centimeters away from the midline to present as unilateral, parasagittal lesions.

The tumor in Case 219A erodes the petrous apex as it traverses the skull base on the right. The fifth cranial nerve can be identified at the superior margin of the mass *(arrow)*. The region of the internal auditory meatus is occupied and destroyed by neoplasm (compare to the normal left side). Small areas of T1-shortening within the mass may represent hemorrhage, mucinous material, or the effect of localized calcification within the tumor matrix.

Intense enhancement is present throughout most of the lesion in Case 219B. Other chordomas enhance less homogeneously and intensely. Although clearly destructive, the above chordoma is well defined, retaining a mildly lobulated contour.

Chondrosarcomas may also occur at the junction of the petrous and occipital bones, as illustrated on the previous page. These lesions should be considered along with metastases, myeloma, and lymphoma in the differential diagnosis of midline or parasagittal masses eroding the skull base.

The petrous segment of the right internal carotid artery is identified by flow void at the lateral margin of the tumor in Case 219B *(arrow)*.

### Case 220

45-year-old woman presenting with
bitemporal hemianopsia and diplopia.
(sagittal, noncontrast T1-weighted SE scan)

### Case 221

51-year-old woman presenting with
bilateral sixth nerve palsies.
(sagittal, noncontrast T1-weighted SE scan)

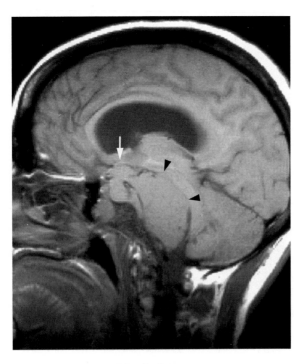

**Meningioma**

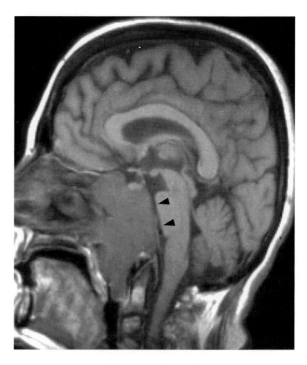

**Nasopharyngeal Carcinoma**

Chordomas and chondrosarcomas are among several benign and malignant neoplasms that can involve the clivus.

In Case 220, a clival meningioma has permeated the basiocciput and basisphenoid. The low signal intensity within the involved bone represents reactive sclerosis. Tumor is present within the sphenoid sinus, sella turcica and suprasellar cistern, in addition to the large prepontine component *(arrowheads)*. The optic chiasm is elevated and thinned *(arrow)*. The brainstem is posteriorly displaced and compressed.

Case 221 demonstrates direct extension of a nasopharyngeal carcinoma through the skull base. The clivus and the body of the sphenoid bone have been destroyed. The tumor crosses the prepontine cistern to flatten the anterior margin of the pons *(arrowheads)*.

Some pituitary adenomas grow predominantly inferiorly, filling the sphenoid sinus and eroding the skull base (see Case 234). Such bone destruction may mimic the skull in-

vasion of a nasopharyngeal neoplasm. The ghost of an expanded sella within the lesion can be an important diagnostic clue in such cases.

An appearance similar to Case 221 could be caused by metastasis, myeloma (or solitary plasmacytoma), or lymphoma involving the skull base, or by a rare carcinoma of the sphenoid sinus. Occasionally the bone destruction of a glomus jugulare tumor mimics a malignant skull base lesion, but the homogeneous texture of the masses in Cases 220 and 221 argues against this possibility.

Osteomyelitis is a rare potential cause of permeation or destruction of the sphenoid bone and/or clivus.

Sagittal and coronal MR scans are valuable for simultaneously defining the pharyngeal and intracranial components of masses involving the skull base. Compare the above images to the midline chordomas in younger patients presented as Cases 168-170.

# DIFFERENTIAL DIAGNOSIS:
## MASS REPLACING THE SPHENOID BONE

### Case 222

51-year-old woman presenting with
bilateral sixth nerve palsies.
(axial, noncontrast T2-weighted SE scan)

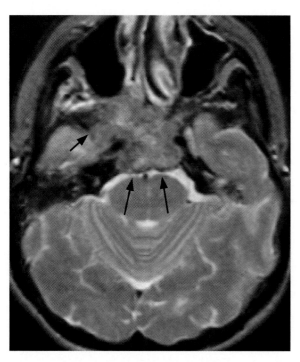

**Nasopharyngeal Carcinoma**
(same patient as Case 221)

### Case 223

26-year-old man presenting with severe headaches.
(coronal, postcontrast T1-weighted SE scan)

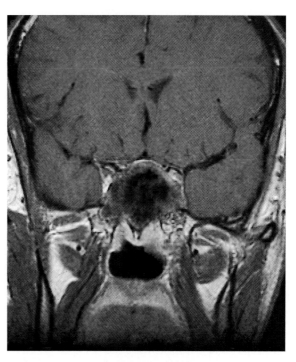

**Fungal Sinusitis**
(aspergillus mycetoma)

---

Metastatic disease is a leading consideration when a destructive lesion of the skull base is discovered in an adult. Case 222 instead represents direct extension of nasopharyngeal carcinoma into the sphenoid bone, as seen in sagittal projection in Case 221. The mass has replaced the clivus, and tumor tissue interfaces with a flattened prepontine cistern *(long arrows)*. The carcinoma has invaded the cavernous sinuses and the pterygopalatine fossae bilaterally, with greater involvement on the right side *(short arrow)*.

Malignancies with dense cellularity and/or a fibrous stroma may be of relatively low intensity on T2-weighted images, as seen in Case 222. The unexciting signal pattern can belie a very aggressive tumor.

Case 223 serves as a reminder to consider inflammatory etiologies when masses are encountered within paranasal sinuses. The nonenhancing tissue with relatively low signal intensity obliterating the sinus in this case proved to be a dense, semisolid mass of fungal hyphae. Mycetomas may

contain paramagnetic ions and calcification, contributing to the characteristic high attenuation on CT scans and low signal intensity on MR images. Chronic fungal sinusitis can cause erosion or sclerosis of adjacent bone, resembling the effects of a malignant or benign neoplasm. Fungal masses of the sphenoid sinus may also extend into the cavernous sinus to surround or invade the internal carotid artery, mimicking the typical vascular encasement of a parasellar meningioma or resembling other parasellar pathologies (such as Case 279).

A mucocele of the sphenoid sinus is a rare cause of a homogeneous mass replacing the central skull base. Such lesions are characteristically well defined and expansile. Their signal intensity may be either high or low on either T1- or T2-weighted images, depending upon the viscosity and inspissation of the contents.

Inferior extension of a pituitary adenoma should also be considered in the differential diagnosis of a mass filling or expanding the sphenoid sinus (see Case 234).

# REFERENCES

Ahn MS, Jackler RK: Exophytic brain tumors mimicking primary lesions of the cerebellopontine angle. *Laryngoscope* 107:466-471, 1997.

Akeson P, Holtas S: Radiological investigation of neurofibromatosis type 2. *Neuroradiology* 38:107-110, 1994.

Allen RW, Harnsberger HR, Shelton C, et al: Low-cost high-resolution fast spin-echo MR of acoustic schwannoma: an alternative to enhanced conventional spin-echo MR? *AJNR* 17:1205-1210, 1996.

Anderson RE, Laskoff JM: Ramsay Hunt Syndrome mimicking intracanalicular acoustic neuroma on contrast-enhanced MR. *ANJR* 11:409, 1990.

Asari S, Katayama S, Itoh T, Tsuchida S, et al: CT and MRI of haemorrhage into intracranial neuromas. *Neurosurgery* 35:247-250, 1993.

Ashley DG, Zee C-S, Chandrasoma PT, Segall HD: Lhermitte-Duclos disease: CT and MR findings. *J Comput Assist Tomgr* 14:984-987, 1990.

Awwad EE, Levy E, Martin DS, Merenda GO: Atypical MR appearance of Lhermitte-Duclos disease with contrast enhancement. *AJNR* 16:1719-1720, 1995.

Baldwin D, King TT, Chevretton E, Morrison AW: Bilateral cerebellopontine angle tumors in neurofibromatosis type 2. *J Neurosurg* 74:910-915, 1991.

Becker RL, Becker AD, Sobel DF: Adult medulloblastoma: review of 13 cases with emphasis on MRI. *Neuroradiology* 37:104-108, 1995.

Beges C, Revel MP, Gaston A, et al: Trigeminal neuromas: assessment of MRI and CT. *Neuroradiology* 34:179-183, 1992.

Bilaniuk LT: Adult infratentorial tumors. *Semin Roentgenol* 25:155-173, 1990.

Bonneville F, Sarrazin J-L, Marsot-Dupuch K, et al: Unusual lesions of the cerebellopontine angle: a segmental approach. *Radiographics* 21:419-438, 2001.

Bourgouin PM, Tampieri D, Grahovac SZ, et al: CT and MR imaging findings in adults with cerebellar medulloblastome: comparison with findings in children. *Am J Roentgenol* 159:609-612, 1992.

Brownlee RD, Sevick RJ, Rewcastle NB, Tranmer BI: Radiologic-pathologic correlation. Intracranial chondroma. *AJNR* 18:889-894, 1997.

Caldemeyer KS, Mathews VP, Azzarelli B, Smith RS: The jugular foramen: a review of anatomy, masses, and imaging characteristics. *Radiographics* 17:1123-1139, 1997.

Caldemeyer KS, Mathews VP, Righi PD, Smith RL: Imaging features and clinical significance of perineural spread or extension of head and neck tumors. *Radiographics* 18:97-110, 1998.

Carvalho GA, Tatagiba M, Samii M: Cystic schwannomas of the jugular foramen: clinical and surgical remarks. *Neurosurgery* 46:560-566, 2000.

Casselman JW, Kuhweide R, Ampe W, Meeus I, et al: Pathology of the menbraneous labyrinth: comparison of T1- and T2-weighted and gadolinium-enhanced spin-echo and 3DFT-CISS imaging. *AJNR* 14:59-69, 1993.

Celli P, Ferrante L, Acqui M, et al: Neuromas of the third, fourth, and sixth cranial nerves: a survey and report of a new fourth nerve case. *Surg Neurol* 38:216-224, 1992.

Chan AW, Tarbell NJ, Black PM, et al: Adult medulloblastoma: prognostic factors and patterns of relapse. *Neurosurgery* 47:623-632, 2000.

Chan, L-L, Singh S, Jones D, et al: Imaging of mucormycosis skull base osteomyelitis. *AJNR* 21:828-830, 2000.

Choyke PL, Glenn GM, Walther MM, et al: Von Hippel-Lindau disease: genetic, clinical, and imaging features. *Radiology* 194:629-642, 1995.

Cohen TI, Powers SK, Williams DW III: MR appearance of intracanalicular eighth nerve lipoma. *AJNR* 13:1188-1190, 1992.

Conway JE, Chou D, Clatterbuck RE, et al: Hemangioblastomas of the central nervous system in von Hippel-Lindau syndrome and sporadic disease. *Neurosurgery* 48:55-63, 2001.

Curati WL, Graif M, Kingsley DPE, et al: Acoustic neuromas: Gd-DTPA enhancement in MR imaging. *Radiology* 158:447-451, 1986.

Curati WL, Graif M, Kingsley DPE, et al: MRI in acoustic neuroma: a review of 35 patients. *Neuroradiology* 28:208-214, 1986.

Curtin HD: Rule out eighth nerve tumor: contrast-enhanced T1-weighted or high-resolution T2-weighted MR? *AJNR* 18:1834-1838, 1997.

Daniels DL, Czervionke LF, Pojunas KW, et al: Facial nerve enhancement in MR imaging. *AJNR* 8:605-607, 1987.

Daniels DL, Czervionke LF, Millen SJ, Haberkamph TJ, et al: MR imaging of facial nerve enhancement inBell palsy or after temporal bone surgery. *Radiology* June 171:807-809, 1989.

Daniels DL, Millen SJ, Meyer GA, et al: MR detection of tumor in the internal auditory canal. *AJNR* 8:249-252, 1987.

Daniels, DL, Pech P, Pojunas KW, et al: Trigeminal nerve: anatomic correlation with MR imaging. *Radiology* 159:577-583, 1986.

Daniels DL, Schenck JF, Foster T, et al: Magnetic resonance imaging of the jugular foramen. *AJNR* 6:699-703, 1985.

DeMonte F, Ginsberg LE, Clayman GL: Primary malignant tumors of the sphenoidal sinus. *Neurosurgery* 46:1084-1092, 2000.

Dietz RR, Davis WL, Harnsberger HR, et al: MR imaging and MR angiography in the evaluation of pulsatile tinnitus. *AJNR* 15:879-889, 1994.

Eisen MD, Yousem DM, Montone KT, et al: Use of preoperative MR to predict dural, perineural, and venous sinus invasion of skull base tumors. *AJNR* 17:1937-1945, 1996.

Eldevik OP, Gabrielsen TO, Jacobsen EA: Imaging findings in schwannomas of the jugular foramen. *AJNR* 21:1939-1144, 2000.

Elster AD, Arthur DW: Intercranial hemangioblastomas: CT and MR findings. *J Comput Assist Tomgr* 12:736-739, 1988.

Engstrom M, Abdsaleh S, Ahlstrom H, et al: Serial gadolinium-enhanced magnetic resonance imaging and assessment of facial nerve function in Bell's palsy. *Otolaryngol Head Neck Surg* 117:559-566, 1997.

Enzmann DR, O'Donohue J: Optimizing MR imaging for detecting small tumors in the cerebellopontine angle and internal auditory canal. *AJNR* 8:99-106, 1987.

Filling-Katz MR, Choyke PL, Patronas NJ, et al: Radiologic screening for von Hippel-Lindau Disease: the role of Gd-DTPA enhanced MR imaging of the CNS. *J Comput Assist Tomogr* 13:743-755, 1989.

Fitzgerald DC, Mark AS: Sudden hearing loss: frequency of abnormal findings on contrast-enhanced MR studies. *AJNR* 19:1433-1436, 1998.

Fukui MB, Weissman JL, Curtin HD, Kanal E: T2-weighted MR characteristics of internal auditory canal masses. *AJNR* 17:1211-1218, 1996.

Gebarski SS, Telian SA, Niparko JK: Enhancement along the normal facial nerve in the facial canal: MR imaging and anatomic correlation. *Radiology* 183:391-394, 1992.

Gebarski SS, Tucci DL, Telian SA: The cochlear nuclear complex: MR location and abnormalities. *AJNR* 14:1311-1318, 1993.

Gentry LR, Jacoby CG, Turski PA, et al: Cerebellopontine angle-retromastoid mass lesions: compatative study of diagnois with MR imaging and CT. *Radiology 162:513-520, 1987.*

Ginsberg LE, DeMonte F: Facial nerve schwannoma with middle cranial fossa involvement. *Radiology* 213:364-368, 1999.

Ginsberg LE, DeMonte F, Gillenwater AM: Greater superficial petrosal nerve: anatomy and MR findings in perineural tumor spread. *AJNR* 17:389-393, 1996.

Greenberg JJ, Oot RF, Wismer GL, et al: Cholesterol granulomas of the petrous apex: MR and CT evaluation. *AJNR* 9:1205-1214, 1988.

Griffin C, De La Paz R, Enzmann D: MR and CT correlation of cholesterol cysts of the petrous bone. *AJNR* 8:825-829, 1987.

Han MH, Jabour BA, Andrews JC, et al: Noneoplastic enhancing lesions mimicking intracanalicular acoustic neuroma on gadolinium-enhanced MR images. *Radiology* 179:795-796, 1991.

Hermans R, Van der Goten A, De Foer B, Baert AL: MRI screening for acoustic neuroma without gadolinium: value of 3DFT-CISS sequence. *Neuroradiology* 39:593-598, 1997.

Ho VT, Rao VM, Doan HT, Mikaelian DO: Low-grade adenocarcinoma of probable endolymphatic sac origin: CT and MR appearance. *AJNR* 17:168-170, 1996.

Ho VB, Smirniotopoulos JG, Murphy FM, Rushing EJ: Radiologic-pathologic correlation: hemangioblastoma. *AJNR* 13:1343-1352, 1992.

Hurst RW, Judkins A, Bolger W, et al: Mycotic aneurysm and cerebral infarction resulting from fungal sinusitis: imaging and pathologic correlation. *AJNR* 22:858-863, 2001.

Hutchins LG, Harnsberger HR, Hardin CW, et al: The radiological assessment of trigeminal neuropathy. *AJNR* 10:1031-1038, 1989.

Isaacson JE, Sismanis A: Cholesterol granuloma cyst of the petrous apex. *Ear Nose Throat J* 75:425-429, 1996.

Iwayama E, Naganawa S, Ito T, et al: High-resolution MR cisternography of the cerebellopontine angle: 2D versus 3D fast spin-echo sequences. *AJNR* 20:889-896, 1999.

Jawahar A, Kondziolka D, Kanal E, et al: Imaging the trigeminal nerve and pons before and after surgical intervention for trigeminal neuralgia. *Neurosurgery* 48:101-107, 2001.

Jee WH, Choi KH, Choe BY, et al: Fibrous dysplasia: MR imaging characteristics with radiopathologic correlation.0*Am J Roentgenol* 167:1523-1527, 1996.

Kamel HAM, Toland J: Trigeminal nerve anatomy: illustrated using examples of abnormalities. *Am J Roentgenol* 176:247-251, 2001.

Kingsley, DPE, Brooks GB, Leung AW-L, Johnson MA: Acoustic neuromas: evaluation by magnetic resonance imaging. *AJNR* 6:1-5, 1985.

Klisch J, Juengling F, Spreer J, et al: Lhermitte-Duclos disease: assessment with MR imaging, positron emission tomography, single photon emission CT, and MR spectroscopy. *AJNR* 22:824-830, 2001.

Koci TM, Chiang F, Mehringer CM, et al: Adult cerebellar medulloblastoma: imaging features with emphasis on MR. *AJNR* 14:929-939, 1993.

Krainik A, Cyna-Gorse F, Bouccara D, et al: MRI of unusual lesions in the internal auditory canal. *Neuroradiology* 43:52-57, 2001.

Larson TL, Wong ML: Primary mucocele of the petrous apex: MR appearance. *AJNR* 13:203-204, 1992.

Lee SR, Sanches J, Mark AS, et al: Posterior fossa hemangioblastomas: MR imaging. *Radiology* 171:463-469, 1989.

Levy RA, Blaivas M, Muraszko K, Robertson PL: Desmoplastic medulloblastoma: MR findings. *AJNR* 18:1364:1366, 1997.

Lhuillier FM, Doyon DL, Halimi PhM, et al: Magnetic resonance imaging of acoustic neuromas: pitfalls and differential diagnosis. *Neuroradiology* 34:144-149, 1992.

Mafee MF: MR imaging of intralabyrinthine schwannoma, labyrinthitis, and other labyrinthine pathology. *Otolaryngol Clin N Am* 28:407-430, 1995.

Majoie CBLM, Verbeeten B, Dol JA, Peeters FLM: Trigeminal neuropathy; evaluation with MR imaging. *Radiographics* 15:795-811, 1995.

Mark, AS, Blake P, Atlas SW, et al: Gd-DTPA enhancement of the cisternal portion of the oculomotor nerve on MR imaging. *ANJR* 13:1463-1470, 1992.

Mark AS, Fitzgeerald D: Segmental enhancement of the cochlea on contrast-enhanced MR: correlation with the frequency of hearing loss and possible sign of perilymphatic fistula and autoimmune labyrinthitis. *AJNR* 14:991-996, 1993.

Mark AS, Seltzer S, Harnsberger HR: Sensorineural hearing loss: more than meets the eye? *AJNR* 14:37-46, 1993.

Martin N, Sterkers O, Mompoint D, Nahum H: Facial nerve neuromas: MR imaging. *Neuroradiology* 34:62-67, 1992.

Martin-Duverneuil N, Sola-Martinez MT, Miaux Y, et al: Contrast enhancement of the facial nerve on MRI: normal or pathological? *Neuroradiology* 39:207-212, 1997.

McCormick PC, Bella JA, Post KD: Trigeminal schwannoma. *J Neurosurg* 69:850-860, 1988.

Meltzer CC, Smirniotopoulos JG, Jones RV: The striated cerebellum: an MRI imaging sign in Lhermitte-Duclos disease (dysplastic gangliocytoma). *Radiology* 194:699-703, 1995.

Michael CB, Lee AG, Patrinely JR, et al: Visual loss associated with fibrous dysplasia of the anterior skull base. Case report and review of the literature. *J Neurosurg* 92:350-354, 2000.

Mikhael MA, Ciric IS, Wolff AP: Differentiation of cerebellopontine angle neuromas and meningiomas with MR imaging. *J Comput Assist Tomogr* 9:852-856, 1985.

Mikhael MA, Ciric IS, Wolff AP: MR diagnosis of acoustic neuromas. *J Comput Assist Tomogr* 11:232-235, 1987.

Moore KR, Davidson HC, Harnsberger HR, Shelton C: A practical imaging approach to petrous apex lesions. *Int J Neurorad* 5: 166-184, 1999.

Moore KR, Harnsberger HR, Shelton C, Davidson HC: 'Leave me alone' lesions of the petrous apex. *AJNR* 19:733-738, 1998.

Mukherji SK, Albernaz VS, Lo WWM: Papillary endolymphatic sac tumors: CT, MR imaging, and angiographic findings in 20 patients. *Radiology* 202:801-808, 1997.

Mulkens TH, Parizel PM, Martin JJ, et al: Acoustic schwannoma: MR findings in 84 tumors. *Am J Roentgenol* 160:395-398, 1993.

Nemzek WR, Hecht S, Gandour-Edwards R, et al: Perineural spread of head and neck tumors: how accurate is MR imaging? *AJNR* 19:701-706, 1998.

Neumann HP, Eggert HR, Scheremet R, et al: Central nervous system lesions in von Hippel-Lindau syndrome. *J Neurol Neurosurg Psychiatry* 55:898-901, 1995.

Noble ER, Smoker WRK, Ghatak NR: Atypical skull base paragangliomas. *AJNR* 18:986-990, 1997.

Olsen, WL, Dillon WP, Kelly WM, et al: MR imaging of paragangliomas. *AJNR* 7:1039-1042, 1986.

Pollack IR, Sekhar LN, Jannetta PF, Janecka JP: Neurilemmomas of the trigeminal nerve. *J Neurosurg* 70:737-745, 1989.

Press GA, Hesselink JR: MR imaging of cerebellopontine angle and internal auditory canal lesions at 1.5 T. *AJNR* 9:241-252, 1988.

Rao AB, Koeller KK, Adair CF: Paragangliomas of the head and neck: radiologic-pathologic correlation. *Radiographics* 19:1605-1632, 1999.

Remley KB, Coit WE, Harnsberger HR, et al: Pulsatile tinnitus and the vascular tympanic membrane: CT, MR, and angiographic findings. *Radiology* 174:383-390, 1990.

Robert Y, Carcasset S, Rocourt N, et al: Congenital cholesteatoma of the temporal bone: MR findings and comparison with CT. *AJNR* 16:755-762, 1995.

Robinson S, Cohen AR: Cowden disease and Lhermitte-Duclos disease: characterization of a new phakomatosis. *Neurosurg* 46:371-383, 2000.

Sartoretti-Schefer S, Brandle P, Wichmann W, Valavanis A: Intensity of MR contrast enhancement does not correspond to clinical and electroneurographic findings in acute inflammatory facial nerve palsy. *AJNR* 17:1229-1236, 1996.

Sartoretti-Schefer S, Wichmann W, Valavanis A: Idiopathic, herpetic, and HIV-associated facial nerve palsies: abnormal MR enhancement patterns. *AJNR* 15:479-486, 1994.

Sato Y, Wazir M, Smith W, et al: Hippel-Lindau disease: MR imaging. *Radiology* 166:241, 1988.

Schmalbrock P, Chakeres DW, Monroe JW, et al: Assessment of internal auditory canal tumors: a comparison of contrast-enhanced T1-weighted and steady-state T2-weighted gradient-echo MR imaging. *AJNR* 20:1207-1214, 1999.

Seltzer S, Mark AS: Contrast enhancement of the labyringh on MR scans in patients with sudden hearing loss and vertigo: evidence of Labyrinthine disease. *AJNR* 12:13-16, 1991.

Sevick RJ, Dillon WP, Engstrom J, et al: Trigeminal neuropathy: Gd-DTPA enhanced MR imaging. *J Comput Assist Tomogr* 15:605-611, 1991.

Shanley DJ, Vassallo CJ: Atypical presentation of Lhermitte-Duclos disease: preoperative diagnois with MRI. *Neuroradiology* 34:102-103, 1992.

Smirniotopoulos JG, Yue NC, Rushing EJ: Cerebellonpontine angle masses: radiologic-pathologic correlation. *Radiographics* 13:1131-1146, 1993.

Smith M, Castillo M, Campbell J, et al: Baseline and follow-up MRI of the internal auditory canal after suboccipital resection of acoustic schwannoma: appearances and clinical correlations. *Neuroradiology* 37: 317-320, 1995.

Smith RR, Grossman RI, Goldberg HI, et al: MR imaging of Lhermitte-Duclos disease: a case report. *AJNR* 10:187-189, 1989.

Som PM, Dillion WP, Sze G, et al: Benign and malignant sinonasal lesions with intracranial extension: differentiatio with MR imaging. *Radiology* 172:763-766, 1989.

Stuckey SL, Harris AJ, Mannolini SM: Detection of acoustic schwannoma: use of constructive interference in the steady state of three-dimensional MR. *AJNR* 17:1219-1225, 1996.

Swartz JD: Sensorineural hearting deficit: a systematic approach based on imaging findings. *Radiographics* 16:516-574, 1996.

Tach RR, Sze G, Leslie DR: Trigeminal neuralgia: MR imaging features. *Radiology* 172:767-770, 1989.

Tali ET, Yuh WTC, Nguyen HD, et al: Cystic acoustic schwannoma: MR characteristics. *AJNR* 14:1241-1247, 1993.

Tien RD, Dillon WP, Jackler RK: Contrast-enhanced MR imaging of the facial nerve in 11 patients with Bell's palsy. *AJNR* 11:735-741, 1990.

Valvassori GE, Morales FJ, Palacios E, Dobben GE: MR of the normal and abnormal internal auditory canal. *AJNR* 9:115-120, 1988.

Vieco PT, Del Carpio-O'Donovan R, Melanson D, et al: Dysplastic gangliocytoma (Lhermitte-Duclos disease): CT and MR imaging. *Pediatr Radiol* 22: 366-369, 1992.

Vogl T, Bruning R, Schedel H, et al: Paraganglioma of the jugular bulb and carotid body: MR imaging with short sequences and Gd-DTPA enhancement. *AJNR* 10:823-827, 1989.

Vogl TJ, Juergens M, Balzer JO, et al: Glomus tumors of the skull base: combined use of MR angiography and spin-echo imaging. *Radiology* 192:103-110, 1994.

Von Gils APG, Van Den Berg R, Falke THM, et al: MR diagnosis of paraganglioma of the head and neck: value of contrast enhancement. *Am J Roentgenol* 162:147-153, 1994.

Weissman JL: A pain in the ear: the radiology of otalgia. *AJNR* 18: 1641-1652, 1997.

Weissman JL: Hearing loss. *Radiology* 199:593-611, 1996.

Weissman JL, Hirsch BE: Beyond the promontory: the multifocal origin of glomus tympanicum tumors. *AJNR* 19:119-122, 1998.

Weissman JL, Hirsch BE: Imaging of tinnitus: a review. *Radiology* 216:342-350, 2000.

West MS, Russell EJ, Breit R, et al: Calvarial and skull base metastases: comparison of nonenhanced and Gd-DTPA-enhanced MR images. *Radiology* 174:85-92, 1990.

Williams Dw, Elster AD, Ginsberg LE, Stanton C: Recurrent Lhermitte-Duclos disease: report of two cases and association with Cowden's disease. *AJNR* 13:287-290, 1992.

Yuh WT, Wright DC, Barloon TJ, et al: MR imaging of primary tumors of the trigeminal nerve and Meckel's cave. *ANJR* 9:665-670, 1988.

# CHAPTER 6

# Pituitary, Suprasellar, and Parasellar Masses

### Case 224

77-year-old man complaining that "the side vision in both eyes has gone."
(sagittal, noncontrast T1-weighted SE scan)

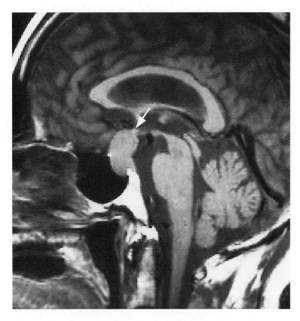

**Pituitary Adenoma**

### Case 225

53-year-old man presenting with bitemporal hemianopsia.
(sagittal, noncontrast T1-weighted SE scan)

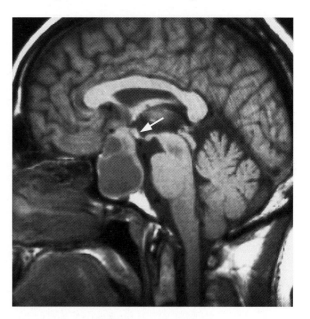

**Pituitary Adenoma**

---

The most reliable CT or MR feature of pituitary adenomas is their origin within the sella turcica. Large adenomas may have confusing suprasellar or parasellar components, heterogeneous signal intensity, and variable enhancement patterns. When a complex lesion is encountered at the skull base, expansion of the sella turcica near the geographic center of the mass is a key clue to pituitary etiology.

On T1-weighted images, the signal intensity of uncomplicated pituitary adenomas is comparable to that of brain parenchyma, as seen in Case 224. Even large tumors may remain very homogeneous (see Case 234 for an example). However, other large adenomas contain cystic or necrotic areas that demonstrate longer T1 values than the surrounding tumor tissue, as illustrated by Case 225. A third pattern of signal intensity is seen when subacute hemorrhage causes areas of T1-shortening within an adenoma (see Cases 228 and 229).

In Case 224, the sella is moderately enlarged. A suprasellar component of the tumor elevates the optic chiasm *(arrow)*, causing bitemporal hemianopsia.

Case 225 demonstrates gross expansion of the sella. The adenoma bulges into the sphenoid sinus and erodes the clivus. Suprasellar extension of the tumor has elevated and flattened the anterior recesses of the third ventricle and the optic chiasm *(arrow)*.

Pathologies other than pituitary adenomas may cause cystic-appearing masses within the sella turcica. Intrasellar craniopharyngiomas, Rathke's pouch cysts, and rare pituitary abscesses can present in this manner.

The relative severity of optic nerve compression or bitemporal hemianopsia (from pressure on the optic chiasm) depends on the congenitally variable proximity of the optic chiasm to the optic canals as well as on the size and location of a suprasellar mass.

## Case 226

49-year-old man presenting with diplopia.
(axial, noncontrast T2-weighted FSE scan)

## Case 227

65-year-old man presenting with headaches.
(coronal, noncontrast T2-weighted FSE scan)

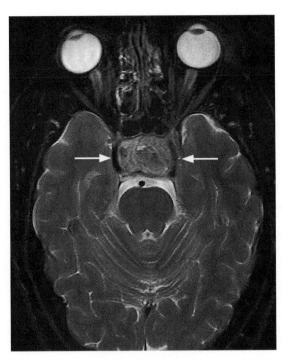

**Pituitary Adenoma**

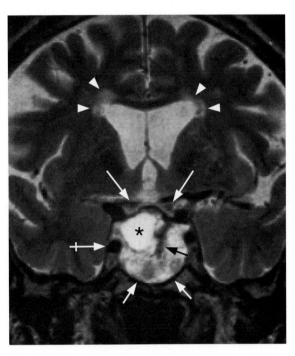

**Pituitary Adenoma**

Nonhemorrhagic pituitary adenomas usually demonstrate intermediate or high signal intensity on T2-weighted images. Focal low intensity may be noted in the presence of hemorrhage or dense calcification. Adenomas with homogenously low intensity on long TR spin echo sequences (as in Case 226) are often more fibrous and more difficult to resect than adenomas with high intensity on such sequences.

The tumor in Case 226 is a large mass that has caused lateral displacement of the internal carotid arteries *(arrows)*. Such lateral extension of pituitary adenomas may distort cranial nerves III through VI, leading to ophthalmoplegia and diplopia, as in this case.

In Case 227, a complex mass has expanded the sella turcica, with depression of the floor *(short white arrows)*. The cavernous sinuses are laterally displaced, with probable in-

tracavernous extension of the tumor on the right, superior to the internal carotid artery which is mildly inferiorly displaced *(crossed white arrow)*. Modest suprasellar growth of the mass is centered between the intracranial segments of the optic nerves *(long white arrows)*. Heterogeneity within the adenoma includes the uniformly high intensity of a cystic component *(asterisk)* and a band of low signal intensity suggesting hemorrhage or calcification *(black arrow)*.

The small zones of prolonged T2 values lateral to the frontal horns in Case 227 *(arrowheads)* are a common nonspecific finding in older adults. Potential contributing factors include the normally "loose" myelin and relatively high concentration of interstitial fluid at this site, superimposed age-related subependymal gliosis, and/or small periventricular infarcts.

## Case 228

35-year-old woman presenting with
bitemporal hemianopsia.
(coronal, noncontrast T1-weighted SE scan)

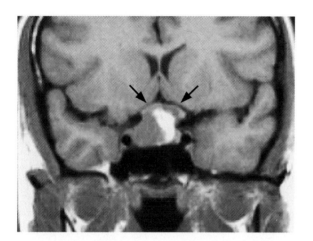

**Pituitary Adenoma**

## Case 229

38-year-old man presenting with headaches.
(coronal, noncontrast T1-weighted SE scan)

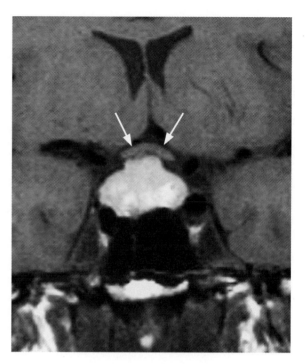

**Pituitary Adenoma**

Hemorrhage is commonly noted within pituitary adenomas at the time of diagnosis or during treatment. Some observers suggest an increased incidence of pituitary hemorrhages in patients receiving bromocriptine therapy.

Active bleeding into an adenoma may cause sudden enlargement of the tumor, with compression of the optic apparatus and adenohypophysis. The associated rapid development of visual impairment and endocrine dysfunction (usually accompanied by headache) has been termed "pituitary apoplexy." (Acute infarction can also cause rapid swelling of an adenoma, leading to sudden visual or endocrine compromise.)

Much more commonly, hemorrhage within an adenoma is small and subclinical. That is, the presence of blood products in a pituitary adenoma is usually *not* correlated with a catastrophic or even recognizable clinical event.

The pattern of hemorrhage within pituitary adenomas is variable. Both of the above cases demonstrate T1-shortening due to methemoglobin, localized to the left side of the tu-

mor in Case 228 and diffuse (and unusually homogeneous) in Case 229. A postcontrast scan of Case 228 demonstrated a nonenhancing zone corresponding exactly to the area of precontrast T1-shortening.

Homogeneous T1-shortening normally occurs within the moderately enlarged pituitary glands of pregnant women. This physiological change should not be mistaken for hemorrhage when such patients present with headaches or other nonspecific symptoms. (The pituitary glands of newborn infants demonstrate similar T1-shortening, probably reflecting the intrauterine hormonal environment.)

Craniopharyngiomas and Rathke's cleft cysts can also present as intrasellar and suprasellar masses of high signal intensity on T1-weighted images (see Cases 251 and 256).

The optic chiasm is stretched over the superior pole of the adenoma in Case 228 *(arrows)*, accounting for the patient's presentation with bitemporal visual field cuts. The superior margin of the tumor in Case 229 lies immediately inferior to the chiasm *(arrows)*.

## Case 230

41-year-old man presenting with
bitemporal hemianopsia.
(sagittal, postcontrast T1-weighted SE scan)

## Case 231

67-year-old man being followed
for a known pituitary adenoma.
(coronal, postcontrast T1-weighted SE scan)

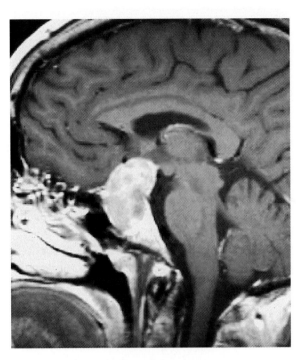

**Pituitary Adenoma**

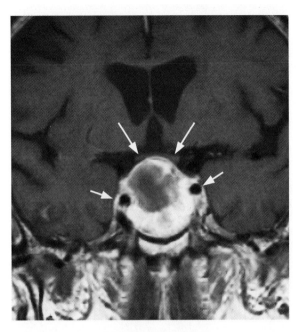

**Pituitary Adenoma**
(same patient as Case 227, two years later)

Many pituitary adenomas demonstrate uniform, intense contrast enhancement, as in Case 230. The superior extension of such tumors may resemble other enhancing suprasellar masses (e.g., meningioma, germinoma, or hypothalamic glioma). However, the lesion in Case 230 arises from an expanded sella turcica, establishing the correct diagnosis. (It is rarer for a suprasellar meningioma to grow inferiorly and enlarge the sella turcica; see Case 237).

Case 231 presents a follow-up postcontrast scan of the cystic/necrotic adenoma shown in Case 227. Large adenomas often contain nonenhancing regions due to cysts, hemorrhage, or necrosis. Sometimes the entire tumor has this appearance, with only a rim of contrast enhancement. The suprasellar extension of a rim-enhancing adenoma can mimic a craniopharyngioma like Case 259.

Pituitary abscesses may closely resemble a cystic or necrotic intrasellar neoplasm. Abscesses may be relatively indolent, causing few symptoms and no systemic signs of infection. However, they are usually smaller than the lesion

in Case 231 and are typically very round with a uniformly thin rim of enhancement.

Coronal MR scans demonstrate the position and caliber of the parasellar internal carotid arteries, seen as flow voids within the cavernous sinus in Case 231 *(short arrows)*. The medial margin of the cavernous sinus is often difficult to define on precontrast or postcontrast scans of pituitary macroadenomas. For this reason, encasement of the parasellar internal carotid artery can be important evidence of cavernous sinus invasion by tumor.

In Case 230, the suprasellar portion of the tumor has elevated the floor of the third ventricle. The optic chiasm, which resides in a notch between the ventricle's optic and infundibular recesses, can be presumed to be displaced and stretched, accounting for the patient's bitemporal hemianopsia.

The superior margin of the adenoma in Case 231 contacts the inferior border of the optic nerves *(long arrows)* as they approach the chiasm.

147

## Case 232

46-year-old man presenting with
headaches and diplopia.
(axial, noncontrast T2-weighted SE scan)

## Case 233

36-year-old woman presenting with diplopia.
(coronal, postcontrast T1-weighted SE scan)

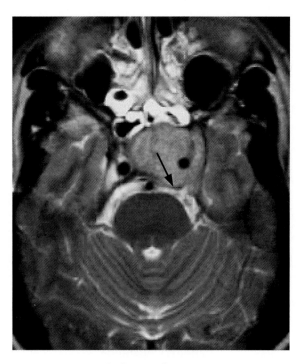

**Pituitary Adenoma**

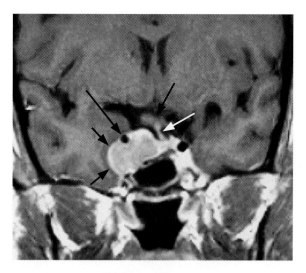

**Pituitary Adenoma**

Pituitary adenomas may grow laterally to involve the cavernous sinus, sometimes with little expansion of the sella itself. Such tumors may mimic other parasellar masses such as meningioma, trigeminal schwannoma, lymphoma, or metastasis.

It may be difficult to distinguish displacement and compression of the cavernous sinus from actual tumor invasion. Invasion is suspected when the signal intensity of the adenoma extends to the lateral wall of the cavernous sinus, when the sinus is widened with convex margins, and when the cavernous segment of the internal carotid artery is largely encased. These features are demonstrated on the left in Case 232 and on the right in Case 233.

Coronal MR scans such as Case 233 provide excellent definition of the optic chiasm *(medium length black ar-*

*row)* and pituitary infundibulum *(white arrow)*, which are key suprasellar landmarks. Eccentric origin of the adenoma in this case causes contralateral displacement of the infundibulum. The optic chiasm is not deformed.

The right internal carotid artery in Case 233 *(longest black arrow)* is elevated and mildly narrowed by intracavernous extension of the tumor. Like parasellar meningiomas, pituitary adenomas may be associated with encasement of adjacent arteries.

Note the mild left retrosellar extension of the adenoma in Case 232, eroding the dorsum sella to indent the prepontine cistern *(arrow)*. Mucosal thickening and fluid largely opacify the ethmoid and sphenoid sinuses in this case.

## Case 234

54-year-old woman presenting with
bitemporal hemianopsia.
(sagittal, noncontrast T1-weighted SE scan)

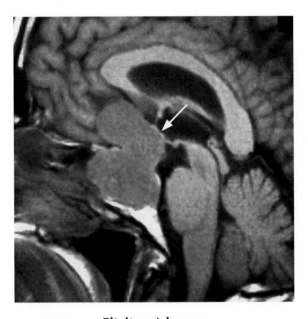

**Pituitary Adenoma**

## Case 235

38-year-old man presenting with
blurred vision and headaches.
(sagittal, noncontrast T1-weighted SE scan)

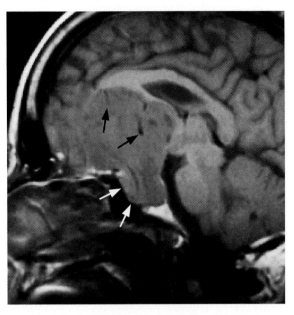

**Pituitary Adenoma**

---

Pituitary adenomas may extend inferiorly through the floor of the sella turcica to occupy the sphenoid sinus. Further growth can erode the skull base, resembling the bone destruction of a metastasis or a nasopharyngeal carcinoma.

The tumor in Case 234 is an example of a transellar adenoma. The mass has filled and expanded the sphenoid sinus and also extends superiorly to displace and elevate the optic chiasm and anterior recesses of the third ventricle *(arrow)*. Despite its size, the lesion is very homogeneous. The correct diagnosis is suggested by recognizing that that the geographic center of the tumor is at the level of the sella turcica. In other cases, a residual ghost of an expanded sella is faintly visible within a mass at the skull base to indicate pituitary origin.

In Case 235, a large subfrontal mass is continuous with an expanded sella turcica *(white arrows)*. Flow voids of low signal intensity near the superior margin of the mass *(black arrows)* represent encased branches of the anterior

cerebral arteries. Encasement of basal arteries is characteristic of parasellar meningiomas (see Cases 39, 61, and 237) but can also be associated with pituitary adenomas, more commonly involving the cavernous segments of the internal carotid arteries (see Cases 232 and 233).

Enhancement of the tumor in Case 235 was intense and uniform. On coronal postcontrast scans, the large subfrontal component of the mass was indistinguishable from a meningioma.

Esthesioneuroblastoma or "olfactory neuroblastoma" is a rare tumor that can also present as an enhancing subfrontal mass in young patients (see Case 337). The characteristic origin of this neoplasm from the region of the cribriform plate and ethmoid roof usually differentiates such tumors from meningiomas or pituitary adenomas.

The above cases demonstrate that nonsecreting pituitary adenomas may become very large before symptoms occur from compression of the optic chiasm.

# DIFFERENTIAL DIAGNOSIS:
## UNIFORMLY ENHANCING INTRASELLAR AND SUPRASELLAR MASS

### Case 236

50-year-old woman presenting with
impaired vision in the left eye.
(coronal, postcontrast T1-weighted SE scan)

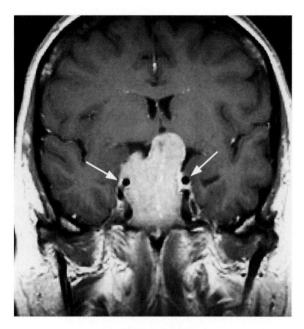

**Pituitary Adenoma**

### Case 237

58-year-old woman presenting with
decreased visual acuity.
(coronal, postcontrast T1-weighted SE scan)

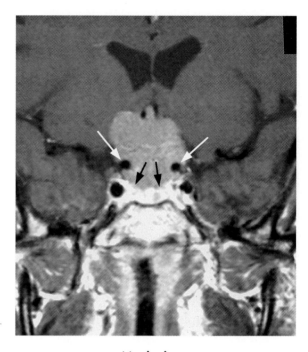

**Meningioma**

The distinction between a pituitary tumor with suprasellar extension and a suprasellar mass growing into the sella may be difficult.

The large intrasellar and suprasellar lesion in Case 236 enhances intensely and uniformly, comparable to the meningiomas illustrated in Chapter 2. However, the wide separation of the cavernous segments of the internal carotid arteries *(arrows)* is typical of an originally intrasellar tumor, providing a clue to the diagnosis. The marked enlargement of the sella and the broad continuity between the intrasellar and suprasellar components also favor a pituitary adenoma in this case.

Enhancement within the suprasellar meningioma in Case 237 is homogeneous but less intense than that of the pituitary gland, defining the intrasellar extension of the tumor *(black arrows)*. Contrast enhancement of other suprasellar meningiomas may be indistinguishable from pituitary tissue, resulting in an appearance similar to Case 236. The width of the waist of the tumor and the degree of sellar expansion are then important clues for distinguishing between intrasellar and suprasellar origin.

The adenoma in Case 236 has grown inferiorly through the sphenoid sinus and eroded the sphenoid bone, presenting substantial risk for postoperative CSF leak.

The meningioma in Case 237 surrounds and mildly narrows the supraclinoid segments of the internal carotid arteries bilaterally *(white arrows)*. Arterial encasement is characteristic of meningiomas at the skull base, but lateral extension of a pituitary adenoma may also surround and narrow the internal carotid artery.

Compare the size of the tumor in Case 237 to the small tuberculum meningioma in Case 55. The size of a tumor at the time of clinical presentation depends on the location of the lesion with respect to adjacent neural structures.

## Case 238

22-year-old woman presenting with amenorrhea
and high serum prolactin levels.
(sagittal, noncontrast T1-weighted SE scan)

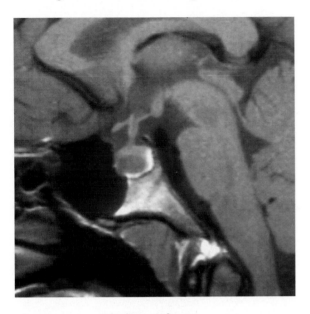

**Pituitary Adenoma**

## Case 239

24-year-old woman presenting with
amenorrhea and galactorrhea.
(coronal, noncontrast T2-weighted FSE scan)

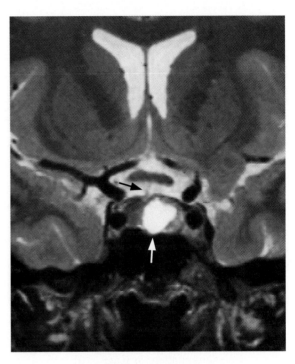

**Pituitary Adenoma**

Secreting adenomas of the pituitary may cause significant endocrine symptoms even when small. (Compare the size of the above tumors to the nonsecreting adenomas in Cases 234 and 235.) Tumors less than ten millimeters in diameter have been termed *microadenomas.* Prolactinomas are the most frequent microadenomas to produce symptoms, usually amenorrhea and/or galactorrhea in a young woman.

Axial CT and MR scans are often normal in the presence of microadenomas. Sagittal and coronal MR scans without contrast material may demonstrate the tumors as focal zones of altered T1 and/or T2 values.

In Case 238, a mass with uniformly low signal intensity occupies the inferior portion of the sella turcica. Coronal scans localized the lesion within pituitary tissue. (Postcon-

trast scans of this patient are presented as Case 242.) Other small adenomas are nearly isointense and not definable on noncontrast T1-weighted images.

Microadenomas may have either higher or lower signal intensity than the surrounding pituitary gland on T2-weighted scans, with the former pattern being more common. Low intensity within adenomas on T2-weighted images may reflect blood products, calcification, or densely fibrous texture.

The small adenoma in Case 239 is unusually well defined by uniform prolongation of T2 values. The mass is associated with focal erosion of the sellar floor *(white arrow)* and contralateral displacement of the pituitary infundibulum *(black arrow).* Case 240 presents a postcontrast scan of this lesion.

## Case 240

24-year-old woman presenting with
amenorrhea and galactorrhea.
(coronal, postcontrast T1-weighted SE scan)

## Case 241

40-year-old woman with elevated
serum prolactin levels.
(coronal, postcontrast T1-weighted SE scan)

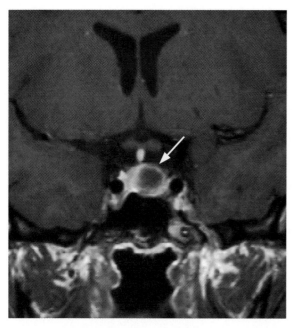

**Pituitary Adenoma**
(same patient as Case 239)

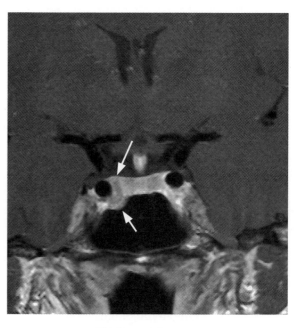

**Pituitary Adenoma**

---

Pituitary microadenomas are often best defined by coronal scans performed immediately after the injection of contrast material. The tumors are usually outlined on such images as filling defects within otherwise enhancing pituitary tissue, as illustrated above. This appearance must be correlated with secondary findings and the clinical presentation, since other nonenhancing regions (e.g., small cysts) are common within the gland.

Secondary findings of a pituitary microadenoma on coronal scans include increased height of the gland, eccentric superior convexity, deviation of the pituitary infundibulum, and focal erosion of the sellar floor. Each of these features can be an isolated normal finding, but their association suggests a responsible mass.

Case 240 presents a postcontrast scan of the microadenoma in Case 239. The mass is large enough to expand the left side of the gland, and the infundibulum is displaced to the right.

The prolactinoma in Case 241 *(long arrow)* is positioned at the lateral margin of the pituitary gland, adjacent to the cavernous sinus. It has caused prominent focal erosion and

depression of the sellar floor *(short arrow)* but has little effect on the superior margin of the gland. Lateral location is common for microadenomas, and careful attention to the periphery of the gland is important in patients with symptoms of pituitary dysfunction. Microadenomas even smaller than Case 241 may be clinically manifested as Cushing's disease, acromegaly, or amenorrhea/galactorrhea.

Note the normally intense enhancement of the pituitary infundibulum in these cases, reflecting both the surrounding hypothalamic/hypophyseal venous plexus and the absence of a blood-brain barrier. The width of normal infundibular enhancement is variable, with the stalk usually tapering smoothly from the hypothalamus (maximum normal diameter about three millimeters) to the sella (maximum normal diameter about two millimeters). Unusually wide or irregular infundibular enhancement can reflect a variety of pathologies (see Cases 270 to 273).

A small area of artifact is often encountered at the junction of the sphenoid sinus septum and the sellar floor on CT and MR scans. This localized abnormality can mimic or obscure a microadenoma. The pseudolesion is best identified by recognizing its relationship to the septum.

## Case 242A

22-year-old woman presenting with amenorrhea.
(coronal, T1-weighted GRE scan performed
60 seconds after injection of contrast)

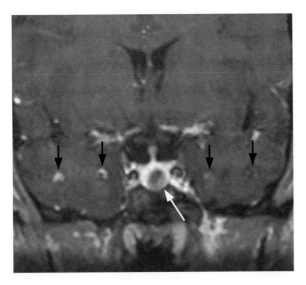

**Pituitary Adenoma**

## Case 242B

Same patient.
(coronal, T1-weighted SE scan performed
8 minutes after injection of contrast)

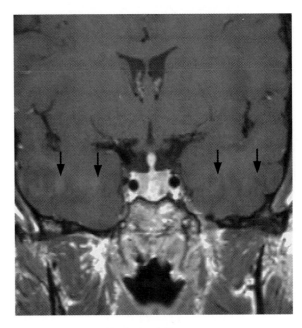

**Pituitary Adenoma**

Scans performed during the early phases of pituitary enhancement may demonstrate microadenomas more clearly than images obtained several minutes after the injection of contrast material. The signal intensity of many microadenomas increases steadily on delayed postcontrast scans, with the tumor becoming progressively less distinct from surrounding pituitary tissue.

Case 242 illustrates this pattern. The majority of the adenoma is nonenhancing on the early scan (Case 242A), with a tiny nodule of active enhancement at the left inferior margin of the lesion *(white arrow)*. However, within a few minutes the adenoma accumulates contrast to a level slightly exceeding the enhancement of surrounding pituitary tissue (Case 242B; note the small nodule of early enhancement is now seen as a relative filling defect).

Occasional microadenomas demonstrate the reverse pattern, with more rapid and more intense enhancement than normal pituitary tissue. This differential may be appreciable for only a brief period (about a minute) during the arrival of contrast material, so that dynamic scans are necessary to convincingly document the finding.

Bands of phase misregistration artifact extend horizontally across the temporal lobes bilaterally in the above images *(black arrows)*. Signal intensity that belongs within the parasellar internal carotid arteries has been mismapped along the phase-encoding axis because of phase changes accumulated by protons in the blood as they flow across magnetic field gradients. This artifact is most prominent on postcontrast scans, because intravascular contrast increases the signal intensity within arterial or venous channels.

### Case 243

8-year-old boy being evaluated for small stature.
(coronal, postcontrast T1-weighted SE scan)

### Case 244

54-year-old woman complaining of diminished
visual acuity in the right eye.
(coronal, postcontrast T1-weighted SE scan)

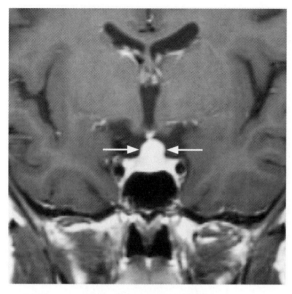

**Pituitary Hyperplasia**
(due to hypothyroidism)

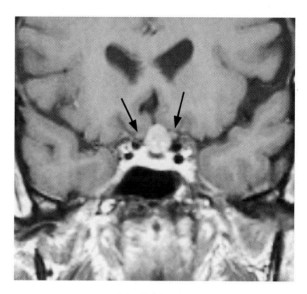

**Meningioma**

Adenomas of the pituitary gland are among several uniformly enhancing masses that may be encountered in the suprasellar region. Case 243 demonstrates that pituitary hyperplasia may also present with suprasellar extension and a mass-like contour *(arrows)*. This possibility should be considered when a symmetrical pituitary "mass" is found in appropriate clinical settings (e.g., hypothyroidism or pregnancy). The snowman contour of hypertrophic pituitary tissue in Case 243 resolved within months of treatment with thyroid hormone.

Lymphocytic adenohypophysitis, an idiopathic (probably autoimmune) inflammatory process usually occurring in women during the peripartum period, may cause an appearance very similar to Case 243. Suprasellar extension and diabetes insipidus are common in this disorder, which has been reported in all ages and in both sexes. Other masses involving the pituitary infundibulum should also be considered in the differential diagnosis, as illustrated in Cases 270-273.

Meningiomas are among the extrapituitary masses to present as midline, suprasellar lesions. The tumor in Case 244 lies between the optic nerves *(arrows)*. In contrast to Case 243, the meningioma is separated from the pituitary gland.

In children, chiasmatic/hypothalamic gliomas, unusual craniopharyngiomas, and histiocytosis should be considered when a uniformly enhancing suprasellar mass is encountered. In adolescents or young adults, germinomas may present in this manner. Optic neuritis occasionally causes a similar appearance (see Case 499).

# CHORISTOMAS (GRANULAR CELL TUMORS)

### Case 245A

49-year-old woman presenting with memory loss.
(axial, noncontrast T2-weighted SE scan)

### Case 245B

Same patient.
(coronal, postcontrast T1-weighted SE scan)

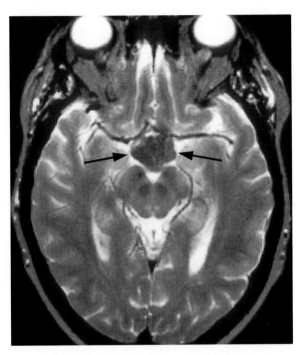

**Choristoma (Granular Cell Tumor)**

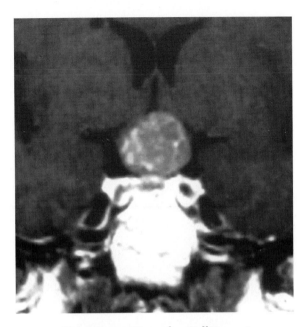

**Choristoma (Granular Cell Tumor)**

---

Choristomas are unusual tumors of the suprasellar and/or posterior pituitary region. These masses have been described under many different names, including *granular cell tumor, myoblastoma,* and *pituicytoma.* The classification of choristomas is controversial: both neuronal and astrocytic origins have been suggested.

The tumors may be intrasellar and/or suprasellar in location. They are slow-growing lesions, causing symptoms by compression of the adenohypophysis or optic chiasm.

The few reported MR scans of choristomas have had variable appearances. The tumor in Case 245 demonstrates impressively low signal intensity on the T2-weighted image. Enhancement is somewhat nodular and subdued. The pattern differs from pituitary adenomas and craniopharyngiomas, but overlaps the spectrum of optic/hypothalamic gliomas.

Choristomas can be highly vascular tumors. If this diagnosis is suggested preoperatively, the surgeon may consider a craniotomy rather than a transsphenoidal approach to the mass.

Recent reports have defined *chordoid gliomas* as a separate unusual and distinctive suprasellar lesion. These masses typically arise from the hypothalamus and anterior third ventricle. Histologically they resemble a chordoma, with cords or clusters of epithelioid cells and a mucinous background. However, the tumor cells stain positively for glial fibrillary acidic protein, indicating glial origin.

MR scans of chordoid gliomas demonstrate oval, well-defined, and intensely and homogeneously enhancing suprasellar masses. The tumors are usually intermediate in signal intensity on T2-weighted scans (resembling Case 245A) and often displace the pituitary infundibulum posteriorly.

### Case 246

10-year-old girl presenting with small stature.
(sagittal, noncontrast T1-weighted SE scan)

### Case 247

6-year-old boy with panhypopituitarism.
(coronal, noncontrast T1-weighted SE scan)

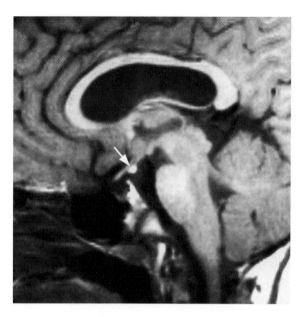

"Ectopic" Neurohypophysis

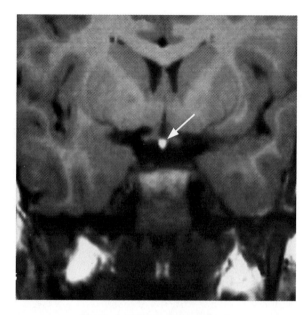

"Ectopic" Neurohypophysis

The normal neurohypophysis demonstrates high signal intensity on T1-weighted images. This finding reflects enhanced relaxation of water protons in the vicinity of neurosecretory vesicles, which function in the storage and secretion of oxytocin and vasopressin. On sagittal MR images, the neurohypophyseal focus of T1-shortening lies immediately anterior to the dorsum sella and has been referred to as the "posterior pituitary bright spot." (See Cases 138, 143, and 151 for normal examples.)

In both of the above cases, an ectopic zone of T1-shortening representing the functional neurohypophysis is seen along the floor of the third ventricle at the base of the infundibulum (arrows). This "bright spot" has failed to develop in the normal intrasellar location due to impaired formation of or damage to the pituitary infundibulum, which normally transmits carrier-bound neuropeptide hormones from the hypothalamus to the neurohypophysis. Similar development of an "ectopic posterior pituitary gland" along the floor of the third ventricle may occur in cases of posttraumatic transsection of the infundibulum.

Failure of development of the pituitary infundibulum and hypoplasia of the adenohypophysis may be isolated abnormalities or part of a midline dysgenesis syndrome (see Cases 863 and 864). In Case 246, the pituitary gland and sella turcica are small. The optic chiasm is also small and the septum pellucidum was absent, suggesting the diagnosis of septooptic dysplasia (de Morsier's syndrome). Associated pituitary insufficiency is often the most clinically significant component of this syndrome.

## Case 248

36-year-old woman with a history of
transsphenoidal hypophysectomy.
(sagittal, noncontrast T1-weighted SE scan)

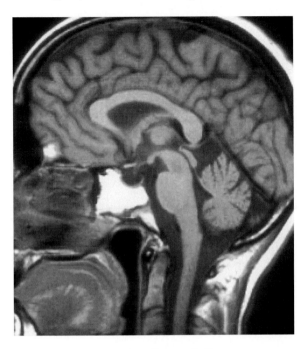

**Secondary Empty Sella**

## Case 249

20-year-old woman complaining of headaches.
(coronal, noncontrast T1-weighted SE scan)

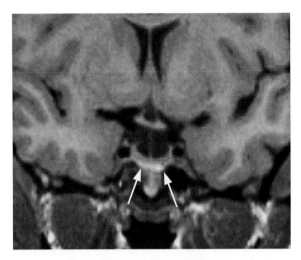

**Primary Empty Sella**

---

After removal of a pituitary macroadenoma, residual normal pituitary tissue may occupy only small portion of the large sella turcica. The remainder of the sella is then filled with CSF, resulting in an "empty" appearance. Case 248 demonstrates this situation. The high signal intensity of fat packing within the sphenoid sinus identifies this empty sella as postsurgical.

Case 249 illustrates a primary empty sella. This "syndrome" is often discovered in otherwise healthy, middle-aged, overweight patients (especially women) with vague complaints (especially headache). Associated pituitary dysfunction is rare. Occasional visual symptoms may be caused by prolapse of the optic chiasm, more commonly seen with secondary empty sellas after necrosis or removal of pituitary tumors.

Primary empty sella syndrome is caused by an unusually large aperture in the diaphragma sellae, allowing spinal fluid from the suprasellar cistern to extend into the sella. The intrasellar cistern participates in normal CSF pulsations and can cause gradual expansion of the sella, closely resembling the enlargement seen with pituitary adenomas.

A number of cystic-appearing lesions can occur within the sella turcica, including some pituitary adenomas, abscesses, cysts, craniopharyngiomas, and dermoid cysts. A primary empty sella can be distinguished from these potential intrasellar masses if the thin pituitary infundibulum is seen to traverse the intrasellar fluid space, reaching the pituitary gland at the floor of the sella (*arrows,* Case 249).

A transsphenoidal meningocele or encephalocele could superficially resemble an empty sella, with CSF values filling the midsphenoid region. Distorted optic nerves may traverse the cephalocele, mimicking a thick pituitary infundibulum. Associated traction deformity of the hypothalamic region should establish the correct diagnosis in such cases.

Occasionally a small pituitary adenoma may be found within an otherwise empty sella. The latter does not exclude the former, and symptomatic cases of empty sella need to be carefully analyzed.

### Case 250

4-year-old boy presenting with headaches.
(sagittal, noncontrast T1-weighted SE scan)

### Case 251

8-year-old girl presenting with weight gain.
(sagittal, noncontrast T1-weighted SE scan)

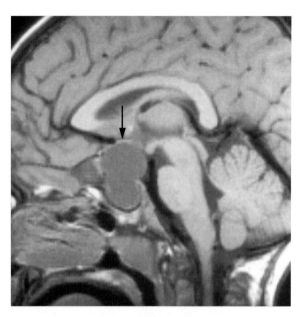

**Craniopharyngioma**

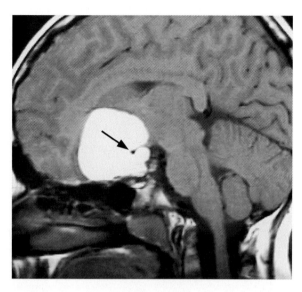

**Craniopharyngioma**

Craniopharyngiomas can present a variety of signal intensities and morphologies on MR scans. These masses most commonly involve the suprasellar region, alone or in combination with intrasellar components. Although midline location is typical, laterally eccentric tumors do occur (see Case 260).

The signal intensity of craniopharyngiomas on T1-weighted scans may be low, intermediate, or high. Low intensity often reflects a cystic lesion, as was true of the craniopharyngioma in Case 250. Solid tumors may be relatively isointense to brain tissue and are variably uniform.

Short T1 components within craniopharyngiomas most often represent high protein content within cystic regions of the tumor. Experimental studies and analysis of fluid from tumor cysts have suggested that protein concentrations up to 10% (10,000 mg/dl) have little effect on T1 relaxation. Appreciable T1-shortening is usually correlated with protein concentrations in the range of 10% to 30%. The mass in Case 251 contained viscous material with no evidence of hemorrhage or cholesterol.

Case 250 emphasizes that the stereotype of craniopharyngiomas as heterogeneous suprasellar lesions is exaggerated. Many craniopharyngiomas are surprisingly homogeneous, and up to 70% demonstrate an intrasellar component. The continuity between the suprasellar tumor and an expanded sella turcica in Case 250 could raise the possibility of a pituitary adenoma, although this would be a rare diagnosis in a child.

Marked elevation of the floor of the third ventricle and optic chiasm is present in Case 250 *(arrow)*. Superior enlargement of craniopharyngiomas may obstruct the foramina of Monro to cause hydrocephalus.

The tumor in Case 251 encases the elevated A1 segment of the anterior cerebral artery *(arrow)*.

Craniopharyngiomas demonstrating prominent lobulation and cysts with short T1 values usually have adamantinous histology (common in children). Spherical tumors that are solid or contain cysts with long T1 values more often represent the squamous-papillary subtype (common in adults).

### Case 252

2-year-old boy presenting with failure to thrive.
(axial, noncontrast T2-weighted FSE scan)

### Case 253

11-year-old boy presenting with impaired vision.
(axial, noncontrast T2-weighted FSE scan)

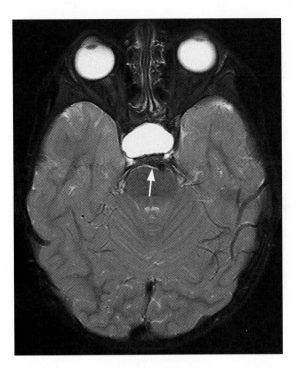

**Craniopharyngioma**

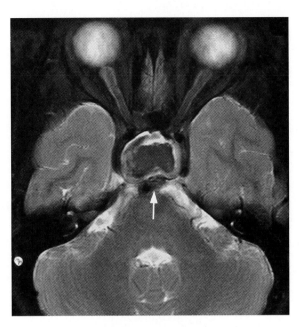

**Craniopharyngioma**

On T2-weighted images, the signal intensity of craniopharyngiomas may be homogeneously high or complex and heterogeneous. Homogeneity may reflect a uniformly solid tumor or a cystic lesion, as was found in Case 252. Large zones of low signal intensity within craniopharyngiomas like Case 253 may be due to blood products causing T2-shortening. Thickly proteinaceous material can also result in low signal intensity on T2-weighted scans, analogous to the appearance of inspissated secretions in chronically obstructed paranasal sinuses.

Calcification, a hallmark of craniopharyngiomas on CT scans, is more difficult to appreciate on MR studies. When detectable, tumor calcifications are usually seen as punctate or coarse foci of sharply defined low signal intensity within the mass.

Both of the above tumors fill the sella turcica, with lateral displacement of the cavernous sinuses. Occasional craniopharyngiomas are completely intrasellar in location. Infrasellar craniopharyngiomas are very rare but do occur (see Case 171).

Retrosellar extension is also present in Cases 252 and 253 *(arrows)*. A lobulation growing posteriorly into the interpeduncular cistern is a common feature of craniopharyngiomas and may be a helpful clue in the differential diagnosis of an intrasellar/suprasellar mass.

The optic nerves in Case 253 can be followed posteriorly from the globes through the orbits and optic canals to the ventral margin of the tumor. Like suprasellar extension of pituitary adenomas, craniopharyngiomas cause visual compromise by distorting the intracranial segment of the optic nerves and the optic chiasm.

Suprasellar craniopharyngiomas often span the distance between the supraclinoid internal carotid arteries. The anterior cerebral and posterior communicating arteries are frequently stretched along the margins of such masses. Tumor adherence to these vessels (and to the optic chiasm) makes complete resection difficult. Postsurgical recurrence is a recognized tendency of craniopharyngiomas, and postoperative radiation therapy may be recommended for these benign lesions.

### Case 254

14-year-old girl presenting with decreased
vision and diabetes insipidus.
(sagittal, noncontrast T1-weighted SE scan)

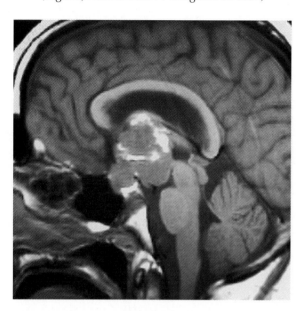

**Germinoma**

### Case 255

59-year-old woman presenting with
a third nerve palsy.
(sagittal, noncontrast T1-weighted SE scan)

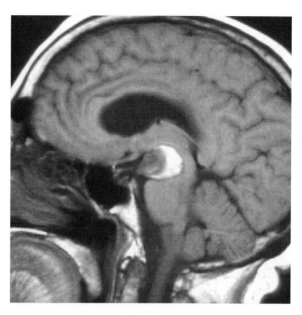

**Thrombosed Aneurysm of the Basilar Artery**

---

The differential diagnosis of a suprasellar mass containing high signal intensity on T1-weighted scans includes many lesions in addition to craniopharyngiomas, as illustrated above and on the next page.

The appearance of Case 254 resembles a craniopharyngioma, with patchy T1-shortening and prominent retrosellar extension. The center of the mass is suprasellar, arguing against pituitary adenoma (although the lesion does have an intrasellar component). At surgery, the tumor was found to be a suprasellar germinoma containing hemorrhage. (Compare to the hemorrhagic pituitary adenoma in Case 228 and to an axial scan of this patient presented as Case 311.)

Suprasellar germinomas are most common in adolescent girls. A clinical clue to the diagnosis is the common presentation with diabetes insipidus, which is rarely an initial symptom of craniopharyngiomas or hypothalamic gliomas. A general discussion of germinomas is presented in Case 294.

Patent aneurysms are easily distinguished from other suprasellar masses on MR scans by their characteristic absence of signal. (This differential diagnosis is much more difficult on CT studies.) However, thrombosed aneurysms can present a pattern of mixed signal intensity that may resemble heterogeneous suprasellar tumors such as craniopharyngiomas.

In Case 255, a thrombosed aneurysm arising from the tip of the basilar artery occupies the interpeduncular fossa. Layers of varying signal intensity within the mass are due to thrombus of differing age. This laminated internal architecture is a hallmark of thrombosed aneurysms and is usually most apparent on T2-weighted scans (see Case 734).

Cavernous angiomas occasionally involve the suprasellar region and optic chiasm. Evidence of T2-shortening usually accompanies T1-shortening within these lesions, assisting differential diagnosis (see Cases 761-764).

### Case 256

36-year-old woman presenting with
decreased vision.
(sagittal, noncontrast T1-weighted SE scan)

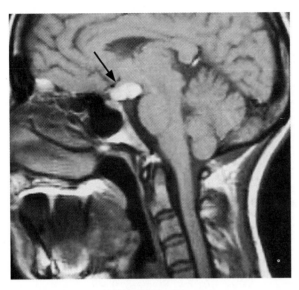

**Rathke's Cleft Cyst**

### Case 257

47-year-old woman presenting with
impaired visual fields.
(sagittal, noncontrast T1-weighted SE scan)

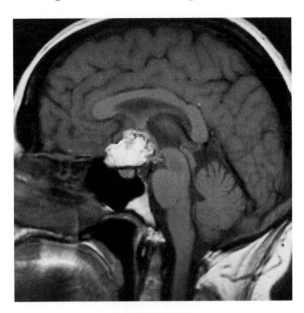

**Dermoid Cyst**

---

Rathke's cleft cysts are related to craniopharyngiomas, since both are derived from remnants of the epithelium embryologically lining Rathke's cleft. Like craniopharyngiomas, these masses can be intrasellar and/or suprasellar. The cysts are usually simple, lined by a single epithelial layer. They may contain thickly mucinous material, serous fluid, or cellular debris. Their signal intensity on T1-weighted images can be correspondingly high, low, or intermediate. Contrast enhancement is usually absent or minimal, which may aid in differential diagnosis.

Case 256 demonstrates T1-shortening within a Rathke's cleft cyst of the suprasellar and retrosellar regions. The optic chiasm is mildly displaced at the anterosuperior margin of the mass *(arrow)*.

The suprasellar region is a common location for intracranial dermoid cysts (see also Case 312). The signal intensity of these masses depends on the proportion of lipid and proteinaceous components within the lesion. When sebaceous material predominates, T1-shortening is apparent, as in Case

257. Fat saturation scans would suppress the high signal intensity in this case, unlike Case 256.

Lipomas may also arise along the floor of the third ventricle and can present as midline masses with short T1 values. Suprasellar lipomas are usually round and homogeneous, more closely resembling Case 256 (but with suppressible signal on fat saturation sequences) than the irregular dermoid cyst in Case 257. Case 276 presents an example.

The normal neurohypophysis demonstrates T1-shortening and is quite round on coronal scans. This appearance may falsely suggest an intrasellar mass such as a Rathke's cleft cyst. The usually midline position of the neurohypophysis in the posterior portion of the sella turcica helps to correctly identify this structure. "Ectopic" neurohypophyseal tissue along the floor of the third ventricle (see Cases 246 and 247) mimics the location and T1-shortening of the above lesions but is typically much smaller.

Compare the morphology and texture of the suprasellar dermoid cyst in Case 257 to the craniopharyngioma in Case 269.

**161**

### Case 258

40-year-old man presenting with headaches
and visual field deficits.
(sagittal, postcontrast T1-weighted SE scan)

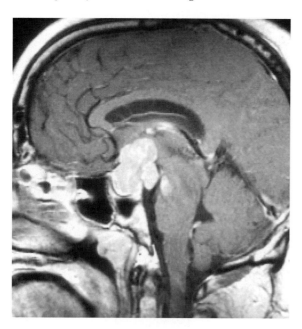

**Craniopharyngioma**

### Case 259

2-year-old boy presenting with failure to thrive.
(coronal, postcontrast T1-weighted
SE scan with MTS)

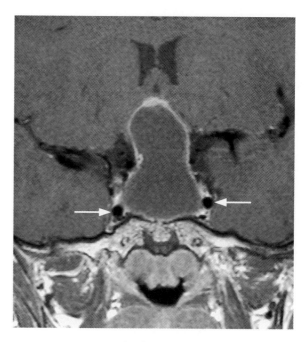

**Craniopharyngioma**
(same patient as Case 252)

Contrast enhancement in craniopharyngiomas may be minimal or intense. Patterns include homogeneous enhancement of solid tumors and rim enhancement surrounding cystic components, as illustrated above. A third common morphology is coarsely heterogeneous enhancement outlining multiple small cyst-like areas within a predominantly solid mass; see Case 269 for an example.

The solid tumor in Case 258 enhances intensely and uniformly. A prominent retrosellar component displaces and partially surrounds the flow void of the distal basilar artery. The suprasellar lobulation of the mass effaces the anterior portion of the third ventricle, nearly reaching the foramina of Monro.

Enhancement in Case 259 is limited to a thin rim at the perimeter of the large craniopharyngioma. The lack of en-

hancement within the mass clearly defines the lateral displacement of the cavernous sinuses, which contain the flow voids of the internal carotid arteries *(arrows)*. The tumor proved to be grossly cystic at surgery.

Both of these cases demonstrate that craniopharyngiomas frequently present as combined intrasellar and suprasellar masses. In adults such as Case 258, the continuity between the suprasellar tumor and an expanded sella turcica can resemble the morphology of a pituitary adenoma (compare to Case 230).

Together, Cases 258 and 259 also emphasize that craniopharyngiomas should be considered in the differential diagnosis of solid or cystic suprasellar masses in all age groups.

# DIFFERENTIAL DIAGNOSIS:
## LOBULATED, ENHANCING INTRASELLAR AND PARASELLAR MASS

### Case 260

40-year-old man presenting with
bitemporal hemianopsia.
(coronal, postcontrast T1-weighted SE scan)

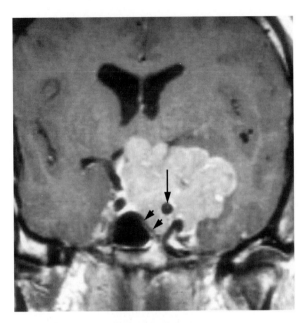

**Craniopharyngioma**
(same patient as Case 258)

### Case 261

46-year-old man presenting with
headaches and diplopia.
(coronal, postcontrast T1-weighted SE scan)

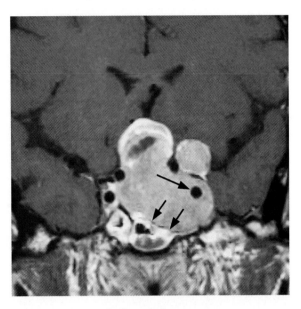

**Pituitary Adenoma**
(same patient as Case 232)

---

These cases demonstrate that both craniopharyngiomas and pituitary adenomas may grow laterally with eccentric, lobulated morphology. Both tumors have surrounded the left internal carotid artery within the cavernous sinus *(long arrows).* Both extend superiorly and laterally into the middle cranial fossa and along the proximal middle cerebral artery.

The intrasellar component of the craniopharyngioma in Case 260 has depressed the floor of the sella turcica on the left *(short arrows).* The entire sella is expanded by the adenoma in Case 261, although erosion and displacement of bone are greater on the left *(short arrows).* Bulky suprasellar growth of the masses occupies the expected location of the optic chiasm in each case.

Hypothalamic gliomas often present as suprasellar masses with eccentric lateral extension demonstrating solid, cystic, or mixed morphology (see Cases 262 and 265). Such tumors can closely resemble asymmetrical suprasellar craniopharyngiomas. However, gliomas of the hypothalamus rarely extend into the sella turcica or cavernous sinus like the masses in Cases 260 and 261.

Proton spectroscopy can contribute to the differential diagnosis of intrasellar and suprasellar masses. A lipid peak (at 1.3 ppm) is often demonstrated in craniopharyngiomas but would be unusual in a pituitary adenoma or a hypothalamic glioma without necrosis.

Compare the above scans to the tumors in Cases 236 and 237.

### Case 262

4-year-old girl complaining of headaches.
(sagittal, noncontrast T1-weighted SE scan)

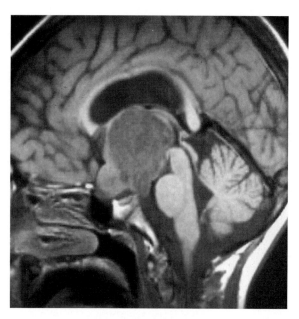

**Hypothalamic Glioma**

### Case 263

48-year-old woman presenting with
a visual field deficit.
(coronal, noncontrast T1-weighted SE scan)

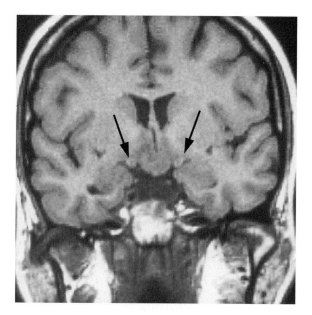

**Hypothalamic Glioma**

Hypothalamic gliomas rank with optic gliomas and craniopharyngiomas as the most common suprasellar masses in children. They are rarer in adults.

Case 262 illustrates that some hypothalamic gliomas are bulky, complex lesions. (See Case 267 for another example.) A mixture of solid and cystic components is common, with the latter demonstrating longer T1 values than the former. The lobulation and heterogeneity of hypothalamic gliomas like Case 262 may resemble the appearance of a craniopharyngioma. These two pathologies should both be considered in the differential diagnosis of a complex suprasellar mass in a child.

Other hypothalamic gliomas are low grade, homogeneous lesions with minimally abnormal signal intensity and little contrast enhancement, as illustrated in Case 263. The CT attenuation values of such tumors may be low, making them difficult to distinguish from the adjacent third ventricle. Evidence of mass effect may be subtle, best demonstrated on coronal and sagittal MR scans.

In Case 263, the floor of the third ventricle is abnormally bulbous, with obliteration of the normal slit of CSF in the anterior recesses. The optic tracts *(arrows)* are well seen on either side of the tumor.

The mass in Case 263 demonstrated high signal intensity on a T2-weighted scan, as well as increased size and enhancement on a follow-up study. These features help to distinguish a low-grade hypothalamic glioma from hypothalamic hamartomas (see Cases 274 and 275). Clinical correlation (i.e., the presence or absence of hypothalamic and chiasmal symptoms) may assist in this differential diagnosis.

The hypothalamus is the second most common site for pilocytic astrocytomas in children, accounting for 25% to 30% of these low grade neoplasms. About two-thirds of pilocytic astrocytomas are cerebellar, as discussed in Cases 142-147.

## Case 264

52-year-old man presenting with
reduced visual fields and acuity.
(axial, noncontrast T2-weighted FSE scan)

## Case 265

4-year-old boy presenting with increasing
irritability and clumsiness.
(axial, noncontrast T2-weighted SE scan)

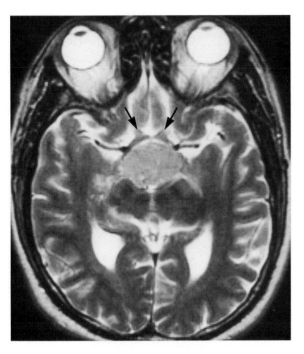

**Hypothalamic Glioma**

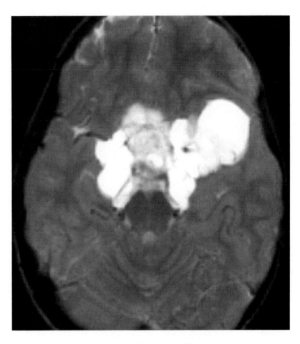

**Hypothalamic Glioma**

As discussed in Chapter 3, low-grade gliomas are usually better defined on MR scans than on CT studies. Such tumors differ more from surrounding normal brain in magnetic relaxation behavior than they do in x-ray absorption. T2-weighted images are particularly helpful in defining these lesions.

The signal intensity of hypothalamic gliomas may be intermediate to high on long TR spin echo images. In Case 264, the homogeneous suprasellar component of the tumor is only slightly higher in signal intensity than adjacent brain. The mass spans the distance between the supraclinoid internal carotid arteries. The optic chiasm is draped across the anterior margin of the tumor *(arrows)*. A postcontrast scan of this glioma closely resembled Case 245B.

Case 265 demonstrates multiple, bilateral, high intensity cysts extending into the parasellar and retrosellar regions.

Some of the cysts enhanced peripherally after contrast injection while others did not, suggesting reactive loculations of the subarachnoid space. (Compare to the cysts seen adjacent to acoustic schwannomas, as discussed in Case 192.) The solid midline component of the mass demonstrates less marked hyperintensity.

Although hypothalamic gliomas are intraaxial tumors, they frequently extend exophytically into basal cisterns as seen above. This tendency may combine with lobulated morphology to closely mimic the appearance of craniopharyngiomas.

The biological behavior of hypothalamic gliomas in children is age-dependent. Pilocytic astrocytomas in patients less than 5 years of age demonstrate rapid growth and/or recurrence more often than tumors in older children.

### Case 266

6-year-old boy presenting with
decreased visual acuity.
(coronal, postcontrast T1-weighted SE scan)

### Case 267

10-year-old boy presenting with
headaches and papilledema.
(sagittal, postcontrast T1-weighted SE scan)

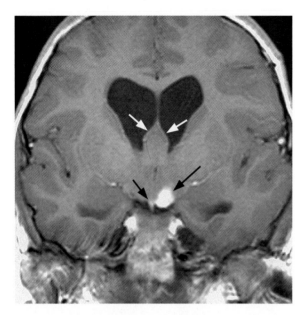

**Hypothalamic Glioma**

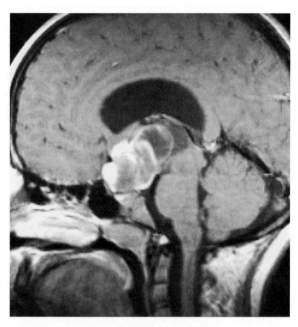

**Hypothalamic Glioma**

The nearly isointense tumor in Case 266 is much larger than the nodule of enhancement in the left suprasellar region *(long black arrow)*. Mass effect surrounds and effaces the third ventricle and extends superiorly to expand the region of the fornix at the inferomedial margin of the frontal horns *(white arrows)*. The base of the pituitary infundibulum *(short black arrow)* lies medial to the small focus of enhancement within the otherwise nonenhancing glioma.

More aggressive hypothalamic gliomas may enhance relatively homogeneously or in complex patterns, as shown in Case 267. Multiple rims of enhancement as in this lesion could also be seen in a craniopharyngioma. The tumor fills both the suprasellar cistern and the majority of the third ventricle, causing obstructive hydrocephalus.

Intense, homogeneous contrast enhancement is often seen in pilocytic astrocytomas of the hypothalamus. As is true of cerebellar pilocytic astrocytomas, extensive enhancement in these tumors does not necessarily imply high histological grade or clinical aggressiveness.

It may be difficult or impossible to distinguish between hypothalamic and chiasmatic origin of a large, lobulated, suprasellar glioma. Eccentric location suggests a tumor arising along the wall of the third ventricle (i.e., hypothalamus), while erosion of the chiasmatic sulcus favors a mass originating in the chiasm. Such distinctions are often not meaningful, since bulky tumors arising from either the chiasm or the hypothalamus usually invade the adjacent structures.

High signal intensity on T2-weighted images and/or abnormal contrast enhancement extending from a suprasellar mass along the optic tracts is not specific for optic/hypothalamic gliomas. Craniopharyngiomas may involve the optic chiasm and follow the optic tracts posteriorly. Rarely, meningeal seeding by CNS tumors (e.g., medulloblastoma) or inflammatory disease (e.g., sarcoidosis) presents a similar appearance.

## Case 268

2-year-old girl, one year after biopsy
of a suprasellar tumor.
(axial, postcontrast T1-weighted SE scan)

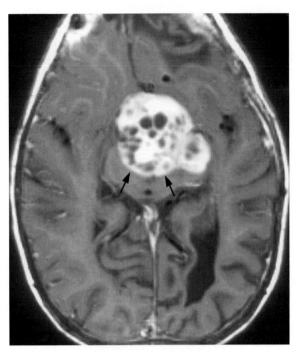

**Hypothalamic Glioma**

## Case 269

32-year-old man presenting with
bitemporal hemianopsia.
(sagittal, postcontrast T1-weighted SE scan with MTS)

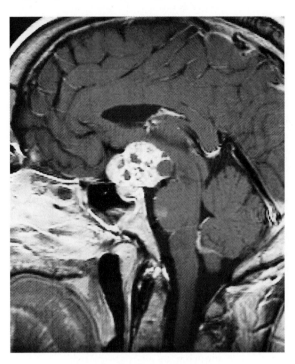

**Craniopharyngioma**

---

Both hypothalamic gliomas and craniopharyngiomas can present as predominantly solid suprasellar masses containing multiple small, nonenhancing cysts or zones of necrosis.

The glioma in Case 268 is centered in the region of the hypothalamus and optic chiasm. Posterior extension of the tumor has caused substantial compression and deformity of the midbrain *(arrows)*. The lobulation at the left posterolateral margin of the mass may represent growth along the optic tract.

Prominent retrosellar extension into the interpeduncular fossa is also characteristic of craniopharyngiomas, as demonstrated in Case 269. This mass is clearly suprasellar in origin, with the inferior margin at the level of the sellar diaphragm. The dorsum sella has been eroded.

The age of the above patients does not narrow the differential diagnosis in either case. Both hypothalamic gliomas and craniopharyngiomas can present in children or adults. Ger-

minomas or teratomas should also be considered among the possible causes of an irregularly enhancing suprasellar mass in either age group (compare the above scans to Cases 309-311).

Occasional hypothalamic hamartomas are associated with cysts and present as complex masses on precontrast scans. The absence of contrast enhancement usually distinguishes such lesions from other suprasellar tumors.

Chordoid gliomas (see discussion of Case 245) could be considered in the differential diagnosis, but these rare lesions usually demonstrate homogeneous enhancement.

An area of long T1 values in the inferior left frontal lobe in Case 268 reflects previous surgery. The poorly defined pattern of increased signal intensity projected over the ventral pons in Case 269 was artifactual. A precontrast scan in Case 269 resembled the suprasellar dermoid cyst presented as Case 257, with slightly less extensive T1-shortening.

# LANGERHANS CELL HISTIOCYTOSIS INVOLVING THE INFUNDIBULUM

### Case 270

3-year-old girl presenting with
polyuria and polydipsia.
(sagittal, noncontrast T1-weighted SE scan)

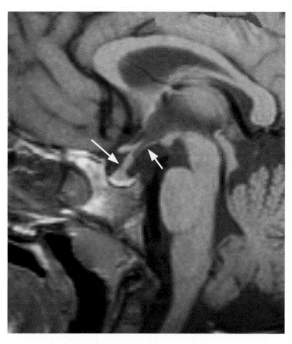

**Langerhans Cell Histiocytosis**

### Case 271

13-year-old boy presenting with
growth hormone deficiency.
(coronal, postcontrast T1-weighted GRE scan)

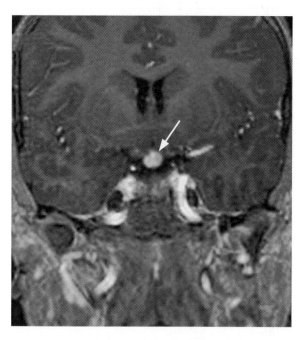

**Langerhans Cell Histiocytosis**

Langerhans cell histiocytosis (previously designated *histiocytosis X*) is a proliferative disorder of the reticuloendothelial system, usually presenting in childhood. The disease commonly causes lytic lesions of the skull and other bones (formerly labelled "eosinophilic granuloma"). Intracranial involvement most commonly affects the pituitary infundibulum and/or hypothalamus, usually manifesting as diabetes insipidus.

The symptoms and scans in the above cases are typical. The infundibulum in Case 270 is abnormally thick and mildly irregular *(long arrow)*. The normal posterior pituitary "bright spot" is absent, implying disruption of the infundibular transport or neurohypophyseal storage of antidiuretic hormone.

Case 271 demonstrates an intensely enhancing mass at the base of the pituitary stalk *(arrow)*. Such tumor-like lesions are within the spectrum of Langerhans cell histiocytosis, which should be considered in the differential diagnosis of pediatric suprasellar masses. Skull films in Case 271 demonstrated a lytic lesion of the mandible, helping to establish the diagnosis.

The position of the lesion in Case 271 mimics a hypothalamic hamartoma (see Cases 274 and 275), but the latter should not enhance to this degree. An optic/hypothalamic glioma could be considered, but the clinical presentation would be unusual for this diagnosis. Suprasellar germinomas can mimic both the imaging features and the clinical presentation of histiocytosis (see Cases 272 and 273). Lymphocytic hypophysitis may extend superiorly to reach the hypothalamus and is frequently associated with diabetes insipidus, but this disorder is rare in children.

Histiocytosis may also involve the cerebral hemispheres, with single or multiple lesions and a tendency to affect the temporal lobes. Some of the parenchymal lesions in histiocytosis may represent a secondary autoimmune pathophysiology.

Note the clearly defined infundibular recess of the third ventricle in Case 270 *(short arrow)*. This thin inferior projection of CSF is mildly truncated by the superior margin of thickened infundibular tissue.

# DIFFERENTIAL DIAGNOSIS:
## THICKENING OF THE PITUITARY INFUNDIBULUM IN A CHILD

### Case 272

15-year-old boy presenting with diabetes insipidus.
(coronal, postcontrast T1-weighted SE scan)

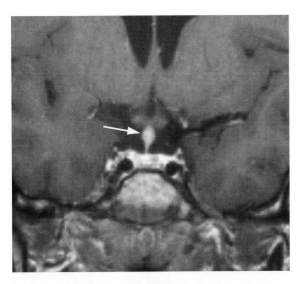

**Langerhans Cell Histiocytosis**

### Case 273

8-year-old boy presenting with diabetes insipidus.
(axial, postcontrast T1-weighted SE scan)

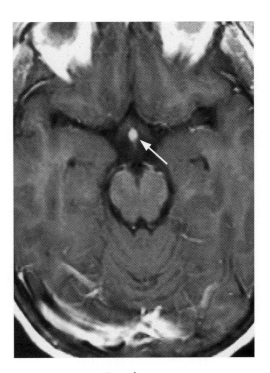

**Germinoma**

---

The normal pituitary stalk enhances intensely due to the lack of a blood-brain barrier and the presence of a surrounding plexus of veins. The diameter of the stalk varies from patient to patient, but the width normally tapers smoothly from a maximum of three millimeters superiorly to a maximum of two millimeters inferiorly. Abnormal thickness or morphology of the infundibulum can be a subtle but important indication of inflammatory or neoplastic disease in children or adults.

The above cases illustrate the major differential diagnosis of infundibular thickening in children. Both Langerhans cell histiocytosis and suprasellar germinomas can present with widening of the stalk in the setting of diabetes insipidus.

In Case 272, the bulging morphology of the superior portion of the infundibulum is distinctly abnormal. Case 273 illustrates more subtle expansion of the infundibulum, with a diameter of four millimeters.

Both Langerhans cell histiocytosis and germinomas can

cause either diffuse thickening of the pituitary stalk or mass-like lesions. The differential diagnosis often rests on the presence of an associated abnormality: lytic skull lesions in histiocytosis, or additional masses involving the posterior third ventricle/pineal region in germinomas (see Case 254).

Diabetes insipidus may precede perceptible thickening of the infundibulum by several months with either of the above pathologies (and/or persist after a mass has resolved). Follow-up scans are indicated if initial studies are negative.

The differential diagnosis of infundibular thickening or masses in adults includes sarcoidosis (see Case 487), tuberculosis, meningitis, lymphocytic adenohypophysitis (see discussion of Case 243), metastasis (most commonly from carcinoma of the breast), lymphoma, germinoma, and choristoma (see Case 245).

Prominent veins near the tentorium bilaterally in Case 273 are a normal variant (see discussion of Case 154).

**169**

### Case 274

32-year-old man complaining of headaches.
(sagittal, noncontrast T1-weighted SE scan)

### Case 275

41-year-old man presenting with seizures.
(coronal, noncontrast T2-weighted FSE scan)

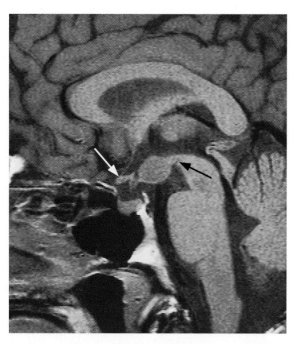

Hypothalamic Hamartoma

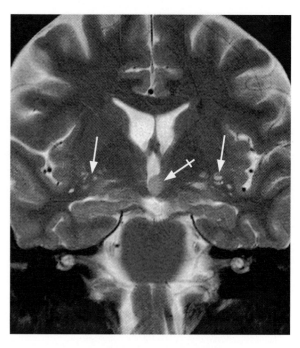

Hypothalamic Hamartoma

Hypothalamic hamartomas are typically midline or paramedian masses that arise along the floor of the third ventricle. They may be sessile, expanding the ventricular floor as in Case 274, or pedunculated, projecting inferiorly into the suprasellar and retrosellar cisterns.

These low grade lesions are frequently asymptomatic. In children (especially boys), hypothalamic hamartomas (especially pedunculated tumors) are often associated with precocious puberty. "Gelastic" seizures (laughing spells) are another typical clinical manifestation of these lesions, seeming to be associated with broadly based tumors deforming the hypothalamus and mamillary bodies. Such spells may be intractable preoperatively but cured by resection of the mass.

Hamartomas of the hypothalamus are typically quite round and are located anterior to the mamillary bodies (*black arrow,* Case 274; the *white arrow* indicates the optic chiasm). These masses consist predominantly of mature ganglion cells and are nearly isointense to gray matter on T1-weighted sequences. They do not demonstrate abnormal contrast enhancement.

In Case 275, a small, round mass deforms the inferior third ventricle *(crossed white arrow).* The lesion is homogeneous, with signal intensity comparable to gray matter. The location, morphology, uniformity, and isointensity of the tumor (together with lack of abnormal enhancement on postcontrast images) are characteristic of a hypothalamic hamartoma. However, a low-grade hypothalamic glioma could not be excluded (compare to Case 263), and a follow-up scan would be indicated.

Mildly increased signal intensity is seen within some hypothalamic hamartomas on T2-weighted scans and does not rule out the diagnosis. Slight eccentricity of the mass, as in Case 275, is common.

The multiple small foci of T2 prolongation inferior to the lentiform nuclei bilaterally in Case 275 *(white arrows)* are attributable to prominent perivascular spaces. These collections of fluid along the course of the lenticulostriate arteries are considered a developmental variant, although they become increasingly prominent with age. The perivascular cystic spaces can be up to two centimeters in diameter and are frequently asymmetrical or unilateral (see Case 838).

### Case 276A

36-year-old woman presenting with headaches.
(sagittal, noncontrast T1-weighted SE scan)

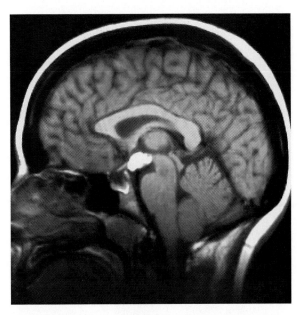

**Lipoma**

### Case 276B

Same patient.
(axial, noncontrast scan; SE 2500/45)

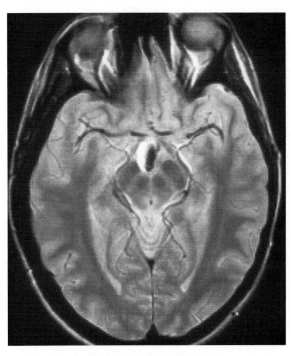

**Lipoma**

Like hamartomas, lipomas may occur along the floor of the third ventricle, as illustrated in this case. They are usually midline masses that are slightly retrosellar. Short T1 values reflecting lipid protons characterize the lesion on short TR spin echo sequences; this high signal intensity would be suppressed on a fat saturation study. As demonstrated in Case 257, suprasellar dermoid cysts can present an appearance similar to a lipoma in this location.

The MR distinction between lipid material and other causes of T1-shortening within a cerebral lesion can be based on (1) the use of pulse sequences that selectively suppress the signal from water or lipid protons or (2) the presence of chemical shift artifact.

Chemical shift artifact is encountered when a fatty mass is "shifted" or misregistered in space with respect to its aqueous surroundings. Because lipid protons resonate at a slightly lower frequency than water protons, the computer has erroneously placed the lipoma in Case 276B a little closer to the low end of the frequency axis than its true location. As a result, the right side of the lipoma appears to overlap the aqueous tissue along its right margin, while a false gap is created between the left side of the lipoma and the adjacent parenchyma.

### Case 277A

17-year-old boy presenting with right-sided
orbital pain and ophthalmoplegia.
(coronal, noncontrast T1-weighted SE scan)

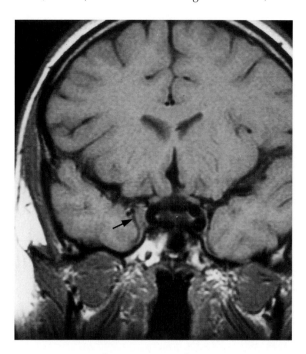

**Tolosa-Hunt Syndrome**

### Case 277B

Same patient.
(coronal, postcontrast T1-weighted SE scan)

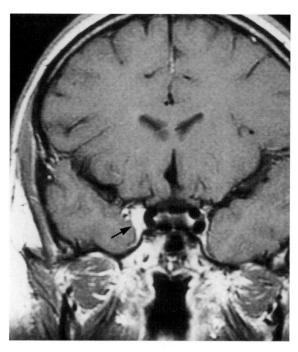

**Tolosa-Hunt Syndrome**

Idiopathic inflammation of the cavernous sinus causing painful ophthalmoplegia is a condition known as "Tolosa-Hunt" syndrome. The disorder is probably related to orbital pseudotumor. (In some cases, orbital and parasellar inflammation communicates through the superior orbital fissure.) Like orbital pseudotumor, Tolosa-Hunt syndrome usually responds to treatment with steroids.

MR scans of patients with Tolosa-Hunt syndrome often demonstrate mild but definite widening of the ipsilateral cavernous sinus, as seen in Case 277A *(arrow)*. The homogeneous tissue within the sinus is relatively isointense to gray matter on T1-weighted scans and usually hypointense on T2-weighted images. The later appearance is nonspecific and can be noted in parasellar meningiomas, metastases, and lymphoma. Conversely, such a mass within the cavernous sinus should not be presumed to represent neoplasm without a trial of steroid therapy.

Intense contrast enhancement within the thickened parasellar tissue is usual, as illustrated in Case 277B. Again this appearance does not distinguish Tolosa-Hunt syndrome from intracavernous tumors. Encasement of the internal carotid artery may be present, comparable to parasellar meningiomas or lateral extension of pituitary adenomas.

The peak age incidence of Tolosa-Hunt syndrome is 40 to 60 years. Sex incidence is equal. Bilateral involvement of the cavernous sinuses is seen in about 5% of cases. Both the development of symptoms and the response to steroids typically occur within days.

Other inflammatory processes that can involve the cavernous sinus and produce similar MR findings include sarcoidosis and Wegener's granulomatosis.

## Case 278

40-year-old woman presenting with
right facial numbness.
(coronal, noncontrast T1-weighted SE scan)

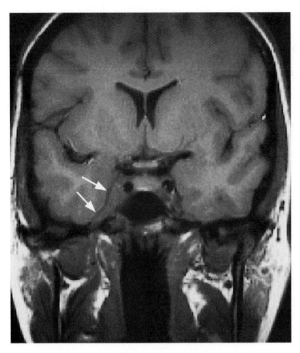

**Adenoid Cystic Carcinoma of the Pharynx**

## Case 279

38-year-old man presenting with diplopia.
(axial, noncontrast T2-weighted FSE scan)

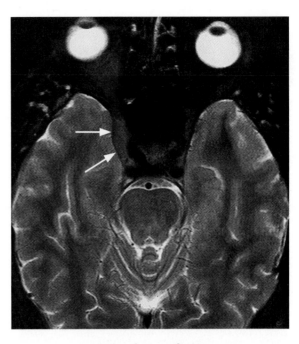

**Systemic Lymphoma**

---

Extracranial tumors of the head and neck may extend intracranially by direct invasion and/or perineural spread. Case 278 illustrates the latter mechanism: a pharyngeal carcinoma has tracked back along branches of the fifth cranial nerve to involve the cavernous sinus *(arrows)*, which demonstrates abnormal thickness and signal intensity.

The foramen ovale and the cavernous sinus should be closely examined in all cases of pharyngeal tumor for evidence of perineural spread. Similarly, enlargement of the foramen ovale or obliteration of adjacent fat planes should be sought on scans demonstrating a parasellar mass as clues to perineural extension of a pharyngeal neoplasm. Adenoid cystic carcinoma is particularly prone to perineural growth, but the more common squamous cell carcinomas of the pharynx may exhibit similar behavior. Melanomas of the head and neck can also traverse the skull base in this manner.

In Case 279, the right cavernous sinus is mildly thickened with an abnormally convex lateral margin *(arrows)*. The relatively low signal intensity of the homogeneous lesion on this T2-weighted scan falls within the spectrum of meningi-

omas, lymphoma, and metastases, and each should be considered in the differential diagnosis. Intracranial involvement by systemic lymphoma is often dural-based (see Cases 24 and 26 for additional examples).

Both of the above lesions demonstrated intense contrast enhancement. The MR features in such cases are not specific, and clinical correlation is required.

In addition to meningioma, metastasis, and lymphoma, lesions to be considered in the differential diagnosis of a homogeneous parasellar mass include lateral extension of a pituitary adenoma, cranial nerve schwannoma, Tolosa-Hunt syndrome (see Case 277), sarcoidosis, Wegener's granulomatosis, and lateral extension of sphenoid sinusitis or mucocele. Chordomas, chondrosarcomas, and cavernous angiomas occur in the parasellar region but typically demonstrate signal characteristics distinct from the above cases. Similarly, distention of the cavernous sinus by an aneurysm or a carotid/cavernous fistula is usually accompanied by characteristic patterns of signal change (see Cases 280 and 281).

### Case 280

54-year-old woman presenting with diplopia.
(axial, noncontrast scan; SE 2800/30)

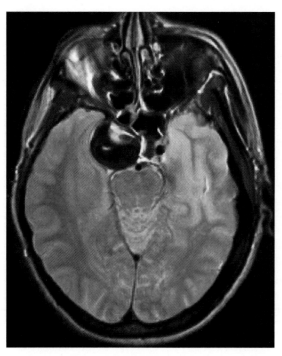

**Aneurysm of the Internal Carotid Artery**
(largely thrombosed)

### Case 281

23-year-old man presenting with proptosis and
chemosis after a "four-wheeler" accident.
(coronal, postcontrast T1-weighted SE scan)

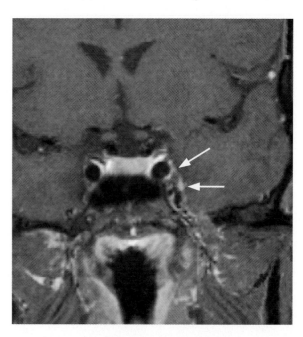

**Carotid-Cavernous Fistula**
(indirect, low flow)

---

Vascular lesions are another important cause of parasellar masses. Aneurysms of the cavernous segment of the internal carotid artery may expand the sinus while demonstrating variable morphology and intensity.

The low signal occupying most of the lumen of the giant aneurysm in Case 280 was proven to represent T2-shortening due to deoxyhemoglobin (and/or intracellular methemoglobin) within thrombus, not flow void. MR angiography can distinguish between patent and thrombosed portions of an aneurysm when the nature of a low intensity zone is ambiguous on routine scans.

Case 281 is an example of an indirect, low flow carotid-cavernous fistula. These lesions are vascular malformations of the dura, often occurring spontaneously in middle-aged or elderly patients. Small meningeal branches of the internal and external carotid arteries supply a network of abnormal channels along the medial wall of the middle cranial fossa, shunting blood into the cavernous sinus.

The left cavernous sinus in Case 281 is mildly expanded, with an abnormally convex lateral margin (*arrows;* compare to Case 279). Within the enhancing sinus are multiple filling defects, reflecting arterialized flow through venous compartments due to the shunt from adjacent arteries.

High flow (direct) carotid-cavernous fistulae due to tears of the parasellar internal carotid artery can cause much greater distention of one or both cavernous sinuses. The low signal intensity and variable enhancement (depending on flow characteristics) of such lesions can resemble a parasellar mass or aneurysm on MR studies. However, clinical manifestations of anterior drainage through one or both superior ophthalmic veins (proptosis, conjunctival injection, and a bruit) usually establish the diagnosis.

Extradural cavernous angiomas may also occur in the parasellar region. Such lesions often demonstrate homogeneously long T1 and T2 values, more closely resembling orbital hemangiomas than the characteristic reticular or honeycomb morphology of intradural angiomas illustrated in Cases 761-768. Uniformly enhancing parasellar cavernous angiomas can mimic other extradural pathologies (e.g., meningioma or metastasis).

# REFERENCES

Abrahams JJ, Trefelner E, Boulware SD: Idiopathic growth hormone deficiency: MR findings in 35 patients. *AJNR* 12:155-160, 1991.

Ahmadi J, Destian S, Apuzzo MLJ, et al: Cystic fluid in craniopharyngiomas: MR imaging and quantitative analysis. *Radiology* 182:783-785, 1992.

Ahmadi J, Meyers GS, Segall HD, et al: Lymphocytic adenohypophysitis: contrast-enhanced MR imaging in five cases. *Radiology* 195:30-34, 1995.

Ahmadi J, North CM, Segall HD, et al: Cavernous sinus invasion by pituitary adenomas. *Am J Neuroradiol* 6:893-898, 1985.

Albright AL, Lee PA: Neurosurigical treatment of hypothalamic harmartomas causing precocious puberty. *J Neurosurg* 78:77-82, 1993.

Appignani B, Landy H, Barnes P: MR in idiopathic central diabetes insipidus of childhood. *AJNR* 14:1407-1410, 1993.

Barkovich AJ, Fram EK, Norman D: Septo-optic dysplasia: MR imaging. *Radiology* 171:189-192, 1989.

Barral V, Brunelle F, Brauner R, et al: MRI of lypothalamic hamartomas in children. *Pediatr Radiol* 18:449, 1988.

Bartynski WS, Lin L: Dynamic and conventional spin-echo MR of pituitary microlesions. *AJNR* 18:965-972, 1997.

Beningfield SJ, Bonnici F, Cremin BJ: Magnetic resonance imaging of hypothalamic hamartomas. *Br J Radiol* 61:1177, 1988.

Benshoff ER, Katz BH: Ectopia of the posterior pituitary gland as a normal variant: assessment with MR imaging. *ANJR* 11:709, 1990.

Boecher-Schwartz HG, Fries G, Bornemann A, et al: Suprasellar granular cell tumor. *Neurosurgery* 31:751-754, 1992.

Bonawitz CA, Castillo M, Mukherji SK: Panhypopituitarism: magnetic resonance imaging findings in children and adults. *Int J Neurorad* 4:431-438, 1998.

Boyko OB, Curnes JT, Oakes Wj, Burger PC: Hamartomas of the tuber cinereum: CT, MR, and pathologic findings. *AJNR* 12:309-314, 1991.

Bronen RA, Fulbright RK, Reynders CS, et al: Magnetic resonance imaging of central precocious puberty: the importance of hypothalamic abnormalities. *Int J Neurorad* 1:145-153, 1995.

Brooks BS, Gammal TE, Allison JD, et al: Frequency and variation of the posterior pituitary bright signal on MR images. *AJNR* 10:943-948, 1989.

Buchfelder M, Nistor R, Fahlbusch R, Huk WJ: The accuracy of CT and MR evaluation of the sella turcica for detection of adrenocorticotropic hormone-secreting adenomas in Cushing disease. *AJNR* 14:1183-1190, 1993.

Burton EM, Ball WS Jr, Crone K, Dolan LM: Hamartoma of the tuber cinereum: a comparison of MR and CT findings in four cases. *AJNR* 10:497-502, 1989.

Byun WM, Kim OL, Kim DS: MR imaging findings of Rathke's cleft cysts: significance of intracystic nodules. *AJNR* 2:485-488, 2000.

Cappabianca P, Cirillo S, Alfieri A, et al: Pituitary macroadenoma and diaphragma sellae meningioma: differential diagnosis. *Neuroradiology* 41:22-26, 1999.

Chakares DW, Curtin A, Ford G: Magnetic resonance imaging of pituitary and parasellar abnormalities. *Radiol Clin North Am* 27:265-282, 1989.

Chong BW, Kucharczyk W, Singer W, George S: Pituitary gland MR: a comparative study of healthy volunteers and patients with microadenomas. *AJNR* 15:675-679, 1994.

Chong BW, Newton TH: Hypothalamic and pituitary pathology. *Radiol Clin North Am* 31:1147-1184, 1993.

Colombo N, Berry I, Kucharczyk J, et al: Posterior pituitary gland: appearance on MR imaging in normal and pathological states. *Radiology* 165:481-485, 1987.

Colombo N, Loli P, Vignati F, Scialfa G: MR of corticotropin-secreting pituitary microadenomas. *AJNR* 15:1591-1595, 1994.

Cone L, Srinivasan M, Romanul FCA: Granular cell tumor (choristoma) of the neurohypophysis: two cases and a review of the literature. *AJNR* 11:403-406, 1990.

Cottier JP, Destrieux C, Brunereau L, et al: Cavernous sinus invasion by pituitary adenoma: MR imaging. *Radiology* 215:463-469, 2000.

Cox, TD, Elster AD: Normal pituitary gland: changes in shape, size, and signal intensity during the 1st year of life at MR imaging. *Radiology* 179:721-724, 1991.

Crenshaw WB, Chew FS: Rathke's cleft cyst. *Am J Roentgenol* 158:1312, 1993.

Daniels EL, Czervonike LF, Bonneville JF, et al: MRI of the cavernous sinus value on spin-echo and gradient recalled echo images. *Am J Roentgenol* 1009-1014, 1988.

Daniels DL, Pech, P, Mark L, et al: Magnetic resonance imaging of the cavernous sinus. *AJNR* 6:187-192, 1985.

Daniels PL, Pojunas KW, Kilgore DP, et al: MR of the diaphragm sellae. *AJNR* 7:765-769, 1986.

Davis P, Hoffman J, Malko J, et al: Gd-DTPA and MR imaging of pituitary adenoma. *AJNR* 8:817, 1987.

Davis PC, Hoffman JC, Spencer T, et al: MR imaging of pituitary adenoma. CT, clinical, and surgical consideration. *AJNR* 8:107-112, 1987.

Davis WL, Lee JN, M.D., King BD, Harnsberger HR: Dynamic contrast-enhanced MR imaging of the pituitary gland with fast spin-echo technique. *JMRI* 4:509-511, 1994.

Dietrich RB, Lis LE, Greensite FS, Pitt D: Normal MR appearance of the pituitary gland in the first 2 years of life. *AJNR* 16:1413-1420, 1995.

Dina TS, Feaster SH, Laws ER Jr, Davis DO: MR of the pituitary gland postsurgery: serial MR studies following transsphenoidal resection. *AJNR* 14:763-769, 1993.

Donovan JL, Nesbit GM: Distinction of masses involving the sella and suprasellar space: specificity of imaging features. *Am J Roentgenol* 167:597-603, 1996.

Doppman JL, Frank JA, Dwyer AJ, et al: Gadolinium-DTPA-enhanced MR imaging of ACTH-secreting microadenomas of the pituitary gland. *J Comput Assist Tomogr* 12:728-736, 1988.

Doraiswamy PM, Potts JM, Axelson DA, et al: MR assessment of pituitary gland morphology in healthy volunteers: age- and gender related differences. *AJNR* 13:1295-1300, 1992.

Downs DM, Damiano TR, Rubinstein D: Gasserian ganglion: appearance on contrast-enhanced MR. *AJNR* 17:237-242, 1996.

Dwyer AJ, Frank JA, Doppman JL, et al: Pituitary adenomas in patients with Cushing disease: initial experience with Gd-DTPA-enhanced MR imaging. *Radiology* 163:421-426, 1987.

Eldevik OP, Blaivas M, Gabrielsen TO, et al: Craniopharyngioma: radiologic and histologic findings and recurrence. *AJNR* 17:1427-1439, 1996.

El Gammal T, Brooks BS, Hoffman WH: MR imaging of the ectopic bright signal of posterior pituitary regeneration. *AJNR* 10:323-328, 1989.

El-Kalliny M, Van Loveren H, Keller JT, Tew Jr J: Tumors of the lateral wall of the cavernous sinus. *Neurosurgery* 77:508-514, 1992.

Elster AD: Imaging of the sella: anatomy and pathology. *Semin US CT MR* 14:182-194, 1993.

Elster AD: Modern imaging of the pituitary. *Radiology* 187:1-14, 1993.

Elster AD: Sellar susceptibility artifacts: theory and implications. *AJNR* 14:129-136, 1993.

Elster AD, Chen MV, Williams D III, Key LL: Pituitary gland: MR imaging of physiologic hypertrophy in adolescents. *Radiology* 174:681-686, 1990.

Elster AD, Chen MYM, Richardson DM, Yeatts PR: Dilated intercavernous sinuses: an MR sign of carotid-cavernous and carotid-dural fistulas. *AJNR* 12:641-645, 1991.

Finelli DA, Kaufman B: Varied microcirculation of pituitary adenomas at rapid, dynamic, contrast-enhanced MR imaging. *Radiology* 189:205-210, 1993.

Freeman MP, Kessler RM, Allen JH, Price AC: Craniopharyngioma: CT and MR imaging in nine cases. *J Comput Assist Tomogr* 11:810-814, 1987.

Fujisawa I, Asato R, Okumura R, et al: Magnetic resonance imaging of neurohypophyseal germinomas. *Cancer* 68:1009-1014, 1991.

Fujisawa I, Kikuchi K, Nishimura K, et al: Transection of the pituitary stalk. Development of an ectopic posterior lobe assessed with MR imaging. *Radiology* 165:487-489, 1987.

Fujisawa I, Nishimura K, Asato R, et al: Posterior lobe of the pituitary in diabetes insipidus: MR findings. *J Comput Assist Tomogr* 11:221-225, 1987.

Giacometti AR, Joseph GJ, Peterson JE, Davis PC: Comparison of full-and half-dose Gadolinium-DTPA: MR imaging of the normal sella. *AJNR* 14:123-128, 1993.

Goyal M, Kucharczyk W, Keystone E: Granulomatous hypophysitis due to Wegener's granulomatosis. *AJNR* 21:1466-1469, 2000.

Grois N, Barkovich AJ, Rosenau W, Ablin AR: Central nervous system disease associated with Langerhans cell histiocytosis. *Am J Pediatr Hematol Oncol* 15:245-254, 1993.

Gudinchet F, Brunelle F, Barth MO, et al: MR imaging of the posterior hypophysis in children. *AJNR* 10:511-514, 1989.

Hahn FJ, Leibrock LG, Huseman CA, et al: The MR appearance of hypothalamic hamartoma. *Neuroradiology* 30:65-68, 1988.

Halimi P, Sigal R, Doyon D, et al: Post-traumatic diabetes insipidus: MR demonstration of pituitary stalk rupture. *J Comput Assist Tomogr* 12:135-140, 1988.

Hamilton J, Blaser S, Daneman D: MR imaging in idiopathic growth hormone deficiency. *AJNR* 19:1609-1616, 1998.

Harrison MJ, Morgello S, Post KD: Epithelial cystic lesions of the sella and parasellar region: a continuum of ectodermal derivatives? *J Neurosurg* 80:1018-1025, 1994.

Hashimoto M, Yanaki T, Nakahara N, Masuzawa T: Lymphocytic adenohypophysitis: an immunohistochemical study. *Surg Neurol* 36:137-144, 1991.

Hershey BL: Suprasellar masses: diagnosis and differential diagnosis. *Semin US CT MR* 14:215-231, 1993.

Hirai T, Korogi Y, Hamatake S, et al: Three-dimensional FISP imaging in the evaluation of carotid cavernous fistula: comparison with contrast-enhanced CT and spin-echo MR. *AJNR* 19:253-260, 1998.

Hirsch WI, Hryshko FG, Sekhar LN, et al: Comparison of MR imaging. CT and angiography in the evaluation of the enlarged cavernous sinus. *AJNR* 9:907-915, 1988.

Hoyt WF, Kaplan S, Grumbach MM, et al: Septo-optic dysplsia and pituitary dwarfism. *Lancet* 1:893-894, 1970.

Hua F, Asato R, Miki Y, et al: Differentiation of suprasellar non-neoplastic cysts from cystic neoplasms by Gd-DTPA MRI. *J Comput Assist Tomogr* 16:747-749, 1992.

Hutchins WW, Crues JV III, Miya P, Pojunas KW: MR demonstration of pituitary hyperplasia and regression after therapy for hypothyroidism. *AJNR* 11:410, 1990.

Ji CH, Teng, MMH, Chang T: Granular cell tumour of the neurohypophysis. *Neuroradiology* 37:451-452, 1995.

Johnson DE, Woodruff WW, Allen IS, et al: MR imaging of the sellar and juxtasellar regions. *Radiographics* 11:727-758, 1991.

Kaard HP, Khangure MS, Waring P: Extraaxial parasellar cavernous hemangioma. *AJNR* 11:1259-1261, 1990.

Kamel HAM, Toland J: Trigeminal nerve anatomy: illustrated using examples of abnormalities. *Am J Roentgenol* 176:247-251, 2001.

Kanungo N, Just N, Black M, et al: Nasopharyngeal craniopharyngioma in an unusual location. *AJNR* 16:1372-1374, 1995.

Karnaze MG, Sartor K, Winthorp JD, et al: Suprasellar lesions: evaluation with MR imaging. *Radiology* 161:77-82, 1986.

Katzman GL, Langford CA, Sneller MC, et al: Pituitary involvement by Wegener's granulomatosis: a report of two cases. *AJNR* 20:519-523, 1999.

Kaufman B, Kaufman BA, Arafah B, et al: Large pituitary gland adenomas evaluated with magnetic resonance imaging. *Neurosurgery* 21:540-546, 1987.

Kaufman B, Tomsak RL, Kaufman BA, et al: Herniation of the suprasellar visual system and third ventricle into empty sellae: Morphologic and clinical considerations. *AJNR* 10:65-76, 1989.

Kelly WM, Kucharczyk J, et al: Posterior pituitary ectopia: an MR feature of pituitary dwarfism. *AJNR* 9:453-460, 1988.

Kobayashi S, Ikeda H, Yoshimoto T: A clinical and histopathological study of factors affecting MRI signal intensities of pituitary adenomas. *Neuroradiology* 36:298-302, 1994.

Komiyama M, Hakuba A, Yasui T, et al: Magnetic resonance imaging of intracavernous pathology. *Neurol Med Chir (Tokyo)* 29:573-578, 1989.

Kornreich L, Horev G, Lazar L, et al: MR findings in hereditary isolated growth hormone deficiency. *AJNR* 18:1743-1748, 1997.

Kucharczyk W, Davis DO, Kelly WM, et al: Pituitary adenoma: high-resolution MRI at 1.5 T. *Radiology* 161:761-765, 1986.

Kucharczyk, W, Peck WW, Kelly WM, et al: Rathke cleft cysts: CT, MR imaging, and pathologic features. *Radiology* 165: 491-495, 1987.

Kucharczyk W, Lenkinski RE, Kucharczyk J, Henkelman RM: The effect of phospholipid vesicles on the NMR relaxation of water: an explanation for the MR appearance of the neurohypophysis? *AJNR* 11:693-700, 1990.

Kulkarni MV, Lee KF, McArdle CB, et al: 1.5 T MR imaging of pituitary microadenomas: technical considerations and CT correlation. *AJNR* 9:5-12, 1988.

Kuo JS, Casey SO, Thompson L, Truwit CL: Pallister-Hall syndrome: clinical and MR features. *AJNR* 20:1839-1841, 1999.

Kuroiwa T, Okabe Y, Hasuo K, et al: MR imaging of pituitary dwarfism. *AJNR* 12:161-164, 1991.

Kuroiwa T, Okabe Y, Hasuo K, et al: MR imaging of pituitary hypertrophy due to juvenile primary hypothyroidism: a case report. *Clin Imaging* 15:202-205, 1991.

Kwan ESK, Wolpert SM, Hedges TR III, Laucella M: Tolosa-Hunt syndrome revisited: not necessarily a diagnosis of exclusion. *AJNR* 8:1067-1072, 1987.

Kyle CA, Laster RA, Burton EM, Sanford RA: Subacute pituitary apoplexy: MR and CT appearance. *J Comput Assist Tomogr* 14:40-44, 1990.

Laine FJ, Braun IF, Jensen ME, et al: Perineural tumor extension through the foramen ovale: evaluation with MR imaging. *Radiology* 174:65-71, 1990.

Lavallee G, Morcos R, Palardy J, et al: MR of nonhemorrhagic postpartum pituitary apoplexy. *AJNR* 16:1939-1941, 1995.

Lazaro CM, Guo WY, Sami M, et al: Haemorrhagic pituitary tumours. *Neuroradiology* 38:111-114, 1994.

Lee BCP, Deck MDF: Sellar and juxtasellar lesion detection with MR. *Radiology* 157:143-148, 1985.

Lenthall RK, Dean JR, Bartlett JR, Jeffree MA: Intrapituitary fluid levels following haemorrhage: MRI appearances in 13 cases. *Neuroradiology* 41:167-170, 1999.

Levine SN, Benzel EC, Fowler MR, et al: Lymphocytic adenohypophysitis: clinical, radioloical, and magnetic resonance imaging characterization. *Neurosurgery* 22:937-941, 1988.

Lohle PNM, Wurzer HAL, Seelen PJ, et al: Cystic lesions accompanying extra-axial tumours. *Neuroradiology* 41:13-17, 1999.

Lundin P, Bergstrom K, Nyman R, et al: Macroprolatinomas: serial MR imaging in long-term bromocriptine therapy. *AJNR* 13:1279-1291, 1992.

Lundin P, Nyman R, Burmas P, et al: MRI of pituitary microadenomas with reference to hormonal activity. *Neuroradiology* 34:43-51, 1992.

Maggio WW, Cail WS, Brookeman JR, et al: Rathke's cleft cyst: computed tomographic and magnetic resonance imaging appearances. *Neurosurgery* 21:60-62, 1987.

Maghnie M, Arico M, Villa A, et al: MR of the hypothalamic-pituitary axis in Langerhans cell histiocytosis. *AJNR* 13:1365-1371, 1992.

Maintz D, Benz-Bohm G, Gindele A, et al: Posterior pituitary ectopia: another hint toward a genetic etiology. *AJNR* 21:1116-1118, 2000.

Majos C, Coll S, Aguilera C, et al: Imaging of giant pituitary adenomas. *Neuroradiology* 40:651-655, 1998.

Mark AS, Phister SH, Jackson DE Jr, Kolsky MP: Traumatic lesions of the suprasellar region: MR imaging. *Radiology* 182:49-52, 1992.

Marro B, Zouaoui A, Sahel M, et al: MRI of pituitary adenomas in acromegaly. *Neuroradiology* 39:394-399, 1997.

Meyer FB, Lombari D, Scheithauer B, Nichols DA: Extra-axial cavernous hemangiomas involving the dural sinuses. *J Neurosurg* 73:187-192, 1990.

Meyer JR, Quint DJ, McKeever PE, et al: Giant Rathke cleft cyst. *AJNR* 15:533-536, 1994.

Meyer JS, Harty MP, Mahboubi S, et al: Langerhans cell histiocytosis: presentation and evolution of radiologic findings with clinical correlation. *Radiographics* 15:1135-1146, 1995.

Michael AS, Paige ML: MR imaging of intrasellar meningiomas simulating pituitary adenomas. *J Comput Assist Tomogr* 12:944, 1988.

Mikhael, MA, Ciric IS: MR imaging of pituitary tumors before and after surgical and/or medical treatment. *J Comput Assist Tomogr* 12:441-445, 1988.

Miki Y, Asato R, Okumura R, et al: Anterior pituitary gland in pregnancy: hyperintensity at MR. *Radiology* 187:229-231, 1993.

Millar WS, Tartaglino LM, Sergott RC, et al: MR of malignant optic glioma of adulthood. *AJNR* 16:1673-1676, 1995.

Moses AM, Clayton B, Hochhauser L: Use of T1-weighted MR imaging to differentiate between primary polydipsia and central diabetes insipidus. *AJNR* 13:1273-1278, 1992.

Mucelli RSP, Frezza F, Magnaldi S, Proto G: Magnetic resonance imaging in patients with panhypopituitarism. *Eur J Radiol* 2:42-46, 1992.

Murray RA, Maheshwari HG, Russell EJ, Baumann G: Pituitary hypoplasia in patients with a mutation in the growth hormone-releasing hormone receptor gene. *AJNR* 21:685-689, 2000.

Nagahata M, Hosoya T, Kayama T, Yamaguchi K: Edema along the optic tract: a useful MRI finding for the diagnosis of craniopharyngiomas. *AJNR* 19: 1753-1757, 1998.

Naheedy MH, Haag JR, Azar-Kia B, et al: MRI and CT of sellar and parasellar disorders. *Radiol Clin North Am* 25:819-848, 1987.

Nakumura T, Schorner W, Bittner RC, et al: Value of paramagnetic contrast agent gadolinium-DTPA in the diagnosis of pituitary adenomas. *Neuroradiology* 30:481, 1988.

Nemoto Y, Inoue Y, Fukuda T, et al: MR appearance of Rathke's cleft cysts. *Neuroradiology* 30:155-159, 1988.

Newton DR, Dillion WP, Norman D, et al: Gd-DTPA-enhanced MR imaging of pituitary adenomas. *AJNR* 10:949-954, 1989.

Nichols DA, Laws ER Jr, Houser OW, Abboud CP: Comparison of magnetic resonance imaging and computed tomography in the preoperative evaluation of pituitary adenomas. *Neurosurgery* 22:380-385, 1988.

Ostrov SG, Quencer RM, Hoffman JC Jr, et al: Hemorrhage within pituitary adenomas: how often associated with pituitary apoplexy syndrome? *AJNR* 10:503-510, 1989.

Peck WW, Dillon WP, Norman D, et al: High resolution MR imaging of microadenomas at 1.5 T: experience with Cushing's disease. *AJNR* 9:1085-1991, 1988.

Pigeau I, Sigal R, Halimi P, et al: MRI features of craniopharyngiomas at 1.5 Tesla: a series of 13 cases. *J Neuroradiol* 15:276, 1988.

Pojunas KW, Daniels DL, Williams AL, Haughton VM: MR imaging of prolactin-secreting microadenoma. *AJNR* 7:209-213, 1986.

Pomper MG, Passe TJ, Burger PC, et al: Chordoid glioma: a neoplasm unique to the hypothalamus and anterior third ventricle. *AJNR* 22:464-469, 2001.

Poussaint TY, Barnes PD, Anthony DC, et al: Hemorrhagic pituitary adenomas of adolescence. *AJNR* 17:1907-1912, 1996.

Poussaint TY, Gudas T, Barnes PD: Imaging of neuroendocrine disorders of childhood. *Neuroimaging Clin North Am* 9:157-176, 1999.

Prasad S, Shah J, Patkar D, et al: Giant hypothalamic hamartoma with cystic change: report of two cases and review of the literature. *Neuroradiology* 42:648-650, 2000.

Pusey E, Kortman KE, Flannigan BD, et al: MR of craniopharyngiomas: tumor delineation and characterization. *AJNR* 8:439-444, 1987.

Rand T, Kink E, Sator M, et al: MRI of microadenomas in patients with hyperprolactinaemia. *Neuroradiology* 38:744-746, 1996.

Rodriguez LA, Edwards MSB, Levin VA: Management of hypothalamic gliomas in children: an analysis of 33 cases. *Neurosurgery* 26:242-247, 1990.

Rodriguez O, Mateos B, de la Pedraja R, et al: Postoperative follow-up of pituitary adenomas after trans-sphenoidal resection: MRI and clinical correlation. *Neuroradiology* 38:747-754, 1996.

Rosenfeld JV, Harvey AS, Wrennall J, et al: Transcallosal resection of hypothalamic hamartomas, with control of seizures in children with gelastic epilepsy. *Neurosurgery* 48:108-118, 2001.

Ross DA, Norman D, Wilson CB: Radiologic characteristics and results of surgical management of Rathke's cysts in 43 patients. *Neurosurgery* 30:173-179, 1992.

Rubinstein D, Symonds D: Gas in the cavernous sinus. *AJNR* 15:561-566, 1994.

Saeki N, Iuchi T, Isono S, et al: MRI of growth hormone-secreting pituitary adenomas: factors determining pretreatment hormone levels. *Neuroradiology* 41:765-771, 1999.

Saiwai S, Inoue Y, Ishihara T, et al: Lymphocytic adenohypophysitis: skull radiographs and MRI. *Neuroradiology* 40:114-120, 1998.

Sakamoto Y, Takahashi M, Korogi Y, et al: Normal and abnormal pituitary glands: gallopentetate dimeglumine-enhanced MR imaging. *Radiology* 178:441-445, 1991.

Sakurai K, Fujita N, Harada K, et al: Magnetic susceptibility artifact in spin-echo MR imaging of the pituitary gland. *AJNR* 13:1301-1308, 1992.

Sartor K, Karnaze MG, Winthrop JD, et al: MR imaging in infra-, para- and retrosellar mass lesions. *Neuroradiology* 29:19-29, 1987.

Sartoretti-Schefer S, Wichmann W, Aguzzi A, Valavanis A: MR differentiation of adamantinomatous and squamous-papillary craniopharyngiomas. *AJNR* 18:77-87, 1997.

Sato N, Sze G, Endo K: Hypophysitis: endocrinologic and dynamic MR findings. *AJNR* 19:439-444, 1998.

Satoh H, Arita K, Kurisu K, et al: Intrasellar meningioma: characteristic imaging findings. *Neuroradiology* 38:328-329, 1996.

Savino PJ, Grossman RI, Schatz NJ, et al: High-field magnetic resonance imaging in the diagnosis of cavernous sinus thrombosis. *Arch Neurol* 43: 1081-1082, 1986.

Schubiger O, Haller D: Metastases to the pituitary hypothalamic axis. *Neuroradiology* 34:131-134, 1992.

Schuknecht B, Simmen D, Wichmann W, Valavanis A: MR identification of carotid artery involvement in septic cavernous sinus thrombosis. *Int J Neurorad* 2:290-295, 1996.

Schwartzberg DG: Imaging of pituitary gland tumors. *Semin US CT MR* 13:207-223, 1992.

Scotti G, Yu CY, Dillon WP, et al: MR imaging of cavernous sinus involvement by pituitary adenomas. *AJNR* 9:657-664, 1988.

Scotti G, Yu CY, Dillon WP, et al: MR imaging of cavernous sinus involvement by pituitary adenomas. *Am J Roentgenol* 151:799-806, 1988.

Shimono T, Hatabu H, Kasagi K, et al: Rapid progression of pituitary hyperplasia in humans with primary hypothyroidism: demonstration with MR imaging. *Radiology* 213:383-398, 1999.

Sigal R, Monnet O, De Baere T, et al: Adenoid cystic carcarinoma of the head and neck: evaluation with MR imaging and clinical-pathologic correlation in 27 patients. *Radiology* 184:95-102, 1992.

Simmons GE, Suchnicki JE, Rak KM, Damiano TR: MR imaging of the pituitary stalk: size, shape, and enhancement pattern. *AJNR* 159:375-377, 1992.

Simonetta AB: Imaging of suprasellar and parasellar tumors. *Neuroimaging Clin North Am* 9:717-732, 1999.

Stadnik T, Stevenaert A, Beckers A, et al: Pituitary microadenomas: diagnosis with two and three dimensional MR imaging at 1.5 T before and after injection of gadolinium. *Radiology* 176:419-428, 1990.

Steiner E, Imhof H, Knosp E: Gd-DTPA-enhanced high resolution MR imaging of pituitary adenomas. *Radiographics* 9:587-598, 1989.

Steiner E, Knosp E. Herold CJ, et al: Pituitary adenomas: findings of postoperative MR imaging. *Radiology* 185:521-527, 1992.

Sumida M, Uozumi T, Mukada K, et al: MRI of pituitary adenomas: the position of the normal pituitary gland. *Neuroradiology* 36: 295-297, 1994.

Sumida M, Uozumi T, Mukada K, et al: Rathke cleft cysts: correlation of enhanced MR and surgical findings. *AJNR* 15:525-532, 1994.

Sumida M, Uozumi T, Yamanaka M, et al: Displacement of the normal pituitary gland by sellar and juxtasellar tumours: surgical-MRI correlation and use in differential diagnosis. *Neuroradiology* 36:372-375, 1994.

Takano K, Utsunomiya H, Ono H, et al: Normal development of the pituitary gland: assessment with three-dimensional MR volumetry. *AJNR* 20:312-315, 1999.

Teramoto A, Hirakawa K, Sanno N, Osamura Y: Incidental pituitary lesions in 1,000 unselected autopsy specimens. *Radiology* 193:161-164, 1994.

Tien R, Dillon WP: MR imaging of cavernous hemangioma of the optic chiasm. *J Comput Assist Tomogr* 13:1087, 1989.

Tien R, Kurcharczyk J, Kucharczyk W: MR imaging of the brain in patients with diabetes insipidus. *AJNR* 12:533-542, 1991.

Tien RD, Newton TH, McDermott MW, et al: Thickened pituitary stalk on MR images in patients with diabetes insipidus and Langerhans cell histiocytosis. *AJNR* 11:703-708, 1990.

Tsunoda A, Okuda O, Sato K: MR height of the pituitary gland as a function of age and sex: especially physiological hypertrophy in adolescence and in climacterium. *AJNR* 18:551-554, 1997.

Vasile M, Marsot-Dupuch K, Kujas M, et al: Idiopathic granulomatous hypophysitis: clinical and imaging features. *Neuroradiology* 39:7-11, 1997.

Voelker JL, Campbell RL, Muller J: Clinical radiographic and pathological features of Rathke's cleft cysts. *J Neurosurg* 74:535-544, 1991.

Vogl TJ, Stemmler J, Scriba PC, et al: Sarciodosis of the hypothalamus and pituitary stalk. *Eur J Radiol* 2:76-78, 1992.

Vogler R, Castillo M: Dural cavernous angioma: MR features. *AJNR* 16:773-774, 1995.

Weissbuch SS: Explanation and implications of MR signal changes within pituitary adenomas after bromocriptime therapy. *AJNR* 7:214-216, 1986.

Whyte AM, Sage, MR, Brophy BP: Imaging of large Rathke's cleft cysts by CT and MRI: report of two cases. *Neuroradiology* 35:258-260, 1993.

Wolansky LJ, Gallagher JD, Heary RF, et al: MRI of pituitary abscess: two cases and review of the literature. *Neuroradiology* 39:499-503, 1997.

Wolansky LJ, Leavitt GD, Elias BJ, et al: MRI of pituitary hyperplasia in hypothyroidism. *Neuroradiology* 38: 50-52, 1996.

Wolansky LJ, Rao SB, Schulder M, et al: Extrasellar extension of pituitary lesions: comparison of T2-weighted fast spin-echo MRI with T1-weighted sequences. *Int J Neurorad* 2:147-152, 1996.

Wolpert SM, Osborne M, Anderson M, et al: The bright pituitary gland—a normal MR appearance in infancy. *AJNR* 9:1-3, 1988.

Yoon P-H, Kim D-I, Jeon P, et al: Pituitary adenomas: early postoperative MR imaging after transsphenoidal resection. *AJNR* 22:1097-1104, 2001.

Young SC, Grossman RI, Goldberg HI, et al: MR of vascular encasement in parasellar masses: comparison with angiography and CT. *AJNR* 9:35-38, 1988.

Yousem DM, Atlas SW, Grossman RI, et al: MR imaging of Tolosa-Hunt syndrome. *AJNR* 10:1181-1184, 1989.

Yuh WTC, Fisher DJ, Nguyen HD, et al: Sequential MR enhancement pattern in normal pituitary gland and in pituitary adenoma. *AJNR* 15:101-108, 1994.

Zimmerman RA: Imaging of intrasellar, suprasellar and parasellar tumors. *Semin Roentgenal* 25:174-197, 1990.

Zournas C, Trakadas S, Kapaki E, et al: Gadopentetate dimeglumine-enhanced MR in the diagnosis of the Tolosa-Hunt syndrome. *AJNR* 16:942-944, 1995.

# CHAPTER 7

# Other Masses

### Case 282

27-year-old man with a history of sudden collapse.
(coronal, noncontrast T1-weighted SE scan)

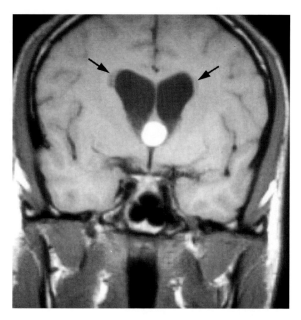

**Colloid Cyst**

### Case 283

44-year-old man presenting with headaches.
(coronal, noncontrast T1-weighted SE scan)

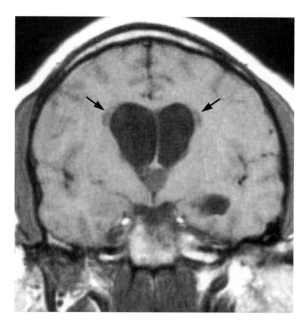

**Colloid Cyst**

Colloid cysts of the third ventricle characteristically present as round, midline masses at the foramina of Monro. These lesions arise from the anterior roof of the third ventricle. They are typically about one centimeter in diameter at the time of diagnosis, although larger cysts are occasionally encountered (see Case 289).

The signal intensity of colloid cysts may be high, low, or intermediate on either T1-weighted or T2-weighted scans. Short T1 values, as in Case 282, may reflect thickly proteinaceous material and/or the presence of paramagnetic metals. Low intensity on T1-weighted images, seen in Case 283, usually correlates with a more watery content.

Coronal and sagittal MR scans add anatomical detail and new tissue contrast to the CT evaluation of lesions near the foramina of Monro. The coronal examinations in the above cases precisely localize the lesions to the junction of the lateral and third ventricles, differentiating the cysts from other potential suprasellar or hypothalamic masses. (Compare to Cases 263 and 275.)

The strategic position of colloid cysts leads to hydrocephalus as the masses enlarge. The lateral ventricles are distended in both of the above cases, and periventricular edema is present *(arrows)*.

Colloid cysts of the third ventricle are occasionally associated with single or recurrent episodes of explosive headache or collapse, as in Case 282. Such sudden events are probably due to a rapid increase in intracranial pressure, caused by acute ventricular obstruction by a somewhat mobile cyst.

## Case 284

59-year-old man complaining of
severe, intermittent headaches.
(axial, noncontrast T2-weighted SE scan)

## Case 285

19-year-old woman presenting with headaches.
(axial, noncontrast scan; SE 2500/45)

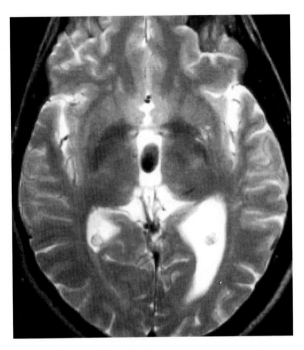

**Colloid Cyst**

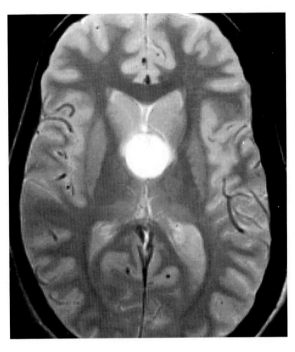

**Colloid Cyst**

The content of colloid cysts varies from liquid to gelatinous to caseous in consistency. Together with variable amounts of paramagnetic materials, this range of hydration and inspissation can cause a variety of signal intensities on long TR spin echo images.

The cyst in Case 284 is well-defined as a low intensity filling defect within the superior portion of the third ventricle. By contrast, the larger cyst of Case 285 demonstrates uniformly high intensity.

Occasional colloid cysts are nearly isointense to surrounding tissues on both T1-weighted and T2-weighted MR scans. Such lesions may be more easily diagnosed as high attenuation masses on CT studies.

In a young patient with a relatively large midline mass as in Case 285, the possibility of craniopharyngioma, hypo-thalamic glioma, suprasellar germinoma, or suprasellar extension of a pituitary adenoma could be considered. Coronal and sagittal views assist in the differential diagnosis by demonstrating that a colloid cyst arises from the superior margin of the third ventricle, above other potential suprasellar masses.

The size of a colloid cyst does not correlate precisely with the presence or severity of hydrocephalus. The large cyst in Case 285 is not associated with ventricular enlargement or periventricular edema.

The origin of colloid cysts is controversial. Recent studies have suggested that these lesions probably arise from ectopic endoderm rather than from neuroepithelium.

### Case 286

34-year-old man presenting with hydrocephalus.
(sagittal, postcontrast T1-weighted SE scan)

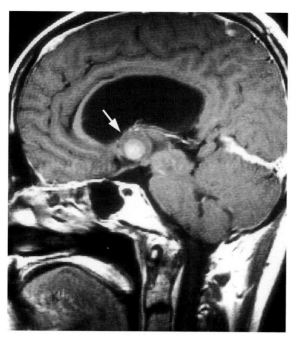

**Colloid Cyst**

### Case 287

41-year-old man presenting with
loss of consciousness.
(axial, noncontrast scan; SE 2500/45)

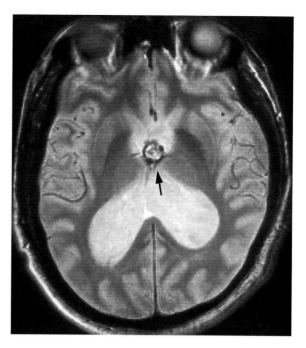

**Colloid Cyst**

Many colloid cysts are simple, round masses of uniform signal intensity. Occasional lesions have a more complex character, as illustrated above.

Concentric layering of different signal intensities may cause a target-like appearance within some colloid cysts, as seen in Case 286. The central zone of short T1 values was apparent on precontrast scans. (Contrast enhancement within colloid cysts is unusual; see Case 289.)

Case 287 demonstrates a colloid cyst with mixed signal intensity and irregular margins. At surgery, the cyst was found to have ruptured, with partial evacuation of its contents and presumed collapse of previously bulging contours.

A number of tumors may occur near the foramen of Monro and should be considered in the differential diagnosis of colloid cysts. Ependymomas, subependymomas, oligodendrogliomas, and astrocytomas can all arise at the ventricular margin and project into the frontal horn (see Cases 123, 129, and 344). Central neurocytomas regularly occupy the anterior body and/or frontal horn of the lateral ventricle (see Cases 342 and 343). Chordoid gliomas are well-defined, homogeneous, intensely enhancing, and histologically distinct tumors that typically involve the third ventricle (see discussion of Case 245). Patients with tuberous sclerosis often demonstrate subependymal tubers and giant cell astrocytomas along the lateral margin of the foramen of Monro (see Cases 896 and 897), in contrast to the medial location of colloid cysts.

Prominent enhancement of the dura and deep venous system in Case 286 had no clinical correlation apart from hydrocephalus and increased intracranial pressure.

### Case 288

5-year-old boy presenting with headaches.
(coronal, noncontrast T1-weighted SE scan)

### Case 289

19-year-old woman presenting with headaches.
(coronal, postcontrast T1-weighted SE scan)

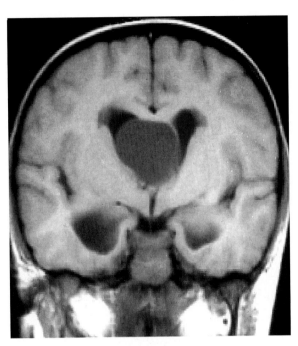

**Cystic Astrocytoma of the Septum Pellucidum**

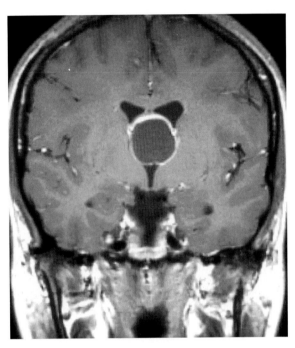

**Colloid Cyst of the Third Ventricle**
(same patient as Case 285)

Not all cystic masses at the foramen of Monro are colloid cysts. Suprasellar or third ventricular cysts (e.g., craniopharyngiomas or cysticercosis) can enlarge superiorly to occupy a similar location (see Cases 250 and 259).

Deep frontal lesions may also involve the midline. Gliomas commonly arise near the frontal horns and frequently extend into the septum pellucidum. In Case 288, the midline cystic tumor resembles Case 289 but is located superior to the foramina of Monro.

Conversely, large colloid cysts can mimic other midline masses. The rim of peripheral contrast enhancement in Case 289 combines with the size of the cyst to suggest a neoplasm. Peripheral contrast enhancement is occasionally associated with colloid cysts on CT or MR scans, usually reflecting surrounding reactive tissue rather than enhancement of the cyst's epithelium. Central contrast enhancement is rare.

Despite its somewhat unusual size and enhancement, the lesion in Case 289 is clearly centered at the level of the foramina of Monro. Recognition of this characteristic location helps to establish the diagnosis.

## Case 290

21-year-old woman complaining of dizziness.
(sagittal, noncontrast T1-weighted SE scan)

## Case 291

76-year-old woman presenting with
a transient ischemic attack.
(axial, noncontrast FLAIR scan)

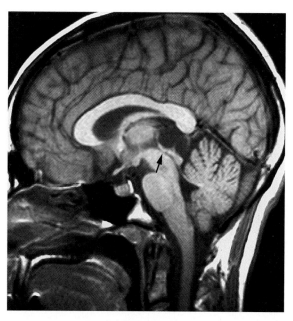

**Pineal Cyst**

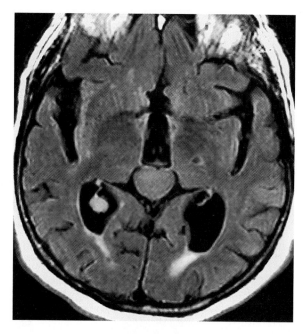

**Pineal Cyst**

Pineal cysts are commonly encountered as incidental findings on MR studies. Small cysts within the substance of the pineal gland rarely cause diagnostic concern. Larger cysts may replace and expand the gland, causing localized mass effect and raising the question of a pineal neoplasm.

The signal intensity of pineal cysts is typically somewhat higher than that of ventricular CSF. This difference may be difficult to appreciate on T1-weighted scans such as Case 290 or on T2-weighted images (see Case 292).

However, FLAIR sequences usually demonstrate that the content of a pineal cyst is not simple cerebrospinal fluid, as illustrated in Case 291. Such images distinguish pineal cysts from arachnoid cysts of the quadrigeminal cistern (see Cases 818 and 819).

Large pineal cysts commonly cause moderate compression of the underlying midbrain tectum, as illustrated by Case 290 (notice the aqueductal narrowing; *arrow*). The majority of patients with this finding have no related symptoms. Rarely, clinical evidence of dorsal midbrain dysfunction (Parinaud's syndrome) or radiographic signs of aqueductal compromise are encountered.

A small, old infarct is present at the lateral margin of the left thalamus in Case 291. Age-related changes cause high signal intensity along the margins of the occipital horns.

**Case 292**

67-year-old woman presenting with
a transient ischemic attack.
(axial, noncontrast T2-weighted FSE scan)

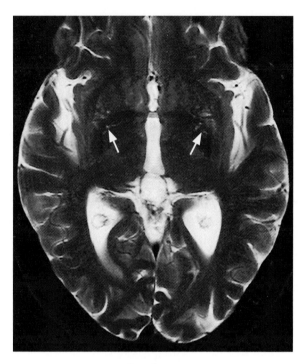

**Pineal Cyst**

**Case 293**

21-year-old woman being evaluated for dizziness.
(axial, postcontrast T1-weighted SE scan with MTS)

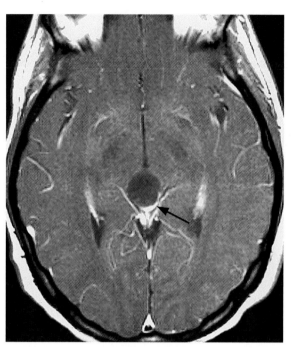

**Pineal Cyst**
(same patient as Case 290)

Pineal cysts are usually homogeneous and nearly isointense with surrounding CSF on T2-weighted images, as in Case 292. Hemorrhage into a cyst occasionally causes shortening of T1 and T2 values. Sedimentation levels of blood products may be noted within hemorrhagic cysts.

Contrast enhancement is often seen at the perimeter of the cyst (*arrow,* Case 293), due to displaced residual parenchyma and/or adjacent vessels. Contrast material may accumulate within the center of a pineal cyst on delayed scans and may remain for a day or more.

Benign pineal cysts are typically simple, round lesions with uniform peripheral enhancement as illustrated in Cases 290 to 293. However, heterogeneous cysts with eccentric, nodular contrast enhancement (presumably representing displaced pineal tissue) have been reported. Such features raise the possibility of a cystic pineal neoplasm (e.g., pineocytoma) and warrant follow-up observation.

Prominent perivascular spaces are present at the inferior margin of the lentiform nuclei bilaterally in Case 292 *(arrows).*

## Case 294A

19-year-old man presenting with
blurred vision and headaches.
(sagittal, noncontrast T1-weighted SE scan)

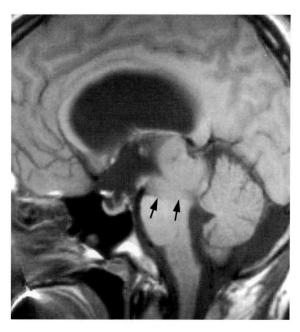

**Germinoma**

## Case 294B

Same patient.
(axial, noncontrast T2-weighted SE scan)

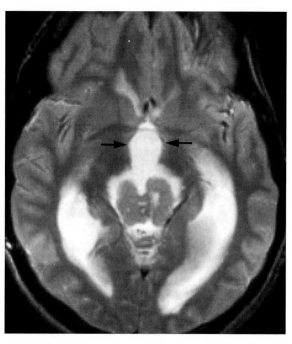

**Germinoma**

---

Germ cell tumors are the most common pineal masses. Within this category, germinomas are the most frequent pathology. (Other pineal germ cell tumors include teratoma, choriocarcinoma, embryonal cell carcinoma, and endodermal sinus tumor.) Pineal germinomas occur with a 9 to 1 male predominance. (Girls more often have suprasellar versions of this tumor; see Cases 254 and 311.) Germinomas may also present in the basal ganglia, particularly in boys and young men.

Pineal germinomas are often quite homogeneous in signal intensity, as seen above. The T2-weighted scan in Case 294B demonstrates the tumor to be nearly isointense to gray matter. This finding is associated with highly cellular neoplasms and has been noted in germinomas, medulloblastomas, primary CNS lymphomas, and densely cellular gliomas. Hemorrhage may occur within germinomas, as in other germ cell tumors of the pineal gland (see Cases 297 and 298).

Germinomas are unencapsulated tumors that may invade adjacent parenchyma. In particular, pineal germinomas often grow anteriorly along the walls of the third ventricle. Bilobed anterior extensions of the mass in Case 294B are well outlined by a halo of intense edema. This pattern of ventral growth may mimic an intraaxial lesion of the diencephalon or hypothalamus.

The clinical presentation of pineal tumors usually reflects hydrocephalus from obstruction of the posterior third ventricle and aqueduct, as in this case. The sagittal view of Case 294A demonstrates inferior bulging of the floor of the third ventricle and stretching of the corpus callosum. The axial plane in Case 294B documents widening of the third ventricle *(arrows)* and dilatation of the temporal and occipital horns of the lateral ventricles. Occasional germinomas are associated with precocious puberty, predominantly in males.

Germinomas are usually radiosensitive. Even bulky masses may disappear completely without recurrence after a course of radiation therapy.

# DIFFERENTIAL DIAGNOSIS:
## HOMOGENEOUS MASS IN THE PINEAL REGION

### Case 295

25-year-old woman presenting with
headaches and weight loss.
(sagittal, noncontrast T1-weighted SE scan)

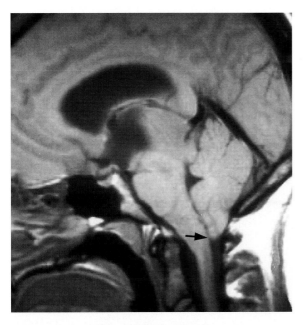

**Diencephalic Glioma**

### Case 296

43-year-old woman presenting with headaches
following an automobile accident.
(sagittal, noncontrast T1-weighted SE scan)

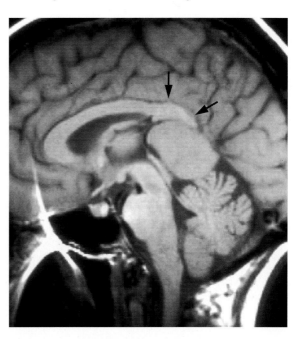

**Subsplenial Meningioma**

---

The differential diagnosis of pineal region masses includes a number of intraaxial and extraaxial pathologies. Gliomas of the brainstem or thalamus may extend into the pineal region to mimic a primary pineal tumor. For example, Case 295 is quite similar in appearance to Case 294A. The potential resemblance of pineal tumors and gliomas is increased by the tendency of the former to invaginate ventrally into adjacent parenchyma (see Case 294B).

A number of clues can contribute to distinguishing gliomas from pineal tumors: (1) eccentricity is more typical of gliomas arising in the pineal region than of true pineal neoplasms; (2) gliomas often demonstrate higher signal intensity than pineal tumors on T2-weighted images; and (3) contrast enhancement of pineal tumors is usually intense, while that of deep gliomas may be much less impressive. None of these considerations is individually reliable, but their combination can be helpful.

Meningiomas are among the extrapineal lesions that may occur in the quadrigeminal region. The tumor in Case 296 is clearly extraaxial, with elevation of the splenium *(arrows)* and flattening of the quadrigeminal plate. Homogeneous contrast enhancement within a meningioma may resemble that of a germinoma.

On CT scans, a patent vein of Galen "aneurysm" would also be included in this differential diagnosis. The characteristic appearance of flow in such lesions is diagnostic on MR studies (see Cases 746 and 747). However, a thrombosed vein of Galen aneurysm may resemble a hemorrhagic pineal neoplasm on MR images.

The cerebellar tonsils in Case 295 extend below the plane of the foramen magnum with peg-like morphology *(arrow)*, suggesting a Chiari I hindbrain malformation as well as caudal displacement. (Compare to Case 294A, where the posterior fossa is not "tight" despite comparable hydrocephalus and mesencephalic mass effect.)

**187**

### Case 297

12-year-old boy presenting with headaches, papilledema, and markedly elevated serum levels of human chorionic gonadotropin.
(axial, noncontrast T2-weighted SE scan)

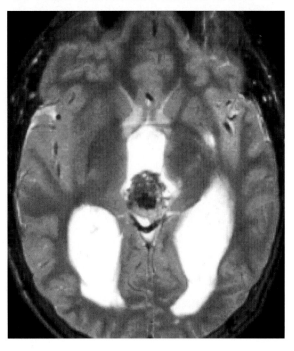

**Choriocarcinoma**

### Case 298

4-year-old girl presenting with increased intracranial pressure.
(axial, noncontrast T2-weighted SE scan)

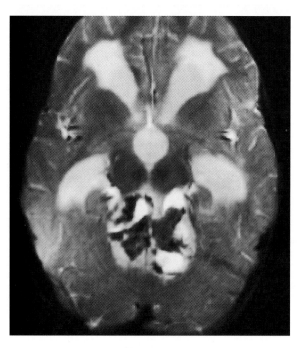

**Teratoma**

Germ cell tumors of the pineal gland other than germinomas are uncommon masses of variable appearance. They are often more heterogeneous than germinomas, with frequent cysts, calcification, and hemorrhage. Lipid components may be present in pineal teratomas.

The choriocarcinoma in Case 297 occupies the typical position of a pineal neoplasm in the midline at the posterior margin of the third ventricle. Obstruction of the aqueduct has caused hydrocephalus. Areas of T2-shortening within the mass suggest hemorrhage or calcification. (T1-shortening indicating subacute blood products was present on T1-weighted scans.)

The teratoma in Case 298 is even more complex. Multiple cysts with high signal intensity are intermixed with solid tissue and low intensity foci suggesting hemorrhage and/or calcification. This coarse, heterogeneous texture is typical of intracranial teratomas (see Case 309). Similar complexity can occur within pineoblastomas (see Case 306).

It is not possible to reliably distinguish among the several types of pineal germ cell tumors on the basis of MR characteristics. Even pathological determinations are difficult, since mixed histologies are frequent in these masses. Serum levels of human chorionic gonadotropin (HCG) and alpha fetoprotein (AFP) can assist in the differential diagnosis: choriocarcinomas are often associated with high HCG levels (as in Case 297), while teratomas may cause elevation of serum AFP.

# DIFFERENTIAL DIAGNOSIS:
## PINEAL REGION MASS CONTAINING BLOOD PRODUCTS

### Case 299

27-year-old man presenting with a sixth nerve palsy.
(axial, noncontrast T2-weighted SE scan)

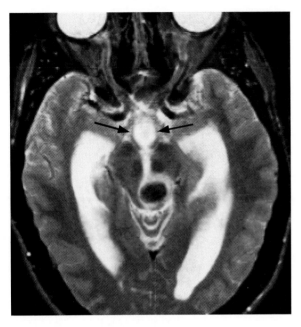

**Metastatic Melanoma**
(hemorrhagic)

### Case 300

68-year-old woman complaining of headaches.
(axial, noncontrast T2-weighted FSE scan)

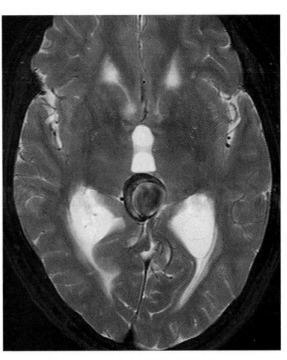

**Aneurysm**
(of the posterior cerebral artery)

---

As illustrated on the previous page, hemorrhage is common within germ cell tumors of the pineal gland. Tumors of pineal cell origin are occasionally hemorrhagic. Several additional pathologies can also present as pineal region masses containing blood products.

In Case 299, a mass within the dorsal midbrain demonstrates homogeneously low signal intensity outlined by a rim of edema. Metastases from melanoma are commonly hemorrhagic, as discussed in Cases 7 and 8. T2-shortening in such lesions is usually attributable to the presence of blood products (see Chapter 13); the paramagnetic effect of melanin itself causes T1-shortening but only a mild decrease in T2 values.

Crescentic layers of variably low signal intensity are present along the anterior and right lateral margins of the mass in Case 300. Such laminated morphology suggests thrombus adherent to the wall of a vascular structure (see Cases 732 and 734). The low intensity occupying the majority of the mass was proven to represent flow void by subsequent MR angiography.

The location of the mass in Case 300 raises the possibility of an "aneurysm" of the vein of Galen (see Cases 746 and 747). However, presentation of a patent vein of Galen aneurysm at age 68 would be highly unusual. Angiography in this case instead demonstrated a dysplastic aneurysm arising from the retromesencephalic segment of a posterior cerebral artery.

Both the intraaxial mass in Case 299 and the extraaxial lesion in Case 300 cause obstructive hydrocephalus. The dilated anterior recesses of the third ventricle in Case 299 *(arrows)* lie immediately posterior to the convergence of the optic nerves and divergence of the optic tracts at the optic chiasm.

**Case 301**

19-year-old man presenting with headaches. (coronal, postcontrast T1-weighted SE scan)

**Case 302**

12-year-old boy presenting with headaches. (coronal, postcontrast T1-weighted SE scan)

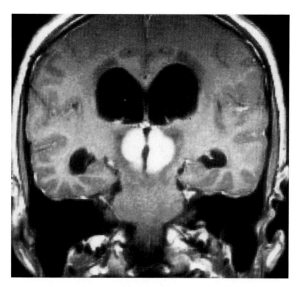

**Germinoma**
(same patient as Case 294)

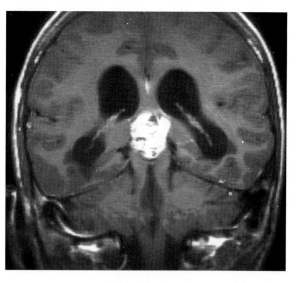

**Choriocarcinoma**
(same patient as Case 297)

Germinomas usually demonstrate intense, homogeneous contrast enhancement, as in Case 301. Parenchymal invasion along the margins of the third ventricle in this case is well demonstrated by the coronal plane.

The enhancement pattern of nongerminomatous germ cell tumors of the pineal gland is typically more heterogeneous. In Case 302, the overall appearance remains one of solid enhancement. In other cases, particularly of teratoma, enhancement may be less prominent. Large, nonenhancing regions in such tumors may reflect cysts, lipid material, coarse calcification, and/or necrosis.

Germinomas are among the primary CNS neoplasms associated with distant meningial or ventricular implants from CSF seeding. A search for isointense or enhancing cisterns and sulci is therefore appropriate in these patients. Contrast-enhanced MR scans are more sensitive than CT studies for the detection of meningeal dissemination of tumor (see Cases 165-167).

Hydrocephalus is present in both of the above cases, with prominent periventricular edema in Case 301.

## Case 303

13-year-old boy presenting with diabetes
insipidus and decreased visual acuity.
(sagittal, noncontrast T1-weighted SE scan)

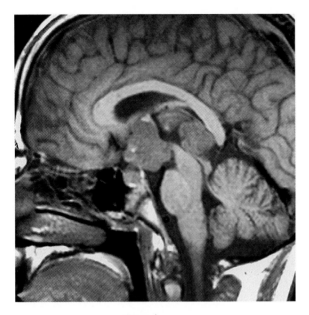

**Germinoma**

## Case 304

19-year-old man admitted after
an automobile accident.
(axial, postcontrast T1-weighted SE scan with MTS)

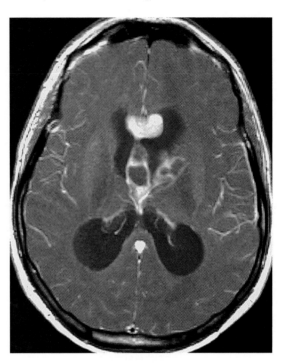

**Germinoma**

Intracranial germinomas occur in several locations outside of the pineal gland. Suprasellar germinomas may be solitary masses (see Cases 254 and 311) or arise in association with a tumor in the pineal region, as in Case 303. In the latter instance it is likely that the simultaneous involvement of the anterior and posterior portions of the third ventricle reflects CSF dissemination of tumor cells from one site to the other.

By itself, the lobulated suprasellar and retrosellar mass in Case 303 could raise consideration of a craniopharyngioma or optic/hypothalamic glioma. The presence of an accompanying lesion within the pineal region narrows the differential diagnosis, strongly suggesting germinoma.

Germinomas occasionally arise in the basal ganglia and/or periventricular regions of the cerebral hemispheres, as illustrated in Case 304. The multifocal tumor in this case demonstrates both solid and peripheral patterns of enhancement. The uniformly enhancing component at the anterior margin of the frontal horns was homogeneously low in intensity on T2-weighted images (comparable to Case 294B), implying dense cellularity.

CSF spread of germinomas may lead to meningeal implants as well as multiple masses along ventricular margins. The entire spinal canal should be examined when a potential intracranial germinoma is discovered.

Note the absence of the normal neurohypophyseal "bright spot" in Case 303, correlating with the history of diabetes insipidus (see discussion in Cases 246 and 247).

### Case 305

9-year-old boy presenting with
headaches and diplopia.
(sagittal, noncontrast T1-weighted SE scan)

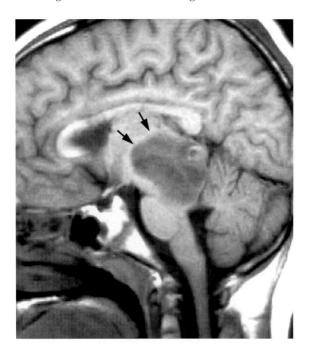

**Pineoblastoma**

### Case 306

2-year-old boy presenting with decreased level of
consciousness on the morning of admission.
(axial, postcontrast T1-weighted SE scan)

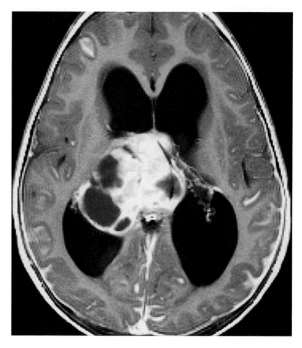

**Pineoblastoma**

---

Tumors of true pineal cell origin are much less common than germ cell tumors. Pineocytomas are relatively well-differentiated pineal cell neoplasms. They may be homogeneously solid or grossly cystic masses. Intense contrast enhancement is usual and comparable to germinomas, although pineocytomas are more likely to have lobulated margins.

Pineoblastomas are less well-differentiated and more malignant. Many neuropathologists classify these lesions in the category of primitive neuroectodermal tumors. They often present as bulky and heterogeneous masses.

Case 305 demonstrates mixed signal intensity, with areas of subacute hemorrhage interspersed among long T1 components. On T2-weighted scans, pineoblastomas may be relatively isointense, reflecting dense cellularity and analogous to germinomas, or high in intensity. A mixed appearance comparable to Case 298 may be encountered. Contrast enhancement is usually prominent and heterogeneous, as in Case 306.

Like germinomas, pineocytomas and pineoblastomas frequently demonstrate CSF spread. Ventricular and meningeal metastases may be present at the time of diagnosis or on follow-up studies. Many sulci in Case 306 are filled with enhancing tumor.

## Case 307

5-year-old-girl being followed after presenting with bilateral retinoblastomas at age 18 months. (coronal, postcontrast T1-weighted SE scan)

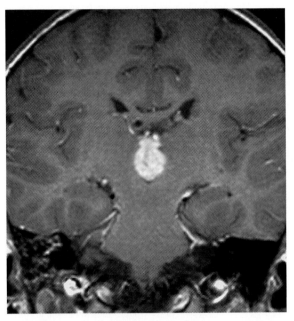

**Pineoblastoma**
*(trilateral retinoblastoma)*

## Case 308

8-year-old boy presenting with precocious puberty. (axial, postcontrast T1-weighted SE scan)

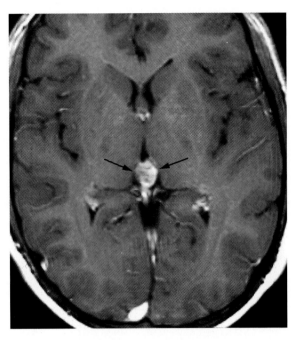

**Germinoma**

The enhancing tumors in these cases have comparable imaging characteristics, emphasizing the difficulty in distinguishing between masses of pineal cell origin and germ cell neoplasms on MR studies. Both masses are located at the posterior-superior margin of the third ventricle. Both are mildly heterogeneous and slightly lobulated. Both are small, and neither has caused hydrocephalus. There is no evidence of intraventricular or meningeal seeding on either scan.

CT images are occasionally helpful in the differential diagnosis of a pineal region mass. Pineal cell tumors tend to "explode" or disperse preexisting calcification of the gland, whereas germinomas tend to surround or engulf previous calcification.

The clinical context strongly suggests the correct diagnosis in both of the above cases. Children who present with bilateral retinoblastomas as infants or toddlers carry an autosomal dominant mutation that frequently leads to development of a pineoblastoma several years later. Case 307 is an example of this condition, often called *trilateral retinoblastoma*. Such children may alternatively present with a primitive neuroectodermal tumor in the suprasellar region. Both pineal and suprasellar masses occur in some cases *(quadrilateral retinoblastoma)*.

Germinomas are occasionally associated with precocious puberty, especially in boys, as illustrated by Case 308. Hypothalamic hamartomas (see Cases 274 and 275) can also cause this syndrome. The region of the third ventricle should be closely examined on MR scans of children with premature sexual development.

Like germinomas, pineoblastomas are typically unencapsulated, with frequent invasion of adjacent parenchyma and/or leptomeningeal dissemination.

**Case 309A**

16-year-old girl presenting with
worsening headaches.
(sagittal, noncontrast T1-weighted SE scan)

**Case 309B**

Same patient.
(axial, postcontrast T1-weighted SE scan)

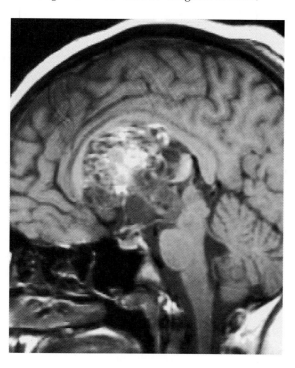

**Teratoma**

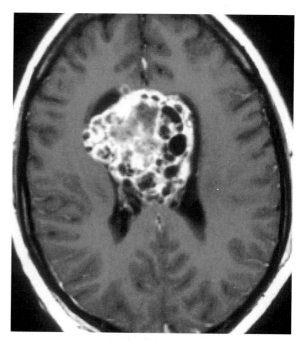

**Teratoma**

Teratomas are among the germ cell tumors that may originate in the pineal region. Teratomas may also occur in hemispheric locations, sometimes presenting as congenital tumors in neonates.

The mass in Case 309 does involve the posterior portion of the third ventricle, but the bulk of the midline lesion is centered at the level of the lateral ventricles. The extensive areas of T1-shortening on the noncontrast scan (Case 309A) may represent lipid components and/or subacute hemorrhage, both of which are common in teratomas. A fat saturation MR sequence or correlation with a CT scan would distinguish between these possibilities.

Contrast enhancement within the lesion is intense (Case 309B), outlining multiple cysts or necrotic areas. Cysts are frequently found within teratomas, combining with hemorrhage, fat, and calcification to cause the striking heterogeneity characteristic of these tumors.

Malignant rhabdoid tumors (also called *atypical teratoid/rhabdoid tumors*) have recently been defined as a clinical entity distinct from other teratomas. These aggressive lesions may arise from neuroectodermal stem cells or germ cells, typically presenting by age two or three as large, heterogeneous masses. Malignant rhabdoid tumors may involve the brain primarily or as a metastasis from an extracranial site, most commonly the kidney. The lesions are similar to primitive neuroectodermal tumors (PNETs) in imaging characteristics (see Case 336) and resemble PNETs or rhabdomyosarcomas histologically. Malignant rhabdoid tumors carry a very poor prognosis, with frequent meningeal dissemination at the time of diagnosis.

# DIFFERENTIAL DIAGNOSIS:
## HETEROGENEOUS, SUPRASELLAR MASS IN A CHILD

### Case 310

2-year-old girl presenting with irritability.
(axial, postcontrast T1-weighted SE scan)

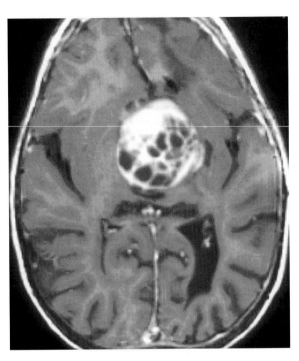

**Hypothalamic Glioma**

### Case 311

14-year-old girl presenting with decreased
vision and diabetes insipidus.
(axial, noncontrast T2-weighted SE scan)

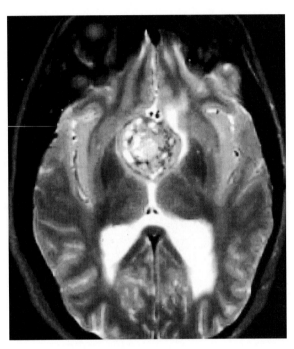

**Suprasellar Germinoma**
(same patient as Case 254)

As discussed in Cases 262-267, hypothalamic gliomas may demonstrate complex morphology with multiple cystic components. The heterogeneous architecture of the tumor in Case 310 closely resembles the appearance of the teratoma in Case 309 (as well as mimicking more common craniopharyngiomas).

Case 311 presents a T2-weighted scan of the hemorrhagic suprasellar germinoma seen in Case 254. The relatively low signal intensity of the tumor is due to dense cellularity and T2-shortening associated with blood products within the mass. The margin of the lesion is defined by a zone of surrounding edema. Central cystic areas are seen as high intensity foci, with an overall pattern resembling Cases 309 and 310.

As noted earlier, germinomas are the most common tumors of the pineal region. In a suprasellar location these lesions have been called *ectopic pinealomas* or *atypical teratomas*. Most patients with suprasellar germinomas are teenagers or young adults presenting with diabetes insipidus or visual impairment. The sex incidence for germinomas in this location is nearly equal, in contrast to the 9:1 male predominance in the pineal region.

The characteristic association of suprasellar germinomas with diabetes insipidus can assist in differential diagnosis. This symptom is rarely part of the initial presentation of craniopharyngiomas or hypothalamic gliomas.

# DERMOID CYSTS

## Case 312

51-year-old woman presenting with headaches.
(sagittal, noncontrast T1-weighted SE scan)

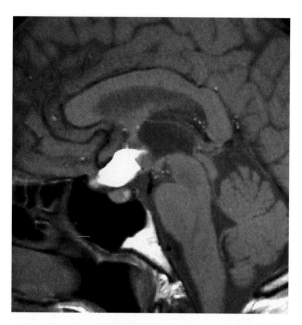

**Dermoid Cyst**

## Case 313

71-year-old woman presenting with
seizures and confusion.
(sagittal, noncontrast T1-weighted SE scan)

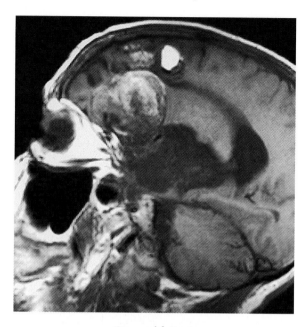

**Dermoid Cyst**

---

Dermoid tumors or "cysts" are benign masses arising from ectodermal cells enclosed intracranially during embryogenesis. In addition to squamous epithelium, dermoid cysts may contain skin appendages such as hair follicles, sweat glands, and sebaceous glands. Slow proliferation of these tissues leads to gradual accumulation of a pilosebaceous mass, with the congenital lesions often presenting in adulthood.

The lipid content of dermoid cysts causes high signal intensity on T1-weighted scans. This T1-shortening may entirely fill the lesion, as in Case 312, or be mixed with lower intensity proteinaceous material, as illustrated in Case 313. The internal architecture of a dermoid cyst may be correspondingly simple or complex.

The above cases also demonstrate that dermoid cysts vary greatly in size. Some lesions remain very circumscribed, while others enlarge to occupy major portions of the intracranial compartment.

Many dermoid cysts are found in the suprasellar or parasellar region, as illustrated by Case 312 (see also Case 257). Other common locations include the posterior fossa, near the fourth ventricle or between the cerebellar hemispheres. Lesions invaginating into the cerebral hemispheres, as in Case 313, are less frequent.

The occurrence of T1-shortening within a parasellar lesion is not specific for dermoid cysts. Craniopharyngiomas, Rathke's pouch cysts, hemorrhage into pituitary adenomas, cavernous hemangiomas, or an "ectopic" neurohypophysis can present a similar appearance (see Cases 254-257). Lipomas may also be located along the floor of the third ventricle in the retrosellar region, with prominent T1-shortening (see Case 276).

The specific diagnosis in Case 312 is enabled by the multiple tiny foci of high signal intensity within subarachnoid spaces some distance from the main mass (e.g., in the interpeduncular fossa, the cistern of the velum interpositum, and the pericallosal region). These small nodules represent droplets of lipid material that have leaked from the suprasellar dermoid cyst (see Cases 316 and 317).

A fat saturation pulse sequence was performed in Case 312 and demonstrated markedly reduced signal intensity throughout the mass.

## Case 314

67-year-old man presenting with a seizure.
(coronal, noncontrast T1-weighted SE scan)

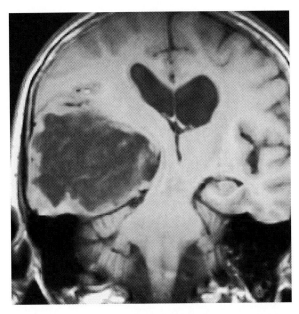

**Dermoid Cyst**

## Case 315

71-year-old woman presenting with confusion.
(axial, noncontrast T2-weighted FSE scan)

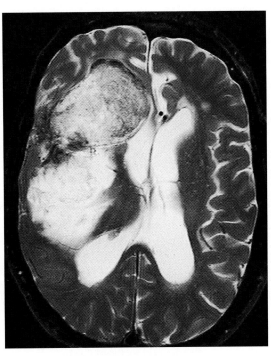

**Dermoid Cyst**
(same patient as Case 313)

Not all cranial (or spinal) dermoid cysts demonstrate T1-shortening. Mixed or low intensity may be noted on T1-weighted images, depending on the amount of contained hair and proteinaceous material and on the proportion of liquid and solid components.

The large dermoid cyst in Case 314 originated in the right parasellar region and invaginated far into the adjacent temporal and frontal lobes. Small areas of T1-shortening were present on more anterior scans, but the majority of the lesion was of low signal intensity on T1-weighted images. Dermoid cysts combining low signal intensity and lobulated margins may resemble the typical MR appearance of an epidermoid cyst (see Cases 320 and 321).

Case 315 provides a T2-weighted scan of the dermoid cyst in Case 313. Mixed intensity is apparent, with the posterior lobulation of the mass demonstrating more aqueous character. The textured low intensity within the anterior component of the lesion may reflect lipid material or hair; hemorrhage within dermoid cysts is rare. The posterior half of the tumor in Case 315 resembles an epidermoid cyst (compare to Cases 322 and 327), but the relative isointen-

sity seen more anteriorly would be unusual in an epidermoid tumor.

CT scans often demonstrate peripheral calcification surrounding a dermoid cyst. This characteristic feature is rarely appreciated on MR studies. Teratomas can also demonstrate both lipid material and calcification, but the latter is usually more dense and central. Lipomas are a third type of lesion in which lipid material may be seen with adjacent calcification apparent on CT scans but poorly demonstrated on MR studies.

The relatively minor midline shift associated with the large masses shown above indicates that they have grown very slowly. These congenital lesions typically do not present until well into adulthood.

The center of an uncomplicated dermoid cyst does not enhance on postcontrast scans. A thin layer of enhancement may be seen at the margin of the mass, reflecting displaced vascular structures and/or a reactive layer of fibrous tissue or thickened meninges. Enhancement within a dermoid cyst suggests superimposed infection and raises the question of an associated dermal sinus tract (see Cases 917-919).

### Case 316

45-year-old woman presenting with headaches.
(sagittal, noncontrast T1-weighted SE scan)

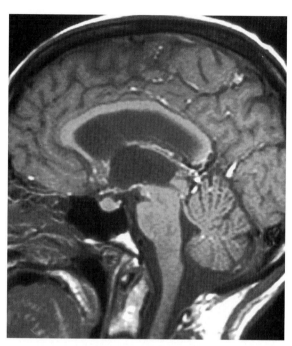

**Ruptured Dermoid Cyst**

### Case 317

47-year-old woman presenting with
a right visual field cut.
(axial, noncontrast scan; SE 2500/20)

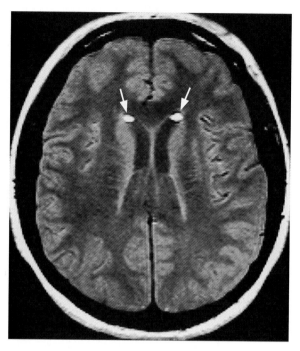

**Ruptured Dermoid Cyst**

Dermoid cysts may leak or rupture, releasing their content into the subarachnoid space and/or ventricular system. The resulting appearance of scattered lipid droplets within sulci and cisterns is demonstrated in Case 316. (The primary tumor in this case was located within the trigone of the left lateral ventricle.) A similar pattern can be caused by intracranial droplets of Pantopaque, an oily contrast material previously used for myelography and posterior fossa cisternography.

Cisternal fat droplets demonstrate low attenuation on CT scans and may be mistaken for pneumocephalus. An MR study such as Case 316 clearly distinguishes between air bubbles and fat droplets within the subarachnoid space when the clinical context is ambiguous (e.g., following head trauma).

In Case 317, small layers of lipid material float at the anterior margin of the frontal horns (arrows), reflecting rupture of a suprasellar dermoid cyst. Similar fat/fluid levels may rarely be seen within ventricles or cisterns in association with leaking teratomas.

Intraventricular rupture or leakage of fatty material is often clinically silent. Some patients experience a severe chemical meningitis, particularly when the contents of a ruptured cyst extend beyond the ventricles to involve the subarachnoid spaces.

### Case 318

10-year-old boy presenting with headaches.
(axial, noncontrast T1-weighted SE scan)

### Case 319

82-year-old woman presenting with left
body seizures following head trauma.
(coronal, noncontrast T1-weighted SE scan)

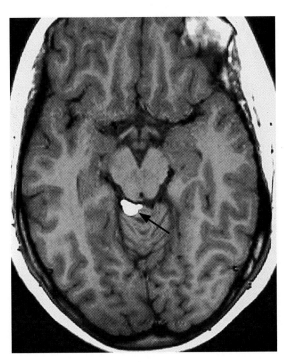

**Lipoma**

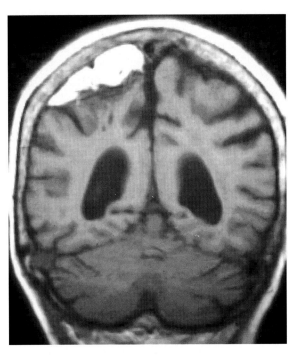

**Lipoma**

Lipomas present as high intensity lesions on T1-weighted images, potentially resembling dermoid cysts or other pathologies associated with T1-shortening. Several characteristic locations of intracranial lipomas may assist in differential diagnosis.

Interhemispheric lipomas are common, often associated with hypoplasia or agenesis of the corpus callosum (see Cases 859-862). Lipomas bordering the floor of the third ventricle have been illustrated in Case 276.

A third common location for intracranial lipomas is the quadrigeminal cistern, demonstrated in Case 318. Lipomas at this site may be unilateral or bilateral, usually measuring only a few millimeters in diameter. The absence of lipid material in other CSF spaces helps to distinguish small cisternal lipomas from free fat due to rupture of a dermoid cyst. The

mass in Case 318 demonstrated uniformly low signal intensity on a T2-weighted scan.

The convexity location of the lipoma in Case 319 is unusual. Such a lesion could be mistaken for a subacute subdural hematoma in the setting of recent head trauma and relevant symptoms. Although the overall morphology of the lipoma is plaque-like, the mild lobulation of the margins suggests the diagnosis (and would be atypical for subdural hemorrhage). The nature of the lesion was confirmed by homogeneously decreased signal intensity on a T2-weighted scan and on a fat saturation sequence.

Blood products within a small mass (e.g., hemorrhage in a trochlear schwannoma or thrombus in an unusual aneurysm) could be considered as rare alternatives in the differential diagnosis of Case 318.

### Case 320

51-year-old man presenting with facial numbness
and incoordination of the right arm.
(sagittal, noncontrast T1-weighted SE scan)

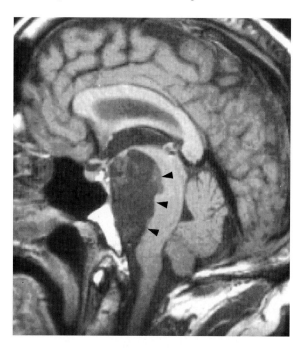

**Epidermoid Cyst**

### Case 321

47-year-old man presenting with
temporal lobe seizures.
(axial, postcontrast T1-weighted SE scan)

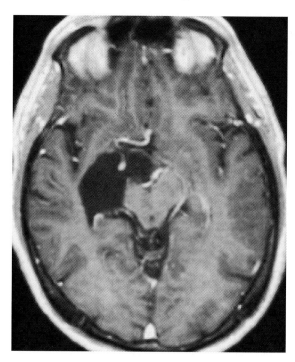

**Epidermoid Cyst**

The signal intensity of most epidermoid cysts is close to that of CSF on a variety of pulse sequences. However, subtle differences are usually apparent. In Case 320, the large prepontine lesion is slightly but definitely higher and less homogeneous in intensity than the CSF within the third ventricle.

Rare epidermoid cysts demonstrate short T1 values (and associated T2-shortening) resembling dermoid cysts. Such masses usually contain viscous liquid components rather than lipid material, with high signal intensity on T1-weighted scans due to enhanced relaxation of *water* protons.

MR is helpful in defining the characteristically lobulated surface of epidermoid cysts. In Case 320, the interface between the lesion and the brainstem is notably irregular, a feature that would be unusual for an arachnoid cyst. The

slow growth of this benign mass has led to impressive displacement and deformity of the brainstem (see Case 322) as well as marked superior bowing of the floor of the third ventricle.

The prepontine and cerebellopontine angle cisterns are common sites for epidermoid cysts. Another frequent location is the suprasellar and parasellar area, demonstrated in Case 321. Masses in this region may be midline or eccentric. Associated compression of the medial temporal lobes may present clinically as seizures or impairment of memory.

Note the lack of contrast enhancement in Case 321, which is characteristic of epidermoid cysts. This expanding extraaxial mass within the choroid fissure has invaginated into the adjacent temporal lobe and could be mistaken for a low grade glioma (compare to Case 81).

### Case 322

51-year-old man presenting with facial numbness
and incoordination of the right arm.
(axial, noncontrast T2-weighted SE scan)

### Case 323

50-year-old man presenting with a seizure.
(axial, noncontrast T2-weighted FSE scan)

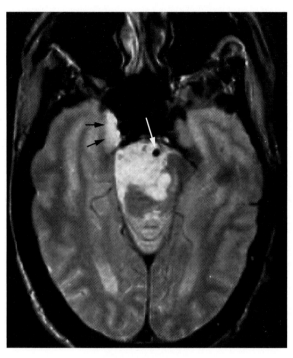

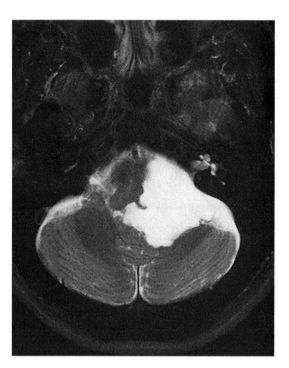

**Epidermoid Cyst**
(same patient as Case 320)

**Epidermoid Cyst**

---

The signal intensity of epidermoid cysts is typically high on T2-weighted scans.

In Case 322, prolonged T2 values within the lesion clearly define its lobulated contour and the marked deformity of the brainstem. Both of these features are hallmarks of a prepontine epidermoid tumor. Even more characteristic is the manner in which the mass has surrounded the vessels and cranial nerves in the region, insinuating itself between the basilar artery *(white arrow)* and the displaced midbrain.

The large epidermoid cyst in Case 323 has expanded the anterolateral recess of the fourth ventricle (compare to Cases 161, 164, and 327). The degree of compression of the left cerebellar hemisphere combines with the lack of reactive edema to suggest a long-standing, slow-growing mass. Lobulation at the margins of the lesion is typical of an epidermoid cyst.

The posterior fossa mass in Case 322 has grown into Meckel's cave on the right *(black arrows)*. Epidermoid cysts are among the lesions with a tendency to span the petrous apex (compare to Cases 61 and 203) and among the masses that may be responsible for trigeminal neuralgia or facial numbness.

### Case 324

55-year-old man with a history
of temporal lobe seizures.
(axial, noncontrast FLAIR scan)

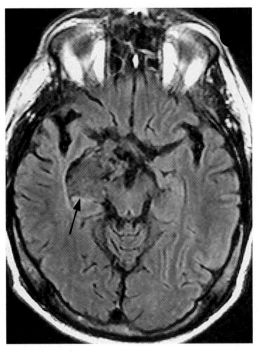

**Epidermoid Cyst**
(recurrent; same patient as Case 321)

### Case 325

Same patient.
(axial, noncontrast diffusion-
weighted echoplanar scan)

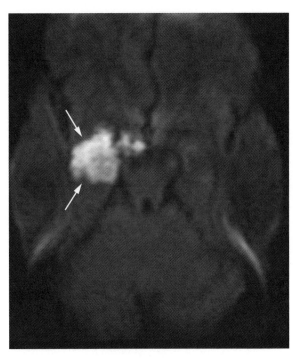

**Epidermoid Cyst**

---

The long T1 and T2 values characteristic of epidermoid inclusion cysts make these lesions difficult to distinguish from CSF by standard spin echo sequences. On such images, small epidermoid tumors may be hidden within cisterns, while larger epidermoid masses may resemble arachnoid cysts. FLAIR sequences and diffusion-weighted scans provide much better definition of epidermoid cysts, as illustrated above.

The medial right temporal mass in Cases 324 and 325 had been discovered and subtotally removed eight years earlier. (Case 321 is a T1-weighted scan of the lesion at that time.) Routine T1-weighted images of the recurrent epidermoid cyst closely resembled Case 321, with long T1 values mimicking CSF.

The FLAIR image in Case 324 shows intermediate signal intensity throughout the lesion *(arrow)*, distinguishing the content from aqueous fluid. The mass is clearly demarcated from the displaced temporal horn laterally and from the suprasellar cistern medially. Fine lobulation, typical of epidermoid cysts, is well demonstrated at the anteromedial margin of the lesion.

High signal intensity is apparent within the same mass in Case 325. This typical finding may represent restricted diffusion and/or "T2-shine through." The calculated apparent diffusion coefficient within some epidermoid cysts is low, but nearly normal values are demonstrated in other cases.

Although the signal-to-noise ratio of the echoplanar study in Case 325 is relatively low, high contrast between the lesion and surrounding tissue clearly defines the boundaries of pathology. A simple CSF-containing cyst within the choroid fissure, which could be considered on T1- and T2-weighted images in this case, should evidence rapid diffusion and is excluded from the differential diagnosis by the above scan.

Susceptibility artifact is present superior to the petrous ridges in Case 325.

## Case 326

36-year-old man presenting with
headaches and papilledema.
(sagittal, noncontrast T1-weighted SE scan)

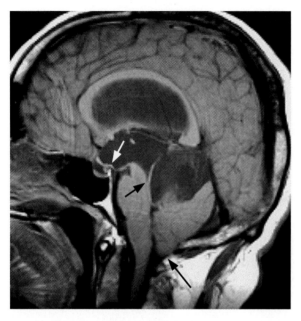

**Epidermoid Cyst**

## Case 327

44-year-old man presenting with
intractable hiccups.
(axial, noncontrast T2-weighted SE scan)

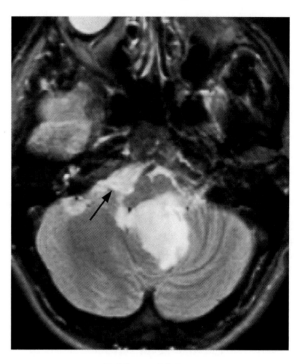

**Epidermoid Cyst**

The mass occupying the quadrigeminal region in Case 326 demonstrates T1 values that are close to CSF, but the lesion is mildly heterogeneous. Contours of the tumor are slightly lobulated. The marked thinning of the quadrigeminal plate and the prominent inferior displacement of the cerebellar vermis imply that the mass has grown slowly. Together, these features (and lack of enhancement on a postcontrast scan) suggest an epidermoid cyst, which was confirmed at surgery.

Epidermoid cysts are occasionally found within the fourth ventricle. Although rarely associated with hydrocephalus, such masses can grow to distort the brainstem. The dorsal medulla is deformed in Case 327, correlating with the patient's presenting symptoms. His hiccups resolved following resection of the lesion.

The differential diagnosis of an intraventricular mass with signal intensity similar to CSF includes tumors such as pilocytic astrocytomas and cysts such as cysticercosis. Most glial and neuroectodermal neoplasms occupying the fourth ventricle would demonstrate areas of contrast enhancement, unlike epidermoid (or dermoid) masses. The margins of cysticercosis cysts are usually smoothly rounded rather than finely lobulated (see Case 806).

Note the aqueductal obstruction in Case 326 *(short black arrow)* causing obstructive hydrocephalus. The floor of the third ventricle is inferiorly displaced, draping over the dorsum sella *(white arrow)*. The stretched corpus callosum arches over the lateral ventricles. These two findings can be helpful in distinguishing more subtle cases of communicating hydrocephalus from atrophic enlargement of the ventricles. Herniation of the cerebellar tonsils is also present *(long black arrow)*.

A small component of the lobulated tumor in Case 327 has extended through the right foramen of Luschka into the cerebellopontine angle *(arrow;* compare to the ependymoma in Case 161).

203

**Case 328**

6-month-old boy presenting with an enlarging head.
(sagittal, noncontrast T1-weighted SE scan)

**Case 329**

4-year-old boy presenting with developmental delay.
(axial, noncontrast T2-weighted SE scan)

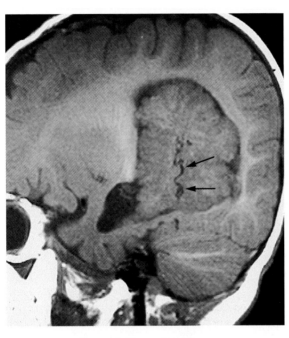

**Choroid Plexus Papilloma**

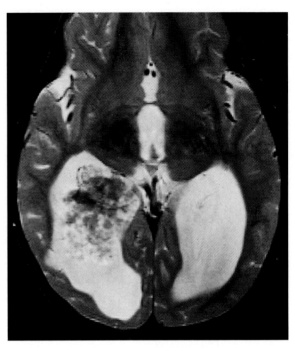

**Choroid Plexus Papilloma**

Choroid plexus papillomas in children are most common in the lateral ventricles, particularly on the left. They usually rise from the trigone and are often massive when discovered.

The homogeneous mass in Case 328 fills and expands the atrium of the lateral ventricle. Finely lobulated margins of the lesion qualify to be described as "papillary." These features strongly suggest the correct diagnosis, which is further supported by the presence of a large vessel extending into the tumor *(arrows)*. Choroid plexus papillomas are highly vascular neoplasms, and arterial supply from enlarged choroidal branches is usual. Angiography in Case 328 demonstrated a hypertrophied anterior choroidal artery corresponding to the flow void within the mass.

Case 329 presents a smaller choroid plexus papilloma outlined by CSF on a T2-weighted scan. The tumor itself is relatively low in signal intensity, reflecting dense cellularity (compare to the germinoma in Case 294 and lymphoma in Cases 348 and 349). Other potential causes of low intensity within choroid plexus tumors on long TR images include calcification and hemorrhage, both of which are common in these masses.

Choroid plexus papillomas and carcinomas are among the intracranial tumors that may be present at birth. They are often associated with hydrocephalus, sometimes due to excessive production of spinal fluid. More commonly, secondary communicating hydrocephalus develops after repeated tumor hemorrhages with high CSF loads of protein and cells.

### Case 330

6-month-old boy presenting with an enlarging head.
(axial, postcontrast T1-weighted SE scan with MTS)

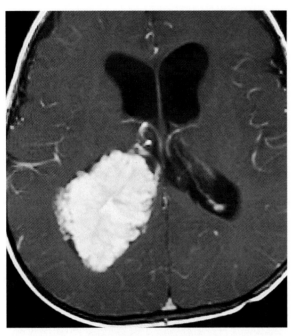

**Choroid Plexus Papilloma**
(same patient as Case 328)

### Case 331

76-year-old woman presenting with headaches.
(axial, postcontrast T1-weighted SE scan)

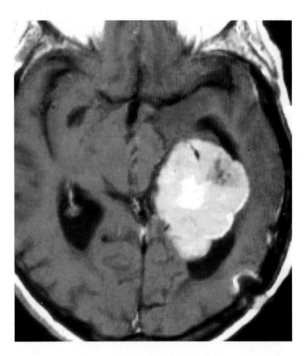

**Meningioma**

---

The age of the patient establishes the likely diagnosis in each of the above cases, although the location and morphology of the lesions are comparable. The lateral ventricle is the most common site for choroid plexus tumors in children, but papillomas in adults are usually infratentorial (see Case 335). Conversely, intraventricular meningiomas are often discovered in adults (see Cases 67-69) but are rarely encountered in pediatric patients.

Case 330 presents a postcontrast image of the choroid plexus papilloma in Case 328. Intense enhancement is typical of choroid plexus tumors. These neoplasms are highly vascular, with prominent angiographic stains fed by the anterior and posterior choroidal arteries.

The appearance and location of the mass in Case 331 are typical for an intraventricular meningioma. Other diagnostic possibilities include metastasis, astrocytoma, oligodendroglioma, ependymoma (see Case 123), central neurocytoma (see Cases 342 and 343), arteriovenous malformation, or an inflammatory lesion (e.g., granuloma, parasitic or fungal mass).

### Case 332

10-week-old boy presenting with seizures.
(axial, noncontrast T2-weighted SE scan)

### Case 333

2-year-old girl presenting with hemiparesis.
(coronal, noncontrast T2-weighted FSE scan)

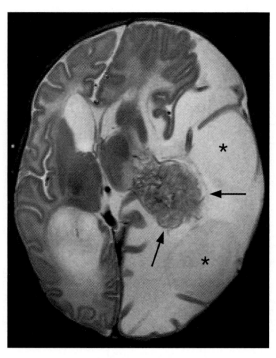

**Choroid Plexus Papilloma**

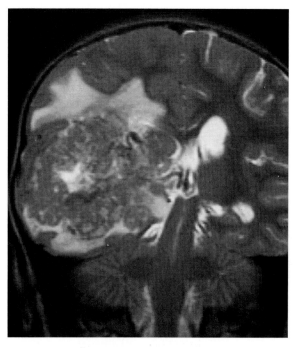

**Choroid Plexus Carcinoma**

---

Histologically benign choroid plexus papillomas may grow into the cerebral hemispheres. Parenchymal extension is often associated with large cysts, as illustrated in Case 332. The cellular tumor itself is relatively small and low in intensity *(arrows)*, while the majority of the abnormal signal within the hemisphere represents cysts *(asterisks)* and edema. Aggressive-appearing choroid plexus papillomas in children can be indistinguishable on CT or MR studies from choroid plexus carcinomas or from malignant ependymomas (compare to Case 124).

The lobulated, heterogeneous mass in Case 333 is centered in the region of the right lateral ventricular trigone. The tumor fills the ventricle and extends into adjacent cerebral parenchyma, with surrounding edema. Diffuse calcification was apparent within the lesion on a CT scan.

Meningeal seeding was demonstrated on a postcontrast scan of Case 333, providing a clue to malignant histology. CSF-borne dissemination of choroid plexus papillomas occurs but is not common.

### Case 334

2-month-old boy with hydrocephalus.
(sagittal, noncontrast T1-weighted SE scan)

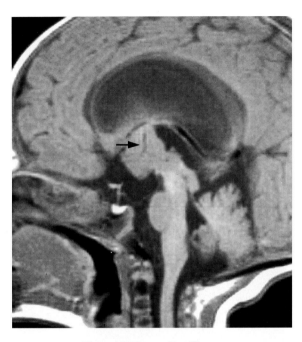

**Choroid Plexus Papilloma**

### Case 335

46-year-old woman presenting with
neck pain and nausea.
(coronal, noncontrast T1-weighted SE scan)

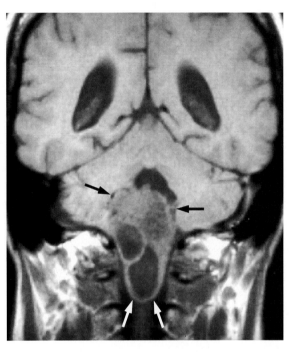

**Choroid Plexus Papilloma**

Choroid plexus papillomas are occasionally encountered in the third ventricle, as illustrated in Case 334. The fleshy or papillary character of the homogeneous mass and the presence of prominent flow voids *(arrow)* implying high vascularity are clues to the diagnosis, even in this unusual location. The associated hydrocephalus probably is due to obstruction of the third ventricle.

In adults, choroid plexus papillomas occur most commonly in the fourth ventricle, particularly caudally. This location and the frequent presence of calcification can suggest the correct diagnosis.

The scan in Case 335 shows a lesion with two components. The superior half of the tumor *(black arrows)* de-forms the fourth ventricle. Dense calcification was seen in this tissue on a CT scan but causes only mild reduction in signal intensity on MR. The caudal half of the tumor *(white arrows)* is a bilocular cyst extending into the cervical spinal canal. This component was inapparent on the patient's CT scan, again demonstrating the superiority of MR for evaluation of lesions involving or traversing the skull base.

The differential diagnosis of a fourth ventricular mass in an adult also includes ependymoma (see Case 157), sub-ependymoma, hemangioblastoma, unusual astrocytoma, metastases to the brainstem or cerebellar vermis, epidermoid or dermoid tumor (see Case 327), arteriovenous malformation, and an inflammatory mass or cyst (see Case 806).

### Case 336A

9-year-old boy presenting with behavioral
changes and headaches.
(sagittal, noncontrast T1-weighted SE scan)

### Case 336B

Same patient.
(axial, noncontrast scan; SE 3000/45)

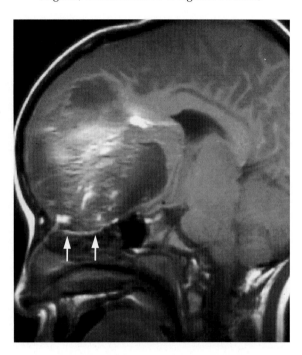

**Primitive Neuroectodermal Tumor**

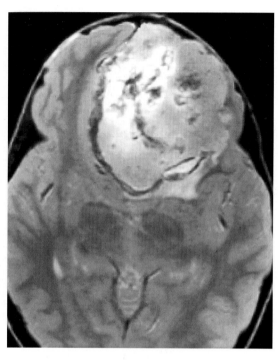

**Primitive Neuroectodermal Tumor**

Primitive neuroectodermal tumors (PNETs) arise from undifferentiated neuroepithelial cells with the capacity for glial and/or neuronal maturation. Pathologists group a number of malignancies under this heading, including medulloblastomas (see Cases 150-156) and and pineoblastomas (see Cases 305-307).

PNETs of the cerebral hemispheres are rare. These lesions, which have also been called *cerebral neuroblastomas,* are usually seen in children. Bulky, heterogeneous masses like Case 336 are typical. Intratumoral hemorrhage, indicated by the patchy zones of T1-shortening in Case 336A, is common. Cysts and calcification are also frequent, with the latter feature better appreciated on CT scans. The

mixture of cystic and solidly enhancing components of a PNET may closely resemble the lobulations of a teratoma like Case 309 or a malignant glioma like Case 99.

Although the heterogeneous character of the mass in Case 336 suggests an aggressive malignancy, the large size of the lesion with little surrounding edema indicates that the tumor may have been enlarging slowly for some time. Supporting this possibility is bony remodeling with depression of the cribriform plate (*arrows,* Case 336A).

Like medulloblastomas and pineoblastomas, cerebral PNETs may be associated with CSF dissemination. Multiple intradural, extramedullary spinal masses developed within months in this case.

# ESTHESIONEUROBLASTOMAS (OLFACTORY NEUROBLASTOMAS)

### Case 337A

3-year-old boy presenting with
headaches and papilledema.
(sagittal, noncontrast T1-weighted SE scan)

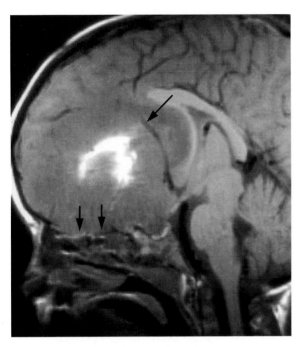

**Esthesioneuroblastoma**

### Case 337B

Same patient.
(axial, noncontrast T2-weighted SE scan)

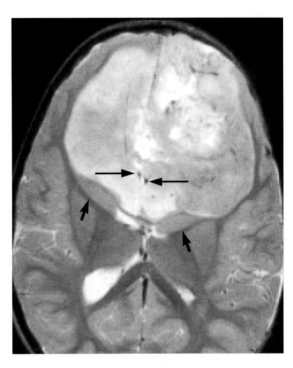

**Esthesioneuroblastoma**

---

Esthesioneuroblastomas or *olfactory neuroblastomas* are uncommon tumors originating from neuroepithelial sensory cells of the olfactory system. These masses arise near the cribriform plate and may present in the ethmoid/nasal region and/or intracranially. In either case, the tumors can be centered in the midline or predominantly unilateral. Esthesioneuroblastomas are seen in both children and adults.

The MR appearance of esthesioneuroblastomas is variable. The tumors may be homogeneous or heterogeneous, with short or long T2 values and mild or intense contrast enhancement. Small cysts are often found at the margins of the lesion. Characteristic location is the most helpful diagnostic clue.

In Case 337A, a very large subfrontal mass is based in the region of the cribriform plate *(short arrows)*. The corpus callosum is markedly displaced, and the anterior cerebral artery *(long arrow)* is encased by tumor. Hemorrhage is present at the center of the lesion.

Marked invagination of the mass into the frontal lobes is apparent in Case 337B. There is posterior displacement and splaying of the caudate nuclei *(short arrows)* and extreme thinning of surrounding white and gray matter of the frontal lobes. The anterior cerebral arteries are seen in cross-section, surrounded by tumor *(long arrows)*. The impressive lack of reactive edema and the marked cerebral deformity argue for a slow-growing lesion of extraaxial origin.

The differential diagnosis for a subfrontal mass in a child is quite limited. Meningiomas would be unusual in this location at this age. Subfrontal extension of pituitary adenomas occurs in adults (see Case 235) but would be rare in a child. Craniopharyngiomas tend to expand laterally or posteriorly rather than anteriorly (see Cases 258 and 260), although this diagnosis would be considered here since the mass does involve the suprasellar region. An exophytic glioma of the hypothalamus/optic chiasm could be included in the differential diagnosis for the same reason.

### Case 338

28-year-old man with a long history of seizures.
(axial, postcontrast T1-weighted SE scan with MTS)

### Case 339

21-year-old woman presenting with seizures.
(coronal, noncontrast T1-weighted GRE scan)

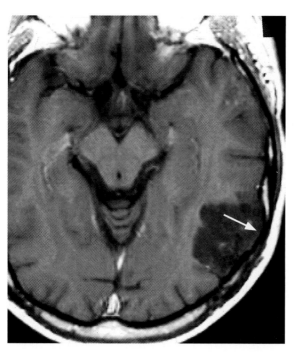

**Dysembryoplastic Neuroepithelial Tumor**

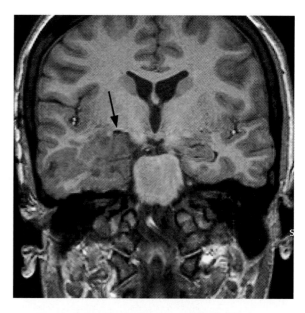

**Dysembryoplastic Neuroepithelial Tumor**

Dysembryoplastic neuroepithelial tumors (DNETs) are low grade masses with features intermediate between those of dysplasia and neoplasm. The lesions are usually cerebral and superficial (i.e., cortical), with the majority involving the temporal lobes. Most patients with DNETs are adolescents or young adults presenting with epilepsy. Some authors assert that DNETs are the most common structural lesion in children with partial seizures.

The superficial location and slow growth of DNETs often cause erosion of the adjacent calvarium with scalloping of the inner table, as seen in Case 338 *(arrow)*. The tumor itself typically demonstrates long T1 values with nodular or thickened gyriform morphology. Case 338 demonstrates a combination of both multinodular and "megagyric" architecture.

DNETs are frequently associated with adjacent cortical dysplasia. Aberrant neuronal organization is noted microscopically in most cases and may be apparent on MR studies. The pattern of gray matter within the right temporal lobe of Case 339 suggests heterotopia, superimposed on which are small nodular and cyst-like masses. The aggregate mass effect has displaced the temporal horn *(arrow)*.

DNETs are typically nonenhancing, as seen in Case 338.

### Case 340

28-year-old man with a long history of seizures.
(coronal, noncontrast T2-weighted FSE scan)

### Case 341

21-year-old woman presenting with seizures.
(coronal, noncontrast T2-weighted FSE scan)

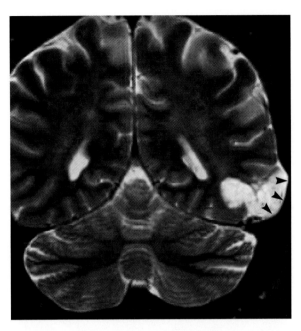

**Dysembryoplastic Neuroepithelial Tumor**
(same patient as Case 338)

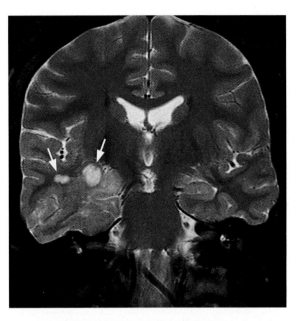

**Dysembryoplastic Neuroepithelial Tumor**
(same patient as Case 339)

DNETs are typically well defined by high signal intensity on T2-weighted scans. Thickened gyriform or multinodular morphology is often more easily appreciated on such images than on T1-weighted sequences. Case 340 again illustrates the features noted in Case 338: multiple small nodules coalescing to cause gyral expansion with erosion of the overlying inner table *(arrowheads).*

Many DNETs appear to contain small cysts, which are best defined on T2-weighted scans. Case 341 demonstrates several areas of focally prolonged T2 values *(arrows)* superimposed on less pronounced signal changes. These "cysts" usually represent zones of homogeneous tissue with high water content (often myxoid or microcystic) rather than actual fluid compartments. In any event, a multicystic appearance of a cortical mass found in a young patient with seizures should suggest a DNET.

The clinical and MR features of DNETs (superficial location, slow growth, temporal lobe involvement in a young patient with seizures, lack of enhancement) overlap those of several other tumors. Low grade glial or glial-neuronal neoplasms (particularly infiltrating astrocytoma, oligodendroglioma, and ganglioglioma) must be considered in the differential diagnosis. Calcification may be seen within DNETs (and in the other tumors listed) on CT scans. Large tumor cysts are rare in DNETs and suggest an alternative diagnosis (e.g., ganglioglioma; see Case 128).

## Case 342

31-year-old man presenting with headaches,
most severe on awakening.
(sagittal, noncontrast T1-weighted SE scan)

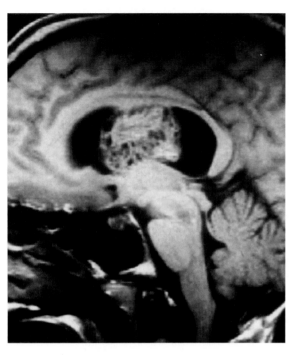

**Central Neurocytoma**

## Case 343

38-year-old man presenting with headaches.
(axial, postcontrast T1-weighted SE scan)

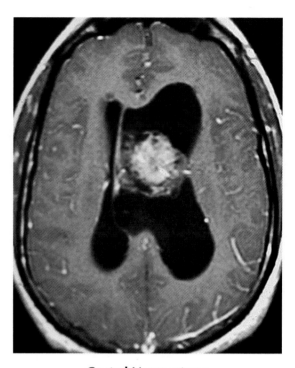

**Central Neurocytoma**

A group of intraventricular tumors with characteristic imaging features and generally favorable prognosis has been recognized over the past two decades. These masses, called *central neurocytomas*, resemble oligodendrogliomas at traditional light microscopy. However, when examined by electron microscopy or immunohistochemical staining, the lesions demonstrate neuronal differentiation. The tumors are comprised of small, uniform cells and may be considered to be a mature intraventricular form of neuroblastoma.

Central neurocytomas are typically heterogeneous masses containing multiple cysts and calcifications and occasional hemorrhage. The tumors are most often located within the body of a lateral ventricle, usually attached to the septum pellucidum. Cases 342 and 343 illustrate these features.

Contrast enhancement in central neurocytomas is variable but often less uniform or extensive than might be expected in a glioma of corresponding size. The majority of

the tumor in Case 343 does enhance, but the typically heterogeneous texture of the neurocytoma is still apparent. The mass has obstructed the left foramen of Monro to cause unilateral hydrocephalus.

Central neurocytomas may simultaneously involve both lateral ventricles. Occasional tumors arise within or extend into the third ventricle.

Unlike intraventricular gliomas, neurocytomas usually do not recur after resection. Adjunctive radiation therapy may therefore not be required, at least initially. For this reason, it is important to recognize the imaging clues to the diagnosis, alerting the pathologist to perform electron microscopy and/or specific immunohistochemical stains for accurate classification.

Compare Case 343 to the heterogeneously enhancing ependymoma in Case 123.

### Case 344

63-year-old man presenting with headaches.
(axial, noncontrast T2-weighted FSE scan)

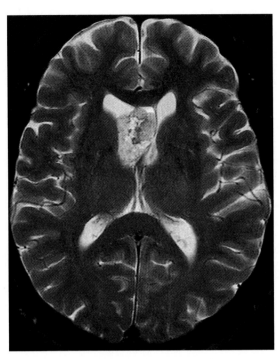

**Subependymoma**

### Case 345

66-year-old man presenting with
headaches and confusion.
(axial, noncontrast T2-weighted SE scan)

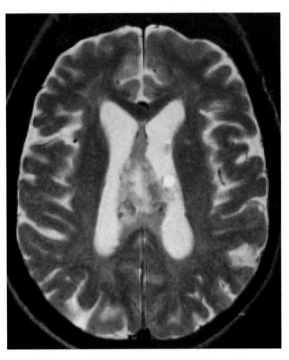

**Grade III Astrocytoma**

Central neurocytomas are among several tumors that can originate from or grow into the septum pellucidum.

Ependymomas and subependymomas can arise from the lateral or medial margins of the lateral ventricles. The mass in Case 344 spans the right frontal horn and displaces the septum pellucidum; it is difficult to determine the site of origin. The heterogeneity of the tumor is comparable to the usual complexity of central neurocytomas like Cases 342 and 343 (and resembles the typical morphology of ependymomas, as in Case 123).

See Case 129 for a general discussion of subependymomas. The mass in Case 344 demonstrated small rings and arcs of contrast enhancement in the mid-anterior portion of the lesion.

Case 345 illustrates invasion of the septum pellucidum by a malignant glioma of the corpus callosum. Although the lesion is heterogeneous, the diffuse septal infiltration and thickening in this case are distinct from the more focal, eccentric and mass-like morphology of most central neurocytomas.

Gliomas commonly occur near the lateral ventricles and frequently invade the septum pellucidum. Thickening of the septum suggests intraaxial origin of an otherwise ambiguous deep frontal lobe lesion. This finding is most commonly associated with gliomas but can also be seen with other pathologies (e.g., primary CNS lymphoma).

Subependymal giant cell astrocytomas (see Cases 896 and 897) are typically attached to the caudate nucleus along the lateral margin of the frontal horn. Large tumors may span the width of the ventricle, displacing the septum pellucidum and resembling Case 344.

### Case 346

38-year-old man with AIDS,
presenting with confusion.
(sagittal, noncontrast T1-weighted SE scan)

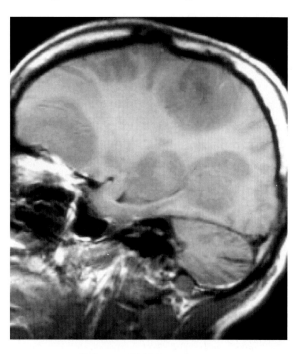

**Primary CNS Lymphoma**

### Case 347

74-year-old woman presenting with blurred
vision and impaired memory.
(coronal, noncontrast T1-weighted SE scan)

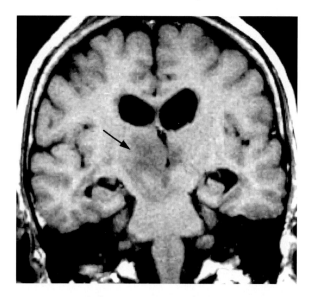

**Primary CNS Lymphoma**

---

Primary CNS lymphoma *(reticulum cell sarcoma, microglioma, immunoblastic lymphoma)* is an increasingly common cause of single or multiple intracranial masses. Primary CNS lymphomas are infrequent in otherwise healthy individuals. They are much more common in patients who are immunosuppressed due to disease (e.g., AIDS) or medication (e.g., transplant regimens). Primary lymphoma of the CNS is more common than parenchymal involvement by systemic lymphoma, which more typically infiltrates the meninges or the ventricular surface (see Cases 26, 29, and 433).

Primary CNS lymphomas can assume a variety of appearances and may mimic other pathologies. Both lobar and deep hemispheric lesions may occur. Frequent areas of involvement include the basal ganglia, corpus callosum, cerebellum, and periventricular white matter.

On T1-weighted scans, the signal intensity of CNS lymphomas is usually low to intermediate, as illustrated above. The multiple lesions in Case 346 are predominantly lobar and demonstrate well-defined T1-prolongation. The deep hemispheric mass in Case 347 is less well demarcated from surrounding parenchyma. (Compare the involvement along the margins of the third ventricle in Case 347 to the ventral extension of a pineal germinoma in Cases 294 and 301.)

The lesions of primary CNS lymphoma often regress (temporarily) in response to steroid therapy and may wax and wane spontaneously. Clues to the diagnosis include involvement of deep hemispheric structures, multicentricity, steroid response, and a clinical association with immunosuppression.

## Case 348

31-year-old woman presenting with ataxia.
(axial, noncontrast T2-weighted SE scan)

## Case 349

73-year-old man presenting with a seizure.
(axial, noncontrast T2-weighted SE scan)

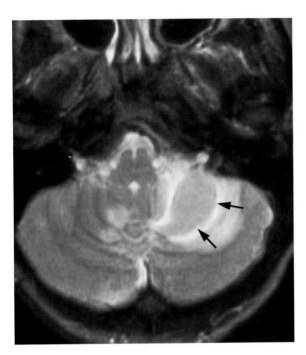

**Primary CNS Lymphoma**

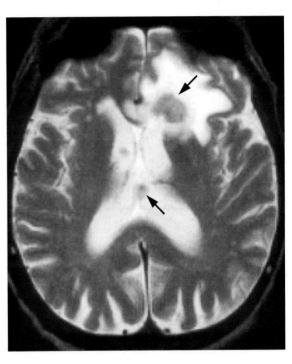

**Primary CNS Lymphoma**

In both of these cases, a rim of high intensity edema surrounds a tumor *(arrows)* that is nearly isointense to gray matter. This lack of T2-prolongation is characteristic of primary CNS lymphoma, reflecting the dense cellularity and high nuclear to cytoplasmic ratio of these tumors. (Compare to medulloblastomas and germinomas, such as Cases 152, 153, and 294.)

The relatively small amount of intracellular and extracellular water in primary CNS lymphoma also correlates with restricted diffusion on diffusion-weighted images. In fact, increasing values of the apparent diffusion coefficient can be the earliest MR evidence of response to treatment in these tumors.

As seen above and on the previous page, primary CNS lymphomas are usually homogeneous lesions. An exception to this rule occurs in AIDS patients, when central necrosis is commonly observed, reflecting rapid tumor growth (see Cases 356 and 357).

Lymphoma should be one of the diagnoses considered when a cerebellar mass is encountered in a young adult, such as Case 348. Other possibilities include lateral medulloblastoma, hemangioblastoma, and astrocytoma (see Cases 177, 181, and 185).

The periventricular location of the frontal lesion in Case 349 is typical for CNS lymphoma. Additional nodules along the septum pellucidum were more easily seen on a postcontrast scan of this patient.

Cerebral aspergillosis should be considered in the differential diagnosis with primary CNS lymphoma when one or more relatively isointense masses are found within the brain of an immunosuppressed patient. Both of these pathologies may be nonenhancing due to vascular invasion and occlusion.

### Case 350

69-year-old man presenting with confusion.
(axial, postcontrast T1-weighted SE scan)

### Case 351

76-year-old man presenting with right hemiparesis.
(coronal, postcontrast T1-weighted SE scan)

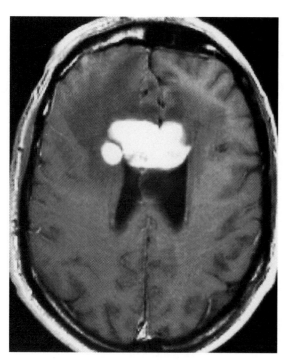

**Primary CNS Lymphoma**

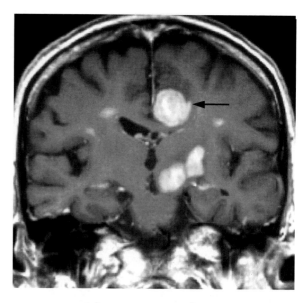

**Primary CNS Lymphoma**

Contrast enhancement within CNS lymphoma may be solid or peripheral. Intense, uniform enhancement is common, as seen in these cases.

CNS lymphoma is among the pathologies that may involve and cross the corpus callosum. (Other tumors in this category are gliomas and occasional metastases.) The large mass occupying the genu and anterior body of the corpus callosum in Case 350 is surrounded by bifrontal edema. A malignant glioma could cause an identical appearance, although central necrosis with irregular rim enhancement would be more common (see Case 98).

The multiple enhancing nodules in Case 351 predominantly involve the basal ganglia and periventricular regions. This deep distribution is typical for CNS lymphoma and would be less common for metastatic disease (compare to Case 15).

The faintly laminated or target-like morphology within the largest mass in Case 351 *(arrow)* is a frequent feature of primary CNS lymphoma.

In rare instances, cerebral masses due to primary CNS lymphoma do not enhance. Pathological examination of such lesions may demonstrate intraluminal tumor obstructing arteries within the neoplasm. In any event, the absence of contrast enhancement does not exclude the diagnosis of CNS lymphoma.

Nonenhancing lymphoma occasionally mimics progressive multifocal leukoencephalopathy in an immunocompromised patient. Fungal disease (e.g., aspergillosis) may also present as multiple nonenhancing masses in this context.

## DIFFERENTIAL DIAGNOSIS:
## ENHANCING MASS INVOLVING THE THIRD VENTRICLE

### Case 352

80-year-old woman presenting with dizziness.
(axial, postcontrast T1-weighted SE scan)

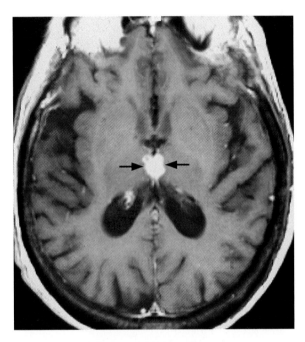

**Primary CNS Lymphoma**

### Case 353

70-year-old man presenting with headaches.
(axial, postcontrast T1-weighted SE scan with MTS)

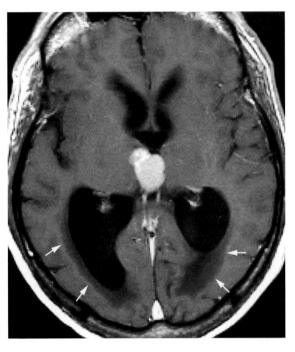

**Metastatic Melanoma**

---

Periventricular involvement by primary CNS lymphoma is common. It may take the form of localized masses or more diffuse infiltration along ventricular margins. A uniform layer of subependymal tumor can mimic inflammatory ventriculitis (see Case 434).

The solid appearance of the third ventricular lesion in Case 352 represents the meeting in the midline of bilateral tumor layers involving the walls of the third ventricle. Reactive edema is present in the thalamus bilaterally.

Case 353 serves as a reminder that metastatic disease must be considered in the differential diagnosis of any intracranial mass in an adult. The midline tumor in this case may have arisen in periventricular tissue or from hematogenous seeding of choroid plexus in the roof of the third ventricle. Intraventricular metastases most frequently occur within the lateral ventricles, potentially resembling intraventricular meningiomas like Cases 68 and 69.

An unusual ependymoma or astrocytoma could be considered in the differential diagnosis of the above scans. Choroid plexus papillomas in adults rarely occur above the fourth ventricle (see Case 335). Germinoma would be a diagnostic possibility in a younger patient (compare to Case 308).

Like the paramedian involvement along the walls of the third ventricle in Case 352, primary CNS lymphoma often affects the periaqueductal region of the dorsal midbrain (see Case 776).

The tumor in Case 353 has obstructed the posterior third ventricle, causing hydrocephalus. Periventricular edema is present along the margins of the trigones and occipital horns of the lateral ventricles *(arrows)*.

# DIFFERENTIAL DIAGNOSIS:
## MULTIFOCAL DEEP HEMISPHERIC MASSES

### Case 354

58-year-old woman presenting with
personality change.
(axial, postcontrast T1-weighted SE scan)

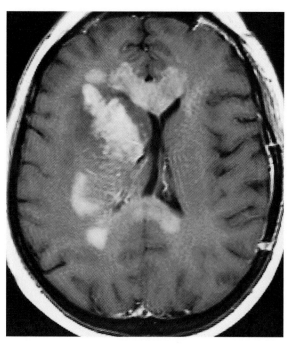

**Primary CNS Lymphoma**
(recurrent)

### Case 355

86-year-old woman presenting with confusion.
(axial, postcontrast T1-weighted SE scan with MTS)

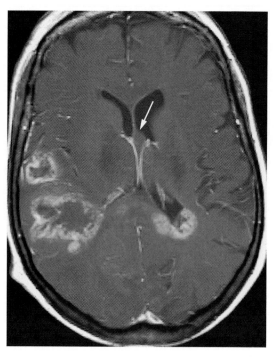

**Gliomatosis Cerebri**

Multicentric involvement of the basal ganglia and periventricular white matter by primary CNS lymphoma may closely resemble the extensive bihemispheral infiltration of gliomatosis cerebri. The cases above demonstrate that these pathologies should both be considered in the differential diagnosis of bilateral cerebral disease. Metastases or inflammatory processes rarely display the infiltrating character or the predominantly periventricular involvement illustrated in these cases.

Tumor in Case 354 occupies both the genu and the splenium of the corpus callosum. Splenial involvement is documented by abnormal enhancement in Case 355.

Nonenhancing tumor extension is common in gliomatosis cerebri, illustrated in Case 355 by expansion of the fornix on the left *(arrow)*. Such widening of fiber tracts is an important clue to the diagnosis in cases of predominantly isointense tumor with little or no abnormal enhancement (see discussion of Case 112).

Widespread cerebral involvement by primary CNS lymphoma occasionally demonstrates little enhancement (see discussion of Cases 350 and 351).

A left-sided craniotomy flap in Case 354 reflects an earlier exploration and biopsy. Although primary CNS lymphoma may initially respond to treatment with steroids or radiation, recurrence is usual.

## Case 356

28-year-old man.
(axial, noncontrast T2-weighted SE scan)

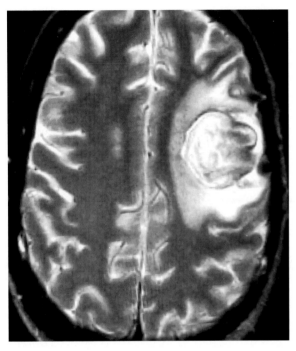

**Primary CNS Lymphoma**

## Case 357

38-year-old man.
(axial, postcontrast T1-weighted SE scan)

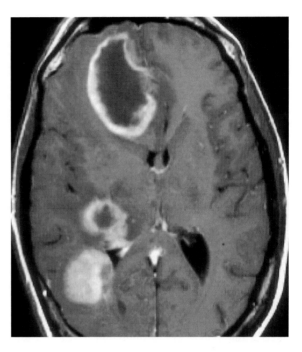

**Primary CNS Lymphoma**

---

Patients with AIDS have a high incidence of primary CNS lymphoma. This diagnosis should be considered (along with toxoplasmosis; see Cases 473-477) whenever a cerebral mass is discovered in an HIV-positive individual. Deep hemispheric involvement and multiple masses are common, as in the simultaneous presence of inflammatory lesions.

CNS lymphoma in AIDS patients is often inhomogeneous, with large areas of central necrosis. The masses may contain zones of high signal intensity on T2-weighted scans, as seen in Case 356. This heterogeneity and T2-prolongation differ from the appearance of typical primary CNS lymphoma, as illustrated in Cases 348 and 349.

Masses due to CNS lymphoma in AIDS patients frequently demonstrate peripheral contrast enhancement, as in Case 357. Similar lesions are occasionally seen as solitary tumors in nonimmunocompromised adults, closely resembling a malignant glioma. (Compare the frontal mass in Case 357 to Cases 100 and 101.) Perfusion-weighted images can contribute to the differential diagnosis in such cases; relative cerebral blood volume (rCBV) is usually lower in primary CNS lymphoma than in high grade gliomas.

The combination of solid and rim-enhancing lesions in Case 357 could represent either variation in the appearance of CNS lymphoma or the coexistence of inflammatory lesions and tumor. The clinical course usually makes this distinction. None of the masses in Case 357 responded to therapy for toxoplasmosis, while all subsequently "melted" with steroids.

# REFERENCES

Ahmadi J, Savabi F, Apuzzo MLJ, et al: Magnetic resonance imaging and quantitative analysis of intracranial cystic lesions: surgical implication. *Neurosurgery* 35:199-207, 1994.

Anderson DR, Falcone S, Bruce JH, et al: Congenital choroid plexus papillomas. *AJNR* 16:2072-2076, 1995.

Armao D, Castillo M, Chen H, Kwock L: Colloid cyst of the third ventricle: imaging-pathologic correlation. *AJNR* 21:1470-1477, 2000.

Bagley LJ, Hurst RW, Zimmerman RA, et al: Imaging in the trilateral retinoblastoma syndrome. *Neuroradiology* 38:166-170, 1996.

Barboriak DP, Lee L, Provenzale JM: Serial MR imaging of pineal cysts: implications for natural history and follow-up. *Am J Roentgenol* 176:737-743, 2001.

Bataille B, Delwail V, Menet E, et al: Primary intracerebral malignant lymphoma: report of 248 cases. *J Neurosurg* 92:261-266, 2000.

Bolen JW, Lipper MH, Caccamo D: Juxtaventricular central neurocytoma: CT and MR findings. *J Comput Assist Tomogr* 13:495-497, 1989.

Boyd MC, Steinbok P: Choroid plexus tumors: problems in diagnosis and management. *J Neurosurg* 66:800-805, 1987.

Buetow PC, Smirniotopoulos JG, Done S: Congenital brain tumors: a review of 45 cases. *AJNR* 11:793-799, 1990.

Carlson BA: Rapidly progressive dementia caused by nonenhancing primary lymphoma of the central nervous system. *AJNR* 17:1695-1698, 1996.

Casadei GP, Komori T, Scheithauer BW, et al: Intracranial parenchymal schwannoma. *J Neurosurg* 79:217-222, 1993.

Castillo M, Chung C, Mukherji SK: Imaging features of atypical teratoid rhabdoid tumors of the central nervous system. *Int J Neurorad* 3:185-191, 1997.

Chang KH, Han MH, Kim DG, et al: MR appearance of central neurocytoma. *Acta Radiologica* 34:520-526, 1993.

Chang SM, Lillis-Hearne PK, Larson DA, et al: Pineoblastoma in adults. *Neurosurgery* 37:383-390, 1995.

Chen C-Y, Zimmerman RA, Faro S, et al: Childhood leukemia: central nervous system abnormalities during and after treatment. *AJNR* 17:295-310, 1996.

Chen S, Ikawa F, Kurisu K, et al: Quantitative MR evaluation of intracranial epidermoid tumors by fast fluid-attenuated inversion recovery imaging and echo-planar diffusion-weighted imaging. *AJNR* 22:1089-1096, 2001.

Cheng PW, Leung SY, Hung KN, et al: Atypical features of dysembryoplastic neuroepithelial tumor with pathologic-radiologic correlation. *Int J Neurorad* 4:268-276, 1998.

Chiechi MV, Smirniotopoulos JG, Mena H: Pineal parenchymal tumors: CT and MR features. *J Comput Assist Tomogr* 19:509-517, 1995.

Coates TL, Hinshaw DBJ, Peckman N, et al: Pediatric choroid plexus neoplasms: MR, CT, and pathologic correlation. *Radiology* 173:81-88, 1989.

Cordoliani, Y-S, Derosier C, Pharaboz C, et al: Primary cerebral lymphoma in patients with AIDS: MR findings: 17 cases. *AJNR* 159:841-847, 1992.

Dahger AP, Smirniotopoulos J: Intracranial dermoid cysts with and without rupture. *Int J Neurorad* 1:134-144, 1995.

Daumas-Duport C, Scheithauer BW, Chodkiewicz JP, et al: Dysembryoplastic neuroepithelial tumor: a surgically curable tumor of young patients with intractable partial seizures: report of 39 cases. *Neurosurgery* 23:545-556, 1988.

Davis PC, Wichman RD, Takei Y, Hoffman JCJ: Primary cerebral neuroblastoma: CT and MR findings in 12 cases. *AJNR* 11:115-120, 1990.

DeAngelis LM: Cerebral lymphomas presenting as a nonenhancing lesion on computed tomographic/magnetic resonance scan. *Ann Neurol* 33:308-311, 1993.

Dina TS: Primary central nervous system lymphoma versus toxoplasmois in AIDS. *Radiology* 179:823-838, 1991.

Donati F, Vasella F, Kaiser G, Blumberg A: Intracranial lipomas. *Neuropediatrics* 23:32-38, 1992.

Edwards MSB, Hudgins RJ, Wilson CB, et al: Pineal region tumors in children. *J Neurosurg* 68:689-697, 1988.

Eghwrudjakpor PO, Kurisaka M, Fukuoka M, Mori K: Intracranial lipomas. *Acta Neurochir (Wien)* 110:124-128, 1991.

El Khoury C, Brugieres P, Decq P, et al: Colloid cysts of the third ventricle: are MR imaging patterns predictive of difficulty with percutaneous treatment? *AJNR* 21:489-492, 2000.

Ellenbogen RG, Winston KR, Kupsky WJ: Tumors of the choroid plexus in children. *Neurosurgery* 25:327-335, 1989.

Engel U, Gottschalk S, Niehaus L, et al: Cystic lesions of the pineal region—MRI and pathology. *Neuroradiology* 42:399-402, 2000.

Erdag N, Bhorade RM, Alberico RA, et al: Primary lymphoma of the central nervous system: typical and atypical CT and MR imaging appearances. *Am J Roentgenol* 176:1319-1326, 2001.

Faerber EN, Roman NV: Central nervous system tumors of childhood. *Radio Clin North Am* 35:1301-1328, 1997.

Fain JS, Tomlinson FH, Bernd W, et al: Symptomatic glial cysts of the pineal gland. *J Neurosurg* 80:454-460, 1994.

Figueroa RE, El Gammal T, Brooks BS, et al: MR findings on primitive neuroectodermal tumors. *J Comput Assist Tomogr* 13:773-778, 1989.

Finelli DA, Shurin SB, Bardenstein DS: Trilateral retinoblastoma: two variations. *AJNR* 16:166-170, 1995.

Fleege MA, Miller GM, Fletcher GP, et al: Benign glial cysts of the pineal gland: imaging characteristics with histologic correlation. *AJNR* 15:161-166, 1994.

Friedman DP: Extrapineal abnormalities of the tectal region: MR imaging findings. *Am J Roentgenol* 159:859-866, 1992.

Gao, P, Osborn AG, Smirniotopoulos JG, Harris CP: Epidermoid tumor of the cerebellopontine angle. *AJNR* 13:863-872, 1992.

Goergen SK, Gonzales, MF, McLean CA: Intraventricular neurocytoma: radiologic features and review of the literature. *Radiology* 182:787-792, 1992.

Golzarian J, Baleriaux D, Bank WO, et al: Pineal cyst: normal or pathological? *Neurosurgery* 35:251-253, 1993.

Gormley WB, Tomecek FJ, Qureshi N, Malik GM: Craniocerebral epidermoid and dermoid tumours: a review of 32 cases. *Acta Neurochir* 128:115-121, 1994.

Gualdi GF, Biasi C, Trasimeni G, et al: Unusual MR and CT appearance of an epidermoid tumor. *AJNR* 12:771-772, 1991.

Hahn FJ, Ong E, McComb RD, et al: MR imaging of ruptured intracranial dermoid. *J Comput Assist Tomogr* 10:888-892, 1986.

Hassoun J, Soylemezoglu F, Gambarelli D, et al: Central neurocytoma: a synopsis of clinical and histological features. *Brain Pathol* 3:297-306, 1993.

Higano S, Takahashi S, Ishii K, et al: Germinoma originating in the basal ganglia and thalamus. MR and CT evaluation. *AJNR* 15:1435-1442, 1994.

Hoffman HJ, Otsubo H, Hendrick EB, et al: Intracranial germ cell tumors in children. *J Neurosurg* 74:545-551, 1991.

Hopper KD, Foley LC, Nieves NL, Smirniotopoulos JG: The intraventricular extension of choroid plexus papillomas: *AJNR* 8:469-472, 1987.

Horowitz BL, Chari MV, James R: MR of intracranial epidermoid tumors: correlation of in vivo imaging with in vitro C-13 spectroscopy. *AJNR* 11:299-302, 1990.

Howlett DC, King AP, Jarosz JM, et al: Imaging and pathological features of primary malignant rhabdoid tumours of the brain and spine. *Neuroradiology* 39:719-723, 1997.

Hunt SJ, Johnsen PC, Coons SW, Pittman HW: Neonatal intracranial teratomas. *Surg Neurol* 34:336-342, 1990.

Ikushima I, Korogi Y, Hirai T, et al: MR of epidermoids with a variety of pulse sequences. *AJNR* 18:1359-1363, 1997.

Jelinek J, Smirniotopoulos JG, Parisi JE, Kanzer M: Lateral ventricular neoplasms of the brain: differential diagnosis based on clinical, CT, and MR findings. *AJNR* 11:567-574, 1990.

Johnson BA, Fram EK, Johnson PC, Jacobowitz R: The variable MR appearance of primary lymphoma of the central nervous system: comparison with histopathologic features. *AJNR* 18:563-572, 1997.

Kallmes DF, Provenzale PM, Cloft HJ, McClendon RE: Typical and atypical MR imaging features of intracranial epidermoid tumors. *Am J Roentgenol* 169:883-888, 1997.

Ken JG, Sobel DF, Copeland B, et al: Choroid plexus papillomas of the foramen of Luschka: MR appearance. *AJNR* 12:1201-1203, 1991.

Kilgore DP, Strother CM, Starshak RJ, Haughton VM: Pineal germinoma: MR imaging. *Radiology* 158:435-438, 1986.

Kim DI, Yoon PH, Ryu YH, et al: MRI of germinomas arising from the basal ganglia and thalamus. *Neuroradiology* 40:507-511, 1998.

Kirsch CFE, Smirniotopoulos JG, Olan WJ, Koeller KK: Colloid cysts: radiologic-pathologic correlation with review of the Armed Forces Institute of Pathology experience and world literature. *Int J Neurorad* 3:460-469, 1997.

Klein P, Rubinstein LJ: Benign symptomatic glial cysts of the pineal gland: a report of seven cases and review of the literature. *J Neurol Neurosurg Psychiatr* 52:991-995, 1989.

Koeller KK, Dillon WP: Dysembryoplastic neuroepithelial tumors: MR appearance. *AJNR* 13:1319-1325, 1992.

Koeller KK, Smirniotopoulos JG, Jones RV: Primary central nervous system lymphoma: radiologic-pathologic correlation. *Radiographics* 17:1497-1510, 1997.

Komatsu Y, Narushima K, Kobayashi E, et al: CT and MR of germinoma in the basal ganglia. *AJNR* 10:59, 1989.

Kuroiwa T, Bergey GK, Rothman MI, et al: Radiologic appearance of the dysembryoplastic neuroepithelial tumor. *Radiology* 197:233-238, 1995.

Latack JT, Kartush JM, Kemink JL, et al: Epidermoidomas of the cerebellopontine angle and temporal bone: CT and MR aspects. *Radiology* 157:361-366, 1985.

Lee DH, Norman D, Newton TH: MR imaging of pineal cysts. *J Comput Assist Tomogr* 11:586-690, 1987..

Li C, Yousem DM, Hayden RE, Doty RL: Olfactory neuroblastoma: MR evaluation. *AJNR* 14:1167-1171, 1993.

Lunardi P, Missori P: Supratentorial dermoid cysts. *J Neurosurg* 75:262-266, 1991.

Maeder PP, Holtas SL, Basibuyuk LN, et al: Colloid cysts of the third ventricle: correlation of MR and CT findings with histology and chemical analysis. *AJNR* 11:575-581, 1990.

Mamourian AC, Cromwell LD, Harbaugh RE: Colloid cyst of the third ventricle: sometimes more conspicuous on CT than MR. *AJNR* 19:875-878, 1998.

Mamourian AC, Towfight J: Pineal cysts: MR imaging. *AJNR* 7:1081-1086, 1986.

Mamourian AC, Yarnell T: Enhancement of pineal cyst of MR images. *AJNR* 12:773-774, 1991.

Markus H, Kendall BE: MRI of a dermoid cyst containing hair. *Neuroradiology* 35:256-257, 1993.

Matthews VP, Broome DR, Smith RR, et al: Neuroimaging of disseminated germ cell neoplasms. *AJNR* 11:319-324, 1990.

Miyazawa N, Yamazaki H, Wakao T, Nukul H: Epidermoid tumors of Meckel's cave: case report and review of the literature. *Neurosurgery* 25:951-954, 1989.

Moon WK, Chang KH, Han MH, Kim I-O: Intracranial germinomas: correlation of imaging findings with tumor response to radiation therapy. *Am J Roentgenol* 172:713-716, 1999.

Moon WK, Chang KH, Kim IO, et al: Germinomas of the basal ganglia and thalamus: MR findings and a comparison between MR and CT. *Am J Roentgenol* 162:1413-1417, 1994.

Morita A, Ebersold MJ, Olsen KD, et al: Esthesioneuroblastoma: prognosis and management. *Neurosurgery* 32:706-715, 1993.

Muller-Forell W, Schroth G, Egan PJ: MR imaging in tumors of the pineal region. *Neuroradiology* 30:224-231, 1988.

Musolino A, Cambria S, Rizzo G, Cambria M: Symptomatic cysts of the pineal gland: stereotactic diagnosis and treatment of two cases and review of the literature. *Neurosurgery* 32:315-321, 1993.

Nakagawa H, Iwasaki S, Kichikawa K, et al: MR imaging of pineocytome: report of two cases. *AJNR* 11:185, 1990.

Nakamura M, Saeki N, Iwadate Y, et al: Neuroradiological characteristics of pineocytoma and pineoblastoma. *Neuroradiology* 42:509-514, 2000.

Newton DR, Larson TC III, Dillon WP, Newton TH: Magnetic resonance characteristics of cranial epidermoid and teratomatous tumors. *AJNR* 8:945, 1987.

Olson JJ, Beck DW, Crawford SC, Menezes AH: Comparative evaluation of epidermoid tumors with computed tomography and magnetic resonance imaging. *Neurosurgery* 21:357-360, 1987.

Ostertun B, Wolf HK, Campos MG, et al: Dysembryoplastic neuroepithelial tumors: MR and CT evaluation. *AJNR* 17:419-430, 1996.

Packer RJ, Perilongo G, Johnson D, et al: Choroid plexus carcinoma of childhood. *Cancer* 69:580-585, 1992.

Pomper MG, Passe TJ, Burger PC, et al: Chordoid glioma: a neoplasm unique to the hypothalamus and anterior third ventricle. *AJNR* 22:464-469, 2001.

Provenzale J, Weber AL, Klintworth GK, McLendon RE: Radiologic-pathologic correlation. Bilateral retinoblastoma with coexistent pineoblastoma (trilateral retinoblastoma). *AJNR* 16:157-165, 1995.

Reiche W, Feiden W, Eymann R, et al: Dysembryoplastic neuroepithelial tumor: neuroradiologic findings in common and uncommon sites. *Int J Neurorad* 3:428-434, 1997.

Robles HA, Smirniotopoulos JG, Fegueroa RE: Understanding the radiology of intracranial primitive neuroectodermal tumors from a pathological perspective: a review. *Semin US CT MR* 13:170-181, 1992.

Roman-Goldstein SM, Goldman DL, Howieson J, et al: MR in primary CNS lymphoma in immunologically normal patients. *AJNR* 13:1207-1213, 1992.

Roosen N, Gahlen D, Stork W, et al: Magnetic resonance imaging of colloid cysts of the third ventricle. *Neuroradiology* 29:10-14, 1987.

Ruiz A, Donovan Post MJ, Bundschu C, et al: Primary central nervous system lymphoma in patients with AIDS. *Neuroimaging Clin North Am* 7:281-296, 1997.

Satoh H, Uozumi T, Kiya K, et al: MRI of pineal region tumours: relationship between tumours and adjacent structures. *Neuroradiology* 37:624-630, 1995.

Savader SJ, Murtagh FR, Savader BL, et al: Magnetic resonance imaging of intracranial epidermoid tumors. *Clin Radiol* 40:282, 1989.

Schuster JJ, Phillips CD, Levine PA: MR of esthesioneuroblastoma (olfactory neuroblastoma) and appearance after craniofacial resection. *AJNR* 15:1169-1177, 1994.

Schwaighofer BW, Hesselink JR, Press GA, et al: Primary intracranial CNS lymphoma: MR manifestations. *AJNR* 10:725-730, 1989.

Scotti G, Scialfa G, Colombo N, et al: MR in the diagnosis of colloid cysts of the third ventricle. *AJNR* 8:370-372, 1987.

Shen WC, Yang CF: Epidermoid cyst with variable contents shown on CT and MRI. *Neuroradiology* 33(suppl):317-318, 1991.

**221**

Shoemaker EI, Romano AS, Gado M: Neuroradiology case of the day: choroid plexus papilloma, third ventricle. *Am J Roentgenol* 152:1333-1338, 1989.

Skulski M, Egelhoff JC, Kollias SS, et al: Trilateral retinoblastoma with suprasellar involvement. *Neuroradiology* 39:41-43, 1997.

Smirniotopoulos JG, Chiechi MV: Teratomas, dermoids and epidermoids of the head and neck. *Radiographics* 15:1437-1455, 1995.

Smirniotopoulos JG, Rushing EJ, Mena H: Pineal region mass: differential diagnosis. *Radiographics* 12:577-595, 1992.

Smith AS, Benson JE, Blaser SI, et al: Diagnosis of ruptured intacranial dermoid cyst: value of MR over CT. *AJNR* 12:175-180, 1991.

Smoker WRK, Townsend JJ, Reichman MV: Neurocytoma accompanied by intraventricular hemorrhage: case report and literature review. *AJNR* 12:765-770, 1991.

Som PM, Lidov M. Brandwein M, et al: Sinonasal esthesioneuroblastomas with intracranial extension: marginal tumor cysts as a diagnostic MR finding. *AJNR* 15:1259-1262, 1994.

Steffev DJ, Filipp GJ, Spera T, Gabrielsen TO: MR imaging of primary epidermoid tumors. *J Comput Assist Tomogr* 12:438-440, 1988.

Stephenson TF, Spitzer RM: MR and CT appearance of ruptured intracranial dermoid tumors. *Comput Radiol* 11:249, 1987.

Sumida M, Uozumi T, Kiya K, et al: MRI of intracranial germ cell tumors. *Neuroradiology* 37:32-37, 1995.

Tampieri D, Melanson D, Ethier R: MR imaging of epidermoid cysts. *AJNR* 10:351-356, 1989.

Tatler GLV, Kendall BE: The radiological diagnosis of epidermoid tumors. *Neuroradiology* 33(suppl):324-325, 1991.

Terae S, Ogata A: Nonenhancing primary central nervous system lymphoma. *Neuroradiology* 38:34-37, 1996.

Thurnher MM, Rieger A, Kleibl-Popov C, et al: Primary central nervous system lymphoma in AIDS: a wider spectrum of CT and MRI findings. *Neuroradiology* 43:29-35, 2001.

Tien RD:Intraventricular mass lesions of the brain: CT and MR findings. *Am J Roentgenol* 157:1283-1290, 1991.

Tien RD, Barkovich AJ, Edwards MSB: MR imaging of pineal tumors. *AJNR* 11:557-565, 1990.

Todo T, Kondo T, Shinoura N, Yamada R: Large cysts of the pineal gland: report of two cases. *Neurosurgery* 29:101-106, 1992.

Tortori-Donati P, Fondelli MP, Rossi A, et al: Atypical teratoid rhabdoid tumors of the central nervous system in infancy: neuroradiologic findings. *Int J Neurorad* 3:327-338, 1997.

Truwit CL, Barkovich AJ: Pathogenesis of intracranial lipoma: an MR study in 42 patients. *AJNR* 11:665-674, 1990.

Urso JA, Ross GJ, Parker RK, et al: Colloid cyst of the third ventricle: radiologic-pathologic correlation. *J Comput Assist Tomog* 22:524-527, 1998.

Vion-Dury J, Vincentilli F, Jiddane M, et al: MR imaging of epidermoid cysts. *Neuroradiology* 29:333-338, 1987.

Waggenspack GA, Guinto FC Jr: MR and CT of masses of the anterosuperior third ventricle. *AJNR* 10:105-110, 1989.

Wagle WA, Jaufmann B, Mincy JE: Magnetic resonance imaging of fourth ventricular epidermoid tumors. *Arch Neurol* 48:438-440, 1991.

Wichmann W, Schubiger O, Von Demling A, et al: Neuroradiology of central neurocytoma. *Neuroradiology* 33:143-148, 1991.

Williams RL, Meltzer CC, Smirniotopoulos JG, et al: Cerebral MR in intravascular lymphomatosis. *AJNR* 19:427-432, 1998.

Wilms G, Casselman J, Demaerel Ph, et al: CT and MRI of ruptured intracranial dermoids. *Neuroradiology* 33:149-151, 1991.

Wilms G, Marchal G, Van Hecke P, et al: Colloid cysts of the third ventricle: MR findings. *J Comput Assist Tomogr* 14:527-531, 1990.

Yasargil MG, Von Ammon K, Von Deimling A, et al: Central neurocytoma: histopathological variants and therapeutic approaches. *J Neurosurg* 76:32-37, 1992.

Yuh WTC, Barloon TJ, Jacoby CG, et al: MR of fourth vertricular epidermoid tumors. *ANJR* 9:794-798, 1988.

Zee C-S, Segall H, Apuzzo M, et al: MR imaging of pineal region neoplasms. *J Comput Assist Tomogr* 15:56-63, 1991.

Zimmerman RA: Central nervous system lymphoma. *Radiol Clin North Am* 28:697-722, 1990.

Zimmerman RA: Pediatric supratentorial tumors. *Semin Roentgenol* 25:225-248, 1990.

# CHAPTER 8

# Disorders of White Matter

### Case 358

37-year-old woman presenting with a two-day
history of worsening hemiparesis.
(sagittal, noncontrast T1-weighted SE scan)

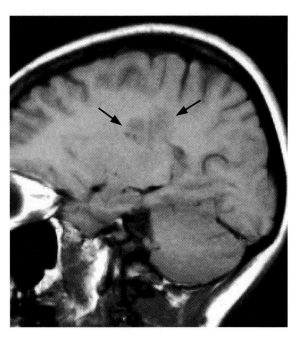

**Multiple Sclerosis**

### Case 359

51-year-old woman with a ten-year
history of multiple sclerosis.
(sagittal, noncontrast T1-weighted SE scan)

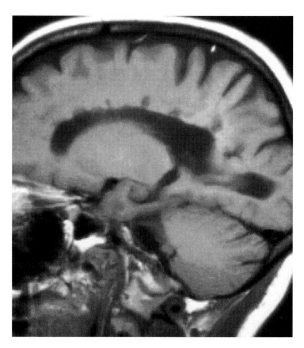

**Multiple Sclerosis**

The MR appearance of multiple sclerosis is widely variable, depending on acuity and extent of disease. Active demyelination usually presents as a zone of moderate T1 prolongation, as in Case 358 *(arrows)*. Such lesions are typically 1 to 2 cm in diameter, with mildly indistinct margins due to associated edema. Relatively rapid onset of related symptoms may mimic cerebral ischemia.

Older multiple sclerosis plaques are typically smaller, more sharply defined, and somewhat lower in signal intensity on T1-weighted scans. Periventricular lesions in Case 359 illustrate this appearance. The characteristically prominent T1 prolongation of established demyelinating foci can be a useful feature in differential diagnosis (on ei-

ther T1-weighted spin echo or inversion recovery pulse sequences). If multiple small lesions seen on a T2-weighted scan are not well defined on a T1-weighted image, they are unlikely to represent multiple sclerosis.

Both of the above cases demonstrate the typical involvement of periventricular white matter by demyelinating disease. Sagittal scans (T1- or T2-weighted) are particularly useful for assessing lesions within the corpus callosum (see Cases 363, 366, and 367).

Cases 374, 378, and 386 illustrate additional variations in the appearance of multiple sclerosis on T1-weighted images.

## Case 360

44-year-old woman presenting with
numbness of the legs and feet.
(axial, noncontrast scan; SE 2500/45)

## Case 361

35-year-old woman presenting with
right body numbness and right leg weakness.
(axial, noncontrast T2-weighted SE scan)

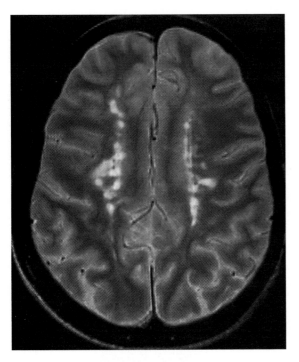

**Multiple Sclerosis**

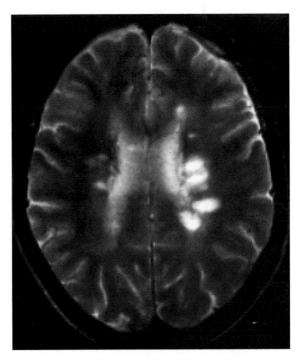

**Multiple Sclerosis**

The detection of plaques in multiple sclerosis was one of the first and most dramatic demonstrations of the contrast sensitivity of magnetic resonance imaging. Although CT scans may disclose many abnormalities in patients with demyelinating disease, MR is the procedure of choice for evaluating these cases. Negative MR scans are rare in a setting of clinically documented multiple sclerosis. (Spinal cord involvement should be considered in such instances.)

Areas of demyelination are well defined as foci of high signal intensity on long TR spin echo scans. T2 prolongation in the lesions probably reflects a variable mixture of inflammatory edema, gliosis, and axonal loss, as well as reduced myelin density. Periventricular involvement is characteristic. However, lesions due to multiple sclerosis may be found in any area of white matter, including myelinated tracts within gray matter nuclei such as the basal ganglia.

Deep hemispheric lesions often demonstrate a relatively elliptical shape, with the long axis directed toward the ventricular margin. This characteristic morphology ("Daw-

son's finger"), which can be helpful in differential diagnosis, has been attributed to the perivenular pathophysiology of demyelination. (See Cases 362 and 590 for additional examples of this appearance.)

The above cases illustrate two commonly encountered types of lesions. The small, uniform, sharply defined foci of high signal intensity in Case 360 and predominating in the right corona radiata of Case 361 are typical of old plaques demonstrated during quiescent clinical periods. The larger lesions with less distinct margins found in the left corona radiata of Case 361 suggest active demyelination with associated edema. Such lesions often demonstrate contrast enhancement (see Cases 382 and 384) and may correlate with new symptoms.

As can be surmised from these cases, the MR pattern of multiple sclerosis can vary from strikingly symmetrical to markedly asymmetrical, depending on the number and activity of individual lesions.

### Case 362

42-year-old woman presenting with
scattered paresthesias.
(axial, noncontrast FLAIR scan)

### Case 363

41-year-old woman presenting with blurred vision.
(sagittal, noncontrast FLAIR scan; 2 mm thickness)

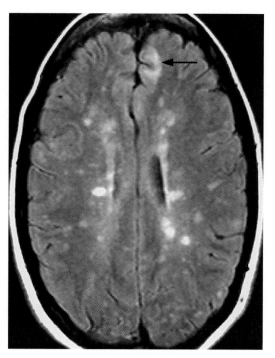

**Multiple Sclerosis**

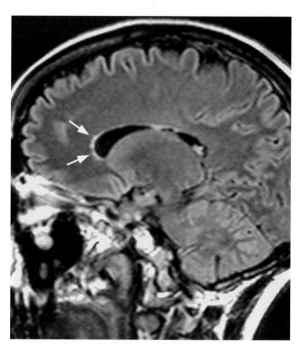

**Multiple Sclerosis**

Fluid-attenuated inversion recovery (FLAIR) pulse sequences have proven to be useful in increasing the conspicuity of small demyelinating foci, particularly within the cerebral hemispheres. The T2-weighting of such images produces abnormally high signal intensity within new or old multiple sclerosis plaques, while the low signal intensity of simple fluid prevents CSF from obscuring small lesions adjacent to ventricles or sulci.

Case 362 illustrates a number of well-defined periventricular plaques measuring a few millimeters in diameter. The larger lesions have typical elliptical morphology, with the long axis oriented perpendicular to the margin of the lateral ventricle. Subcortical lesions with more irregular shape are present in the medial left frontal lobe *(arrow)*, demonstrating the potential variation among multiple sclerosis plaques in location and morphology.

Thin sagittal FLAIR images can help detect subtle demyelinating disease involving the corpus callosum and periventricular white matter. Small lesions along the "callososeptal interface" at the inferior margin of the corpus

callosum may be the earliest indication of multiple sclerosis on MR scans.

Case 363 illustrates a few "subependymal striations" in the frontal region *(arrows)*. FLAIR images normally demonstrate a thin, smooth stripe of subependymal hyperintensity along the margin of the lateral ventricle; nodularity or striation of this hyperintensity is an early sign of perivenular inflammation/demyelination.

White matter that appears normal on conventional MR images of patients with multiple sclerosis may be demonstrably abnormal when assessed by magnetization transfer measurements, diffusion-weighted imaging, or proton spectroscopy. Reduced magnetization transfer presumably reflects decreased concentration or altered structure of myelin-related macromolecules. Decreased anisotropy on diffusion-weighted tensor images is attributable to lessening of structural barriers to the diffusion of water molecules across the myelinated margins of axons. Abnormally low concentrations of *N*-acetyl aspartate at spectroscopy imply that axonal damage may occur as an early concomitant of the demyelinating process.

### Case 364

40-year-old woman presenting with numbness of the right arm and face.
(axial, noncontrast FLAIR scan)

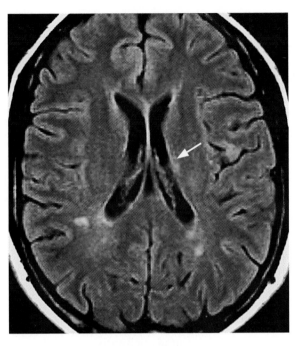

**Multiple Sclerosis**

### Case 365

18-year-old woman presenting with dizziness.
(axial, noncontrast T2-weighted SE scan)

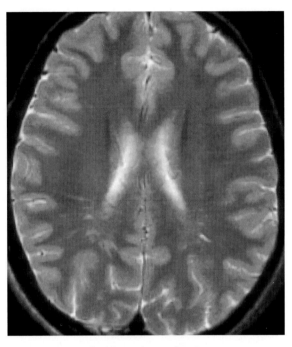

**Prominent Perivascular Spaces**
(normal variant)

---

A number of pathologies can cause multiple small lesions within cerebral white matter. The periventricular clustering of high signal foci in the parietal lobes Case 364 is typical for demyelinating disease but not specific. Other inflammatory processes (e.g., sarcoidosis, systemic lupus erythematosus, and Lyme disease; see Cases 495 and 496) or small infarcts (see Case 606) could present similarly.

The subtle lesion in the mid left corona radiata of Case 364 *(arrow)* would likely be overlooked on a standard T2-weighted scan with high signal intensity CSF filling the adjacent ventricle. "Intermediate" or "balanced" spin echo sequences with long TR and short TE values or FLAIR images (as above) are best able to distinguish small plaques from neighboring fluid-containing structures.

Case 365 illustrates a normal developmental variant. Unusually wide sleeves of CSF often accompany small arter-

ies from the cerebral surface into the hemisphere, representing giant Virchow-Robin spaces. Such perivascular spaces have a linear, radial pattern on scans paralleling the direction of penetrating arteries, as is usually true on axial images in the deep parietal region.

Scans perpendicular to penetrating arteries (e.g., axial images at the vertex) demonstrate prominent perivascular spaces as a field of tiny dots that are smaller, more uniform, and more peripheral than typical plaques of multiple sclerosis (or than typical "lacunar" infarcts). Prominent perivascular spaces are usually inconspicuous on long TR short TE spin echo or FLAIR images, in contrast to the clear definition of demyelinating foci on such scans.

See Case 413 for a more subtle presentation of prominent perivascular spaces in deep parietal white matter.

# MULTIPLE SCLEROSIS: INVOLVEMENT OF THE CORPUS CALLOSUM

### Case 366

46-year-old man presenting with facial numbness.
(sagittal, noncontrast T1-weighted SE scan)

### Case 367

27-year-old woman presenting with paresthesias.
(sagittal, noncontrast T2-weighted FSE scan)

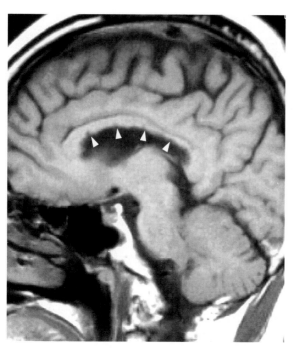

**Multiple Sclerosis**

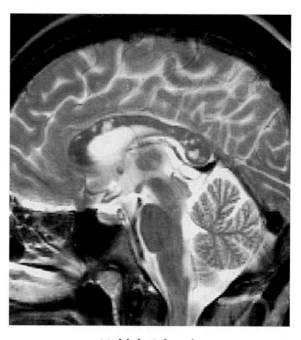

**Multiple Sclerosis**

The corpus callosum is routinely involved by multiple sclerosis. Demyelinating foci within the transversely oriented commissure are often better demonstrated on sagittal or coronal views than on axial images.

A particularly common location for plaques is the inferior surface of the corpus callosum or "callososeptal interface" (see Case 363). Case 366 is a good example, demonstrating thinning of the corpus callosum in association with a series of small lesions causing marked irregularity along its inferior margin *(arrowheads)*.

Lesions within the substance of the corpus callosum or spanning its diameter are also encountered, as in Case 367. Such plaques are usually apparent on axial T2-weighted scans as short, transversely oriented zones of increased signal intensity immediately superior to the bodies of lateral ventricles (see Case 370).

Long-standing multiple sclerosis is typically associated with callosal atrophy, reflecting both direct involvement and secondary loss of volume due to hemispheric disease.

The presence of callosal lesions can be a helpful clue to the diagnosis of multiple sclerosis when hemispheric abnormalities are nonspecific. Foci of ischemic change may mimic multiple sclerosis in the centrum semiovale or periventricular regions (see Cases 606 and 607) but less commonly involve the corpus callosum.

### Case 368

28-year-old woman.
(axial, noncontrast scan; SE 3000/20)

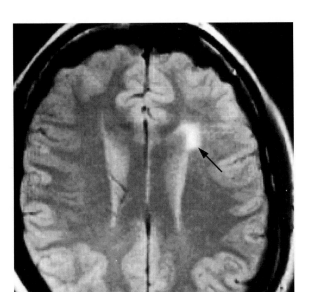

**Multiple Sclerosis**

### Case 369

37-year-old woman.
(axial, noncontrast scan; 3000/25)

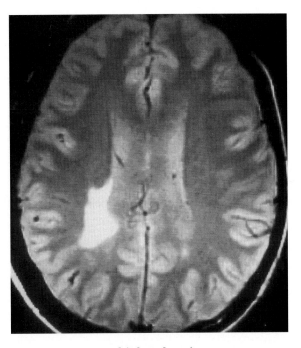

**Multiple Sclerosis**

These patients illustrate a characteristic morphology occasionally demonstrated by lesions of multiple sclerosis. In both cases, a plaque is based along a corner of the ventricular margin. Despite the otherwise convex borders of the lesion, there is little effacement or compression of the ventricle. This lack of ventricular deformity is distinct from the appearance of a true subependymal mass (compare to Case 349) and can suggest the diagnosis of multiple sclerosis.

### Case 370

25-year-old woman presenting with
scattered paresthesias.
(axial, noncontrast T2-weighted FSE scan)

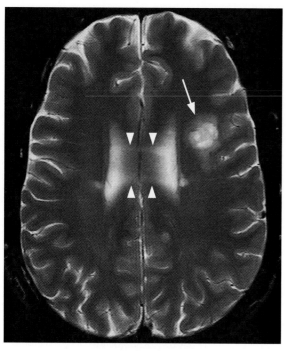

**Multiple Sclerosis**

### Case 371

30-year-old woman complaining of patchy
bilateral arm and leg numbness.
(axial, noncontrast T2-weighted SE scan)

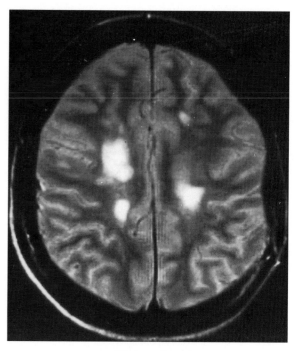

**Multiple Sclerosis**

Although small lesions within periventricular white matter are characteristic of multiple sclerosis, larger and more peripheral plaques are commonly encountered. The left frontal focus in Case 370 is an example *(arrow)*. Without the associated periventricular plaques, this mass-like morphology could suggest granulomatous inflammation or neoplasm. Correlation with clinical findings and a careful search for accompanying lesions may be necessary for diagnosis in such cases.

Multiple sclerosis is one of several pathologies to be considered in the presence of multiple subcortical lesions, as demonstrated in Case 371. A similar pattern may be seen in acute disseminated encephalomyelitis (see Cases 390-392), progressive multifocal leukoencephalopathy (see Cases 398-401), systemic lupus erythematosus (see Cases 481-483), and metastatic disease (see Cases 6, 8, 11, and 15).

Case 370 illustrates the typical transversely oriented or striated appearance of T2 prolongation due to demyelinating disease within the corpus callosum as seen on axial images *(arrowheads)*.

### Case 372

23-year-old woman presenting with
vague paresthesias.
(axial, noncontrast scan; SE 3000/28)

### Case 373

39-year-old man complaining of headaches.
(axial, noncontrast scan; SE 3000/25)

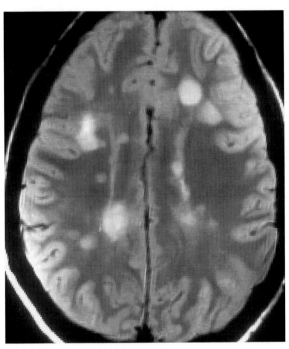

**Multiple Sclerosis**

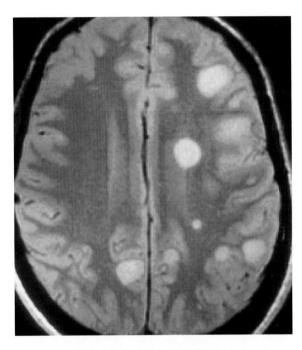

**Metastatic Adenocarcinoma**
(unknown primary)

Demyelinating foci may be sufficiently numerous and nodular to mimic metastatic lesions, as in Case 372. Prominent involvement of periventricular regions and the clinical context are clues to the correct diagnosis.

Metastatic disease should be included in the differential diagnosis of multiple white matter lesions, even in young adults. The majority of the metastases in Case 373 are subcortical, with less involvement of periventricular areas.

Both multiple sclerosis and cerebral metastases may also present with a "miliary" pattern of smaller, more numerous foci of signal abnormality throughout cerebral white matter. Such lesions may demonstrate contrast enhancement and mimic infectious etiologies (see Cases 384 and 385).

### Case 374

21-year-old woman presenting with optic neuritis.
(sagittal, noncontrast T1-weighted SE scan)

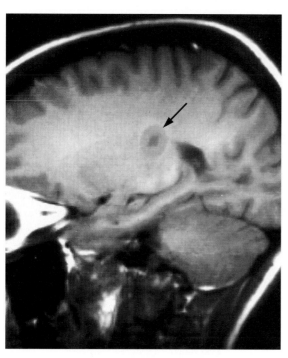

**Multiple Sclerosis**

### Case 375

29-year-old woman presenting with
"trouble controlling my right side."
(axial, noncontrast T2-weighted SE scan)

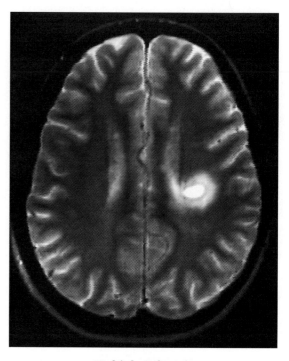

**Multiple Sclerosis**

---

Active plaques sometimes demonstrate a variably thick ring or band of altered signal intensity within a larger lesion. This feature is most commonly appreciated as a rim of relatively low intensity within an edematous zone on T2-weighted scans, as in Case 375 (see also Case 471). Alternatively, a peripheral band of long T1 and T2 values may marginate the remainder of a lesion, as illustrated in Case 374 (and in Case 471). These findings may correlate with a rim of enhancement on postcontrast scans.

The ring structure likely represents a zone of inflammation and reaction that corresponds to an intermediate stage of demyelination. The finding can suggest the diagnosis of multiple sclerosis in ambiguous cases. However, a thin rim can also be seen on MR studies of cerebral abscesses (see Cases 459-462). Target morphologies have been noted within masses due to toxoplasmosis and primary CNS lymphoma (especially in AIDS patients).

Cases 374 and 375 illustrate that multiple sclerosis may present as a single focus of acute demyelination. The large size and indistinct margins of these lesions suggest active inflammation.

A form of rapidly progressive demyelination in young patients causing large lesions that contain parallel arcs of alternating signal intensity has been recognized and labelled as *concentric sclerosis of Balo.*

### Case 376

18-year-old woman presenting with
worsening left hemiparesis.
(axial, noncontrast scan; SE 3000/28)

### Case 377

29-year-old woman presenting with numbness
and clumsiness of the right arm.
(axial, noncontrast scan; SE 3000/28)

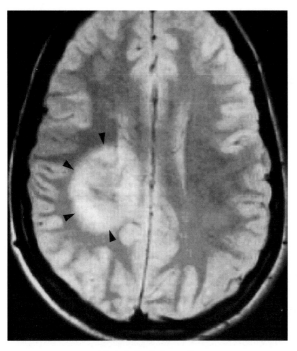

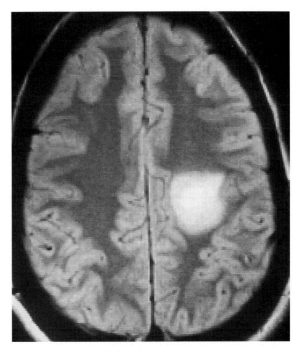

**Multiple Sclerosis**

**Multiple Sclerosis**

Regions of active demyelination in multiple sclerosis may measure several centimeters in diameter, mimicking cerebral neoplasms on CT and MR scans. Such lesions are usually located in the centrum semiovale, as in the above cases. They may also occur within the corpus callosum. Associated contrast enhancement is typically present and may be solid or peripheral. Marginal enhancement is often asymmetrical (see Case 383).

A giant focus of demyelinating disease should be considered whenever a deep hemispheric "tumor" is encountered in a young adult. A round shape and relative lack of mass effect (see Cases 368 and 369) can be clues to the correct diagnosis.

Perfusion-weighted imaging may help distinguish between a large demyelinating lesion and a primary neoplasm. Cerebral blood volume (CBV) is normal or slightly reduced (due to capillary compression by edema) in a zone of demyelination, whereas even low grade gliomas typically demonstrate an increase in rCBV.

The morphology within giant plaques can also be characteristic on dynamic T2*-weighted perfusion images. Parallel stripes or bands of transiently decreased signal intensity may be seen coursing through edematous tissue in a direction perpendicular to the ventricular margin, probably representing engorgement of medullary veins in the inflamed region. This accentuation (rather than distortion) of anatomy favors a reactive process over a neoplastic one.

### Case 378

15-year-old girl presenting with abnormal gait.
(sagittal, noncontrast T1-weighted SE scan)

### Case 379

39-year-old man presenting with diplopia.
(axial, noncontrast T2-weighted SE scan)

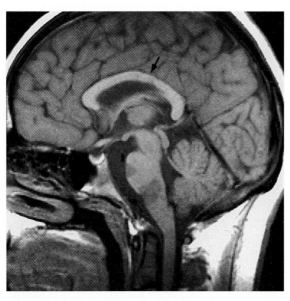

**Multiple Sclerosis**

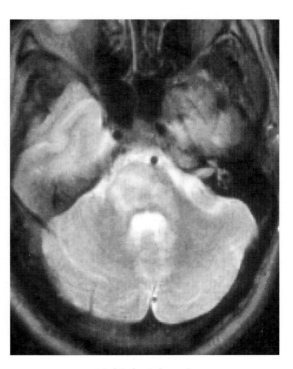

**Multiple Sclerosis**

Multiple sclerosis frequently involves the brainstem and cerebellar peduncles. The pattern of demyelinating foci in these locations may be multinodular or confluent.

In Case 378, well-defined zones of localized edema are present at the ventral margin of the pons and at the pontomedullary junction. Mass effect from the latter lesion causes slight deformity of the floor of the fourth ventricle.

Case 379 illustrates patchy prolongation of T2 values involving most of the pons and extending to the brachium pontis bilaterally. Such large areas of confluent brainstem demyelination and edema may mimic a neoplasm. This appearance can be especially confusing in adolescents or young children, who present with brainstem gliomas more commonly than demyelinating disease. (Also compare Case 379 to the appearance of the central pontine myelinolysis in Case 406.)

The middle cerebellar peduncle is a common site for demyelinating plaques. One or more small lesions within the brachium pontis in a young patient should suggest the possibility of multiple sclerosis. (See Case 405 for another example.)

Small plaques are faintly seen within the body of the corpus callosum in Case 378 *(arrow)*.

# DIFFERENTIAL DIAGNOSIS:
## FOCAL MIDBRAIN LESION

### Case 380

52-year-old man presenting with headaches.
(axial, noncontrast scan; SE 3000/45)

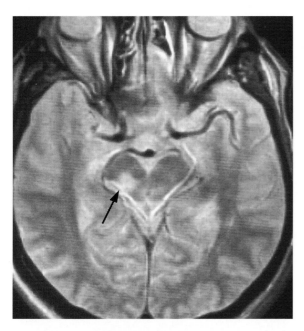

**Metastatic Melanoma**

### Case 381

15-year-old girl presenting with abnormal gait.
(axial, noncontrast T2-weighted FSE scan)

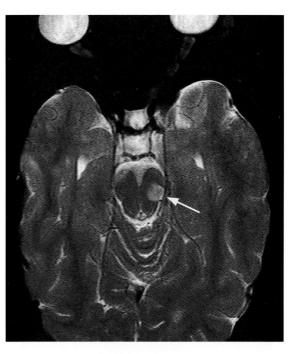

**Multiple Sclerosis**
(same patient as Case 378)

---

Metastatic disease should be considered whenever focal brainstem lesions are encountered in adults. MRI has demonstrated that the incidence of metastasis to the brainstem (and spinal cord) is higher than appreciated by prior imaging techniques (see also Cases 21 and 22). The appearance of the small metastasis in Case 380 is nonspecific, and demyelinating disease could be considered in the differential diagnosis.

Case 381 illustrates a demyelinating plaque within the midbrain of the patient presented as Case 378 (*arrow*; a small amount of abnormal signal is also present at the an-

terior margin of the right cerebral peduncle). By itself, this lesion is also nonspecific. However, the association with other foci of signal abnormality in the brainstem and corpus callosum (see Case 378) suggests a multifocal disorder of white matter. The main differential diagnosis in this young patient then becomes multiple sclerosis versus acute disseminated encephalomyelitis.

Both of the above lesions demonstrated focal enhancement on postcontrast images.

Compare these cases to the differential diagnosis in Cases 614 and 615.

## Case 382

24-year-old woman presenting with
incoordination and imbalance.
(axial, postcontrast T1-weighted SE scan)

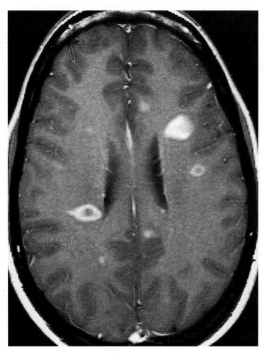

**Multiple Sclerosis**

## Case 383

34-year-old man presenting with a seizure.
(axial, postcontrast T1-weighted SE scan with MTS)

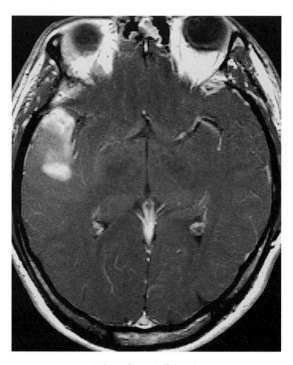

**"Singular" Sclerosis**

Active demyelinating plaques may demonstrate solid or peripheral patterns of contrast enhancement, as illustrated in Case 382. Relatively homogeneous enhancement can be seen throughout lesions ranging from a few millimeters to several centimeters in size. Rim enhancement may form complete rings or partial arcs and can be found within multiple small plaques or at the margin of giant lesions. Occasional "target" lesions are seen with both central and peripheral enhancement.

Either pattern of enhancement may cause confusion if demyelinating foci are few or solitary. The unusual clinical presentation and nonspecific MRI appearance of the temporal lobe mass in Case 383 led to a biopsy, which documented only demyelination.

Such solitary demyelinating foci have been referred to as "singular sclerosis." When large, they may closely resemble a neoplasm. Demyelinating disease should be included

in the differential diagnosis of such lesions in a young patient (see discussion of Cases 376 and 377).

Serial scans may demonstrate evolution of a plaque from an active enhancing phase to a quiescent, nonenhancing lesion over a period of several weeks. Occasional plaques continue to enhance for several months. Although the presence of contrast enhancement within a plaque presumably indicates active inflammation, the majority of enhancing lesions are clinically silent.

Restricted diffusion on diffusion-weighted scans has been reported to be a more sensitive marker of active demyelination than contrast enhancement. However, established lesions of multiple sclerosis (and acute disseminated encephalomyelitis) often demonstrate facilitated diffusion, correlating with the usual prolongation of T1 values and suggesting focal loss of tissue with an increased fluid compartment.

# DIFFERENTIAL DIAGNOSIS:
## MULTIPLE ENHANCING CEREBRAL NODULES

### Case 384

21-year-old woman presenting with blurred vision.
(axial, postcontrast T1-weighted SE scan)

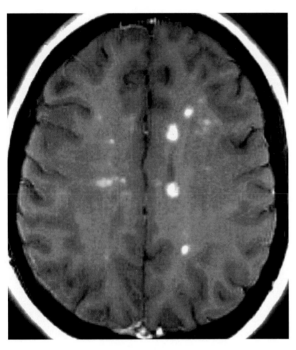

**Multiple Sclerosis**

### Case 385

40-year-old woman presenting with
nausea and dizziness.
(axial, postcontrast T1-weighted SE scan)

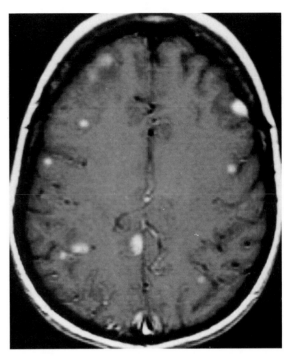

**Metastatic Carcinoma of the Breast**

---

The enhancing plaques of multiple sclerosis may be numerous and relatively uniform in size, as in Case 384. The pattern of such lesions can resemble the appearance of multiple metastases, illustrated by Case 385.

Plaques usually occupy a midhemispheric location. This distribution is more central than the peripheral position of most metastases near the gray-white matter junction. The clinical setting often distinguishes these two processes when overlapping MR patterns are encountered.

Additional pathologies in the differential diagnosis of multiple enhancing nodules include acute disseminated encephalomyelitis (see Case 397), disseminated infection (e.g., cysticercosis, tuberculosis, histoplasmosis, or toxoplasmosis), sarcoidosis (see Case 487), primary CNS lymphoma (see Case 351), subacute multifocal infarction (arterial or venous; see Case 587), vasculitis, and multiple cavernous angiomas.

237

## Case 386

49-year-old woman.
(sagittal, noncontrast T1-weighted SE scan)

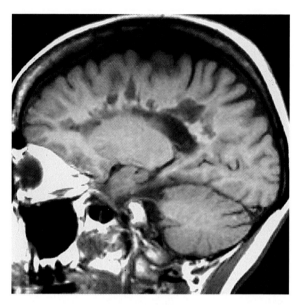

**Multiple Sclerosis**

## Case 387

41-year-old man.
(axial, noncontrast scan; SE 2500/28)

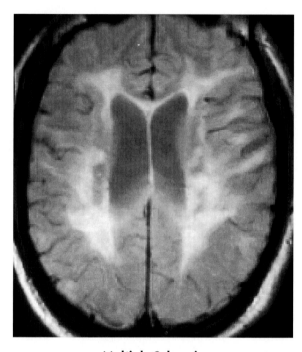

**Multiple Sclerosis**

Long-standing multiple sclerosis is often associated with ventricular and sulcal enlargement, as seen in the above cases. This diagnosis is among the potential causes of prominent CSF spaces in a young patient (see discussion of Cases 534 and 535).

The sagittal scan in Case 386 demonstrates abnormally large sulci and ventricles for the patient's age. In addition, multiple irregular zones of very well-defined low signal intensity occupy the periventricular region, representing areas of old demyelination. A thin rim of high intensity is present at the margins of these lesions, an occasional finding on short TR scans of MS plaques. The basis of such peripheral T1-shortening is undetermined but may relate to accumulation of myelin degradation products. The finding is normally noted in the context of chronic disease.

Case 387 demonstrates large areas of abnormal intensity throughout the white matter, reflecting long-standing mul-

tiple sclerosis. Ventricular enlargement indicates associated volume loss. The pattern is bilateral and extensive, resembling a diffuse leukoencephalopathy (see Cases 408-410), severe vascular insufficiency (as in Cases 608 and 609), or radiation change (see Case 548).

Another MRI finding in some cases of chronic multiple sclerosis is abnormally prominent or extensive low signal intensity within the basal ganglia and thalamus on T2-weighted images. This appearance has been suggested to reflect the accumulation of iron due to impaired peripheral axonal transport.

In an elderly patient and in an ambiguous clinical context, chronic demyelinating disease can be distinguished from ischemic white matter changes by involvement of subcortical "U" fibers and the corpus callosum in the former disorder. These regions are typically spared from ischemic change, as discussed in Chapter 11.

### Case 388

11-year-old boy who developed somnolence
and hemiparesis over a four-day period,
two weeks after a viral illness.
(coronal, postcontrast T1-weighted scan)

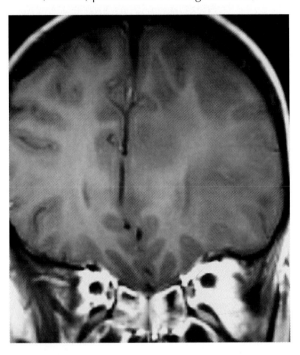

**Acute Disseminated Encephalomyelitis**

### Case 389

23-year-old woman presenting with
rapidly worsening hemiparesis,
three weeks after "the flu."
(axial, noncontrast T1-weighted SE scan)

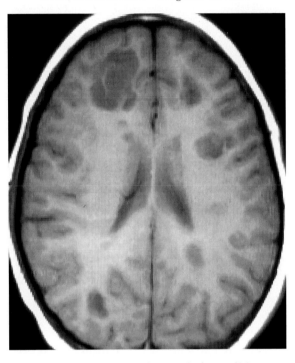

**Acute Disseminated Encephalomyelitis**

---

Acute disseminated encephalomyelitis (ADEM) is alternatively called *immune-mediated encephalitis* because the pathophysiology is believed to involve autoimmune demyelination. Patients typically give a history of antigenic challenge (e.g., virus or vaccination) days or weeks prior to the onset of symptoms.

ADEM primarily affects white matter, but deep gray matter is often involved. The pattern is highly variable. Large, geographical regions of edema and mass effect may develop, as seen in the left frontal lobe in Case 388. (See Case 390 for a T2-weighted axial scan of this patient.) Both symmetrical and asymmetrical presentations may be encountered.

In other cases of ADEM, smaller and more nodular lesions are scattered throughout the hemispheres, illustrated by Case 389 (see also Cases 391 and 392). Such lesions are typically a little larger than quiescent plaques of multiple sclerosis and have a more random distribution.

The demyelinating lesions of ADEM usually present as variably defined foci of low signal intensity on T1-weighted scans. Some cases of immune-mediated encephalitis are associated with hemorrhage, which can cause T1-shortening due to the presence of methemoglobin. This entity, previously called *acute hemorrhagic leukoencephalitis*, progresses rapidly and carries a poor prognosis.

Contrast enhancement in ADEM is variable (see Cases 396 and 397). Many lesions demonstrate little or no enhancement, as in Case 388. Other foci of ADEM enhance prominently, resembling the active plaques of multiple sclerosis.

239

### Case 390

11-year-old boy presenting with
somnolence and hemiparesis.
(axial, noncontrast T2-weighted SE scan)

### Case 391

3-year-old girl with rapidly decreasing mental status.
(axial, noncontrast T2-weighted SE scan)

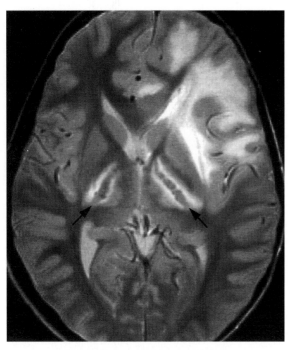

**Acute Disseminated Encephalomyelitis**
(same patient as Case 388)

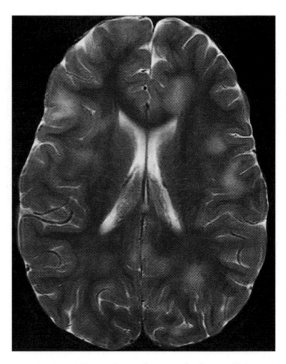

**Acute Disseminated Encephalomyelitis**

---

Zones of inflammation in ADEM are well demonstrated as regions of high signal intensity on long TR images. The size and symmetry of hemispheric lesions are variable.

Case 390 demonstrates symmetrical involvement of the internal capsules *(arrows)*, with grossly asymmetrical demyelination in the left frontal lobe. In Case 391, multiple patchy areas of T2 prolongation are predominantly subcortical. Case 392 presents a third morphology in ADEM, with a multinodular appearance, and Case 409 illustrates confluent hemispheric edema.

Nonhemorrhagic cases of ADEM usually respond well to steroids. Clinical improvement often precedes resolution of the MR abnormalities, which may continue to evolve while symptoms are regressing. Both of the above children were clinically normal within a month after presentation.

Like multiple sclerosis, ADEM frequently involves the brainstem, cerebellar peduncles, and cerebellum.

# DIFFERENTIAL DIAGNOSIS:
## MULTIPLE ROUND LESIONS WITHIN CEREBRAL WHITE MATTER

### Case 392

23-year-old woman presenting with
the rapid onset of hemiparesis.
(axial, noncontrast T2-weighted SE scan)

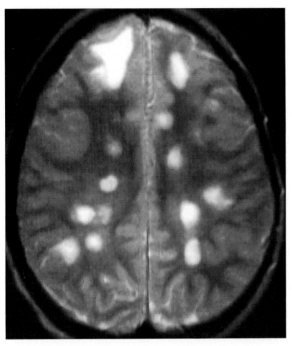

**Acute Disseminated Encephalomyelitis**

### Case 393

39-year-old man presenting with headaches.
(axial, noncontrast T2-weighted SE scan)

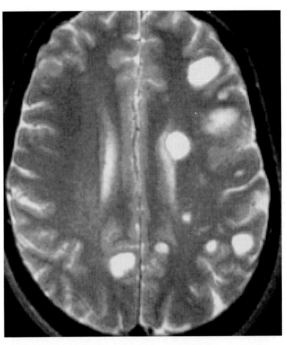

**Metastatic Adenocarcinoma**
(unknown primary)

---

ADEM may present as multiple nodular lesions scattered throughout the cerebral hemispheres, as in Case 392. The corpus callosum is commonly involved.

Such an appearance can resemble the pattern of cerebral metastases within subcortical and periventricular white matter, illustrated in Case 393. As discussed in Chapter 1, metastases are characteristically sharply defined and occasionally incite little edema. In such instances, metastatic disease in a young patient may resemble a demyelinating disorder.

The lesions of ADEM are typically larger and more scattered than the plaques of multiple sclerosis. However, the appearance of these two disorders can clearly overlap (compare Case 392 to Case 372). Characteristic associated findings of multiple sclerosis may assist in differential diagnosis. In other cases, clinical correlation and follow-up studies are necessary to distinguish between the two pathologies.

Unlike the typical relapsing course of multiple sclerosis, ADEM is usually monophasic. However, an episode of ADEM may extend over a period of four to six weeks.

### Case 394

3-year-old girl presenting with decreased
level of consciousness.
(axial, noncontrast T2-weighted FSE scan)

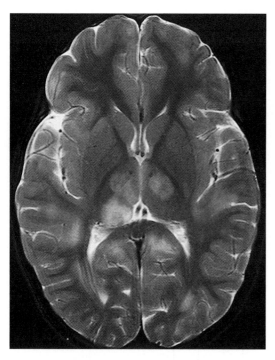

**Acute Disseminated Encephalomyelitis**
(same patient as Case 391)

### Case 395

4-year-old boy presenting with a one-day
history of left hemiparesis.
(axial, noncontrast FLAIR scan)

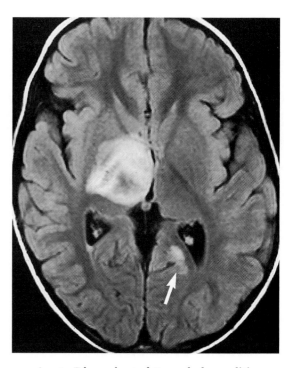

**Acute Disseminated Encephalomyelitis**

Because white matter tracts extend among the neuronal masses of deep nuclei, demyelinating disorders may affect these structures. ADEM commonly causes lesions in the basal ganglia and thalami. Areas of nuclear edema may be accompanied by lesions within peripheral white matter or be relatively solitary.

Case 394 demonstrates bilateral but asymmetrical thalamic lesions. Multiple areas of signal abnormality were present within subcortical white matter on other images (see Case 391).

A large zone of confluent edema involves the majority of the right thalamus in Case 395, extending across the posterior limb of the internal capsule to reach the lentiform nucleus. The mass effect of the lesion displaces and compresses the third ventricle, resembling the thalamic gliomas in Cases 79 and 80. The presence of a smaller second lesion medial to the trigone of the left lateral ventricle *(arrow)* is a clue to consider a multifocal inflammatory process in the differential diagnosis. Another clue is the characteristic morphology of edema outlining (but not displacing) the descending corticospinal tract within the internal capsule (compare to Case 390).

See Cases 396 and 415 for other examples of thalamic lesions in ADEM. Compare Case 394 to the thalamic involvement by Wernicke's encephalopathy in Case 515 and by viral encephalitis in Case 656.

# ACUTE DISSEMINATED ENCEPHALOMYELITIS: CONTRAST ENHANCEMENT

### Case 396

6-year-old girl presenting with bilateral
arm and leg numbness.
(axial, postcontrast T1-weighted SE scan)

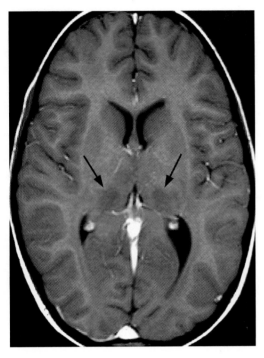

**Acute Disseminated Encephalomyelitis**

### Case 397

5-year-old girl presenting with
drowsiness and a seizure.
(axial, postcontrast T1-weighted SE scan)

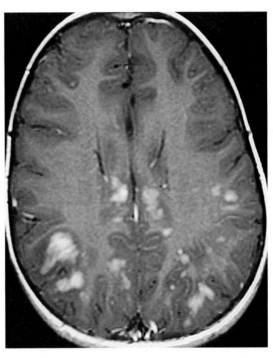

**Acute Disseminated Encephalomyelitis**

Lesions of acute disseminated encephalomyelitis often demonstrate little or no contrast enhancement, as illustrated by the symmetrical thalamic involvement in Case 396 *(arrows)*. Alternatively, ADEM may cause intense, multifocal enhancement, as seen in Case 397.

Variation in the extent of enhancement probably reflects differing stages in the evolution of inflammation/demyelination, as well as varying severity of injury to the blood-brain barrier. Since ADEM is a monophasic illness, the lesions in any individual case usually progress together and demonstrate comparable enhancement at any given time. (Compare to the common presence of lesions with differ-

ing degrees of enhancement in patients with multiple sclerosis.)

The enhancing foci in Case 397 resemble a disseminated infectious process such as tuberculosis or histoplasmosis (see Cases 472 and 479). However, the morphology of enhancing lesions in ADEM is usually more irregular and patchy than the rounded nodules and/or rims of multifocal bacterial or fungal infection. The subcortical predominance of enhancement in Case 397 is also distinct from the typical patterns of viral encephalitis (see Chapter 9).

Case 415 presents an example of enhancing thalamic lesions in ADEM.

### Case 398

60-year-old man presenting with hemiparesis.
(sagittal, noncontrast T1-weighted SE scan)

### Case 399

57-year-old man presenting with confusion.
(coronal, noncontrast T1-weighted SE scan)

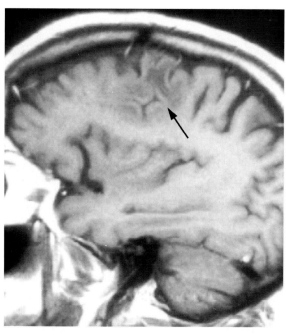

**Progressive Multifocal Leukoencephalopathy**

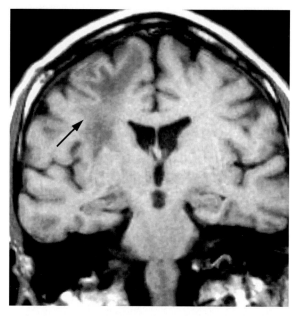

**Progressive Multifocal Leukoencephalopathy**

Progressive multifocal leukoencephalopathy (PML) is a demyelinating disorder representing infection by a papovavirus. The lesion is usually seen in immunocompromised hosts. Lymphoma and leukemia have been common predisposing conditions, but a rapidly increasing proportion of PML cases now occurs in AIDS patients. Iatrogenic immunosuppression may also be implicated. (Compare with the epidemiology of primary CNS lymphoma, discussed in Cases 346 and 347.)

The multifocal demyelination of PML often involves subcortical white matter, as seen in the above cases. Mass effect is rare, and hemorrhage is very uncommon. Contrast enhancement is notably absent in most cases.

Notice the relative sparing of the cortical ribbon in involved areas. This "heart of the gyrus" pattern with discretely subcortical edema is even more striking on T2-weighted images (see Case 401).

Cerebral involvement in PML is often bilateral but asymmetrical. Unlike multiple sclerosis or ADEM, PML rarely involves the spinal cord.

### Case 400

28-year-old woman with systemic lymphoma.
(axial, noncontrast scan; SE 3000/45)

### Case 401

57-year-old man presenting with confusion.
(axial, noncontrast T2-weighted SE scan)

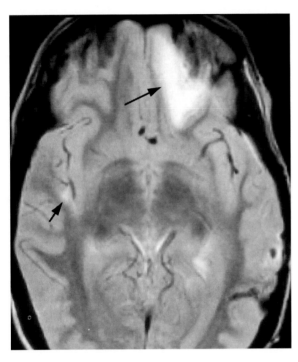

**Progressive Multifocal Leukoencephalopathy**

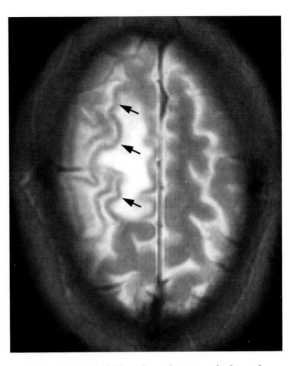

**Progressive Multifocal Leukoencephalopathy**
(same patient as Case 399)

---

PML may cause signal abnormality in subcortical or deep hemispheric white matter. Case 400 illustrates the variable size of such lesions. A large focus is present in the left frontal lobe *(long arrow)*, with much smaller lesions in the right superior temporal gyrus *(short arrow)*, and near the apex of the left sylvian cistern.

A prominent finding on many CT and MR scans in PML is the "heart of the gyrus" involvement demonstrated in Case 401. Individual gyri are thickened by edema of central white matter, with conspicuous sparing and margination of the overlying cortical ribbon *(arrows)*.

Although subcortical edema is characteristic of PML, the finding is not specific. Edema associated with metastases near the gray/white junction may produce an appearance similar to Case 401 on noncontrast scans. The injection of

contrast material should help to narrow the diagnosis: metastases inciting edema would be expected to enhance, whereas the lesions of PML usually do not.

The asymmetrical and multifocal appearance of PML may also resemble early cerebritis or venous infarction (due to thrombosis of a dural sinus). The correct diagnosis in such cases is aided by the concentration of findings in PML within white matter and the usual lack of contrast enhancement.

Another potential cause of multifocal subcortical signal abnormality in the clinical setting of immunosuppression is cyclosporin A toxicity in transplant patients (see Case 546). Cerebral vasculitis (e.g., primary angiitis of the CNS) is an additional pathology that may present with scattered areas of subcortical edema (see Cases 486, 641, and 642).

## Case 402

29-year-old man presenting with
ataxia and known AIDS.
(axial, noncontrast T2-weighted SE scan)

## Case 403

41-year-old woman presenting with confusion
and a history of lymphoma.
(axial, noncontrast T2-weighted SE scan)

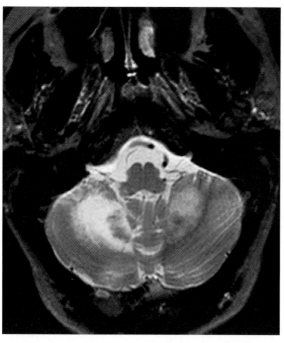

**Progressive Multifocal Leukoencephalopathy**

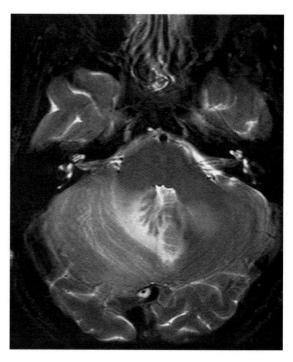

**Progressive Multifocal Leukoencephalopathy**

Progressive multifocal leukoencephalopathy may cause unilateral or bilateral lesions within cerebellar white matter. The most common appearance is a variably defined zone of T2 prolongation surrounding the dentate nucleus, as illustrated above. (Compare this margination of the dentate nucleus to the cortical sparing by supratentorial lesions such as Case 401.)

Bilateral cerebellar involvement is usually asymmetrical, as seen in Cases 402 and 403. Edema in Case 403 extends into the vermis and is associated with mass effect compressing the fourth ventricle.

Multiple sclerosis can also cause one or more lesions of infratentorial white matter in young adults, but involvement of the brainstem and brachium pontis is more common than cerebellar plaques (see Cases 378 and 379).

Cerebellar lesions may be found in acute disseminated encephalomyelitis, but the clinical context usually differs from PML, and the pattern of accompanying supratentorial lesions often helps to distinguish between these pathologies.

Several other processes can present images similar to the above cases. Edema within cerebellar white matter may be seen in hypertensive encephalopathy (see Cases 544 and 545), alone or in combination with supratentorial abnormality. Infarction in the distribution of the superior cerebellar artery can involve white matter surrounding the dentate nucleus. Symmetrical prolongation of T1 and T2 values in cerebellar white matter has also been reported in occasional cases of Langerhans cell histiocytosis.

# DIFFERENTIAL DIAGNOSIS:
## LESIONS WITHIN THE BRACHIUM PONTIS

### Case 404

29-year-old-man with AIDS.
(axial, noncontrast T2-weighted SE scan)

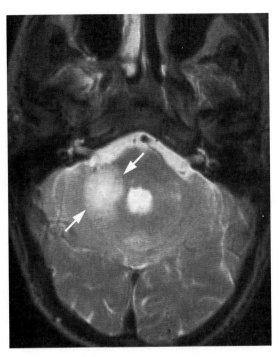

**Progressive Multifocal Leukoencephalopathy**

### Case 405

37-year-old-man presenting with left facial pain.
(axial, noncontrast T2-weighted SE scan)

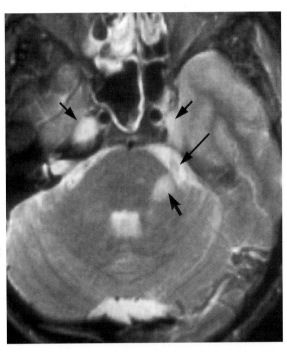

**Multiple Sclerosis**

---

The size and hazy definition of the lesion in Case 404 are compatible with active demyelination (compare to Cases 358 and 375). Multiple sclerosis and acute disseminated encephalomyelitis would be included in the differential diagnosis. Although the edema does not outline the dentate nucleus in this instance (as in Cases 402 and 403), PML should be considered as the etiology of any focal demyelination in an immunocompromised patient.

As discussed in Cases 378 and 379, the middle cerebellar peduncle is a common site of demyelination in multiple sclerosis. The lesion in Case 405 *(wide arrow)* is located at the junction of the pons and brachium pontis. The patient's facial pain probably indicates dysfunction of axons entering the pons from the trigeminal nerve *(long arrow)*. Multiple sclerosis is among the potential etiologies of trigeminal neuralgia.

A rare cause of focal edema within the lateral pons is trigeminal neuritis (e.g., herpes) extending from the nerve into the brainstem.

CSF within Meckel's caves is well seen as areas of high signal intensity occupying the posterior portion of the cavernous sinuses in Case 401 *(small arrows)*. Head tilt can cause asymmetrical prominence of Meckel's cave on one side, falsely suggesting a posterior parasellar lesion on the side with better visualization.

### Case 406A

46-year-old man presenting with decreased level of consciousness and a history of alcohol abuse.
(sagittal, noncontrast T1-weighted SE scan)

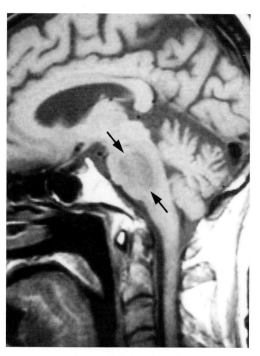

**Central Pontine Myelinolysis**

### Case 406B

Same patient.
(axial, noncontrast T2-weighted SE scan)

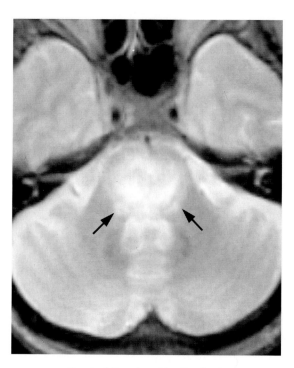

**Central Pontine Myelinolysis**

Central pontine myelinolysis (CPM) is an acute demyelinating process affecting the brainstem. It is incompletely understood but seems to correlate with the rapid correction (or overcorrection) of severe electrolyte abnormalities. The condition has also been called *osmotic demyelination syndrome* or *osmotic myelinolysis*. Other factors (e.g., nutritional) may contribute.

CT scans may be abnormal in cases of CPM, but definition of the lesion is often vague. MR provides unequivocal documentation of this pathology, as seen above. The pons is expanded by a central zone of long T1 and T2 values suggesting edema. Pontine involvement is symmetrical, unlike most brainstem infarcts. Transverse pontine fibers are most affected, with relative sparing of peripheral tissue and descending tracts. The morphology of the involved region on axial images may be round, triangular, or butterfly shaped. Contrast enhancement in CPM is unusual.

A similar demyelinating pathology ("extrapontine myelinolysis") can occur within the basal ganglia and cerebral hemispheres, together with or independent of pontine involvement (see Case 530). Conversely, other white matter disorders (e.g., PML) may involve the pons.

The characteristic MR findings of CPM may not develop until several days after the onset of symptoms. Symptoms usually begin a few days after the correction of hyponatremia.

### Case 407A

48-year-old woman, four months after admission
for central pontine myelinolysis.
(sagittal, noncontrast T1-weighted SE scan)

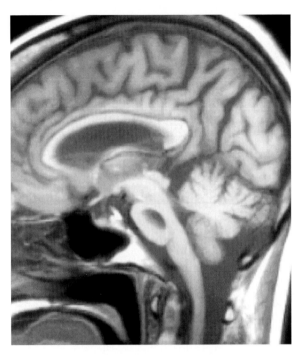

**Central Pontine Myelinolysis**

### Case 407B

Same patient.
(axial, noncontrast T2-weighted SE scan)

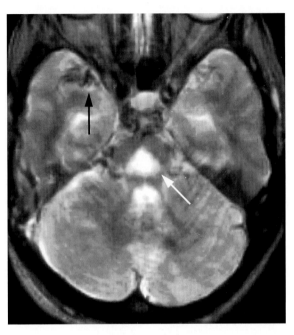

**Central Pontine Myelinolysis**

Some cases of CPM progress inexorably to death. Other patients recover completely, with resolution of scan abnormalities. A third group of patients demonstrates partial or complete clinical recovery with residual abnormality of the pons on follow-up MR studies.

In this case the pontine lesion is smaller and better defined than in Case 406, reflecting demarcation of old encephalomalacia. Involvement of the central pons with sparing of peripheral tracts may result in a distinctive trian-

gular shape of myelinolysis on axial images in early or late stages, as seen here (*white arrow*, Case 407B).

A prominent tangle of vessels in the anterior portion of the right middle cranial fossa (*black arrow*, Case 407B) represents proximal branches of the middle cerebral artery (with adjacent CSF pulsation). This normal finding should not be mistaken for an arteriovenous malformation (compare to Cases 738-741).

### Case 408A

10-year-old boy with a one-year history of
deteriorating school performance, behavior
problems, and diminished reflexes.
(sagittal, noncontrast T1-weighted SE scan)

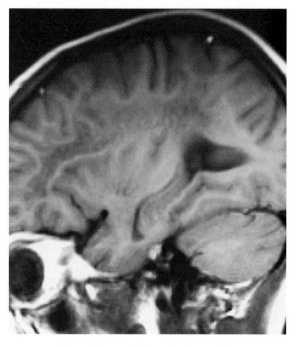

**Metachromatic Leukodystrophy**

### Case 408B

Same patient.
(axial, noncontrast T2-weighted SE scan)

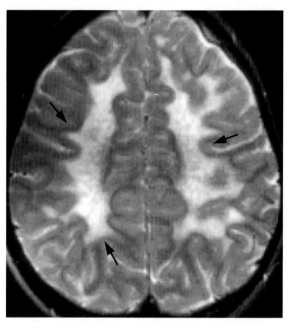

**Metachromatic Leukodystrophy**

The demyelinating disorders described in the previous portion of this chapter are characterized by destruction of normally formed myelin. A number of other pathological conditions can be classified as "dysmyelinating," in that they cause abnormal or incomplete development of myelin.

Metachromatic leukodystrophy, one of the relatively common dysmyelinating disorders, is caused by insufficient activity of the enzyme arylsulfatase A. Most cases of metachromatic leukodystrophy present in infancy. The patient above represents the less frequent "juvenile" variant of the disease.

Unlike adrenoleukodystrophy (see Case 411), metachromatic leukodystrophy involves white matter throughout the cerebral hemispheres. Extensive, scalloped zones with long T1 and long T2 values typically fill the centrum semiovale. Subcortical "U" fibers (*arrows*, Case 408B) are usu-

ally spared. A spotted or striped appearance caused by islands or bands of relatively normal white matter within involved regions has been noted in some cases, as seen above. Contrast enhancement is rare.

The prognosis in untreated metachromatic leukodystrophy is poor. Bone marrow transplantation is considered for early cases to restore adequate enzyme levels.

When white matter abnormality is patchy or multifocal rather than diffuse, congenital and metabolic disorders should be included in the differential diagnosis along with leukodystrophy. (See the discussions of mitochondrial encephalomyopathy in Case 510 and tuberous sclerosis in Cases 900-902.)

Proton spectroscopy in metachromatic leukodystrophy has been reported to demonstrate an increased concentration of myoinositol.

## Case 409

4-year-old girl presenting with a three-day
history of increasing obtundation.
(axial, noncontrast scan; SE 2500/45)

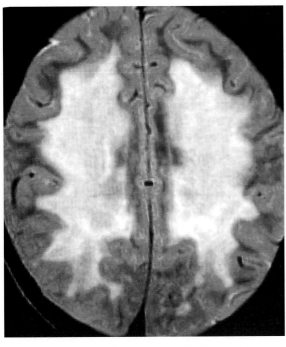

**Acute Disseminated Encephalomyelitis**

## Case 410

14-year-old girl previously treated
for acute lymphocytic leukemia.
(axial, noncontrast FLAIR scan)

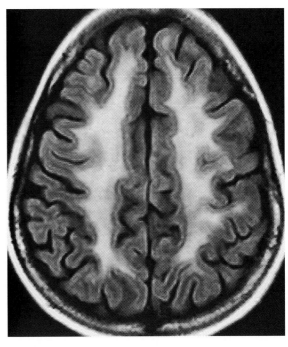

**Diffuse Necrotizing Leukoencephalopathy**

---

Widespread abnormality of cerebral white matter may
be the result of demyelinating, dysmyelinating, or toxic disorders. Case 409 represents the first of these categories as
an unusually severe and symmetrical example of ADEM
(compare to Cases 388-392).

Case 408B on the previous page demonstrates diffuse
dysmyelinating involvement of the cerebral hemispheres.
Overall volume of white matter is mildly reduced, in contrast to the swelling reflecting edema in Case 409.

Case 410 illustrates confluent signal abnormality
throughout the centrum semiovale in association with reduced white matter volume. Subcortical "U" fibers are relatively spared. Sulci are abnormally large for the patient's
age.

The child in Case 410 received both cerebral radiation
and intrathecal methotrexate during treatment for acute

leukemia. Extensive white matter damage has been noted
pathologically and on follow-up imaging studies in such
children. The phrase *disseminated necrotizing leukoencephalopathy* has been used for methotrexate-associated
disease but may apply to other combinations of chemotherapy and/or radiation. Histological analysis of such
cases suggests the primary damage is astrocytic rather than
neuronal. See Case 421 for another example of diffuse
necrotizing leukoencephalopathy.

The time course of neurological deterioration is a useful
clue to the categorization of white matter diseases. Demyelinating disorders are typically more rapidly progressive than dysmyelinating disease.

Compare the diffuse white matter damage in the above
cases to the adult scans in Cases 422 and 423.

## Case 411A

8-year-old boy presenting with bilateral hearing loss.
(axial, noncontrast T2-weighted SE scan)

## Case 411B

Same patient.
(axial, postcontrast T1-weighted SE scan)

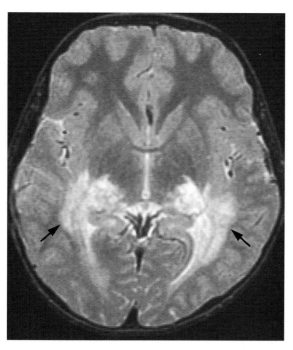

**Adrenoleukodystrophy**

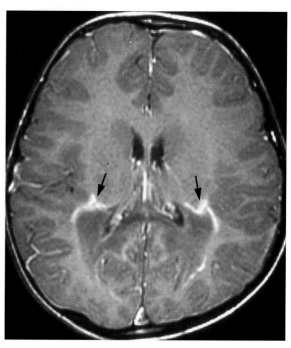

**Adrenoleukodystrophy**

Adrenoleukodystrophy is an X-linked recessive dysmyelinating disease caused by inadequate metabolism of very long chain fatty acids. Affected boys typically present between 5 and 10 years of age with progressive school problems and gait abnormality. Involvement of visual pathways in the temporal and occipital lobes or of auditory pathways within the brainstem (see Case 504) may lead to visual or hearing loss, as in this case. Associated adrenal hypofunction varies widely in severity.

Most cases of adrenoleukodystrophy demonstrate symmetrical abnormality of white matter beginning within the parietooccipital regions and spreading anteriorly. In Case 411, large, scalloped zones with long T1 and long T2 values are confined to the posterior portion of the cerebral hemispheres. (Compare this appearance to the more diffuse involvement of metachromatic leukodystrophy in Case 408.) The margins or center of the white matter lesions occasionally demonstrate high signal intensity on precontrast T1-weighted scans, possibly reflecting lipid products of myelin metabolism (see Case 386).

The pattern of contrast enhancement in adrenoleukodystrophy is usually characteristic, as demonstrated in Case 411B. A flame-shaped zone of enhancement is defined at the advancing edge of involvement *(arrows)*. The presence of contrast enhancement in a patient with adrenoleukodystrophy is strongly associated with subsequent clinical progression of the disease.

Many atypical appearances of adrenoleukodystrophy have been reported, including frontal lobe predominance and unilateral, holohemispheric patterns.

## Case 412

21-month-old girl presenting with
developmental delay.
(axial, noncontrast T2-weighted SE scan)

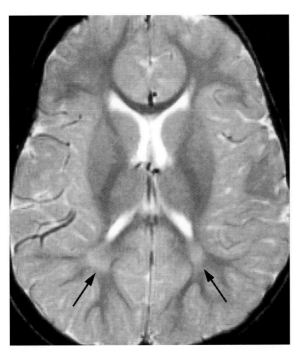

**Slow Myelination**

## Case 413

60-year-old woman presenting with confusion.
(axial, noncontrast T2-weighted SE scan)

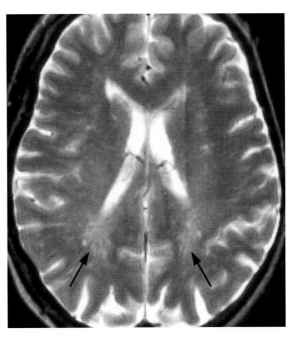

**Prominent Perivascular Spaces**

Two normal variants can cause symmetrical high signal intensity in deep parietal white matter on T2-weighted scans. These developmental features should not be confused with demyelinating or dysmyelinating disorders.

The periventricular parietal region is the last zone of the cerebral hemispheres to become fully myelinated during normal maturation. At ages 2 or 3, this residual unmyelinated tissue (containing more water and demonstrating longer T2 values than myelinated areas) contrasts with the uniform background of surrounding white matter. Case 412 is a typical example *(arrows)*.

In adults, a hazy appearance of increased signal within the deep parietal regions can be seen normally due to prominent perivascular spaces. These sleeves of CSF surrounding penetrating vessels are often most prominent in the parietal lobes. If the individual perivascular spaces are large, they may be resolved as fine, radial, or linear structures (see Case 365). When the perivascular spaces are smaller (or spatial resolution of the scan is lower), the fluid within the spaces is averaged with adjacent tissue to cause a zone of high signal on T2-weighted scans. Case 413 illustrates this appearance *(arrows)*.

## Case 414

7-year-old boy presenting with left hemiparesis
and bilateral ankle clonus.
(axial, postcontrast T1-weighted SE scan)

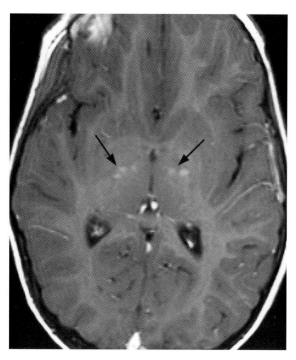

**Adrenoleukodystrophy**

## Case 415

5-year-old boy who presented ten days earlier
with decreased level of consciousness.
(axial, postcontrast T1-weighted SE scan with MTS)

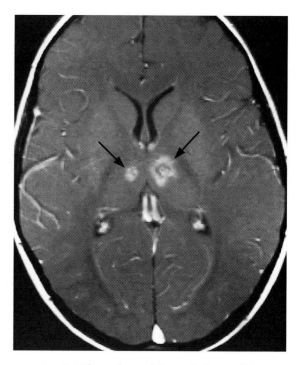

**Acute Disseminated Encephalomyelitis**

---

Symmetrical lesions deep in the cerebral hemispheres may represent pathology involving the internal capsule or disorders affecting the basal ganglia or thalami.

Case 414 falls in the former category as an unusual presentation of adrenoleukodystrophy, with enhancement along the course of the corticospinal tract *(arrows)*. Adrenoleukodystrophy more commonly causes focal signal abnormality and abnormal enhancement within the optic radiations or the auditory pathways of the brainstem (see Case 504). Amyotrophic lateral sclerosis can demonstrate symmetrical signal abnormality within the corticospinal tract in adults (see Cases 528 and 529), but contrast enhancement would be unusual.

In Case 415, the bilateral enhancement is due to mildly asymmetrical involvement of the thalami by ADEM. As discussed in Cases 394 and 395, thalamic or ganglionic lesions are commonly noted in ADEM and occasionally dominate the presentation. Like the plaques of multiple sclerosis, the lesions of ADEM may enhance during their acute or subacute stage. The affected areas in Case 415 had demonstrated no enhancement on a scan one week earlier.

## Case 416

21-year-old man presenting with
adrenal insufficiency.
(axial, noncontrast T2-weighted SE scan)

## Case 417

36-year-old man presenting with paraparesis.
(axial, noncontrast T2-weighted SE scan)

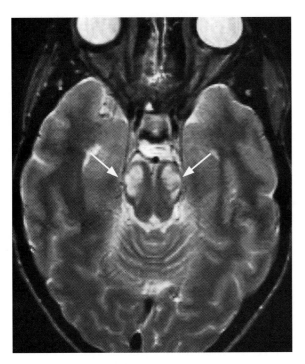

Adrenomyeloneuropathy

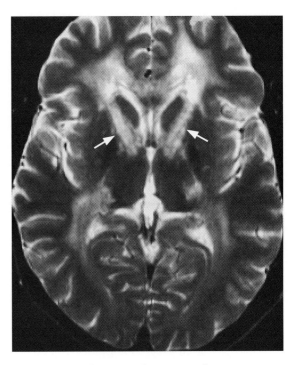

Adrenomyeloneuropathy

Adrenomyeloneuropathy is considered to be a less severe variant of adrenoleukodystrophy, typically presenting in young adulthood. Both disorders reflect deficient function of peroxisomal enzymes (mainly acyl-CoA synthetase) leading to impaired degradation of very long chain fatty acids. Although the gene for the enzyme is X-linked and adrenoleukodystrophy is seen only in boys, some women present with adrenomyeloneuropathy and are presumably heterozygous.

Patients with adrenomyeloneuropathy typically seek medical attention in their 20's or 30's due to myelopathy, peripheral neuropathy, or adrenal insufficiency. MR scans in such cases have demonstrated more frequent intracranial involvement than had been previously appreciated.

Case 416 illustrates striking T2 prolongation throughout the corticospinal tracts within the cerebral peduncles (*arrows;* compare to the symmetrical lesions of the internal capsules in Case 414 and contrast with the more dorsal involvement of auditory pathways in Case 504). Higher

scans showed confluent demyelination crossing through the splenium and major forceps, as well as symmetrical lesions within the posterior corona radiata.

Symmetrical demyelination and edema are most marked in the frontal lobes of Case 417, occupying the genu of the corpus callosum and minor forceps. Prominent involvement of the anterior limb of the internal capsule (*arrows*) outlines the head of the caudate nucleus bilaterally. (Compare to the edema within the posterior limbs of the internal capsules in Case 390.) Less impressive signal abnormality is present in peritrigonal white matter, the site usually most extensively involved in childhood adrenoleukodystrophy. Symmetrical lesions are also seen at the lateral margin of the thalami.

Paired lesions within the brainstem may be caused by disorders involving white matter tracts (as in Case 416) or by pathologies affecting brainstem nuclei (see discussion of Leigh disease in Cases 501-503).

## Case 418A

10-month-old girl presenting with
developmental delay.
(sagittal, noncontrast T1-weighted SE scan)

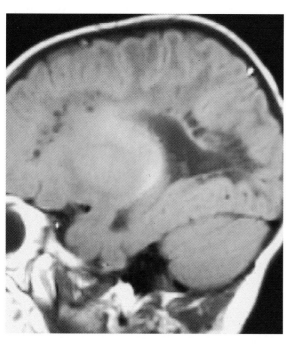

**Canavan's Disease**

## Case 418B

Same patient.
(coronal, noncontrast T1-weighted SE scan)

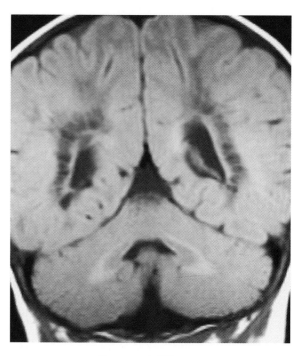

**Canavan's Disease**

Canavan's disease is an autosomal recessive disorder caused by deficiency of the enzyme *N*-acetyl aspartase. The condition is also known as *spongiform leukoencephalopathy* because normal white matter is replaced by a meshlike network of small cysts. This vacuolization is often very fine, causing homogeneously prolonged T1 and T2 values throughout cerebral white matter.

In some cases the cysts are large enough to be individually resolved, as seen above. This finding can be a clue to the diagnosis in an infant with otherwise nonspecific "watery" white matter. The concentration of cysts in the periventricular white matter of Case 418 is similar to several other pathologies (compare to Cases 519 and 520).

The typically diffuse and symmetrical involvement of Canavan's disease often causes T2-weighted images that resemble Cases 408 and 409. Subarcuate "U" fibers are char-

acteristically involved, unlike metachromatic leukodystrophy. The internal capsule may be relatively spared.

Canavan's disease usually presents within the first year of life. Hypotonia and seizures typically accompany developmental delay. Prognosis is poor, with death occurring by age 2 or 3.

Head size can be a useful clinical discriminator in children with leukodystrophy. Patients with metachromatic leukodystrophy and adrenoleukodystrophy are usually normocephalic. If the affected child presents with a large head, Alexander's disease (characterized by frontal lobe predominance) or Canavan's disease (with more diffuse abnormality) should be considered.

Canavan's disease is associated with an abnormally large peak of *N*-acetyl aspartate at proton spectroscopy.

# DIFFERENTIAL DIAGNOSIS:
## LACK OF NORMAL MYELINATION IN AN INFANT

### Case 419

11-month-old boy presenting with nystagmus, head bobbing, and chorea.
(axial, noncontrast T2-weighted SE scan)

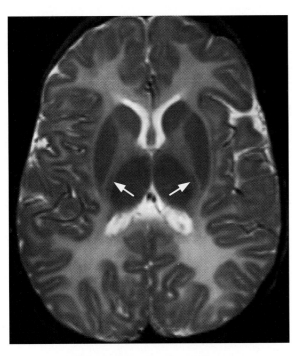

**Pelizaeus-Merzbacher Disease**

### Case 420

14-month-old girl presenting with developmental delay.
(axial, noncontrast T2-weighted SE scan)

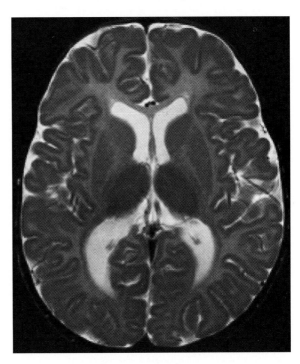

**Niemann-Pick Disease**

---

Lack of normal myelination in a child may be due to metabolic abnormalities specifically affecting white matter or to systemic disorders with neuronal toxicity.

Case 419 is an example of a specific leukodystrophy. Pelizaeus-Merzbacher disease is an X-linked disorder caused by deficiency of proteolipid protein, one of the components of myelin. It is categorized as one of the "sudanophilic" leukodystrophies because of the characteristic presence of macrophages containing increased amounts of lipid material. Severe cases demonstrate no progression of myelination after birth.

In Case 419, the only apparent myelin is the small zone of reduced intensity within the posterior limbs of the internal capsule *(arrows)*. (In a normal infant, unequivocal myelin should be visible on T2-weighted scans within the anterior limb of the internal capsule by 4-7 months, within the splenium of the corpus callosum by 4-6 months, and within the genu of the corpus callosum by 5-8 months.) Unusually low signal intensity is present throughout the basal ganglia and thalami, possibly reflecting abnormal accumulation of iron due to impaired axonal transport.

The scan in Case 420 is almost identical to Case 419. Near total lack of myelin is strikingly abnormal for the infant's age, and the low signal intensity of the thalami suggests a disturbance in normal transport and/or storage of paramagnetic metal ions. However, in this case the cause of impaired myelination is an autosomal recessive systemic disorder.

Niemann-Pick disease, also called *lipid histiocytosis,* is produced by an enzyme deficiency (sphingomyelinase), which leads to the accumulation of phospholipid in histiocytes of the liver, spleen, lymph nodes, and bone marrow. Neuronal and glial toxicity is part of the spectrum of the disorder, with cell loss and secondary demyelination. (Compare to the discussion of mucopolysaccharidoses in Cases 519 and 520.)

A lack of myelination similar to the above cases may be demonstrated in infants with carbohydrate-deficient glycoprotein syndrome, typically accompanied by microcephaly and cerebellar atrophy (see Case 536).

## Case 421A

4-year-old boy being treated for acute lymphocytic leukemia, presenting with change in personality and behavior.
(axial, noncontrast T2-weighted FSE scan)

## Case 421B

Same patient.
(single voxel proton spectroscopy, PRESS technique, SE 1500/135, from more affected *[top]* and less affected *[bottom]* regions)

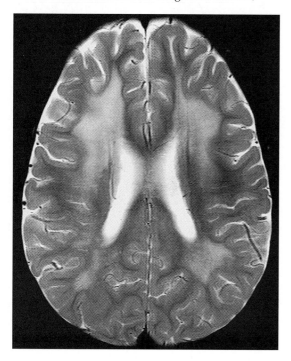

**Diffuse Necrotizing Leukoencephalopathy**

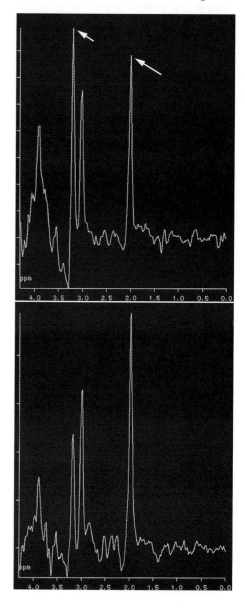

Symmetrical abnormality within white matter can be caused by toxicity of physical or chemical agents as well as by demyelinating and dysmyelinating disorders.

The child in Case 421 had received multiple courses of intrathecal methotrexate during treatment for acute leukemia. (There was no history of CNS radiation.) Damage to white matter is a recognized complication of such chemotherapy and has been termed *diffuse necrotizing leukoencephalopathy.* Patchy areas of T2 prolongation as illustrated above may progress to involve the entire hemisphere, with eventual loss of white matter volume (see Case 410).

The proton spectrum from right frontal white matter (Case 421B, *top*) demonstrates reduced *N*-acetyl aspartate *(long arrow)* and elevated choline *(short arrow)* as compared to the more normal spectrum from the right occipital lobe (Case 421B, *bottom*). (See discussion of Case 83 for an overview of major peaks in proton spectroscopy.) These findings suggest decreased neuronal/ axonal density and increased breakdown or turnover of cell membranes.

A very similar spectroscopic pattern can be seen within primary brain tumors. It is important to recognize that elevated choline levels (and reduced NAA peaks) are not specific for lesions with neoplastic cellular proliferation.

# DIFFERENTIAL DIAGNOSIS:
## DIFFUSELY ABNORMAL WHITE MATTER IN AN ADULT

### Case 422

46-year-old woman presenting with
memory loss and ataxia.
(axial, noncontrast T2-weighted FSE scan)

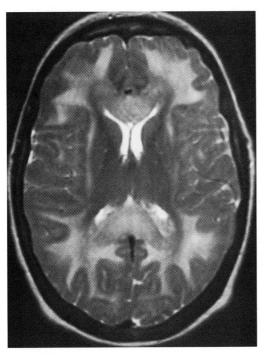

**Metronidazole Toxicity**

### Case 423

57-year-old woman presenting with
visual hallucinations.
(axial, noncontrast T2-weighted SE scan)

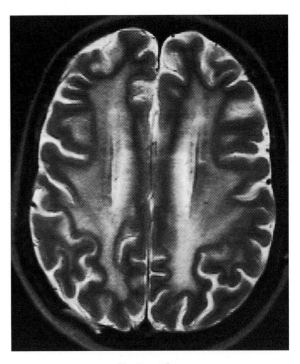

**Radiation Change**

Widespread injury to cerebral white matter in adults is most commonly the result of aging and presumed ischemic change, as illustrated in Cases 608 and 609. However, toxicity from chemical or physical agents should also be considered (along with demyelinating and dysmyelinating disorders) when diffuse changes are found within white matter.

Case 422 demonstrates symmetrical prolongation of T2 values in subcortical regions of the frontal and parietal lobes and within the external capsules. The genu and splenium of the corpus callosum are also involved and expanded. This pattern of edema within white matter has been reported in cases of toxicity from metronidazole *(Flagyl)*, a widely used antibiotic. The patient in Case 422 had been taking a high dose of this medication for a prolonged period, and the diagnosis of toxicity was presumed when symptoms and MR findings resolved within weeks after the drug was discontinued.

Physical injury from radiation therapy can also cause diffuse abnormality of cerebral white matter, as seen in Case 423. This patient had received cranial radiation during treatment for small cell carcinoma of the lung. In adults, the extent of radiation damage as depicted by MR and its clinical significance appear to increase with patient age at the time of treatment. (See Cases 549-551 for other possible presentations of radiation change.)

Some cases of carbon monoxide poisoning result in extensive damage to white matter. Mitochondrial encephalopathy (see Case 510) can also lead to an appearance resembling the above the scans.

Gliomatosis cerebri (see Cases 112 and 484) is an additional pathology that can present as bilateral signal abnormality involving large regions of white matter with little mass effect and no contrast enhancement.

# REFERENCES

Andreula CF, Recchia Luciani ANM, Milella D: Magnetic resonance imaging in the diagnosis of acute disseminated encephalomyelitis (ADEM). *Int J Neurorad* 3:21-34, 1997.

Atlas SW, Grossman RI, Goldberg HI, et al: MR diagnosis of acute disseminated encephalomyelitis. *J Comput Assist Tomogr* 10: 798-801, 1986.

Baram TZ, Goldman AM, Percy AK: Krabbe's disease: specific MR and CT findings. *Neuroradiology* 36:111, 1986.

Barkhof F, Karas GB, van Walderveen MAA: T1 hypointensities and axonal loss. *Neuroimaging Clin North Am* 10:739-752, 2000.

Barkhof F, Scheltens P, Freguin STFB, et al: Relapsing-remitting multiple sclerosis: sequential enhanced MR imaging vs clinical findings in determining disease activity. *Am J Roentgenol* 159:1041-1047, 1992.

Barkhof F, Thompson AJ, Kappos L, et al: Database for serial magnetic resonance imaging in multiple sclerosis. *Neuroradiology* 35:362-366, 1993.

Barkhof F, Valk J, Hommes OR, Scheltens P: Meningeal Gd-DTPA enhancement in multiple sclerosis. *AJNR* 13:397-400, 1992.

Barkhof F, Valk J, Hommes OR, et al: Gadopentetate Dimeglumine enhancement of multiple sclerosis lesions on long TR spin-echo images at 0.6T. *AJNR* 13:1257-1260, 1992.

Barkovich AJ: Concepts of myelin and myelination in neuroradiology. *AJNR* 21:1099-1109, 2000.

Barkovich AJ, Ferriero DM, Bass N, Boyer R: Involvement of the pontomedullary corticospinal tracts: a useful finding in the diagnosis of X-linked adrenoleukodystrophy. *AJNR* 18:95-100, 1997.

Barkovich AJ, Lyon G, Evrard P: Formation, maturation and disorders of white matter. *AJNR* 13:447-461, 1992.

Bastianello S, Gasperini C, Paolillo A: Sensitivity of enhanced MR in multiple sclerosis: effects of contrast dose and magnetization transfer contrast. *AJNR* 19:1863-1868, 1998.

Baum PA, Barkovich AJ, Koch TK, Berg BD: Deep gray matter involvement in acute disseminated encephalomyelitis. *AJNR* 15: 1275-1283, 1994.

Besenski N, Bosnjak V, Cop S, et al: Neuroimaging and clinically distinctive features in van der Knaap megalencephalic leukoencephalopathy. *Int J Neurorad* 3:244-249, 1997.

Bewermeyer H, Bamborschke S, Ebhardt G, et al: MR imaging in adrenoleukomyeloneuropathy. *J Comput Assist Tomogr* 9:793-796, 1985.

Boggild MD, Williams R, Haq N, Hawkins CP: Cortical plaques visualised by fluid-attenuated inversion recovery imaging in relapsing multiple sclerosis. *Neuroradiology* 38:S10-S13, 1996.

Bourgouin PM, Chalk C, Richardson J, et al: Subcortical white matter lesions in osmotic demyelination syndrome. *AJNR* 16:1495-1497, 1995.

Brismar J, Brismar G, Gascon G, Oznan P: Canavan disease: CT and MR imaging of the brain. *AJNR* 11:805-810, 1990.

Brown MS, Stemmer SM, Simon JH, et al: White matter disease induced by high-dose chemotherapy: longitudinal study with MR and proton spectroscopy. *AJNR* 19:217-222, 1998.

Butman JA, Frank JA: Overview of imaging in multiple sclerosis and white matter disease. *Neuroimaging Clin North Am* 10:669-685, 2000.

Caldemeyer KS, Edwards MK, Smith RR, Moran CC: Viral and postviral demyelination central nervous system infection, neuroimaging. *Radiol Clin North Am* 3:305-317, 1993.

Caldemeyer KS, Harris TM, Smith RR, Edwards MK: Gadolinium enhancement in acute disseminated encephalomyelitis. *J Comput Assist Tomogr* 15:673-675, 1991.

Caldemeyer KS, Smith RR, Harris TM, Edwards MK: MRI in acute disseminated encephalomyelitis. *Neuroradiology* 36:216-220, 1994.

Caracciolo JT, Murtagh RD, Rojiani AM, Murtagh FR: Pathognomonic MR imaging findings in Balo concentric sclerosis. *AJNR* 22:292-293, 2001.

Castellote A, Vera J, Vasquez E, et al: MR in adrenoleukodystrophy: atypical presentation as bilateral frontal demyelination. *AJNR* 16:814-815, 1995.

Cha S, Pierce S, Knopp EA, et al: Dynamic contrast-enhanced T2*-weighted MR imaging of tumefactive demyelinating lesions. *AJNR* 22:1109-1116, 2001.

Chen CJ, Ro LS, Wang LJ, Wong YC: Balo's concentric sclerosis: MRI. *Neuroradiology* 38:322-324, 1996.

Choi S. Enzmann DR: Infantile Krabbe disease: complementary CT and MR findings. *AJNR* 14:1164-1166. 1993.

Chrysikopoulos HS, Press GA, Grafe MR, et al: Encephalitis caused by human immunodeficiency virus: CT and MR imaging manifestations with clinical and pathologic correlation. *Radiology* 175:185-191, 1990.

Cure' JK, Cromwell LD, Case JL, et al: Auditory dysfunction caused by multiple sclerosis: detection with MR imaging. *AJNR* 11:817-820, 1990.

Dagher AP, Smirniotopoulos J: Tumefactive demyelinating lesions. *Neuroradiology* 38:560-565, 1996.

Demaerel P, Faubert C, Wilms G, et al: MR findings in leukodystrophy. *Neuroradiology* 33:368-371, 1991.

Dietrich R, Bradley WG, Zaragoza EG, et al: MR evaluation of early myelination patterns in normal and developmentally delayed infants. *AJNR* 9:69-76, 1988.

Drayer BP, Burger P, Hurwitz B, Dawson D, et al: Reduced signal intensity on MR images of thalamus and putamen in multiple sclerosis: increased iron content? *AJNR* 8:413-419, 1987.

Dunn V, Bale JF Jr, Zimmerman RA, et al: MRI in children with post-infectious disseminated encephalomyelitis. *Magn Reson Imaging* 4:25-32, 1986.

Ebner F, Millner MM, Justich E: Multiple sclerosis in children: value of serial MR studies to monitor patients. *AJNR* 11:1023-1027, 1990.

Edwards MK, Farlow MR, Stevens JC: Multiple sclerosis: MRI and clinical correlation. *AJNR* 7:595-598, 1986.

Edwards-Brown MK, Farlow MR, Bognanno J, et al: Clinical utility of inversion recovery magnetic resonance imaging in the diagnosis of multiple sclerosis. *Int J Neurorad* 3:13-17, 1997.

Engelbrecht V, Rassek M, Gartner J, et al: The value of new MRI techniques in adrenoleukodystrophy. *Pediatr Radiol* 27:207-210, 1997.

Farina L, Bizzi A, Finocchiaro G, et al: MR imaging and proton MR spectroscopy in adult Krabbe disease. *AJNR* 21:1478-1482, 2000.

Farley TJ, Ketonen LM, Bodensteiner JB, Wang DD: Serial MRI and CT findings in infantile Krabbe disease. *Pediatr Neurol* 8:455-458, 1992.

Farlow MR, Markand ON, Edwards MK, et al: Multiple sclerosis: magnetic resonance imaging, evoked responses, and spinal fluid electrophoresis. *Neurology* 36:828-831, 1986.

Fazekas F, Offenbacher H, Fuchs S, et al: Criteria for an increased specificity of MRI interpretation in elderly subjects with suspected multiple sclerosis. *Neurology* 38:1822-1825, 1988.

Filippi M, Rossi P, Campi A, et al: Serial contrast-enhanced MR in patients with multiple sclerosis and varying levels of disability. *AJNR* 18:1549-1556, 1997.

Finelli DA, Tarr RW, Sawyer, RN, Horwitz SJ: Deceptively normal MR in early infantile Krabbe disease. *AJNR* 15:167-171, 1994.

Fulton JC, Grossman RI, Udupa J, et al: MR lesion load and cognitive function in patients with relapsing-remitting multiple sclerosis. *AJNR* 20:1951-1955, 1999.

Garrels K, Kucharczyk W, Wortzman G, Shandling M: Progressive multifocal leukoencephalopathy: clinical and MR response to treatment. *AJNR* 17:597-600, 1996.

Gasperini C, Bastianello S, Ristori G, et al: MRI in the differential diagnosis of multiple sclerosis without CSF abnormalities. *Int J Neurorad* 2:117-122, 1996.

Gean-Marton AD, Vezina LG, Martin KL, et al: Abnormal corpus callosum: a sensitive and specific indicator of multiple sclerosis. *Radiology* 180:215-221, 1991.

Gebarski SS, Gabrielsen TO, Gilman S, et al: The initial diagnosis of multiple sclerosis: clinical impact of magnetic resonance imaging. *Ann Neurol* 17:469-474, 1985.

Gerard D, Healy ME, Hesselink JR: MR demonstration of mesencephalic lesions in osmotic demyelination syndrome (central pontine myelinolysis). *Neuroradiology* 29:582-584, 1987.

Giang DW, Poduri KR, Eskin TA, et al: Multiple sclerosis masquerading as a mass lesion. *Neuroradiology* 34:150-154, 1992.

Glasier CM, Robbins MB, Davis PC, et al: Clinical, neurodiagnostic, and MR findings in children with spinal and brain stem multiple sclerosis. *AJNR* 16:87-96, 1995.

Grossman RI, Braffman BH, Bronson JR, et al: Multiple sclerosis: serial studies of gadolinium-enhanced MR imaging. *Radiology* 169:117-122, 1988.

Grossman RI, Gonzalez-Scarano F, Atlas SW, et al: Multiple sclerosis: Gadolinium enhancement in MR imaging. *Radiology* 161:721-725, 1986.

Grossman RI, McGowan JC: Review article: perspectives on multiple sclerosis. *AJNR* 19:1251-1266, 1998.

Guilleux MH, Steiner RE, Young IR: MR imaging of progressive multifocal leukoencephalopathy. *AJNR* 7:1033-1035, 1986.

Guttmann CRG, Ahn SS, Hsu L, et al: The evolution of multiple sclerosis lesions on serial MR. *AJNR* 16:1481-1491, 1995.

Haas G, Schroth G, Krageloh-Mann I, et al: Magnetic resonance imaging of the brain of children with multiple sclerosis. *Dev Med Child Neurol* 29:586, 1985.

Hashemi RH, Bradley WG, Chen DY, et al: Suspected multiple sclerosis: MR imaging with a thin-section fast FLAIR pulse sequence. *Radiology* 196:505-510, 1995.

He J, Grossman RI, Ge Y, Mannon LJ: Enhancing patterns in multiple sclerosis: evolution and persistence. *AJNR* 22:644-669, 2001.

Heier LA, Bauer CJ, Schwarts L, et al: Large Virchow-Robin spaces: MR-clinical correlation. *AJNR* 10:929-936, 1989.

Hirabuki N, Fujita N, Fujii K, et al: MR appearance of Virchow-Robin spaces along lenticulostriate arteries: spin-echo and two-dimensional fast low-angle shot imaging. *AJNR* 15:277-282, 1994.

Hirsch JA, Lenkinski RE, Grossman RI: MR spectroscopy in the evaluation of enhancing lesions in the brain in multiple sclerosis. *AJNR* 17:1829-1836, 1996.

Ho VB, Fitz CR, Yoder CC, Geyer CA: Resolving MR features in osmotic myelinolysis (central pontine and extrapontine myelinolysis). *AJNR* 14:163-167, 1993.

Holland BA, Haas DK, Norman D: MRI of normal brain maturation. *AJNR* 7:201, 1986.

Horowitz AL, Kaplan RD, Grewe G, et al: The ovoid lesions a new MR observation in patients with multiple sclerosis. *AJNR* 10:303-305, 1989.

Honkaniemi J, Dastidar P, Kähärä V, Haapasalo H: Delayed MR imaging changes in acute disseminated encephalomyelitis. *AJNR* 22:1117-1124, 2001.

Huckman MS, Wong PWK, Sullivan T, et al: Magnetic resonance imaging compared with computed tomography in adrenoleukodystrophy. *Am J Dis Child* 150:1001-1003, 1986.

Jackson A, Fitzgerald JB, Gillespie JE: The callosal-septal interface lesion in multiple sclerosis: effect of sequence and imaging plane. *Neuroradiology* 35:573-577, 1993.

Jackson JA, Leake DR, Schneiders NJ, et al: Magnetic resonance imaging in multiple sclerosis: results in 32 cases. *AJNR* 6:171-176, 1985.

Jensen ME, Sawyer, RW, Braun IF, Rizzo WB: MR imaging appearance in childhood adrenoleukodystrophy with auditory, visual, and motor pathway involvement. *Radiographics* 10:53-66, 1990.

Kepes JJ: Large focal tumor-like demyelinating lesions of the brain: intermediate entity between multiple sclerosis and acute disseminated encephalomyelitis. A study of 31 patients. *Ann Neurol* 33:18-27, 1993.

Kermode AG, Thompson AJ, Tofts P, et al: Breakdown of the blood-brain barrier precedes symptoms and other MRI signs of new lesions in multiple sclerosis: pathogenetic and clinical implications. *Brain* 113:1477-1489, 1990.

Kesselring J, Miller DH, Robb SA, et al: Acute disseminated encephalomyelitis. MRI findings and the distinction from multiple sclerosis. *Brain* 113:291, 1990.

Kim TS, Kim IO, Kim WS, et al: MR of childhood metachromatic leukodystrophy. *AJNR* 18:733-738, 1997.

Kimura H, Grossman RI, Lenkinski RE, Gonzalez-Scarano F: Proton MR spectroscopy and magnetization transfer ratio in multiple sclerosis: correlative findings of active versus irreversible plaque disease. *AJNR* 17:1539-1548, 1996.

Kimura S, Unayama T, Mori T: The natural history of acute disseminated leukoencephalitis: a serial magnetic resonance imaging study. *Neuropediatrics* 23:192-195, 1992.

Koci TM, Chiang F, Chow P, et al: Thalamic extrapontine lesions in central pontine myelinolysis. *AJNR* 11:1229-1233, 1990.

Korogi Y, Takashashi M, Shinzato J, et al: MR findings in two presumed cases of mild central pontine myelinolysis. *AJNR* 14:651-654, 1993.

Korte JH, Bom EP, Vos LD, et al: Balo concentric sclerosis: MR diagnosis. *AJNR* 15:1284-1285, 1994.

Krupp LB, Lipton RB, Swerdlow ML, et al: Progressive multifocal encephalopathy: clinical and radiographic features. *Ann Neurol* 17:344-349, 1985.

Kumar AJ, Kohler W, Kruse B, et al: MR findings in adult-onset adrenoleukodystrophy. *AJNR* 16:1227-1237, 1995.

Kumar AJ, Rosenbaum AE, Naidu S, et al: Adrenoleukodystrophy: correlating MR imaging with CT. *Radiology* 165:497-504, 1987.

Lee KH, Hashimoto SA, Hooge JP, et al: Magnetic resonance imaging of the head in the diagnosis of multiple sclerosis: a prospective 2-year follow-up with comparison of clinical evaluation, evoked potentials, oligoclonal banding, and CT. *Neurology* 41:657-660, 1991.

Levy JD, Cottingham KL, Campbell RJ, et al: Progressive multifocal leukomalacia and magnetic resonance imaging. *Ann Neurol* 19:399-401, 1986.

Li DKB, Zhao G, Paty DW: T2 hyperintensities: findings and significance. *Neuroimaging Clin North Am* 10:717-738, 2000.

Loes DJ, Hite S, Moser H, et al: Adrenoleukodystrophy: a scoring method for brain MR observations. *AJNR* 15:1761-1766, 1994.

Loes DJ, Peters C, Krivit W: Globoid cell leukodystrophy: distinguishing early-onset from late-onset disease using a brain MR imaging scoring method. *AJNR* 20:316-323, 1999.

Loevner LA, Grossman RI, McGowan JC, et al: Characterization of multiple sclerosis plaques with T1-weighted MR and quantitative magnetization transfer. *AJNR* 16:1473-1479, 1995.

Lukes SA, Norman D, Mills C: Acute disseminated encephalomyelitis: CT and NMR findings. *J Comput Assist Tomogr* 7:182, 1983.

Mader I, Stock KW, Ettlin T, Probst A: Acute disseminated encephalomyelitis: MR and CT features. *AJNR* 17:104-109, 1996.

Mark AS, Atlas SW: Progressive multifocal leukoencephalopathy in patients with AIDS: appearance of MR images. *Radiology* 173:517-520, 1989.

McAdams HP, Geyer CA, Done SL, et al: CT and MR imaging of Canavan disease. *AJNR* 11:397, 190.

McArdle CB, Richardson CJ, Nicholas DA, et al: Developmental features of the neonatal brain: MR imaging. *Radiology* 162:223-229, 1987.

McFarland HF: Correlation between MR and clinical findings of disease activity in multiple sclerosis. *AJNR* 20:1777-1778, 1999.

McGraw P, Edwards-Brown MK: Reversal of MR findings of central pontine myelinolysis. *J Comput Assist Tomog* 22:989-991, 1998.

Mehta RC, Pike GB, Enzmann DR: Improved detection of enhancing and nonenhancing lesions of multiple sclerosis with magnetization transfer. *AJNR* 16:1771-1778, 1995.

Melhem ER, Barker PB, Raymond GV, Moser HW: X-linked adrenoleukodystrophy in children: review of genetic, clinical, and MR imaging characteristics. *Am J Roentgenol* 173:1575-1582, 1999.

Melhem ER, Loes DJ, Georgiades CS, et al: X-linked adrenoleukodystrophy: the role of contrast-enhanced MR imaging in predicting disease progression. *AJNR* 21:839-844, 2000.

Miller GM, Baker HL, Okazaki H, Whisnant JP: Central pontine myelinolysis and its imitators: MR findings. *Radiology* 168:795-802, 1988.

Mirfakhraee M, Hardjasudarma M, Boudreaux B, El Gammal T: Semilunar and ring-like enhancing plaques: imaging features in patients with multiple sclerosis. *Int J Neurorad* 5:232-239, 1999.

Mirsen TR: Clinical correlates of white-matter changes on magnetic resonance imaging scans of the brain. *Arch Neurol* 48:1015, 1991.

Moriwaka F, Tashiro K. Maruo Y, et al: MR imaging of pontine and extrapontine myelinolysis. *J Comput Assist Tomogr* 12:446-449, 1988.

Nesbit GM, Forbes GS, Scheithauer BW, et al: Multiple sclerosis: histopathologic and MR and/or CT correlation in 37 cases at biopsy and three cases at autopsy. *Radiology* 180:467-474, 1991.

Niebler G, Harris T, Davis T, Ross K: Fulminant multiple sclerosis. *AJNR* 13:1547-1551, 1992.

Nowell MA, Grossman RI, Hackney DB, et al: MR imaging of white matter diseases in children. *AJNR* 9:503, 1988.

Nyul LG, Udupa JK: MR image analysis in multiple sclerosis. *Neuroimaging Clin North Am* 10:799-815, 2000.

Olsen WL, Longo FM, Mills CM, Norman D: White Matter disease in AIDS: findings at MR imaging. *Radiology* 169:445-448, 1988.

Osborn AG, Harnsberger HR, Smoker WRK, et al: Multiple sclerosis in adolescents: CT and MR Findings. *AJNR* 11:489-494, 1990.

Palmer S, Bradley WG, Chen D-Y, Patel S: Subcallosal striations: early findings of multiple sclerosis on sagittal, thin-section, fast FLAIR MR images. *Radiology* 210:149-154, 1999.

Paty DW, Oger JJF, Kastrukoff LF, et al: MRI in the diagnosis of multiple sclerosis: a prospective study with comparison of clinical evaluation. Evoked potentials, oligoclonal banding, and CT. *Neurology* 38:180, 1988.

Petrella JR, Grossman RI, McGowan JC, et al: Multiple sclerosis lesions: relationship between MR enhancement pattern and magnetization transfer effect. *AJNR* 17:1041-1050, 1996.

Phillips MD, Grossman RI, Miki Y, et al: Comparison of T2 lesion volume and magnetization transfer ratio histogram analysis and of atrophy and measures of lesion burden in patients with multiple sclerosis. *AJNR* 19:1055-1060, 1998.

Pike GB, de Stefano N, Narayanan S, et al: Combined magnetization transfer and proton spectroscopic imaging in the assessment of pathologic brain lesions in multiple sclerosis. *AJNR* 20:829-838, 1999.

Pike GB, de Stefano N, Narayanan S, et al: Multiple sclerosis: magnetization transfer MR imaging of white matter before lesion appearance on T2-weighted images. *Radiology* 215:824-830, 2000.

Post MJD, Yiannoutsos C, Simpson D, et al: Progressive multifocal leukoencephalopathy in AIDS: are there any MR findings useful to patient management and predictive of patient survival? *AJNR* 20:1896-1906, 1999.

Powell T, Sussman JG, Davies-Jones GAB: MR imaging in acute multiple sclerosis: ring-like appearance in plaques suggesting the presence of paramagnetic free radicals. *AJNR* 13:1544-1546, 1992.

Quint DJ: Multiple sclerosis and imaging of the corpus callosum. *Radiology* 180:15-17, 1991.

Ragland RL, Duffis AW, Gendelman S, et al: Central pontine myelinolysis with clinical recovery: MR documentation. *J Comput Assist Tomogr* 13:316-318, 1989.

Rippe DJ, Edwards MK, D'Amour PG, et al: MR imaging of central pontine myelinolysis. *J Comput Assist Tomogr* 11:724-726, 1987.

Rovaris M, Comi G, Rocca MA, et al: Relevance of hypointense lesions on fast fluid-attenuated inversion recovery MR images as a marker of disease severity in cases of multiple sclerosis. *AJNR* 20:813-820, 1999.

Rovaris M, Filippi M: Contrast enhancement and the acute lesion in multiple sclerosis. *Neuroimaging Clin North Am* 10:705-715, 2000.

Rovaris M, Filippi M, Minicucci L, et al: Cortical/subcortical disease burden and cognitive impairment in patients with multiple sclerosis. *AJNR* 21:402-408, 2000.

Rovira A, Alonso J, Cucurella G, et al: Evolution of multiple sclerosis lesions on serial contrast-enhanced T1-weighted and magnetization-transfer MR images. *AJNR* 20, 1939-1945, 1999.

Roychowdhury S, Maldjian JA, Grossman RI: Multiple sclerosis: comparison of trace apparent diffusion coefficients with MR enhancement pattern of lesions. *AJNR* 21:869-874, 2000.

Runge VM, Price AC, Kirshner HS, et al: The evaluation of multiple sclerosis by magnetic resonance imaging. *Radiographics* 6:203-212, 1986.

Runge VM, Price AC, Kishner HS, et al: Magnetic resonance imaging of multiple sclerosis: a study of pulse-technique efficacy. *AJNR* 5:691-702, 1984.

Russo C, Smoker WRK, Kubal W: Cortical and subcortical T2 shortening in multiple sclerosis. *AJNR* 18:124-126, 1997.

Sasaki M, Sakuragawa N, Takashima S, et al: MRI and CT findings in Krabbe disease. *Pediatr Neurol* 7:283-288, 1991.

Scanderbeg AC, Tomaiuolo F, Sabatini U, et al: Demyelinating plaques in relapsing-remitting and secondary-progressive multiple sclerosis: assessment with diffusion MR imaging. *AJNR* 21:862-868, 2000.

Scotti G, Scialfa G, Biondi A, et al: Magnetic resonance in multiple sclerosis. *Neuroradiology* 28:319-323, 1986.

Sheldon JJ, Siddharthan R, Tobias J, et al: MR imaging of multiple sclerosis: comparison with clinical and CT examination in 74 patients. *AJNR* 6:683-690, 1985.

Simon JH: Brain and spinal cord atrophy in multiple sclerosis. *Neuroimaging Clin North Am* 10:753-769, 2000.

Simon JH, Holtas SL, Schiffer RB, et al: Corpus callosum and subcallosal-periventricular lesions in multiple sclerosis: detection with MR. *Radiology* 160:363-368, 1986.

Simon JH, Schiffer RB, Rudick RA, Herndon RM: Quantitative determination of MS-induced corpus callosum atrophy in vivo using MR imaging. *AJNR* 8:599-604, 1987.

Singh S, Alexander M, Korah IP: Acute disseminated encephalomyelitis: MR imaging features. *Am J Roentgenol* 173: 1101-1108, 1999.

Takanashi J, Sugita K, Osaka H, et al: Proton MR spectroscopy in Pelizaeus-Merzbacher disease. *AJNR* 18:533-535, 1997.

Takeda K, Sakuta M, Saeki F: Central Pontine myelinolysis diagnosed by magnetic resonance imaging. *Ann Neurol* 17:310, 1985.

Tas MW, Barkhol F, van Walderveen MAA, et al: The effect of gadolinium on the sensitivity and specificity of MR in the initial diagnosis of multiple sclerosis. *AJNR* 16:259-264, 1995.

Thompson AJ, Brown MM, Swash MM, et al: Autopsy validation of MRI in central pontine myelinolysis. *Neuroradiology* 30:175, 1988.

Thurnher MM, Thurnher SA, Muhlbauer B, et al: Progressive multifocal leukoencephalopathy in AIDS: initial and follow-up CT and MRI. *Neuroradiology* 39:611-618, 1997.

Tintore M, Rovira A, Martinez MJ, et al: Isolated demyelinating syndromes: comparison of different MR imaging criteria to predict conversion to clinically definite multiple sclerosis. *AJNR* 21:702-706, 2000.

Tubridy N, Barker GJ, MacManus DG, et al: Optimisation of unenhanced MRI for detection of lesions in multiple sclerosis: a comparison of five pulse sequences with variable slice thickness. *Neuroradiology* 40: 293-297, 1998.

Uchiyama M, Hata Y, Tada S: MR imaging of adrenoleukodystrophy. *Neuroradiology* 33:25-29, 1991.

Uhlenbrook D, Seidel D, Genlen W, et al: MR imaging in multiple sclerosis: comparison with clinical, CSF, and visual evoked potential findings. *AJNR* 9:59-68, 1988.

Uhlenbrook D, Sehlen S: The value of T1-weighted images in the differentiation between MS, white matter lesions, and subcortical arteriosclerotic encephalopathy (SAE). *Neuroradiology* 31:203-212, 1989.

Van der Knaap MS, Naidu S, Breiter SN, et al: Alexander disease: diagnosis with MR imaging. *AJNR* 22:541-552, 2001.

Van der Knaap MS, Valk J: MR of adrenoleukodystrophy: histopathologic correlations. *AJNR* 10:512-514, 1989.

Van der Knaap MS, Valk J: The reflection of histology in MR imaging of Pelizaeus-Merzbacher disease. *AJNR* 10:99-103, 1989.

Van der Knaap MS, Valk J, DeNeeling N, Nauta JJP: Pattern recognition in magnetic resonance imaging of white matter disorders in children and young infants. *Neuroradiology* 33:478-493, 1991.

van der Meyden CH, de Villiers JFK, Middlecote BD, Terblanche J: Gadolinium ring enhancement and mass effect in acute disseminated encephalomyelitis. *Neuroradiology* 36:221-223, 1994.

van Waesberghe JHTM, van Walderveen MAA, Castelijns JA, et al: Patterns of lesion development in multiple sclerosis: longitudinal observations with T1-weighted spin-echo and magnetization transfer MR. *AJNR* 19:675-684, 1998.

Wallace CJ, Seland TP, Fong TC: Multiple sclerosis: the impact of MR imaging. *Am J Roentgenol* 158:849-857, 1992.

Wheeler AL, Truwit CL, Kleinschmidt-DeMasters BK, et al: Progressive multifocal leukoencephalopathy: contrast enhancement on CT scans and MR images. *Am J Roentgenol* 161:1049-1051, 1993.

Whiteman MLH, Post MJD, Berger JR, et al: Progressive multifocal leukoencephalopathy in 47 HIV-seropositive patients: neuroimaging with clinical and pathologic correlation. *Radiology* 187:233-240, 1993.

Wilms G, Marchal G Kersschot E, et al: Axial vs sagittal T2-weighted brain MR images in the evaluation of multiple sclerosis. *J Comput Assist Tomogr* 15:359-364, 1991.

Yetkin Z, Haughton VM: Atypical demyelinating lesions in patients with multiple sclerosis. *Neuroradiology* 37:284-286, 1995.

Yetkin FZ, Houghton, VM, et al: Multiple sclerosis: specificity of MR for diagnosis. *Radiology* 178:447-451, 1991.

Yousry TA, Filippi M, Becker, et al: Comparison of MR pulse sequences in the detection of multiple sclerosis lesions. *AJNR* 18:959-964, 1997.

Yuh WTC, Simonson TM, D'Alessandro MP, et al: Temporal changes of MR findings in central pontine myelinolysis. *AJNR* 16:975-977, 1995.

# CHAPTER 9

# Inflammatory Disorders

### Case 424

1-year-old girl presenting with a two-day history of fever and increasing irritability.
(axial, noncontrast scan; SE 3000/30)

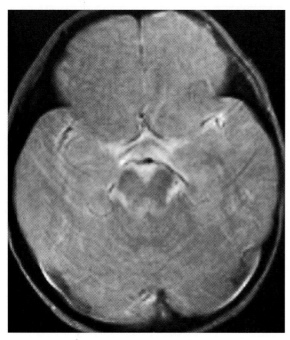

**Bacterial Meningitis**
*(Haemophilus influenzae)*

### Case 425

11-month-old girl presenting with fever and decreased level of consciousness.
(coronal, postcontrast FLAIR scan)

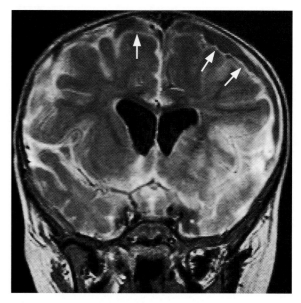

**Bacterial Meningitis**
*(Streptococcus pneumoniae)*

---

MR scans may be negative in the clinical setting of meningitis. In some cases, communicating hydrocephalus is the only clue to meningeal pathology.

In other cases, cells, protein, and reactive tissue alter the signal intensity within sulci and cisterns. This finding may be obvious or subtle on noncontrast scans.

In Case 424, basal cisterns are too bright for normal CSF given the intermediate weighting (long TR, short TE) of the pulse sequence. Abnormal signal intensity within cisterns due to meningitis is most often associated with bacterial, fungal, or granulomatous pathogens and most commonly found near the base of the brain.

FLAIR sequences are currently the most sensitive MR technique for detecting the presence of cells or protein within spinal fluid. (See Case 718 for discussion of FLAIR images in the diagnosis of subarachnoid hemorrhage.) Normal CSF should be dark on such scans, as seen within the lateral ventricles in Case 425. The high signal intensity throughout the subarachnoid spaces in Case 425 represents increased content of cells and protein with superimposed contrast enhancement. Meninges of the head or spinal canal frequently leak contrast material into adjacent CSF spaces when involved by an inflammatory or neoplastic process, and postcontrast FLAIR scans are particularly sensitive for detection of meningeal pathology.

The subdural fluid collections over the superior frontal regions in Case 425 *(arrows)* were found to be sterile effusions. Subdural effusions are common in bacterial meningitis, particularly in cases due to *Streptococcus pneumoniae* or *Haemophilus influenzae,* the leading causes of meningitis in the United States. The effusions typically contain large amounts of protein but few cells. Their appearance is nonspecific and often indistinguishable from subdural empyemas on routine noncontrast or postcontrast images (compare to Case 437).

Increased signal intensity may be seen routinely within subarachnoid spaces on FLAIR images performed during general anesthesia. Increased CSF oxygen content has been suggested as the etiology of this false positive finding.

## Case 426

11-month-old girl presenting with fever
and decreased level of consciousness.
(axial, noncontrast T2-weighted FSE scan)

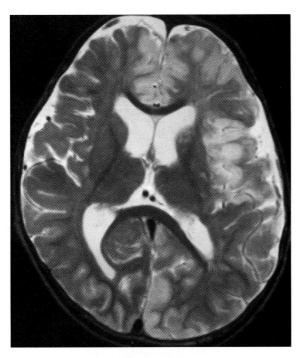

**Bacterial Meningitis**
*(Streptococcus pneumoniae;*
same patient as Case 425)

## Case 427

5-year-old girl who suffered a seizure after
admission for viral meningitis.
(coronal, noncontrast T2-weighted SE scan)

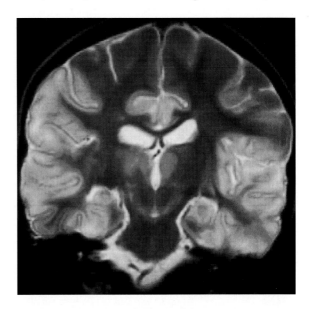

**Viral Meningitis**

---

Meningeal inflammation may extend to the cerebral parenchyma, causing localized or generalized cerebritis. In many cases, encephalitis and meningitis are concurrent. Another mechanism of parenchymal damage associated with meningitis is subacute cerebral infarction, due to spasm or occlusion of arteries or veins traversing the infected subarachnoid space.

Case 426 demonstrates multifocal cortical edema predominantly bordering the interhemispheric fissure and the left sylvian fissure. Although the pattern resembles the gyriform morphology characteristic of recent infarction, the involved regions occupy only portions of major arterial distributions. Small areas of infarction may contribute to the findings, but inflammatory edema reflecting superficial cerebritis is probably the major component.

Extensive superficial edema in Case 427 is nearly symmetrical. Increased water content causes swelling of affected gyri, partially effacing adjacent sulci. Note the involvement of the cingulate gyri (immediately superior to the corpus callosum).

Viral encephalitis often involves deep hemispheric regions near the skull base (see Cases 441 and 442). Poorly defined areas of mildly prolonged T2 values are present within the hypothalamus and midbrain bilaterally in Case 427.

Gyriform contrast enhancement may accompany the superficial pattern of edema illustrated in the above scans.

## Case 428

18-year-old man presenting with headaches.
(axial, postcontrast T1-weighted SE scan with MTS)

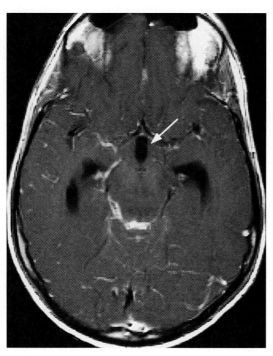

**Meningitis**
(coccidioidomycosis)

## Case 429

3-year-old boy adopted from Eastern
Europe, presenting with a seizure.
(axial, postcontrast T1-weighted SE scan)

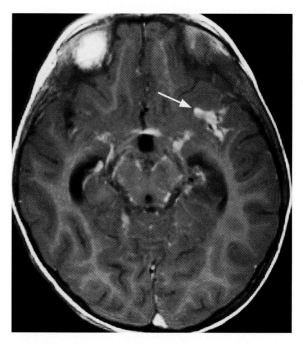

**Meningitis**
(tuberculosis)

Superficial contrast enhancement may confirm the suspicion of meningitis raised clinically or on noncontrast studies. Involvement may be generalized or localized. The pattern may be predominantly dural (linear, paralleling the calvarium) or pia-arachnoidal (with invaginations into cerebral sulci and cisterns).

In Case 428, abnormal leptomeningeal enhancement is thickest in the quadrigeminal and right ambient cisterns. Less prominent pial enhancement is present along the medial margins of the temporal lobes, in the inferior frontal region, and within superior vermian sulci. Dilatation of the temporal horns and the anterior recesses of the third ventricle *(arrow)* indicates associated communicating hydrocephalus.

Case 429 demonstrates a finely nodular layer of abnormal pial enhancement on the surface of the midbrain and along the medial margin of the uncus bilaterally. The left

sylvian cistern is filled with enhancing material near the genu of the middle cerebral artery *(arrow;* compare to Case 450). Moderate communicating hydrocephalus is present, due to impaired cisternal circulation of CSF.

Contrast-enhanced MR scans (particularly using magnetization transfer suppression or FLAIR techniques) are more sensitive than CT studies in detecting inflammatory meningeal pathology. However, the degree of abnormal enhancement varies among the multiple potential etiologies of meningitis. For example, coccidioidomycosis typically provokes an intense inflammatory response, while cryptococcus often incites minimal meningeal enhancement.

Sarcoidosis or syphilis in an adult could cause an appearance very similar to Case 429 (see Case 487). Meningeal carcinomatosis should also be included in the differential diagnosis of leptomeningeal enhancement (see Cases 29, 30, and 165-167).

### Case 430

11-month-old girl presenting with fever
and decreased level of consciousness.
(coronal, postcontrast T1-weighted
SE scan with MTS)

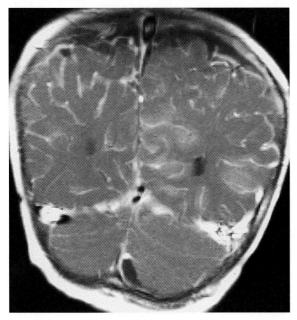

**Bacterial Meningitis**
*(Streptococcus pneumoniae;*
same patient as Cases 425 and 426)

### Case 431

7-year-old girl presenting with a seizure.
(coronal, postcontrast T1-weighted SE scan)

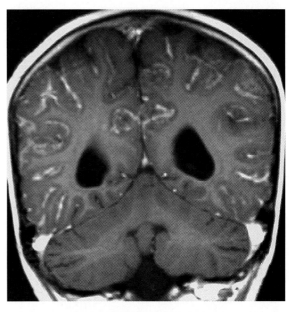

**Acute Lymphocytic Leukemia**

---

Case 430 illustrates diffuse leptomeningeal enhancement due to pneumococcal meningitis. Virtually all supratentorial sulci are filled with enhancing tissue or exudate. Hazy cortical enhancement is also present, particularly in the left occipital region. Compare the widespread leptomeningeal changes in this case to the more localized findings in Cases 428 and 429.

Several noninflammatory pathologies can cause abnormal enhancement of the leptomeninges resembling meningitis. Localized or generalized meningeal infiltration by tumor may be seen in association with systemic leukemia or lymphoma (as in Case 431), metastatic solid tumors (see Cases 29, 30, and 167), or seeding from primary intracranial malignancies (see Cases 165 and 166).

Vascular congestion of the meninges can result in superficial enhancement similar to meningitis. Possible etiologies include meningeal hyperemia in an area of acute cerebral infarction (see Cases 578 and 579), meningeal congestion due to thrombosis of dural sinuses, and leptomeningeal angiomas in Sturge-Weber syndrome (see Cases 32, 910, and 911).

Contrast enhancement at the cerebral surface may also represent cortical pathology. Compare the images on this page to Cases 449-451.

Intracranial involvement by leukemia or lymphoma may alternatively present as dural-based masses resembling meningiomas or metastases from solid tumors (see Cases 24 and 26).

### Case 432A

49-year-old man with AIDS and
systemic CMV infection.
(axial, noncontrast scan; SE 2500/25)

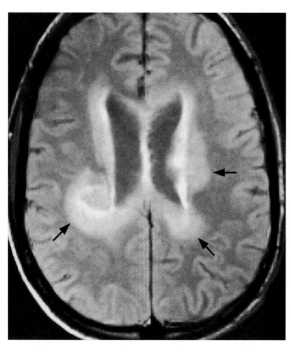

**Ventriculitis**
(cytomegalovirus)

### Case 432B

Same patient.
(sagittal, postcontrast T1-weighted SE scan)

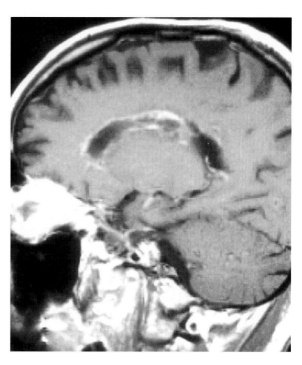

**Ventriculitis**
(cytomegalovirus)

---

Bacterial, fungal, viral, or parasitic infections may involve the ventricular lining. Fungal or viral ventriculitis most commonly occurs in immunosuppressed patients, as in this case. Bacterial ventriculitis may develop in previously healthy individuals when organisms are introduced through trauma or surgery. Pyogenic ventriculitis may also accompany a cerebral abscess (see Case 463).

Case 432A demonstrates the thick rind of subependymal inflammation and edema associated with ventriculitis. (Compare to the periventricular edema in Cases 786 and 787.) The inflammatory process is beginning to "bud" or extend away from the ventricular system into the deep white matter of both hemispheres *(arrows)*.

Intraventricular sedimentation levels may occur in cases of ventriculitis, representing cells, proteinaceous debris, and/or leakage of contrast material from inflamed epen-

dyma or choroid plexus. The visualization of intracranial sedimentation levels requires a period of limited head movement prior to a CT or MR scan. A patient who is actively shaking his or her head will disperse sediment and make detection more difficult.

Prominent ependymal/subependymal enhancement is seen in Case 432B. Postcontrast scans may also highlight inflammatory septations and loculations within the ventricular chambers. Such adhesions can cause focal cysts or generalized hydrocephalus.

Cytomegalovirus (CMV) is recognized as a cause of intrauterine encephalitis and ventriculitis but is rarely associated with cerebritis in healthy adults. Patients with AIDS or other immunodeficiency states are susceptible to infection by opportunistic pathogens, and CMV encephalitis and ventriculitis may be encountered in such cases.

### Case 433

79-year-old woman presenting with confusion.
(sagittal, postcontrast T1-weighted SE scan)

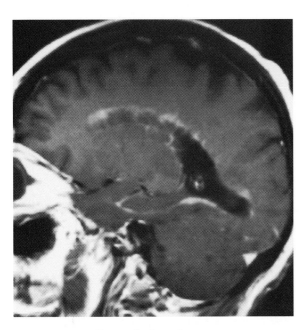

**Systemic Lymphoma**

### Case 434

67-year-old woman presenting with diplopia.
(axial, postcontrast T1-weighted SE scan)

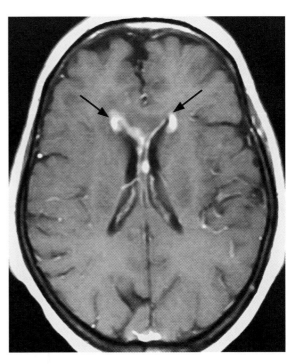

**Primary CNS Lymphoma**

Enhancing ventricular margins may be caused by ependymal-based tumor as well as by inflammatory processes. Case 433 is an example of ependymal/subependymal metastasis from a systemic neoplasm. Melanoma and carcinomas of the breast and lung can cause a similar appearance.

Primary CNS lymphoma frequently arises near ventricular borders and extends subependymally (see Cases 350-352). Case 434 illustrates linear and nodular tumor at the margin of the frontal horns, including disease of the septum pellucidum.

Other CNS tumors may involve ventricular margins through direct extension or by CSF seeding and colonization. Malignant gliomas often infiltrate through cerebral white matter to reach the ventricular margin, with subsequent subependymal spread. Medulloblastomas and germinomas are among the primary intracranial tumors that frequently demonstrate CSF-borne metastases along ventricular or meningeal surfaces.

Ependymal/subependymal enhancement is occasionally seen in patients with noninfectious inflammatory disease (e.g., sarcoidosis).

### Case 435

14-year-old girl presenting with severe headaches
and a history of mastoiditis.
(sagittal, noncontrast T1-weighted SE scan)

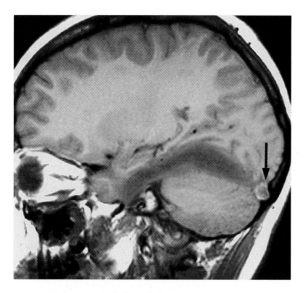

**Subdural Empyema**

### Case 436

15-year-old boy presenting with fever, aphasia,
and a history of frontal sinusitis.
(axial, noncontrast T2-weighted SE scan)

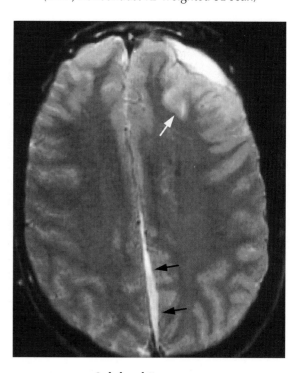

**Subdural Empyema**

---

Sinusitis or mastoiditis may cause intracranial infection by direct extension across the skull base or by septic thrombophlebitis traversing otherwise intact bone. Epidural and/or subdural abscesses may result.

In Case 435, a homogeneous layer of fluid-like signal intensity extends along the superior surface of the tentorium from the petrous bone to the thrombosed transverse sinus *(arrow)*. This compartment was one of several loculations of subdural empyema associated with mastoiditis and septic thrombophlebitis in this case (see Case 438).

Subdural fluid collections are present in the left frontal region and posterior interhemispheric fissure *(black arrows)* in Case 436. An area of cerebral edema is seen deep to the frontal collection *(white arrow)*.

The narrow subdural collection adjacent to the posterior falx in Case 436 is typical of subdural empyemas. These abscesses are often very thin and easily overlooked as symptoms begin. Involvement of the interhemispheric fissure and the tentorial surface is common, as is extension of infection along the dura to distant portions of the intracranial compartment.

Subdural empyemas are often considered to be a surgical emergency. The course in nonoperated cases can lead to rapid morbidity and mortality. One or more re-explorations may be necessary to remove persistent or recurrent locations of subdural infection. The boy in Case 436 underwent several craniotomies for recurrent empyemas but eventually recovered completely.

### Case 437

15-year-old boy presenting with fever,
aphasia, and a history of frontal sinusitis.
(coronal, postcontrast T1-weighted SE scan)

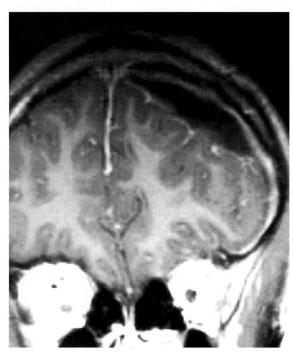

**Subdural Empyema**
(same patient as Case 436)

### Case 438

14-year-old girl presenting with severe headaches
and a history of mastoiditis.
(coronal, postcontrast T1-weighted
SE scan with MTS)

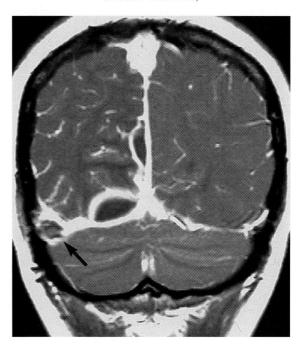

**Subdural Empyemas**
(same patient as Case 435)

Contrast enhancement usually outlines the margins of subdural empyemas, increasing the conspicuity of even thin collections and establishing their extraaxial location. Peripheral enhancement may be surprisingly thin, as in Case 437, or quite thick, as in Case 438.

The distinction between a sterile subdural effusion associated with meningitis (see Case 425) and a subdural empyema is usually indicated by the clinical condition of the patient. Patients with even large subdural effusions are often remarkably well, while patients with even small subdural empyemas are usually remarkably ill. The relative amount of contrast enhancement within the membranes of the subdural collection is an inexact index of the degree of infection. In general, membranes surrounding subdural empyemas tend to enhance more than those bordering subdural effusions, but Case 437 demonstrates the unreliability of this criterion.

Diffusion-weighted images are a more dependable means to distinguish the thickly purulent content of a subdural empyema (demonstrating restricted diffusion) from the simpler fluid within a subdural effusion (characterized by unrestricted diffusion).

Case 438 illustrates the multiloculated morphology of many subdural empyemas. Thrombus within the right transverse sinus *(arrow)* causes the filling defect surrounded by enhancement at the lateral margin of the tentorium.

Thin convexity subdural empyemas are more easily detected by MR than by CT due to the absence of artifact from adjacent bone and the availability of the coronal scan plane.

### Case 439

15-year-old boy presenting with fever
and decreased mental status.
(coronal, postcontrast T1-weighted SE scan)

### Case 440

17-year-old boy after a craniotomy (and multiple
lumbar punctures) for medulloblastoma.
(sagittal, postcontrast T1-weighted SE scan)

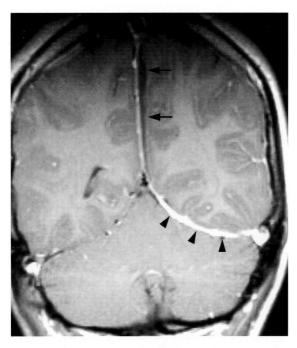

**Inflammatory Meningeal Thickening**
(associated with subdural empyema)

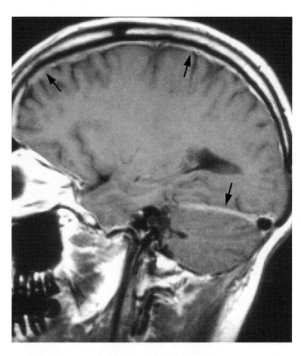

**Dual Hyperemia**
(due to intracranial hypotension)

The differential diagnosis of thick dural enhancement includes inflammatory disease (e.g., pyogenic meningitis, tuberculosis, fungal infections such as coccidioidomycosis, cysticercosis, Lyme disease, and sarcoidosis), meningeal tumor (e.g., en plaque meningioma, carcinomatosis, seeding from a primary CNS malignancy, lymphoma, and leukemia), and vascular congestion or hyperemia (e.g., secondary to recent surgery, dural sinus thrombosis, or intracranial hypotension).

Case 439 again illustrates the subtle appearance of an interhemispheric subdural empyema *(arrows),* which is associated with asymmetrical thickening of the tentorium of the left *(arrowheads).*

In Case 440, abnormal tentorial enhancement *(lower arrow)* is part of a more generalized process including convexity dura *(upper arrows).* Uniform dural thickening as seen here can be noted shortly after craniotomy or shunt placement and is often surprisingly diffuse. The rapid occurrence and widespread nature of this finding suggest a reactive phenomenon, probably reflecting an increase in dural blood volume.

A similar appearance is encountered in patients with intact skulls who experience low intracranial pressure due to spinal loss of CSF (after lumbar puncture or spontaneously). Such patients characteristically present with positional headaches (worse when upright). MR scans may demonstrate inferior sagging of the brainstem and posterior fossa structures (see Case 540).

It is important to recognize that uniform thickening of dural enhancement can be a normal consequence of craniotomy and/or lumbar punctures in patients with cranial or spinal neoplasms or infection. The finding does not necessarily imply recurrent or persistent tumor or meningitis.

### Case 441

33-year-old man presenting with
progressive somnolence.
(coronal, noncontrast T1-weighted SE scan)

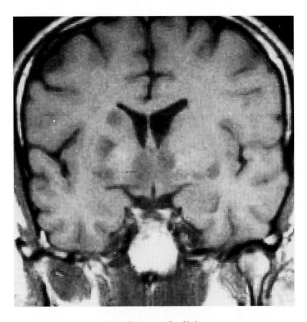

**Viral Encephalitis**

### Case 442

9-year-old boy presenting with fever and lethargy.
(axial, noncontrast T2-weighted SE scan)

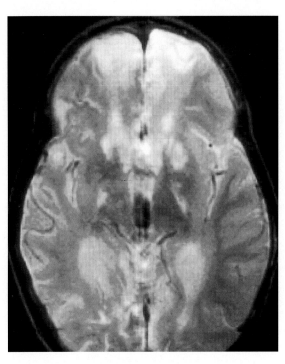

**Viral Encephalitis**

---

The MR appearance of viral encephalitis is widely variable, reflecting the age of the patient and the specific infectious agent.

Infants and young children often demonstrate panencephalitis. Herpes simplex virus type 2 is particularly likely to cause such widespread infection in a neonate (see Cases 451 and 836).

Older children and adults often present with more localized involvement by viral encephalitis. Although any area of the brain may be affected, deep hemispheric regions near the skull base are often most severely involved.

The scans above illustrate this appearance. In Case 441, zones of edema with mass effect and prolonged T1 values are present in the hypothalamus and basal ganglia bilaterally. Case 442 demonstrates similar bilateral deep hemis-

pheric involvement in association with more superficial lesions in the frontal lobes. (The low signal intensity within the third ventricle is due to CSF pulsations.)

Another possible etiology for inflammatory lesions near the third ventricle is the extension of basal meningitis into the hypothalamus (see Case 455). Bacterial or fungal pathogens (e.g., cryptococcus) may ascend along Virchow-Robin spaces accompanying penetrating arteries at the base of the brain to present at the hypothalamic level. Sarcoidosis may similarly spread from the suprasellar region into the brain to cause bilateral hypothalamic lesions.

Infants sometimes present with inflammation localized to the cerebellum. Several viruses (e.g., varicella and adenovirus) may cause such acute cerebellitus, which is often complicated by hydrocephalus and brainstem compression.

## Case 443

56-year-old woman presenting with
fever and somnolence.
(axial, noncontrast T2-weighted SE scan)

## Case 444

68-year-old woman presenting with
rapidly increasing confusion.
(axial, noncontrast FLAIR scan)

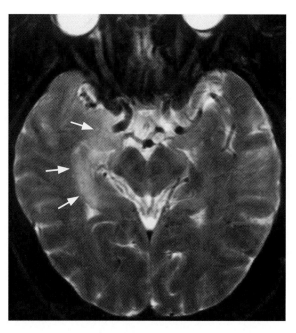

**Herpes Encephalitis**

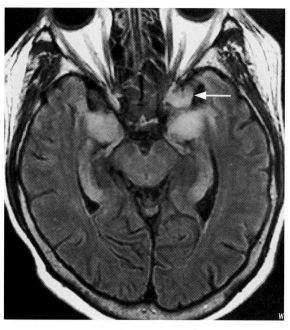

**Herpes Encephalitis**

Neonatal or perinatal herpes encephalitis is usually due to infection by type 2 (genital) herpes simplex virus (see Cases 451, 688, and 836). Herpes encephalitis in older children and adults is caused by type 1 (orofacial) herpes simplex.

Adult herpes encephalitis typically begins in the medial anterior temporal and posterior-inferior frontal lobes. Early scan findings are limited to subtle edema and mass effect in these locations, much better demonstrated by MR than by CT.

In Case 443, a poorly defined zone of mildly prolonged T2 values is present within the right uncus and anterior hippocampus *(arrows)*. Although the appearance is nonspecific, the characteristic location in the medial temporal lobe suggests herpes encephalitis in the appropriate clinical context. The diagnosis in this case was confirmed by biopsy, and the patient made a good recovery on antiviral therapy.

Case 444 demonstrates symmetrically increased signal intensity in the medial temporal lobes, predominantly involving the amygdala and hippocampal formations. Edema is also present within the small visualized portion of the posterior-inferior frontal lobe on the left *(arrow)*. Bilateral involvement is apparent on initial scans in about one-third of cases of herpes encephalitis.

As encephalitis due to type 1 herpes simplex progresses, patchy hemorrhage and abnormal contrast enhancement are common. Small hemorrhages within the edematous tissue may be apparent on MR scans as zones of T1- and/or T2-shortening. A rare alternative cause of rapidly progressive edema and patchy hemorrhage in the temporal lobe is thrombosis of the transverse sinus or vein of Labbé with venous infarction.

Gliomatosis cerebri may involve the frontal and temporal lobes unilaterally or bilaterally, resembling the MR appearance of herpes encephalitis (see Case 484).

# DIFFERENTIAL DIAGNOSIS:
## MASS EFFECT AND EDEMA INVOLVING THE MEDIAL TEMPORAL LOBE

### Case 445

4-year-old boy presenting with seizures.
(axial, noncontrast T2-weighted SE scan)

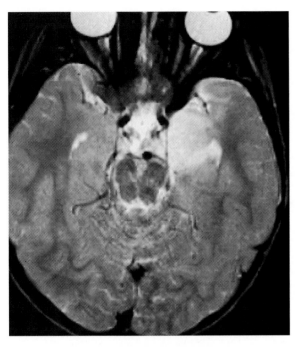

**Low-Grade Astrocytoma**

### Case 446

72-year-old man with a several month history of
memory loss and partial complex seizures.
(coronal, noncontrast T2-weighted FSE scan)

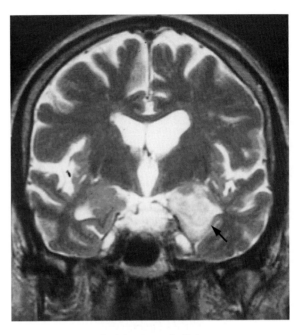

**Limbic Encephalitis**

---

The uncus is a characteristic site for herpes encephalitis, but other pathologies may also be encountered in this location.

Low or intermediate grade gliomas frequently involve the medial portion of the temporal lobe, as in Case 445. (See also Cases 72, 74, and 526.) The MR features of glial tumors and localized encephalitis may be identical, with variably defined margins and infiltration. Contrast enhancement in either entity may be minimal or striking. Diffusion-weighted images can contribute to the differential diagnosis by demonstrating more restricted diffusion in herpes encephalitis (due to cytotoxic edema; see Case 448) than in glial neoplasms.

A relatively acute clinical context often distinguishes viral encephalitis from a long-standing mass lesion. However, occasional adult cases of herpes encephalitis present with a surprisingly long history of smoldering dysfunction. The diagnosis should still be considered in such cases if scan findings are suggestive.

Limbic encephalitis is a rare paraneoplastic disorder in which cerebral inflammation is associated with a systemic

tumor, most frequently oat cell carcinoma of the lung. The presence of antineuronal nuclear antibodies within the CSF of affected patients presumably indicates the etiology of this cerebritis. Predilection for the medial temporal lobes mimics herpes encephalitis, but no viral inclusions are present in affected tissue. Bilateral involvement is common with frequent marked asymmetry, as was true in Case 446. Contrast enhancement may be absent or extensive, probably reflecting differing phases of inflammation.

Symptoms of limbic encephalitis may precede evidence of the primary neoplasm. The course of the disorder is usually more gradual than that of herpes encephalitis, evolving over weeks to months.

The clinical presentation, histological pattern, and antibody studies in Case 446 were all characteristic of limbic encephalitis. However, despite a thorough work-up, an associated tumor has not been identified.

Neurosyphilis is an additional pathology that can affect the medial temporal lobe and mimic herpes encephalitis.

### Case 447

68-year-old woman presenting with
rapidly increasing confusion.
(coronal, noncontrast FLAIR scan)

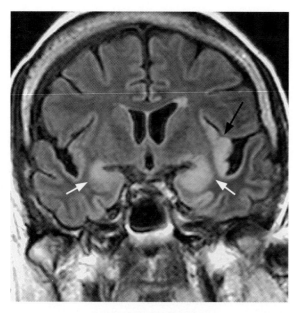

**Herpes Encephalitis**
(same patient as Case 444)

### Case 448

66-year-old woman presenting with a seizure.
(axial, noncontrast diffusion-weighted scan)

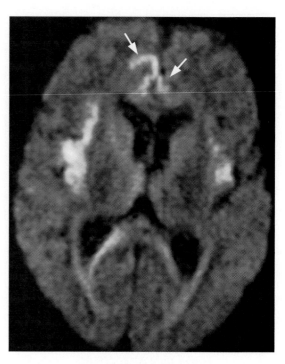

**Herpes Encephalitis**

---

Involvement of the insula and white matter lateral to the lentiform nucleus is characteristic of herpes encephalitis. Edema sharply marginating the lateral border of the putamen should suggest this diagnosis.

Case 447 demonstrates signal abnormality involving the left insula *(black arrow)*, as well as within the medial temporal lobes bilaterally *(white arrows)*.

The diffusion-weighted scan in Case 448 illustrates bilateral (but asymmetrical) insular lesions. Restricted diffusion is also noted within cortex of the cingulate gyri *(arrows)*, another characteristic site of early involvement in herpes encephalitis.

Case 448 makes the point that gyriform cortical abnormality on diffusion-weighted scans is not specific for recent infarction. Multiple sclerosis can also cause foci of restricted diffusion within cerebral white matter, resembling recent deep hemisphere infarcts.

Embolic infarction affecting only the cortical distribution of the middle cerebral artery can present as peri-insular abnormality resembling herpes encephalitis. The clinical context and absence of accompanying medial frontal-temporal involvement usually clarify the diagnosis in such cases.

# DIFFERENTIAL DIAGNOSIS:
## SUPERFICIAL CONTRAST ENHANCEMENT IN THE SYLVIAN REGION

### Case 449

61-year-old man with a two-week
history of increasing confusion.
(axial, postcontrast T1-weighted SE scan)

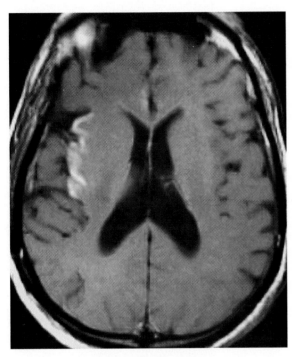

**Herpes Encephalitis**

### Case 450

25-year-old man presenting with mild
aphasia and right hemiparesis.
(axial, postcontrast T1-weighted SE scan)

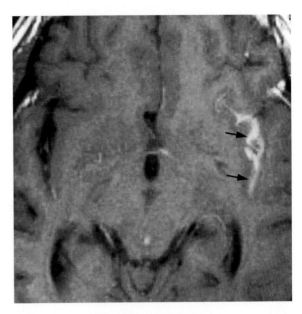

**Tuberculous Meningitis**

---

Superficial contrast enhancement may represent cortical or meningeal pathology, or a combination of the two.

Case 449 illustrates intense, gyriform enhancement of insular cortex involved by herpes encephalitis. (Compare to the gyriform enhancement seen in subacute infarcts such as Cases 579 and 580.) Involvement of the insula is characteristic of this disorder and should suggest the diagnosis. Edema and enhancement of the cingulate gyrus (faintly seen in Case 449) are also common and distinctive features of encephalitis due to herpes.

The superficial enhancement in Case 450 is meningeal in origin. Enhancing tissue fills the left sylvian cistern (com-
pare to the normal right side), surrounding vascular structures. Fungal or granulomatous meningitis often localizes to a small portion of the subarachnoid space, as illustrated here. (Compare to the more extensive tuberculous meningitis in Case 429.)

Cisternal or sulcal enhancement on MR scans is often more easily detected and more extensive than appreciated on CT studies. The absence of masking artifact from the adjacent calvarium, multiplanar display, and the higher sensitivity to small amounts of contrast material contribute to the advantage of MR in cases of enhancing superficial pathology.

## Case 451

1-month-old girl presenting with
fever and seizures.
(coronal, postcontrast T1-weighted SE scan)

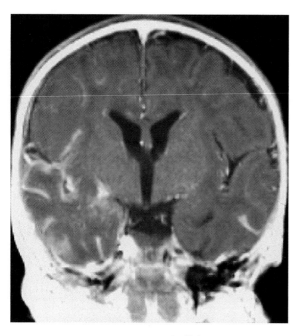

**Herpes Encephalitis**
(type 2)

## Case 452

64-year-old man presenting with
fever and obtundation.
(axial, postcontrast T1-weighted SE scan)

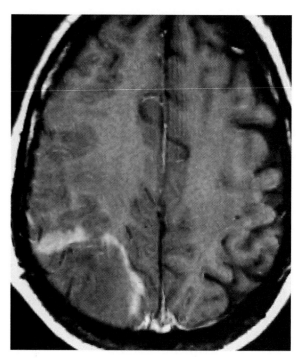

**Bacterial Cerebritis**
(presumed)

---

The MR spectrum of cerebritis includes a wide range of pathogens and patterns. Neonatal encephalitis due to herpes simplex type 2 is often diffuse and devastating, as illustrated in Case 451. Initial multifocal or symmetrical cerebral edema with loss of gray/white discrimination evolves to a phase of intense, gyriform contrast enhancement, as seen above. Rapid loss of parenchymal volume leads to generalized or patchy encephalomalacia, dystrophic calcification, and secondary ventricular enlargement (see Case 836).

No organism was cultured from CSF or brain biopsy in Case 452. However, the patient recovered on broad-spectrum antibiotics, and a presumptive diagnosis of pyogenic cerebritis was made.

Pyogenic or fungal cerebritis may initially present as a nonspecific region of edema and swelling similar to that seen in viral encephalitis. Patchy contrast enhancement is more common than the gyriform pattern typical of herpes encephalitis.

Case 452 demonstrates a prominent band of enhancement at the margin of inflammation in the right parietal region. This peripheral zone represents the brain's attempt to contain the infection. Peripheral enhancement typically precedes the development of a true abscess capsule by days or weeks. Clues that a lesion is still in the cerebritis stage (i.e., lacks an organized capsule) include nonvisualization of the capsule on precontrast scans (see Cases 459-462) and progressive diffusion of contrast material into the center of the lesion on postcontrast images.

### Case 453

77-year-old woman presenting with TIAs and fever.
(coronal, noncontrast T2-weighted FSE scan)

### Case 454

50-year-old man presenting with headaches.
(sagittal, postcontrast T1-weighted SE scan)

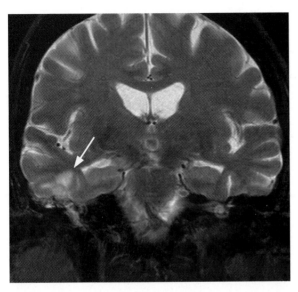

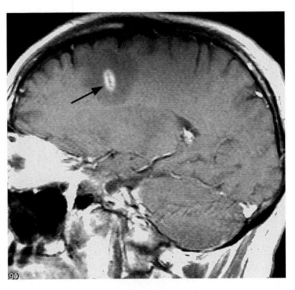

**Bacterial Cerebritis**
(due to mastoiditis)

**Bacterial Cerebritis**
(due to a previous shunt catheter)

Bacterial cerebritis may be localized to a small region at the site of infection.

Case 453 demonstrates focal edema within the inferior right temporal lobe *(arrow)*, immediately adjacent to mucosal thickening and/or fluid within mastoid air cells. The possibility of an inflammatory process related to mastoiditis should be considered whenever a lesion is discovered in the temporal lobe (see also Case 467). (Another potential etiology for patchy mid-temporal edema and enhancement is venous infarction due to occlusion of the vein of Labbé or an equivalent vessel.)

Infection is a well-recognized complication of ventricular shunts. Such cases may present with ventriculitis or meningitis. In Case 454, the shunt track itself is infected *(arrow)*, with enhancing margins and surrounding edema.

# DIFFERENTIAL DIAGNOSIS:
## MILIARY ENHANCEMENT IN THE BASAL GANGLIA

### Case 455

10-year-old boy being treated for a PNET, now presenting with impaired consciousness.
(axial, postcontrast T1-weighted SE scan)

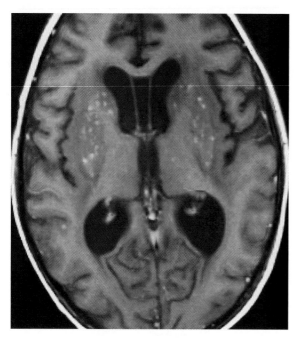

**Encephalitis Secondary to
Streptococcal Meningitis**

### Case 456

35-year-old woman presenting with headaches.
(axial, postcontrast T1-weighted SE scan)

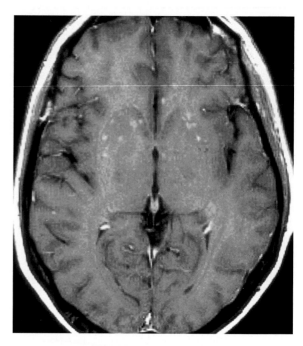

**Carcinomatous Encephalitis**
(metastatic carcinoma of the breast)

---

Case 455 illustrates miliary encephalitis developing as a consequence of streptococcal meningitis in an immuno-suppressed patient. The predominance of lesions in the basal ganglia may reflect hematogenous seeding to these well-perfused nuclei, comparable to the presumably blood-borne distribution of metastatic disease in Case 456.

Alternatively, ganglionic infection may reflect direct extension of basal meningitis. Organisms can ascend along the Virchow-Robin spaces accompanying lenticulostriate arteries into the base of the brain. This route of spread is characteristic of cryptococcal meningitis, with small "gelatinous pseudocysts" developing in the same distribution as the enhancing foci of Case 455. Ascending infection from the skull base may account for the deep hemispheric involvement in some patients with viral encephalitis (see Cases 441 and 442). Ganglionic lesions in the setting of meningitis may also represent sterile infarcts.

Cerebral involvement by multiple tiny metastases, as in Case 456, is sometimes termed *carcinomatous encephalitis*. Enhancement of such lesions produces a miliary pattern that resembles disseminated infection, vasculitis, or noninfectious inflammatory processes (e.g., multiple sclerosis or sarcoidosis). In some cases, numerous tiny metastases do not enhance significantly and are detected only as a finely granular texture within the basal ganglia and/or cerebral cortex, best appreciated on T2-weighted images.

Hypertrophied lenticulostriate arteries (e.g., moya moya disease, as illustrated in Case 582) can also cause an appearance similar to the above scans.

Ventricular enlargement in Case 455 probably represents a combination of radiation effect and low-grade communicating hydrocephalus.

## Case 457

38-year-old man presenting with confusion.
(axial, noncontrast T2-weighted FSE scan)

## Case 458

33-year-old man with a history of AIDS.
(axial, noncontrast T2-weighted SE scan)

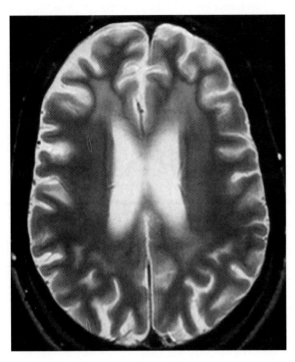

HIV Encephalitis

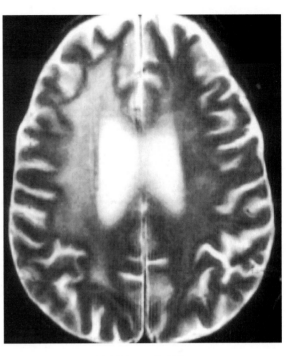

HIV Encephalitis

Most of the cerebral masses seen in patients with AIDS are well demonstrated by CT scans. MR is helpful to characterize lesions or detect additional masses that are more easily biopsied than those apparent on a CT study.

Another imaging advantage of MR in AIDS is the detection of subtle white matter disease. Infection of glial and macrophage-derived cells by the human immunodeficiency virus (HIV) or by an opportunistic pathogen (e.g., CMV) can cause extensive leukoencephalopathy with little or no CT abnormality.

The MR study in Case 457 demonstrates large areas of mildly abnormal signal intensity within white matter of the frontal and parietal lobes. This soft, symmetrical pattern of white matter pathology is a common finding in HIV encephalitis. CMV can cause a similar appearance.

Case 458 illustrates that white matter involvement by HIV encephalitis may be strikingly asymmetrical. The affected region of the right centrum semiovale demonstrates the same hazy quality seen bilaterally in Case 457.

Extension into the corpus callosum can occur with either unilateral or bilateral disease. A similar combination of hemispheric and callosal lesions in a patient with AIDS can be caused by progressive multifocal leukoencephalopathy.

In both of the above cases, the ventricles and sulci are abnormally large for the patient's age. This is a common finding on cerebral scans of patients with AIDS and may be the only apparent abnormality (see Case 534).

Cranial CT and MR studies in AIDS patients may also demonstrate sinusitis, multicystic enlargement of the parotid glands, and cervical adenopathy. These findings support the diagnosis in the appropriate clinical context.

### Case 459

2-year-old boy presenting with hemiparesis.
(sagittal, noncontrast T1-weighted SE scan)

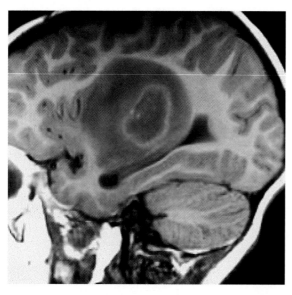

**Bacterial Abscess**

### Case 460

13-year-old boy, one year after resection of
a medulloblastoma, now presenting with
increasing ataxia and facial weakness.
(sagittal, noncontrast T1-weighted SE scan)

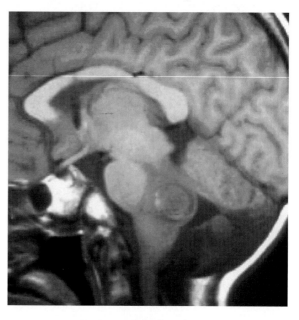

**Bacterial Abscess**

Cerebral abscesses are characterized by three distinct zones of signal abnormality on MR scans. Centrally, a necrotic cavity often demonstrates long T1 and T2 values. This feature is more obvious in Case 459 than in Case 460, where the abscess content is relatively isointense due to the presence of cells and/or protein. Peripherally, a zone of extensive edema surrounds the lesion. This area is well seen in both of the above cases as a region of reduced signal intensity, clearly defined in Case 459 and more amorphous in Case 460.

Separating the abscess cavity from surrounding edema is the abscess capsule, which can often be identified as a discrete structure on noncontrast MR images. The capsule is typically smoothly rounded in shape and uniform in thickness. It may appear to be unilaminar or bilaminar.

Segments of the abscess capsule often demonstrate shortening of both T1 and T2. As a result, all or part of the capsule may be seen as a high signal intensity rim on T1-weighted sequences and as a low intensity rim on T2-weighted images. This appearance does not correlate well with the presence of blood products in the wall of the abscess. Other etiologies (e.g., the presence of free radicles produced by activated macrophages) have been suggested as the source of the paramagnetic effect.

The abscess capsule is well defined in each of the above cases as a uniformly thin layer of distinct signal intensity, with some areas of T1-shortening. These features are all useful in distinguishing abscesses from necrotic cerebral neoplasms. The wall of a tumor infrequently demonstrates T1-shortening and is usually thicker, less uniform, and less round than the capsule of an abscess.

The child in Case 459 had been hospitalized several weeks earlier for streptococcal pneumonia, and culture of material aspirated from the abscess cavity grew streptococci.

## Case 461

8-year-old boy presenting with increasing
headaches and vomiting.
(axial, noncontrast T2-weighted SE scan)

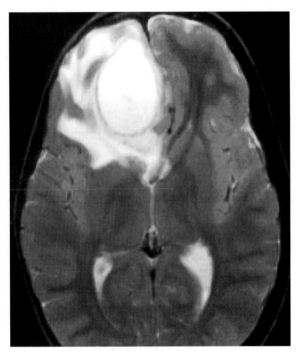

**Bacterial Abscess**

## Case 462

13-year-old boy presenting with
ataxia and facial weakness.
(axial, noncontrast T2-weighted SE scan)

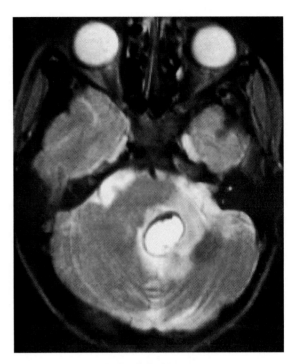

**Bacterial Abscess**
(same patient as Case 460)

---

The capsule of an abscess is usually defined on T2-weighted scans as a thin and round zone of isointensity or low signal intensity separating surrounding edema from the central cavity. The wall of many abscesses is uniformly thin, as in Case 461. In other cases, irregular thickening of tissue is encountered along portions of the abscess capsule (as seen anteriorly in Case 462), but the overall morphology remains suggestive of the correct diagnosis.

Uniformly thin and spherical rims of tissue are occasionally seen at the perimeter of cerebral neoplasms. The margin of some gliomas is surprisingly round and regular (see Case 100), and metastases can be centrally necrotic with a uniform rim of surrounding viable tumor (see Cases 13, 14,

and 16). As discussed on the preceding page, T1- and T2-shortening within the wall of a cystic lesion raise the possibility of inflammatory origin, but hemorrhage at the margin of a tumor can produce similar changes. Supplemental MR techniques (proton spectroscopy and diffusion-weighted scans) may help to distinguish pyogenic cerebral abscesses from neoplasms when standard images are indeterminate (see discussion of Cases 465 and 466).

Many abscesses can be aspirated with CT or MR guidance and/or followed to resolution by serial scans during antibiotic therapy. Repeated drainage may be necessary. Enhancement of the abscess capsule often persists for weeks or months during successful treatment.

## Case 463

62-year-old woman presenting with a
presumed cerebrovascular accident.
(coronal, postcontrast T1-weighted SE scan)

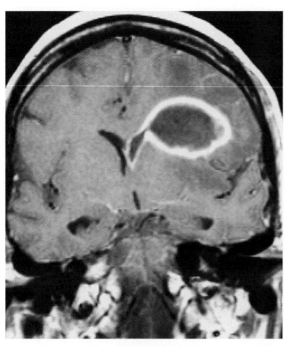

**Bacterial Abscess**

## Case 464

2-year-old boy presenting with hemiparesis.
(axial, postcontrast T1-weighted SE scan)

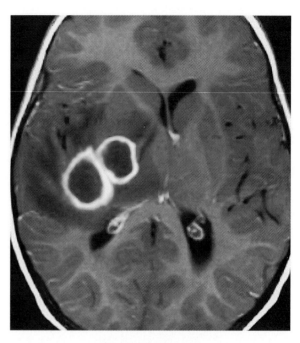

**Bacterial Abscess**
(same patient as Case 459)

---

The capsule of an abscess enhances intensely, demonstrating the same features of uniform thinness and round contours seen on noncontrast scans. The appearance of the above cases is typical.

Slight thickening and irregularity of the capsule is well within the spectrum of observed abscess morphologies. Occasional pyogenic abscesses develop a thicker and more irregular capsule, which resembles the periphery of a high-grade glioma or metastasis. Fungal abscesses may also demonstrate thick-walled, loculated, or semisolid morphology.

The lesion in Case 463 has reached the margin of the lateral ventricle. Associated ependymal enhancement indicates ventriculitis (see Case 432). This finding has been reported to be a warning sign of potential intraventricular rupture.

The abscess in Case 464 is strikingly lobulated. More subtle "budding" morphology is common, as daughter abscesses form at the margin of the original collection. Although suggestive of an abscess, such loculations are not specific; occasional tumors present a similar appearance.

The relatively poor inflammatory response of deep hemispheric white matter may cause the capsule of an abscess to be less developed along the medial wall than along the superficial margin. When present, this feature can help to distinguish an abscess from a tumor.

Abscesses may rupture into the ventricular system. This event can cause dramatic clinical deterioration (from dissemination of infection) or temporary improvement (from reduction of mass effect). The mortality associated with intraventricular rupture of a cerebral abscess has been reduced by aggressive diagnosis and treatment but remains high (about 40% in most series).

# DIFFERENTIAL DIAGNOSIS:
## CEREBRAL MASS WITH A THIN, ENHANCING WALL

### Case 465

8-year-old boy presenting with increasing
headaches and vomiting.
(coronal, postcontrast T1-weighted SE scan)

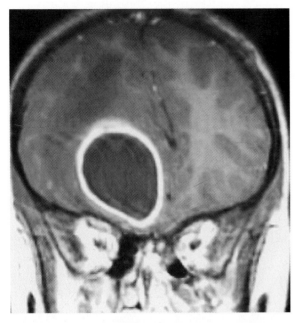

**Bacterial Abscess**
(same patient as case 461)

### Case 466

52-year-old man presenting with
headaches and left hemiparesis.
(coronal, postcontrast T1-weighted SE scan)

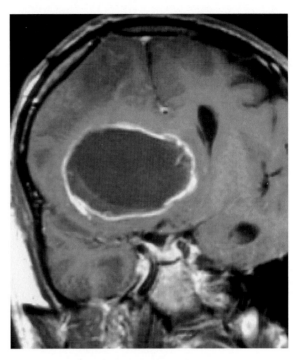

**Glioblastoma Multiforme**

---

The enhancing rim of some primary and metastatic tumors is quite uniform and may mimic the capsule of an abscess. The border of the malignant glioma in Case 466 is only a little more irregular than the margin of the abscess in Case 465. An abscess should always be considered when a thin-walled cystic lesion is encountered, but other clues should be sought to support the diagnosis.

In Case 465, the inferior pole of the abscess points toward the cribriform plate. A history of old trauma was retrospectively obtained, and a fracture of the cribriform plate was identified at surgery as a likely route of infection.

Specialized MR techniques can help to distinguish between abscesses and necrotic tumors when routine images are ambiguous. Proton spectroscopy typically demonstrates organic acids (e.g., acetate at 1.9 ppm and succinate at 2.4 ppm) and proteolyzed amino acids (e.g., valine and leucine at 0.9 ppm, alanine at 1.5 ppm) within pyogenic abscesses. Organic acids are rarely found within cystic or necrotic neoplasms, while amino acids occur at lower (often undetectable) concentrations. Both abscesses and necrotic tumors may demonstrate elevated lactate levels at 1.3 ppm.

Diffusion-weighted scans can also assist in this differential diagnosis. Restricted diffusion is usually apparent within the thickly proteinaceous and cellular content of a pyogenic abscess, and usually absent in the cystic/necrotic cavity of a tumor. (In fact, diffusion in the latter is often facilitated.)

Diffusion-weighted scans do not distinguish all tumors from all abscesses. Densely cellular neoplasms (e.g., primary CNS lymphoma, primitive neuroectodermal tumors, and some cerebral metastases) without central necrosis may demonstrate restricted diffusion. Also, diffusion is less commonly restricted in abscesses due to fungi or toxoplasmosis than in pyogenic lesions.

Extensive frontal edema and subfalcial herniation are present in each of the above cases.

### Case 467

38-year-old woman presenting with a seizure.
(axial, postcontrast T1-weighted SE scan with MTS)

### Case 468

38-year-old man presenting with
transient receptive aphasia.
(axial, postcontrast T1-weighted SE scan with MTS)

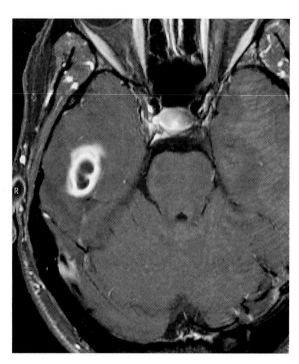

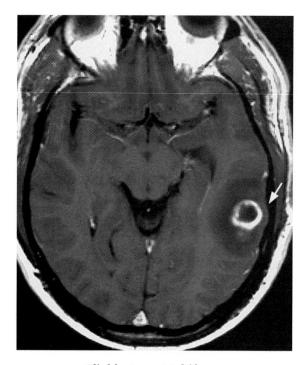

**Bacterial Abscess**

**Glioblastoma Multiforme**

---

The ages and MR features of the above cases are nearly identical, again demonstrating the potential overlap in the presentation of inflammatory lesions and cerebral neoplasms.

The abscess in Case 467 was caused by direct extension of infection from the petrous bone. (The patient gave a history of right mastoid surgery for cholesteatoma as a child.) The possibility of an inflammatory process secondary to mastoiditis should be considered whenever a lesion is encountered at the inferior aspect of the temporal lobes. Coronal scans are useful in establishing this relationship (see Case 453).

The relatively thin and uniform enhancing rim of the small mass in Case 468 combines with extensive surrounding edema and the young age of the patient to suggest an abscess. One clue to the correct diagnosis is the subtle but definite erosion of the adjacent inner table *(arrow)*, implying localized superficial mass effect of some duration at this site. Another clue was the absence of restricted diffusion within the lesion on diffusion-weighted images. As discussed on the previous page, the thickly proteinaceous and cellular content of a bacterial abscess typically impairs diffusion of water molecules more than the fluid in a cystic or necrotic neoplasm.

A solitary parasitic cyst (e.g., cysticercosis or toxoplasmosis), fungal abscess (e.g., histoplasmosis or candidiasis), or caseating granuloma (i.e., tuberculosis) would be included in the differential diagnosis for the above lesions (see Cases 469, 477, and 478), together with a rare solitary demyelinating plaque.

# CYSTICERCOSIS

## Case 469A

33-year-old man presenting with a seizure.
(axial, noncontrast T2-weighted SE scan)

## Case 469B

Same patient.
(axial, postcontrast T1-weighted SE scan)

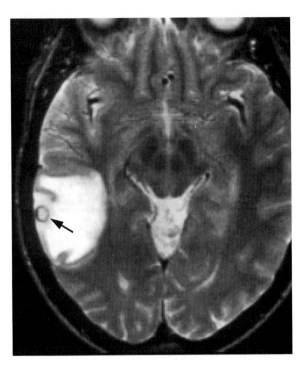

**Cysticercosis**

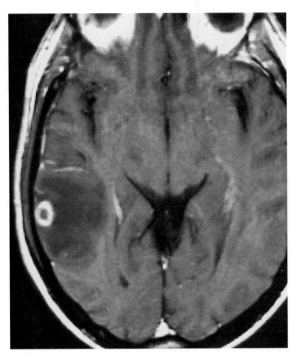

**Cysticercosis**

---

Cysticercosis is the most important parasitic infection of the CNS in this hemisphere. The disease occurs when man serves as an intermediate host for the larval form of the pork tapeworm, *Taenia solium.*

Cysts of cysticercosis may present as solitary lesions or clustered aggregates. "Racemose cysts" are commonly found in the suprasellar, sylvian, or cerebellopontine angle cisterns. Intraventricular cysts are common in all ventricles and may blend with surrounding spinal fluid while obstructing the ventricular system (see Cases 525, 806, and 807).

Typical parenchymal cysts measure about one centimeter in diameter, as seen in this case *(arrow)*. A small nodule may be visible along the perimeter of the cyst, representing the scolex of the parasite (see Case 525).

The cyst wall in Case 469A is well defined by extensive surrounding edema. Intense peripheral enhancement of the lesion is demonstrated in Case 469B. Enhancement becomes smaller and more solid as cysts degenerate and involute.

Contrast enhancement is observed when cysticerical larvae have incited a host response. Since living larvae are immunologically invisible and do not provoke cerebral edema or enhancement, the presence of these features usually implies larval death. In fact, edema and contrast enhancement may be correlates of successful treatment of cysticercosis.

An enhancing granulomatous stage follows the cystic form of parenchymal cysticercosis. A solitary lesion in this stage may resemble primary or metastic tumors. Cysticercosis should also be included (along with tuberculosis and other potentially "miliary" infections) in the differential diagnosis of multiple focal enhancing lesions in an adult (see Cases 472 and 479).

Calcification is the final result of the host's response to the death of the larva. This appearance marks the end of the granulomatous phase in cysticercal infection. Lesions of variable activity (e.g., nonenhancing and calcified) may be seen in the same patient.

### Case 470

14-year-old boy presenting with lethargy
following a respiratory illness.
(axial, noncontrast T2-weighted SE scan)

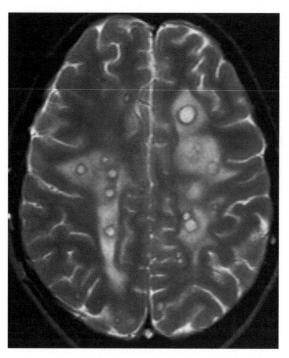

**Histoplasmosis**

### Case 471

24-year-old woman presenting with
scattered paresthesias.
(axial, noncontrast T2-weighted FSE scan)

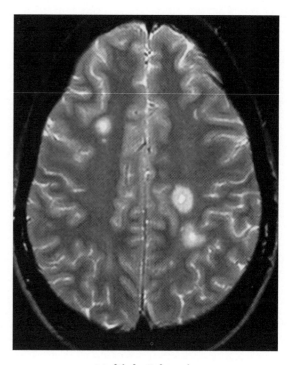

**Multiple Sclerosis**

The characteristic appearance of cerebral cysticercosis as illustrated on the previous page can be mimicked by several other pathologies.

Fungal abscesses are often small and multiple, as seen in Case 470. Like pyogenic lesions, the capsules of fungal abscesses are clearly outlined on T2-weighted scans as isointense or low intensity structures separating the contents from reactive edema. Abscesses similar to Case 470 could be caused by other fungi (e.g., *Candida*), parasites (e.g., toxoplasmosis; see Case 477), or caseating granulomas (i.e., tuberculosis; see Case 478). The multiple lesions in Case 470 probably represent hematogenous dissemination of the yeast form of histoplasmosis following primary pulmonary infection.

Case 471 serves as a reminder that demyelinating disease can produce ring-like lesions of any diameter. The target morphology of these plaques correlates with concentric tissue zones reflecting stages of demyelination and secondary reactive edema (see Cases 374 and 375).

Histoplasmosis is one of the fungal families that can be encountered in immunologically normal hosts. (Others include *Blastomyces, Cryptococcus,* and *Coccidioides.*) Cerebral infection by *Aspergillus, Mucor,* and *Candida* species is usually limited to patients who are immunocompromised.

# CEREBRAL TUBERCULOSIS

## Case 472A

19-year-old woman from Somalia
presenting with a seizure.
(axial, noncontrast T2-weighted FSE scan)

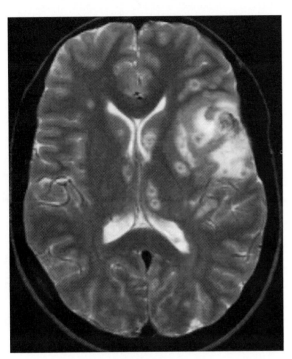

**Cerebral Tuberculosis**

## Case 472B

Same patient.
(axial, postcontrast T1-weighted SE scan)

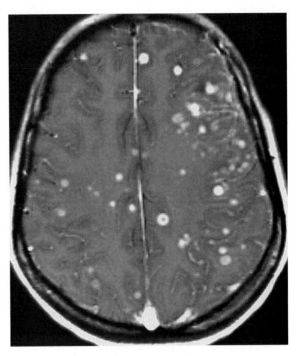

**Cerebral Tuberculosis**

---

Intracranial involvement by tuberculosis can take many forms. Tuberculous meningitis has been previously illustrated in Cases 429 and 450. Parenchymal lesions of tuberculosis may be solitary or multiple, abscesses or granulomas.

The majority of the lesions in Case 472 are individual, although coalescence is present in the posterior left frontal lobe. Collars of edema outline the isointense central nodules in Case 472A. The small masses demonstrate both solid and peripheral enhancement in Case 472B.

The pattern and distribution of lesions in this patient resemble Case 470, reflecting hematogenous seeding. Dis-

seminated tuberculosis frequently involves cortex, subcortical white matter, and deep nuclei. Multiple or solitary tuberculomas of the cerebellum or brainstem are common in children or adults.

Solitary tuberculomas may be much larger than the nodules in this case. Contrast enhancement of such masses can be solid or peripheral, with rim enhancement reflecting central caseous necrosis. Large tuberculomas may mimic a primary or metastatic tumor or a pyogenic abscess.

Case 472B demonstrates widespread abnormal leptomeningeal enhancement in addition to the parenchymal lesions.

### Case 473

37-year-old man with AIDS,
presenting with headaches.
(sagittal, noncontrast T1-weighted SE scan)

### Case 474

44-year-old man with AIDS, presenting with
left hemiparesis and headaches.
(axial, postcontrast T1-weighted SE scan)

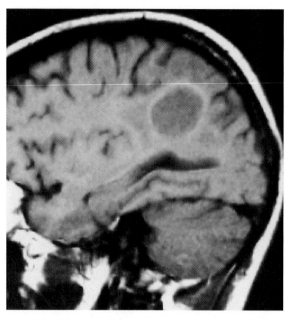

**Toxoplasmosis**

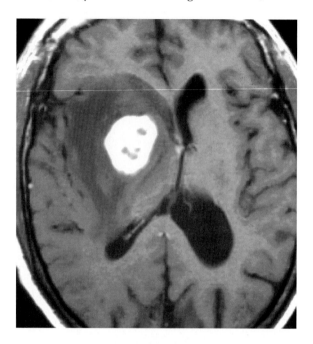

**Toxoplasmosis**

Intracranial masses are reported in 10% to 20% of AIDS patients. Toxoplasmosis ranks as the most common etiology in most series (followed by primary CNS lymphoma). The disease is caused by *Toxoplasma gondii*, an environmentally common protozoan that produces mild or subclinical infection in immunocompetent individuals.

Toxoplasmosis usually presents as multiple lesions of variable size and depth. Solitary masses are found in about 20% of cases. (A solitary cerebral mass in a patient with AIDS is more likely to represent primary CNS lymphoma than toxoplasmosis.) Lesions are most commonly located within the basal ganglia or near the gray/white matter junction. Individual masses may appear solid or demonstrate central necrosis. Hemorrhage is common.

The subcortical lesion in Case 473 has a uniformly smooth and thin rim of mild T1-shortening that suggests an abscess cavity (compare to Cases 459 and 460). A postcontrast scan of this patient demonstrated the expected thin rim of peripheral enhancement.

Other masses due to toxoplasmosis enhance more solidly, as in Case 474. Neither pattern is specific: the broad spectrum of morphology seen in cerebral toxoplasmosis is over-

lapped by many other pathologies. Multiloculated abscesses are uncommon in toxoplasmosis and should suggest other diagnostic possibilities (e.g., tuberculosis or fungal disease).

The hemispheric masses in the above cases could equally well represent primary CNS lymphoma (see Cases 356 and 357). Metabolic studies (i.e., PET or SPECT scans), MR spectroscopy (elevated choline in lymphoma, not in toxoplasmosis), and perfusion-weighted sequences (lower cerebral blood volume in toxoplasmosis than in lymphoma) may help to distinguish between these pathologies. Because of the high incidence of toxoplasmosis in patients with AIDS, antibiotic therapy is often begun empirically when masses are discovered. Biopsy is reserved for nonresponding lesions.

Cerebral toxoplasmosis may wax and wane over several months in response to courses of antimicrobial therapy. Treatment usually causes regression of toxoplasmosis within weeks but does not eradicate the pathogen. When treatment is discontinued (e.g., due to toxicity), recurrence is expected.

# DIFFERENTIAL DIAGNOSIS:
## HETEROGENEOUS GANGLIONIC MASS WITH EXTENSIVE EDEMA

### Case 475

44-year-old man presenting with
left hemiparesis and headaches.
(axial, noncontrast T2-weighted SE scan)

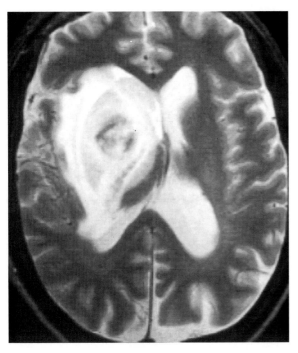

**Toxoplasmosis**
(same patient as Case 474)

### Case 476

46-year-old woman presenting with a seizure.
(axial, noncontrast T2-weighted FSE scan)

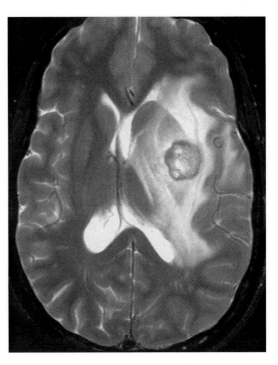

**Metastatic Carcinoma of the Breast**

---

These patients of nearly the same age have similar MRI scans. In each case a heterogeneous mass containing regions of both high and low signal intensity is centered in the area of the lentiform nucleus. Marked surrounding edema occupies the internal and external capsules and contributes to mass effect that exaggerates the size of the inciting nodules.

Solitary or multiple ganglionic lesions like Case 475 are common in toxoplasmosis, resembling the frequent periventricular distribution of primary CNS lymphoma (see Cases 347 and 349-354). Like the latter pathology, toxoplasmosis may also involve the corpus callosum.

Case 476 is a reminder that metastatic disease must be included in the differential diagnosis of any cerebral mass, even in young adults.

Toxoplasmosis and primary CNS lymphoma are among the pathologies to be considered when multiple ganglionic lesions are discovered. Mucor mycosis can cause extensive ganglionic edema (usually with little contrast enhancement) in immunocompromised patients or intravenous drug users. Venous infarction due to thrombosis of the internal cerebral vein(s) should also be included in the differential diagnosis (see Case 654).

The heterogeneity of the above lesions is somewhat similar to that of cavernous angiomas (see Cases 761-764), but the surrounding edema would be very unusual for a hemangioma without significant recent hemorrhage.

### Case 477

38-year-old man with AIDS presenting with
fever and lethargy.
(sagittal, postcontrast T1-weighted SE scan)

### Case 478

47-year-old woman presenting with
mild difficulty swallowing.
(axial, postcontrast T1-weighted SE scan)

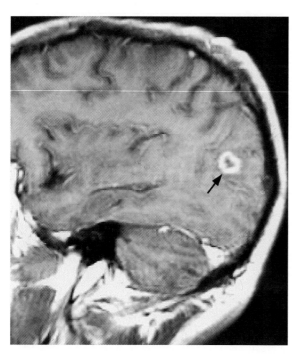

**Toxoplasmosis**

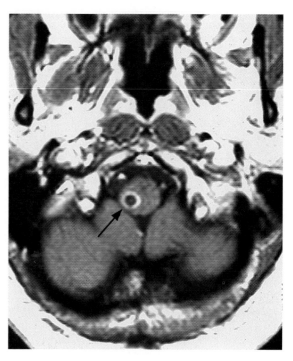

**Tuberculosis**

---

Toxoplasmosis may cause smaller masses than illustrated on the previous pages. The thick-walled abscess in Case 477 resembles the size and morphology of typical lesions in cysticercosis (see Case 469) or fungal cerebritis (see Case 470).

Case 478 is an example of a solitary tuberculoma, contrasting with the miliary involvement illustrated in Case 472. Other tuberculomas may be much larger, with solid and/or peripheral enhancement. The lesion in Case 478 was resected and found to contain caseous debris. The patient recovered completely.

In addition to dysphagia, lateral medullary dysfunction (Wallenberg syndrome) may include hoarseness, hiccups, vertigo, nystagmus, diplopia, ataxia, ipsilateral facial pain or numbness, diminished taste, and contralateral numbness or decreased sensation of pain and temperature. This syndrome is most commonly caused by infarction in the distribution of the posterior inferior cerebellar artery (see Cases 618 and 620).

# DIFFERENTIAL DIAGNOSIS:
## MULTIPLE SMALL, RING-ENHANCING MASSES

### Case 479

14-year-old boy presenting with lethargy
following a respiratory illness.
(axial, postcontrast T1-weighted SE scan)

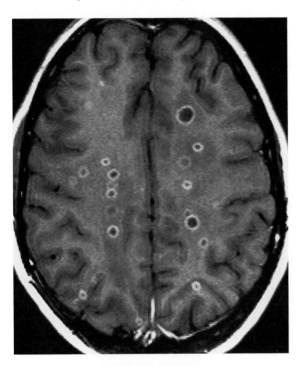

**Histoplasmosis**
(same patient as Case 470)

### Case 480

36-year-old woman presenting with rapidly
progressive weakness and numbness.
(axial, postcontrast T1-weighted SE scan)

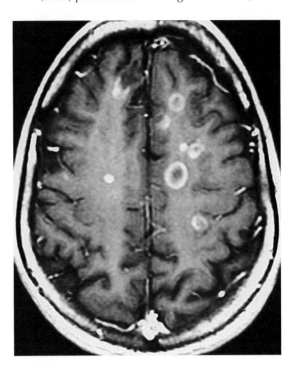

**Multiple Sclerosis**

---

The above images present the postcontrast equivalent of the differential diagnosis in Cases 470 and 471. Both infectious and demyelinating foci can present as multiple small, rim-enhancing masses.

Additional possible etiologies in the former category include other fungi (e.g., candidiasis), cysticercosis, toxoplasmosis, and tuberculosis. The child in Case 479 was systemically ill, with pulmonary and hepatic involvement.

Case 480 demonstrates that a flare of multiple sclerosis can cause many lesions to develop synchronously, progressing together through a stage of inflammation/demyelination associated with a ring of enhancement. The patient in this case was known to have demyelinating disease and

presented clinically with an acute relapse. Occasional patients experience a similarly fulminant episode at the onset of multiple sclerosis, the so-called "Marburg" variant.

The history in Case 479 raises the possibility of acute disseminated encephalomyelitis, which can cause multiple areas of parenchymal enhancement (see Case 397). However, ring-enhancing lesions are less common in ADEM than in multiple sclerosis; an appearance resembling Case 479 would be highly unusual.

In an older adult, multiple small cystic or necrotic metastases (e.g., from carcinoma of the breast or lung) would be included in the differential diagnosis of these cases.

### Case 481

13-year-old girl presenting with confusion.
(axial, noncontrast FLAIR scan)

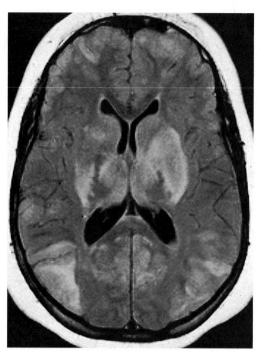

**Systemic Lupus Erythematosus**

### Case 482

68-year-old woman presenting with
right hemiparesis.
(axial, noncontrast T2-weighted SE scan)

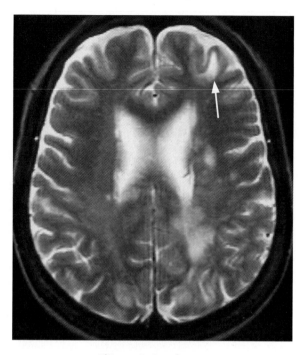

**Sjögren's Syndrome**

Systemic lupus erythematosus (SLE) is a condition of unknown etiology in which autoantibodies and the deposition of immune complexes cause damage to tissues. Although the great majority of patients (90%) with SLE are women, men and children can be affected. SLE may involve any area of the central or peripheral nervous system as a solitary or multifocal process, with or without concurrent disease in other organs. Cerebral lesions may represent primary inflammation, resembling encephalitis of other etiologies, and/or ischemia or infarction due to SLE-associated vasculitis or coagulopathy.

As a result, SLE can present a wide variety of MR appearances. Scans in many patients with clinically definite disease are normal. In other cases, nonspecific atrophy is seen with or without a history of steroid treatment.

Case 481 illustrates multiple patchy areas of edema involving cortex, subcortical white matter, and deep nuclei. Although this combination of scattered superficial and deep lesions is nonspecific (compare to primary angiitis of the CNS in Cases 486 and 641), it is typical of an autoimmune disorder. Such lesions are often rapidly and completely reversible, with no clinical or MR residual.

Sjögren's syndrome is a chronic, slowly progressive autoimmune disorder, primarily affecting exocrine glands and typically presenting with xerostomia and dry eyes. CNS lesions are probably attributable to associated vasculitis.

Small areas of subcortical (arrow) and periventricular signal abnormality in Case 482 have an appearance intermediate between focal infarction and demyelinating plaques. This combined inflammatory/ischemic character is a common feature of large or small parenchymal lesions due to autoimmune disease and can suggest the diagnosis.

In a child such as Case 481, the pattern of multifocal, patchy, and partially reversible lesions could alternatively represent a mitochondrial encephalomyelopathy (see Case 510) or acute disseminated encephalomyelitis (see Cases 388-395).

Cases 483 and 485 present additional examples of cerebral involvement by systemic lupus erythematosus.

### Case 483

43-year-old woman presenting with aphasia.
(coronal, noncontrast T2-weighted SE scan)

### Case 484

36-year-old man presenting with increasing
confusion and seizures.
(coronal, noncontrast T2-weighted SE scan)

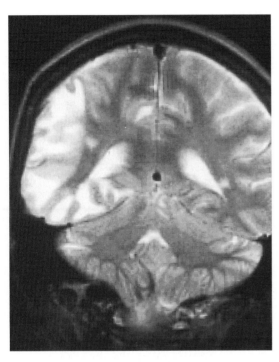

**Systemic Lupus Erythematosus**

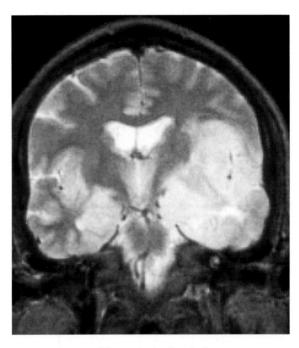

**Gliomatosis Cerebri**

Several pathologies can cause scattered areas of patchy signal abnormality affecting both cortex and subcortical tissue of the brain.

The extensive zone of superficial edema in Case 483 spans two major arterial distributions (the middle and posterior cerebral arteries) and demonstrates substantial sparing of cortex. These features argue against simple infarction. The geographic, nonvascular morphology of the edema and the association with smaller lesions elsewhere suggest the alternative possibility of an autoimmune disorder (or cerebritis of some other cause). The same pattern in a child would raise the question of a mitochondrial encephalomyopathy such as MELAS (see Case 510).

Case 484 demonstrates that infiltrating neoplasms can also cause multiple areas of extensive but poorly defined signal abnormality involving both superficial and deep regions of the cerebral hemispheres. This possibility should be considered along with inflammatory and metabolic disorders in the differential diagnosis of one or more large, patchy zones of prolonged T2 values crossing the boundaries of arterial distributions.

Vasculitis (e.g., primary angiitis of the CNS; see Cases 486 and 641) is also included among possible etiologies of multifocal cortical and subcortical edema, as is intravascular lymphomatosis or "angiocentric lymphoma."

# DIFFERENTIAL DIAGNOSIS:
## MULTIFOCAL CORTICAL AND SUBCORTICAL EDEMA WITH MENINGEAL ENHANCEMENT

### Case 485

28-year-old woman presenting with
left homonymous hemianopsia.
(axial, postcontrast T1-weighted SE scan)

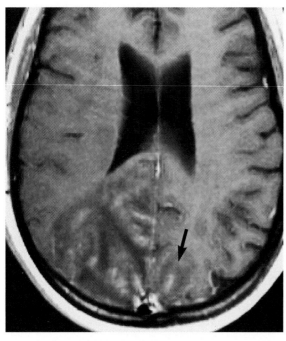

**Systemic Lupus Erythematosus**

### Case 486

74-year-old man presenting with rapidly
progressing motor and sensory deficits.
(axial, postcontrast T1-weighted SE scan)

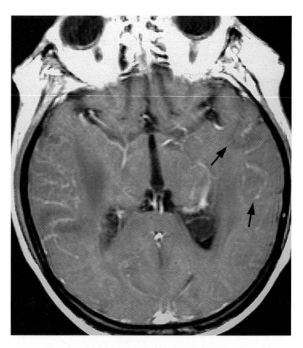

**Primary Angiitis of the CNS**
(Granulomatous Angiitis)

---

As discussed in Case 481, parenchymal lesions of systemic lupus erythematosus can take many forms. Case 485 demonstrates a large zone of cortical and subcortical edema in the right parieto-occipital region, extending laterally beyond the distribution of the posterior cerebral artery. Overlying leptomeningeal enhancement is present. A smaller lesion with similar character is noted at the left occipital pole *(arrow)*. Although nonspecific, this appearance is typical of acute lupus cerebritis. The patient's visual field deficit and the MR abnormalities resolved following treatment with steroids.

The scan in Case 486 presents similar zones of poorly defined superficial edema in association with increased meningeal enhancement. The right sylvian region is most prominently affected, with additional abnormality in the left temporal lobe *(arrows)*. T2-weighted scans confirmed multiple regions of predominantly subcortical edema (see Case 641). As in Case 485, the involved areas have features intermediate between infarction and inflammation.

In particular, the zones of prolonged T1 (and T2) values are less well defined than most simple infarcts and do not conform to the boundaries of major arterial distributions. This pattern, especially when multifocal, should suggest an inflammatory process, with autoimmune disease and acute vasculitis included in the differential diagnosis along with infectious possibilities (i.e., encephalitis). The diagnosis in Case 486 was established by biopsy.

Antiphospholipid antibodies are often present in patients with SLE, and infarcts due to coagulopathy can cause irreversible cerebral lesions in such cases.

A discussion of cerebral arteritis is presented in Cases 641-644.

## Case 487

67-year-old woman presenting with
decreased vision.
(coronal, postcontrast T1-weighted SE scan)

## Case 488

41-year-old woman presenting with
headaches and confusion.
(axial, postcontrast T1-weighted SE scan)

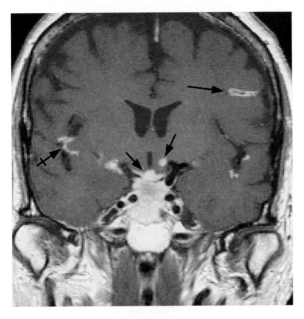

**Sarcoidosis**

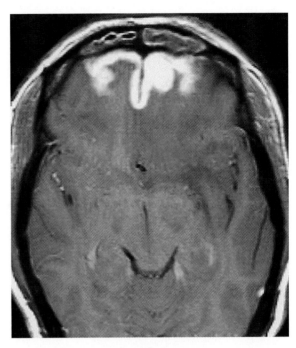

**Sarcoidosis**

Sarcoidosis is an idiopathic multisystem inflammatory disorder characterized by noncaseating granulomas in affected tissues. The disease may be acute or chronic, self-limited or recurrent and progressive. Sarcoidosis can involve the brain, meninges, spinal cord (see Cases 1142-1144), and cranial nerves (most often nerves II and VII).

Case 487 illustrates a combination of parenchymal and leptomeningeal disease. Small nodules of enhancement are present at the inferior margin of the hypothalamus *(short arrows)*. Sarcoidosis frequently involves the suprasellar region, thickening the pituitary infundibulum and deforming or surrounding the optic chiasm. This diagnosis should be considered (along with basal meningitis such as tuberculosis and syphilis) when a hypothalamic/infundibular mass is discovered in an adult. (Compare to the differential diagnosis of infundibular thickening in children discussed in Cases 272 and 273.)

Parenchymal involvement by sarcoidosis can alternatively take the form of small, deep hemispheric lesions resembling multiple sclerosis (see Case 496) or larger subcortical patches of abnormal signal and enhancement (see Case 489).

Scattered leptomeningeal enhancement is present within the sylvian cisterns *(crossed arrow)* and in cortical sulci *(long arrow)* in Case 487. Sarcoidosis is among the etiologies of localized or generalized meningitis and is often most apparent in the depths of sulci. Axial scans in Case 487 closely resembled the appearance of Case 429.

Another common presentation of sarcoidosis is uniform dural thickening, as illustrated anteriorly in Case 488. Extensive edema of underlying white matter is typical and is usually the cause of symptoms. Both the dural reaction and the frontal edema in this patient responded gradually to treatment with steroids but recurred when the medication was tapered.

Inflammatory changes in the frontal sinus in Case 488 were unrelated to the intracranial disease.

Meningovascular syphilis should be considered in the differential diagnosis of multifocal enhancing gyral and/or leptomeningeal lesions.

**299**

# DIFFERENTIAL DIAGNOSIS:
## MULTIPLE ENHANCING SUBCORTICAL LESIONS

### Case 489

63-year-old woman presenting with disorientation.
(axial, postcontrast T1-weighted SE scan)

### Case 490

36-year-old woman presenting with
rapidly progressive weakness and
numbness of all extremities.
(axial, postcontrast T1-weighted SE scan)

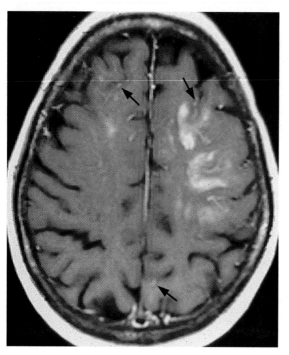

**Sarcoidosis**

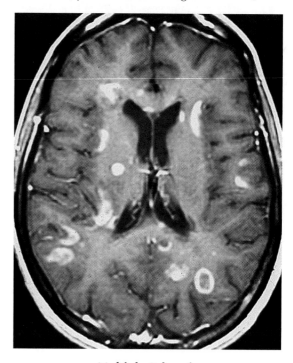

**Multiple Sclerosis**

In addition to hypothalamic/infundibular masses, sarcoidosis may cause lesions within the cerebral hemispheres. Small foci of prolonged T2 values in periventricular or subcortical white matter can closely resemble multiple sclerosis (see Case 496). Larger areas of patchy signal abnormality and contrast enhancement are occasionally encountered, as in Case 489.

Some of the enhancing subcortical lesions in Case 490 are solid and irregular, resembling the appearance of Case 489. Others are clearly ring-shaped, a morphology that would be very unusual in sarcoidosis but is a familiar feature of multiple sclerosis (see Cases 382 and 480). The

large number of actively inflamed sites in this case correlated with an acute exacerbation of the patient's known demyelinating disease.

A small amount of leptomeningeal enhancement accompanies the parenchymal lesions in Case 489 *(arrows)*. This feature is common in sarcoidosis but rare in multiple sclerosis and can help to distinguish between these disorders in otherwise ambiguous cases.

The differential diagnosis of multiple enhancing subcortical lesions also includes hematogenously distributed infection or metastases.

# DIFFERENTIAL DIAGNOSIS:
## FOCAL DURAL THICKENING

### Case 491

41-year-old woman presenting with
headaches and confusion.
(axial, postcontrast T1-weighted SE scan with MTS)

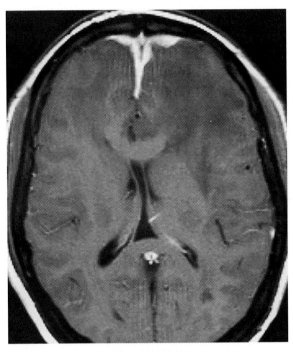

**Sarcoidosis**
(same patient as Case 488)

### Case 492

50-year-old woman presenting with
right-sided hearing loss.
(axial, postcontrast T1-weighted SE scan with MTS)

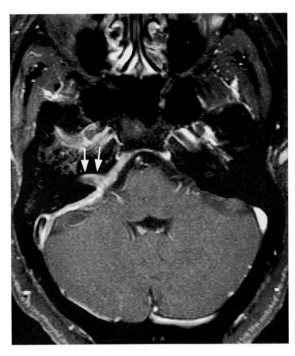

**Systemic Lymphoma**

---

Case 491 demonstrates the interhemispheric extension of the dural-based process presented in Case 488. Sarcoidosis is one of several possible inflammatory etiologies for pachymeningitis. Others include tuberculosis, syphilis, and fungal infections. Wegener granulomatosis and Langerhans cell histiocytosis can also present with focal or more generalized dural thickening.

Neoplastic infiltration should be considered in the differential diagnosis of plaque-like dural thickening. In Case 492, systemic lymphoma presented as hearing loss due to extension of dural-based disease into the internal auditory canal *(arrows)*. Dural infiltration by leukemia or dural metastases from solid tumors could cause similar findings. (Compare Case 492 to the similar presentation of metastatic breast carcinoma in Case 202.)

The prominent bifrontal edema in Case 491 is not specific and by itself could raise the question of cerebritis, autoimmune disorders (compare to Case 485), or arteritis (see Case 486). Contrast administration was essential to narrow the diagnosis.

Dural thickening due to sarcoidosis typically demonstrates low signal intensity on T2-weighted scans.

## Case 493

67-year-old woman presenting with headaches.
(axial, noncontrast FLAIR scan)

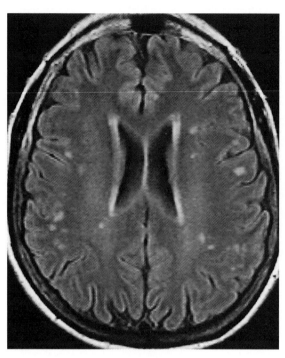

**Lyme Disease**

## Case 494

42-year-old man presenting with headaches,
leg paresthesias, and transient diplopia.
(axial, postcontrast T1-weighted SE scan)

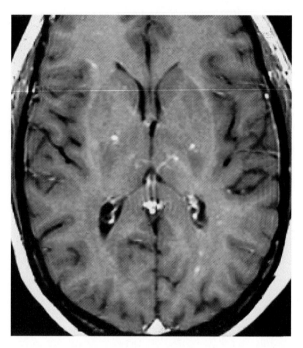

**Lyme Disease**

Lyme disease, due to infection by the spirochete *Borrelia burgdorferi,* is among the inflammatory disorders that have been associated with multiple small, subcortical lesions on MR studies. Case 493 illustrates a patient with clinically definite Lyme disease and no other known explanation for the foci of long T2 in subcortical white matter. However, as emphasized on the next page, this is a nonspecific appearance.

The multiple small enhancing foci in the white matter and basal ganglia of Case 494 are similarly nonspecific (compare to Cases 455 and 456). However, the clinical presentation and serology strongly supported the diagnosis of Lyme disease in this patient.

Other neurological presentations of Lyme disease include meningitis and cranial neuritis, especially optic neuritis and Bell's palsy. Postcontrast scans may demonstrate abnormal enhancement of meninges and/or involved nerves (see Case 497).

# DIFFERENTIAL DIAGNOSIS:
## SMALL FOCI OF SUBCORTICAL SIGNAL ABNORMALITY

### Case 495

53-year-old woman presenting with fatigue,
myalgias, and arm numbness.
(axial, noncontrast T2-weighted SE scan)

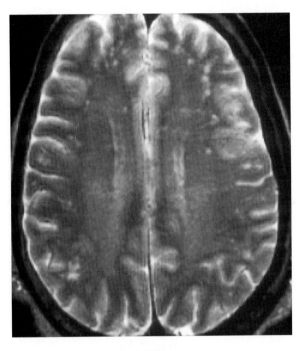

**Lyme Disease**

### Case 496

58-year-old woman presenting with
hilar adenopathy.
(axial, noncontrast T2-weighted SE scan)

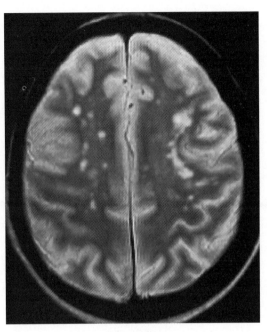

**Sarcoidosis**

A number of pathologies can involve subcortical white matter. Relatively large lesions in this location may be seen in progressive multifocal leukoencephalopathy, acute disseminated encephalomyelitis, multiple sclerosis, cerebral metastases, arterial or venous infarction, and tuberous sclerosis.

Smaller foci of subcortical signal abnormality may likewise arise in a variety of contexts. Case 495 is another example of miliary lesions within the white matter of a patient with clinically established Lyme disease.

Case 496 illustrates that parenchymal involvement by sarcoidosis can closely mimic multiple sclerosis. Foci of signal abnormality may be found in periventricular regions or in subcortical white matter. Localized contrast enhancement may occur.

Like sarcoidosis, systemic lupus erythematosus may involve subcortical white matter to cause patchy or punctate lesions, with or without contrast enhancement.

Another inflammatory disorder that may cause multiple small foci of signal abnormality is Behçet disease. This multisystem immune-mediated vasculitis presents clinically with the triad of oral and genital ulceration and ocular inflammation. Some of the cerebral lesions in such cases may demonstrate focal contrast enhancement.

Miliary subcortical metastases should also be considered in the differential diagnosis on this page. Postcontrast scans with high contrast dose and/or magnetization transfer suppression may demonstrate confirmatory enhancement. Many focal, subcortical metastases do not significantly prolong T2 values and are poorly seen on noncontrast images.

Shearing injuries (diffuse axonal injury) can present as multiple subcortical foci of high signal intensity on T2-weighted images (see Case 695). Multifocal infarction should also be included among diagnostic possibilities (see Cases 602, 606, and 696).

**Case 497**

33-year-old woman presenting with
bilateral facial pain.
(coronal, postcontrast T1-weighted SE scan)

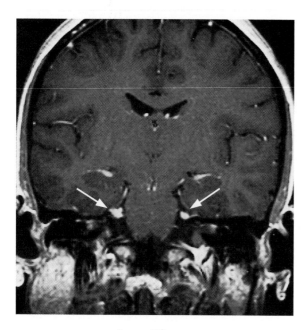

**Lyme Disease**

**Case 498**

40-year-old man presenting with
left peripheral facial palsy.
(axial, postcontrast T1-weighted SE scan
with fat saturation)

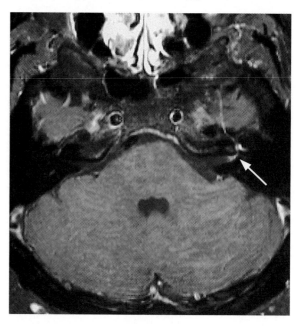

**Bell's Palsy**

Inflammation of a cranial nerve may cause both clinical dysfunction and abnormal enhancement. Lyme disease and sarcoidosis are among the well-recognized etiologies of cranial neuritis, most commonly affecting the optic or facial nerves. Many other agents can cause inflammation of cranial nerves, and any nerve can be involved.

Case 497 illustrates intense, bilateral enhancement of the trigeminal nerves *(arrows)* due to Lyme disease. The appearance is similar to that of meningeal tumor coating the fifth nerves in Case 206. Together, these cases demonstrate that both inflammatory and neoplastic conditions of either the nerve or the meninges must be considered in the differential diagnosis of enhancing cranial neuropathy.

A small amount of enhancement is also seen at the medial margin of the cerebral peduncles and in the lateral portion of the internal auditory canals bilaterally in Case 497, reflecting concomitant neuritis of the oculomotor and facial nerves.

Bell's palsy has long been categorized as an idiopathic inflammation of the facial nerve, but there is increasing evidence to implicate infection by a herpes virus. Imaging is performed to exclude other potential etiologies for facial paresis, including schwannomas or hemangiomas of the fa-

cial nerve, destructive lesions of the petrous bone (e.g., cholesteatoma or metastasis), or retrograde perineural extension of extracranial tumor (e.g., adenoid cystic carcinoma).

Mild contrast enhancement can normally be seen on MR scans along the geniculate, tympanic, and descending portions of the facial nerve canal, probably reflecting the vascular epineurium in these locations. However, asymmetrically intense enhancement of the fundal, labyrinthine, and geniculate segments of the nerve, as seen in Case 498 *(arrow)*, is abnormal and compatible with the diagnosis of neuritis. The lack of expansion of the enhancing segments argues against the alternative possibilities of schwannoma or hemangioma. Perineural spread of tumor along the facial nerve remains as a possible consideration.

Other inflammatory causes of enhancement and dysfunction of the facial nerve include herpes zoster (Ramsey-Hunt syndrome), Lyme disease, sarcoidosis, and syphilis.

Bell's palsy is usually unilateral. Symptoms typically develop acutely and resolve in two to three months. A different time course of onset or resolution raises the suspicion of an alternative diagnosis.

## Case 499

30-year-old woman presenting with
rapidly progressive visual loss.
(axial, postcontrast T1-weighted SE scan with MTS)

## Case 500

75-year-old woman presenting with
decreased visual acuity.
(coronal, postcontrast T1-weighted SE scan)

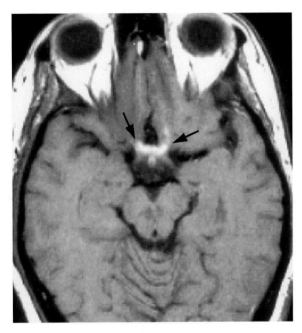

**Optic Neuritis**
(due to multiple sclerosis)

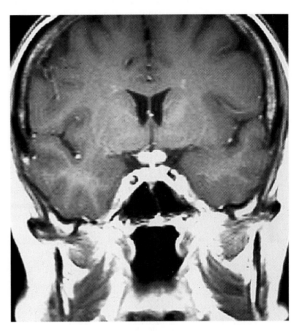

**Glioblastoma**
(of the optic chiasm)

---

The optic nerves and chiasm normally demonstrate little or no enhancement on postcontrast images. The presence of enhancement is nonspecific and may reflect inflammatory, neoplastic, or vascular processes.

Multiple sclerosis is the most common cause of optic neuritis. Optic nerve involvement may precede, accompany, or follow cerebral or spinal symptoms. Inflammation may be unilateral or bilateral, affecting nerve and/or chiasm. Examination of the accompanying cerebral scan for evidence of demyelinating disease is warranted in patients with clinical optic neuritis, whether or not nerve lesions are apparent on MR images.

Case 499 demonstrates intense enhancement of the chiasm and the posterior portion of the optic nerves. As with parenchymal plaques, the intensity of enhancement in optic neuritis varies with the stage of demyelination and associated inflammation. Coronal postcontrast scans with fat saturation are useful for detecting subtle enhancement of the optic nerves and/or chiasm.

Gliomas involving the optic chiasm and hypothalamus are among the suprasellar masses encountered in children

(see Cases 262-268). Optic gliomas are much less common in adults, and malignant gliomas, as in Case 500, are rare. The chiasm in this case is expanded but retains its characteristic bi-lobed or dumbbell morphology. Intense enhancement extended anteriorly into the optic nerves bilaterally. CSF dissemination was present at the time of diagnosis, with several small enhancing meningeal lesions.

Other potential etiologies of optic neuritis include sarcoidosis, Lyme disease, and acute disseminated encephalomyelitis. Vasculitis due to systemic lupus erythematosus, syphilis, rheumatoid arthritis, or Sjögren's syndrome can also present as optic neuritis. Rapidly progressive optic neuritis may develop after radiation of a suprasellar or anterior temporal neoplasm (with a latency period of six months to three years). Many cases of optic neuritis are idiopathic.

The optic chiasm is an occasional site of cavernous hemangiomas and craniopharyngiomas, which should be included in the differential diagnosis of an enhancing chiasmal mass.

# REFERENCES

Aisen AM, Gabrielsen TO, McCune WJ: MR imaging of systemic lupus erythematosus involving the brain. *AJNR* 6:197-202, 1985.

Aladro Y, Ponce P, Santullano V, et al: Cerebritis due to Listeria monocytogenes: CT and MR findings. *Eur Radiol* 6:188-191, 1996.

Ashdown BC, Tien RD, Felsberg GJ: Aspergillosis of the brain and paranasal sinuses in immunocompromised patients: CT and MR imaging findings. *Am J Roentgenol* 162:155-159, 1994.

Baganz MD, Dross PE, Reinhardt JA: Rocky Mountain spotted fever encephalitis: MR findings. *AJNR* 16:919-920, 1995.

Balakrishnan J, Becker PS, Kumur AJ, et al: Acquired immunodeficiency syndrome: correlation of radiologic and pathologic findings in the brain. *Radiographics* 10:201-215, 1990.

Bale JF, Anderson RD, Grose C: Magnetic resonance imaging of the brain in childhood herpesvirus infections. *Pediatr Infect Dis J* 6:644-647, 1987.

Bargallo N, Berenguer J, Tomas X, et al: Intracranial tuberculosis: CT and MRI. *Eur J Radiol* 3:123-128, 1993.

Barkovich AJ, Lindan CE: Congenital cytomegalovirus infection of the brain: imaging analysis and embryologic considerations. *AJNR* 15:703-715, 1994.

Barloon TJ, Yuh WTC, Knepper LE, et al: Cerebral ventriculitis: MR findings. *J Comput Assist Tomogr* 14:272-275, 1990.

Bash S, Hathout GM, Cohen S: Mesiotemporal T2-weighted hyperintensity: neurosyphilis mimicking herpes encephalitis. *AJNR* 22:314-316, 2001.

Bazan C III, Rinaldi MG, Rauch RR, Jinkins JR: Fungal infections of the brain. *Neuroimaging Clin N Amer* 1:57-88, 1991.

Becker LE: Infections of the developing brain. *AJNR* 13:537-549, 1992.

Bell CL, Partington C, Robbins M, et al: Magnetic resonance imaging of central nervous system lesions in patients with lupus erythematosus. *Arthritis Rheum* 34:437-441, 1991.

Berkefeld J, Enzensberger W, Lanfermann H: Cryptococcus meningoencephalitis in AIDS: parenchymal and meningeal forms. *Neuroradiology* 41:129-133, 1999.

Boesch C, Issakainen J, Kewitz G, et al: Magnetic resonance imaging of the brain in congenital cytomegalovirus infection. *Pediatr Radiol* 19:91-93, 1989.

Brightbill TC, Ihmeidan IH, Post MJD, et al: Neurosyphilis in HIV-positive and HIV-negative patients: neuroimaging findings. *AJNR* 16:703-711, 1995.

Brismar J, Gascon GG, von Steyern KV, Bohlega S: Subacute sclerosing panencephalitis: evaluation with CT and MR. *AJNR* 17:761-772, 1996.

Brodsky MC, Beck RW: The changing role of MR imaging in the evaluation of acute optic neuritis. *Radiology* 192:22-23, 1994.

Burke JW, Mathews VP, Elster AD, et al: Contrast-enhanced magnetization transfer saturation imaging improves MR detection of herpes simplex encephalitis. *AJNR* 17:773-776, 1996.

Burke JW, Podrasky AE, Bradley WG Jr: Meninges: benign postoperative enhancement on MR images. *Radiology* 174:99, 1990.

Burtscher IM, Holtas S: In vivo proton MR spectroscopy of untreated and treated brain abscesses. *AJNR* 20:1049-1053, 1999.

Caldemeyer KS, Mathews VP, Edwards-Brown MK, Smith RR: Central nervous system cryptococcosis: parenchymal calcification and large gelatinous pseudocysts. *AJNR* 18:107-110, 1997.

Callebaut J, Dormant D, Dubois B, et al: Contrast-enhanced MR imaging of tuberculous pachymeningitis cranialis hypertrophica: case report. *AJNR* 11:821-822, 1990.

Carmody RF, Mafee MF, Goodwin JA, et al: Orbital and optic pathway sarcoidosis: MR findings. *AJNR* 15:775-783, 1994.

Castillo M: Imaging brain abscesses with diffusion-weighted and other sequences. *AJNR* 20:1193-1194, 1999.

Castillo M: Magnetic resonance imaging of meningitis and its complications. *Topics Magn Res Imag* 6:53-58, 1994.

Castillo M, Salgado P, Rojas R, et al: Unusual imaging manifestations of neurocysticercosis. *Int J Neurorad* 2:168-175, 1996.

Cerna F, Mehrad B, Luby JP, et al: St. Louis encephalitis and the substantia nigra: MR imaging evaluation. *AJNR* 20:1281-1283, 1999.

Chamberlain MC, Nichols SL, Chase CH: Pediatric AIDS: comparative cranial MRI and CT scans. *Pediatr Neurol* 7:357-362, 1992.

Chanalet S, Gense de Beaufort D, Greselle JF, et al: Clinical and radiological aspects of extracerebral empyemas: 39 cases. *Neuroradiology* 33 (suppl):225-228, 1991.

Chang KH, Cho SY, Hesselink JR, et al: Parasitic diseases of the central nervous system. *Neuroimaging Clin N Amer* 1:159-178, 1991.

Chang K-H, Han M-H, Roh J-K, et al: Gd-DTPA-enhanced MR imaging in intracranial tuberculosis. *Neuroradiology* 238:340-344, 1991.

Chang KH, Han MH, Roh JK, et al: Gd-DTPA-enhanced MR imaging of the brain in patients with meningitis: comparison with CT. *AJNR* 11:69-76, 1990.

Chang KH, Lee JH, Han MH, Han MC: The role of contrast-enhanced MR imaging in the diagnosis of neurocysticerosis. *AJNR* 12:509-512, 1991.

Chang L, Cornford ME, Chiang FL, et al: Radiologic-pathologic correlation. Cerebral toxoplasmosis and lymphoma in AIDS. *AJNR* 16:1653-1664, 1995.

Chapelon C, Zisa JM, Piette JC, et al: Neurosarcoidosis: signs, course and treatment in 35 confirmed cases. *Radiology* 179:887, 1991.

Cheng PW, Ho SL, Chan FL, Leong L: Abscess: real or mimic? *Int J Neurorad* 3:18-20, 1997.

Cho IC, Chang KH, Kim YH, et al: MRI features of choroid plexitis. *Neuroradiology* 40:303-307, 1998.

Christoforidis GA, Spickler EM, Recio MV, Mehta BM: MR of CNS sarcoidosis: correlation of imaging features to clinical symptoms and response to treatment. *AJNR* 20:655-669, 1999.

Cohen WA, Maravilla KR, Gerlach R, et al: Prospective cerebral MR study of HIV seropositive and seronegative men: correlation of MR findings with neurologic, neuropsychologic, and cerebrospinal fluid analysis. *AJNR* 13:1231-1240, 1992.

Cooper SD, Brady MB, Williams JP, et al: Neurosarcoidosis: evaluation using CT and MRI. *J Comput Assist Tomogr* 12:96-99, 1988.

Cox J, Murtagh FR, Wilfong A, Brenner J: Cerebral aspergillosis: MR imaging and histopathologic correlation. *AJNR* 13:1489-1492, 1992.

Creasy JL, Alarcon JJ: Magnetic resonance imaging of neurocysticercosis. *Topics Mag Res Imag* 6:59-68, 1994.

Davenport C, Dillon WP, Sze G: Neuroradiology of the immunosuppressed state. *Radiol Clin North Am* 30:611-638, 1992.

Davidson HD, Steiner RE: Magnetic resonance imaging of infections of the central nervous system. *AJNR* 6:499-504, 1985.

De Castro CC, Hesselink JR: Tuberculosis. *Neuroimaging Clin North Amer* 1:119-139, 1991.

Deliganis AV, Fisher DJ, Lam AM, Maravilla KR: Cerebrospinal fluid signal intensity increase on FLAIR MR images in patients under general anesthesia: the role of supplemental $O_2$. *Radiology* 218:152-156, 2001.

Del Brulto OH, Zenbeno MA, Salgado P, et al: MR imaging of cysticercotic encephalitis. *AJNR* 10:518, 1989.

DeLone DR, Goldstein RA, Petermann G, et al: Disseminated aspergillosis involving the brain: distribution and imaging characteristics. *AJNR* 20:1597-1604, 1999.

Demaerel Ph, Wilms G, Robberecht W, et al: MRI of herpes simplex encephalitis. *Neuroradiology* 34:490-493, 1992.

Demaerel P, Wilms G, Van Lierde S, et al: Lyme disease in childhood presenting as primary leptomeningeal enhancement without parenchymal findings on MR. *AJNR* 15:302-304, 1994.

Desprechins B, Stadnik T, Koerts G, et al: Use of diffusion-weighted MR imaging in differential diagnosis between intracerebral necrotic tumors and cerebral abscesses. *AJNR* 20:1252-1258, 1999.

Dumas J-L, Valeyre D, Chapelon-Abric C, et al: Central nervous system sarcoidosis: follow-up at MR imaging during steroid therapy. *Radiology* 214:411-420, 2000.

Dumas JL, Visy JM, Belin C, et al: Parenchymal neurocysticercosis: follow-up and staging by MRI. *Neuroradiology* 39:12-18, 1997.

Enzmann D, Chang Y, Augustyn G: MR findings in neonatal herpes simplex encephalitis type II. *J Comput Assist Tomogr* 14:453-457, 1990.

Erly WK, Bellon RJ, Seeger JF, Carmody RF: MR imaging of acute coccidioidal meningitis. *AJNR* 20:509-514, 1999.

Ernst T, Chang L, Witt M, et al: Progressive multifocal leukoencephalopathy and human immunodeficiency virus-associated white matter lesions in AIDS: magnetization transfer MR imaging. *Radiology* 210:539-544, 1999.

Falcone S, Post MJD: Encephalitis, cerebritis, and brain abscess: pathophysiology and imaging findings. *Neuroimaging Clin North Am* 10:333-354, 2000.

Fernandez RE, Rothberg M, Ferencz G, et al: Lyme disease of the CNS: MR imaging findings in 14 cases. *AJNR* 11:479-481, 1990.

Filippi CG, Ulug AM, Lin D, et al: Hyperintense signal abnormality in subarachnoid spaces and basal cisterns of children anesthetized with propofol: new fluid-attenuated inversion recovery findings. *AJNR* 22:394-399, 2001.

Fitz CR: Inflammatory diseases of the brain in childhood. *AJNR* 13:551-567, 1992.

Flowers CH, Mafee MF, Crowell R, et al: Encephalopathy in AIDS patients: evaluation with MR imaging. *AJNR* 11:1235-1245, 1990.

Friedman D, Flanders A, Tartaglino L: Contrast-enhanced MR imaging of idiopathic hypertrophic craniospinal pachymeningitis. *Am J Roentgenol* 160:900-901, 1993.

Friedman SD, Stidley CA, Brooks WM, et al: Brain injury and neurometabolic abnormalities in systemic lupus erythematosus. *Radiology* 209:79-84, 1998.

Gee GT, Bazan C III, Jinks JR: Miliary tuberculosis involving the brain: MR findings. *Am J Roentgenol* 159:1075-1076, 1992.

Georgy BA, Snow RD, Brogdon BG, Wertelecki W: Neuroradiologic findings in Marinesco Sjögren syndrome. *AJNR* 19:281-283, 1998.

Ginier BL, Porier VC: MR imaging of intraventricular cysticercosis. *AJNR* 13:1247-1248, 1992.

Go JL, Kim PE, Ahmadi J, et al: Fungal infections of the central nervous system. *Neuroimaging Clin North Am* 210:409-426, 2000.

Govindappa SS, Narayanan JP, Krishnamoorthy VM, et al: Improved detection of intraventricular cysticercal cysts with the use of three-dimensional constructive interference in steady state MR sequences. *AJNR* 21:679-684, 2000.

Goyal M, Malik A, Mishra NK, Gaikwad SB: Idiopathic hypertrophic pachymeningitis: spectrum of the disease. *Neuroradiology* 39:619-623, 1997.

Goyal M, Sharma A, Mishra NK, et al: Imaging appearance of pachymeningeal tuberculosis. *Am J Roentgenol* 169:1421-1424, 1997.

Grafe MR, Press GA, Berthofy DP, et al: Abnormality of the brain in AIDS patients: correlation of postmortem MR findings with neuropathology. *AJNR* 11:905-911, 1990.

Grand S, Passaro G, Ziegler A, et al: Necrotic tumor versus brain abscess: importance of amino acids detected at 1H spectroscopy—initial results. *Radiology* 213:785-793, 1999.

Greco A, Steiner R: Magnetic resonance imaging in neurosarcoidosis. *Magn Reson Imaging* 5:15-21, 1987.

Gupta RK, Gupta S, Singh D, et al: MR imaging and angiography in tuberculous meningitis. *Neuroradiology* 38:87-92, 1994.

Gupta RK, Jena A, Sharma A: MR imaging of intracranial tuberculomas. *J Comput Assist Tomogr* 12:280-285, 1988.

Gupta RK, Kohli A, Gaur V, et al: MRI of the brain in patients with miliary pulmonary tuberculosis without symptoms or signs of central nervous system involvement. *Neuroradiology* 39:699-704, 1997.

Haimes AB, Zimmerman RD, Morgello S, et al: MR imaging of brain abscesses. *AJNR* 10:279-291, 1989.

Harris DE, Enterline DS: Fungal infections of the central nervous system. *Neuroimaging Clin North Am* 7:187-198, 1997.

Harris DE, Enterliine DS, Tien RD: Neurosyphilis in patients with AIDS. *Neuroimaging Clin North Am* 7:215-221, 1997.

Harris TM, Edwards MK: Meningitis. *Neuroimaging Clin N Amer* 1:39-56, 1991.

Hatta S, Mochizuki H, Kuru Y, et al: Serial neuroradiological studies in focal cerebritis. *Neuroradiology* 36:285-288, 1994.

Hawkins CP, McLaughlin JE, Kendall BE, McDonald WI: Pathological findings correlated with MRI in HIV infection. *Neuroradiology* 35:264-268, 1993.

Hayes WS, Sherman JL, Stern BJ, et al: MR and CT evaluation of intracranial sarcoidosis. *AJNR* 8:841-848, 1987.

Holland BA, Perrett LV, Mills CM: Meningovascular syphillis: CT and MR findings. *Radiology* 158:439-442, 1986.

Jackson A, Sheppard S, Laitt RD, et al: Optic neuritis: MR imaging with combined fat- and water-suppression techniques. *Radiology* 206:57-64, 1998.

Jarvik JG, Hesselink JR, Kennedy C, et al: Acquired immunodeficiency syndrome: magnetic resonance patterns of brain involvement with pathologic correlation. *Arch Neurol* 45:731-736, 1988.

Jensen MC, Brant-Zawadzki M: MR imaging of the brain in patients with AIDS: value of routine use of IV gadopentetate dimeglumine. *Am J Roentgenol* 160:153-157, 1993.

Jinkins JR, Gupta R, Chang KH, Rodriguez-Carbajal J: MR imaging of central nervous system tuberculosis. *Radiol Clin North Am* 33:771-786, 1995.

Jordan J, Enzmann DR: Encephalitis. *Neuroimaging Clin N Amer* 1:17-38, 1991.

Kanamalla US, Ibarra RA, Jinkins JR: Imaging of cranial meningitis and ventriculitis. *Neuroimaging Clin North Am* 10:309-332, 2000.

Kaufman WM, Sivit CJ, Fitz CR, et al: CT and MR evaluation of intracranial involvement in pediatric HIV infection: a clinical-imaging correlation. *AJNR* 13:949-957, 1992.

Ketonen L, Oksanen U, Kuuliala I: Preliminary experience of magnetic resonance imaging in neurosarcoidosis. *Neuroradiology* 29:127-129, 1987.

Kieburtz KD, Ketonen L, Zettelmaier AE, et al: Magnetic resonance imaging findings in HIV cognitive impairment. *Arch Neurol* 47:643-645, 1990.

Kim SH, Chang KH, Song IC, et al: Brain abscess and brain tumor: discrimination with in vivo H-1 MR spectroscopy. *Radiology* 204:239-245, 1997.

Kim TK, Chang KH, Kim CJ, et al: Intracranial tuberculoma: comparison of MR with pathologic findings. *AJNR* 16:1903-1908, 1995.

Kim YJ, Chang K-H, Song IC, et al: Brain abscess and necrotic or cystic brain tumor: discrimination with signal intensity on diffusion-weighted MR imaging. *Am J Roentgenol* 171:1487-1490, 1998.

Kocer N, Islak C, Siva A, et al: CNS involvement in Neuro-Behçet syndrome: an MR study. *AJNR* 20:1015-1024, 1999.

Kodama T, Numagredri Y, Gella FE, et al: Magnetic resonance imaging of limbic encephalitis. *Neuroradiology* 33:520-523, 1991.

Koelfen W, Freund M, Guckel F, et al: MRI of encephalitis in children: comparison of CT and MRI in the acute stage with long-term follow-up. *Neuroradiology* 38:73-79, 1996.

Kornbluth CM, Destian S: Imaging of rickettsial, spirochetal, and parasitic infections. *Neuroimaging Clin North Am* 10:375-390, 2000.

Kumar S, Misra UK, Kalita J, et al: MRI in Japanese encephalitis. *Neuroradiology* 39:180-184, 1997.

Kupfer M, Zee CS, Colleti PM, et al: MRI evaluation of AIDS-related encephalopathy: toxoplasmoisis vs lymphoma. *Magn Reson Imaging* 8:51-57, 1990.

Lacomis D, Koshbin S, Schick RM: MR imaging of paraneoplastic limbic encephalitis. *J Comput Assist Tomogr* 14:155-117, 1990.

Lai P-H, Lin S-M, Pan H-B, Yang C-F: Disseminated miliary cerebral candidiasis. *AJNR* 18:1303-1306, 1997.

Leonard JR, Moran CJ, Cross DT III, et al: MR imaging of herpes simplex type I encephalitis in infants and young children: a separate pattern of findings. *Am J Roentgenol* 174:1651-1656, 2000.

Lester JW, Carter MP, Reynolds TL: Herpes encephalitis: MR monitoring of response to acyclovir therapy. *J Comput Assist Tomogr* 12:941-943, 1988.

Lexa FJ, Grossman RI: MR of sarcoidosis of the head and spine: spectrum of manifestations and radiographic response to steroid therapy. *AJNR* 15:973-982, 1994.

Liem MD, Gzesh DJ, Flanders AE: MRI and angiographic diagnosis of lupus cerebral vasculitis. *Neuroradiology* 38:134-136, 1996.

Lim CCT, Sitoh YY, Hui F, et al: Nipah viral encephalitis or Japanese encephalitis? MR findings in a new zoonotic disease. *AJNR* 21:455-461, 2000.

Lim, MK, Suh CH, Kim JH, et al: Systemic lupus erythematosus: brain MR imaging and single-voxel hydrogen 1 MR spectroscopy. *Radiology* 217:43-49, 2000.

Lizerbram EK, Hesselink JR: Viral infections. *Neuroimaging Clin North Am* 7:261-280, 1997.

Lotz J, Hewlett R, Alheit B, Bowen R: Neuroysticercosis: correlative pathomorphology and MR imaging: *Neuroradiology* 30:35-41, 1988.

Mamelak AN, Kelly WM, Davis RL, Rosenblum ML: Idiopathic hypertrophic cranial pachymeningitis. *J Neurosurg* 79:270-276, 1993.

Martinez HR, Rangel-Guerra R, Elizondo G, et al: MR imaging in neurocysticercosis: a study of 56 cases. *AJNR* 10:1011-1019, 1989.

Mathews VP, Alo PL, Glass JD, et al: AIDS-related CNS cryptococcosis: radiologic-pathologic correlation. *AJNR* 13:1477-1486, 1992.

Mathews VP, Smith RR, Bognanno JR, et al: Gd-DTPA-enhanced MR of meningitis: initial clinical experience. *AJNR* 10:1290, 1989.

Meltzer CC, Fukui MB, Kanal E, Smirniotopoulos JG: MR imaging of the meninges. Part I. Normal anatomic features and non-neoplastic disease. *Radiology* 201:297-308, 1996.

Miller DH, Kendall BE, Barter S, et al: MRI in central nervous system sarcoidosis. *Neurology* 38:378-383, 1988.

Miller RF, Lucas SB, Hall-Craggs MA, et al: Comparison of magnetic resonance imaging with neuropathological findings in the diagnosis of HIV and CMV associated CNS disease in AIDS. *J Neurol Neurosurg Psych* 62:346-351, 1997.

Murphy JM, Gomez-Anson B, Gillard JH, et al: Wegener granulomatosis: MR imaging findings in brain and meninges. *Radiology* 213:794-799, 1999.

Neils EW, Lukin R, Romsick TA, Tew JM: Magnetic resonance imaging and computerized tomography scanning of herpes simplex encephalitis: report of two cases. *J Neurosurg* 67:592-594, 1987.

Noguchi K, Watanabe N, Nagayoshi T, et al: Role of diffusion-weighed echo-planar MRI in distinguishing between brain abscess and tumour: a preliminary report. *Neuroradiology* 41:171-174, 1999.

Noujaim SE, Rossi MD, Rao SK, et al: CT and MR imaging of neurocysticercosis. *Am J Roentgenol* 173:1485-1490, 1999.

Offenbacher H, Fazekas F, Schmidt R, et al: MRI in tuberculous meningoencephalitis: report of four cases and review of the neuroimaging literature. *J Neurol* 238:340-344, 1991.

Osborn RE, Byrd SE: Congenital infections of the brain. *Neuroimaging Clin N Amer* 1:105-118, 1991.

Park S-W, Chang K-H, Cho SY, et al: Long-term follow-up of neurocysticercosis: changes in computed tomographic and magnetic resonance imaging findings compared with results of enzyme-linked immunosorbent assay. *Int J Neurorad* 4:425-430, 1998.

Post MJD: Fluid-attenuated fast spin-echo MR: a clinically useful tool in the evaluation of neurologically symptomatic HIV-positive patients. *AJNR* 18:1611-1616, 1997.

Post MJD: Neuroimaging in various stages of human immunodeficiency virus infections. *Curr Opin Radiol* 2:73-79, 1990.

Post MJD, Berger JR, Duncan R, et al: Asymptomatic and neurologically symptomatic HIV-seropositive subjects: results of long-term MR imaging and clinical follow-up. *Radiology* 188:727-733, 1993.

Post MJD, Berger JR, Quencer HM: Asymptomatic and neurologically symptomatic HIV-seropositive individuals: prospective evaluation with cranial MR imaging. *Radiology* 178:131-139, 1991.

Post MJD, Levin BE, Berger JR, et al: Sequential cranial MR findings of asymptomatic and neurologically symptomatic HIV + subjects. *AJNR* 13:359-370, 1992.

Post MJD, Tate LG, Quencer RM, et al: CT, MR and pathology in HIV encephalitis and meningitis. *AJNR* 9:469-476, 1988.

Press GA, Weindling SM, Hesselink JR, et al: Rhinocerebral mucormycosis: MR manifestations. *J Comput Assist Tomogr* 12:744-749, 1988.

Provenzale JM, Allen NB: Wegener Granulomatosis: CT and MR findings. *AJNR* 17:785-792, 1996.

Provenzale JM, Jinkins JR: Brain and spine imaging findings in AIDS patients. *Radiol Clin North Am* 35:1127-1166, 1997.

Rafto SE, Milton WJ, Galetta SL, et al: Biopsy-confirmed CNS Lyme disease: MR appearance at 1.5 T. *AJNR* 11:482-484.

Rajshekhar V, Haran RP, Prakash S, Chandy MJ: Differentiating solitary small cysticercus granulomas and tuberculomas in patients with epilepsy. *J Neurosurg* 78:402-406, 1993.

Ramsey RG, Gean AD: Neuroimaging of AIDS; I: central nervous system toxoplasmosis. *Neuroimaging Clin North Am* 7:171-185, 1997.

Ramsey RG, Geremia GK, CNS complications of AIDS: CT and MR findings. *Am J Roentgenol* 151:449-454, 1988.

Ressler JA, Nelson M: Central nervous system infections in the pediatric population. *Neuroimaging Clin North Am* 210:427-444, 2000.

Rhee RS, Kumasaki DY, Sarwar M, et al: MR imaging of intraventricular cysticercosis. *J Comput Assist Tomogr* 11:598, 1987.

Riccio TJ, Hesselink JR: Gd-DTPA-enhanced MR of multiple cryptococcal brain abscesses. *AJNR* 10:565-566, 1989.

Rosenblum JD, Kim T, Ramsey RG: Neuroradiologic evaluation of complications of AIDS: a review. *Postgrad Radiol* 10:245-262, 1990.

Rovira MJ, Post MJD, Bowen BC: Central nervous system infections in HIV-infected persons. *Neuroimaging Clin N Amer* 1:179-200, 1991.

Runge VM, Wells JW, Williams NM, et al: Detectability of early brain meningitis with magnetic resonance imaging. *Invest Radiol* 30:484-489, 1995.

Sartoretti-Schefer S, Kollias S, Valavanis A: Ramsay Hunt syndrome associated with brain stem enhancement. *AJNR* 20:278-280, 1999.

Sartoretti-Schefer S, Kollias S, Wichmann W, Valavanis A: T2-weighted three-dimensional fast spin-echo MR in inflammatory peripheral facial nerve palsy. *AJNR* 19:491-495, 1998.

Sartoretti-Schefer S, Wichman W, Valvanis A: Idiopathic, herpetic, and HIV-associated facial nerve palsies: abnormal MR enhancement patterns. *AJNR* 15: 479-485, 1994.

Sartoretti-Schefer S, Wichmann W, Valavanis A: Optic neuritis: characteristic magnetic resonance imaging features and differential diagnosis. *Int J Neurorad* 3:417-427, 1997.

Schnider P, Trattnig S, Kollegger H, Auff E: MR of cerebral Whipple disease. *AJNR* 16:1328-1330, 1995.

Schoeman J, Hewlett R, Donald P: MR of childhood tuberculous meningitis. *Neuroradiology* 30:473, 1988.

Schroth G, Gawehn J, Thron A, et al: Early diagnosis of herpes simplex encephalitis by MRI. *Neurology* 37:179-183, 1987.

Schroth G, Kretzschmar K, Gawehn J, Voight K: Advantages of magnetic resonance imaging in the diagnosis of cerebral infections. *Neuroradiology* 29:120-126, 1987.

Schumacher DJ, Tien RD, Lane K: Neuroimaging findings in rare amebic infections of the central nervous system. *AJNR* 16:930-935, 1995.

Seltzer S, Mark AS, Atlas SW: CNS sarcoidosis: evaluation with contrast-enhanced MR imaging. *AJNR* 12:1227-1233, 1991.

Shah GV: Central nervous system tuberculosis: imaging manifestations. *Neuroimaging Clin North Am* 10:355-374, 2000.

Shaw DWW, Cohen WA: Viral infections of the CNS in children: imaging features. *Am J Roentgenol* 160:125-133, 1993.

Shen W-C, Cheng T-Y, Lee S-K, et al: Disseminated tuberculoms in spinal cord and brain demonstrated by MRI with gadolinium-DTPA. *Neuroradiology* 35:213-215, 1993.

Shen W-C, Chiu H-H, Chow K-C, Tsai C-H: MR imaging findings in enteroviral encephalomyelitis: an outbreak in Taiwan. *AJNR* 20:1889-1895, 1999.

Sherman JL, Stern BJ: Sarcoidosis of the CNS: comparison of unenhanced and enhanced MR images. *AJNR* 11:915-923, 1990.

Sheth TN, Pilon L, Keystone J, Kucharczyk W: Persistent MR contrast enhancement of calcified neurocysticercosis lesions. *AJNR* 19:79-82, 1998.

Singer MB, Atlas SW, Drayer BP: Subarachnoid space disease: diagnosis with fluid-attenuated inversion-recovery MR imaging and comparison with gadolinium-enhanced spin-echo MR imaging-blinded reader study. *Radiology* 208:417-422, 1998.

Smith AS, Meisler DM, Tomsak RL, et al: High signal periventricular lesions in patients with sarcoidosis: neurosarcoidosis or multiple sclerosis? *AJNR* 10:898-891, 1989.

Smith MM, Anderson JC: Neurosyphilis as a cause of facial and vestibulocochlear nerve dysfunction: MR imaging features. *AJNR* 21:1673-1675, 2000.

States, IJ, Rutstein RM, Zimmerman RA, Vezina LG: Imaging of pediatric central nervous system HIV infection. *Int J Neurorad* 3:42-56, 1997.

Sugita K, Ando M, Makino M, et al: Magnetic resonance imaging of the brain in congenital rubella virus and cytomegalovirus infections. *Neurorad* 33:239-242, 1991.

Suss RA, Maravilla KR, Thompson J: MR imaging of intracranial cysticercosis: comparison with CT and anatomopathologic features. *AJNR* 7:235-242, 1986.

Sze G: Diseases of the intracranial meninges: MR imaging features. *Am J Roentgenal* 160:727-733, 1993.

Sze G, Brant-Zawadzki M, Norman D, Newton TH: The neuroradiology of AIDS. *Semin Roentgenol* 22(1):42-53, 1987.

Sze G, Zimmerman RD: Magnetic resonance imaging of infectious and inflammatory disease. *Radiol Clin North Am* 26:839-860, 1988.

Takeshita M, Kawamata T, Izawa M, Hori T: Prodromal signs and clinical factors influencing outcome in patients with intraventricular rupture of purulent brain abscess. *Neurosurgery* 48:310-317, 2001.

Taoka T, Yuh WTC, White ML, et al: Sulcal hyperintensity on fluid-attenuated inversion recovery MR images in patients without apparent cerebrospinal fluid abnormality. *Am J Roentgenol* 176:519-524, 2001.

Teitelbaum GP, Otto RJ, Lin M, et al: MR imaging of neurocysticercosis. *AJNR* 10:709-718, 1989.

Thurnher MM, Schindler EG, Thurnher SA, et al: Highly active antiretroviral therapy for patients with AIDS dementia complex: effect on MR imaging findings and clinical course. *AJNR* 21:670-678, 2000.

Tien RD, Chu RK, Hesselink JR, et al: Intracranial crytocroccosis in immunocompromised patients: CT and MR findings in 29 cases. *AJNR* 12:283-289, 1991.

Tien RD, Dillon WP: Herpes trigeminal neuritis and rhombencephalitis on Gd-DTPA-enhanced MR imaging. *AJNR* 11:413, 1990.

Tien RD, Dillon WP: Herpes trigeminal neuritis and rhombencephalitis on Gd-DTPA-enhanced MR imaging. *AJNR* 11:413-414, 1990.

Tien RD, Felsberg GJ, Osumi AK: Herpesvirus infections of the CNS: MR findings. *Am J Roentgenol* 161:167-176, 1993.

Tien RD, Gean-Marton AD, Mark AS: Neurosyphilis in HIV carriers: MR findings in six patients. *Am J Roentgenol* 158:1325-1328, 1992.

Tishler S, Williamson T, Mirra SS, et al: Wegener granulomatosis with meningeal involvement. *AJNR* 14:1248-1252, 1993.

Trotot PM, Gray F: Diagnostic imaging contribution in the early stages of HIV infection of the brain. *Neuroimaging Clin North Am* 7:243-260, 1997.

Tsuchiya K, Inaoka S, Mitzutani Y, Hachiya J: Fast fluid-attenuated inversion-recovery MR of intracranial infections. *AJNR* 18:909-914, 1997.

Tsuchiya K, Katase S, Yoshino A, Hachiya J: Diffusion-weighted MR imaging of encephalitis. *Am J Roentgenol* 173:1097-1100, 1999.

Tsuchiya K, Makita K, Furui S, et al: Contrast-enhanced magnetic resonance imaging of sub- and epidural empyemas. *Neuroradiology* 34:494-496, 1992.

Tsuchiya K, Yamakami N, Hachiya J, et al: Multiple brain abscesses: differentiation from cerebral metastases by diffusion-weighted magnetic resonance imaging. *Int J Neurorad* 4:258-262, 1998.

Tuite M, Ketonen L. Keiburtz K, Handy B: Efficacy of gadolinium in MR brain imaging of HIV infected patients. *AJNR* 14:257-263 1993.

Tuncay R, Akman-Demir G, Gokyigit A, et al: MRI in subacute sclerosing panencephalitis. *Neuroradiology* 38:636-640 1996.

Van Mieghem F, Van Goethem JWM, Parizel PM, et al: MR of the brain in Sjögren-Larsson syndrome. *AJNR* 18:1561-1564, 1997.

Vanzieleghem B, Lemmerling M, Carton D, et al: Lyme disease in a child presenting with bilateral facial nerve palsy: MRI findings and review of the literature. *Neuroradiology* 40:739-742, 1998.

When SM, Heinz ER, Burger PC, Boyko OB: Dilated Virchow-Robin spaces in cryptococcal meningitis associated with AIDS: CT and MR findings. *J Comput Assist Tomogr* 13:756-762, 1989.

Weingarten K, Zimmerman RD, Becker RD, et al: Subdural and epidural empyemas: MR imaging. *AJNR* 10:81-87, 1989.

Whiteman MLH: Neuroimaging of central nervous system tuberculosis in HIV-infected patients. *Neuroimaging Clin North Am* 7:199-214, 1997.

Whiteman MLH, Post MJD, Bowen BC, Bell MD: AIDS-related white matter diseases. *Neuroimaging Clin N Amer* 3:331-359, 1993.

Whiteman M, Espinoza L, Post MJD, et al: Central nervous system tuberculosis in HIV-infected patients: clinical and radiographic findings. *AJNR* 16:1319-1327, 1995.

Williams DW III, Elster AD, Kramer SI: Neurosarcoidosis: Gadolimium-enhanced MR imaging. *J Comput Assist Tomogr* 14:704, 1990.

Wood BP: Children with acquired immune deficiency syndrome. *Invest Radiol* 27:964-970, 1992.

Wrobel CJ, Meyer S, Johnson RH, Hesselink JR: MR findings in acute and chronic coccidioidmycosis meningitis. *AJNR* 13:1241-1245, 1992.

Yuh WTC, Drew JM, Rizzo M, et al: Evaluations of pachymeningitis by contrast-enhanced MR imaging: a patient with rheumatoid disease. *AJNR* 11:1247-1248, 1990.

Zee C-S, Go JL, Kim PE, DiGiorgio CM: Imaging of neurocysticercosis. *Neuroimaging Clin North Am* 10:391-408, 2000.

Zee C-S, Segall HD, Boswell W, et al: MR imaging of neurocysticercosis. *J Comput Assist Tomogr* 12:927-934, 1988.

Zimmerman RD, Becker RD, Devinsky O, et al: Magnetic resonance features of cerebral abscesses and other intracranial inflammatory lesions. *Acta Radiol* (Suppl) 369:754, 1986.

Zimmerman RD, Weingarten K: Neuroimaging of cerebral abscesses. *Neuroimaging Clin N Amer* 1:1-16, 1991.

# CHAPTER 10

# Metabolic, Degenerative, and Reactive Disorders

### Case 501

10-month-old girl examined because
of diffuse hypotonia.
(sagittal, noncontrast T1-weighted SE scan)

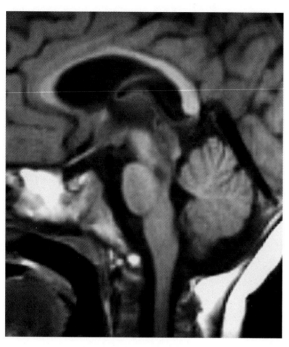

**Leigh Disease**

### Case 502

1-year-old boy presenting with truncal
instability and nystagmus.
(axial, noncontrast T2-weighted SE scan)

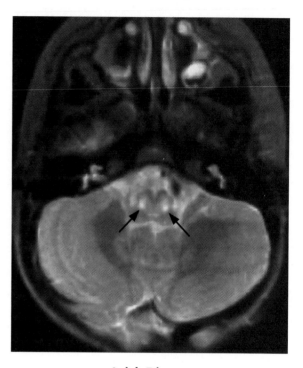

**Leigh Disease**

Leigh disease (also called *subacute necrotizing encephalomyelopathy*) is a metabolic disorder caused by deficiency in one of the enzymes necessary for oxidative metabolism within mitochondria (e.g., cytochrome *c* oxidase, pyruvate carboxylase, and pyruvate dehydrogenase). Infants with this disease typically present during the first two years of life with ataxia, nystagmus, dystonia, and/or motor weakness. High levels of pyruvate and lactic acid are present in the serum and spinal fluid of affected individuals.

Brainstem lesions are found on MR scans in the majority of children with Leigh disease, typically affecting nuclei and/or periaqueductal gray matter. Case 501 demonstrates involvement of the dorsal midbrain and pons, with abnormally low signal intensity and moderate mass effect surrounding the aqueduct. Brainstem lesions are usually strikingly symmetrical on axial images, with high signal intensity on T2-weighted scans. Paired lesions are seen within the medullary olives in Case 502 *(arrows)*.

All levels of the brainstem can be involved separately or simultaneously in Leigh disease. Associated spinal cord lesions are common.

Recent reports of enterovirus encephalitis have demonstrated symmetrical edema of the dorsal brainstem with a pattern resembling Leigh disease. Accompanying lesions of the basal ganglia and spinal cord have also been noted in these cases.

# DIFFERENTIAL DIAGNOSIS:
## SYMMETRICAL BRAINSTEM LESIONS IN A CHILD

### Case 503

1-month-old boy presenting with hypotonia.
(axial, noncontrast T2-weighted SE scan)

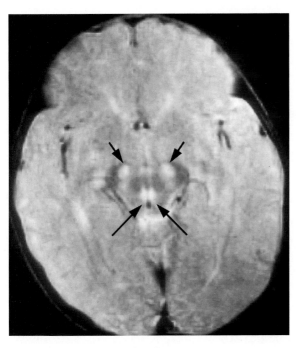

**Leigh Disease**

### Case 504

8-year-old boy presenting with bilateral hearing loss.
(axial, noncontrast scan; SE 2900/30)

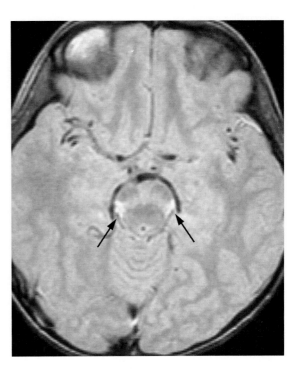

**Adrenoleukodystrophy**
(same patient as Case 411)

---

Paired, bilateral brainstem foci of signal abnormality are characteristic of Leigh disease, as seen in Case 503. Lesions within the cerebral peduncles *(short arrows)* accompany the more typical involvement of the midbrain tegmentum *(long arrows)* in this instance.

Demyelinating and dysmyelinating disorders can also cause symmetrical zones of abnormal signal intensity within the brainstem, reflecting involvement of specific tracts. The ascending auditory pathways are often affected by adrenoleukodystrophy, as illustrated in Case 504. The bilateral foci of high signal intensity along the lateral margin of the brainstem represent the lateral lemnisci, which carry auditory information from the cochlear nuclei to the inferior colliculi. More rostral involvement of the auditory pathways (inferior colliculus, brachium of the inferior colliculus, and medial geniculate body) can be demonstrated in many cases.

Sites of active dysmyelination in adrenoleukodystrophy may demonstrate intense contrast enhancement (see Case 414), unlike the lesions of Leigh disease. The usual age of onset also distinguishes between these disorders: adrenoleukodystrophy typically presents between 5 and 10 years of age, while Leigh disease becomes apparent during infancy.

### Case 505

10-month-old girl presenting with hypotonia.
(axial, noncontrast T2-weighted SE scan)

### Case 506

1-year-old boy presenting with hypotonia and ataxia.
(axial, noncontrast T2-weighted SE scan)

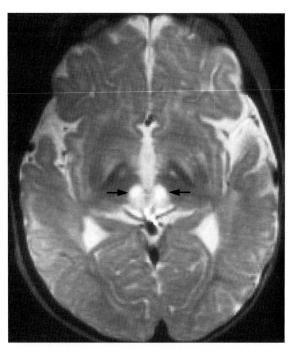

**Leigh Disease**
(same patient as Case 501)

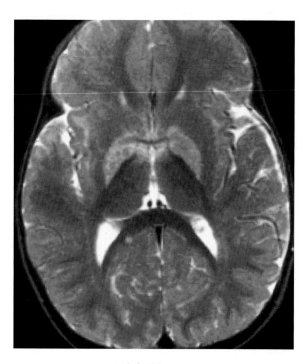

**Leigh Disease**

---

The basal ganglia and/or thalami often demonstrate symmetrical signal abnormality in Leigh disease, usually accompanying brainstem involvement but occasionally in isolation.

In Case 505, prominent symmetrical lesions are present within the thalami *(arrows)*. The pathological findings in Leigh disease resemble those of Wernicke's encephalopathy in adults (see Cases 515 and 516), which frequently causes thalamic abnormalities.

Case 506 illustrates the common involvement of the lentiform nuclei in Leigh disease. The globus pallidus is often most prominently affected, as in this patient. Mild, hazy T2 prolongation is also present within the lentiform nuclei in Case 505.

The lesions of Leigh disease may demonstrate increased signal intensity on diffusion-weighted scans, but the degree of abnormality is usually less than that of acute cerebral infarcts.

Symmetrical lesions within the basal ganglia of a child or an adult suggest an anoxic, toxic, or metabolic etiology. Leigh disease is only one example in this category. Carbon monoxide poisoning and other impairments of oxidative phosphorylation typically present with bilateral findings in the globus pallidus (see Cases 671 and 672). Kernicterus (bilirubin encephalopathy) is another cause of symmetrical prolongation of T2 values (and initial shortening of T1 values) within the globus pallidus in newborns and infants.

Occasional cases of Leigh disease demonstrate symmetrical, confluent areas of T2 prolongation in cerebral white matter, resembling a leukodystrophy.

See Case 510 for discussion of other mitochondrial encephalopathies.

# DIFFERENTIAL DIAGNOSIS:
## SYMMETRICAL LESIONS OF THE BASAL GANGLIA IN A CHILD

### Case 507

10-month-old boy presenting with seizures
and decreased level of consciousness.
(axial, noncontrast T2-weighted SE scan)

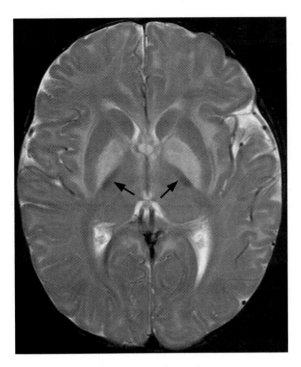

**Maple Syrup Urine Disease**

### Case 508

7-year-old boy presenting with
bilateral ankle clonus.
(axial, noncontrast T2-weighted SE scan)

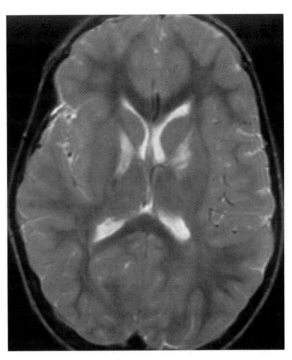

**Adrenoleukodystrophy**
(same patient as Case 414)

---

Symmetrical lesions deep within the cerebral hemispheres may be due to pathology involving nuclear structures and/or white matter tracts.

Case 507 is another example of a metabolic disorder affecting the globus pallidus (compare to Case 506). Maple syrup urine disease (MSUD) is an aminoacidopathy caused by enzymatic deficiency in decarboxylation of leucine, isoleucine, and valine. Ketoacids accumulate in the blood, with urinary excretion of metabolites that have a characteristic sweet odor. The disorder usually presents in infancy, with symptoms including vomiting, dystonia, seizures, and lethargy. In addition to symmetrical edema within the globus pallidus (and often also within the adjacent internal capsule), MSUD can cause edema in the dorsal brainstem (closely resembling Leigh disease) and cerebellar white matter. If instituted promptly, dietary control (restricted protein) results in reversal of symptoms and normalization of MR scans, as was true for the patient in Case 507.

The symmetrical prolongation of T2 values in Case 508 primarily involves the internal capsule at the medial margin of the globus pallidus. Edema in either of these structures

can extend to the other, and it is important to consider both nuclear and white matter disorders when symmetrical lesions are encountered deep within the basal ganglia. Note that the well-myelinated posterior limb of the internal capsule is seen as a zone of low signal intensity spared by edema in Case 507 *(arrows)*.

Cases 506 and 507 illustrate that mitochondrial disorders and aminoacidopathies can present similar MR findings and must often be listed together in the differential diagnosis of metabolic diseases affecting deep nuclei. There are more than 70 recognized disorders of amino acid metabolism, many of which can cause dysfunction and imaging abnormalities of the basal ganglia. Among other relatively common organic acidopathies that can produce symmetrical edema within the lentiform nuclei are methylmalonic acidemia/aciduria and propionic acidemia/aciduria.

Unilateral or bilateral zones of T2 prolongation within the globus pallidus may be seen in neurofibromatosis type 1 (see Cases 904 and 905). Systemic lupus erythematosus occasionally causes symmetrical ganglionic edema in adolescents or young adults (see Case 481).

### Case 509A

3-year-old boy presenting with developmental
delay and ankle clonus.
(sagittal, noncontrast T1-weighted SE scan)

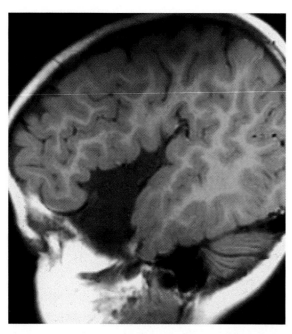

**Glutaric Aciduria Type I**

### Case 509B

Same patient.
(axial, noncontrast T2-weighted SE scan)

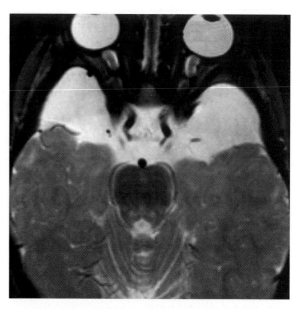

**Glutaric Aciduria Type I**

Glutaric aciduria type I is a metabolic disease that can be characterized as a mitochondrial disorder, an aminoacidopathy, or an organic acidopathy. Deficiency of the mitochondrial enzyme glutaryl-CoA dehydrogenase impairs the normal degradation of lysine, hydroxylysine, and tryptophan, leading to elevated levels of glutaric acid in the blood and urine.

MR scans of affected children may demonstrate prolongation of T1 and T2 values within the basal ganglia, resembling other metabolic disorders. Symmetrical zones of delayed or disturbed myelination can be seen within white matter of the cerebral hemispheres.

A more characteristic finding of the disorder is localized frontotemporal atrophy, with associated enlargement of the Sylvian fissures. Some patients develop large CSF spaces within the middle cranial fossa, having the appearance of bilateral arachnoid cysts. Case 509 is an example of this presentation.

As with simple arachnoid cysts (see Cases 812 and 813), it is not clear whether the cystic temporal collections in glutaric aciduria type I are the cause or the effect of associated hypoplasia of the temporal lobes. In any event, the morphology demonstrated above is highly suggestive of the diagnosis.

# MITOCHONDRIAL ENCEPHALOMYOPATHIES

### Case 510A

16-year-old girl presenting with a stroke.
(axial, noncontrast scan; SE 2500/30)

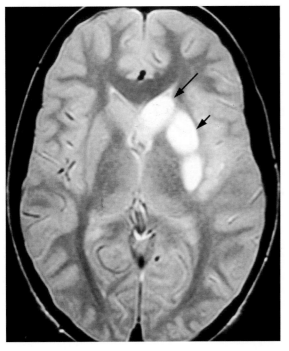

**MELAS**

### Case 510B

Same patient.
(axial, noncontrast T2-weighted SE scan)

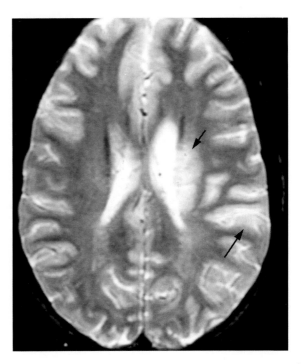

**MELAS**

A number of systemic disorders with prominent neurological components are caused by abnormalities in oxidative metabolism within mitochondria. These multisystem diseases are characterized pathologically by the presence of "ragged red fibers" in muscle biopsies. Among the clinical syndromes in this category are Kearns-Sayre syndrome, mitochondrial myopathy, MERRF or MERRLA (*m*yoclonus, *e*pilepsy, *r*agged *r*ed *f*ibers, and *l*actic *a*cidosis), and MELAS (*m*itochondrial myopathy, *e*ncephalopathy, *l*actic *a*cidosis, and *s*troke-like episodes).

MR findings in patients with mitochondrial encephalopathies are variable. Some cases demonstrate symmetrical signal abnormality within the basal ganglia and brainstem, as previously illustrated in Leigh disease. Scans in other patients evidence diffuse T2 prolongation throughout cerebral white matter, resembling a leukodystrophy. Still other cases present with asymmetrical stroke-like lesions, illustrated by Case 510.

In most cases of MELAS, areas of cerebral "infarction" are seen bilaterally, with predilection for the posterior portions of the hemispheres. The "infarcts" often do not conform precisely to major arterial distributions. Subcortical involvement is common. Lesions frequently demonstrate facilitated rather than restricted diffusion and may prove to be completely reversible. These features, together with multiplicity of lesions in space and time, should suggest the possibility of mitochondrial encephalomyopathy in a young patient.

Case 510 is somewhat unusual in that a single acute infarct is demonstrated involving portions of the distribution of the left middle cerebral artery. The caudate nucleus (*long arrow*, Case 510A) and putamen (*short arrow*, Case 510A) are edematous, with additional zones of signal abnormality within the corona radiata and inferior parietal cortex (*short* and *long arrows*, Case 510B). The subsequent clinical evaluation of this patient documented lactic acidosis and ragged red fibers on muscle biopsy.

Other pathologies that can resemble the MR appearance of mitochondrial encephalomyopathies are hypertensive encephalopathy (see Cases 544 and 545) and systemic lupus erythematosus (see Cases 481 and 483). Type 1 neurofibromatosis may present with patchy areas of signal abnormality in the basal ganglia similar to some cases of mitochondrial disease (see Cases 904 and 905).

See Case 576 for discussion of the differential diagnosis of infarction in children and young adults.

### Case 511

4-year-old boy with "cerebral palsy."
(axial, noncontrast T2-weighted SE scan)

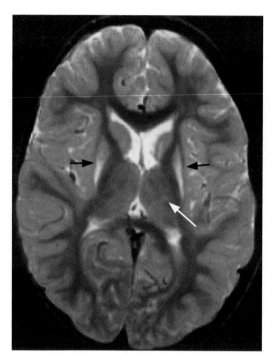

**Hypoxic-Ischemic Injury**

### Case 512

5-year-old girl with a history of perinatal anoxia.
(axial, noncontrast T2-weighted SE scan)

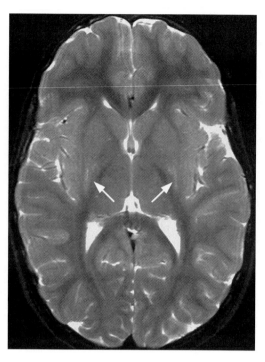

**Hypoxic-Ischemic Injury**

---

Oxidative metabolism within deep neuronal cell masses can be impaired by enzymatic deficiency (e.g., Leigh disease), toxins (e.g., carbon monoxide poisoning), or interruption of the normal flow of oxygenated blood (hypoxic-ischemic insult). Any of these processes or events may cause bilateral damage within the basal ganglia and/or thalami, resulting in a characteristic patten of symmetrical signal abnormality and volume loss.

The putamen is commonly injured in cases of severe perinatal hypoxia/ischemia, often in association with damage to the ventral-lateral thalamus and in the perirolanic regions of the hemispheres (where active myelination is occurring near the time of birth). Case 511 demonstrates striking atrophy and T2 prolongation throughout the putamen bilaterally *(black arrows)*. Less impressive signal abnormality is also present within the caudate nuclei bilaterally and at the ventral-lateral margin of the thalamus, at least on the left *(white arrow)*.

In Case 512, more subtle putaminal damage is limited to the posterolateral portion of the nucleus. This zone of the putamen is often solely or most severely involved in cases

of hypoxic-ischemic injury. Symmetrical volume loss and mildly abnormal signal intensity at this site *(arrows)* have the same etiologic implications as the more extensive change in Case 511, suggesting an earlier hypoxic-ischemic insult.

The symmetrical putaminal abnormality in the above cases differs from the predominant involvement of the globus pallidus in Leigh disease and aminoacidopathies, as illustrated in Cases 506 and 507. However, both hypoxic-ischemic injury and metabolic disorders can primarily involve either the globus pallidus or the putamen. Severe perinatal asphyxia in premature infants often damages the brainstem (ventral pons and inferior olivary nuclei) as well as the basal ganglia, potentially resembling the pattern of a mitochondrial disorder or aminoacidopathy.

The clinical syndrome of "cerebral palsy" has many potential etiologies, including intrauterine events and congenital malformations. Hypoxic-ischemic injury in the perinatal period accounts for only a minority of such cases (see Cases 663 and 664).

### Case 513

43-year-old woman presenting with choreoathetosis.
(coronal, noncontrast scan: SE 2500/45)

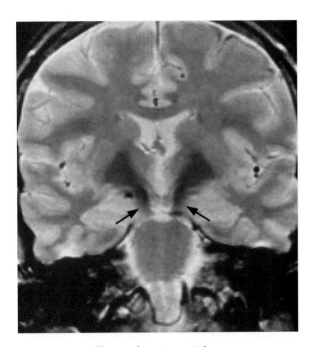

**Hallervorden-Spatz Disease**

### Case 514

6-year-old boy presenting with abnormal gait.
(axial, noncontrast T2-weighted SE scan)

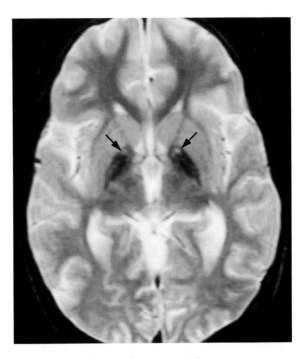

**Hallervorden-Spatz Disease**

Symmetrical lesions within the basal ganglia may reflect a degenerative process as well as toxic, anoxic, and metabolic disorders.

Hallervorden-Spatz disease (HSD) is a degenerative disorder primarily affecting neurons of the globus pallidus, with or without accompanying involvement of the substantia nigra. Both inherited (autosomal recessive) and sporadic cases are encountered. Most patients are recognized in the second or third decade of life. The primary clinical manifestation is motor dysfunction with progressive spasticity, gait abnormality, rigidity, slowing of voluntary movements, posturing, and choreoathetosis.

A characteristic pathological feature of HSD is deposition of iron in the affected tissues. This pigmentation causes prominent T2-shortening on MR scans, as seen in Cases 513 and 514. Smaller zones of T2 prolongation may be apparent within the area of T2-shortening, probably reflecting focal demyelination and necrosis. This so-called "eye of the tiger" appearance is appreciable in Case 514 *(arrows)*.

It is not clear whether iron deposition in HSD is simply a reaction to a primary neurodegenerative process or somehow contributes to the disorder. In any event, the degree of T2-shortening within affected structures has been observed to progress over time. The proportion of dark and bright areas within the globus pallidus on T2-weighted scans in HSD may vary from patient to patient, with the stage of disease in a given patient, and with field strength: at low fields, high signal intensity may predominate on T2-weighted images.

The symmetrical zones of low signal intensity in Case 513 extend inferiorly from the globus pallidus into the midbrain *(arrows)*. In Case 514, abnormality was confined to the globus pallidus, which is much lower in signal intensity than normal for a child.

The differential diagnosis of abnormally low signal intensity within the globus pallidus (and substantia nigra) of a child on T2-weighted scans includes hypothyroidism. A similar appearance can be seen in adults with Wilson's disease (accompanied by *high* intensity within the putamen).

319

## Case 515

38-year-old man presenting with confusion
and a history of alcoholism.
(axial, noncontrast T2-weighted FSE scan)

## Case 516

46-year-old man presenting with
psychiatric symptoms.
(axial, postcontrast T1-weighted SE scan with MTS)

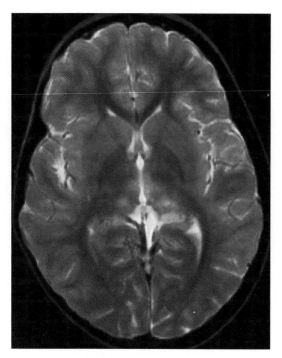

**Wernicke's Encephalopathy**

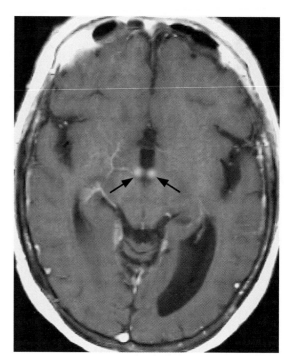

**Wernicke's Encephalopathy**

A number of metabolic diseases can cause symmetrical lesions of the basal ganglia and thalami in adults, resembling the presentation of mitochondrial encephalomyopathies and aminoacidopathies in children.

Wernicke's encephalopathy is due to deficiency of thiamine (Vitamin B1). The most common cause of this disorder is chronic alcoholism, but the disease can be seen in any form of malnutrition. Symptoms may include any of the originally described triad: confusion, ataxia, and ophthalmoplegia.

Wernicke's encephalopathy resembles Leigh disease pathologically and in anatomical distribution. Symmetrical lesions occur in the medial thalami, along the walls and floor of the third ventricle, and within the periaqueductal region of the midbrain. In addition (and in contrast to Leigh disease), the mamillary bodies are characteristically involved, demonstrating signal abnormality, contrast enhancement, and/or atrophy as the disorder progresses.

Case 515 illustrates nearly symmetrical zones of T2 prolongation within the medial and posterior portions of the thalami. Accompanying foci of abnormal signal were present in the tegmentum and tectum of the midbrain.

Enlargement and enhancement of the mamillary bodies in Case 516 *(arrows)* is a characteristic finding of acute Wernicke's encephalopathy. These structures become atrophic if affected patients do not receive supplementary thiamine.

Untreated Wernicke's encephalopathy is fatal. Successful treatment of acute encephalopathy may be followed by Korsakoff's psychosis, characterized by memory disorder.

Primary CNS lymphoma should be considered in the differential diagnosis of multiple lesions near the third ventricle and aqueduct (see Cases 347, 352, and 776), but lymphoma affecting the mamillary bodies would be very unusual.

Behçet's disease, a systemic vasculitis, can present with multiple lesions of the thalami and brainstem and could be included in the differential diagnosis of Case 515. However, the characteristic edema at the diencephalic-mesencephalic junction in Behçet's disease is usually more coalescent than seen above.

Compare Case 515 to the thalamic involvement by ADEM in Case 394 and by viral encephalitis in Case 656.

## Case 517

64-year-old man with a history of alcoholism.
(coronal, noncontrast T1-weighted SE scan)

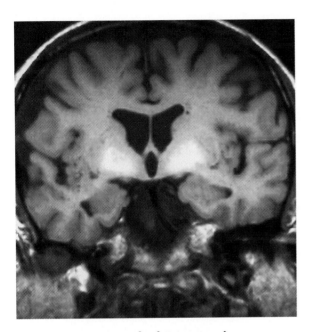

**Hepatocerebral Degeneration**

## Case 518

48-year-old woman with chronic liver disease.
(coronal, noncontrast T1-weighted SE scan)

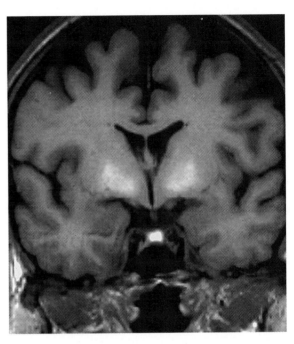

**Hepatocerebral Degeneration**

The most common disorder causing symmetrical signal abnormality within the basal ganglia in adults is chronic hepatic disease, as illustrated in Cases 517 and 518. T1-shortening may be seen within the globus pallidus (as above), putamen, and other deep nuclei in various hepatocerebral syndromes, including alcoholic cirrhosis. The high signal intensity in these regions on noncontrast T1-weighted images is probably due to the deposition of paramagnetic minerals. (CT scans and T2-weighted images in such cases are usually normal.) The finding has been reported to resolve following liver transplantation.

An appearance similar to the above scans may be seen in patients who are receiving total parenteral nutrition. Deposition of manganese is believed to be the responsible factor in this setting. Idiopathic calcification of the basal ganglia can also cause symmetrical T1-shortening.

Among other metabolic disorders that may present with symmetrical lesions of the basal ganglia in adults is Wilson's disease, or *hepatolenticular degeneration*. This autosomal recessive syndrome is caused by low levels of ceruloplasmin, a serum protein that transports copper. Abnormal copper deposition occurs in the deep cerebral and cerebellar nuclei (particularly in the lentiform nucleus), as well as in the liver. Symmetrical involvement of the caudate nucleus, putamen, globus pallidus, thalamus, rostral brainstem, and dentate nucleus may be seen in variable combinations. High signal intensity and eventual atrophy of the putamen are typically apparent on T2-weighted scans.

A rare cause of increased signal intensity within the basal ganglia of adults on T2-weighted scans is Creutzfeldt-Jakob disease, a transmissible spongiform encephalopathy. Symmetrical T2 prolongation within the caudate nucleus and putamen (accompanied by restricted diffusion on diffusion-weighted images) can be a clue to this diagnosis as the etiology of a rapidly progressive dementia.

See Cases 532 and 533 for discussion of basal ganglia changes in Huntington's disease.

### Case 519

3-year-old boy presenting with a large head.
(sagittal, noncontrast T1-weighted SE scan)

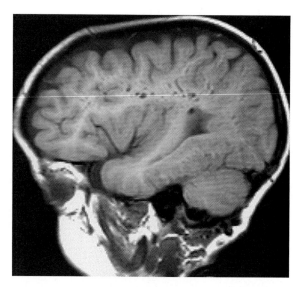

**Maroteaux-Lamy Syndrome**
(MPS type VI)

### Case 520

14-month-old girl presenting with
developmental delay.
(coronal, noncontrast T1-weighted SE scan)

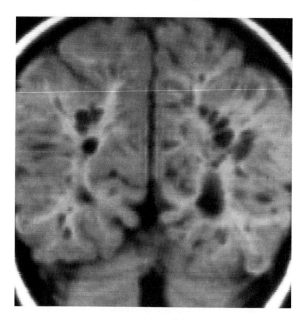

**Hurler's Syndrome**
(MPS type I-H)

The mucopolysaccharidoses are systemic metabolic disorders with major neurological components. Although these syndromes are characterized by neuronal damage, they also involve white matter and may resemble traditional leukodystrophies.

Deficiencies of various lysosomal enzymes in these diseases impair degradation of mucopolysaccharides (glycosaminoglycans), leading to toxic intracellular accumulation or "storage" of these materials. Several of the mucopolysaccharidoses present with prominent visceral and skeletal abnormalities, including spinal involvement with potential compression of the spinal cord (e.g., Morquio's disease, or mucopolysaccharidosis type IV).

Cerebral involvement in the mucopolysaccharidoses may be manifested as atrophy, patchy areas of prolonged T1 and T2 values within white matter resembling a leukodystrophy (see Case 521), and/or focal cysts or cavities within the corpus callosum and periventricular tissue.

Cases 519 and 520 demonstrate the latter finding. Such "cribriform changes" or "gargoyle bodies" are characteristic of the mucopolysaccharidoses, reflecting expansion of perivascular spaces by vacuolar cells containing glycosaminoglycans. These "cysts" may increase in size and number as the disease progresses.

Similar cystic areas within deep hemispheric white matter can also be seen among the leukodystrophies (e.g., Canavan's disease; see Case 418) and in the group of aminoacidopathies (e.g., maple syrup urine disease). There is considerable potential overlap in the MR appearance of disorders from different categories of metabolic disease.

The severity of neurological impairment varies substantially among the mucopolysaccharidoses, typically mild in Maroteaux-Lamy disease and severe in Hurler's disease. Macrocephaly is common, reflecting increased parenchymal volume and/or hydrocephalus. Dural thickening is usually present and may combine with vertebral deformity and/or subluxation to compromise the foramen magnum.

Untreated patients with Hurler's syndrome usually die before age 10 due to cardiac or pulmonary failure. Bone marrow transplantation is currently considered in newly diagnosed cases.

# DIFFERENTIAL DIAGNOSIS:
## PATCHY AREAS OF ABNORMAL SIGNAL IN SUBCORTICAL WHITE MATTER OF A CHILD

### Case 521

3-year-old boy presenting with macrocephaly.
(axial, noncontrast T2-weighted SE scan)

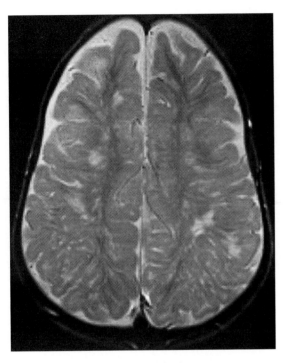

**Mucopolysaccharidosis Type VI**
(same patient as Case 519)

### Case 522

2-year-old boy presenting with seizures.
(axial, noncontrast T2-weighted FSE scan)

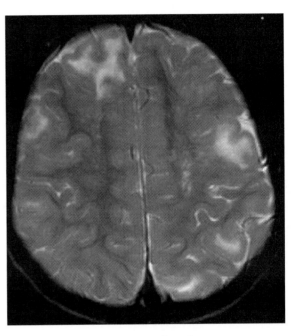

**Tuberous Sclerosis**

---

In addition to the focal, cyst-like "gargoyle bodies" illustrated on the previous page, mucopolysaccharidoses may present with patchy or diffuse zones of T2 prolongation in cerebral white matter. This finding probably reflects impaired myelination or damage to myelinated axons due to the lysosomal accumulation of large macromolecules.

Case 521 illustrates several small areas of signal abnormality within subcortical white matter, which is also reduced in volume. A background of mild, diffuse enlargement of perivascular spaces is present, and cortical atrophy is apparent.

Subcortical lesions are common in tuberous sclerosis, which is discussed in Cases 896-902. When associated subependymal nodules are few or inconspicuous, scattered areas of abnormal white matter may be the dominant

MR finding. Such lesions are often irregular or stellate in morphology and one to two centimeters in diameter, as illustrated in Case 522. "Migration lines" of immature or dysplastic tissue radiating outward from the lateral ventricles may be seen in tuberous sclerosis (see Cases 898 and 899), superficially resembling the distended perivascular spaces of a mucopolysaccharidosis.

Acute disseminated encephalomyelitis can also cause multiple areas of focal edema and/or demyelination within cerebral white matter, including subcortical involvement (see Cases 391 and 392). The morphology of such lesions is often more rounded or more confluent than the abnormalities in the above cases, and the clinical context is usually distinctive.

### Case 523

26-year-old man with seizures.
(coronal, noncontrast T1-weighted GRE scan)

### Case 524

42-year-old woman with seizures.
(coronal, noncontrast T2-weighted FSE scan)

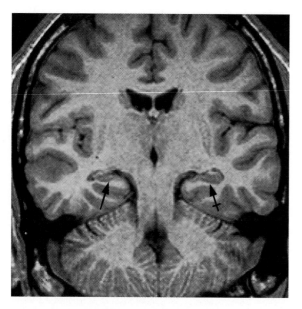

**Mesial Temporal Sclerosis**

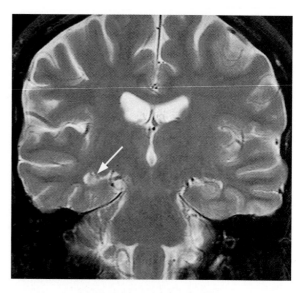

**Mesial Temporal Sclerosis**

Magnetic resonance imaging is routinely used to screen for structural lesions of the brain in patients with seizures.

A second goal of MR scans in the context of epilepsy is careful assessment of the hippocampal formations. Many patients suffer from seizures of temporal lobe origin that are associated with neuronal loss and gliosis of the ipsilateral hippocampus. The etiology of such hippocampal "sclerosis" is not well established, but the relationship to subsequent seizures is strong. As a result, resection of the anterior temporal lobe may be recommended to epileptic patients whose seizures are correlated with structural changes in the hippocampus. Current studies indicate that seizures can be controlled or reduced by surgery in the majority of such cases.

Traditional reference to this entity as "mesial temporal sclerosis" should probably be replaced by the more specific name of "hippocampal sclerosis." The benign degenerative changes in this syndrome are largely confined to the hippocampus. More generalized abnormality in the medial temporal region should suggest an alternative diagnosis (see Cases 525 and 526).

The hippocampal formations are well visualized in cross section on thin, coronal scans that are angled so as to be perpendicular to the long axis of the temporal lobe. Hippocampal sclerosis may present two major features on such studies.

A characteristic finding is reduced hippocampal volume. Thin, oblique coronal images (at approximately the level of the red nucleus) will provide several sections over which the bulk of the left and right hippocampus can be visually compared and/or measured. Case 523 demonstrates mild but definite atrophy of the right hippocampal formation *(arrow)* as compared to the left *(crossed arrow)*.

Focal signal abnormality (with prolonged T2 values) may be directly demonstrated within the sclerotic hippocampus, as seen on the right in Case 524 *(arrow)*. On thick sections partial volume of the temporal horn, enlarged due to hippocampal atrophy, may contribute to perceived hippocampal brightness.

An additional corollary finding in some cases of hippocampal sclerosis is secondary atrophy of the ipsilateral fornix and mamillary body due to deafferentation.

# DIFFERENTIAL DIAGNOSIS:
## FOCAL LESION IN THE MEDIAL TEMPORAL LOBE OF A PATIENT WITH SEIZURES

### Case 525

15-year-old girl presenting with a seizure.
(coronal, postcontrast T1-weighted
SE scan with MTS)

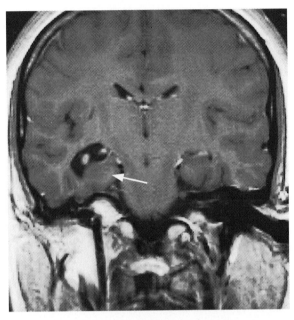

**Cysticercosis**
(within the temporal horn)

### Case 526

24-year-old woman with recurrent seizures.
(coronal, noncontrast T2-weighted FSE scan)

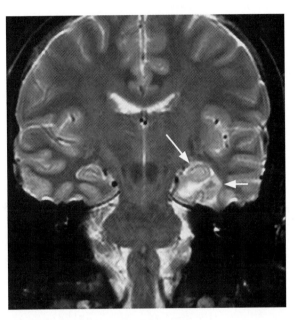

**Grade II Astrocytoma**

---

Awareness of mesial temporal sclerosis as a potential diagnosis in epileptic patients may confuse the interpretation of small mass lesions in the medial temporal lobe. Signal abnormality in true mesial temporal sclerosis should be localized to the hippocampus (with possible involvement of subjacent collateral white matter) and associated with hippocampal atrophy.

The right temporal horn in Case 525 is expanded due to an intraventricular mass, not because of hippocampal atrophy. The hippocampal formation *(arrow)* is displaced medially and inferiorly but is normal in volume.

Cysticercosis commonly causes one or more intraventricular cysts. Cysts within the third or fourth ventricle may lead to obstructive hydrocephalus while being difficult to distinguish from surrounding ventricular enlargement (see Cases 806 and 807). In Case 525, focal enhancement within the cyst represents the scolex of the parasite and

suggests the etiology of the localized ventricular enlargement.

Case 526 illustrates a small, infiltrating neoplasm within the medial temporal lobe *(short arrow)*. The volume and internal architecture of the adjacent hippocampal formation are preserved *(long arrow)*, excluding the diagnosis of hippocampal sclerosis.

The presence of mesial temporal sclerosis does not preclude the possibility of a second, coexisting structural lesion. Careful examination of the temporal lobes in a patient with seizures should not stop with identification of hippocampal atrophy.

Transient edema may be demonstrated within one or both hippocampal formations during status epilepticus and occasionally following single seizures. That is, mild swelling and signal abnormality within the hippocampus may represent the effect rather than the cause of seizures in the acute setting.

### Case 527

26-year-old man presenting with
"loss of muscle control."
(axial, noncontrast scan; SE 2500/45)

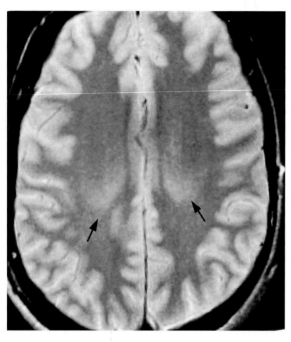

**Amyotrophic Lateral Sclerosis**

### Case 528

48-year-old man presenting with
bilateral leg weakness.
(axial, noncontrast scan; SE 2500/45)

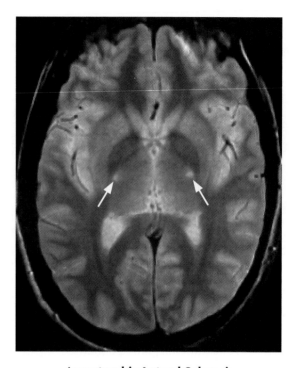

**Amyotrophic Lateral Sclerosis**

Amyotrophic lateral sclerosis (ALS) is an idiopathic degenerative disorder of upper and lower motor neurons. The clinical presentation is characterized by progressive dysfunction of the corticospinal tracts.

MR scans may be surprisingly negative in the presence of major neurological impairment. Other ALS patients demonstrate bihemispheral abnormality extending from the motor cortex to the brainstem.

In Case 527, vague areas of increased signal intensity are seen at the junction of the centrum semiovale and the corona radiata bilaterally *(arrows)*. This appearance reflects loss of myelin and increased water content along the course of the motor axons originating from the frontoparietal cortex. Compare this appearance to that of HIV encephalitis in Cases 457 and 458.

Signal abnormality within the corticospinal tract becomes increasingly concentrated and better defined as it passes inferiorly into the hemisphere. Case 528 illustrates strikingly sharp and symmetrical foci of abnormal intensity within the posterior limb of the internal capsule bilaterally *(arrows).*

This finding should be correlated with ascending and descending extension along the corticospinal tracts to suggest the diagnosis of ALS. Other etiologies can cause symmetrical foci of abnormal signal limited to the level of the internal capsule (see Cases 529 and 530). Progressive multifocal leukoencephalopathy and adult-onset Krabbe's disease (globoid cell leukodystrophy) may produce unilateral or bilateral zones of abnormal intensity within the corticospinal tracts, resembling the appearance of ALS. Wallerian degeneration can also cause signal abnormality along the course of the corticospinal tract, as illustrated in Case 541.

Some cases of ALS demonstrate reduced signal intensity within involved cortex on T2-weighted images. This finding is typically uniform and laminar but localized, often affecting the precentral gyrus. The low cortical intensity may reflect an increased concentration of minerals associated with neuronal degeneration.

The average age at presentation of ALS is near 50. The disease is usually progressive and fatal.

# DIFFERENTIAL DIAGNOSIS:
## SYMMETRICAL HIGH SIGNAL FOCI NEAR THE POSTERIOR LIMBS OF THE INTERNAL CAPSULES ON T2-WEIGHTED IMAGES

### Case 529

15-year-old girl presenting with headaches.
(axial, noncontrast T2-weighted SE scan)

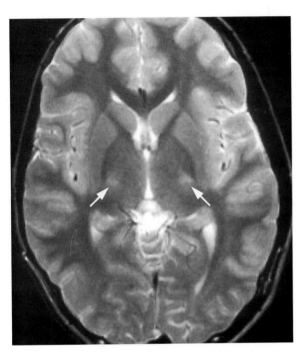

**Normal Variant**
(corticospinal tract)

### Case 530

46-year-old man with a history of alcoholism, now presenting with obtundation.
(axial, noncontrast T2-weighted SE scan)

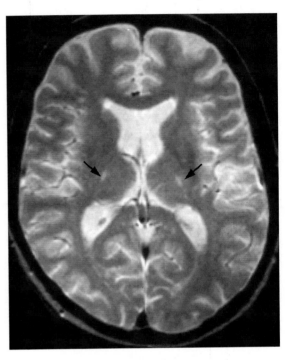

**Extrapontine Myelinolysis**
(same patient as Case 406)

---

A small area of a relatively high signal intensity may be seen within the posterior limb of the internal capsule on T2-weighted scans (including FLAIR images) as a normal variant. This focal zone of relatively long T2 values occupies the posterior portion of the posterior limb and is bilaterally symmetrical (*arrows*, Case 529). The finding has been ascribed to relatively lower myelin density in the region of large axons constituting the corticospinal tract.

Clues to distinguish this incidental variant from bilateral capsular pathology (as in Case 528) include (1) relative isointensity of the variant on long TR, short TE images, on which true capsular lesions are usually well appreciated and (2) lack of contiguous extension of the abnormality to adjacent sections (see discussion of Case 528).

The symmetrical foci of signal abnormality in Case 530 (*arrows*) are caused by osmotic myelinolysis affecting the lateral portions of the thalami. Extrapontine myelinolysis occurs in the same clinical context as central pontine myelinolysis (see Case 406) and may be found in association with or independent of brainstem disease. Symmetrical hemispheric involvement may include the basal ganglia and/or thalami.

As illustrated on the preceding page, ALS often causes small, symmetrical lesions within the posterior limb of the internal capsule. However, the paired abnormalities of ALS can be followed caudally into the cerebral peduncles and pons, unlike the findings in the above cases.

### Case 531A

78-year-old woman presenting with
tremor, rigidity, and akinesia.
(axial, noncontrast scan; SE 2800/45)

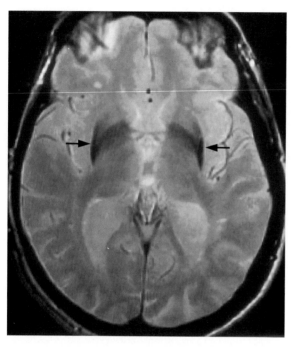

**Parkinson's Disease**

### Case 531B

Same patient.
(axial, noncontrast T2-weighted SE scan)

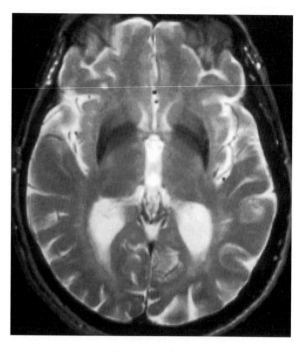

**Parkinson's Disease**

MR scans in most patients with Parkinson's disease demonstrate only atrophy and nonspecific age-related changes. Careful attention to the midbrain may define abnormal thinning of the pars compacta of the substantia nigra, a relatively high signal intensity band interposed between the lower signal intensity of the pars reticulata anteriorly and the red nucleus posteriorly on axial T2-weighted scans. This thinning correlates with the pathological loss of dopaminergic neurons in the substantia nigra, which is the primary cause of the disease.

Some patients with severe or drug-resistant Parkinson's disease and others with "Parkinson's plus" syndromes (e.g., striatonigral degeneration, Shy-Drager syndrome, and progressive supranuclear palsy) may show abnormally prominent low signal intensity within the basal ganglia on long TR images. Case 531 demonstrates this finding. The globus pallidus is unusually dark bilaterally, even allowing for the patient's age. More important and specific is the prominent low intensity within the posterior and lateral portions of the putamen bilaterally (*arrows*, Case 531A). This signal loss likely reflects susceptibility effects due to degenerative deposition of pigment and/or metals, especially iron.

Susceptibility effects are less prominent on MR scans performed at lower field strengths. On such studies, symmetrically *increased* signal intensity may be seen in the putamen on T2-weighted scans of patients with Parkinson's syndromes. This appearance presumably reflects neuronal loss and gliosis, analogous to changes that typically occur in Wilson's disease.

The above patient was clinically categorized as having uncomplicated but severe Parkinson's disease, which proved to be unresponsive to therapy with dopamine agonists.

## Case 532

61-year-old man presenting with dementia.
(coronal, noncontrast T1-weighted SE scan)

## Case 533

57-year-old woman presenting with
choreoathetosis and confusion.
(coronal, noncontrast T1-weighted SE scan)

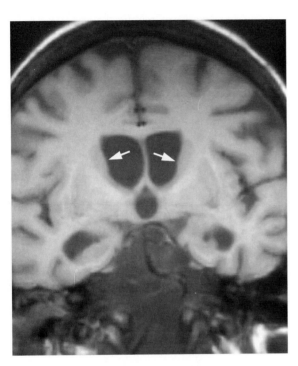

**Huntington's Disease**

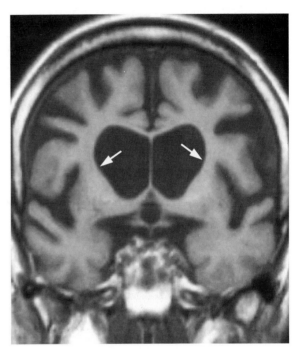

**Huntington's Disease**

The normal caudate head bulges into the lateral aspect of the frontal horn to cause a medially convex margin. Atrophy of the caudate nucleus in advanced Huntington's disease causes the curvature to flatten or reverse, as seen above *(arrows)*. The putamen may also be severely atrophic in patients with this disorder. Associated ventricular and sulcal enlargement is often present.

On long TR images of patients with Huntington's disease, the caudate nucleus and putamen may demonstrate either high or low signal intensity, depending on the predominance of neuronal loss and gliosis versus degenerative deposition of minerals and pigment. The signal intensity of these structures also depends to some extent on field

strength, with low intensity due to susceptibility effects more prominent at higher fields. Huntington's disease should be considered among the degenerative and metabolic disorders producing symmetrical signal abnormality within the basal ganglia.

The characteristic CT/MR finding of caudate atrophy is a late development in Huntington's disease and is not seen in presymptomatic carriers. Positron emission tomography can identify abnormal caudate metabolism before atrophy appears on CT or MR scans. A genetic marker for Huntington's disease has also been found and may enable screening of individuals at risk for inheriting this autosomal dominant disorder.

### Case 534

38-year-old man with AIDS,
presenting with confusion.
(sagittal, noncontrast T1-weighted SE scan)

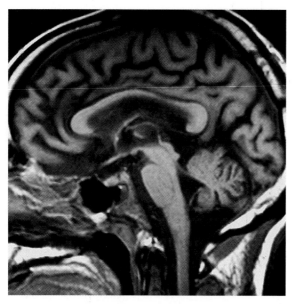

**Cerebral Atrophy**
(AIDS)

### Case 535

67-year-old woman presenting with dementia.
(axial, noncontrast T2-weighted FSE scan)

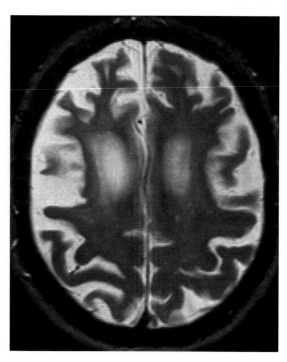

**Cerebral Atrophy**
(Alzheimer's disease)

Cerebral atrophy is demonstrated on CT and MR scans by diffuse enlargement of ventricles and subarachnoid spaces. The relative degree of ventricular and sulcal enlargement is usually similar. Disproportionate prominence of the ventricular component raises the question of hydrocephalus.

A number of conditions other than aging may cause enlargement of intracranial CSF spaces. Atrophy is a common finding in patients with AIDS, as illustrated in Case 534, with or without apparent parenchymal lesions (see Cases 457 and 458). Alcoholic "atrophy" is frequent, possibly due to nutritional or hydration factors as well as to direct effects of ethanol. In some patients the enlarged sulci return to a more normal size after successful treatment.

Other circumstances associated with abnormal enlargement of cerebral sulci include malnutrition (e.g., anorexia nervosa), high doses of exogenous or endogenous steroids, multiple sclerosis, lupus cerebritis, chronic renal disease, radiation therapy, prior head trauma, anoxia, and presenile dementing disorders. When a young patient presents with enlarged sulci, these possibilities should be considered.

Localized atrophy of the hippocampus, amygdala, and temporal lobe is characteristic of Alzheimer's disease, the major cause of dementia in this country. Affected patients usually demonstrate enlargement of the temporal horns and subarachnoid spaces (e.g., hippocampal fissure) in the medial temporal region. Conversely, absence of temporal lobe atrophy argues against the diagnosis of Alzheimer's disease as an explanation for dementia. Evidence of medial temporal volume loss is more useful than generalized measures of atrophy in separating patients with Alzheimer's disease from cognitively normal patients of the same age.

Pick's disease (or "frontotemporal dementia") may be suggested when localized frontal atrophy is associated with prominent atrophy of the inferior and middle temporal gyri. Classic Pick's disease demonstrates strikingly thin gyri separated by gaping sulci in the frontal and temporal lobes. However, these "knife-like" gyri are not present in all cases. Furthermore, most cases with gross pathology suggesting Pick's disease are found to represent Alzheimer's disease microscopically.

## Case 536

1-year-old girl presenting with developmental delay.
(sagittal, noncontrast T1-weighted SE scan)

## Case 537

14-year-old girl with a long history
of seizures and dilantin therapy.
(coronal, noncontrast T2-weighted SE scan)

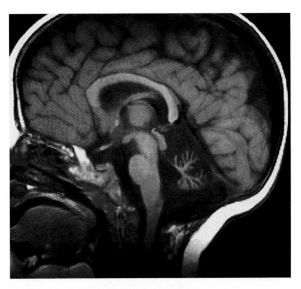

**Cerebellar Atrophy**
(metabolic)

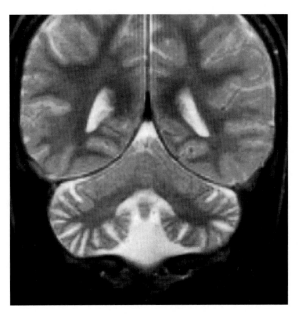

**Cerebellar Atrophy**
(seizures/dilantin)

A number of familial syndromes (e.g., spinocerebellar atrophy types 1 to 8 and Marie's ataxia) may cause cerebellar degeneration with or without brainstem atrophy. Friedreich's ataxia, an autosomal recessive disorder that may present in childhood, usually includes spinal cord and medullary involvement, with less prominent cerebellar findings. Ataxia telangiectasia, another autosomal recessive syndrome with pediatric presentation, is characterized by oculocutaneous telangiectasia accompanying ataxia and cerebellar atrophy.

The infant in Case 536 suffers from carbohydrate deficient glycoprotein syndrome type I, an autosomal recessive metabolic abnormality. This multisystem disease causes prominent cerebellar atrophy due to complete loss of Purkinje cells and subtotal loss of granular cells. Accompanying neuronal loss occurs in the pons but is less severe. The marked reduction of cerebellar volume in Case 536 results in expansion of the fourth ventricle and striking enlargement of infratentorial cisterns.

Acquired cerebellar atrophy may be associated with alcohol abuse, paraneoplastic syndromes, degenerative disorders (e.g., multisystem atrophy), and the phenytoin/seizure combination, as in Case 537. Alcoholic cerebellar atrophy primarily involves the vermis and is often more impressive than related symptoms.

Paraneoplastic cerebellar degeneration is probably an autoimmune disorder, most commonly associated with carcinomas of the lung, breast, and colon in adults and with neuroblastoma in children. Loss of Purkinje cells in this condition is usually not associated with recognizably decreased cerebellar volume.

### Case 538

59-year-old man presenting with ataxia.
(sagittal, noncontrast T1-weighted SE scan)

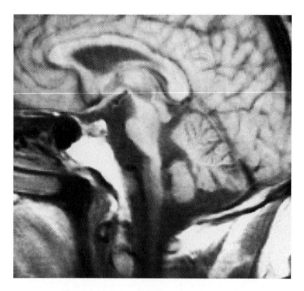

**Olivopontocerebellar Degeneration**

### Case 539

44-year-old man presenting with gait abnormality.
(axial, noncontrast T2-weighted SE scan)

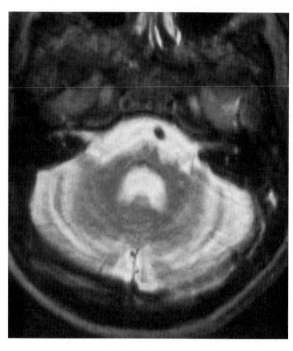

**Idiopathic Brainstem Atrophy**

Atrophy of the brainstem usually occurs in association with cerebellar atrophy, as in Case 538. The midbrain in this patient is normal in size. However, the bulk of the pons is markedly reduced. A characteristically flat and angular contour replaces the normally convex ventral margin. The prepontine cistern and fourth ventricle are large. Associated atrophy of the cerebellum and medulla is present, due to degeneration of tracts passing through the middle and inferior cerebellar peduncles.

This combination of morphological features is helpful in establishing the diagnosis of olivopontocerebellar degeneration (OPCD), which is clinically nonspecific. OPCD may be inherited as an autosomal dominant trait but is more commonly sporadic. Primary degeneration of pontine nuclei is believed to lead to secondary involution of the cerebellum and cerebellar peduncles. The sporadic form of the disease typically presents in the fifth or sixth decade and evolves over ten to twenty years.

T2-weighted MR scans in OPCD may demonstrate increased signal intensity involving transverse pontine tracts, with sparing of ascending and descending fiber bundles. Olivopontocerebellar degeneration is among the "Parkinson's plus" syndromes that are often correlated with abnormal T2-shortening in the lentiform nucleus (see Case 531).

The relatively isolated brainstem atrophy in Case 539 is rare. The cross section of the brainstem at the pontomedullary junction is tiny, with marked enlargement of the prepontine cistern and fourth ventricle.

# SPONTANEOUS INTRACRANIAL HYPOTENSION

## Case 540A

40-year-old woman presenting with
severe postural headaches.
(sagittal, noncontrast T1-weighted SE scan)

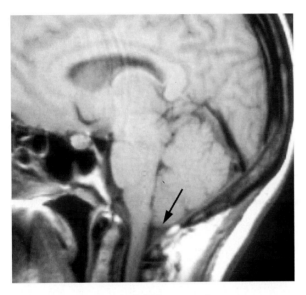

**Intracranial Hypotension**

## Case 540B

Same patient.
(axial, postcontrast T1-weighted SE scan)

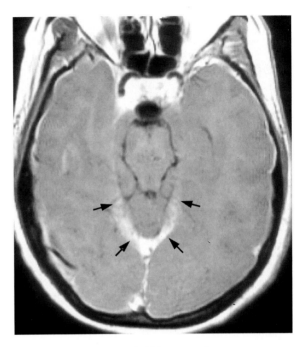

**Intracranial Hypotension**

Some patients present with postural headaches (worse when standing) due to low intracranial pressure caused by loss of fluid from the spinal subarachnoid space. The CSF leakage may be spontaneous (e.g., due to rupture of a root sleeve cyst) or posttraumatic (e.g., following lumbar puncture).

When contrast-enhanced MR scans are performed in such cases, diffuse dural thickening and enhancement may be demonstrated (see Case 440). This finding probably represents an increase in dural blood volume secondary to the low intracranial pressure. The uniform dural thickening can be misinterpreted as meningeal pathology causing the patient's symptoms.

Sagittal scans such as Case 540A often provide an important clue to the correct diagnosis. The brainstem and cerebellum sag inferiorly, reflecting the low pressure within the spinal subarachnoid space. The ventral margin of the pons is flatter than normal, the cerebellar tonsils approach the foramen magnum *(arrow)*, and the fourth ventricle looks narrowed in anteroposterior dimension. These find-

ings are all reversible when the cause of low spinal fluid pressure is corrected.

Case 540B demonstrates thick enhancement of the tentorium *(arrows)* and the convexity dura. Intracranial hypotension should be considered in any patient with diffuse dural thickening, whether or not there is accompanying caudal displacement of the brainstem and cerebellum.

Crowding of tissue at the tentorial hiatus in Case 540B resembles the appearance of a Chiari II hindbrain malformation. Unusually prominent signal loss from CSF pulsation ventral to the brainstem reflects the obstruction of more dorsal incisural CSF pathways by the caudal displacement of the brain.

Additional potential MR findings in cases of intracranial hypotension include unusually prominent enhancement of choroid plexus, enlarged dural veins and sinuses, and subdural effusions.

The etiology of intracranial hypotension in Case 540 was not established. Symptoms gradually improved over a period of several weeks.

## Case 541A

48-year-old man, one year after severe head trauma.
(axial, noncontrast T2-weighted SE scan)

## Case 541B

Same patient.
(axial, noncontrast T2-weighted SE scan)

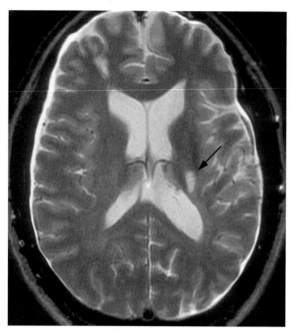

**Wallerian Degeneration**

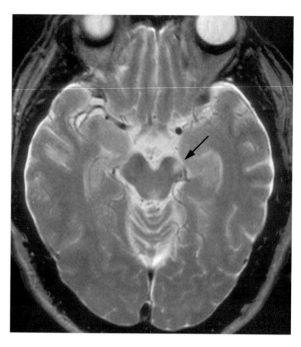

**Wallerian Degeneration**

The phrase "Wallerian degeneration" is used to describe degeneration of an axon secondary to injury to the body (or more proximal axon) of a nerve cell. When tissue damage involves a group of neurons that serves as the source of a major fiber tract, the aggregate degeneration of clustered axons may become apparent on CT and MR scans.

MR studies have shown biphasic intensity changes during Wallerian degeneration. An initial period of T2-shortening within the fiber tract (lasting approximately from week four to week ten) is possibly related to predominance of hydrophobic myelin lipids. This is followed by permanent prolongation of T2, reflecting cell death and gliosis. Accompanying volume loss of the affected tract is often apparent.

Case 541A demonstrates a focal zone of signal abnormality at the junction of the posterior corona radiata and the posterior limb of the internal capsule. This "lesion" represents the cross-section of axonal degeneration along the corticospinal tract, which began more superiorly in a large area of frontoparietal encephalomalacia. High signal intensity within this tract could be followed sequentially

across every section of the scan, with an increasingly compact area at more inferior levels.

Case 541B illustrates the appearance of Wallerian degeneration involving the corticospinal tract within the cerebral peduncle *(arrow)*. Lower sections documented extension of localized T2 prolongation into the pyramid of the medulla.

The cross-sectional appearance of Wallerian degeneration on any one axial image resembles focal infarction. However, the continuity of the finding across adjacent levels establishes the diagnosis. Coronal scans confirm the cephalo-caudal course of tract degeneration in such cases.

Involvement of the corticospinal tract by Wallerian degeneration is analogous to the MR findings in some cases of amyotrophic lateral sclerosis, illustrated in Cases 527 and 528.

Small subdural hygromas are present bilaterally in Case 541. The left lateral ventricle is mildly enlarged due to posttraumatic loss of volume in the superior left cerebral hemisphere. A small area of posttraumatic encephalomalacia is also seen in the right frontal lobe.

334

## Case 542

26-year-old man with a history of left pontine hemorrhage from a vascular malformation.
(axial, noncontrast T2-weighted FSE scan)

## Case 543

40-year-old man being followed for a growing cavernous angioma involving the left pontine tegmentum and the left superior cerebellar peduncle.
(axial, noncontrast T2-weighted SE scan)

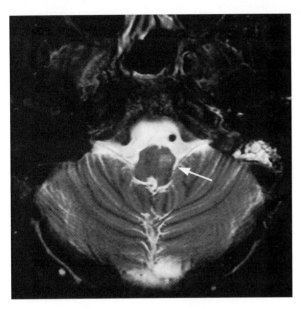

**Hypertrophic Olivary Degeneration**

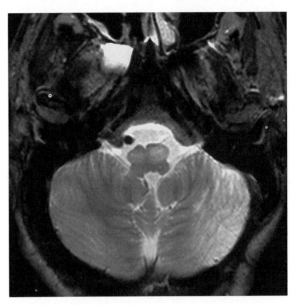

**Hypertrophic Olivary Degeneration**

Degeneration of a nucleus may occur if the neurons lose afferent input. Hypertrophic olivary degeneration is an example of such transsynaptic degeneration.

The olivary nucleus of the medulla receives afferent fibers from the ipsilateral red nucleus via the central tegmental tract, which vertically traverses the pons. The red nucleus in turn receives input from the contralateral dentate nucleus of the cerebellum via cerebellorubral fibers that pass through the superior cerebellar peduncle before decussating at the level of the inferior colliculus. This relationship among the contralateral dentate nucleus, the ipsilateral red nucleus, and the olive has been called the *Guillain-Mollaret triangle.*

A lesion destroying axons of the ipsilateral central tegmental tract or the contralateral superior cerebellar peduncle causes denervation and subsequent degeneration of the olivary nucleus. Prolonged T2 values (and occasionally short T1 values) are first noted within the olive about a month after axonal damage. Focal swelling of the nucleus develops six to eighteen months after injury to the ipsilateral pontine tegmentum or contralateral dentate nucleus or superior cerebellar peduncle. This "hypertrophy" corre-

lates histologically with vacuolization of neurons and reactive enlargement of astrocytes. The resulting lateral medullary lesion may mimic a subacute infarct (see Case 618), demyelinating plaque, or small mass. The presence of coexisting pathology and the typical clinical presentation with palatal myoclonus and dysarthria help to establish the diagnosis. Olivary hypertrophy may persist for more than a year after the event interrupting synaptic input to the nucleus.

Both of the above cases demonstrate abnormal T2 prolongation and enlargement of the olivary nucleus. The unilateral involvement in Case 542 reflects damage to the ipsilateral central tegmental tract. Bilateral olivary hypertrophy is present in Case 543, because the angioma and associated hemorrhages affected both the left central tegmental tract (causing denervation of the left olive) and the left superior cerebellar peduncle (interrupting input to the right olive).

Compare the enlarged olives in Cases 542 and 543 to the olivary involvement without hypertrophy in Leigh disease illustrated in Case 502.

335

# HYPERTENSIVE ENCEPHALOPATHY
## (REVERSIBLE POSTERIOR EDEMA SYNDROME)

### Case 544

20-year-old woman presenting with eclampsia, headaches, and impaired vision.
(axial, noncontrast T2-weighted FSE scan)

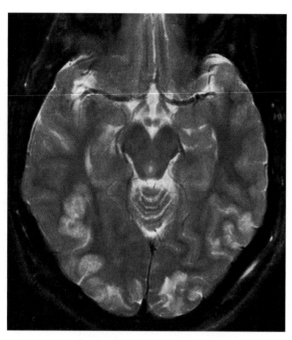

**Hypertensive Encephalopathy**

### Case 545

67-year-old woman presenting with a seizure.
(coronal, noncontrast FLAIR scan)

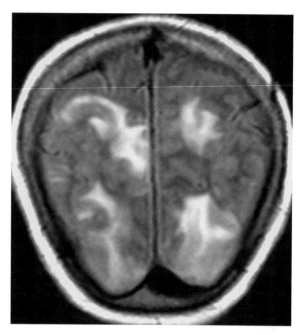

**Hypertensive Encephalopathy**

Severe hypertension may be associated with patchy or coalescent areas of superficial edema in the cerebral and/or cerebellar hemispheres. Involvement of subcortical white matter is characteristic, with lesions most common in the parieto-occipital regions. Case 545 illustrates typical multifocal subcortical edema involving the posterior parietal and occipital lobes.

Cortical edema is often also present, as demonstrated in the posterior temporal and occipital lobes in Case 544. This finding is often best seen on FLAIR images.

An appearance similar to hypertensive encephalopathy has been encountered in uremia, thrombotic thrombocytopenic purpura, cyclosporine toxicity (see Case 546), and following seizures. In each of these circumstances, the clinical and MR findings have been shown to be potentially reversible. The name *reversible posterior edema syndrome* or *posterior reversible encephalopathy/edema syndrome* (PRES) has been applied to this clinical/radiological entity.

There is usually no evidence of restricted diffusion in the involved regions on diffusion-weighted scans, indicating that the zones of prolonged T2 values likely represent increased extracellular fluid rather than cytotoxic edema.

That is, the findings probably reflect transient leakage of plasma across a disrupted blood-brain barrier. Elevation of cerebral blood flow and cerebral blood volume has been documented in affected regions, supporting the concept of "hyperperfusion encephalopathy." The predominant involvement of the parieto-occipital regions has been suggested to reflect the relatively lower autoregulatory reserve (due to less sympathetic innervation) of arteries in the vertebrobasilar distribution, making the supplied tissues more prone to hyperperfusion and associated dysfunction of the blood-brain barrier.

Edema of the cerebellum (or brainstem) may accompany parieto-occipital lesions and is occasionally the most prominent MR finding. The basal ganglia are involved in some cases. Lesions of PRES may be nonenhancing or demonstrate patchy enhancement. Leptomeningeal enhancement was present in the involved regions on a postcontrast scan in Case 544.

Multifocal patches of edema can also be seen in many other conditions, such as lupus cerebritis (see Cases 481 and 483), mitochondrial encephalopathies (see Case 510), arteritis (see Cases 641 and 642), and dural venous sinus thrombosis (see Cases 649 and 650).

### Case 546

58-year-old woman with a history of cardiac transplantation, presenting with a seizure.
(axial, noncontrast T2-weighted SE scan)

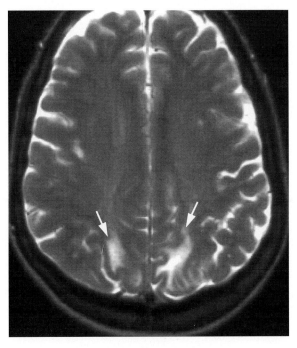

**Cyclosporine Toxicity**
(reversible posterior edema syndrome)

### Case 547

45-year-old truck driver presenting with impaired vision.
(axial, noncontrast T2-weighted SE scan)

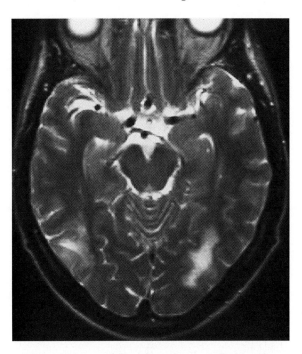

**Progressive Multifocal Leukoencephalopathy**

---

Multifocal, predominantly subcortical edema is a characteristic feature of the *reversible posterior edema* or *posterior reversible encephalopathy syndrome* (PRES), as discussed on the previous page. Cyclosporine toxicity is one of the recognized causes of this entity, illustrated by Case 546.

Neurotoxicity from cyclosporin A may present within days (or even hours) after the initiation of treatment. The most common symptoms are confusion, seizures, and cortical blindness. MR scans demonstrate reversible zones of nodular or scalloped subcortical edema, most often in the parieto-occipital regions and cerebellum.

The subcortical predominance of edema, multifocality, and usual absence of contrast enhancement in PRES mimic the features of progressive multifocal leukoencephalopathy. The lesions in Case 547 closely resemble those of Case 546. However, none of the clinical conditions associated with PRES was present, and the patient was found to be HIV positive. PML was diagnosed by biopsy. (See Cases 398-403 for other examples and general discussion of PML.)

The mechanism of reversible white matter edema in cyclosporine toxicity has not been established. Some form of endothelial injury is likely, as in other cases of PRES. Associated hypertension is usually not high enough to implicate loss of autoregulation, which is believed to underlie hypertensive encephalopathy as discussed in Cases 544 and 545.

Seizures have been suggested as the common clinical factor among the various conditions associated with PRES, but this relationship may be effect rather than cause. (PRES is rare in patients with idiopathic epilepsy or seizures related to structural lesions.)

Edema associated with subcortical metastases should also be considered in the differential diagnosis of the above cases. Thrombosis of the superior sagittal sinus is another potential cause of multifocal parasagittal edema.

### Case 548

57-year-old woman treated for
carcinoma of the lung.
(axial, noncontrast T2-weighted SE scan)

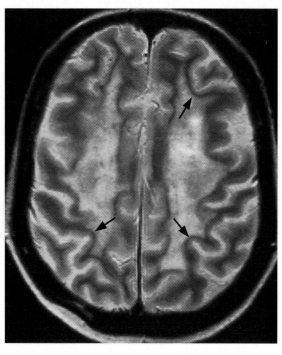

**Radiation Leukoencephalopathy**

### Case 549

8-year-old girl, four years after surgery and radiation
therapy for a right occipital ependymoma, now
presenting with homonymous hemianopsia.
(axial, noncontrast T2-weighted SE scan)

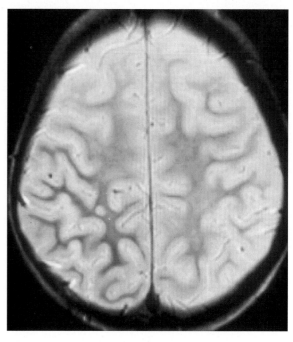

**Mineralizing Microangiopathy**

---

A spectrum of MR changes may be seen following cerebral radiation. Alterations can range from mild, generalized atrophy to the focal mass lesions of radiation necrosis (see Cases 550 and 551). Intermediate patterns may be encountered, with localized or multifocal abnormalities that are not mass-like.

Case 548 illustrates diffuse T2 prolongation throughout white matter of the centrum semiovale. Subcortical "U" fibers *(arrows)* are largely spared. This appearance is typical for postradiation change, but not specific: other end-stage leukoencephalopathies could present similarly (compare to Cases 422 and 423).

The mechanism of radiation toxicity to normal parenchyma probably involves vascular injury. Endothelial cells are among the most radiosensitive tissues in the brain. Damage to small vessels may lead to thickening of the wall, thrombosis, ischemia, and infarction. In some cases, calcium and other minerals are deposited in perivascular spaces. Such "mineralizing microangiopathy" may lead to coarse multifocal calcifications apparent at the gray/white matter junction or within the basal ganglia on CT scans.

Case 549 illustrates a more subtle MR presentation of microangiopathy within a radiation field. Low signal intensity suggesting mild mineralization is present throughout white matter of the right parietooccipital region. Subcortical iron accumulation in an area of recent infarction may contribute to this appearance.

Another pattern of parenchymal abnormality after radiation therapy is "hemorrhagic radiation vasculopathy," resembling scattered cavernous angiomas (see discussion of Cases 761-768). This appearance, probably reflecting multiple small hemorrhages from damaged vessels, may become increasingly prominent over time.

Some cases of radiation microangiopathy respond to steroid therapy, while others are progressive. The patient illustrated in Case 549 recovered almost completely within one month.

## Case 550

45-year-old man with worsening
hemiparesis one year after treatment for
a glioma of the right temporal lobe.
(axial, postcontrast T1-weighted SE scan)

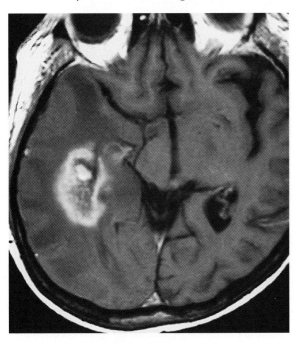

**Radiation Necrosis**

## Case 551

43-year-old woman, two years after treatment for a
malignant oligodendroglioma of the left frontal lobe.
(coronal, postcontrast T1-weighted SE scan)

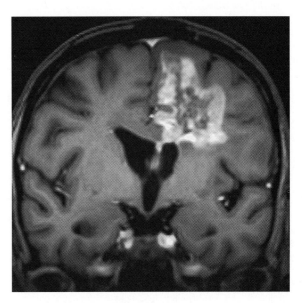

**Radiation Necrosis**

In both of the above cases, irregular peripheral enhancement of a lesion near the site of prior surgery suggests recurrent neoplasm. Associated edema and mass effect are apparent. In each case, subsequent surgery demonstrated only radiation necrosis.

Delayed tissue damage following radiation is predominantly due to fibrinoid necrosis of small arteries. White matter is typically affected more severely than gray matter. Most series suggest a threshold dose for cerebral radiation necrosis in the range of 5,500 to 6,000 cGy. Although latency of presentation may range from a few months to decades, most cases occur within two years after treatment.

The morphology, contrast enhancement, and associated edema of enlarging masses due to radiation necrosis can be indistinguishable from a tumor on standard MR images. In many cases, a combination of radiation necrosis and recurrent tumor is present. Low metabolic activity within the lesion demonstrated by positron emission tomography or single photon emission CT or reduced cerebral blood volume on perfusion-weighted MR images supports the possibility of radiation necrosis, but some recurrent tumors are also hypometabolic.

Proton spectroscopy can help to distinguish radiation necrosis from recurrent neoplasm. The spectrum from a region of necrosis is usually dominated by a lactic acid peak at 1.3 ppm, with few other definable resonances. The spectrum of recurrent tumor tissue demonstrates several recognizable molecules, usually including an abnormally large choline peak reflecting increased metabolism of cell membranes (see Case 83). A grid of small spectroscopic volumes covering the region of interest (chemical shift imaging) often discloses a mixture of necrotic and neoplastic voxels.

The granular texture of abnormal enhancement within the mass in Case 550 is a characteristic (but nonspecific) feature of radiation necrosis.

# REFERENCES

Abodollah A, Tampieri D, Melanson D: Wilson's disease: Computed tomography and magnetic resonance imaging findings. *Can Assoc Radiol J* 42:130-134, 1991.

Aisen AM, Martel LW, Gabrielsen TO, et al: Wilson's disease of the brain: MR imaging. *Radiology* 157:137-142, 1985.

Akaboshi S, Ohno K, Takeshita K: Neuroradiological findings in the carbohydrate-deficient glycoprotein syndrome. *Neuroradiology* 37:491-495, 1995.

Allard JC, Tilak S, Carter AP: CT and MR of MELAS syndrome. *AJNR* 9:1234-1238, 1988.

Angelini L, Nardocci N, Rumi V, et al: Hallervorden-Spatz disease: clinical and MR study of 11 cases diagnosed in life. *J Neurol* 239: 417-425, 1992.

Antunez E, Estruch R, Cardenal C, et al: Usefulness of CT and MR imaging in the diagnosis of acute Wernicke's encephalopathy. *Am J Roentgenol* 171:1131-1138, 1998.

Arii J, Tanabe Y: Leigh syndrome: serial MR imaging and clinical follow-up. *AJNR* 21:1502-1510, 2000.

Ashtari M, Barr WB, Schaul N, Bogerts B: Three-dimensional fast low-angle shot imaging and computerized volume measurement of the hippocampus in patients with chronic epilepsy of the temporal lobe. *AJNR* 12:941-947, 1991.

Aylward EH, Li Q, Stine OC, et al: Longitudinal change in basal ganglia volume in patients with Huntington's disease. *Neurology* 48:394-399, 1997.

Ball WS Jr, Prenger EC, Ballard ET: Neurotoxicity of radio/chemotherapy in children: pathologic and MR correlation. *AJNR* 13:761, 1992.

Barboriak DP, Provenzale JM, Boyko OB: MR diagnosis of Creutzfeldt-Jakob disease: significance of high signal intensity of the basal ganglia. *Am J Roentgenol* 162:137-140, 1994.

Barkovich AJ, Ali FA, Rowley HA, Bass N: Imaging patterns of neonatal hypoglycemia. *AJNR* 19:523-528, 1998.

Barkovich AJ, Good WV, Koch TK, Berg BO: Mitochondrial disorders: analysis of their clinical and imaging characteristics. *AJNR* 14:1119-1138, 1993.

Becker LD: Lysosomes, peroxisomes, and mitochondria: function and disorder. *AJNR* 13:609-620, 1992.

Bowen BC, Pattany PM, Bradley WG, et al: MR imaging and localized proton spectroscopy of the precentral gyrus in amyotrophic lateral sclerosis. *AJNR* 21:647-658, 2000.

Bradley WG, Shey RB: MR imaging evaluation of seizures. *Radiology* 214:651-656, 2000.

Braffman BH, Gussman RI, Goldberg HI, et al: MR imaging of Parkinson disease with spin-echo and gradient-echo sequence. *AJNR* 9:1093-1099, 1988.

Brismar J, Ozand PT: CT and MR of the brain in disorders of the propionate and methylmalonate metabolism. *AJNR* 15:1459-1473, 1994.

Brismar J, Ozand PT: CT and MR of the brain in glutaric acidemia type I: a review of 59 published cases and a report of 5 new patients. *AJNR* 16:675-684, 1995.

Brismar J, Ozand PT: CT and MR of the brain in the diagnosis of organic acidemias. Experiences from 107 patients. *Brain Dev* 16:104-124, 1994.

Bronen RA: Epilepsy: the role of imaging. *Am J Roentgenol* 159:1165-1174, 1992.

Bronen RA: MR of mesial temporal sclerosis: how much is enough? *AJNR* 19:15-18, 1998.

Bronen RA&lt; Cheung G, Charles JT, et al: Imaging findings in hippocampal sclerosis: conrrelation with pathology. *AJNR* 12:933-940, 1991.

Bronen RA, Fulbright RK, Kim JH, et al: A systematic approach for interpreting MR imaging of the seizure patient. *Am J Roentgenol* 169:241-248, 1997.

Bronen RA, Fulbright RK, Kim JH, et al: Regional distribution of MR findings in hippocampal sclerosis. *AJNR* 16:1193-1200, 1995.

Bronen RA, Fulbright RK, King D, et al: Qualitative MR imaging of refractory temporal lobe epilepsy requiring surgery: correlation with pathology and seizure outcome after surgery. *Am J Roentgenol* 169:875-882, 1997.

Bronen RA, Fulbright RK, Spencer DD, et al: Refractory epilepsy: comparison of MR imaging, CT, and histopathologic findings in 117 patients. *Radiology* 201:97-105, 1996.

Bronen RA, Fulbright RK, Spencer SS, et al: Comparison of magnetic resonance and computed tomographic imaging of refractory epilepsy: correlation with postoperative seizure outcome in 109 patients. *Int J Neurorad* 3:140-146, 1997.

Brooks BS, King DW, el Gammal T, et al: MR imaging in patients with intractable complex partial seizures. *Am J Roentgenol* 154:577-583, 1990.

Brunberg J, Kanal E, Hirsch W, Van Thiel DH: Chronic acquired hepatic failure: MR imaging of the brain at 1.5 T: *AJNR* 12:909-914, 1991.

Casey SO, Sampaio R, Michel E, Truwit CL: Posterior reversible encephalopathy syndrome: utility of fluid-attenuated inversion recovery MR imaging in the detection of cortical and subcortical lesions. *AJNR* 21:1199-1206, 2000.

Castillo M, Kwock L, Green C: MELAS syndrome: imaging and proton MR spectroscopic findings. *AJNR* 16:233-239, 1995.

Castillo M, Smith JK, Kwock L: Proton MR spectroscopy in patients with acute temporal lobe seizures. *AJNR* 22:152-157, 2001.

Cendes F, Leproux F, Melanson D, et al: MRI of amygdala and hippocampus in temporal lobe epilepsy. *J Comput Assist Tomogr* 16:206-210, 1993.

Chang KH, Han MH, Kim HS, et al: Delayed encephalopathy after acute carbon monoxide intoxication: MR imaging features and distribution of cerebral white matter lesions. *Radiology* 184: 117-122, 1992.

Chan S, Chin SSM, Kartha K, et al: Reversible signal abnormalities in the hippocampus and neocortex after prolonged seizures. *AJNR* 17:1725-1732, 1996.

Chan S, Erickson JK, Yoon SS: Limbic system abnormalities associated with mesial temporal sclerosis. *Radiographics* 17:1095-1110, 1997.

Chen JC, Hardy PA, Kucharczyk W, et al: MR of human postmortem brain tissue: correlative study between T2 and assay of iron and ferritin in Parkinson and Huntington disease. *AJNR* 14:275-282, 1993.

Cheon J-E, Chang K-H, Kim HD, et al: MR of hippocampal sclerosis: comparison of qualitative and quantitative assessments. *AJNR* 19:465-468, 1998.

Cheon J-E, Chang K-H, Won HJ, et al: Magnetic resonance imaging findings in temporal lobe epilepsy. *Int J Neurorad* 3:199-205, 1997.

Cheung G, Gawal MJ, Cooper PW, et al: Amyotrophic lateral sclerosis: correlation of clinical and MR imaging findings. *Radiology* 194:263-270, 1995.

Choi KH, Yoon YD, Jung SL, et al: Imaging and clinical findings in idiopathic intracranial hypotension. *Int J Neurorad* 4:227-232, 1998.

Chong VF-H, Fan Y-F, Mukherji SK: Radiation-induced temporal lobe changes: CT and MR imaging characteristics. *Am J Roentgenol* 175:431-436, 2000.

Christoforidis GA, Mehta BA, Landi JL, et al: Spontaneous intracranial hypotension: report of four cases and review of the literature. *Neuroradiology* 40:636-643, 1998.

Constine L, Konski A, Ekholm S, et al: Adverse effects of brain irradiation correlated with MR and CT. *Int J Radiat Oncol Biol Phys* 13:88, 1987.

Cooney MJ, Bradley WG, Symko C, et al: Hypertensive encephalopathy: complication in children treated for myeloproliferative disorders-report of three cases. *Radiology* 214:711-716, 2000.

Curnes JT, Laster DW, Ball MR, et al: Magnetic resonance imaging of radiation injury to the brain. *AJNR* 7:389-394, 1986.

D'Aprile P, Farchi G, Pagliarulo R, Carella A: Thrombotic thrombocytopenic purpura: MR demonstration of reversible brain abnormalities. *AJNR* 15:19-20, 1994.

D'Aprile P, Gentile MA, Carella A: Enhanced MR in the acute phase of Wernicke encephalopathy. *AJNR* 15:591-593, 1994.

Davis PC, Hoffman JC Jr, Braun IF, et al: MR of Leigh's disease (subacute) necrotizing encephalomyelopathy). *AJNR* 8:71-75, 1987.

De Haan J, Grossman RI, Civitello L, et al: High-field magnetic resonance imaging of Wilson's disease. *J Comput Assist Tomogr* 11:132-135, 1987.

DeLeon MJ, George AE, Golomb J, et al: Frequency of hippocampal formation atrophy in normal aging and Alzheimer's disease. *Neurobiol Aging* 18:1-11, 1997.

De Leon MJ, Golomb J, George AE, et al: The radiologic prediction of Alzheimer disease: the atrophic hippocampal formation. *AJNR* 14:897-906, 1993.

de Seze J, Mastain B, Stojkovic T, et al: Unusual MR findings of the brain stem in arterial hypertension. *AJNR* 21:391-394, 2000.

Digre KB, Varner MV, Osborn AG, Crawford S: Cranial magnetic resonance imaging in severe pre-eclampsia versus eclampsia. *Arch Neurol* 50:399-406, 1993.

Dillon WP: The reversible posterior cerebral edema syndrome. *AJNR* 19:591-592, 1998.

Dillon WP, Fishman RA: Some lessons learned about the diagnosis and treatment of spontaneous intracranial hypotension. *AJNR* 19:1001-1002, 1998.

DiRocco A, Molinari S, Stollman AL, et al: MRI abnormalities in Creutzfeldt-Jakob disease. *Neuroradiology* 35:584-585, 1993.

Donnal JF, Heinz ER, Burger PC: MR of reversible thalamic lesions in Wernicke syndrome. *AJNR* 11:893-894, 1990.

Dooms GC, Hecht S, Brant-Zawadski M, et al: Brain radiation lesions: MR imaging. *Radiology* 158:149-156, 1986.

Drayer BP: Based ganglia:significance of signal hypointensity on T2-weighted MR images. *Radiology* 173:311-312, 1989.

Drayer BP: Imaging of the aging brain. Part II. Pathologic conditions. *Radiology* 166:797-806, 1988.

Drayer BP, Olanow W, Burger P, et al: Parkinson plus syndrome: diagnosis using high field MR imaging of brain iron. *Radiology* 159:493-498, 1986.

Duguid JR, DeLa Paz R, DeGroot J: Magnetic resonance imaging of the midbrain in Parkinson's disease. *Ann Neurol* 20:744-747, 1986.

Edwards-Brown MK, Jakacki RI: Imaging the central nervous system effects of radiation and chemotherapy of pediatric tumors. *Neuroimaging Clin North Am* 9:177-194, 1999.

Erbetta A, Ciceri E, Chiapparini L, et al: Magnetic resonance imaging findings in bilirubin encephalopathy. *Int J Neurorad* 4:161-164, 1998.

Falcone S, Quencer RM, Bowen B, et al: Creutzfeldt-Jakob disease: Focal symmetrical cortical involvement demonstrated by MR imaging. *AJNR* 13:403-406, 1992.

Fazekas F, Chawluk JB, Alavi A, et al: MR signal abnormalities at 1.5 T in Alzheimer's dementia and normal aging. *AJNR* 8:421-426, 1987.

Feliciani M, Curatolo P: Early clinical and imaging (high-field MR) diagnosis of Hallervorden-Spatz disease. *NeuroRadiology* 36:247-248, 1994.

Finkenstaedt M, Szudra A, Zerr I, et al: MR imaging of Creutzfeldt-Jakob disease. *Radiology* 199:793-798, 1996.

Fishman RA, Dillon WP: Dural enhancement and cerebral displacement secondary to intracranial hypotenion. *Neuroradiology* 43:609-611, 1993.

Galluci M, Bozzao A, Splendiani A, et al: Follow-up in Wernicke's encephalopat. *Neuroradiology* 33 (Suppl):594-595, 1991.

Galluci M, Bozzao A, Splendiani A, et al: Wernicki enceophalopathy: MR finding in five patients. *AJNR* 11:887-892, 1990.

Galluci M, Cardona F, Arachi M, et al: Follow-up MR studies in Hallervorden-Spatz disease. *J Comput Assist Tomogr* 14:118-120, 1990.

Gaul HP, Wallace CJ, Auer RN, Fong TC: MR findings in methanol intoxication. *AJNR* 16:1783-1786, 1995.

Genovese E, Maghnie M, Maggiore G, et al: MR imaging of CNS involvement in children affected by chronic liver disease. *AJNR* 21:845-851, 2000.

George AE, de Leon MJ, Golomb J, et al: Imaging the brain in dementia: expensive and futile? *AJNR* 18:1847-1849, 1997.

George AE, DeLeon MV, Kalnin A, et al: Leukoencephalopathy in normal and pathologic aging. 2. MRI of brain lucencies. *AJNR* 7:567-570, 1986.

Gertz HJ, Henkes H, Cervos-Navarro J: Creutzfeldt-Jakob disease: correlation of MRI and neuropathologic findings. *Neurology* 38:1481-1482, 1988.

Geyer CA, Sartor KH, Prensky AJ, et al: Leigh disease (subacute necrotizing encephalomyelopathy): CT and MR in five cases. *J Comput Assist Tomogr* 12:40-44, 1988.

Gibby WA, Stecker MM, Goldberg HI, et al: Reversal of white matter edema in hypertensive encephalopathy. *AJNR* 10:578, 1989.

Goodin DS, Rowley Ha, Olney RK: Magnetic resonance imaging in amyotrophic lateral sclerosis. *Ann Neurol* 23:418-420, 1988.

Goyal M, Versnick E, Tuite P, et al: Hypertrophic olivary degeneration: metaanalysis of the temporal evolution of MR findings. *AJNR* 21:1073-1077, 2000.

Grattan-Smith JD, Harvey AS, Desmond PM, Chow CW: Hippocampal sclerosis in children with intractable temporal lobe epilepsy: detection with MR imaging. *Am J Roentgenol* 161:1045-1048, 1993.

Grunewald RA, Jackson GD, Connelly A, Duncan JS: MR detection of hippocampal disease in epilepsy: factors influencing T2 relaxation time. *AJNR* 15:1149-1156, 1994.

Hanner JS, Li KCP, Davis GL: Acquired hepatocerebral degeneration: MR similarity with Wilson disease. *J Comput Assist Tomogr* 12:1076-1077, 1988.

Harris GJ, Pearlson GD, Peyser CE, et al: Putamen volume reduction on magnetic resonance imaging exceeds caudate changes in mild Huntington's disease. *Ann Neurol* 31:69-75, 1992.

Harter SB, Nokes SR: Gadolinium-enhanced MR findings in a pediatric case of Wernicke encephalopathy. *AJNR* 16:700-702, 1995.

Hayman LA, Fuller GN, Cavazos JE, et al: The hippocampus: normal anatomy and pathology. *Am J Roentgenol* 171:1139-1146, 1998.

Hecht-Leavitt C, Grossman R, Curran W, et al: MR of brain radiation injury. *AJNR* 8:427, 1987.

Heckmann JM, Eastman R, Handler L, et al: Leigh disease (subacute necrotizing encephalomyelopathy): MR documentation of the evolution of an acute attack. *AJNR* 14:1157-1159, 1993.

Heinz E, Heinz R, et al: Efficacy of MR vs. CT in epilepsy. *AJNR* 9:1123, 1988.

Heinz R, Ferris N, Lee EK, et al: MR and position emission tomography in the diagnosis of surgically correctable temporal lobe epilepsy. *AJNR* 15:1341-1348, 1994.

Hirai T, Korogi Y, Yoshizumi K, et al: Limbic lobe of the human brain: evaluation with turbo fluid-attenuated inversion-recovery MR imaging. *Radiology* 215:470-475, 2000.

Ho VB, Chuang HS, Rovira MJ, Koo B: Juvenile Huntington disease: CT and MR features. *AJNR* 16:1405-1412, 1995.

Ho VB, Fitz CR, Chuang SH, Geyer CA: Bilateral basal ganglia lesions: pediatric differential considerations. *Radiographics* 13:269-292, 1993.

Hofmann E, Ochs G, Pelzl A, Warmuth-Metz M: The corticospinal tract in amyotrophic lateral sclerosis: an MRI study. *Neuroradiology* 40:71-75, 1998.

Holodny AI, George AE, Golomb J, et al: The perihippocampal fissures: normal anatomy and disease states. *Radiographics* 18:653-665, 1998.

Huber SJ, Chakeres DW, Paulson GW, Khanna R: Magnetic resonance imaging in Parkinson's disease. *Arch Neurol* 47:735-737, 1990.

Huber SJ, Shuttleworth EC, Christy JA, et al: Magnetic resonance imaging in dementia of Parkinson's disease. *J Neurol Neurosug Psychiatr* 52:1221-1227, 1989.

Hughes DG, Chadderton RD, Cowle RA, et al: MRI of the brain and craniocervical junction in Morquio's disease. *Neuroradiology* 39:381-385, 1997.

Hutchinson M, Raff U: Structural changes of the substantia nigra in Parkinson's disease as revealed by MR imaging. *AJNR* 21:697-701, 2000.

Inoue E, Hori S, Narumi Y, et al: Portal-systemic encephalopathy: presence of basal ganglia lesions with high signal intensity on MR images. *Radiology* 179:551-555, 1991.

Inoue Y, Matsumura Y, Fukuda T, et al: MR imaging of the Wallerian degeneration in the brainstem: temporal relationships. *AJNR* 11:897-902, 1990.

Jack CR, Petersen RC, O'Brien PC, Tangalos, EG: MR-based hippocampal volumetry in the diagnosis of Alzheimer's disease. *Neurology* 42:183, 1992.

Jack CR Jr, Krecke KN, Luetmer PH, et al: Diagnosis of mesial temporal sclerosis with conventional versus fast spin-echo MR imaging. *Radiology* 192:123-128, 1994.

Jack CR Jr, Rydberg CH, Krecke KN, et al: Mesial temporal sclerosis: diagnosis with fluid-attenuated inversion-recovery versus spin-echo MR imaging. *Radiology* 199:367-374, 1996.

Jackson GD, Berkovic SF, Duncan JS, Connelly A: Optimizing the diagnosis of hippocampal sclerosis using MR imaging. *AJNR* 14:753-762, 1993.

Jarosz JM, Howlett DC, Cox TCS, Bingham JB: Cyclosporine-related reversible posterior leukoencephalopathy: MRI. *Neuroradiology* 39:711-715, 1997.

Jensen PR, Hansen FJ, Skovby F: Cerebellar hypoplasia in children with the carbohydrate-deficient glycoprotein syndrome. *Neuroradiology* 37:328-330, 1995.

Jones BV, Egelhoff JC, Patterson RJ: Hypertensive encephalopathy in children. *AJNR* 18:101-106, 1997.

Kantarci K, Jack CR, Xu YC, et al: Mild cognitive impairment and Alzheimer disease: regional diffusivity of water. *Radiology* 219:101-107, 2001.

Kendall BE: Disorders of lysosomes, peroxisomes, and mitochomdria. *AJNR* 13:621-653, 1992.

Kido DK, Tien RD, Lee B, Bahn MM: Hippocampal pathology. *Neuroimaging Clin North Am* 7:51-66, 1997.

Kim J-A, Chung JI, Yoon PH, et al: Transient MR signal changes in patients with generalized tonicoclonic seizure or status epilepticus: periictal diffusion-weighted imaging. *AJNR* 22:1149-1160, 2001.

Kim JH, Tien RD, Felsberg GJ, et al: Clinical significance of asymmetry of the fornix and mamillary body on MR in hippocampal sclerosis. *AJNR* 16:509-516, 1995.

Kim I-O, Kim JH, Kim WS, et al: Mitochondrial myopathy-encephalopathy-lactic acidosis-and strokelike episodes (MELAS) syndrome: CT and MR findings in seven children. *Am J Roentgenol* 166:641-646, 1996.

King AD, Walshe JM, Kendall BE, et al: Cranial MR imaging in Wilson's disease. *Am J Roentgenol* 167:1579-1584, 1996.

Kitajima M, Korogi Y, Shimomura O, et al: Hypertrophic olivary degeneration: MR imaging and pathologic findings. *Radiology* 192:539-544, 1994.

Kodama K, Murakami A, Yamanouchi N, et al: MR in temporal lobe epilepsy: early childhood onset versus later onset. *AJNR* 16:523-530, 1995.

Koskinen T, Valanne L, Ketonen LM, Pihko H: Infantile-onset spinocerebellar ataxia: MR and CT findings. *AJNR* 16:1427-1434, 1995.

Kovanen J, Erkinjuntti T, Iivanainen M, et al: Cerebral MR and CT imaging in Creutzfeldt-Jakob disease. *J Comput Assist Tomogr* 9:125-128, 1985.

Krageloh-Mann I, Grodd W, Niemann G, et al: Assessment and therapy monitoring of Leigh disease by MRI and proton spectroscopy. *Pediatr Neuro* 8:60-64, 1992.

Kuhn MJ, Johnson KA, Davis KK: Wallerian degeneration: evaluation with MR imaging. *Radiology* 168:199-202, 1988.

Kuhn MJ, Mikulis DJ, Ayoub DM, et al: Wallerian degeneration after cerebral infarction: evaluation with sequential imaging. *Radiology* 172:179-182, 1989.

Kulisevsky J, Pugol J, Balanzo J: Pallidal hyperintensity on magnetic resonance imaging in cirrhotic patients: clinical correlations. *Hepatology* 16:1382-1388, 1992.

Kulisevsky J, Ruscalleda J, Grau JM:MR imaging of acquired hepatocerebral degeneration. *AJNR* 12:527-528, 1991.

Kuteifan K, Oesterle H, Tajahmady T, et al: Necrosis and haemorrhage of the putamen in methanol poisoning shown on MRI. *Neuroradiology* 40:158-160, 1998.

Lai PH, Chen C, Liang HL, Pan HB: Hyperintense basal ganglia on T1-weighted MR imaging. *Am J Roentgenol* 172:1109-1116, 1999.

Lee BCP: Magnetic resonance imaging of metabolic and primary white matter disorders in children. *Neuroimaging Clin N Amer* 3:267-289, 1993.

Lee C, Dineen TE, Brack M, et al: The mucopolysaccharidoses: characterization by cranial MR imaging. *AJNR* 14:1285-1292, 1993.

Lee DH, Gao F-Q, Rogers JM, et al: MR in temporal lobe epilepsy; analysis with pathologic confirmation. *AJNR* 19:19-28, 1998.

Lee HK, Chang KH, Na DG, Han MH: MR imaging findings of Wernicke's encephalopathy in non-alcoholic patients. *Int J Neurorad* 2:210-215, 1996.

Lee J, Lacomis D, Comu S, Jacobsohn J, Kanal E: Acquired hepatocerebral degeneration: MR and pathologic findings. *AJNR* 19:485-487, 1998.

Lehericy S, Semah F, Hasboun D, et al: Temporal lobe epilepsy with varying severity: MRI study of 222 patients. *Neuroradiology* 39:788-796, 1997.

Littrup PJ, Gebarski SS: MR imaging of Hallervorden-Spatz disease. *J Comput Assist Tomogr* 9:491, 1985.

Maeda H, Sato M, Yoshikawa A, et al: Brain MR imaging in patients with hepatic cirrhosis: relationship between high intensity signal in basal ganglia on T1-weighted images and elemental concentrations in brain. *Neuroradiology* 39:546-555, 1997.

Mamourian AC, Cho CH, Saykin AJ, Poppito NL: Association between size of lateral ventricle and asymmetry of the fornix in patients with temporal lobe epilepsy. *AJNR* 19:9-14, 1998.

Mamourian AC, Rodichok L, Towfiahi J: The asymmetric mamillary body: association with medial temporal lobe disease demonstrated with MR. *AJNR* 16:517-522, 1995.

Martich-Kriss V, Kollias SS, Ball WS Jr: MR findings in kernicterus. *AJNR* 16:819-820, 1995.

Mascalchi M, Simonelli P, Tessa C, et al: Do acute lesions of Wernicke's encephalopathy show contrast enhancement? Report of three cases and review of the literature. *Neuroradiology* 41:249-254, 1999.

Medina L, Chi TL, DeVivo DC, Hilal SK: MR findings in patients with subacute necrotizing encephalomyelopathy (Leigh syndrome): correlation with biochemical defect. *AJNR* 11:379-384, 1990.

Meiners LC, van Gils A, Jansen GH, et al: Temporal lobe epilepsy: the various MR appearances of histologically proven medial temporal sclerosis. *AJNR* 15:1547-1555. 1994.

Men S, Lee DH, Barron JR, Munoz DG: Selective neuronal necrosis associated with status epilepticus: MR findings. *AJNR* 21:1837-1840, 2000.

Mirowitz S, Sartor K, Gado MG, et al: Focal signal-intensity variations in the posterior internal capsule: normal MR findings and distinction from pathologic findings. *Radiology* 172:535-539, 1989.

Mirowitz SA, Westric TJ: Basal ganglial signal intensity alterations: reversal after discontinuation of parenteral manganese administration. *Radiology* 185:525-526, 1992.

Miyamoto A, Oki J, Takahashi S, et al: Serial imaging in MELAS. *Neuroradiology* 39:427-430, 1997.

Mokri B, Piepgras DG, Miller GM: Syndrome of orthostatic headache and diffuse pachymeningeal gadolinium enhancement. *Mayo Clin Proc* 72:400-413, 1997.

Moore KR, Osborn AG, Townsend JJ, et al: The imaging and pathologic spectrum of hemolytic-uremic syndrome-thrombotic thrombocytopenic purpura (HUS-TTP syndrome). *Int J Neurorad* 3:147-159, 1997.

Moore KR, Swallow CE, Tsuruda JS: Incidental detection of hippocampal sclerosis on MR images: is it significant? *AJNR* 20:1609-1612, 1999.

Moser FG, Hilal SK, Abrams G, et al: MR imaging of pseudotumor cerebri. *AJNR* 9:39-46, 1988.

Munoz A, Mateos F, Simon R, et al: Mitochondrial diseases in children: neuroradiological and clinical features in 17 patients. *Neuroradiology* 41:920-928, 1999.

Murata R, Nakajima S, Tanaka A, et al: MR imaging of the brain in patients with mucopolysaccharidosis. *AJNR* 10:1165-1170, 1989.

Naegele T, Grodd W, Viebahn R, et al: MR imaging and 1H spectroscopy of brain metabolites in hepatic encephalopathy: timecourse of renormalization after liver transplantation. *Radiology* 216:683-691, 2000.

Naidu SB, Moser HW: Value of neuroimaging on metabolic diseases in affecting the CNS. *AJNR* 12:413-416, 1991.

Nazer H, Brismar J, Al-Kawi MZ, et al: Magnetic resonance imaging of the brain in Wilson's disease. *Neuroradiology* 35:130-133, 1993.

Norris AM, Carrington BM, Slevin NJ: Late radiation change in the CNS: MR imaging following gadolinium enhancement. *Clin Radiol* 52:356-362, 1997.

Oba H, Araki T, Ohtomo K, et al: Amyotrophic lateral sclerosis: T2 shortening in motor cortex at MR imaging. *Radiology* 189:834-846, 1993.

Oba H, Araki T, Ohtomo K, et al: Amyotrophic lateral sclerosis: T2-shortening in motor cortex at MR imaging. *Radiology* 189:843-846, 1993.

O'Connor MM, Mayberg MR: Effects of radiation on cerebral vasculature: a review. *Neurosurgery* 46:138-151, 2000.

Ogura H, Takaoka M, Kishi M, et al: Reversible MR findings of hemolytic uremic syndrome with mild encephalopathy. *AJNR* 19:1144-1146, 1998.

Oppenheim C, Dormont D, Biondi A, et al: Loss of digitation of the hippocampal head on high-resolution fast spin-echo MR: a sign of mesial temporal sclerosis. *AJNR* 19:457-464, 1998.

Orita T, Tsurutani T, Izumihara A, Matsunaga T: Coronal MR imaging for visualization of Wallerian degeneration of the pyramidal tract. *J Comput Assist Tomogr* 15:802-804, 1991.

Pannullo SC, Reich JB, Krol G, et al: MRI changes in intracranial hypotension. *Neurology* 43:919-926, 1993.

Pastakia B, Polinsky R, DiChiro G, et al: Multiple system atrophy (Shy-Drager syndrome): MR imaging. *Radiology* 159:499-505, 1986.

Pavone L, Fiumara A, Barone R, et al: Olivopontocerebellar atrophy leading to recognition of carbohydrate-deficient glycoprotein syndrome type I. *J Neurol* 243:700-705, 1996.

Pearl GS, Anderson RE: Creutzfeldt-Jakob disease: high caudate signal on magnetic resonance imaging. *South Med J* 82:1177-1180, 1989.

Peretti-Viton P, Azulay JP, Trefouret S, et al: MRI of the intracranial corticospinal tracts in amyotrophic and primary lateral sclerosis. *Neuroradiology* 41:744-749, 1999.

Port JD, Beauchamp NJ: Reversible intracerebral pathologic entities mediated by vascular autoregulatory dysfunction. *Radiographics* 18:353-367, 1998.

Porter-Grenn L, Silbergleit R, Mehta BA: Hallervorden-Spatz disease with bilateral involvement of globus pallidus and substantia nigra: MR demonstration. *J Comput Assist Tomogr* 17:961-963, 1993.

Poussaint TY, Siffert J, Barnes PD, et al: Hemorrhagic vasculopathy after treatment of central nervous system neoplasia in childhood: diagnosis and follow-up. *AJNR* 16:693-699, 1995.

Pujol JA, Pujol J, Graus F, et al: Hyperintense globus pallidus on T1-weighted MRI in cirrhotic patients is associated with severity of liver failure. *Neurology* 43:65-69, 1993.

Rabin BM, Meyer JR, Berlin JW, et al: Radiation-induced changes in the central nervous system and head and neck. *Radiographics* 16:1055-1072, 1996.

Regis J, Semah F, Bryan RN, et al: Early and delayed MR and PET changes after selective temporomesial radiosurgery in mesial temporal lobe epilepsy. *AJNR* 20:213-216, 1999.

Revel MP, Mann M, Brugieres P, et al: MR appearance of hypertrophic olivary degeneration after contraloateral cerebellar hemorrhage. *AJNR* 12:71-72, 1991.

Rosen L, Phillipo S, Enzmann DR: Magnetic resonance imaging in MELAS syndrome. *Neuroradiology* 32:168, 1990.

Rubinstein D, Escott E, Kelly JP: Methanol intoxication with putaminal and white matter necrosis: MR and CT findings. *AJNR* 16:1492-1494, 1995.

Rusinek H, DeLeon MJ, George AE, et al: Alzheimer disease: measuring loss of cerebral gray matter with MR imaging. *Radiology* 178:109-114, 1991.

Rutledge JN, Hilal SK, Silver AJ, et al: Study of movement disorders and brain iron by MR. *AJNR* 8:397-411, 1987.

Salamon-Murayama N, Russell EJ, Rabin BM: Hypertrophic olivary degeneration secondary to pontine hemorrhage. *Radiology* 213:814-818, 1999.

Sandhu FS, Dillon WP: MR demonstration of leukoencephalopathy associated with mitochondrial encephalopathy: case report. *AJNR* 12:385-379, 1991.

Savoiardo M, Grisoli M, Girotti F, et al: MRI in sporadic olivopontocerebellar atrophy and striatonigral degeneration. *Neurology* 48:790-791, 1997.

Savoiardo M, Halliday WC, Nardocci N, et al: Hallervorden-Spatz disease: MR and pathologic findings. *AJNR* 14:155-162, 1993.

Savoiardo M, Strada L, Girotti F, et al: MR imaging in progressive supranuclear palsy and Shy-Drager syndrome. *J Comput Assist Tomogr* 13:555-560, 1989.

Savoiardo M, Strada L, Girotti F, et al: Olivopontocerebellar atrophy: MR diagnosis and relationship to multisystem atrophy. *Radiology* 174:693-696, 1990.

Schaffert DA, Johnsen SD, Johnson PC, et al: Magnetic resonance imaging in pathologically proven Hallervorden-Spatz disease. *Neurology* 39:440-442, 1989.

Schroth G, Wichmann W, Valavanis A: Blood-brain-barrier disruption in acute Wernicke encephalopathy: MR findings. *J Comput Assist Tomogr* 15:1059-1061, 1991.

Schwaighofer BW, Hesselink JR, Healy ME: MR demonstration of reversible brain abnormalities in eclampsia. *J Comput Assist Tomogr* 13:310-312, 1989.

Schwartz RB, Feske SK, Polak JF, et al: Preeclampsia-eclampsia: clinical and neuroradiographic correlates and insights into the pathogenesis of hypertensive encephalopathy. *Radiology* 217:371-376, 2000.

Schwartz RB, Jones KM, Kalina P, et al: Hypertensive encephalopathy: findings on CT, MR imaging and SPECT imaging in 14 cases. *Am J Roentgenol* 159:379-383, 1992.

Schwartz RB, Mulkern RV, Gudbjartsson H, Jolesz F: Diffusion-weighted MR imaging in hypertensive encephalopathy: clues to pathogenesis. *AJNR* 19:859-862, 1998.

Sethi KD, Adams RJ, Loring DW, et al: Hallervorden-Spatz syndrome: clinical and magnetic resonance imaging correlations. *Ann Neurol* 24:692-694, 1988.

Sherman JL, Clawson LL, Citrin CH, et al: MR evaluation of amyotrophic lateral sclerosis (ALS). *AJNR* 8:941, 1987.

Shogry MEC, Curnes JT, Mamillary body enhancement of MR as the only sign of acute Wernicke encephalopathy. *AJNR* 15:172-174, 1994.

Silbergleit T, Junck L, Gebarski S, Hatfield MK: Idiopathic intracranial hypertension (pseudotumor cerebri):MR imaging. *Radiology* 170:207-210, 1989.

Silverstein AW, Alexander JA: Acute postictal cerebral imaging. *AJNR* 19:1485-1488, 1998.

Simmons JT, Pastakia B, Chase TN, Shults CW: Magnetic resonance imaging in Huntington disease. *AJNR* 7:25-28, 1986.

Sishman RA, Dillon WP: Dural enhancement and cerebral displacement secondary to intracranial hypotension. *Neuroradiology* 43:609-611, 1993.

Spar JA, Lewine JD, Orrison WW Jr: Neonatal hypoglycemia: CT and MR findings. *AJNR* 15:1477-1478, 1994.

Starkstein SE, Brandt J, Bylsma F, et al: Neuropsycological correlates of brain atrophy in Huntington's disease: a magnetic resonance imaging study. *Neuroradiology* 34:487-489, 1992.

Stern MB, Braffman BH, Skolnick BE, et al: Magnetic resonance imaging in Parkinson's disease and parkisonian syndromes. *Neurology* 39:1524-1526, 1989.

Suzuki H, Takanashi J-I, Kobayashi K, et al: MR imaging of idiopathic intracranial hypertension. *AJNR* 22:196-199, 2001.

Thuomas KA, Acquilonius SM, Bergstrom K, Westermark K: Magnetic resonance imaging of the brain in Wilson's disease. *Neuroradiology* 35:134-141, 1993.

Tien RD, Felsberg GJ: The hippocampus in status epilepticus: demonstration of signal intensity and morphologic changes with sequential fast spin-echo MR imaging. *Radiology* 194:249-256, 1995.

Tien RD, Felsberg GJ, Compi De Castro C, et al: Complex partial seizures and mesial temporal sclerosis: evaluation with fast spin-echo MR imaging. *Radiology* 189:835-842, 1993.

Tien RD, Felsberg GJ, Ferris NJ, Osumi AK: The dementias: correlation of clinical features, pathophysiology, and neuroradiology. *Am J Roentgenol* 161:245-255, 1993.

Tien RD, Felsberg GJ, Osumi AK, et al: Fast spin-echo MR in hippocampal sclerosis: correlation with pathology and surgery. *AJNR* 16:627-636, 1995.

Truwit CL, Denaro CP, Lake JR, DeMarco T: MR imaging of reversible cyclosporin A-induced neurotoxicity. *AJNR* 12:651-659, 1991.

Tsuruda JS, Kortman KE, Bradley WG, et al: Radiation effects in cerebral white matter: MR evaluation. *AJNR* 8:431-438, 1987.

Uchino A, Hasuo K, Uchida K, et al: Olivary degeneration after cerebellar or brain stem haemorrhage: MRI. *Neuroradiology* 35:335-338, 1993.

Udaka F, Sawada H, Seriu N, et al: MRI and SPECT findings in amyotrophic lateral sclerosis: demonstration of upper motor neuron involvement by clinical neuroimaging. *Neuroradiology* 34:389-393, 1992.

Urbach H, Klisch J, Wolf HK, et al: MRI in sporadic Creutzfeldt-Jakob disease: correlation with clinical and neuropathological data. *Neuroradiology* 40:65-70, 1998.

Valanne L, Ketonen L, Majander A, et al: Neuroradiologic findings in children with mitochondrial disorders. *AJNR* 19:369-377, 1998.

Valk PE, Dillon WP: Review article. Radiation injury of the brain. *AJNR* 12:45-62, 1991.

Valk J, Van der Knapp MS: Toxic encephalopathy. *AJNR* 13:747-760, 1992.

Van der Knapp MS, Valk J: The MR spectrum of peroxisomal disorders. *Neuroradiology* 33:30-37, 1991.

van Wassenaer-van Hall HN, van den Heuvel AG, Algra A, et al: Wilson's disease: findings at MR imaging and CT of the brain with clinical correlation. *Radiology* 198:531-536, 1996.

van Wassenaer-van Hall HN, van den Heuvel AG, Jansen GH, et al: Cranial MR in Wilson disease: abnormal white matter in extrapyramidal and pyramidal tracts. *AJNR* 16:2021-2027, 1995.

Vymazal J, Babis M, Brooks RA, et al: T1 and T2 alterations in the brains of patients with hepatic cirrhosis. *AJNR* 17:333-336, 1996.

Waragai M: MRI and clinical features in amyotrophic lateral sclerosis. *Neuroradiology* 39:847-851, 1997.

Weingarten K, Barbut K, Filippi C, Zimmerman RD: Acute hypertensive encephalopathy: findings on spin-echo and gradient-echo MR imaging. *Am J Roentgenol* 162:665-670, 1994.

Yaffe K, Ferriero D, Barkovich AJ, Rowley H: Reversible MRI abnormalities following seizures. *Neurology* 45:104-108, 1995.

Yagishita A, Nakano I, Oda M, Hirano A: Location of the corticospinal tract in the internal capsule at MR imaging. *Radiology* 191:455-460, 1994.

Yue NC, Arnold AM, Longstreth WT Jr, et al: Sulcal, ventricular, and white matter changes at MR imaging in the aging brain: data from the cardiovascular health study. *Radiology* 202:33-40, 1997.

# CHAPTER 11

# Cerebral Infarction

### Case 552

14-month-old girl presenting with a
one-day history of hemiparesis.
(sagittal, noncontrast T1-weighted SE scan)

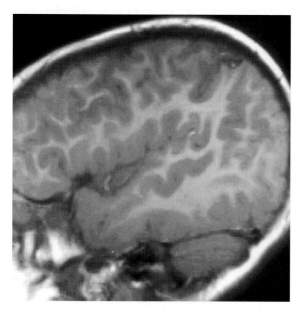

**Acute Infarct**
(MCA distribution)

### Case 553

73-year-old woman presenting one day
after the acute onset of confusion.
(sagittal, noncontrast T1-weighted SE scan)

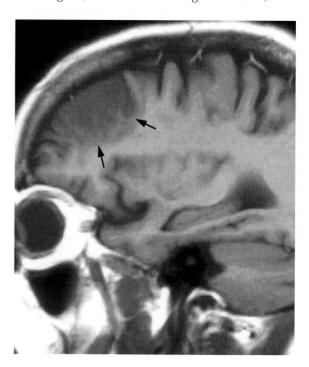

**Acute Infarct**
(MCA branch distribution)

---

The MR appearance of cerebral infarction evolves over time. The rate and nature of these changes are characteristic and may be used to identify an initially ambiguous lesion.

Standard spin echo scans are usually normal within the first few hours after infarction. The rapid development of edema within infarcted cortex soon causes swelling and prolongation of T1 and T2 values. These findings are usually perceptible on routine spin echo images within six hours after the onset of a clinical deficit.

Even earlier MR evidence of acute cerebral infarction can be provided by diffusion and/or perfusion imaging (see Cases 560 to 563), or by findings of reduced flow in major vessels.

The pattern of ischemic edema in an area of recent infarction is often gyriform, as seen in Case 552. Cortex throughout the distribution of the middle cerebral artery is thicker and darker than the normal gray matter at the frontal and occipital poles. This "super normal" appearance reflects the longer T1 values and mild mass effect caused by cortical edema. CT scans at this early stage of infarction would demonstrate blurring of the normal gray/white matter interface by developing edema and indistinct sulcal markings reflecting mild gyral swelling.

In other cases, a zone of ischemic edema appears confluent or solid. This morphology may mimic a mass lesion (compare Case 553 to Case 71). Clues to the correct diagnosis include the clinical context of an acute neurological event and the peripherally based, often wedge-shaped involvement of tissue extending to the termination of a vascular distribution.

### Case 554

34-year-old woman, one day after the
onset of left hemiparesis.
(axial, noncontrast T2-weighted SE scan)

### Case 555

2-month-old boy, twelve hours after
the onset of right hemiparesis.
(axial, noncontrast T2-weighted SE scan)

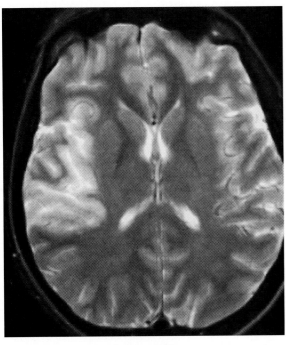

**Acute Infarct**
(MCA distribution)

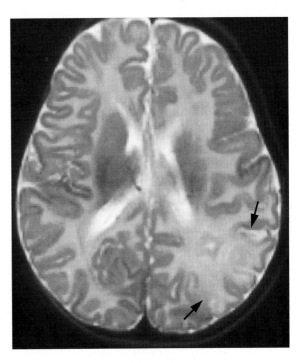

**Acute Infarct**
(MCA branch distribution)

Case 554 presents the T2-weighted equivalent of the pattern demonstrated in Case 552. Cortical edema within a recent infarct is seen as a gyriform increase in signal intensity in the right sylvian region. Involved cortex is thickened or swollen, although there is no overall mass effect.

The MR demonstration of gyral edema may clarify the etiology of ambiguous zones of low attenuation on CT studies. However, a gyriform pattern of signal abnormality can be noted in nonvascular lesions (see Cases 77 and 78).

Ischemic cortical edema in infants may be much less obvious on T2-weighted scans than in older children or adults. The normal high water content of immature white matter provides little contrast to overlying edema within ischemic gray matter. Careful attention is required to recognize cortical infarction in infants as an area of *reduced* cortical

definition. Conversely, preservation of a normally defined cortical ribbon is reassuring evidence that the watery appearance of underlying white matter does not represent edema from an arterial occlusion.

In Case 555, infarcted cortex of the left parietal lobe is "washed-out" or partially "erased" as compared with other areas of the brain *(arrows)*. This finding is most apparent at the depths of sulci in the affected region. (The tops of gyri are normally better perfused than the depths of sulci in the neonatal period.)

The demonstration of ischemic edema does not necessarily imply cerebral infarction. MR has documented reversible prolongation of T1 and T2 values correlating with transient clinical deficits in patients who have suffered temporary vascular insults.

# DIFFERENTIAL DIAGNOSIS:
## GYRIFORM CORTICAL EDEMA

### Case 556

2-year-old girl presenting with irritability and
fever two weeks after adenoidectomy.
(sagittal, noncontrast T1-weighted SE scan)

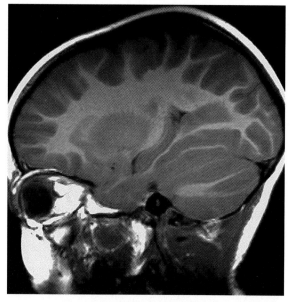

**Bacterial Meningitis**

### Case 557

9-year-old boy presenting with acute hemiparesis.
(sagittal, noncontrast T1-weighted SE scan)

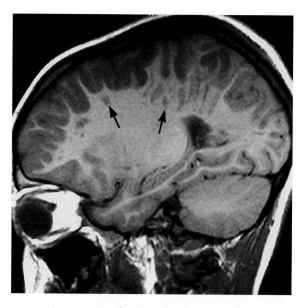

**Border Zone Infarct**

Although gyriform cortical edema is characteristic of recent infarction, other pathologies can cause a similar appearance. Superficial cerebral edema may develop secondary to overlying meningeal disease (i.e., meningitis or
meningeal carcinomatosis), encephalitis, or cortical neoplasms.

The "super normal" cortex in Case 556 indicates increased water content. This edema may be reactive or
reflect accompanying superficial cerebritis, with a possible
additional component of ischemia due to inflammation of
small cortical arteries. Restricted diffusion has been
demonstrated within edematous cortex in regions of
meningitis on diffusion-weighted scans.

The boy in Case 557 has sickle cell anemia, which is often associated with arteriopathy involving the circle of

Willis (see Case 585). His ipsilateral internal carotid artery
was tightly stenotic, and the gyriform cortical edema of the
parasagittal frontal lobe was due to acute border zone or
"watershed" infarction (see Cases 584-587). Old intrahemispheric border zone infarcts *(arrows)* are also apparent (see Cases 588 and 589).

When gyriform edema extends beyond the distribution
of a single major cerebral artery (as in the above cases), the
differential diagnosis includes occlusion or stenosis of the
internal carotid artery, multifocal infarction due to emboli
or vasculitis (see Case 642), anoxia (see Cases 661, 662,
667, and 668), superficial inflammation (as in Case 556; see
also Cases 426 and 427), and infiltrating neoplasm (see
Cases 77, 78, and 558).

# DIFFERENTIAL DIAGNOSIS (CONTINUED): GYRIFORM CORTICAL EDEMA

## Case 558

37-year-old man presenting with
sudden disorientation.
(axial, noncontrast scan; SE 2500/45)

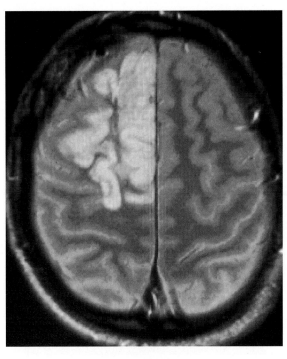

**Grade II Astrocytoma**
(recurrent)

## Case 559

28-year-old woman presenting with acute confusion.
(axial, noncontrast T2-weighted SE scan)

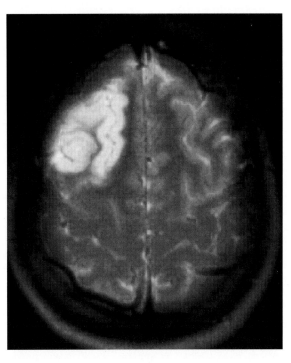

**Infarct**
(anterior division MCA distribution)

---

Gyriform edema is a typical MR finding in subacute infarction and can help to characterize an otherwise ambiguous lesion. Conformity to a vascular distribution is another key distinguishing feature.

Case 558 demonstrates that infiltrating tumors can also present with gyriform morphology (see Cases 77 and 78 for additional examples). The pattern of superficial edema in this case is compatible with infarction, but the lesion crosses the cortical watershed between the anterior and middle cerebral arteries. This lack of conformity to a single arterial territory should raise consideration of carotid occlusion, multifocal infarction due to emboli or arteritis, or nonvascular etiologies. An old right frontal craniotomy flap suggests the diagnosis in this patient.

The subacute infarction in Case 559 demonstrates characteristic cortical edema with relative sparing of subcortical white matter. The lesion is confined to the distribution of the anterior division of the middle cerebral artery. The medial margin of the infarct defines the watershed with the

anterior cerebral artery (see Case 580). This anatomical boundary has been displaced medially by swelling of the involved tissue.

Mass effect develops during the first week after cerebral infarction, most commonly after a few days have elapsed. If the patient is first scanned at this time and the clinical context is ambiguous, the possibility of a neoplasm may be raised on CT studies. MR scans can resolve the issue by demonstrating characteristic gyriform edema and/or laminar necrosis (see Case 572) within subacute infarcts. Diffusion-weighted scans (see Cases 560 and 561) often help to establish an ischemic etiology for nonspecific edema.

Angiography in Case 559 demonstrated a dissection of the distal right internal carotid artery. Embolization of thrombus from the site of a dissection is one of the important causes of cerebrovascular accidents in young patients. Reduced flow due to narrowing of the lumen at the site of a dissection rarely produces symptoms in the absence of emboli.

### Case 560

67-year-old man presenting with left hemiparesis.
(axial, noncontrast diffusion-weighted
echoplanar scan)

### Case 561

80-year-old woman with multiple neurological
deficits after cardiac surgery.
(axial, noncontrast diffusion-weighted
echoplanar scan)

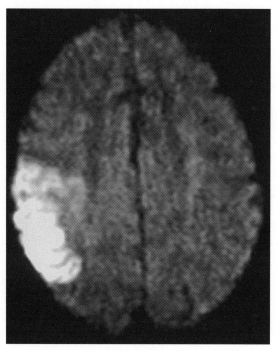

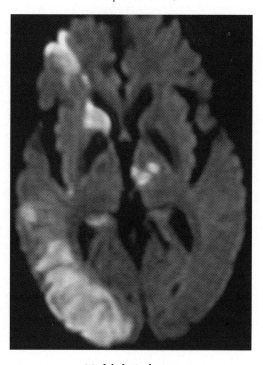

**Infarct**
(posterior division MCA distribution)

**Multiple Infarcts**

Diffusion-weighted scans are more sensitive than T1- or T2-weighted images in demonstrating lesions within the first few hours after cerebral infarction.

Zones of high signal intensity on diffusion-weighted images reflect abnormally restricted movement of water molecules. Note that the measure of molecular diffusion, the "apparent diffusion coefficient" or "ADC," is altered in the direction opposite to the change in signal intensity; in an area of restricted diffusion, the ADC is decreased.

The mechanism of increased diffusion-weighted signal intensity (and reduced ADC) in an area of acute infarction is thought to involve cellular swelling secondary to failure of energy-dependent sodium/potassium pumps of the cell membrane. Cytotoxic edema occurs as water moves from the extracellular space into the intracellular compartment. Since the movement of intracellular water molecules is more restricted by organelles and proteins than the movement of extracellular water, a relative increase in the former and decrease in the latter causes an overall decrease in the net diffusibility of protons in the affected region. An increase of intracellular "viscosity" or "tortuosity" for dif-

fusion of water molecules may also contribute to the decreased ADC of ischemic tissue.

In experimental models, diffusion-weighted scans are abnormal within minutes of cerebral infarction. Clinical studies demonstrate restricted diffusion in nearly all patients with acute infarcts. However, false negative scans occur, particularly when infarcts are small as well as acute. Reversible ischemic abnormalities on diffusion-weighted scans are observed on rare occasions.

Restricted diffusion within infarcted tissue may persist for one to two weeks. This finding overlaps the development of T2 prolongation in the affected region, which can cause a persistent zone of high signal intensity on diffusion-weighted scans due to "T2 shine-through."

The zone of restricted diffusion reflecting cytotoxic edema due to acute cerebral infarction in Case 560 involves cortex of the posterior frontal and parietal lobes, representing the territory of the posterior division of the middle cerebral artery (see Case 565).

Multifocal acute infarction in Case 561 affects deep nuclei (the right caudate nucleus and the left thalamus) in addition to cortex, suggesting multiple emboli.

## Case 562

69-year-old man, five days after
a cerebrovascular accident.
(axial map of relative cerebral blood volume,
calculated from a dynamic, contrast-enhanced
echoplanar sequence)

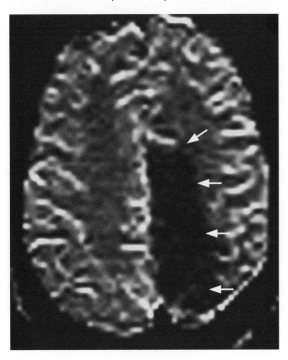

**Infarct**
(ACA distribution)

## Case 563

75-year-old man, one day after
a cerebrovascular accident.
(axial map of relative cerebral blood volume,
calculated from a dynamic, contrast-enhanced
echoplanar sequence)

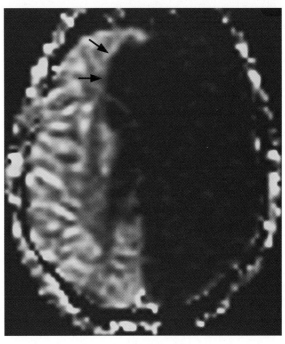

**Infarct**
(left hemisphere and right ACA distribution)

Echoplanar imaging sequences can assess cerebral perfusion by rapidly measuring changes in signal intensity caused by the first pass of injected contrast material through the brain. Perfusion parameters such as relative cerebral blood volume (rCBV), relative cerebral blood flow (rCBF), and mean transit time (MTT) can be calculated for each voxel in the scan plane. The results are often displayed as a map covering the entire section, with low intensity indicating reduced rCBV or rCBF.

The zone of diminished rCBV in Case 562 predominantly involves the distal portion of the distribution of the left anterior cerebral artery. Localized area of infarction suggests embolization in this patient, who had angiographically demonstrated occlusion of the left internal carotid artery.

Case 563 illustrates a much larger perfusion defect, with reduced rCBV throughout the majority of the left hemisphere and within the medial right frontal lobe. MR angiography demonstrated occlusion of the left internal carotid artery; there was no supply to the right anterior cerebral artery from the right carotid system.

Early experience with perfusion-weighted images in acute cerebral infarction has suggested that rCBV is the least sensitive but most specific parameter of reduced perfusion, with the closest correlation to subsequent infarct size. Abnormalities in MTT and rCBF sensitively identify tissue at risk due to hypoperfusion, which may not yet be so severe or prolonged as to cause cell death. For this reason, zones of increased MTT or decreased rCBF overestimate the size of eventual infarcts in most cases.

Stroke investigators emphasize comparison of the area of restricted diffusion and the zone of reduced perfusion in cases of acute cerebral infarction. When the latter is more extensive than the former, the hypoperfused tissue outside of the diffusion abnormality is considered to be potentially salvageable ("ischemic penumbra"), encouraging therapeutic efforts. The ischemic penumbra is dynamic and unstable, both temporally and spatially. Without treatment, the diffusion abnormality often grows over hours or days to match the size of the initial perfusion deficit.

Comparison of the volume of infarcted tissue in the above cases demonstrates the critical role of collateral circulation in determining the extent of infarction when a specific vessel is occluded.

The right frontal infarct in Case 563 *(arrows)* and the left hemispheric infarct in Case 562 together illustrate the normal distribution of the anterior cerebral artery.

## Case 564

3-year-old boy, two days after the onset
of right hemiparesis and aphasia.
(axial, noncontrast T2-weighted SE scan)

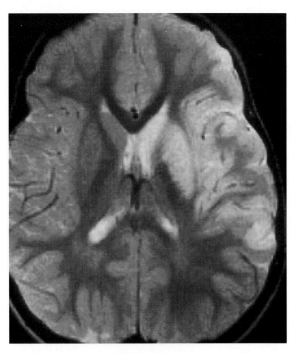

**MCA Infarct**
(anterior division)

## Case 565

5-year-old boy with a history of congenital heart
disease, presenting with confusion.
(axial, noncontrast T2-weighted SE scan)

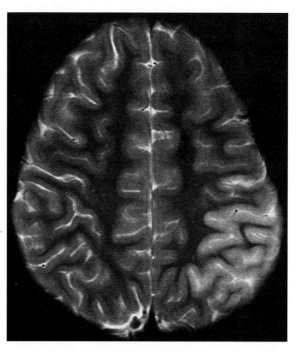

**MCA Infarct**
(posterior division)

---

Infarction within the distribution of the middle cerebral artery (MCA) may present variable morphology, depending on the extent of cortical involvement and the presence or absence of ganglionic components.

When the main trunk of the MCA is occluded, a large zone of mid hemispheric infarction develops. (A similar pattern may occur with occlusion of the internal carotid artery when the ipsilateral anterior cerebral artery is well perfused from the anterior communicating artery.) The anterior and posterior margins of the infarct reflect the anatomical and physiological extent of collateral flow from the anterior and posterior cerebral arteries. The lesion often has a trapezoidal shape based laterally, as demonstrated on axial or coronal images (see Case 575 for an example). If the occlusion compromises the origins of the lenticulostriate arteries, deep nuclei will also be involved.

In Case 564, gyriform cortical edema is present throughout the territory of the anterior division of the MCA. (See Cases 553, 559, and 574 for other examples of anterior division MCA infarcts.) In addition, uniform high signal intensity is seen within the putamen and caudate head. (Compare to the normal definition of the caudate nucleus and frontal horn on the right side.) These nuclei are supplied by lenticulostriate branches arising from the horizontal or M1 segment of the MCA. Occlusion of this segment (e.g., by embolus, dissection, or arteritis) produces a combination of cortical and ganglionic infarction.

Cortical edema in Case 565 predominantly involves the parietal lobe, corresponding to the territory of the posterior division of the middle cerebral artery. (Cases 555 and 560 present other examples of this distribution.) The parasagittal band of spared tissue medial to the lesion is supplied by the posterior cerebral artery.

### Case 566

47-year-old woman presenting with
a one-week history of confusion.
(axial, noncontrast FLAIR scan)

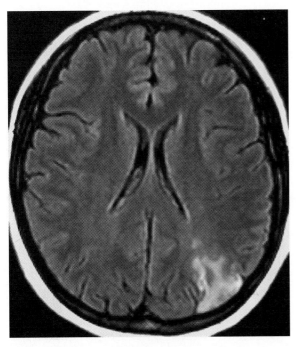

**Cortical Infarct**

### Case 567

64-year-old woman presenting with weakness
and numbness of the left arm.
(axial, noncontrast FLAIR scan)

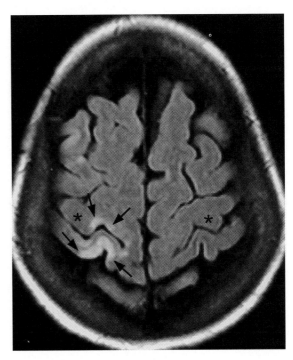

**Cortical Infarct**

---

Occlusion of a single branch of the middle cerebral artery causes focal cortical infarction. Characteristic gyriform morphology of localized cortical edema may suggest the diagnosis of ischemia even when a lesion is very small.

Two other common morphologies of focal infarction are illustrated above. In Case 566, a small wedge of abnormal signal intensity is broadly based at the surface of the brain. This territory represents the distribution of a single cortical artery, corresponding to the most posterior portion of the infarct in Case 565. Gyriform contrast enhancement was present in the involved region.

Case 567 demonstrates laminar and nodular foci of prolonged T2 values within gray matter of the right precentral and postcentral gyri *(arrows)*. Subtle signal abnormality is also present within cortex of the right middle frontal gyrus. Laminar necrosis, a characteristic pathological feature of cerebral infarction, can occasionally be appreciated on high resolution MR studies of small infarcts. (In particular, laminar necrosis may be seen as a distinct subcortical line of T2 prolongation within involved gyri on MR studies of in-

fants and children suffering cerebral infarction; see Case 668.)

FLAIR sequences are a little more sensitive than routine T2-weighted spin echo scans for demonstrating large cerebral infarcts. Small cortical infarcts are substantially better defined on FLAIR sequences than on T2-weighted scans, because the high signal intensity of superficial lesions is more easily distinguished from CSF within adjacent sulci. Case 567 is an example of this application. (In general, FLAIR sequences are less sensitive than diffusion-weighted scans for the detection of cerebral infarcts.)

Case 567 illustrates the characteristic morphology of the superior portion of the precentral and postcentral gyri. The precentral gyrus *(asterisk)* is the thicker of the two and is readily identified by a nodular convexity along its posterior margin correlating with the location of upper motor neurons controlling the contralateral hand. (This typical gyral anatomy is also apparent in Cases 30, 496, 535, and 719.)

## Case 568

57-year-old man presenting two days
after sudden loss of vision.
(axial, noncontrast T2-weighted FSE scan)

## Case 569

34-year-old woman presenting one day after
the abrupt onset of right body numbness
and right homonymous hemianopsia.
(axial, noncontrast FLAIR scan)

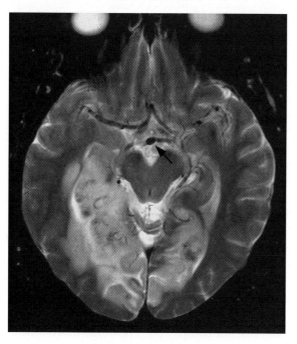

**Bilateral PCA Infarcts**

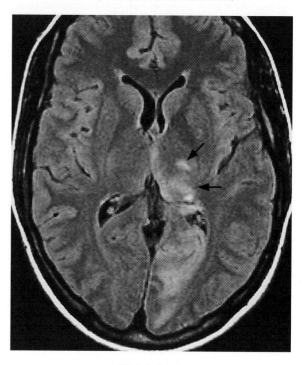

**PCA Infarct**

The posterior cerebral artery (PCA) supplies the medial temporal lobe, the tentorial surface of the temporal and occipital lobes, the occipital pole, and a variably extensive band of the parasagittal parieto-occipital lobes. The superior and lateral extent of this distribution reflects variations in size of the anterior and middle cerebral arteries.

Case 568 demonstrates bilateral PCA infarcts, more extensive on the right. Edematous cortex of the temporal and occipital lobes retains gyriform morphology in some regions, but is more amorphous and mass-like in others. Although the dominant signal abnormality is T2 prolongation, central areas of low intensity are present bilaterally due to deoxyhemoglobin.

Patchy hemorrhage causing areas of T1- and T2-shortening is common within PCA infarcts (see Cases 570 and 573). The presence of blood products can make the lesions appear complex, but this typical feature actually supports the diagnosis of subacute infarction in cases with poorly defined clinical context.

Less confluent and more laminar edema is present in the left temporo-occipital region in Case 569. Subtotal infarction of the PCA territory is frequent and can cause diagnostic confusion, particularly when hemorrhagic components are present. Infarction should be considered whenever a puzzling occipital lesion is encountered.

Thalamo-perforating branches arise from the proximal PCA (as well as from the posterior communicating artery). For this reason, thalamic infarction often accompanies infarcts of the medial temporal and occipital lobes, as illustrated in Case 569 *(arrows)*. The presence of thalamic edema favors PCA infarction as the etiology of an otherwise ambiguous abnormality in the temporo-occipital region.

The lumen of the basilar artery in Case 568 appears patent *(arrow)*. However, the appearance of bilateral PCA infarcts suggests embolization to or through the distal portion of this vessel. The young patient in Case 569 was found to have a dissection of a vertebral artery, which was the source of embolization.

**Case 570**

66-year-old man presenting with impaired vision.
(axial, noncontrast scan; SE 3000/45)

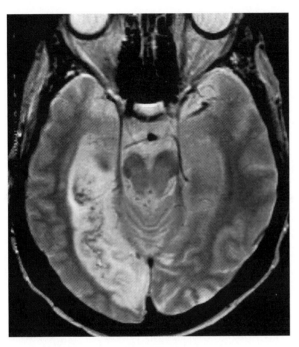

**PCA Infarct**

**Case 571**

14-year-old girl presenting with headaches.
(axial, noncontrast T2-weighted SE scan)

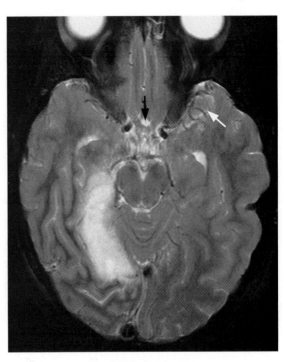

**Subdural Empyema**
(same patient as Cases 435 and 438)

The tentorium shapes the morphology of adjacent parenchymal or extraaxial processes. The medial margin of the PCA infarct Case 570 is defined by the tentorial surface. (The lateral margin of ischemic tissue is often more irregular than in this case, reflecting the watershed with the posterior division of the middle cerebral artery; see Case 568.) The tentorium similarly establishes a smooth *lateral* margin for infarcts of the superior cerebellar hemisphere, while their medial margin may be variable (see Cases 625 and 626).

The subdural empyema in Case 571 is also based along the superior surface of the tentorium. A pattern recognition approach to a similar image in an older patient might mistakenly suggest PCA infarction. Closer attention to the scan demonstrates that medial occipital gyri are not edematous but are compressed and displaced laterally by the extraaxial collection.

Case 570 illustrates a gyriform pattern of low signal intensity within the recently infarcted cortex. This finding often precedes T1-shortening (see Cases 572 and 573), probably reflecting the presence of deoxyhemoglobin within petechial hemorrhages and/or stagnant intravascular compartments. Gyriform T2-shortening in a zone of acute infarction is often predictive of subsequent hemorrhagic transformation of the lesion.

The optic chiasm is well defined within the suprasellar cistern of Case 571 *(black arrow)*. Prominent vessels at the medial margin of the middle cranial fossa, as seen on the left in Case 571 *(white arrow),* are a frequent normal finding and should not be misinterpreted as a vascular malformation.

### Case 572

69-year-old woman, three days after
the acute onset of confusion.
(sagittal, noncontrast T1-weighted SE scan)

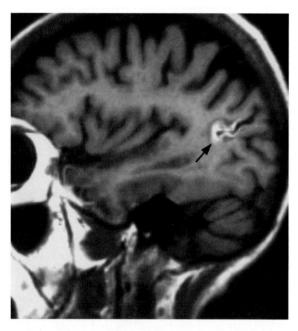

**Subacute Infarct**

### Case 573

74-year-old woman with a four-day history of
worsening homonymous hemianopsia.
(sagittal, noncontrast T1-weighted SE scan)

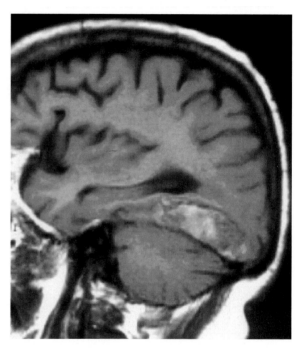

**Subacute Infarct**

Zones of T1-shortening often develop within subacute infarcts, helping to localize and characterize the lesions. Case 572 illustrates a ribbon of high signal intensity following the contour of involved cerebral cortex *(arrow)*. This gyriform pattern may be due to petechial hemorrhage and/or biochemical changes caused by laminar necrosis (e.g., protein denaturation). CT scans in such cases usually do not demonstrate high attenuation values in the area of T1-shortening, and the MR finding does not by itself contraindicate anticoagulation. Compare the morphology of precontrast T1-shortening as in Case 572 to the gyriform enhancement of subacute infarction illustrated in Cases 579 and 580.

Less commonly, recent ischemic infarcts become frankly hemorrhagic, either spontaneously or following therapy with anticoagulants. Dissolution of a cerebral embolus may predispose to hemorrhagic infarction by allowing reperfusion of damaged vessels. Multifocal hemorrhagic infarcts suggest an embolic source such as subacute bacterial endocarditis.

Case 573 demonstrates extensive T1-shortening due to subacute hemorrhage within an occipital infarct. As mentioned in Case 568, hemorrhage is a particularly common component of infarction in the distribution of the posterior cerebral artery.

356

## Case 574

70-year-old woman with known atrial fibrillation,
two days after the acute onset of confusion.
(axial, noncontrast scan; SE 2800/45)

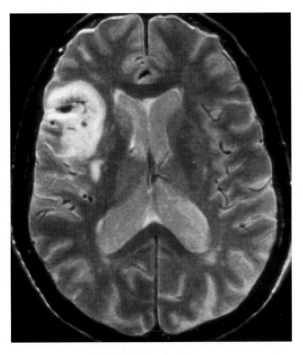

**Hemorrhagic Infarct**

## Case 575

48-year-old man, ten days after
the onset of left hemiparesis.
(axial, noncontrast T2-weighted SE scan)

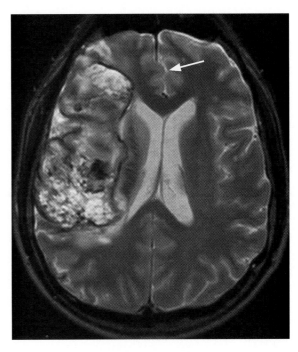

**Hemorrhagic Infarct**

---

Low signal intensity on T2-weighted images is a characteristic feature of acute or early subacute intracerebral hemorrhage (see discussion of Cases 673-676). This finding may add complexity to the MR appearance of recent infarcts, as illustrated above.

The lesion in Case 574 is nonspecific. The combination of hemorrhage and mass effect simulates a tumor (compare to Case 682). However, the clinical context and location of the lesion within the territory of the anterior division of the middle cerebral artery suggest the correct diagnosis. CT scanning might be considered to prove that the focal areas of low signal intensity represent hemorrhage rather than calcification.

Case 575 illustrates a large zone of mixed signal abnormality with trapezoidal morphology matching the distribution of the right middle cerebral artery. Scattered areas of hemorrhage causing T2-shortening are present within the lesion and at its margins. Anticoagulation would carry high risk in this patient due to the size of the infarct, its probable embolic origin, and the apparent hemorrhagic tendency.

Chronic atrial fibrillation is known to be associated with an increased risk of stroke, which can be reduced by anticoagulation. A small focus of high signal abnormality posterior to the main lesion in Case 574 probably represents an additional infarct of undetermined age.

Venous pathology (e.g., dural sinus thrombosis) should also be considered as a cause of hemorrhagic cerebral infarction (see Case 650).

Residual mass effect from the large infarct in Case 575 compresses the right lateral ventricle and causes subfalcial midline shift *(arrow)*.

### Case 576

16-year-old girl, one day after the rapid development
of aphasia and hemiparesis.
(axial, postcontrast T1-weighted SE scan)

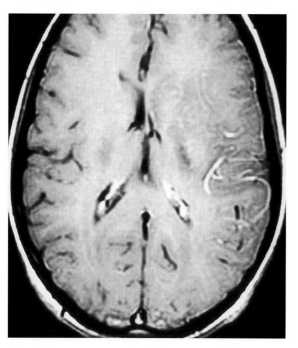

**Acute Infarct**
(MCA distribution)

### Case 577

72-year-old woman, one day
after the onset of aphasia.
(axial, postcontrast T1-weighted SE scan)

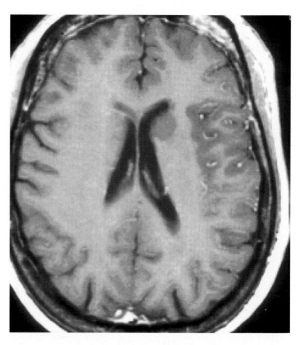

**Acute Infarct**
(MCA distribution)

Rapid blood flow through normal cerebral arteries causes a lack of signal or flow void on routine spin echo images. Slower flow, whether in normal veins or abnormal arteries, is often associated with intraluminal enhancement on postcontrast scans.

Abnormal contrast enhancement within major arteries may be the earliest sign of cerebral infarction on standard MR studies. This finding depends on the presence of slow antegrade or retrograde collateral perfusion of the affected vascular territory. Abnormal arterial enhancement may persist for several days, disappearing as more normal flow velocities are reestablished in the obstructed distribution.

Both of the above cases demonstrate abnormal enhancement of middle cerebral artery branches supplying the left hemisphere. (Compare this finding to the normal lack of arterial enhancement over the right hemisphere in each case.) In both cases, evidence of early parenchymal change

is present, with edema causing swelling and reduced signal intensity of sylvian cortex and deep hemispheric nuclei.

Increasingly sophisticated pulse sequences are becoming available, offering excellent flow compensation with routine demonstration of arterial enhancement. However, this successful rephasing of normal arterial flow may decrease conspicuity of reduced arterial velocities in an area of cerebral infarction.

A cerebrovascular accident in a young patient should suggest the possibility of an embolic source (see also Case 569). Leading causes include spontaneous dissection of the carotid or vertebral arteries or posttraumatic lesions of these vessels (e.g., pseudoaneurysm). Cardiac emboli or coagulopathy should also be considered. The patient in Case 576 was found to have a mitochondrial encephalomyopathy (MELAS; see Case 510) that is associated with stroke-like events.

### Case 578

53-year-old man, two days after the abrupt onset of
headache and left homonymous hemianopsia.
(axial, postcontrast T1-weighted SE scan)

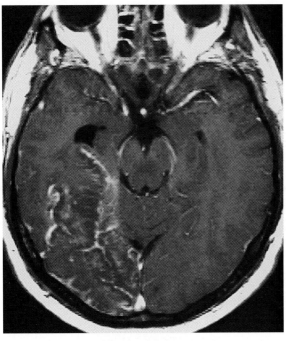

**Acute Infarct**
(PCA distribution)

### Case 579

2-year-old girl with suspected cerebral emboli.
(coronal, postcontrast T1-weighted SE scan)

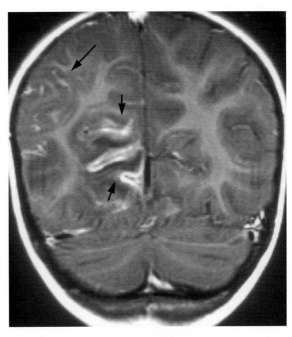

**Recent Infarcts**
(multifocal)

In Case 578, cortex of the right medial posterior temporal and occipital lobes is abnormally prominent, with thickening and T1-prolongation indicating edema. Contrast enhancement within the overlying leptomeninges fills the adjacent sulci.

This combination of features may be observed early in the course of cerebral infarction (day one or two). The phase of superficial pial enhancement is interposed between (and often superimposed on) the periods of arterial enhancement and gyral enhancement. It is important to recognize that this pattern may occur within the MR spectrum of a vascular event, since the appearance could otherwise be interpreted as meningeal disease (e.g., meningitis or meningeal carcinomatosis) with secondary cortical edema.

Parenchymal contrast enhancement in cerebral infarcts is usually confined to gray matter. Several morphologies may be encountered. The most characteristic pattern is band-like, tubular, or gyriform enhancement, as seen in the right occipital region of Case 579 *(short arrows)*. More amor-

phous patterns can occur, and solid enhancement is common when deep nuclei are involved. Ring-enhancing appearances are occasionally noted. In most cases, the enhancing lesion retains the peripherally-based shape typical of a large infarct.

The occipital enhancement in Case 579 involves the gray matter ribbon, with sparing of the intervening sulcal/ meningeal spaces. A different pattern with pial enhancement is present in the posterior parietal region *(long arrow)*. The latter finding represents a more recent infarct, which evolved to gyral enhancement over the subsequent two days.

Gyriform contrast enhancement is a familiar CT hallmark of subacute infarction, seen from the end of week one through week three or four. MR demonstration of this pattern begins a little earlier, often by day two or three following the clinical event. Reactive *luxury perfusion* (hyperperfusion with loss of autoregulation) and breakdown of the blood-brain barrier both contribute to this finding.

# DIFFERENTIAL DIAGNOSIS:
## FOCAL GYRIFORM CONTRAST ENHANCEMENT

### Case 580

55-year-old woman, nine days after
the acute onset of right leg paresis.
(coronal, postcontrast T1-weighted SE scan)

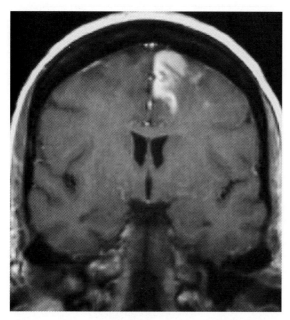

**Subacute Infarct**
(ACA distribution)

### Case 581

61-year-old man with decreased mental status.
(coronal, postcontrast T1-weighted SE scan)

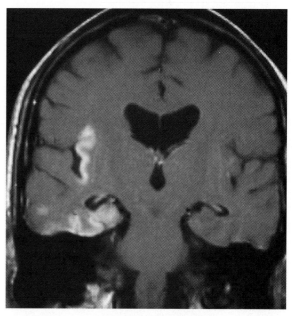

**Herpes Encephalitis**
(same patient as Case 449)

---

A gyriform pattern of contrast enhancement is characteristic but not specific for cerebral infarction. In an ambiguous clinical context, a differential diagnosis of this finding should be considered.

Case 580 demonstrates typical gyriform cortical enhancement within an infarct localized to the distribution of the anterior cerebral artery (ACA). The ACA supplies a parasagittal band of tissue extending from the medial frontal lobe to the parietal vertex. (Compare the area involved by infarction in Case 580 to the territory spared from infarction in Case 559; see Cases 562 and 563 for additional examples of ACA infarcts.) Included in this distribution is the medial portion of the motor cortex supplying the lower extremity, correlating with the leg weakness in this patient. Obstruction of the ACA may be caused by

embolization, spasm following subarachnoid hemorrhage, compression by a subfrontal mass, or marked subfalcial herniation.

Herpes encephalitis characteristically involves cortex of the temporal lobe and insula, as in Case 581. The resultant edema and enhancement following the cortical contour may mimic a subacute cerebral infarct. The diagnosis of infarction in Case 581 is unlikely because the affected areas fall within more than one vascular distribution. The medial temporal lobe is supplied by the anterior choroidal and posterior cerebral arteries, while the insula is perfused by the middle cerebral artery.

Occasional tumors (usually gliomas) infiltrate cortex and can mimic the appearance of cerebral infarction (see Cases 77, 78, and 558).

## Case 582

3-year-old boy, one week after the
acute onset of right hemiparesis.
(axial, postcontrast T1-weighted SE scan)

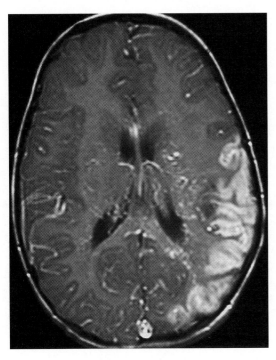

**Subacute Infarct**
(in moyamoya disease)

## Case 583

35-year-old man with a history of epilepsy.
(axial, postcontrast T1-weighted SE scan)

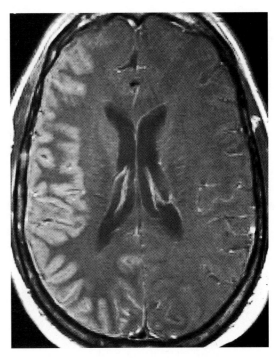

**Cortical Hyperemia Due to Seizures**

Extensive gyriform enhancement is a familiar feature of large, subacute cortical infarcts. Case 582 illustrates this finding throughout the distribution of the posterior division of the left middle cerebral artery. The small zone of spared tissue at the left occipital pole is supplied by the posterior cerebral artery (compare to the areas of infarction in Cases 568 to 570).

In Case 583, the region of cortical enhancement extends beyond the distribution of the MCA. Occlusion of the internal carotid artery with persistent fetal origin of the posterior cerebral artery could conceivably produce this appearance. However, cortical edema or enhancement crossing a major arterial watershed should raise the possibility of pathologies other than arterial infarction. Anoxia, multifocal infarction due to emboli or vasculitis, venous infarction, and meningitis/encephalitis are among the alternatives to be considered in such cases.

Recent or ongoing seizure activity can also cause gyriform cortical edema and enhancement, as illustrated by

Case 583. The latter finding reflects increased blood flow with variable transient alteration of the blood-brain barrier. Gyriform enhancement can be present for several hours after seizures have stopped. It is important to recognize that cortical edema and enhancement may represent the effect rather than the cause of seizure activity in a postictal patient. (Compare to transient postictal edema of the hippocampus, discussed in Cases 525 and 526.)

Cortical edema associated with seizures typically demonstrates near-normal signal intensity on diffusion-weighted scans, but restricted diffusion is occasionally apparent. The abnormalities are usually reversible in either case.

Small arteries within the basal ganglia and periventricular white matter of Case 582 have become hypertrophied as collateral channels in this patient with moyamoya disease (see Case 638 and compare to Cases 455 and 456). Unusually prominent leptomeningeal enhancement probably reflects an accompanying increase in pial vascularity.

## Case 584

33-year-old woman with multiple neurological deficits one day after cardiac surgery.
(axial, noncontrast scan; SE 2500/28)

## Case 585

9-year-old boy with sickle cell anemia, now presenting with acute right hemiparesis.
(axial, noncontrast T2-weighted FSE scan)

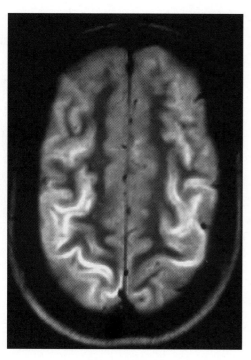

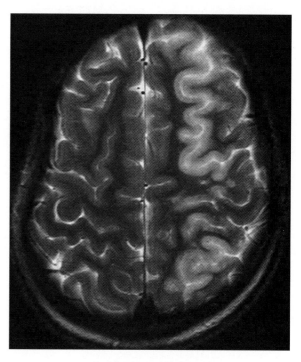

**Border Zone Infarcts**

**Border Zone Infarcts**
(same patient as Case 557)

Infarction occurs along the margins of cerebral vascular territories when flow is impaired on both sides of the boundary. Such border zone or "watershed" ischemia may be caused by generalized hypoperfusion, isolated vascular compromise, or a combination of both factors. For example, stenosis of an internal carotid artery may lead to infarction along the anterior/middle cerebral artery watershed during systemic hypotension.

The location of the cortical border zones has been illustrated by the margins of the infarcts on preceding pages. Watershed infarcts are typically small, patchy lesions aligned along the same parasagittal boundaries, as illustrated on the next page. (The differential diagnosis of this parasagittal pattern of edema includes venous infarction due to thrombosis of the superior sagittal sinus; see Cases 649 and 650.)

The above cases demonstrate unusually extensive border zone infarcts reflecting severe hypoperfusion. In Case 584,

symmetrical high signal intensity is present within gyri throughout the parasagittal zones of the anterior cortical arterial watershed. (Compare the location of the gyral edema in this case to Cases 559 and 565.) Laminar high signal intensity was apparent in the same distribution on T1-weighted scans. The bilateral symmetry of the lesions suggests a diffuse cerebral insult, and the localization to watershed areas indicates a hypoxic/ischemic etiology.

Case 585 illustrates extensive unilateral edema within cortex along the border zone between the territories of the left middle cerebral artery laterally and the anterior and posterior cerebral arteries medially. MR angiography demonstrated high-grade stenosis of the supraclinoid segment of the left internal carotid artery.

Sickle cell arteriopathy probably reflects damage to the endothelium from a combination of high flow velocity, rigidity of erythrocytes, and adhesion of red blood cells to the vessel wall, with superimposed intravascular sludging.

### Case 586

50-year-old woman presenting with
confusion and left hemiparesis.
(axial, noncontrast FLAIR scan)

### Case 587

58-year-old man resuscitated after a cardiac arrest.
(axial, postcontrast T1-weighted SE scan)

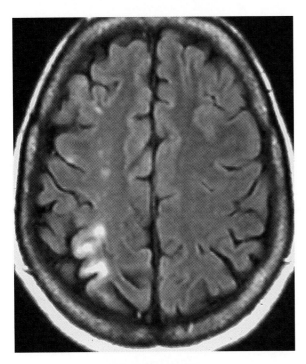

**Border Zone Infarcts**

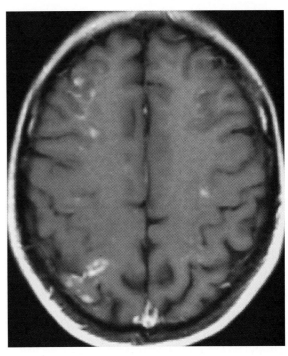

**Border Zone Infarcts**

Infarcts within the cortical border zones are often small and multifocal. When watershed infarcts are due to a proximal stenosis, new lesions may be superimposed on a background of older events.

The small cortical and subcortical foci of signal abnormality in Case 586 are located along the parasagittal border zone between the middle cerebral artery laterally and the anterior and posterior cerebral arteries medially. Multiple cortical infarcts aligned in this manner should prompt close examination of flow characteristics within the ipsilateral internal carotid artery (ICA). In this case, there was lack of flow void within the parasellar ICA, correlating with complete occlusion on MR angiography.

Small areas of infarction often demonstrate focal enhancement, as seen in Case 587. Enhancement defining cortical infarcts is best demonstrated by MR scans, since the cerebral surface is not obscured by artifact from the adjacent calvarium as in CT studies. Postcontrast scans using magnetization transfer suppression are particularly helpful to detect and characterize subacute ischemic foci.

The appearance in Case 587 is nonspecific and could suggest inflammatory or metastatic disease. The correct diagnosis is supported by (1) the location of the lesions along the parasagittal zones of the cortical arterial watersheds and (2) the pial and gyriform components of enhancement within some of the affected areas. Multifocal infarction may also be caused by multiple emboli, cerebral vasculitis (e.g., systemic lupus erythematosus), meningitis, or cortical venous thrombosis.

Border zone infarction is occasionally limited to a single area of mass-like edema located near the anterior or posterior margins of the cortical watersheds. Infarction should be considered in the differential diagnosis of nonspecific lesions near the 1, 5, 7, and 11 o'clock positions on axial CT or MR scans (see Case 589).

Case 586 is another example of the usefulness of FLAIR sequences in distinguishing small cortical lesions from adjacent sulci.

### Case 588

59-year-old woman with occlusion of
the left internal carotid artery.
(axial, noncontrast scan; SE 2500/45)

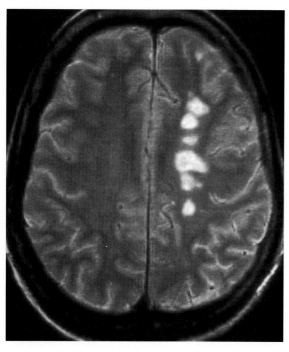

**Border Zone Infarcts**

### Case 589

45-year-old woman with high-grade stenosis
of the right internal carotid artery.
(axial, noncontrast T2-weighted SE scan)

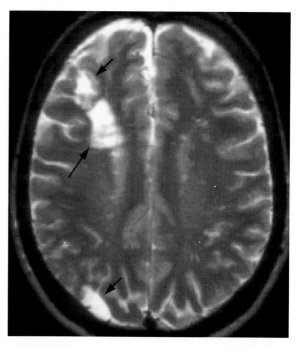

**Border Zone Infarcts**

In addition to the cortical arterial watershed over the cerebral convexity, a border zone exists within each cerebral hemisphere. This area occurs at the junction of centrifugal perfusion from basal perforating arteries (e.g., lenticulostriate arteries) and centripetal perfusion from penetrating branches of the cortical vessels. The location of the intrahemispheric watershed moves peripherally during fetal development. At full term (and thereafter), the border zone is within white matter of the centrum semiovale, slightly lateral and superior to the bodies of the lateral ventricles.

Reduced perfusion of one cerebral hemisphere may cause scattered infarction within the intrahemispheric watershed zone. Such infarcts may occur in isolation or accompany cortical lesions. While cortical border zone infarcts are frequently due to global hypoperfusion from cardiovascular impairment, intrahemispheric watershed infarction often reflects isolated disease of the ipsilateral internal carotid artery.

In Case 588, the parasagittal row of white matter lesions is strikingly unilateral. The appearance would be unusual for inflammatory disorders, and compromise of the ipsilateral internal carotid artery should be suspected. Examination of flow void within arteries at the skull base and/or MR angiography is indicated when lesions resembling unilateral multiple sclerosis are encountered.

Case 589 demonstrates the association of cortical watershed infarcts *(short arrows)* with intrahemispheric border zone infarction *(long arrow)*. The size and number of lesions in either category may be variable, but their position should raise consideration of watershed hemodynamics.

## Case 590

31-year-old woman presenting with
right arm weakness.
(axial, noncontrast scan; SE 2600/45)

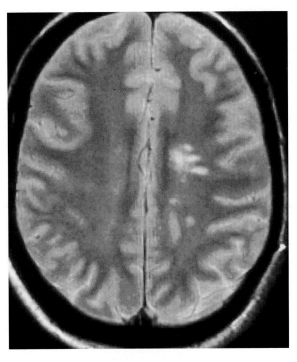

**Multiple Sclerosis**

## Case 591

56-year-old man presenting with left-sided
headaches and right hemiparesis.
(axial, noncontrast scan; SE 2500/45)

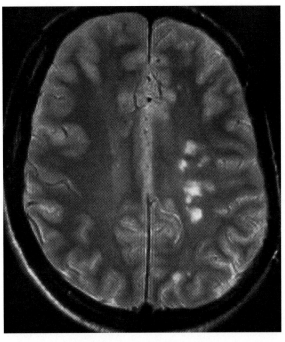

**Border Zone Infarcts**
(due to ICA dissection)

Hemispheric involvement by multiple sclerosis may be asymmetrical, as in Case 590. In some instances, multiple plaques are entirely unilateral. The characteristic elliptical morphology of several lesions in Case 590 combines with the clinical context to suggest the diagnosis (compare to Cases 360 to 362).

Unilateral clustering of small lesions in the centrum semi-ovale should also raise the possibility of intrahemispheric border zone infarction. This diagnosis is favored by a parasagittal, band-like distribution of round foci, as in Case 591. Attention to the presence or absence of normal flow void within basal arteries and/or MR angiography can confirm the vascular etiology of white matter lesions in such cases.

The patient in Case 591 was found to have suffered a dissection of the left internal carotid artery at the skull base (see Cases 632-634).

## Case 592

8-year-old boy presenting with a mildly spastic gait.
(axial, noncontrast T2-weighted SE scan)

## Case 593

5-year-old girl with "cerebral palsy."
(coronal, noncontrast T1-weighted SE scan)

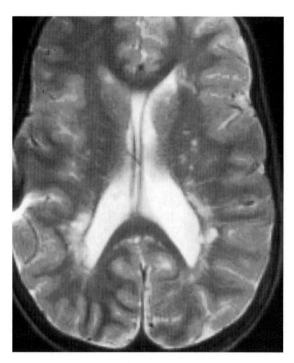

**Periventricular Leukomalacia**

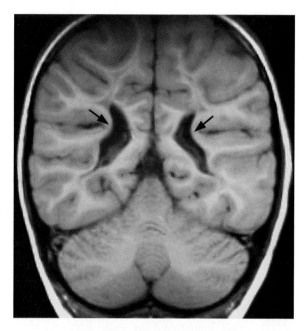

**Periventricular Leukomalacia**

Periventricular leukomalacia (PVL) is a syndrome of multifocal damage within deep hemispheric white matter in premature infants. The etiology of PVL has traditionally been assumed to be a hypoxic/ischemic insult to the intrahemispheric border zones of the developing brain. Other contributing factors (toxic, metabolic, and immune mediated) have been suggested recently.

The perinatal diagnosis of PVL is based on ultrasound studies, which demonstrate abnormal echogenicity and subsequent cyst formation in the periventricular regions. White matter near the posterior bodies and trigones of the lateral ventricles is most frequently and most severely affected.

Areas of focal periventricular necrosis often cavitate. They may persist as independent cysts surrounded by margins of scar tissue. Alternatively, they may become incorporated into the adjacent ventricular body, causing it to acquire an irregular or scalloped lateral margin.

Case 592 illustrates the former appearance. Multiple posterior periventricular foci of signal abnormality indicate sites of white matter necrosis. The posterior bodies of the lateral ventricles are expanded due to the loss of adjacent parenchyma.

The areas of abnormal signal intensity in Case 592 are sharper, smaller, and closer to the ventricular border than the zones of slow myelination frequently seen in deep parietal white matter of young children (compare to Case 412).

Loss of white matter volume is a hallmark of periventricular leukomalacia and may establish the diagnosis even when individual lesions are poorly defined. Case 593 demonstrates marked thinning of white matter which should normally separate the cortical sulci from the ventricular margin *(arrows)* Together with expansion of the posterior portions of the lateral ventricles, this abnormally deep invagination of lateral sulci suggests a hypoxic/ischemic insult before or early in the third trimester of fetal development.

### Case 594

3-year-old boy presenting with
seizures and spasticity.
(axial, noncontrast scan; SE 2800/45)

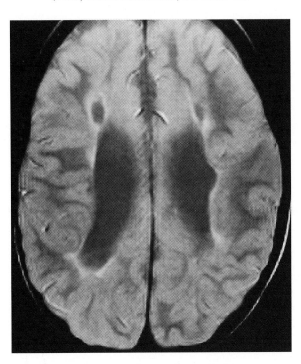

**Periventricular Leukomalacia**

### Case 595

11-month-old girl with "cerebral palsy."
(axial, noncontrast T2-weighted SE scan)

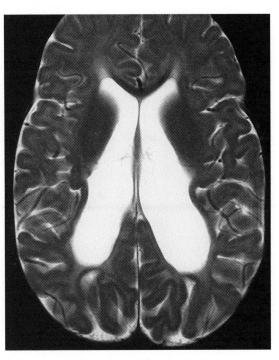

**Periventricular Leukomalacia**

The reactive capability of the immature brain is very limited. Parenchymal damage of any type leads to dissolution of tissue with minimal residual gliosis. As a result, PVL may present as a featureless loss of white matter volume (see Case 593). Alternatively, areas of focal necrosis within periventricular white matter may be incorporated into the adjacent ventricular chamber.

This process results in a typical morphology of the lateral ventricles, as illustrated in the above cases. The posterior portions of the ventricles are symmetrically expanded, reflecting overall loss of deep hemispheric white matter. In addition, the lateral margin of the ventricles is irregular or angular, due to focal loss and cavitation of sub-ependymal parenchyma. Margins of gliosis may line the ventricular contour, as in Case 594.

The dilatation of the posterior portion of the lateral ventricles associated with PVL should be distinguished from the more rounded appearance of colpocephaly, a developmental malformation (see Cases 857 and 858).

The clinical presentation of spastic diplegia or "cerebral palsy" is a common manifestation of PVL. However, PVL (and presumed hypoxic/ischemic encephalopathy) accounts for only a small fraction of such cases. Many infants with "cerebral palsy" attributed to "birth asphyxia" are found to have congenital malformations of the brain such as neuronal migration disorders.

### Case 596

33-year-old woman presenting with
acute weakness of the left arm.
(axial, noncontrast T2-weighted SE scan)

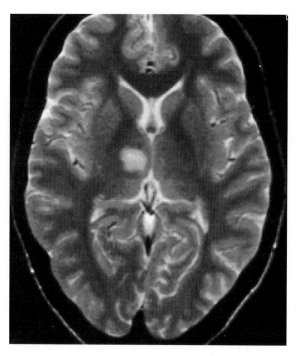

**Infarct**

### Case 597

35-year-old woman who suddenly developed
left hemiparesis four days earlier.
(axial, noncontrast T2-weighted SE scan)

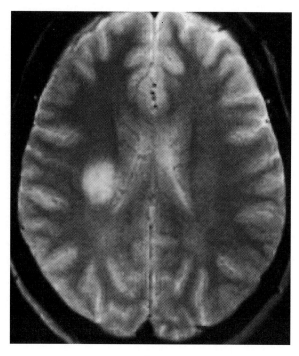

**Infarct**

The basal ganglia, internal capsule, and corona radiata are largely supplied by lenticulostriate branches arising from the horizontal portion of the middle cerebral artery. Other contributions include medial lenticulostriate branches from the anterior cerebral artery, the anterior choroidal artery, and thalamo-perforating branches of the posterior cerebral artery.

Occlusion of these small perforating arteries may cause localized infarction within deep nuclei or periventricular white matter. Such lesions are often quite round and about one centimeter in diameter, as seen in the above cases. Deep hemispheric infarction may accompany extensive cortical ischemia or occur as an isolated event.

Many ganglionic/capsular infarcts are presumed to reflect atherosclerotic disease of small cerebral arteries. Other possible causes include arteritis (e.g., herpes zoster involving the basal cisterns as a complication of trigeminal neuritis). The etiology of infarction in the young adults above was not established (see discussion of Case 576).

Focal infarcts within the basal ganglia may be seen in children after head trauma. It has been suggested that the sharp angle of origin of the lenticulostriate arteries predisposes them to stretch injury and subsequent spasm. As discussed in Cases 600 and 601, ganglionic infarcts in children may also reflect large vessel disease or pathology within the basal cisterns.

### Case 598

51-year-old man.
(axial, noncontrast T2-weighted SE scan)

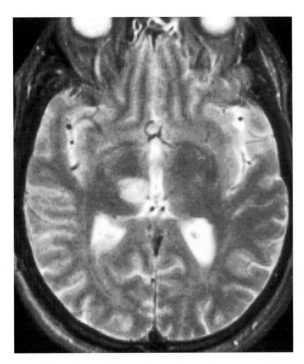

**Metastatic Melanoma**

### Case 599

21-year-old woman with worsening left hemiparesis.
(axial, noncontrast scan; SE 2500/45)

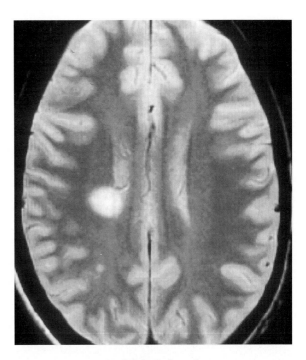

**Multiple Sclerosis**

---

The appearance of the small infarcts on the preceding page is nonspecific. The above cases emphasize the potential resemblance of neoplastic, inflammatory, and vascular lesions deep within the cerebral hemispheres.

As discussed in Chapter 1, metastatic disease typically involves subcortical portions of the brain. Case 598 illustrates that deep hemispheric metastases also occur. The faint visualization of a ring of internal architecture within the lesion would be unusual for a simple infarct and warrants further evaluation with contrast injection.

The lesion in Case 599 is comparable in size, shape, and location to Case 597. The diagnosis of demyelination can be established by a characteristic history, the presence of associated MR findings that are hallmarks for multiple sclerosis (see Chapter 8), or CSF analysis. A ring or target appearance resembling Case 598 is also commonly encountered in an intermediate stage of focal demyelination (see Case 375).

Another cause of focal signal abnormality within the corona radiata, internal capsule, or brainstem is Wallerian degeneration (see Case 541).

### Case 600

3-year-old boy adopted from Eastern Europe, presenting with a stroke.
(axial, noncontrast scan; SE 2800/45)

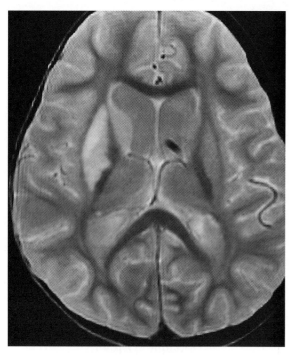

**Tuberculous Meningitis**
(causing MCA compromise)

### Case 601

6-year-old boy presenting with right hemiparesis.
(submentovertex view, maximal intensity projection reconstruction, noncontrast, three-dimensional, time-of-flight GRE scan)

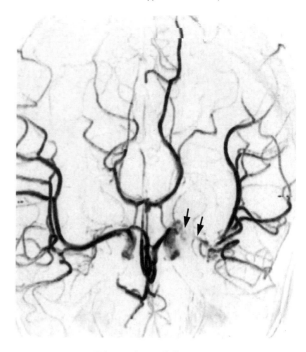

**Dissection of the MCA**

---

The lenticulostriate arteries supplying the basal ganglia arise from the horizontal or M-1 segment of the middle cerebral artery. When this vessel is compromised or occluded, the origins of the lenticulostriate arteries are affected. Because these perforating branches are end arteries without significant collateral anastomoses, their obstruction causes infarction within deep hemispheric nuclei.

Such ganglionic infarction may accompany infarction in the cortical distribution of the MCA (as in Cases 569, 576, and 577). Alternatively, infarction of the basal ganglia may be an isolated finding, as in Case 600.

In young patients, collateral flow across leptomeningeal anastomoses may prevent infarction of midhemispheric cortex despite complete occlusion of the MCA (or internal carotid artery). Ganglionic infarction may be the only manifestation of major arterial compromise in such cases.

Basal meningitis due to tuberculosis in Case 600 had caused focal inflammation and constriction of the MCA and its lenticulostriate branches. Confluent ischemic edema is

seen throughout the putamen; the caudate nucleus is also involved. A shunt is present within the left frontal horn to decompress communicating hydrocephalus, another frequent complication of meningitis.

In Case 601, routine scans showed infarction involving the left caudate nucleus, putamen, and internal capsule. No accompanying cortical edema was present. The MR angiogram demonstrates severely reduced caliber of the proximal left middle cerebral artery *(arrows)*, spanning the origins of lenticulostriate arteries. Dissection of the middle cerebral artery occurs as an infrequent spontaneous event in both children and adults.

Sydenham's chorea has been reported with edema and contrast enhancement of the corpus striatum in children, potentially resembling ganglionic infarction. This syndrome, most commonly a sequela of streptococcal infection, is thought to be caused by immune-mediated cross reactivity.

# DIFFERENTIAL DIAGNOSIS:
## MULTIPLE FOCI OF T2 PROLONGATION WITHIN THE BASAL GANGLIA

### Case 602

62-year-old woman presenting with a TIA.
(axial, noncontrast T2-weighted FSE scan)

### Case 603

95-year-old man being evaluated for confusion.
(axial, noncontrast T2-weighted FSE scan)

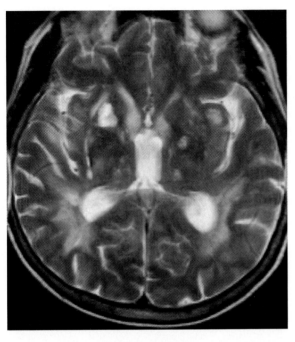

**Multiple Infarcts**

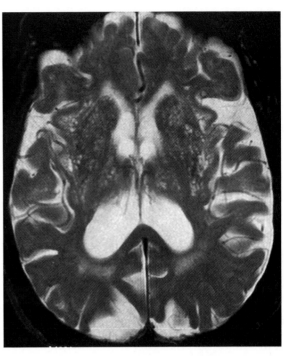

**Prominent Perivascular Spaces**
(normal variant)

Small, deep cerebral infarcts are often called *lacunar infarcts*, using the name that pathologists have given to tiny lesions found in the basal ganglia at autopsy. Large numbers of such infarcts have previously been suggested to be the cause of clinical "lacunar states," with components of dementia or pseudobulbar palsy. These correlations are controversial; the symptoms of patients with multiple deep hemispheric infarcts may range from minimal to profound.

Case 602 illustrates well-defined foci of prolonged T2 values within the basal ganglia and thalami. These presumed deep hemispheric infarcts range in size from one millimeter to about one centimeter. Autopsies in similar cases disclose many more lacunar infarcts of microscopic dimensions. Ischemic lesions of the basal ganglia in elderly patients are typically accompanied by focal and confluent areas of T2 prolongation within white matter, as in Case 602.

The multiple tiny foci of T2 prolongation within the caudate and lentiform nuclei and the thalami in Case 603 are smaller and more uniform than the ischemic lesions of Case 602. The former likely represent enlarged Virchow-Robin spaces surrounding lenticulostriate arteries. This prominence of perivascular spaces is a normal variant accentuated by age and should not be misdiagnosed as multiple lacunar infarcts.

Large perivascular spaces within the basal ganglia may be seen together with or distinct from prominent perivascular spaces within cerebral white matter. Other common locations of enlarged perivascular spaces are the sublentiform region (see Case 838) and the cerebral peduncles.

True lacunar infarcts and prominent perivascular spaces can occur together within deep cerebral nuclei.

## Case 604

73-year-old woman with a history of hypertension.
(axial, noncontrast FLAIR scan)

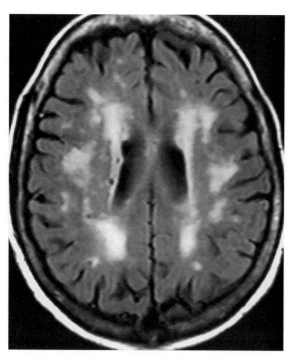

**White Matter "Infarcts"**

## Case 605

89-year-old woman.
(axial, noncontrast scan; SE 2500/45)

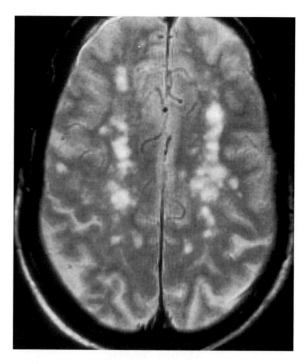

**White Matter "Infarcts"**

Multiple sites of focal and confluent signal abnormality are commonly seen in subcortical and periventricular white matter of patients with disease affecting small arteries. This pattern is frequently present in diabetic and/or hypertensive individuals and is routinely noted in elderly people. The lesions have been pathologically demonstrated to represent a spectrum ranging from atrophy to frank infarction.

MR often demonstrates more ischemic foci than are visible on CT studies. In some cases, these lesions are so large and numerous that they coalesce to form zones of ischemic leukoencephalopathy (see Cases 608 and 609).

The bilaterality and overall symmetry of the lesions in Cases 604 and 605 favor small arterial disease as the etiology. This pattern is distinct from intrahemispheric border zone infarction due to large vessel compromise (compare to Cases 588, 589, and 591).

One specific etiology of multifocal ischemic lesions within white matter is an inherited microangiopathy referred to as *CADASIL* (cerebral autosomal dominant arteriopathy with subcortical infarcts and leukoencephalopathy). This disorder presents as recurrent ischemic episodes leading to progressive cognitive decline in younger patients than are typically affected by small vessel disease. MR scans in patients with CADASIL often demonstrate more involvement of white matter in the superior frontal and anterior temporal lobes than is usually seen in age-related subcortical arteriosclerotic encephalopathy. The mutation causing the disorder has been localized to chromosome 19, manifesting as deposits of granular material within arterial basement membranes.

Like the plaques of demyelinating disease, ischemic lesions within periventricular white matter are well demonstrated by FLAIR sequences, as illustrated in Case 604.

# DIFFERENTIAL DIAGNOSIS:
## MULTIPLE WHITE MATTER LESIONS WITH PERIVENTRICULAR INVOLVEMENT

### Case 606

59-year-old woman presenting with
left body numbness.
(axial, noncontrast scan; SE 2500/45)

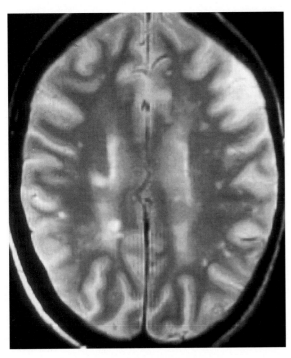

**White Matter Infarcts**
(associated with diabetes mellitus)

### Case 607

38-year-old woman presenting with
left facial numbness.
(axial, noncontrast scan; SE 2500/45)

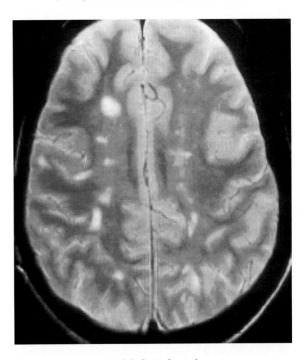

**Multiple Sclerosis**

---

Scattered infarcts in and near the corona radiata as in Case 606 may mimic the appearance of demyelinating plaques in multiple sclerosis, illustrated by Case 607. In both pathologies, periventricular lesions may be accompanied by more peripheral foci of signal abnormality in the centrum semiovale or subcortical white matter.

The periventricular plaques of multiple sclerosis are often elliptical in morphology, with the long axis perpendicular to the ventricular margin (see Cases 360-362). Deep hemispheric infarcts tend to be more rounded or angular in shape. However, this distinction is often difficult, as seen in the above cases.

Prolongation of T1 is usually apparent within established plaques of multiple sclerosis (see Case 359). Low signal in-tensity on T1-weighted scans is usually less impressive and less well defined in zones of focal ischemic change (unless there is central cavitation).

Associated clinical clues (e.g., a history of prior optic neuritis) or scan findings may also help to establish the diagnosis of multiple sclerosis when periventricular lesions are ambiguous. Patient age can assist in separating demyelinating disease from deep hemispheric infarcts, but substantial overlap in the incidence of these pathologies occurs between ages 45 and 60.

Sarcoidosis may cause multifocal white matter lesions similar to the above cases. Intrahemispheric border zone infarcts due to large vessel disease should also be considered in the differential diagnosis (see Cases 588 and 591).

An old cortical infarct is present in the left frontal region in Case 606.

373

## Case 608

82-year-old woman presenting with dementia.
(axial, noncontrast T2-weighted SE scan)

## Case 609

81-year-old woman presenting with confusion.
(axial, noncontrast scan; SE 3000/45)

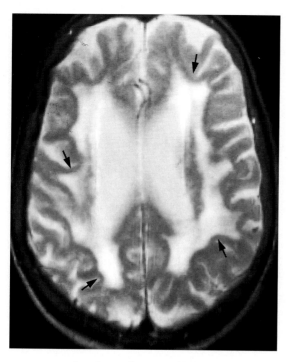

**Ischemic Leukoencephalopathy**

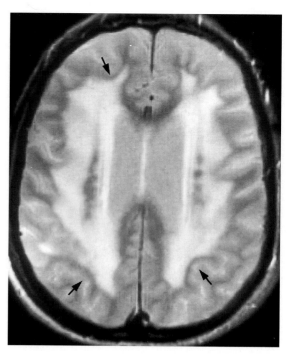

**Ischemic Leukoencephalopathy**

---

The spectrum of ischemic white matter changes extends from focal lesions such as Case 597 through multifocal patterns such as Cases 604-606 to the confluent, diffuse signal abnormality seen above. This common finding in elderly patients represents generalized microvascular white matter disease or "ischemic leukoencephalopathy." Pathological studies demonstrate hyalinization of arterioles in such cases.

Involvement may be limited to periventricular regions near the frontal horns and trigones or may extend diffusely throughout the centrum semiovale, as in Cases 608 and 609. No associated mass effect is present, and no enhancement is seen on postcontrast scans.

There is relative sparing of subcortical "U" fibers (*arrows;* compare to Case 408B), which receive a dual blood supply from recurrent loops and penetrating branches of cortical arteries. The corpus callosum is also usually spared, as seen above. The latter feature has been attrib-

uted to callosal supply from short arterioles that are not as susceptible to the vascular changes developing with age as longer penetrating vessels.

Microvascular white matter disease may present a pattern of scattered, patchy signal abnormality resembling a leukoencephalopathy such as PML. Clues to the correct diagnosis include the general symmetry of ischemic cerebral involvement and the predominant location in midhemispheric and deep hemispheric regions. By contrast, PML frequently affects subcortical white matter and often demonstrates less symmetry than is seen in Cases 608 and 609.

White matter changes in elderly patients correlate clinically with impairment of fine motor control, diminished reflexes, gait abnormality, and an increased incidence of falls. There is little relationship to reduced cognitive ability, which is better correlated with ganglionic lesions and temporal lobe atrophy.

## Case 610

51-year-old woman, two years after
a right hemispheric stroke.
(axial, noncontrast scan; SE 3000/30)

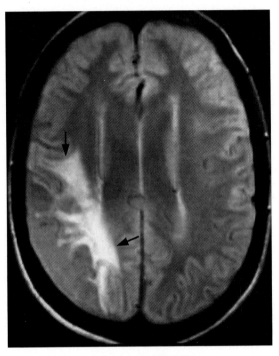

**Old MCA Infarct**
(posterior division)

## Case 611

61-year-old man with bilateral carotid stenosis.
(axial, noncontrast scan; SE 2500/28)

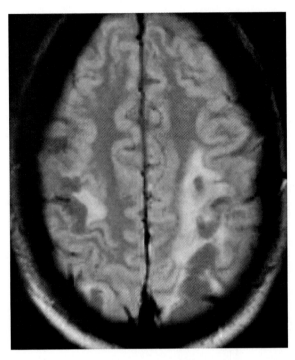

**Old Border Zone Infarcts**

---

FLAIR images or spin echo scans with long TR and short TE values typically demonstrate two zones of signal abnormality within old cerebral infarcts. The above cases illustrate this characteristic appearance.

Scar tissue along the interface between the affected area and normal parenchyma causes a margin of high signal intensity. This border zone is typically irregular and of variable thickness. The more peripheral portion of the infarcted region is homogeneous and comparable to CSF in intensity. This region may be microcystic and/or grossly cavitated, with variable communication to the subarachnoid space.

Volume loss usually accompanies the altered signal intensity of old infarcts, with expansion of adjacent portions of the ventricular system. No enhancement is seen after contrast injection.

The distribution of multiple cerebral infarcts may help to characterize underlying pathophysiology. Multiple infarcts at scattered cortical locations independent of watershed boundaries suggest multifocal occlusion of distal cerebral arteries and raise the possibility of embolization, vasculitis or coagulopathy. On the other hand, multiple infarcts aligned along watershed distributions, as in Case 611, suggest generalized hypoperfusion rather than involvement of individual cortical vessels.

Tissue damage from cortical watershed infarction is often most severe in the parietal regions. This area represents the most distal supply zone of the major cerebral arteries. A generalized reduction in perfusion would be expected to most adversely affect parenchyma that is furthest downstream, while more proximal territories might be relatively spared.

In term infants, this gradient of ischemic damage along the (mature) cortical arterial watershed from anterior to posterior can produce a clinical picture of spastic diplegia. Such presentations may resemble the outcome of periventricular leukomalacia caused by hypoxic/ischemic insult to the immature brain (see Cases 592-595).

# REFERENCES

Aida N, Nishimura G, Hachiya Y, et al: MR imaging of perinatal brain damage: comparison of clinical outcome with initial and follow-up MR findings. *AJNR* 19:1909-1922, 1998.

Amerenco P, Kase CS, Rosengart A, et al: Very small (border zone) cerebellar infarcts. *Brain* 116:161-186, 1993.

Amerenco P, Rosengart A, DeWitt L, et al: Anterior inferior cerebellar artery territory infarcts: mechanisms and clinical features. *Arch Neurol* 50:154-161, 1993.

Anderson CM, Saloner D, Lee RE, et al: Assessment of carotid artery stenosis by MR angiography: comparison with x-ray angiography and color-coded Doppler ultrasound. *AJNR* 13:989-1003, 1992.

Anderson SC, Shah CP, Murtagh FR: Congested deep subcortical veins as a sign of dural venous thrombosis: MR and CT correlation. *J Comput Assist Tomogr* 11:1059-1061, 1987.

Anson JA, Heiserman JE, Drayer BP, Spetzler RF: Surgical decisions on the basis of magnetic resonance angiography of the carotid arteries. *Neurosurgery* 32:335-343, 1993.

Arbelaez A, Castillo M, Mukherji SK: Diffusion-weighted MR imaging of global cerebral anoxia. *AJNR* 20:999-1008, 1999.

Armstrong FD, Thompson RJ Jr, Wang W, et al: Cognitive functioning and brain magnetic resonance imaging in children with sickle cell disease. *Pediatrics* 97:864-870, 1996.

Auer DP, Pütz B, Gössl C, et al: Differential lesion patterns in CADASIL and sporadic subcortical arteriosclerotic encephalopathy: MR imaging study with statistical parametric group comparison. *Radiology* 218:433-451, 2001.

Ayanzen RH, Bird CR, Keller PJ, et al: Cerebral MR venography: normal anatomy and potential diagnostic pitfalls. *AJNR* 21:74-78, 2000.

Baenziger O, Martin E, Steinlin M, et al: Early pattern recognition in severe perinatal asphyxia: a prospective MRI study. *Neuroradiology* 35:437-442, 1993.

Bakac G, Wardlaw JM: Problems in the diagnosis of intracranial venous infarction. *Neuroradiology* 39:566-570, 1997.

Barkhof F, Valk J: "Top of the basilar" syndrome: a comparison of clinical and MR findings. *Neuroradiology* 30:293, 1988.

Barkovich AJ: MR and CT evaluation of profound neonatal and infantile asphyxia. *AJNR* 13:959-972, 1992.

Barkovich AJ, Sargent SK: Profound asphyxia in the premature infant: imaging findings. *AJNR* 16:1837-1846, 1995.

Barkovich AJ, Truwitt CL: Brain damage from perinatal asphyxia: correlation of MR findings with gestational age. *AJNR* 11:1087-1096, 1990.

Barkovich AJ, Westmark K, Partridge C, et al: Perinatal asphyxia: MR findings in the first 10 days. *AJNR* 16:427-438, 1995.

Beaulieu C, de Crespigny A, Tong DC, et al: Longitudinal magnetic resonance imaging study of perfusion and diffusion in stroke: evolution of lesion volume and correlation with clinical outcome. *Ann Neurol* 46:568-578, 1999.

Bell DA, Davis WL Osborn AG, Harnsberger HR: Bithalamic hyperintensity on T2-weighted MR: vascular causes and evaluation with MR angiography. *AJNR* 15:893-899, 1994.

Biller J, Adams HP Jr, Dunn V, et al: Dichotomy between clinical findings and MR abnormalities in pontine infarction. *J Comput Assist Tomogr* 10:379-385, 1986.

Birbamer G, Aichner F, Felber S, et al: MRI of cerebral hypoxia. *Neuroradiology* (suppl):53-55, 1991.

Blankenberg FG, Norbash AM, Lane B, et al: Neonatal intracranial ischemia and hemorrhage: diagnosis with US, CT and MR imaging. *Radiology* 199:253-260, 1996.

Bousson V, Levy C, Brunereau L, et al: Dissections of the internal carotid artery: three-dimensional time-of-flight MR angiography and MR imaging features. *Am J Roentgenol* 173:139-143, 1999.

Bui LN, Brant-Zawadzki M, Verghese P, Gillan G: Magnetic resonance angiography of craniocervical dissection. *Stroke* 24:126-131, 1993.

Bulas DI, Vezina GL: Preterm anoxic injury: radiologic evaluation. *Radiol Clin North Am* 37:1147-1162, 1999.

Castillo M, Falcone S, Naidich TP, et al: Imaging in acute basilar artery thrombosis. *Neuroradiology* 36:426-429, 1994.

Chang KH, Han MH, Kim HS, et al: Delayed encephalopathy after acute carbon monoxide intoxication: MR imaging features and distribution of cerebral white matter lesions. *Radiology* 184:117-122, 1992.

Cormier PJ, Long ER, Russell EJ, et al: MR imaging of posterior fossa infarctions: vascular territories and clinical correlations. *Radiographics* 12:1079-1096, 1992.

Demaerel P, Casaer P, Casteels-Van Daele M, et al: Moyamoya disease: MRI and MR angiography. *Neuroradiology* 33(suppl):50-52, 1991.

Derdeyn CP, Khosla A, Videen TO, et al: Severe hemodynamic impairment and border zone-region infarction. *Radiology* 220:195-201, 2001.

Dormont D, Sag K, Biondi A, et al: Gadolinium-enhanced MR of chronic dural sinus thrombosis. *AJNR* 16:1347-1352, 1995.

Dubowitz DJ, Bluml S, Acinue E, Dietrich RB: MR of hypoxic encephalopathy in children after near drowning: correlation with quantitative proton MR spectroscopy and clinical outcome. *AJNR* 19:1617-1627, 1998.

Elster AD: MR contrast enhancement brainstem and deep cerebral infarctions. *AJNR* 12:1127-1132, 1991.

Elster AD, Richardson DN: Focal high signal on MR scans of the midbrain caused by enlarged perivascular spaces: MR-pathologic correlation. *AJNR* 11:1119-1122, 1990.

Erdman WA, Weinreb JC, Cohen JM, et al: Venous thrombosis: clinical and experimental MR imaging. *Radiology* 161:233-238, 1986.

Falini A, Barkovich AJ, Calabrese G, et al: Progressive brain failure after diffuse hypoxic ischemic brain injury: a seriesl MR and proton MR spectroscopic study. *AJNR* 19:648-652, 1998.

Forbes KPN, Pipe JG, Bird R: Neonatal hypoxic-ischemic encephalopathy: detection with diffusion-weighted MR imaging. *AJNR* 21:1490-1496, 2000.

Fox AJ, Bogousslavsky J, Carey LS, et al: Magnetic resonance imaging of small medullary infarctions. *AJNR* 7:229-234, 1986.

Friedman DP: Abnormalities of the deep medullary white matter veins: MR imaging findings. *Am J Roentgenol* 168:1103-1108, 1997.

Friedman DP: Abnormalities of the posterior inferior cerebellar artery: MR imaging findings. *Am J Roentgenol* 160:1257-1263, 1993.

Fujisawa I, Asato R, Nishimura K et al: Moyamoya disease: MR imaging. *Radiology* 164:103-106, 1987.

Fujita N, Hirabuki N, Fujii K, et al: MR imaging of middle cerebral artery stenosis and occlusion: value of MR angiography. *AJNR* 15:335-342, 1994.

Geijer B, Lindgren A, Brockstedt S, et al: Persistent high signal on diffusion-weighted MRI in the late stages of small cortical and lacunar ischaemic lesions. *Neuroradiology* 43:115-122, 2001.

Goldberg HI, Grossman RI, Gomori JM, et al: Cervical internal carotid artery hemorrhage: diagnosis using MR. *Radiology* 158:157-162, 1986.

Greenan TJ, Grossman RI, Goldbert HI: Cerebral vasculitis: MR imaging and angiographic correlation. *Radiology* 182:65-72, 1992.

Greenberg SM, Vonsattel JPG, Stakes JW, et al: The clinical spectrum of cerebral amyloid angiopathy: presentations without lobar hemorrhage. *Neurology* 43:2073-2079, 1993.

Greenough GP, Mamourian A, Harbaugh RE: Venous hypertension associated with a posterior fossa dural arteriovenous fistula: another cause of bithalamic lesions on MR images. *AJNR* 20:145-148, 1999.

Harris KG, Tran DD, Sickels WJ, Cornel SH: Diagnosing intracranial vasculitis: the roles of MR and angiography. *AJNR* 15:317-330, 1994.

Heinz ER, Yeates AE, Djang WT: Significant extracranial carotid stenosis: detection on routine cerebral MR images. *Radiology* 170:843-848, 1989.

Heiserman JE, Drayer BP, Keller PJ, Fram EK: Intracranial vascular occlusion: evaluation with three dimensional time-of-flight MR angiography. *Radiology* 185:667-673, 1992.

Ho VB, Rovira MJ, Borke RC, Smirniotopoulos JG: Arachnoid granulations in the transverse sinuses: incidence and features on magnetic resonance imaging and magnetic resonance venography. *Int J Neurorad* 3:482-489, 1997.

Horowitz AL, Kaplan R, Sarpel G: Carbon monoxide toxicity: MR imaging in the brain. *Radiology* 162:787-788, 1987.

Hosoya TW, Watanabe N, Yamaguchi K, et al: Intracranial vertebral artery dissection in Wallenberg syndrome. *AJNR* 15:1161-1165, 1994.

Jager HR, Albrecht T, Curati-Alasonatti WL, et al: MRI in neuro-Behcet's syndrome: comparison of conventional spin-echo and FLAIR pulse sequences. *Neuroradiology* 41:750-758, 1999.

Johnson AJ, Lee BCP, Lin W: Echoplanar diffusion-weighted imaging in neonates and infants with suspected hypoxic-ischemic injury: correlation with patient outcome. *Am J Roentgenol* 172:219-226, 1999.

Johnson BA, Heiserman JE, Drayer BP, Keller PJ: Intracranial MR angiograpnhy: its role in the integrated approach to brain infarction. *AJNR* 15:901-908, 1994.

Johnson MH, Christman CW: Posterior circulation infarction: anatomy, pathophysiology, and clinical correlation. *Semin Ultrasound CT, MRI* 16:237-252, 1995.

Jouvet P, Cowan FM, Cox P, et al: Reproducibility and accuracy of MR imaging of the brain after severe birth asphyxia. *AJNR* 20:1343-1345, 1999.

Karonen JO, Kaarina Partanen PL, Vanninen RL, et al: Evolution of MR contrast enhancement patterns during the first week after acute ischemic stroke. *AJNR* 22:103-111, 2001.

Katz BH Quencer RM, Kaplan JO, et al: MR imaging of intracranial carotid occlusion. *AJNR* 10:345-350, 1989.

Keeney SE, Adcock EW, McArdle CB: Prospective observations of 100 high-risk neonates by high field (1.5 Tesla) magnetic resonance imaging of the central nervous system: II. Lesions associated with hypoxic-ischemic encephalopathy. *Pediatrics* 87:431-438, 1991.

Kim JS, Lee JH, Choi CG: Patterns of lateral medullary infarction: vascular lesion-magnetic resonance imaging correlation of 34 cases. *Stroke* 29:645-652, 1998.

Kirsch E, Kaim A, Engelter S, et al: MR angiography in internal carotid artery dissection: improvement of diagnosis by selective demonstration of the intramural haematoma. *Neuroradiology* 40:704-709, 1998.

Knepper L, Biller J, Adams HP Jr, et al: MR imaging of basilar artery occlusion. *J Comput Assist Tomogr* 14:32-35, 1990.

Korogi Y, Takahashi M, Hirai T, et al: The ventral posterolateral thalamus: magnetic resonance findings in healthy neonates and in neonatal asphyxia. *Int J Neurorad* 4:97-104, 1998.

Lafitte F, Boukobza M, Guichard JP, et al: Deep cerebral venous thrombosis: imaging in eight cases. *Neuroradiology* 41:410-418, 1999.

Lane JL, Flanders AE, Doan HT, Bell RD: Assessment of carotid artery patency in routine spin-echo MR imaging of the brain. *AJNR* 12:819-826, 1991.

Lang E, Lang C, Huk W, Neundorfer B: Magnetic resonance imaging of dorsolateral medullary infarction in Wallenberg syndrome. *Neuroradiology* 36:269-270 1994.

Lansberg MG, Thijs VN, O'Brien W, et al: Evolution of apparent diffusion coefficient, diffusion-weighted, and T2-weighted signal intensity of acute stroke. *AJNR* 22:637-644, 2001.

Laster RE Jr, Acker JD, Halford HH III, Nauert TC: Assessment of MR angiography versus arteriography for evaluation of cervical carotid bifurcation disease. *AJNR* 14:681-688, 1993

Lazar EB, Russel EJ, Cohen BA, et al: Contrast-enhanced MR of cerebral arteritis: intravascular enhancement related to flow stasis within areas of focal arterial ectasia. *AJNR* 13:271-276, 1992.

Leach JL, Jones BV, Tomsick TA, et al: Normal appearance of arachnoid granulations on contrast-enhanced CT and MR of the brain: differentiation from dural sinus disease. *AJNR* 17:1523-1532, 1996.

Levy C, Laissy JP, Raveau V, et al: Carotid and vertebral artery dissections: three-dimensional time-of-flight MR angiography and MR imaging versus conventional angiography. *Radiology* 190:97-103, 1994.

Liauw L, van Buchem MA, Spilt A, et al: MR angiography of the intracranial venous system. *Radiology* 214:678-682, 2000.

Litt AW, Eidelman EM, Pinto RS, et al: Diagnosis of carotid artery stenosis: comparison of 2DFT time-of-flight MR angiography with contrast angiography in 50 patients. *AJNR* 12:149-154, 1991.

Macchi PJ, Grossman RI, Gomori JM, et al: High field MR imaging of cerebral venous thrombosis. *J Comput Assist Tomogr* 10:10-15, 1986.

Madan A, Sluzewski M, van Rooij WJJ, et al: Thrombosis of the deep cerebral veins: CT and MRI findings with pathologic correlation. *Neuroradiology* 39:777-780, 1997.

Maeda M, Yamamoto T, Daimon S, et al: Arterial hyperintensity on fast fluid-attenuated inversion recovery images: a stubtle finding for hyperacute stroke undetected by diffusion-weighted MR imaging. *AJNR* 22:632-636, 2001.

Manzione J, Newman GC, Shapiro A, Santo-Ocampo R: Diffusion- and perfusion-weighted MR imaging of dural sinus thrombosis. *AJNR* 21:68-73, 2000.

Mascalchi M, Bianchi MC, Mangiafico S, et al: MRI and MR angiography of vertebral artery dissection. *Neuroradiology* 39:329-340, 1997.

McArdle CB, Mirfakhraee M, Amparo EG, Kulkarni MV: MR imaging of transverse/sigmoid dural sinus and jugular vein thrombosis. *J Comput Assist Tomogr* 11:831-838, 1987.

McArdle CB, Richardson CJ, Hayden CK, et al: Abnormalities of the neonatal brain: MR imaging. Part II. Hypoxic-ischemic brain injury. *Radiology* 163:395-404, 1987.

Medlock MD, Olivero WC, Hanigan WC, et al: Children with cerebral venous thrombosis diagnosed with magnetic resonance imaging and magnetic resonance angiography. *Neurosurgery* 31:870-876, 1992.

Milandre L, Rumeau C, Sangla I, et al: Infarction in the territory of the anterior inferior cerebella artery: report of five cases. *Neuroradiology* 34:500-503, 1992.

Miller DH, Ormerod IEC, Gibson A, et al: MR brain scanning in patients with vasculitis: differentiation from multiple sclerosis. *Neuroradiology* 29:226-231, 1987.

Moran CJ, Siegel MJ, DeBaun MR: Sickle cell disease: imaging of cerebrovascular complications. *Radiology* 206:311-321, 1998.

Morrissey SP, Miller DH, Hermaszewski R, et al: MRI of the CNS in Behcet's disease. *Eur Neurol* 33:287-293, 1993.

Moser FG, Miller ST, Bello JA, et al: The spectrum of brain MR abnormalities in sickle cell disease: a report from the cooperative study of sickle cell disease. *AJNR* 17:965-972, 1996.

Ozawa T, Sasaki O, Sorimachi T, Tanaka R: Primary angiitis of the central nervous system: report of two cases and review of the literature. *Neurosurgery* 36:173-179, 1995.

Ozdoba C, Sturzenegger M, Schroth G: Internal carotid artery dissection: MR imaging features and clinical-radiologic correlation. *Radiology* 199:191-198, 1996.

Padayachee TS, Bingham JB, Graves MJ, et al: Dural sinus thrombosis: diagnosis and follow-up by magnetic resonance angiography and imaging. *Neuroradiology* 33:165-167, 1991.

Pantano P, Toni D, Caramia F, et al: Relationship between vascular enhancement, cerebral hemodynamics, and MR angiography in cases of acute stroke. *AJNR* 22:255-260, 2001.

Phillips MD, Zimmerman RA: Diffusion imaging in pediatric hypoxic ischemia injury. *Neuroimaging Clin North Am* 9:41-52, 1999.

Pomper MG, Miller TJ, Stone JH, et al: CNS vasculitis in autoimmune disease: MR imaging findings and correlation with angiography. *AJNR* 20:75-90, 1999.

Provenzale JM, Allen NB: Neuroradiologic findings in polyarteritis nodosa. *AJNR* 17:1119-1126, 1996.

Provenzale JM, Joseph GJ, Barboriak DP: Dural sinus thrombosis: findings on CT and MR imaging and diagnostic pitfalls. *Am J Roentgenol* 170:777-783, 1998.

Provenzale JM, Loganbill HA: Dural sinus thrombosis and venous infarction associated with antiphospholipid antibodies: MR findings. *J Comput Assist Tomogr* 18:719-723, 1994.

Quint D, Spickler E: Magnetic resonance demonstration of vertebral artery dissection. Report of two cases. *J Neurosurg* 72:964-967, 1990.

Rippe DJ, Boyko OB, Spritzer CE, et al: Demonstration of dural sinus occlusion by the use of MR angiography. *AJNR* 11:199-201, 1990.

Roche J, Warner D: Arachnoid granulations in the transverse and sigmoid sinuses: CT, MR, and MR angiographic appearance of a normal anatomic variation. *AJNR* 17:677-684, 1996.

Seibert JJ, Miller SF, Kirby RS, et al: Cerebrovascular disease in symptomatic and asymptomatic patients with sickle cell anemia: screening with duplex transcranial doppler US–correlation with MR imaging and MR angiography. *Radiology* 189:457-466, 1993.

Shin JH, Suh DC, Choi CG, Lee HK: Vertebral artery dissection: spectrum of imaging findings. *Radiographics* 20:1687-1696, 2000.

Shoemaker EI, Lin Z-S, Rae-Grant AD, Little B: Primary agniitis of the central nervous system: unusual MR appearance. *AJNR* 15:331-334, 1994.

Sie LTL, van der Knaap MS, van Wezel-Meijler G, et al: Early MR features of hypoxic-ischemic brain injury in neonates with periventricular densities on sonograms. *AJNR* 21:852-861, 2000.

Silverman CS, Brenner J, Murtagh FR: Hemorrhagic necrosis and vascular injury in carbon monoxide poisoning: MR demonstration. *AJNR* 14:168-170, 1993.

Simmons Z, Biller J, Adams HP, et al: Cerebellar infarction: Comparison of computed tomography and magnetic resonance imaging. *Ann Neurol* 19:291-293, 1986.

Skehan SJ, Hutchinson M, MacErlaine DP: Cerebral autosomal dominant arteriopathy with subcortical infarcts and leukoencephalopathy: MR findings. *AJNR* 16:2115-2120, 1995.

Stone JH, Pomper MG, Roubenoff R, et al: Sensitivities of noninvasive tests for central nervous system vasculitis: a comparison of lumbar puncture, computed tomography, and magnetic resonance imaging. *J Rheumatol* 21:1277-1282, 1994.

Sue DE, Brant-Zawadzki MN, Chana J: Dissection of cranial arteries in the neck: correlation of MRI and arteriography. *Neuroradiology* 34:273-278, 1992.

Sunshine JL, Bambalidis N, Tarr RW et al: Benefits of perfusion MR imaging relative to diffusion MR imaging in the diagnosis and treatment of hyperacute stroke. *AJNR* 22:915-921, 2001.

Sze C, Simmons B, Krol G, et al: Dural sinus thrombosis: verification with spin-echo techniques. *AJNR* 9:679-686, 1988.

Takahashi S, Higano S, Ishii K, et al: Hypoxic brain damage: cortical laminar necrosis and delayed changes in white matter at sequential MR imaging. *Radiology* 189:449-456, 1993.

Takanashi J, Sugita K, Ishii M, et al: Moyamoya syndrome in young children: MR comparison with adult onset. *AJNR* 14:1139-1142.

Tali ET, Atilla S, Keskin T, et al: MRI in neuro-Behcet's disease. *Neuroradiology* 39:2-6, 1997.

Tatemichi TK, Steinke W, Duncan C, et al: Paramedian thalamopeduncular infarction: clinical syndromes and magnetic resonance imaging. *Ann Neurol* 32:162-171, 1992.

Toyoda K, Ida M, Fukuda K: Fluid-attenuated inversion recovery intraarterial signal: an early sign of hyperacute cerebral ischemia. *AJNR* 22:1021-1029, 2001.

Tsai FY, Wang A, Matovich VB, et al: MR staging of acute dural sinus thrombosis: correlation with venous pressure measurements and implications for treatment and prognosis. *AJNR* 16:1021-1029, 1995.

Vogl TJ, Bergman C, Villringer A, et al: Dural sinus thrombosis: value of venous MR angiography for diagnosis and follow-up. *Am J Roentgenol* 162:1191-1198, 1994.

Wentz KY, Rother J, Schwartz A, et al: Intracranial vertebrobasilar system: MR angiography. *Radiology* 190:105-110, 1994.

Westmark KD, Barkovich AJ, Sola A, et al: Patterns and implications of MR contrast enhancement in perinatal asphyxia: a preliminary report. *AJNR* 16:685-692, 1995.

Yamada I, Matsushima Y, Suzuki S, Childhood moyamoya disease before and after encephalo-duro-arterio-syanangiosis: an angiographic study. *Neuroradiology* 34:318-322, 1992.

Yamada I, Matsushima Y, Suzuki S: Moyamoya disease: diagnosis with three-dimensional time-of-flight MR angiography. *Radiology* 184:773-778, 1992.

Yamada I, Suzuki S, Matsushima Y: Moyamoya disease: comparison of assessment with MR angiography and MR imaging versus conventional angiography. *Radiology* 196,211-215, 1995.

Yamada I, Suzuki S, Matsushima Y: Moyamoya disease: Diagnostic accuracy of MRI. *Neuroradiology* 37:356-361, 1995.

Yasui T, Komiyama M, Nishikawa M, Nakajima H: Subarachnoid hemorrhage from vertebral artery dissecting aneurysms involving the origin of the posteroinferior cerebellar artery: report of two cases and review of the literature. *Neurosurgery* 46:196-200, 2000.

Yuh WTC, Simonson TM, Wang A-M, et al: Venous sinus occlusive disease: MR findings. *AJNR* 15:309-316 1994.

Yuh WTC, Ueda T, Maley JE: Perfusion and diffusion imaging: a potential tool for improved diagnosis of CNS vasculitis. *AJNR* 20:87-88, 1999.

Zimmerman RD, Ernst RJ: Neuroimaging of cerebrovenous thrombosis. *Neuroimaging Clin N Amer* 2:463-485, 1992.

# CHAPTER 12

# Infratentorial Infarction, Arterial Pathology, Venous Thrombosis, and Anoxia

## Case 612

82-year-old woman presenting with dementia.
(axial, noncontrast T2-weighted SE scan)

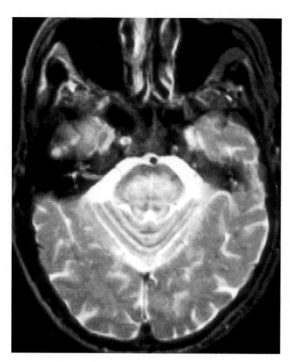

**Brainstem Ischemic Changes**

## Case 613

29-year-old woman presenting with
acute dizziness and diplopia.
(axial, noncontrast FLAIR scan)

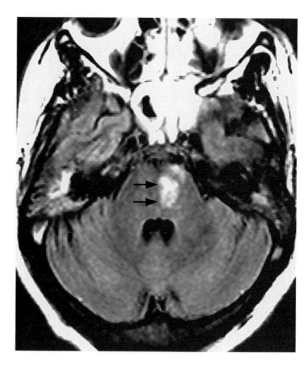

**Brainstem Infarct**

MR is valuable for confirming and localizing the clinical diagnosis of brainstem ischemia. CT scans may fail to define recent brainstem infarcts, since they are often small and their subtle attenuation changes are obscured by interpetrous artifact.

Small arterial disease affecting the brainstem is usually most apparent at the rostral pontine level. Case 612 is a typical example, with multiple hazy foci of increased signal intensity clustered centrally. Scans through the cerebral hemispheres in such cases usually demonstrate associated lacunar infarcts in the basal ganglia and periventricular white matter, comparable to Cases 602 and 604. Patients with this MR appearance may have suprisingly minimal symptoms.

Case 613 illustrates a focal brainstem infarct. Such lesions are usually better defined and less symmetrical than the generalized ischemic changes seen in Case 612. A sharp medial margin of the lesion near the anatomical midline is apparent *(arrows)*. This feature is common in brainstem infarcts and may help to distinguish them from demyelinating foci, central pontine myelinolysis, and other brainstem pathologies.

The status of the basilar artery is of interest in cases of brainstem ischemia. Reduced lumen size and absence of normal flow void may be noted (see Case 628). However, most localized brainstem infarcts are caused by small vessel disease involving the pontine perforating arteries. In the above cases, the basilar artery appears normal.

Clinical studies have demonstrated that FLAIR images are less sensitive in defining small lesions within the brainstem and cerebellum (especially demyelinating plaques) than is true in the supratentorial compartment. Diffusion-weighted scans (see Cases 560, 561, and 623) are useful when conventional spin echo and FLAIR images are not diagnostic in a patient with symptoms of brainstem dysfunction.

Mucosal thickening fills the ethmoid and sphenoid sinuses and mastoid air cells in Case 613.

### Case 614

35-year-old woman presenting with acute ataxia.
(axial, noncontrast T2-weighted SE scan)

### Case 615

68-year-old man presenting with headaches.
(axial, noncontrast T2-weighted FSE scan)

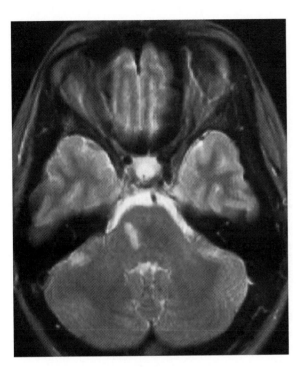

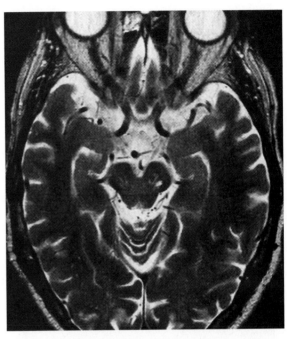

**Brainstem Infarct**

**Prominent Perivascular Spaces**
(normal variant)

---

Case 614 is another example of a typical brainstem infarct. The lesion is smaller than Case 613 but is similarly eccentric and well defined.

Small cysts of developmental origin are occasionally found within the cerebral peduncles, as in Case 615. These tiny CSF collections have been described as prominent perivascular spaces, analogous to similar structures in the sublentiform areas (see Case 838) or cerebral hemispheres (see Case 365). They may be unilateral or bilateral, producing a vague haze of focally increased signal intensity or a clearly defined cystic zone. Their characteristic location within the ventral midbrain and the absence of associated symptoms distinguish these developmental variants from brainstem infarcts, most of which occur more caudally.

Small brainstem infarcts may resemble involvement by multiple sclerosis (see Case 381). The clinical setting and associated lesions help to establish the diagnosis of either pathology. Demyelinating plaques in the brainstem tend to be rounder than focal infarcts.

Brainstem metastases can present a similar appearance and should be considered in the appropriate context (see Case 380). Wallerian degeneration may cause a focal area of signal abnormality resembling brainstem infarction on axial images (see Case 541B). Associated encephalomalacia within the ipsilateral cerebral hemisphere is apparent in such cases, and the lesion can be followed in continuity across several levels of anatomy as it courses along a fiber tract.

Central pontine myelinolysis may also produce abnormal signal intensity within the brainstem, as discussed in Cases 406 and 407. The typical clinical context and symmetrical central involvement of the pons assist in the diagnosis of this disorder.

### Case 616

9-year-old boy presenting with
the acute onset of ataxia.
(axial, noncontrast T2-weighted SE scan)

### Case 617

11-year-old girl with a history
of congenital heart disease.
(coronal, noncontrast T2-weighted SE scan)

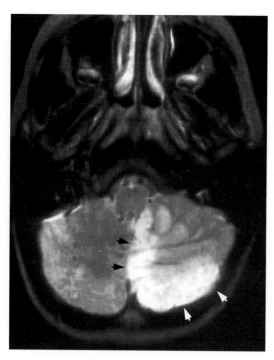

**PICA Infarct**

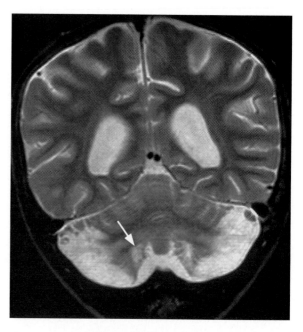

**Bilateral PICA Infarcts**

Infarction of the cerebellum may cause confusing lesions in the posterior fossa. In many cases, the diagnosis can be made by recognizing the distribution of a major cerebellar artery.

The posterior inferior cerebellar artery (PICA) supplies (1) a broad rim of peripheral cerebellar hemisphere along the occipital inner table (*white arrows,* Case 616) and (2) a parasagittal strip of medial hemisphere and inferior vermis extending posteriorly from the fourth ventricle (*black arrows,* Case 616). Infarction in the PICA distribution is suggested when a cerebellar lesion demonstrates a scythe-like configuration, with a curving peripheral crescent of involved hemisphere linked to a parasagittal band that borders the midline. Incomplete infarction in the PICA territory can cause abnormal signal intensity in either the peripheral or the parasagittal component of the distribution.

The localization of a cerebellar lesion within a major arterial distribution may be more easily appreciated on coronal or sagittal scans than on axial images. Case 617 illustrates that the PICA supplies the inferior and lateral portion

of the cerebellar hemispheres posteriorly. (The anterolateral margin of the cerebellum is perfused by the anterior inferior cerebellar artery.) The vermis is often spared in cases of PICA infarction due to collateral anastomoses between the superior vermian artery (a branch of the superior cerebellar artery) and the inferior vermian artery (from the PICA). PICA branches supply the cerebellar tonsil, which is involved by infarction when occlusion of the vessel is proximal (see Case 620). A small amount of tonsillar edema is suggested in Case 617, at least on the right *(arrow).*

Early ischemic edema is seen within the lateral portion of the right cerebellar hemisphere in Case 616. This boy was found to have spontaneous dissection of a vertebral artery, with multiple secondary emboli to the basilar system. Symptoms associated with dissection of carotid or vertebral arteries are more commonly due to secondary embolization than to hypoperfusion from luminal compromise.

The bilateral PICA infarctions in Case 617 were presumed to have resulted from emboli of cardiac origin.

### Case 618

33-year-old woman presenting with
the acute onset of vertigo and ataxia.
(axial, noncontrast T2-weighted FSE scan)

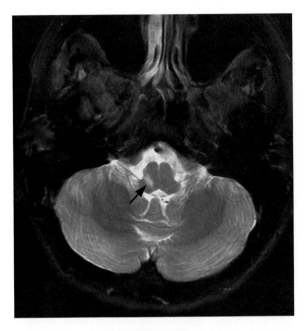

**Medullary Infarct**

### Case 619

73-year-old man presenting with recurrent dizziness.
(axial, noncontrast T2-weighted FSE scan)

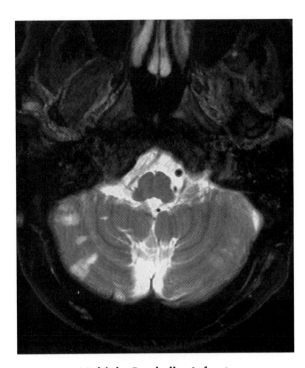

**Multiple Cerebellar Infarcts**

Infarction within the distribution of the PICA may be limited to the territory of a single branch. Such focal lesions imply small emboli that have passed through the proximal portion of the vessel and lodged distally.

A clinically important component of the PICA distribution is the lateral aspect of the medulla. PICA occlusion or embolization regularly leads to lateral medullary infarction, which can accompany cerebellar ischemia (see Case 620) or be an isolated event, as in Case 618 *(arrow)*.

PICA infarction may cause one or more manifestations of "Wallenberg syndrome". This constellation of potential symptoms reflecting dysfunction of the lateral medulla includes dysphagia, hoarseness, nystagmus, diplopia, ataxia, vertigo, nausea, vomiting, hiccups, ipsilateral facial pain or numbness, impaired taste, ipsilateral preganglionic Horner's syndrome and contralateral reduction in pain and temperature sensation.

Case 619 demonstrates multiple small lesions within the cerebellar hemispheres bilaterally. These discrete foci of signal abnormality suggest embolic occlusion of individual PICA branches leading to wedge-shaped, peripherally based

cortical infarcts. (Compare to the morphology of cortical infarction of the cerebral hemisphere in Case 566.)

The great horizontal fissure of the cerebellum is mildly oblique to the plane of axial CT or MR scans. If the fissure is enlarged due to cerebellar atrophy in an elderly patient, it will be noted as a focal zone of prolonged T1 and T2 values at the margin of the cerebellar hemisphere. Mild head tilt can cause the fissure to be asymmetrically more prominent on one side, and the appearance may simulate a peripheral PICA infarct like those in Case 619. Attention to adjacent sections and consideration of cerebellar atrophy and head tilt (or correlation with sagittal and coronal scans) will clarify such pseudolesions.

Compare the lateral medullary infarct in Case 618 to hypertrophic olivary degeneration as illustrated in Cases 542 and 543. In a different clinical context, diagnostic possibilities in Case 618 would include a plaque of multiple sclerosis.

See Case 635 for an MR angiogram of the patient in Case 618.

# DIFFERENTIAL DIAGNOSIS:
## EXTENSIVE CEREBELLAR EDEMA

### Case 620

58-year-old man presenting with ataxia.
(axial, noncontrast T2-weighted FSE scan)

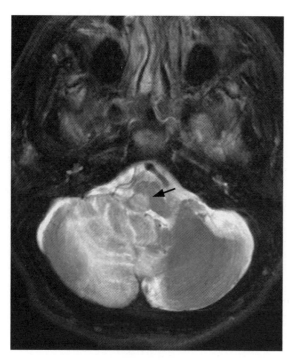

**PICA Infarct**

### Case 621

52-year-old woman presenting with ataxia.
(axial, noncontrast T2-weighted FSE scan)

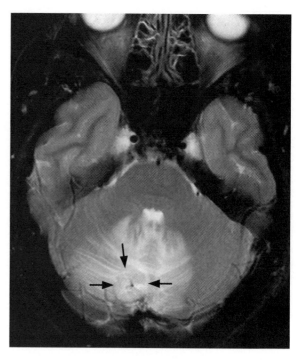

**Hemangioblastoma**

Extensive edema within the right cerebellar hemisphere and tonsil in Case 620 is associated with mass effect causing midline shift. When this displacement of tissue is taken into account, the edema is seen to respect the anatomical midline, now bowed medially by swelling. Sharp medial margination of the lesion at the cerebellar midline is a characteristic feature of PICA infarction (see Case 622) and contrasts with the reactive edema crossing midline in Case 621. Another hallmark of PICA infarction in Case 620 is involvement of the lateral medulla *(arrow),* as discussed previously.

The edema in Case 621 outlines the posterior margin of the dentate nucleus bilaterally. Within the large zone of T2 prolongation is a small tissue nodule containing a prominent central vessel *(arrows).* This mass enhanced intensely on postcontrast images and proved to be a solid hemangioblastoma.

The confluent signal abnormality and convex margins of a subacute PICA infarct may be even more mass-like than Case 620. Ischemic edema should be considered in the differential diagnosis of cerebellar "masses" at any age. Attention to the diagnostic clues listed above, correlation with the clinical context, and further assessment by diffusion-weighted and postcontrast scans will eliminate confusion in most cases.

Tissue swelling from cerebellar infarction may lead to life-threatening pressure on the brainstem. Acute decompression is required in such cases, similar to the urgent evacuation of large cerebellar hematomas. In Case 620, cerebellar mass effect has caused mild deformity of the caudal fourth ventricle and the dorsolateral medulla on the right.

Compare the definition of the dentate nuclei in Case 621 to the appearance of cerebellar involvement by PML in Cases 402 and 403.

## Case 622

45-year-old man presenting with acute
nausea, dizziness, and imbalance.
(axial, noncontrast diffusion-weighted
echo planar scan)

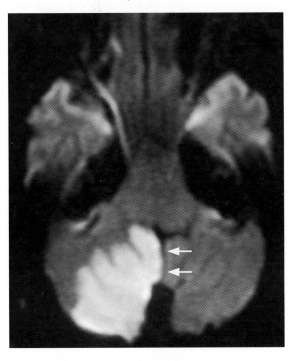

**PICA Infarct**

## Case 623

71-year-old man presenting with the abrupt onset of
right hemiparesis and left facial weakness.
(axial, noncontrast diffusion-weighted
echo planar scan)

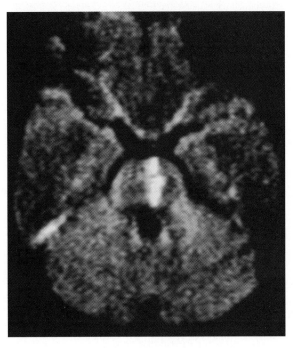

**Brainstem Infarct**

Restricted diffusion of water molecules due to cytotoxic edema is a hallmark of acute infarction, as discussed in Cases 560 and 561. Relatively immobile protons in a zone of infarction generate higher signal intensity (reflecting a lower apparent diffusion coefficient) than adjacent normal tissues on diffusion-weighted images. This feature can be very helpful in detecting and characterizing ischemic lesions, above or below the tentorium.

Although the spatial resolution of the above scans is quite coarse, the contrast of the lesions is high and their morphologies are characteristic. The sharply defined medial margin of the PICA infarct in Case 622 *(arrows)* respects the anatomical midline and establishes the diagnosis of a vascular process. Similarly, the elongated anteroposterior band of abnormal signal intensity in Case 623 demonstrates the typical morphology of infarction following the

course of a parasagittal penetrating artery within the brainstem (compare to Case 613).

The presence of restricted diffusion within a lesion is compatible with recent infarction but not specific. A cerebellar tumor as large as the lesion in Case 622 would rarely demonstrate such prominent abnormality of diffusion. However, demyelinating or inflammatory processes (e.g., multiple sclerosis, abscess, or encephalitis) can cause impaired diffusion and could potentially produce bright lesions within the brainstem or cerebellum on diffusion-weighted scans.

Artifacts near bone interfaces at the skull base are common on echo planar diffusion-weighted images, as seen above at the margins of the middle cranial fossae in Case 622 and near the right petrous ridge in Case 623.

### Case 624

9-year-old boy presenting with the
acute onset of ataxia.
(sagittal, noncontrast T1-weighted SE scan)

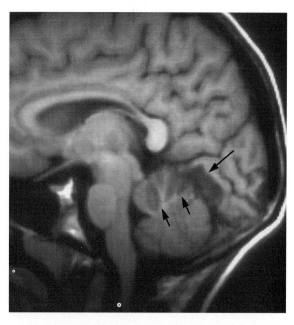

**Superior Cerebellar Artery Infarct**
(same patient as Case 616)

### Case 625

47-year-old woman presenting with headaches.
(axial, noncontrast T2-weighted SE scan)

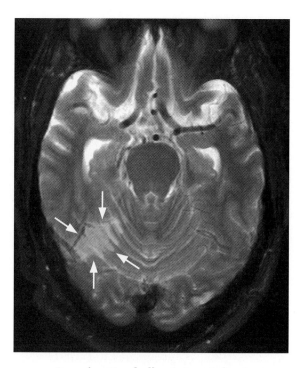

**Superior Cerebellar Artery Infarct**

---

The superior cerebellar artery (SCA) supplies the superior portion of the cerebellar hemisphere and vermis. Infarction in the distribution of this vessel usually involves the hemisphere but may spare the vermis due to collateral circulation from the inferior vermian arteries.

The above cases illustrate the variable medial/lateral extent of SCA infarction. In Case 624, a midsagittal scan demonstrates cortical edema within folia of the superior vermis *(short arrows)*. In Case 625, the midline SCA territory is spared, and infarction is limited to a small portion of the superior cerebellar hemisphere on the right *(arrows)*.

Cerebellar infarcts may accompany lesions in the occipital lobes when embolization has occurred within the vertebrobasilar system. Ischemic occipital edema is present in Case 624 *(long arrow)*. A careful search for cerebellar lesions can help to suggest vertebrobasilar emboli when ambiguous occipital pathology is encountered.

Cerebellar border zone infarction is infrequent. Such lesions are usually intrahemispheric, occurring within the corpus medullaris at the junction of the PICA, AICA, and SCA territories. Cystic encephalomalacia is occasionally seen in this location in children, possibly reflecting intrauterine or perinatal vascular insufficiency of the watershed zone.

# DIFFERENTIAL DIAGNOSIS:
## EDEMA OF SUPERIOR CEREBELLAR FOLIA

### Case 626

24-year-old man presenting with
the acute onset of ataxia.
(axial, noncontrast T2-weighted SE scan)

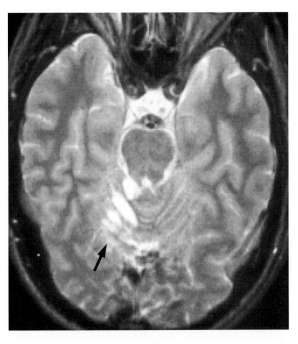

**Superior Cerebellar Artery Infarct**

### Case 627

60-year-old woman presenting with unsteady gait.
(axial, noncontrast T2-weighted SE scan)

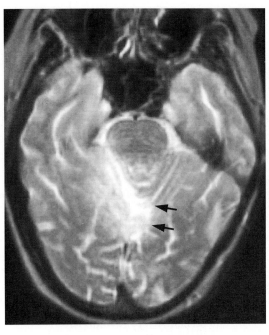

**Leptomeningeal Metastasis**
(from carcinoma of the breast)

---

The small region of high signal intensity involving the superior right cerebellar hemisphere in Case 626 *(arrow)* represents infarction within the distribution of the superior cerebellar artery. Layered edema in this region reflects the parallel structure of cerebellar folia, contrasting with the gyriform pattern of ischemic edema in cerebral cortex.

The straight, diagonal lateral margin of the lesion is a hallmark of infarction in the SCA territory, which is bounded laterally by the tentorium. The medial margin of SCA infarcts is variable and less distinct, depending on collateral flow patterns.

Meningeal seeding of intracranial tumors or systemic neoplasms often affects the superior cerebellar surface (see Cases 165-167 for additional examples). This occurrence resembles the preferential deposition of superficial siderosis in the same region under conditions of chronic subarachnoid hemorrhage (see Case 721). Both phenomena may reflect patterns of CSF flow and stagnation, with subarachnoid cells or hemorrhage settling over superior cerebellar tissue.

The zone of signal abnormality in Case 627 corresponds approximately to the SCA distribution. However, the extension across midline *(arrows)* would be atypical for a vascular etiology.

Postcontrast scans in both of the above cases might show a pattern of parallel, enhancing bands. In Case 626, the enhancement would represent ischemic cortex. In Case 627, a similar morphology could be produced by enhancing layers of meningeal tumor within cerebellar sulci (see Cases 165-167).

Case 627 also illustrates that pathologies other than SCA infarction can be marginated by the tentorium. A subdural empyema or chronic hematoma along the inferior surface of the tentorium could resemble the overall morphology of the above cases. (See discussion of Cases 570 and 571.)

## Case 628

74-year-old man presenting with
loss of consciousness.
(sagittal, noncontrast T1-weighted SE scan)

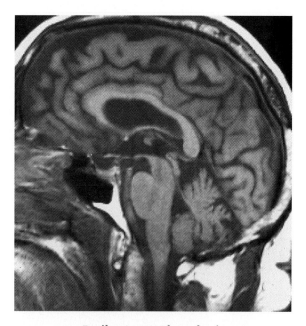

**Basilar Artery Thrombosis**

## Case 629

59-year-old woman presenting with
left hemisphere TIAs.
(axial, noncontrast T2-weighted SE scan)

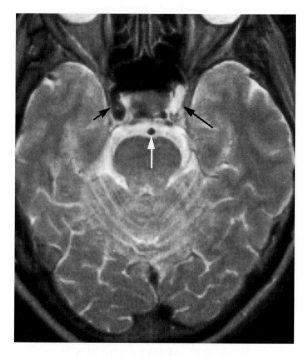

**Internal Carotid Artery Occlusion**

---

The characteristic appearance of rapidly flowing blood on routine spin echo MR scans is an absence of signal. When this expected flow void is replaced by measurable intraluminal intensity, slow flow or thrombus should be suspected. (See the discussion of arterial enhancement in Cases 576 and 577.)

Case 628 demonstrates a column of intermediate signal intensity at the expected position of the basilar artery. Although the possibility of hemorrhage or tissue within the prepontine cistern could be considered, the tubular morphology of the finding suggests an occluded vessel. Angiography confirmed thrombosis of the basilar artery.

In Case 629, high signal within the left supraclinoid internal carotid artery *(long black arrow)* contrasts with the normal flow void of the right paraclinoid internal carotid artery *(short black arrow)* and rostral basilar artery *(white arrow)*. The left parasellar internal carotid artery was found to be completely occluded at angiography.

The signal intensity of intraluminal thrombus is variable. Arterial ("white") thrombi are often isointense to cerebral parenchyma. Venous ("red") thrombi containing more erythrocytes may demonstrate T1-shortening and T2-shortening.

Reduced caliber of patent arteries at the skull base is another MR sign of vascular compromise. This finding may be associated with extracranial or intracranial stenoses (see discussion of moyamoya disease in Case 638).

A band of poorly defined low signal intensity within the pons in Case 628 is due to early ischemic edema, which was more apparent on T2-weighted scans.

## Case 630

54-year-old woman presenting with
diplopia and ataxia.
(axial partition from a noncontrast, three-
dimensional, time-of-flight GRE sequence)

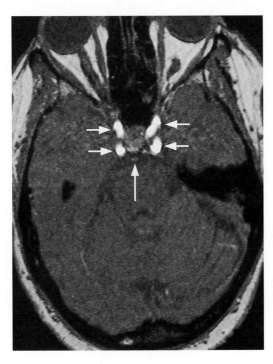

**Basilar Artery Stenosis**

## Case 631

51-year-old man presenting with
acute nausea and ataxia.
(AP view, maximal intensity projection
reconstruction, noncontrast, three-dimensional,
time-of-flight GRE sequence)

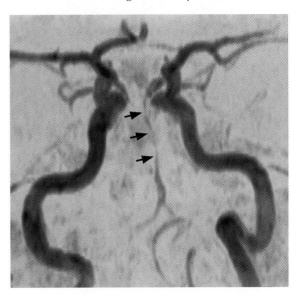

**Basilar Artery Stenosis**

MR angiography provides an excellent noninvasive means of assessing patency of arteries at the skull base. Time-of-flight techniques emphasize the higher signal intensity of "fresh" protons entering the plane of imaging as compared to surrounding stationary tissue.

Case 630 demonstrates strong flow within the parasellar internal carotid arteries *(short arrows)*. However, the rostral basilar artery *(long arrow)* is abnormally small and faint, implying significantly reduced perfusion.

The basilar artery in Case 631 is very narrow and irregular *(arrows)*, whereas the internal carotid arteries are grossly patent. The length of a mid basilar stenosis may be exaggerated by surrounding slow or turbulent flow on noncontrast time-of-flight images. MR angiography performed with intravenous injection of contrast material provides more accurate definition of luminal dimensions in cases of tight stenosis.

The basilar artery may normally be somewhat narrow if one or both posterior cerebral arteries are predominantly supplied from the internal carotid arteries. However, flow signal within the basilar artery should remain strong in such cases.

MR angiography of the vertebrobasilar system is very helpful in assessing elderly patients with suspected brainstem ischemia. The noninvasive documentation of severe arterial stenosis can clarify ambiguous or intermittent symptoms and support a decision to begin anticoagulation.

There is hypoplasia of the A1 segment of the left anterior cerebral artery in Case 631.

## Case 632

47-year-old man presenting with a three-day
history of left neck pain and mild aphasia.
(axial, noncontrast scan; SE 2500/45)

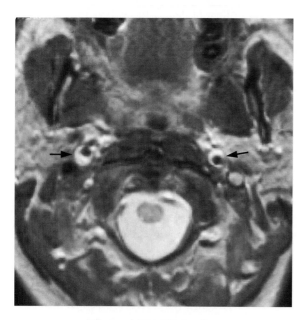

**Bilateral ICA Dissection**

## Case 633

29-year-old woman presenting with left
posterior neck pain and dizziness.
(axial partition from a noncontrast, three-
dimensional, time-of-flight GRE sequence)

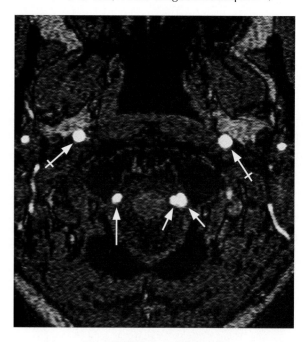

**Vertebral Artery Dissection**

Spontaneous dissections of cervical arteries tend to occur in young to middle-aged adults (mean age 45 years).
The internal carotid arteries are involved four times more
commonly than the vertebral arteries. Dissection of the internal carotid artery usually begins several centimeters distal to the bifurcation. Unusually tortuous or coiled arteries
seem to be prone to this pathology.

MR can diagnose arterial dissection by direct demonstration of the intramural hematoma. Scans perpendicular
to the long axis of an artery define crescentic thickening of
the vessel wall, eccentrically narrowing the lumen at the
level of dissection. Signal intensity of the intramural thrombus is variable but usually high, well demonstrated by noncontrast, axial T1-weighted scans with fat saturation.

Case 632 illustrates bilateral dissection of the internal
carotid arteries near the junction of the cervical and
petrous segments *(arrows)*. The distal cervical internal
carotid artery is frequently involved by dissection, which
often terminates abruptly at the entrance to the carotid
canal in the petrous bone. The patient in Case 632 could
not recall a history of right-sided neck pain or right hemisphere symptoms.

In Case 633, the flow channel of the distal left vertebral
artery is duplicated *(short arrows)*. This morphology
could represent either a false lumen (which occurs when
the dissection reenters the parent lumen distally) or a
pseudoaneurysm adjacent to the main vessel (see Cases
635 and 737). Angiography demonstrated the latter.

About 25% of patients with dissection of one internal
carotid artery or vertebral artery are found to have coexisting dissection of a second cervical vessel. When a single
spontaneous carotid or vertebral artery dissection occurs,
the risk of recurrence (usually in a different neck artery) is
reported to be 5% to 10%. In Case 633, the right vertebral
artery *(long arrow)* and the internal carotid arteries
*(crossed arrows)* are normal.

Among conditions predisposing to dissection of the
carotid or vertebral arteries are fibromuscular dysplasia,
Marfan's syndrome, and Ehlers-Danlos syndrome.

Patients with dissection of the carotid or vertebral arteries have an increased incidence of intracranial aneurysms,
which should be considered as angiograms are reviewed.

## Case 634

45-year-old man presenting with right hemiparesis.
(AP view, maximal intensity projection
reconstruction, noncontrast, three-dimensional,
time-of-flight GRE sequence)

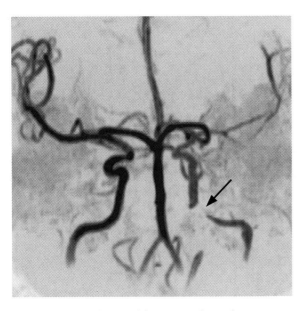

**Internal Carotid Artery Dissection**

## Case 635

33-year-old woman presenting with
the acute onset of vertigo and ataxia.
(rotated AP view, maximal intensity projection
reconstruction, noncontrast, three-dimensional,
time-of-flight GRE sequence)

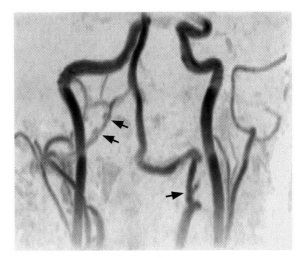

**Bilateral Vertebral Artery Dissection**
(same patient as Case 618)

Angiographic studies may demonstrate stenoses, pseudo-aneurysms, or both at the site of arterial dissection. The tapering, high grade narrowing of the distal left internal carotid artery in Case 634 *(arrow)* is a typical morphology for luminal compromise due to eccentric intramural hematoma.

The location of the lesion is also characteristic. Spontaneous or post-traumatic dissections of the internal carotid artery commonly involve or extend to the petrous segment.

The dissection itself is usually associated with neck pain, headache, and a partial Horner's syndrome (ptosis and miosis without anhydrosis). Accompanying palsies of lower cranial nerves (e.g., hypoglossal paresis) may occur due to distortion within the carotid sheath. Other secondary neurological deficits most often reflect cerebral embolization rather than hypoperfusion due to stenosis.

Dissections of the internal carotid artery usually occur within the media, while dissections of the distal vertebral artery are typically subadventitial. Vertebral artery dissections are more frequently accompanied by pseudo-aneurysms, as seen bilaterally in Case 635 *(arrows)*. Although these weakened areas of the vessel wall occasion-

ally rupture, they more commonly serve as a source of emboli. Dissection of the vertebral artery regularly occurs at the C1-2 level, probably correlating with mobility of the atlantoaxial articulation.

Infarction is the most likely cause of acute cerebellar (and/or brainstem) signs in a young adult. This possibility should be considered (along with labyrinthine disease) when young patients present with vertigo or ataxia. Dissection of a vertebral artery with subsequent embolization of associated thrombus is a leading diagnostic option in such cases.

Intracranial extension of carotid or vertebral artery dissections carries the risk of subarachnoid hemorrhage. Subadventitial dissections of the distal vertebral arteries are particularly prone to present in this manner and should be considered among the causes of hemorrhage within the posterior fossa.

Poor visualization of the left middle cerebral artery in Case 634 implies reduced flow that may be due to severe stenosis at the site of the carotid dissection and/or to secondary embolization.

## Case 636

33-year-old man presenting with
acute right hemiparesis.
(AP view, maximal intensity projection
reconstruction, noncontrast, three-dimensional,
time-of-flight GRE sequence)

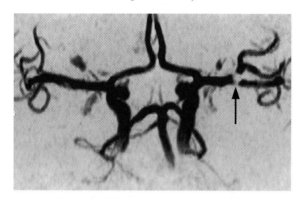

**Middle Cerebral Artery Embolus**

## Case 637

7-year-old boy presenting with right hemiparesis.
(slightly brow-up AP view, maximal intensity
projection reconstruction, noncontrast, three-
dimensional, time-of-flight GRE sequence)

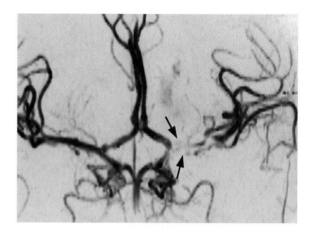

**Middle Cerebral Artery Dissection**

MR angiography provides noninvasive evaluation of the circle of Willis in patients presenting with transient ischemic attacks or cerebrovascular accidents. The morphology of arterial compromise in such cases is often diagnostic.

An embolus lodged at the bifurcation of the left middle cerebral artery is well defined as a filling defect in Case 636 *(arrow)*.

Case 637 illustrates spontaneous dissection of the left middle cerebral artery. The narrowing of the M1 segment *(arrows)* has compromised the origins of the ipsilateral lenticulostriate arteries. Associated hemorrhagic infarction causing T1-shortening within the left basal ganglia is superimposed on vague hyperemia in this region on the image formed by an algorithm recording maximal intensities of pixels along reconstruction rays.

Dissection of the middle cerebral artery is usually idiopathic and not recurrent. The middle cerebral artery in Case 637 returned to normal caliber on follow-up studies.

Unilateral or bilateral segments of arterial narrowing resembling Case 637 may be discovered in patients with moyamoya disease (see Case 638).

# MOYAMOYA DISEASE

## Case 638A

9-year-old boy presenting with bihemispheral TIAs.
(axial, noncontrast T1-weighted SE scan)

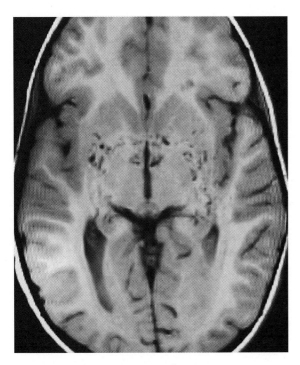

**Moyamoya Disease**

## Case 638B

Same patient.
(axial partition from a noncontrast, three-dimensional, time-of-flight GRE sequence)

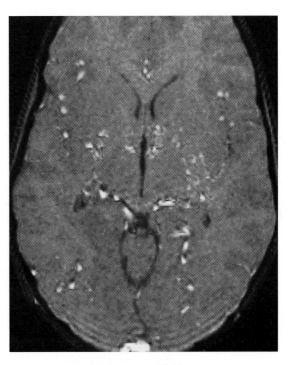

**Moyamoya Disease**

---

Moyamoya disease is a syndrome of progressive, idiopathic occlusion of major cerebral arteries at the skull base. The supraclinoid internal carotid arteries and proximal anterior, middle, and posterior cerebral arteries are commonly involved. Gradually worsening stenosis of these vessels causes hypertrophy of collateral channels. Prominent among these are perforating branches such as the lenticulostriate arteries. Angiography in these cases demonstrates a "cloud" or "puff of smoke" of small collateral arteries at the base of the brain, described historically by the Japanese phrase *moyamoya.*

The diagnosis of moyamoya disease is suggested on routine MR images by: (1) absence or reduced caliber of flow voids within the proximal middle, anterior, and posterior cerebral arteries; (2) abnormal prominence of low signal foci within the basal ganglia; and (3) evidence of hemispheric ischemia.

Case 638A illustrates the appearance of hypertrophied, transganglionic collateral vessels. The small diameter, slight tortuosity, and sublentiform concentration of these channels should distinguish them from lacunar infarcts. (Compare to the prominent perivascular spaces in Case 603 as well as to the miliary lesions in Cases 455 and 456.)

Flow sensitive gradient echo sequences can be used to confirm the vascular nature of such foci. Case 638B demonstrates high flow within small vessels throughout the ganglionic region bilaterally.

The diagnosis of idiopathic arterial occlusion at the base of the brain (i.e., moyamoya disease) should be made only after other possible etiologies are excluded. Basal meningitis, sickle cell disease, Down syndrome, neurofibromatosis, tumors such as meningiomas, and radiation therapy may all be associated with stenosis or occlusion of basal arteries.

The ischemic symptoms in this case are typical for the pediatric presentation of moyamoya disease. (See Case 582 for another example.) Adolescents and adults with this syndrome may present with intracerebral or subarachnoid hemorrhage due to rupture of hypertrophied collateral vessels.

### Case 639

44-year-old woman with a history of systemic lupus erythematosus and recurrent small strokes.
(axial, noncontrast scan; SE 2800/45)

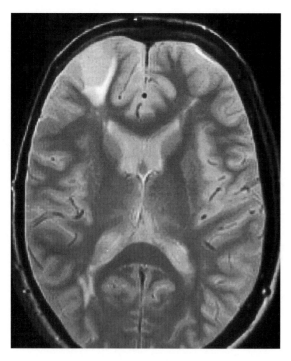

**Antiphospholipid Antibody Syndrome**
(positive lupus anticoagulant)

### Case 640

78-year-old woman presenting with decreased level of consciousness.
(axial, noncontrast T2-weighted FSE scan)

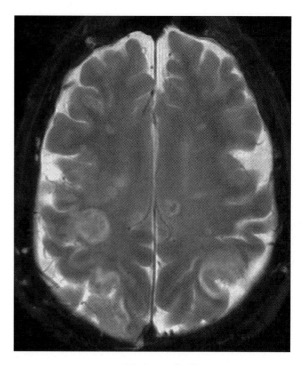

**Multiple Emboli**

Multifocal infarction occurring synchronously or over a period of time suggests a differential diagnosis including coagulopathy, emboli, and vasculitis.

Case 639 is an example of multiple deep and superficial cerebral infarcts due to coagulopathy. The presence of the lupus anticoagulant (an antiphospholipid antibody) in vitro is a marker for a tendency toward thrombosis in vivo. This syndrome may also present clinically as recurrent thrombophlebitis, dural sinus thrombosis, or repeated fetal loss during pregnancy. Cerebral symptoms and edema in systemic lupus erythematosus may be due to cerebritis (see Cases 481, 483, and 485), infarction secondary to vasculitis or coagulopathy, or a combination of these processes.

The heart and carotid arteries are the most likely sources of multiple cerebral emboli. Paradoxical cardiac embolization may be due to congenital heart disease or pulmonary arteriovenous communication, as in the Osler-Weber-Rendu syndrome (hereditary hemorrhagic telangectasia).

The patient in Case 640 presented with evidence of emboli to the arms and legs as well as the brain. The source of the debris proved to be severe atherosclerotic disease of the aortic arch.

Note that several of the small cortical infarcts in Case 640 are located outside of the arterial border zones (compare to Cases 584-587). This pattern of multifocal occlusion of individual cortical arteries (as distinct from regional watershed infarcts) was more apparent on lower sections. Mild T2-shortening within several of the lesions in Case 640 represents focal hemorrhage, which is a common feature of embolic infarction.

Vasculitis, a third major cause of multifocal infarction, is discussed in Cases 641-645. Other etiologies of multifocal infarction include anoxia, moyamoya disease (see Case 638), border zone arterial infarction, and venous infarction secondary to dural sinus thrombosis (see Cases 649 and 650).

## Case 641

74-year-old man presenting with rapidly
progressing motor and sensory deficits.
(axial, noncontrast T2-weighted FSE scan)

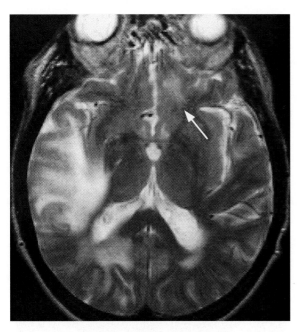

**Primary Angiitis of the CNS**
(same patient as Case 486)

## Case 642

45-year-old man with a three-day history
of decreasing level of consciousness.
(axial, noncontrast scan; SE 3000/45)

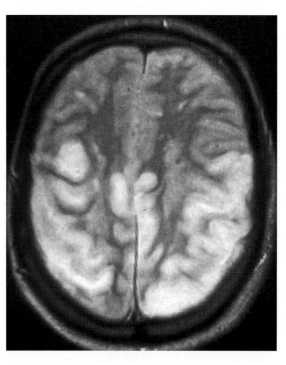

**Primary Angiitis of the CNS**

Primary angiitis of the CNS (PACNS) is an idiopathic inflammatory disorder affecting small cerebral arteries and veins. An alternative name for the disease, *granulomatous angiitis,* reflects the characteristic pathological finding of granulomas, giant cells, leukocytes, and lymphocytes in the walls of involved cerebral and meningeal vessels. PACNS may be immune mediated, and an association with herpes zoster has been suggested. Mean age of onset is between 40 and 50 years, with nearly equal incidence in men and women. The course of the disease is variable: some patients recover completely, whereas other cases are progressive and fatal.

The examples above, both proven by biopsy, demonstrate the spectrum of potential MR findings in PACNS. Edema in Case 641 is predominantly subcortical. The right temporal lobe is severely involved, with additional lesions in the left frontal lobe *(arrow)* and parieto-occipital region bilaterally. In some patients, zones of focal edema in PACNS (like the right temporal lesion in Case 641) are sufficiently mass-like to be biopsied as presumed neoplasms. PACNS should also be considered among the pathologies that can cause multifocal lesions affecting white matter.

The pattern of involvement in Case 642 is mainly cortical. Edema is bilateral and multifocal, affecting several major arterial distributions. PACNS is among the disorders that can present as multifocal cortical infarction (see discussion of Cases 639 and 640). The widespread cortical edema in Case 642 resembles inflammatory processes such as meningitis (see Cases 426 and 427), encephalitis (see Case 448), or autoimmune syndromes (see Cases 481, 483, and 485).

Contrast enhancement in PACNS is variable. No parenchymal enhancement was demonstrated in Case 641, despite the active edema. In other cases, multifocal patchy, linear, or miliary enhancement has been noted, with the latter two patterns presumably representing perivascular inflammation. Leptomeningeal enhancement may also be present.

Vascular involvement by PACNS is segmental rather than diffuse. Premortem biopsies may be negative in autopsy-proven cases due to sampling error. The pathological diagnosis of PACNS has been reported in patients whose cerebral angiograms were normal, reflecting involvement of vessels below the limit of angiographic resolution.

### Case 643

46-year-old woman presenting with
TIAs and hematuria.
(axial, noncontrast diffusion-weighted
echo planar scan)

### Case 644

36-year-old woman presenting with headaches.
(axial, noncontrast FLAIR scan)

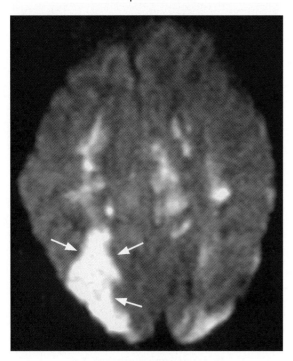

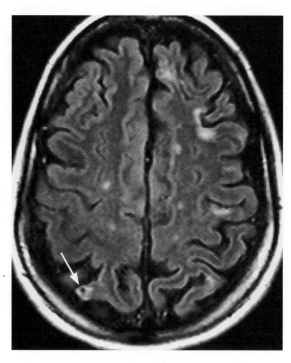

**Polyarteritis Nodosa**

**Vasculitis**
(nonspecific)

Cerebral vessels may be inflamed as an apparently isolated disorder (see discussion of primary angiitis of the CNS on the preceding page) or as a manifestation of systemic disease. Among pathologies in the latter category are systemic lupus erythematosus (see Cases 481, 483, and 485), Sjögren's syndrome (see Case 482), Wegener's granulomatosis, sarcoidosis, and neurovascular syphilis.

The woman in Case 643 presented with multisystem involvement from an exacerbation of polyarteritis nodosa. The diffusion-weighted scan demonstrates scattered bihemispheral sites of cytotoxic edema. Relatively large, cortically based infarcts (e.g., in the right parietal lobe; *arrows*) are accompanied by multiple smaller lesions within white matter.

The MR spectrum of vasculitis also includes many scans resembling Case 644. Multiple foci of signal abnormality are present within cortex and subcortical white matter. Many of the small infarcts have an angular morphology, whereas others are more rounded. Central necrosis is demonstrated in some of the lesions on FLAIR images (*arrow*).

Occasional patients with angiographically convincing and/or biopsy-proven vasculitis have no apparent parenchymal lesions on MR scans. Abnormal leptomeningeal enhancement may be the only positive finding in other cases.

An angiogram in Case 644 demonstrated diffuse cerebral arteritis. There was no evidence of demyelinating disease, sarcoidosis, Lyme disease, or autoimmune disorder. Meningeal or cortical biopsy was not performed.

Intravascular lymphomatosis ("angiocentric lymphoma") can cause multiple cortical and subcortical infarcts resembling vasculitis. Striated contrast enhancement may be seen in the involved regions, reflecting the intravascular or perivascular proliferation of lymphoid cells and/or associated stasis.

Amyloid angiopathy, a noninflammatory cause of multifocal cerebral vasculopathy, is discussed in Case 694.

Coagulopathy (e.g., antiphospholipid antibody syndrome; see Case 639) should also be considered in the differential diagnosis of multiple infarcts of variable size and age.

### Case 645

50-year-old woman presenting with TIAs.
(axial, noncontrast FLAIR scan)

### Case 646

53-year-old woman presenting with
scattered paresthesias.
(axial, noncontrast FLAIR scan)

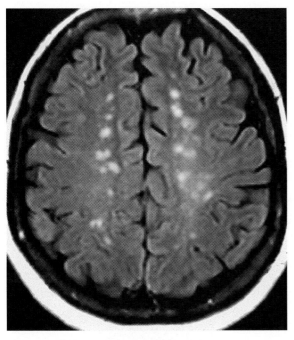

**Vasculitis**

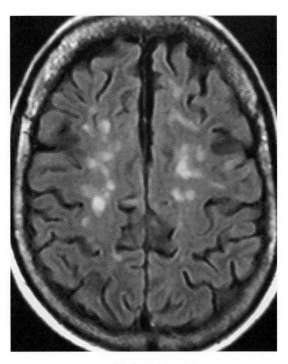

**Multiple Sclerosis**

The pattern of multiple small infarcts due to cerebral vasculitis may closely resemble the appearance of multifocal inflammatory disease. The above cases illustrate this potential similarity.

More inferior sections in Case 645 demonstrated numerous additional round and angular lesions within periventricular tissue. Several of the small foci of T2 prolongation contained central necrosis, resembling the right parietal lesion in Case 644.

Sarcoidosis, Lyme disease, and systemic lupus erythematosus are among other inflammatory disorders that can

present similarly to Case 646 (see Cases 495 and 496). Scattered or miliary metastases could also be included in the differential diagnosis.

Cases 644 and 645 demonstrate that cerebral vasculitis should be considered among the diagnostic possibilities when multiple small areas of signal abnormality are widely distributed throughout the brain. Clinical context and angiography will usually clarify the nonspecific findings on MR scans. Meningeal and/or cortical biopsy are necessary for diagnosis in some cases.

### Case 647

32-year-old woman presenting with a two-day history of worsening headaches and papilledema. (sagittal, noncontrast T1-weighted SE scan)

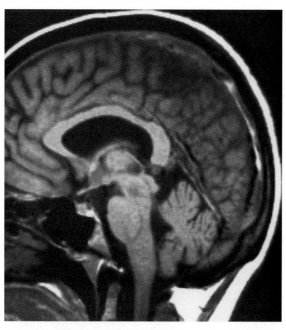

**Superior Sagittal Sinus Thrombosis**

### Case 648

12-day-old girl presenting with seizures. (sagittal, noncontrast T1-weighted SE scan)

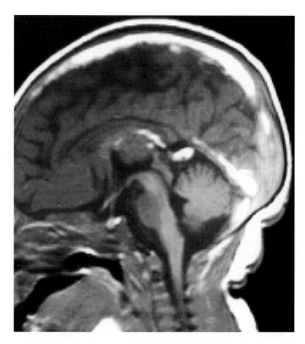

**Superior Sagittal Sinus Thrombosis**

Dural sinus thrombosis can cause a confusing variety of nonspecific symptoms in patients of any age. Standard and angiographic MR images provide a highly accurate, noninvasive method to establish the diagnosis.

On routine noncontrast spin echo scans (away from the margins of the imaging volume), the dural sinuses should contain little signal. Thrombosis and stasis replace this normal flow void with variable intraluminal intensity.

In Case 647, the superior sagittal sinus is filled with a mixture of isointense and high intensity components. Other thrombosed dural sinuses may be completely isointense or strikingly hyperintense (as in Case 648) on T1-weighted images. Gradient echo pulse sequences (maximizing flow-related enhancement) may be used to distinguish between slow flow and thrombus within a vascular structure.

The straight sinus is also thrombosed in Case 647, as was the left transverse sinus. The patient gave a history of chronic otitis and mastoiditis, which likely precipitated thrombophlebitis of the sigmoid sinus. Other factors associated with an increased incidence of dural sinus thrombosis include pregnancy, coagulopathy, dehydration, head trauma, the presence of antiphospholipid antibodies (e.g., lupus anticoagulant and anticardiolipin antibody), and some specific chemotherapeutic agents (e.g., L-asparaginase).

Case 648 demonstrates extensive dural sinus (and deep venous) thrombosis in the neonatal period. This occurrence is more frequent than has been previously recognized. The responsible mechanism may involve hemoconcentration, coagulopathy, and/or mechanical compression of the dural sinuses by calvarial molding during delivery. Affected infants typically present at age one to two weeks with irritability, seizures, or deepening lethargy. MR scans often demonstrate more extensive thrombosis than seen in adults. However, the prognosis for such infants is surprisingly good; most recover completely and develop normally.

MR venography is useful for assessing the patency of dural sinuses in equivocal cases. Either two-dimensional time-of-flight or phase contrast techniques are capable of demonstrating the presence or absence of slow venous flow.

### Case 649

8-year-old boy presenting with headaches,
vomiting, and seizures.
(axial, noncontrast T2-weighted SE scan)

### Case 650

4-year-old boy being treated with L-asparaginase
for leukemia, now presenting with irritability.
(axial, noncontrast T2-weighted FSE scan)

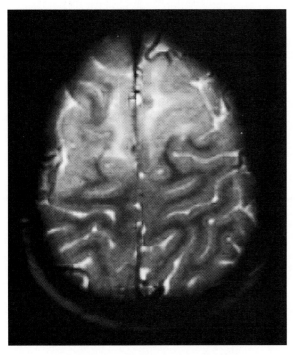

**Superior Sagittal Sinus Thrombosis**

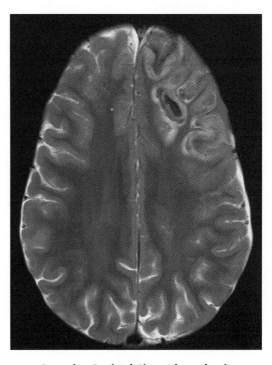

**Superior Sagittal Sinus Thrombosis**

The clinical course of patients with superior sagittal sinus thrombosis (SSST) usually reflects the extent to which thrombus propagates into cortical veins. In about 70% of cases there is no clinical or MR evidence of venous infarction, and a complete recovery is made.

When venous infarction occurs in patients with SSST, parasagittal regions are usually involved. Edema may be predominantly subcortical or involve both cortex and underlying white matter. Superimposed hemorrhage is common and may be patchy or confluent. Subcortical hemorrhage can occur at a considerable distance proximal to the occluded segment of the sinus.

In Case 649, symmetrical edema is present in the medial frontal lobes. Both cortex and subcortical white matter are affected. There is no evidence of hemorrhage. MR venography in this case demonstrated thrombosis of the middle third of the superior sagittal sinus.

Venous infarction in Case 650 is unilateral and hemorrhagic. Cortical edema crosses the watershed between the anterior and middle cerebral arteries. Patchy areas of T2-shortening within cortex and subcortical tissue indicate

the presence of blood products. The anterior half of the superior sagittal sinus was thrombosed in this case (see Case 651 for the corresponding MR venogram).

Discovery of parasagittal edema or hemorrhage should raise the possibility of sagittal sinus thrombosis. Scattered areas of cerebral edema due to SSST may resemble the appearance of primary white matter disease (such as progressive multifocal leukoencephalopathy), multifocal cortical arterial infarction, or "posterior reversible edema syndrome" (see Cases 544-546).

Other potential secondary findings on scans of patients with dural sinus thrombosis include focal or generalized cerebral swelling (which may precede any signal abnormality), areas of restricted diffusion and decreased perfusion (which may be reversible), tentorial/dural congestion/hyperemia, leptomeningeal enhancement, and communicating hydrocephalus due to impaired resorption of CSF.

See Cases 653 and 659 for additional examples of non-hemorrhagic venous infarcts.

### Case 651

4-year-old boy presenting with irritability.
(sagittal view, maximal intensity projection
reconstruction, noncontrast, two-dimensional,
time-of-flight GRE sequence)

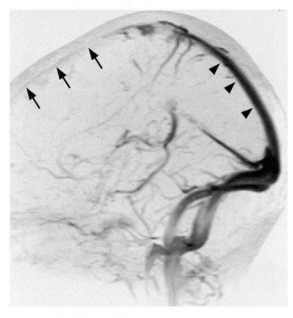

**Superior Sagittal Sinus Thrombosis**
(partial)

### Case 652

13-year-old boy presenting with severe headaches.
(sagittal view, maximal intensity projection
reconstruction, noncontrast, two-dimensional,
time-of-flight GRE sequence)

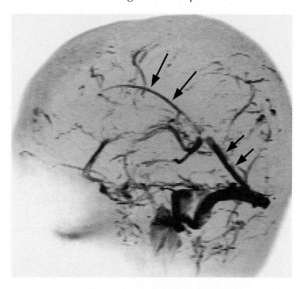

**Superior Sagittal Sinus Thrombosis**
(complete)

The patency of dural sinuses can be noninvasively assessed by MR venography. Both phase contrast and two-dimensional, time-of-flight techniques provide good demonstration of slow venous flow. Contrast administration is usually not needed for evaluation of major dural sinuses but can improve the mapping of cortical veins.

Case 651 presents a venographic study of the patient in Case 650. No flow is seen within the anterior half of the superior sagittal sinus *(arrows)*, whereas the posterior half is normally patent *(arrowheads)*.

The large venous infarct in this case (see Case 650) is somewhat unusual. Most patients can tolerate thrombosis (or surgical sacrifice) of the anterior third of the SSS because (1) it is relatively small, and (2) often large parasagittal veins in the frontal region serve as collateral channels.

In Case 652, the entire length of the SSS is occluded. The inferior sagittal sinus *(long arrows)*, straight sinus *(short arrows)*, and transverse sinuses remain patent. Occlusion or resection of the posterior third of the SSS usually causes significant impairment of cortical venous drainage and precipitates symptoms of venous hypertension. Many

cortical and meningeal veins in Case 652 are tortuous, having been recruited as routes of collateral flow.

Localized areas of reduced flow signal are commonly found within the transverse sinuses on MR venograms. This normal variant may be caused by arachnoid granulations or by complex flow patterns near the entrance of major tributary veins (such as the vein of Labbé).

The syndrome of benign intracranial hypertension or "pseudotumor cerebri" may be considered in young patients with papilledema and symptoms of elevated intracranial pressure. Apart from a few specific associations (e.g., hypervitaminosis A, tetracycline toxic reaction), the cause of the syndrome is undefined and controversial. It is characterized by the typical clinical picture in the absence of specific intracranial pathology. Small ventricles suggesting cerebral swelling may be seen in a minority of cases. In such patients, CT or MR scans serve the primary purpose of excluding a mass lesion, hydrocephalus, or venous thrombosis. MR venography is occasionally useful in this context.

### Case 653A

35-year-old woman presenting with
a seizure, two weeks postpartum.
(sagittal, noncontrast T1-weighted SE scan)

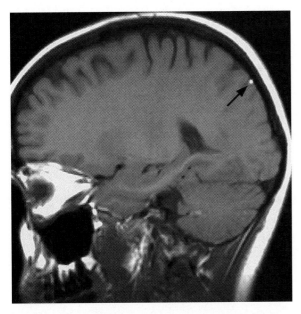

**Cortical Venous Thrombosis**

### Case 653B

Same patient.
(coronal, noncontrast T2-weighted FSE scan)

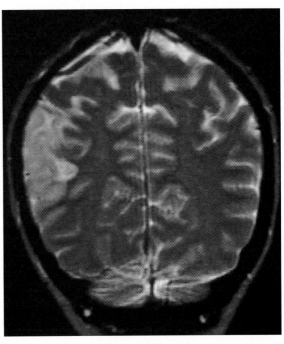

**Venous Infarct**

As discussed earlier, dural sinus thrombosis may not cause venous infarction unless and until there is propagation of clot into cortical veins. Conversely, thrombosis of a cortical vein can cause venous infarction in the absence of dural sinus occlusion.

Case 653 illustrates this occurrence. A single cortical vein in the right parietal region is thrombosed (*arrow,* Case 653A). MR venography documented that the superior sagittal sinus was entirely patent. The cortical and subcortical edema seen in Case 653B represents localized venous infarction in the territory drained by the single thrombosed vein.

Edema due to thrombosis of a cortical vein or dural sinus may be reversible, and it is difficult to predict the extent of permanent damage on initial routine scans. Restricted diffusion on diffusion-weighted images suggests cytotoxic edema, but even lesions with decreased ADC values may

subsequently resolve. Hemorrhage is common in venous infarcts (see Case 650), but none is apparent in Case 653.

Venous infarcts often demonstrate little parenchymal enhancement on postcontrast scans. Leptomeningeal enhancement is common, probably reflecting both congestion and dilatation of small collateral channels.

Thrombosis of the vein of Labbé (or of the transverse sinus) can cause localized venous edema (or hemorrhage) within the temporal lobe (see Case 659). This possibility should be considered in the differential diagnosis of non-specific temporal lesions, including hematomas.

Flow-related enhancement normally produces bright signal within cortical veins on scans at the margin of the imaging volume. The multiplicity of channels with this appearance and the recognition that the scan in question is near the edge of the study should reduce potential confusion with venous thrombosis.

# DEEP VENOUS THROMBOSIS

### Case 654A

3-year-old girl presenting with lethargy.
(mildly rotated sagittal view, maximal intensity projection reconstruction, noncontrast, two-dimensional, time-of-flight GRE sequence)

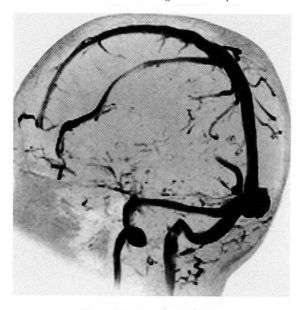

**Deep Venous Thrombosis**

### Case 654B

Same patient.
(axial, noncontrast T2-weighted FSE scan)

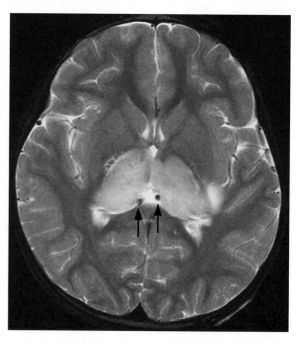

**Deep Venous Thrombosis**

Thrombosis of the straight sinus and vein of Galen may occur in association with thrombosis of other dural sinuses (as in Cases 647 and 648) or as an isolated process. Either event is often accompanied by thrombosis of one or both internal cerebral veins.

The venogram in Case 654A demonstrates gross patency of the superior sagittal sinus and the transverse sinuses. However, there is no visualization of flow in the internal cerebral veins, vein of Galen, or proximal straight sinus.

Case 654B presents one pattern of parenchymal findings in deep venous thrombosis. Symmetrical edema expands the thalami bilaterally and extends laterally into the internal capsules. The combination of mass effect and uniform signal abnormality resembles the bithalamic gliomas in Cases 79 and 80.

Edema within the caudate and lentiform nuclei is commonly encountered in other patients with obstruction of the internal cerebral veins. Although usually bilateral, ganglionic or thalamic abnormality due to deep venous thrombosis may be asymmetrical or unilateral. A third pattern of parenchymal change associated with deep venous thrombosis is asymmetrical hemorrhage within deep nuclei or the medial occipital lobes (see Case 783).

Neonates with deep venous thrombosis may demonstrate multiple hemorrhages in periventricular white matter. Venous congestion represents one of several potential mechanisms for hemorrhagic periventricular damage in the perinatal period—along with germinal matrix hemorrhages and periventricular leukomalacia.

Note that there is low signal intensity within the internal cerebral veins in Case 654B *(arrows)*. This appearance does not necessarily imply patency. T2-shortening due to deoxyhemoglobin within intraluminal thrombus can mimic flow void in a recently occluded sinus or vein (see Case 659 for another example).

# DIFFERENTIAL DIAGNOSIS:
## BITHALAMIC EDEMA

### Case 655

72-year-old man who suddenly
became unresponsive.
(axial, noncontrast T2-weighted SE scan)

### Case 656

38-year-old man presenting with
decreasing level of consciousness.
(axial, noncontrast T2-weighted FSE scan)

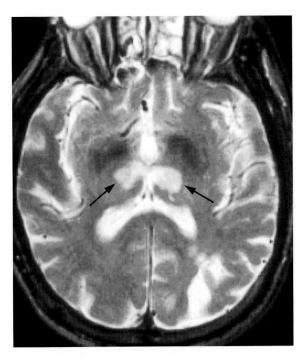

**Occlusion of the Distal Basilar Artery**
(embolic)

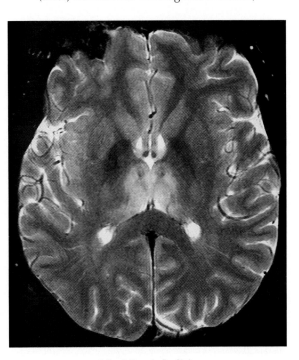

**Viral Encephalitis**

---

A number of pathologies can cause bithalamic edema. Among potential vascular etiologies are deep venous thrombosis (as in Case 654) and arterial infarction due to thrombosis, embolization, or spasm involving the tip of the basilar artery, illustrated by Case 655.

Perforating branches arise near the basilar bifurcation (and from the posterior communicating and proximal posterior cerebral arteries) to supply the diencephalon. Pathology affecting these vessels at the level of the suprasellar and interpeduncular cisterns may cause a characteristic pattern of symmetrical thalamic infarction. Bilateral thalamic infarcts sometimes reflect occlusion of midline vessels that supply the paramedian mesencephalon before branching to perfuse both medial thalami ("artery of Percheron").

Inflammatory processes can also cause bithalamic edema, as in Case 656. A specific viral agent was not established in this patient, but bilateral thalamic involvement has been reported in encephalitis due to arboviruses and in Japanese encephalitis. Acute disseminated encephalomyelitis in children often involves the thalami, occasionally symmetrically (see Cases 394-396). Systemic lupus erythematosus may also present with lesions in deep nuclei (see Case 481).

Anoxic, toxic, and metabolic disorders may produce bilateral thalamic lesions (e.g., Wernicke's encephalopathy as in Case 515, Wilson's disease, and osmotic myelinolysis).

Bithalamic gliomas occur (see Cases 79 and 80) but usually present less acutely than vascular or inflammatory pathologies.

## Case 657

32-year-old woman presenting with
headaches and papilledema.
(axial, noncontrast T2-weighted SE scan)

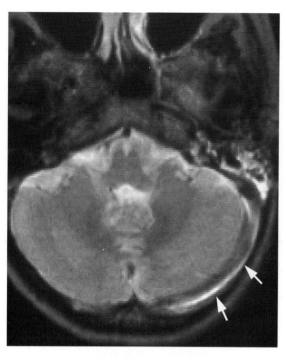

**Transverse Sinus Thrombosis**
(same patient as Case 647)

## Case 658

68-year-old woman presenting with headaches after
surgery for a cholesteatoma of the right ear.
(coronal, postcontrast T1-weighted SE scan)

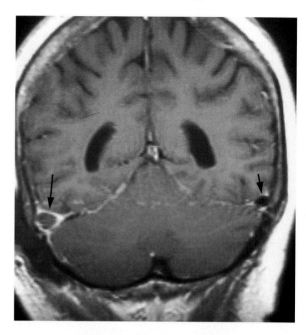

**Transverse Sinus Thrombosis**

---

Superior sagittal sinus thrombosis is often accompanied or precipitated by thrombosis of the transverse sinus.

Propagation of infection from the petrous bone to cause thrombophlebitis of the sigmoid and transverse sinuses was a common cause of increased intracranial pressure ("otitic hydrocephalus") in children prior to the widespread availability of antibiotics. This etiology of dural sinus thrombosis is still observed on occasion, as in Case 657. The patient in this case gave a history of chronic left otitis media, and the scan confirms inflammatory thickening of mucosa in the left mastoid region. The left transverse sinus *(arrows)* demonstrates uniformly high intensity due to thrombus replacing the expected flow void.

On postcontrast scans, the lumen of a thrombosed dural sinus usually fails to enhance. Peripheral enhancement of dura at the margins of the sinus results in a ring or "empty triangle" appearance, first observed on CT scans in cases of

superior sagittal sinus thrombosis. Case 658 illustrates this pattern *(long arrow)*.

The amount of central enhancement normally demonstrated within the transverse sinus, sigmoid sinus, or jugular vein is variable. In some cases, substantial intraluminal signal is present, suggesting relatively slow flow. In other cases (as in the left transverse sinus of Case 658, *short arrow),* flow void is observed even on postcontrast images.

MR angiograms frequently demonstrate artifactual filling defects within the flow pattern of a transverse sinus that can be misinterpreted as intraluminal thrombus. Inflow from large tributary veins (e.g., the vein of Labbé) and large arachnoid granulations are the most common causes of such pseudolesions.

Fluid is present within the scalp in the right retromastoid region of Case 658.

# DIFFERENTIAL DIAGNOSIS:
## LOCALIZED EDEMA ADJACENT TO THE TRANSVERSE SINUS

### Case 659

15-year-old girl presenting with a seizure.
(coronal, noncontrast T2-weighted SE scan)

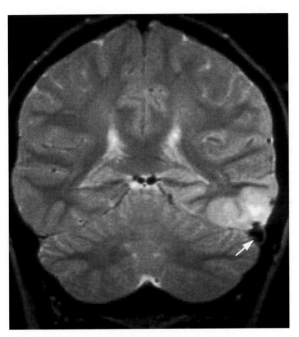

**Venous Infarct**
(due to transverse sinus thrombosis)

### Case 660

36-year-old woman with a long history of seizures.
(coronal, noncontrast T2-weighted SE scan)

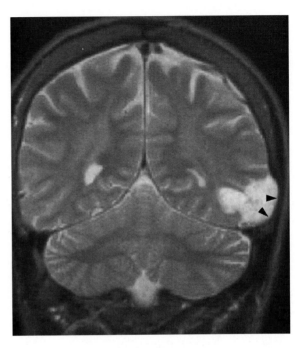

**Grade II Astrocytoma**

---

Localized edema due to acute venous infarction may resemble a superficial mass lesion. The clinical presentation and MR appearance in Case 659 mimic the low grade glioma in Case 660.

T1-weighted scans in Case 659 demonstrated high signal intensity thrombus occluding the left transverse sinus. The low intensity within the distended sinus on the above scan *(arrow)* is due to T2-shortening from deoxyhemoglobin. It is important to realize that low signal intensity within the lumen of a dural sinus on T2-weighted scans does not necessarily represent normal flow void.

The long-standing glioma in Case 660 is associated with localized erosion of the adjacent inner table *(arrowheads)*. This evidence of chronic mass effect may accompany superficial lesions of any kind (compare to Cases 73, 116, 338, 340, and 809).

See Cases 649, 650, and 653 for additional examples of venous infarcts.

### Case 661

7-year-old boy with decreased level of consciousness one day after abdominal surgery. (sagittal, noncontrast T1-weighted SE scan)

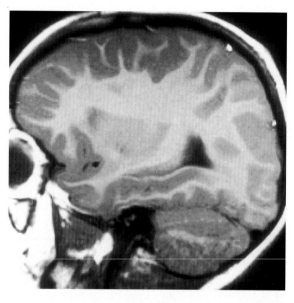

**Anoxia**

### Case 662

4-month-old boy three days after resuscitation for "sudden infant death syndrome." (sagittal, noncontrast T1-weighted SE scan)

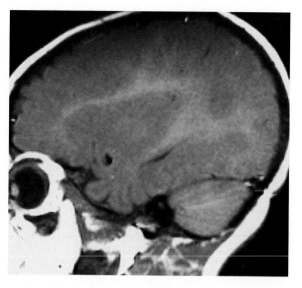

**Anoxia**

Cerebral anoxia may cause edema leading to prolongation of T1 and T2 values and swelling within involved regions. Gray matter is usually more severely affected than white matter, although holohemispheric patterns with diffuse white matter edema may be encountered.

Gray matter damage in anoxia may involve cortex, deep hemispheric nuclei, or both. This variability is probably due to differing combinations of hypoxia and hypoperfusion, as well as variable severity of the anoxic injury.

Another factor in the MR presentation of cerebral anoxia is the time elapsed from the insult. Scans in the first few days after an anoxic episode are characterized by progressively increasing swelling and signal abnormality, which may eventually cause effacement of sulci and ventricles. Later examinations may demonstrate a rapid transition (often within days) to a pattern of parenchymal loss with secondary expansion of ventricles and subarachnoid spaces.

In Case 661, the cortical gray matter is abnormally well defined due to swelling and prolongation of T1. The appearance closely resembles that of acute infarction (compare to Case 552) but involves multiple arterial distributions.

By contrast, cortical definition is diffusely blurred in Case 662. Severe edema has developed in the several days since the profound insult, extending into subcortical white matter and effacing overlying subarachnoid spaces.

### Case 663

2-week-old girl delivered by emergency cesarean section after uterine rupture.
(axial, noncontrast T1-weighted SE scan)

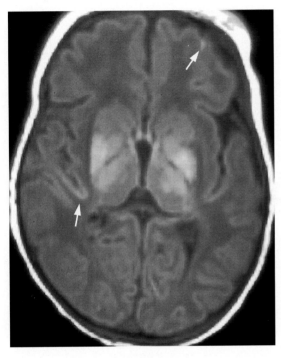

**Neonatal Hypoxia/Ischemia**

### Case 664

1-day-old girl with seizures and decreased level of consciousness.
(coronal, noncontrast T1-weighted SE scan)

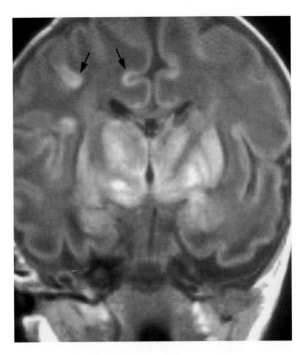

**Neonatal Hypoxia/Ischemia**

Neonatal "anoxia" is probably a multifactorial insult, with components of hypoxia, hypercarbia, acidosis, and hypotension. The newborn brain is actually quite resistant to hypoxia per se, but cerebral autoregulation and cardiac function are significantly impaired under hypoxic conditions. The resulting hypoperfusion is probably more responsible for cerebral damage than the initiating hypoxia. Because ischemia plays a key role in the pathophysiology, this neonatal insult is often called *hypoxic/ischemic encephalopathy* or *HIE.*

Severe neonatal HIE usually damages the deep gray nuclei, with typical involvement of the globus pallidus, posterior putamen, and ventrolateral thalamus. Less severe anoxia often affects watershed regions of cortex and white matter, with relative sparing of the corpus striatum and thalamus.

A characteristic pattern of T1-shortening commonly develops within a few days in affected gray matter of neonates who suffer hypoxic/ischemic insults. Petechial hemorrhage may contribute to this appearance, but other biochemical changes (such as protein denaturation, myelin breakdown products, and/or calcification) probably play a role. The high signal intensity on T1-weighted scans within deep nuclei of neonates with HIE may last for several months.

In the above cases, confluent signal abnormality throughout the deep nuclei dominates the presentation. However, smaller areas of T1-shortening within gyri *(arrows)* are also present in each patient.

The internal capsule is well outlined as a spared zone between the putamen and thalamus in Case 663 and between the caudate and lentiform nuclei in Case 664. This is the reverse of the normal pattern within the newborn brain on T1-weighted scans: the region of the posterior limb of the internal capsule should be the brightest structure visible. Lateral portions of the thalamus are most severely involved in Case 663, as is usual.

Scans of newborns who have experienced severe anoxia may also demonstrate signal abnormality within regions that are myelinating (and therefore metabolically active) at birth. The corticospinal tracts (i.e., perirolandic cortex; see Case 670) and the optic radiations (i.e., occipital cortex) are frequently affected.

**407**

## Case 665

14-year-old boy resuscitated after near hanging.
(axial, noncontrast scan; SE 3000/45)

## Case 666

14-year-old boy resuscitated after near drowning.
(axial, noncontrast T2-weighted SE scan)

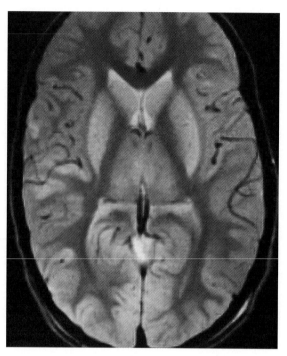

Anoxia

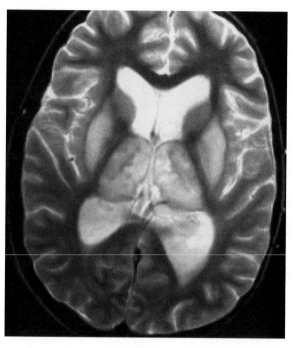

Anoxia

MR findings of cerebral anoxia may be seen within deep nuclei, cortical gray matter, or both. The cases above illustrate predominant ganglionic involvement, whereas those on the next page demonstrate cortical damage. Edema in either region causes swelling and high signal intensity on T2-weighted scans.

In Case 665, homogeneously increased intensity is present throughout the caudate nucleus, lentiform nuclei, and thalami. A few areas of cortical edema are also noted, particularly near the depths of sulci.

Symmetrical edema in Case 666 affects the thalami and putamina more prominently than the caudate nuclei. The thalamic involvement is more heterogeneous than seen in Case 665 or within other nuclei in Case 666. No accompanying cortical injury is apparent.

Anoxic changes within deep nuclei (and in cortex) may be very subtle on MR scans performed within a day or two of the insult. CT examinations sometimes demonstrate convincing low attenuation change in patients whose MR studies are equivocal. This diagnostic disparity is frequently noted in infants.

Proton spectroscopy can confirm the suspicion of anoxic injury when routine MR images are equivocal. A prominent lactate peak (a doublet at 1.3 ppm) indicating hypoxic metabolism may be the most convincing abnormality on early studies.

As discussed in Chapter 10, a variety of metabolic disorders can cause symmetrical abnormalities of the basal ganglia resembling anoxia in pediatric patients (see Cases 505-508). Kernicterus (bilirubin encephalopathy) in newborns characteristically affects the globus pallidus but spares the putamen and thalamus, unlike hypoxic-ischemic insults. Mitochondrial encephalopathies may cause lesions within the caudate and lentiform nuclei but usually do not involve the thalami.

In contrast to the pattern illustrated in Cases 665 and 666, neonates and infants may develop uniform T2-shortening causing *low* signal intensity throughout the corpus striatum and thalamus several days after a severe anoxic insult (usually accompanying T1-shortening like that in Cases 663 and 664).

## Case 667

18-month-old girl with a history
of choking while eating.
(axial, noncontrast T2-weighted FSE scan)

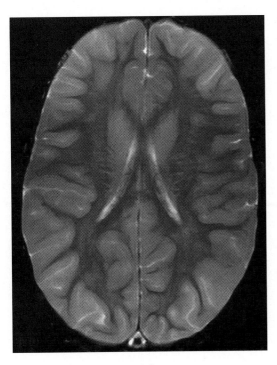

**Anoxia**

## Case 668

13-year-old boy with severe hemolytic
anemia leading to cardiac arrest.
(axial, noncontrast T2-weighted FSE scan)

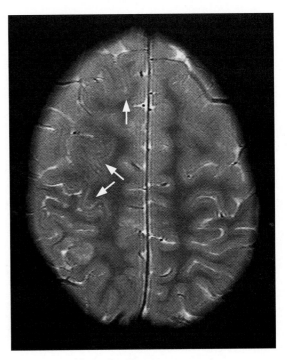

**Anoxia**

Diffuse edema causes swelling and mild T2 prolongation of the entire cortical mantle in Case 667. This appearance is the T2-weighted equivalent of the "super normal" cortex illustrated in Case 661. Symmetry of the changes can hinder diagnosis, particularly on scans performed within a day or two of the insult. Diffuse cortical edema may be much more apparent on CT scans at this stage.

Case 668 demonstrates a thin layer or stripe of T2 prolongation paralleling the gray/white matter junction in several locations *(arrows)*. This finding of layered signal abnormality at the base of the cortex correlates with the pathology of laminar necrosis. When present, this sign can help to distinguish anoxia from other potential causes of cortical edema (e.g., meningitis; compare Case 668 to Case 426).

Contrast enhancement is common within cerebral cortex or nuclei following an anoxic insult. Enhancement of the cortical ribbon may resemble the gyriform pattern seen in subacute cerebral infarction, except that several arterial distributions are involved. In infants, such cortical enhancement may persist for hours or days after contrast injection. This stain indicates severe cortical injury and resembles the appearance in some cases of infantile encephalitis (see Case 451).

### Case 669

11-year-old girl with a history of "cerebral palsy."
(axial, noncontrast T2-weighted SE scan)

### Case 670

2-year-old girl with spastic diplegia.
(axial, noncontrast T2-weighted SE scan)

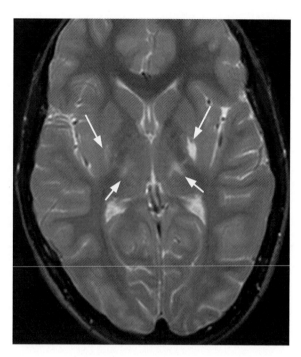

**Old Hypoxic/Ischemic Injury**

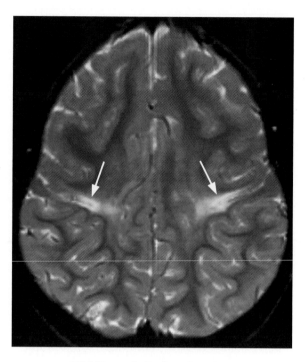

**Old Hypoxic/Ischemic Injury**

The selective vulnerability of specific cerebral tissues to neonatal hypoxic/ischemic injury produces a recognizable pattern of old anoxic damage on subsequent MR studies. Typical findings are illustrated above.

In Case 669, volume loss and signal abnormality are present within the posterior portion of the putamen bilaterally *(long arrows).* Accompanying T2 prolongation is seen within the ventral lateral thalami *(short arrows).* This combination of lesions matches the distribution of acute nuclear damage due to neonatal HIE as illustrated in Case 663. The findings strongly suggest that the patient's symptoms are related to a perinatal insult.

Case 670 documents reduced volume and signal abnormality within tissue bordering the central sulcus bilaterally

*(arrows).* Perirolandic cortex is another characteristic zone of focal injury from neonatal HIE, probably reflecting the relatively high metabolic requirements of active myelination in this region at the time of birth.

It is important to note that the majority of neonates with hypoxic/ischemic encephalopathy do not develop the clinical syndrome of "cerebral palsy." Conversely, perinatal HIE is only one of several potential causes of static encephalopathy with spastic diplegia or quadriplegia. This nonspecific clinical syndrome is more commonly due to periventricular leukomalacia (see Cases 592-595) or malformations of cortical development, as discussed in Chapter 16.

## Case 671

17-year-old woman found unconscious.
(coronal, noncontrast T2-weighted SE scan)

## Case 672

32-year-old man with a history of depression.
(axial, noncontrast T2-weighted SE scan)

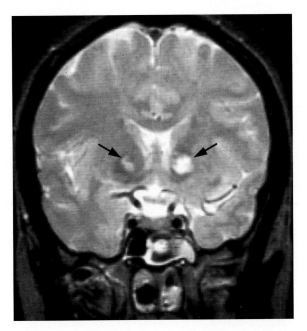

**Carbon Monoxide Poisoning**

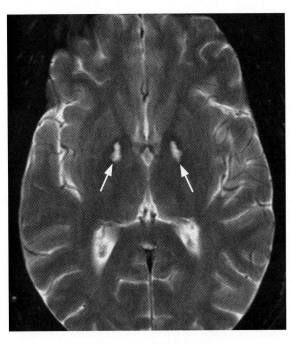

**Carbon Monoxide Poisoning**

Carbon monoxide poisoning characteristically leads to necrosis of the globus pallidus. Typical bilateral lesions in this location are demonstrated in Case 671 *(arrows)*, with central high intensity suggesting cytotoxic edema. (The more peripheral zone of low intensity may simply represent a background of normal T2-shortening in pallidal tissue.)

Case 672 illustrates residual bilateral pallidal necrosis in a patient with previous exposure to carbon monoxide. (Compare this appearance to the findings of Hallervorden-Spatz disease in Case 514.)

Other processes that may cause pallidal necrosis include barbiturate intoxication, cyanide poisoning (which characteristically also affects cerebellar cortex), hydrogen sulfide poisoning, hypoglycemia, hypoxia (e.g., drug overdose), and hypotension. Leigh disease (subacute necrotizing encephalomyelopathy; see Cases 505 and 506) may demonstrate symmetrical foci of signal abnormality in the basal ganglia, usually in children and commonly associated with brainstem involvement. Myelinolysis related to electrolyte disorders (see Case 530) can affect the basal ganglia sym-

metrically or asymmetrically. Unilateral or bilateral zones of signal abnormality in the globus pallidus may also be noted in neurofibromatosis type 1 (see Cases 904 and 905).

Symmetrical foci of T2 prolongation can occur within the posterior limb of the internal capsule (i.e., *adjacent* to the globus pallidus) in amyotrophic lateral sclerosis (see Case 528) and in some leukodystrophies (see Case 508). Wilson's disease may be associated with T2 prolongation in the lentiform nuclei despite the deposition of metals. The scan findings of methanol intoxication are usually seen within the putamen, often including hemorrhagic necrosis.

Hypoxia due to carbon monoxide poisoning can affect susceptible tissue outside of the globus pallidus. Other images in Case 671 demonstrated edema and swelling within gray matter of the hippocampal formations, which are known to be vulnerable to anoxic injury.

Some cases of carbon monoxide poisoning result in extensive damage to white matter. In such instances, initial recovery from an anoxic insult is followed by rapid deterioration after several weeks or months due to delayed postanoxic leukoencephalopathy.

# REFERENCES

Aida N, Nishimura G, Hachiya Y, et al: MR imaging of perinatal brain damage: comparison of clinical outcome with initial and follow-up MR findings. *AJNR* 19:1909-1922, 1998.

Amerenco P, Kase CS, Rosengart A, et al: Very small (border zone) cerebellar infarcts. *Brain* 116:161-186, 1993.

Amerenco P, Rosengart A, DeWitt, et al: Anterior inferior cerebellar artery territory infarcts: mechanisms and clinical features. *Arch Neurol* 50:154-161, 1993.

Anderson CM, Saloner D, Lee RE, et al: Assessment of carotid artery stenosis by MR angiography: comparison with x-ray angiography and color-coded Doppler ultrasound. *AJNR* 13:989-1003, 1992.

Anderson SC, Shah CP, Murtagh FR: Congested deep subcortical veins as a sign of dural venous thrombosis: MR and CT correlation. *J Comput Assist Tomogr* 11:1059-1061, 1987.

Anson JA, Heiserman JE, Drayer BP, Spetzler RF: Surgical decisions on the basis of magnetic resonance angiography of the carotid arteries. *Neurosurgery* 32:335-343, 1993.

Arbelaez A, Castillo M, Mukherji SK: Diffusion-weighted MR imaging of global cerebral anoxia. *AJNR* 20:999-1008, 1999.

Armstrong FD, Thompson RJ Jr, Wang W, et al: Cognitive functioning and brain magnetic resonance imaging in children with sickle cell disease. *Pediatrics* 97:864-870, 1996.

Ayanzen RH, Bird CR, Keller PJ, et al: Cerebral MR venography: normal anatomy and potential diagnostic pitfalls. *AJNR* 21:74-78, 2000.

Baenziger O, Martin E, Steinlin M, et al: Early pattern recognition in severe perinatal asphyxia: a prospective MRI study. *Neuroradiology* 35:437-442, 1993.

Bakac G, Wardlaw JM: Problems in the diagnosis of intracranial venous infarction. *Neuroradiology* 39:566-570, 1997.

Barkhof F, Valk J: "Top of the basilar" syndrome: a comparison of clinical and MR findings. *Neuroradiology* 30:293, 1988.

Barkovich AJ: MR and CT evaluation of profound neonatal and infantile asphyxia. *AJNR* 13:959-972, 1992.

Barkovich AJ, Sargent SK: Profound asphyxia in the premature infant: imaging findings. *AJNR* 16:1837-1846, 1995.

Barkovich AJ, Truwitt CL: Brain damage from perinatal asphyxia: correlation of MR findings with gestational age. *AJNR* 11:1087-1096, 1990.

Barkovich AJ, Westmark K, Partridge C, et al: Perinatal asphyxia: MR findings in the first 10 days. *AJNR* 16:427-438, 1995.

Bell DA, Davis WL Osborn AG, Harnsberger HR: Bithalamic hyperintensity on T2-weighted MR: vascular causes and evaluation with MR angiography. *AJNR* 15:893-899, 1994.

Biller J, Adams HP Jr, Dunn V, et al: Dichotomy between clinical findings and MR abnormalities in pontine infarction. *J Comput Assist Tomogr* 10:379-385, 1986.

Birbamer G, Aichner F, Felber S, et al: MRI of cerebral hypoxia. *Neuroradiology* (suppl):53-55, 1991.

Blankenberg FG, Norbash AM, Lane B, et al: Neonatal intracranial ischemia and hemorrhage: diagnosis with US, CT and MR imaging. *Radiology* 199:253-260, 1996.

Bousson V, Levy C, Brunereau L, et al: Dissections of the internal carotid artery: three-dimensional time-of-flight MR angiography and MR imaging features. *Am J Roentgenol* 173:139-143, 1999.

Bui LN, Brant-Zawadzki M, Verghese P, Gillan G: Magnetic resonance angiography of craniocervical dissection. *Stroke* 24:126-131, 1993.

Bulas DI, Vezina GL: Preterm anoxic injury: radiologic evaluation. *Radiol Clin North Am* 37:1147-1162, 1999.

Castillo M, Falcone S, Naidich TP, et al: Imaging in acute basilar artery thrombosis. *Neuroradiology* 36:426-429, 1994.

Caulo M, Tampieri D, Brassard R, et al: Cerebral amyloid angiopathy presenting as nonhemorrhagic diffuse encephalopathy: neuropathologic and neuroradiologic manifestations in one case. *AJNR* 22:1072-1076, 2001.

Chang KH, Han MH, Kim HS, et al: Delayed encephalopathy after acute carbon monoxide intoxication: MR imaging features and distribution of cerebral white matter lesions. *Radiology* 184:117-122, 1992.

Cormier PJ, Long ER, Russell EJ, et al: MR imaging of posterior fossa infarctions: vascular territories and clinical correlations. *Radiographics* 12:1079-1096, 1992.

Demaerel P, Casaer P, Casteels-Van Daele M, et al: Moyamoya disease: MRI and MR angiography. *Neuroradiology* 33(suppl):50-52, 1991.

Dormont D, Sag K, Biondi A, et al: Gadolinium-enhanced MR of chronic dural sinus thrombosis. *AJNR* 16:1347-1352, 1995.

Dubowitz DJ, Bluml S, Acinue E, Dietrich RB: MR of hypoxic encephalopathy in children after near drowning: correlation with quantitative proton MR spectroscopy and clinical outcome. *AJNR* 19:1617-1627, 1998.

Elster AD: MR contrast enhancement brainstem and deep cerebral infarctions. *AJNR* 12:1127-1132, 1991.

Elster AD, Richardson DN: Focal high signal on MR scans of the midbrain caused by enlarged perivascular spaces: MR-pathologic correlation. *AJNR* 11:1119-1122, 1990.

Erdman WA, Weinreb JC, Cohen JM, et al: Venous thrombosis: clinical and experimental MR imaging. *Radiology* 161:233-238, 1986.

Falini A, Barkovich AJ, Calabrese G, et al: Progressive brain failure after diffuse hypoxic ischemic brain injury: a series 1 MR and proton MR spectroscopic study. *AJNR* 19:648-652, 1998.

Forbes KPN, Pipe JG, Bird R: Neonatal hypoxic-ischemic encephalopathy: detection with diffusion-weighted MR imaging. *AJNR* 21:1490-1496, 2000.

Forbes KPN, Pipe JG, Heiserman JE: Evidence for cytotoxic edema in the pathogenesis of cerebral venous infarction. *AJNR* 22:450-455, 2001.

Fox AJ, Bogousslavsky J, Carey LS, et al: Magnetic resonance imaging of small medullary infarctions. *AJNR* 7:229-234, 1986.

Friedman DP: Abnormalities of the deep medullary white matter veins: MR imaging findings. *Am J Roentgenol* 168:1103-1108, 1997.

Friedman DP: Abnormalities of the posterior inferior cerebellar artery: MR imaging findings. *Am J Roentgenol* 160:1257-1263, 1993.

Fujisawa I, Asato R, Nishimura K, et al: Moyamoya disease: MR imaging. *Radiology* 164:103-106, 1987.

Fujita N, Hirabuki N, Fujii K, et al: MR imaging of middle cerebral artery stenosis and occlusion: value of MR angiography. *AJNR* 15:335-342, 1994.

Goldberg HI, Grossman RI, Gomori JM, et al: Cervical internal carotid artery hemorrhage: diagnosis using MR. *Radiology* 158:157-162, 1986.

Greenan TJ, Grossman RI, Goldbert HI: Cerebral vasculitis: MR imaging and angiographic correlation. *Radiology* 182:65-72, 1992.

Greenberg SM, Vonsattel JPG, Stakes JW, et al: The clinical spectrum of cerebral amyloid angiopathy: presentations without lobar hemorrhage. *Neurology* 43:2073-2079, 1993.

Greenough GP, Mamourian A, Harbaugh RE: Venous hypertension associated with a posterior fossa dural arteriovenous fistula: another cause of bithalamic lesions on MR images. *AJNR* 20:145-148, 1999.

Harris KG, Tran DD, Sickels WJ, Cornel SH: Diagnosing intracranial vasculitis: the roles of MR and angiography. *AJNR* 15:317-330, 1994.

Heinz ER, Yeates AE, Djang WT: Significant extracranial carotid stenosis: detection on routine cerebral MR images. *Radiology* 170:843-848, 1989.

Heiserman JE, Drayer BP, Keller PJ, Fram EK: Intracranial vascular occlusion: evaluation with three dimensional time-of-flight MR angiography. *Radiology* 185:667-673, 1992.

Ho VB, Rovira MJ, Borke RC, Smirniotopoulos JG: Arachnoid granulations in the transverse sinuses: incidence and features on magnetic resonance imaging and magnetic resonance venography. *Int J Neurorad* 3:482-489, 1997.

Horowitz AL, Kaplan R, Sarpel G: Carbon monoxide toxicity: MR imaging in the brain. *Radiology* 162:787-788, 1987.

Hosoya TW, Watanabe N, Yamaguchi K, et al: Intracranial vertebral artery dissection in Wallenberg syndrome. *AJNR* 15:1161-1165, 1994.

Jager HR, Albrecht T, Curati-Alasonatti WL, et al: MRI in neuro-Behcet's syndrome: comparison of conventional spin-echo and FLAIR pulse sequences. *Neuroradiology* 41: 750-758, 1999.

Johnson AJ, Lee BCP, Lin W: Echoplanar diffusion-weighted imaging in neonates and infants with suspected hypoxic-ischemic injury: correlation with patient outcome. *Am J Roentgenol* 172: 219-226, 1999.

Johnson BA, Heiserman JE, Drayer BP, Keller PJ: Intracranial MR angiograpnhy: its role in the integrated approach to brain infarction. *AJNR* 15:901-908, 1994.

Johnson MH, Christman CW: Posterior circulation infarction: anatomy, pathophysiology, and clinical correlation. *Semin Ultrasound CT, MRI* 16:237-252, 1995.

Jouvet P, Cowan FM, Cox P, et al: Reproducibility and accuracy of MR imaging of the brain after severe birth asphyxia. *AJNR* 20:1343-1345, 1999.

Katz BH Quencer RM, Kaplan JO, et al: MR imaging of intracranial carotid occlusion. *AJNR* 10:345-350, 1989.

Keeney SE, Adcock EW, McArdle CB: Prospective observations of 100 high-risk neonates by high field (1.5 Tesla) magnetic resonance imaging of the central nervous system: II. Lesions associated with hypoxic-ischemic encephalopathy. *Pediatrics* 87:431-438, 1991.

Kim JS, Lee JH, Choi CG: Patterns of lateral medullary infarction: vascular lesion-magnetic resonance imaging correlation of 34 cases. *Stroke* 29:645-652, 1998.

Kirsch E, Kaim A, Engelter S, et al: MR angiography in internal carotid artery dissection: improvement of diagnosis by selective demonstration of the intramural haematoma. *Neuroradiology* 40:704-709, 1998.

Knepper L, Biller J, Adams HP Jr, et al: MR imaging of basilar artery occlusion. *J Comput Assist Tomogr* 14:32-35, 1990.

Korogi Y, Takahashi M, Hirai T, et al: The ventral posterolateral thalamus: magnetic resonance findings in healthy neonates and in neonatal asphyxia. *Int J Neurorad* 4:97-104, 1998.

Lafitte F, Boukobza M, Guichard JP, et al: Deep cerebral venous thrombosis: imaging in eight cases. *Neuroradiology* 41:410-418, 1999.

Lane JL, Flanders AE, Doan HT, Bell RD: Assessment of carotid artery patency in routine spin-echo MR imaging of the brain. *AJNR* 12:819-826, 1991.

Lang E, Lang C, Huk W, Neundorfer B: Magnetic resonance imaging of dorsolateral medullary infarction in Wallenberg syndrome. *Neuroradiology* 36:269-270 1994.

Laster RE Jr, Acker JD, Halford HH III, Nauert TC: Assessment of MR angiography versus arteriography for evaluation of cervical carotid bifurcation disease. *AJNR* 14:681-688, 1993

Lazar EB, Russel EJ, Cohen BA, et al: Contrast-enhanced MR of cerebral arteritis: intravascular enhancement related to flow stasis within areas of focal arterial ectasia. *AJNR* 13:271-276, 1992.

Leach JL, Jones BV, Tomsick TA, et al: Normal appearance of arachnoid granulations on contrast-enhanced CT and MR of the brain: differentiation from dural sinus disease. *AJNR* 17:1523-1532, 1996.

Levy C, Laissy JP, Raveau V, et al: Carotid and vertebral artery dissections: three-dimensional time-of-flight MR angiography and MR imaging versus conventional angiography. *Radiology* 190:97-103, 1994.

Liauw L, van Buchem MA, Spilt A, et al: MR angiography of the intracranial venous system. *Radiology* 214:678-682, 2000.

Litt AW, Eidelman EM, Pinto RS, et al: Diagnosis of carotid artery stenosis: comparison of 2DFT time-of-flight MR angiography with contrast angiography in 50 patients. *AJNR* 12:149-154, 1991.

Macchi PJ, Grossman RI, Gomori JM, et al: High field MR imaging of cerebral venous thrombosis. *J Comput Assist Tomogr* 10:10-15, 1986.

Madan A, Sluzewski M, van Rooij WJJ, et al: Thrombosis of the deep cerebral veins: CT and MRI findings with pathologic correlation. *Neuroradiology* 39:777-780, 1997.

Manzione J, Newman GC, Shapiro A, Santo-Ocampo R: Diffusion- and perfusion-weighted MR imaging of dural sinus thrombosis. *AJNR* 21:68-73, 2000.

Mascalchi M, Bianchi MC, Mangiafico S, et al: MRI and MR angiography of vertebral artery dissection. *Neuroradiology* 39:329-340, 1997.

McArdle CB, Mirfakhraee M, Amparo EG, Kulkarni MV: MR imaging of transverse/sigmoid dural sinus and jugular vein thrombosis. *J Comput Assist Tomogr* 11:831-838, 1987.

McArdle CB, Richardson CJ, Hayden CK, et al: Abnormalities of the neonatal brain: MR imaging. Part II. Hypoxic-ischemic brain injury. *Radiology* 163:395-404, 1987.

Medlock MD, Olivero WC, Hanigan WC, et al: Children with cerebral venous thrombosis diagnosed with magnetic resonance imaging and magnetic resonance angiography. *Neurosurgery* 31:870-876, 1992.

Milandre L, Rumeau C, Sangla I, et al: Infarction in the territory of the anterior inferior cerebella artery: report of five cases. *Neuroradiology* 34:500-503, 1992.

Miller DH, Ormerod IEC, Gibson A, et al: MR brain scanning in patients with vasculitis: differentiation from multiple sclerosis. *Neuroradiology* 29:226-231, 1987.

Moran CJ, Siegel MJ, DeBaun MR: Sickle cell disease: imaging of cerebrovascular complications. *Radiology* 206:311-321, 1998.

Morrissey SP, Miller DH, Hermaszewski R, et al: MRI of the CNS in Behçet's disease. *Eur Neurol* 33:287-293, 1993.

Moser FG, Miller ST, Bello JA, et al: The spectrum of brain MR abnormalities in sickle cell disease: a report from the cooperative study of sickle cell disease. *AJNR* 17:965-972, 1996.

Ozawa T, Sasaki O, Sorimachi T, Tanaka R: Primary angiitis of the central nervous system: report of two cases and review of the literature. *Neurosurgery* 36:173-179, 1995.

Ozdoba C, Sturzenegger M, Schroth G: Internal carotid artery dissection: MR imaging features and clinical-radiologic correlation. *Radiology* 199:191-198, 1996.

Padayachee TS, Bingham JB, Graves MJ, et al: Dural sinus thrombosis: diagnosis and follow-up by magnetic resonance angiography and imaging. *Neuroradiology* 33:165-167, 1991.

Phillips MD, Zimmerman RA: Diffusion imaging in pediatric hypoxic ischemia injury. *Neuroimaging Clin North Am* 9:41-52, 1999.

Pomper MG, Miller TJ, Stone JH, et al: CNS vasculitis in autoimmune disease: MR imaging findings and correlation with angiography. *AJNR* 20:75-90, 1999.

Provenzale JM, Allen NB: Neuroradiologic findings in polyarteritis nodosa. *AJNR* 17:1119-1126, 1996.

Provenzale JM, Joseph GJ, Barboriak DP: Dural sinus thrombosis: findings on CT and MR imaging and diagnostic pitfalls. *Am J Roentgenol* 170:777-783, 1998.

Provenzale JM, Loganbill HA: Dural sinus thrombosis and venous infarction associated with antiphospholipid antibodies: MR findings. *J Comput Assist Tomogr* 18:719-723, 1994.

Quint D, Spickler E: Magnetic resonance demonstration of vertebral artery dissection. Report of two cases. *J Neurosurg* 72:964-967, 1990.

Rippe DJ, Boyko OB, Spritzer CE, et al: Demonstration of dural sinus occlusion by the use of MR angiography. *AJNR* 11:199-201, 1990.

Roche J, Warner D: Arachnoid granulations in the transverse and sigmoid sinuses: CT, MR, and MR angiographic appearance of a normal anatomic variation. *AJNR* 17:677-684, 1996.

Seibert JJ, Miller SF, Kirby RS, et al: Cerebrovascular disease in symptomatic and asymptomatic patients with sickle cell anemia: screening with duplex transcranial doppler US–correlation with MR imaging and MR angiography. *Radiology* 189:457-466, 1993.

Shin JH, Suh DC, Choi CG, Lee HK: Vertebral artery dissection: spectrum of imaging findings. *Radiographics* 20:1687-1696, 2000.

Shoemaker EI, Lin Z-S, Rae-Grant AD, Little B: Primary angiitis of the central nervous system: unusual MR appearance. *AJNR* 15:331-334, 1994.

Sie LTL, van der Knaap MS, van Wezel-Meijler G, et al: Early MR features of hypoxic-ischemic brain injury in neonates with periventricular densities on sonograms. *AJNR* 21:852-861, 2000.

Silverman CS, Brenner J, Murtagh FR: Hemorrhagic necrosis and vascular injury in carbon monoxide poisoning: MR demonstration. *AJNR* 14:168-170, 1993.

Simmons Z, Biller J, Adams HP, et al: Cerebellar infarction: comparison of computed tomography and magnetic resonance imaging. *Ann Neurol* 19:291-293, 1986.

Skehan SJ, Hutchinson M, MacErlaine DP: Cerebral autosomal dominant arteriopathy with subcortical infarcts and leukoencephalopathy: MR findings. *AJNR* 16:2115-2120, 1995.

Stone JH, Pomper MG, Roubenoff R, et al: Sensitivities of noninvasive tests for central nervous system vasculitis: a comparison of lumbar puncture, computed tomography, and magnetic resonance imaging. *J Rheumatol* 21:1277-1282, 1994.

Sue DE, Brant-Zawadzki MN, Chana J: Dissection of cranial arteries in the neck: correlation of MRI and arteriography. *Neuroradiology* 34:273-278, 1992.

Sze C, Simmons B, Krol G, et al: Dural sinus thrombosis: verification with spin-echo techniques. *AJNR* 9:679-686, 1988.

Takahashi S, Higano S, Ishii K, et al: Hypoxic brain damage: cortical laminar necrosis and delayed changes in white matter at sequential MR imaging. *Radiology* 189:449-456, 1993.

Takanashi J, Sugita K, Ishii M, et al: Moyamoya syndrome in young children: MR comparison with adult onset. *AJNR* 14:1139-1142.

Tali ET, Atilla S, Keskin T, et al: MRI in neuro-Behcet's disease. *Neuroradiology* 39:2-6, 1997.

Tatemichi TK, Steinke W, Duncan C, et al: Paramedian thalamopeduncular infarction: clinical syndromes and magnetic resonance imaging. *Ann Neurol* 32:162-171, 1992.

Toyoda K, Ida M, Fukuda K: Fluid attenuated inversion recovery intraarterial signal: an early sign of hyperacute cerebral ischemia. *AJNR* 22:1021-1029, 2001.

Tsai FY, Wang A, Matovich VB, et al: MR staging of acute dural sinus thrombosis: correlation with venous pressure measurements and implications for treatment and prognosis. *AJNR* 16:1021-1029, 1995.

Vogl TJ, Bergman C, Villringer A, et al: Dural sinus thrombosis: value of venous MR angiography for diagnosis and follow-up. *Am J Roentgenol* 162:1191-1198, 1994.

Wentz KY, Röther J, Schwartz A, et al: Intracranial vertebrobasilar system: MR angiography. *Radiology* 190:105-110, 1994.

Westmark KD, Barkovich AJ, Sola A, et al: Patterns and implications of MR contrast enhancement in perinatal asphyxia: a preliminary report. *AJNR* 16:685-692, 1995.

Yamada I, Matsushima Y, Suzuki S, Childhood moyamoya disease before and after encephalo-duro-arterio-syanangiosis: an angiographic study. *Neuroradiology* 34:318-322, 1995.

Yamada I, Matsushima Y, Suzuki S: Moyamoya disease: diagnosis with three-dimensional time-of-flight MR angiography. *Radiology* 184:773-778, 1992.

Yamada I, Suzuki S, Matsushima Y: Moyamoya disease: comparison of assessment with MR angiography and MR imaging versus conventional angiography. *Radiology* 196,211-215, 1995.

Yamada I, Suzuki S, Matsushima Y: Moyamoya disease: Diagnostic accuracy of MRI. *Neuroradiology* 37:356-361, 1995.

Yasui T, Komiyama M, Nishikawa M, Nakajima H: Subarachnoid hemorrhage from vertebral artery dissecting aneurysms involving the origin of the posteroinferior cerebellar artery: report of two cases and review of the literature. *Neurosurgery* 46:196-200, 2000.

Yuh WTC, Simonson TM, Wang A-M, et al: Venous sinus occlusive disease: MR findings. *AJNR* 15:309-316 1994.

Yuh WTC, Ueda T, Maley JE: Perfusion and diffusion imaging: a potential tool for improved diagnosis of CNS vasculitis. *AJNR* 20:87-88, 1999.

Zimmerman RD, Ernst RJ: Neuroimaging of cerebrovenous thrombosis. *Neuroimaging Clin N Amer* 2:463-485, 1992.

# CHAPTER 13

# Intracranial Hemorrhage and Trauma

## Case 673

83-year-old woman with a history of a
CVA two days before admission.
(sagittal, noncontrast T1-weighted SE scan)

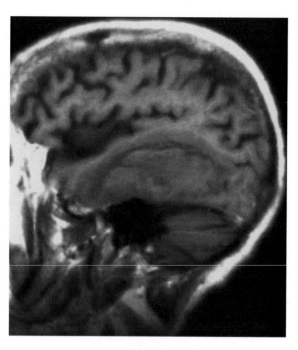

**Intracerebral Hematoma**
(acute)

## Case 674

69-year-old woman, two days after
the acute onset of aphasia.
(axial, noncontrast T2-weighted SE scan)

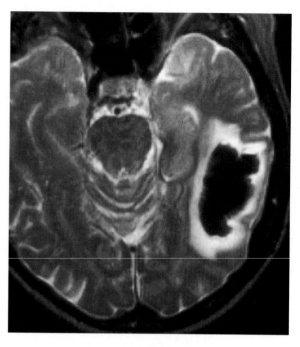

**Intracerebral Hematoma**
(acute)

The appearance of recent intracranial hemorrhage is more complicated and time-dependent on MR scans than on CT studies. A sequence of changes in signal intensity reflects progressive oxidation and breakdown of blood products.

Acute intracerebral hematomas usually present as nearly isointense masses on T1-weighted scans. Mild prolongation of T1 may be present, causing slightly decreased signal intensity within the lesion. In Case 673, a large hematoma in the middle cranial fossa is slightly lower in intensity than adjacent parenchyma. A rim of edema helps to define the perimeter of the hemorrhage.

T2-weighted images of acute hematomas typically demonstrate very low signal intensity, as in Case 674. This signal loss reflects selective T2 relaxation enhancement due to magnetic field inhomogeneity produced when deoxyhemoglobin is compartmentalized within erythrocytes. The finding is less prominent on fast spin echo images than on conventional T2-weighted spin echo scans.

Hyperacute intracerebral hematomas may present a less distinctive MR appearance. Such fresh hemorrhages represent a solution of nonparamagnetic oxyhemoglobin. Their MR behavior resembles that of proteinaceous fluid, with prolongation of T1 and T2. Hyperacute hematomas can therefore mimic other homogeneous cystic or solid masses.

"Spontaneous" lobar hemorrhages in elderly patients are frequently due to amyloid angiopathy. In younger adults, spontaneous intraparenchymal hemorrhages tend to occur in the basal ganglia, thalamus, pons and cerebellum, often correlating with the history of systemic hypertension and angiopathic changes of small arteries. Some of these "hypertensive" hemorrhages are now believed to result from dissections of lenticulostriate arteries.

### Case 675

33-year-old man with a history of hypertension, five days after admission with acute hemiparesis.
(sagittal, noncontrast T1-weighted SE scan)

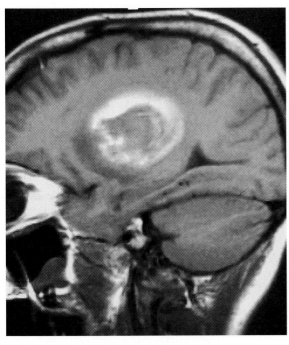

**Intracerebral Hematoma**
(early subacute)

### Case 676

63-year-old man, one month after presentation with acute ataxia.
(axial, noncontrast scan; SE 2800/45)

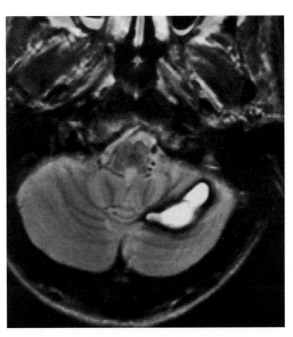

**Cerebellar Hematoma**
(late subacute)

---

The MR appearance of intracerebral hemorrhage on T1-weighted scans changes during the first week of age. Prominent T1-shortening usually begins near the periphery of the lesion, gradually extending toward the center over a period of days to weeks. This alteration in signal intensity reflects the oxidation of deoxyhemoglobin to methemoglobin, which acts as a paramagnetic agent shortening T1.

The thick rind of high signal intensity surrounding an isointense center in Case 675 is a typical presentation for an early subacute hematoma on a T1-weighted scan. A follow-up scan with the same parameters after an additional week showed uniformly high signal intensity throughout the lesion.

Cell lysis and watery dilution of blood products accompany the oxidation of intracerebral hematomas, progressing inward from the periphery of the lesion. The combination of these events converts the initially low signal intensity of acute hematomas on T2-weighted scans to high signal intensity over a period of weeks, as illustrated in Case 676. Case 681 presents a hematoma midway through this transition.

The rim of low signal intensity surrounding the lesion in Case 676 is due to the accumulation of old blood products (mainly hemosiderin) within macrophages at the perimeter of the organizing hematoma. This intracellular debris causes selective T2-relaxation enhancement. The presence of a low intensity rim on T2-weighted scans implies that a hematoma has reached the late subacute or chronic stage. The lack of surrounding edema also suggests that the hemorrhage is not a recent event; compare to Case 674. (Note that the relative position of the high and low signal components of the late subacute hematoma in Case 676 is reversed from the acute hematoma in Case 674.)

About 10% to 15% of spontaneous and/or hypertensive hematomas occur in the posterior fossa. They may involve the cerebellum or the brainstem, usually the pons. Cerebellar hemorrhages often originate near the dentate nucleus, as in Case 676. It is important to distinguish between cerebellar and brainstem hematomas in patients with symptoms of brainstem compromise, since the former may be evacuated with life-saving results.

### Case 677

4-year-old boy presenting with irritability.
(sagittal, noncontrast T1-weighted SE scan)

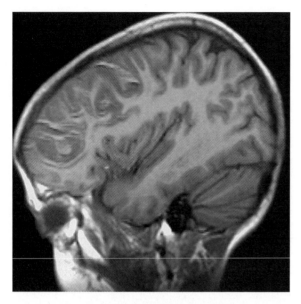

**Acute Subcortical Hemorrhage**
(due to sagittal sinus thrombosis)

### Case 678

41-year-old woman presenting with
fever and confusion.
(axial, noncontrast T2*-weighted GRE scan)

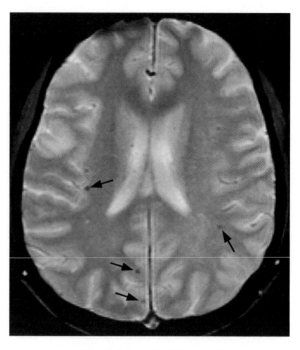

**Multifocal Subacute Hemorrhages**
(due to emboli from subacute
bacterial endocarditis)

Magnetic field alterations associated with intracerebral hemorrhages can help to detect and/or characterize these lesions. Focal field inhomogeneities reflecting the presence of diamagnetic or paramagnetic substances within a hematoma can cause both geometric distortion and misregistration along the frequency-encoding axis.

The latter effect, resembling the appearance of chemical shift artifact, is illustrated in Case 677. Arcs of high and low intensity paralleling the contours of frontal gyri represent spatially mismapped signal due to a layer of acute subcortical hemorrhage. A follow-up scan five days later (see Case 782) demonstrated a thick band of gyriform T1-shortening in the same location.

The misregistration artifact illustrated by Case 677 may be seen at the margins of acute hematomas before any of the other characteristic intensity changes caused by blood products. The finding can be an important clue that an otherwise ambiguous mass represents recent hemorrhage.

Spatial variations in magnetic susceptibility due to deoxyhemoglobin or hemosiderin produce local field gradients that decrease the phase coherence of adjacent protons. The resultant loss of signal intensity can be used to detect even small hemorrhages. In Case 678, multiple tiny subcortical foci of low intensity probably represent microhemorrhages at the sites of small septic emboli.

Susceptibility effects are proportional to the strength of the applied magnetic field and become increasingly prominent as the band width of an imaging sequence is decreased. These distortions are most apparent on gradient echo sequences, which lack the 180-degree refocusing RF pulses that reduce local field effects in spin echo sequences. For this reason, gradient echo sequences are useful to screen for small hemorrhagic lesions, as in Case 678.

Compare the pattern of multiple small hemorrhagic lesions in Case 678 with Cases 693 and 694.

## Case 679

39-year-old man with a history of an old stroke.
(axial, noncontrast scan; SE 3000/45)

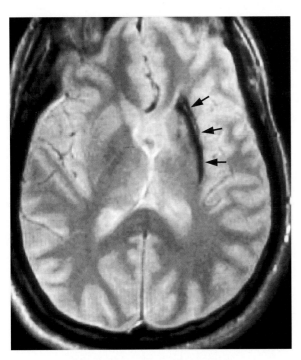

**Old Intracerebral Hematoma**

## Case 680

47-year-old man, one year after
a left hemispheric CVA.
(coronal, noncontrast T2*-weighted GRE scan)

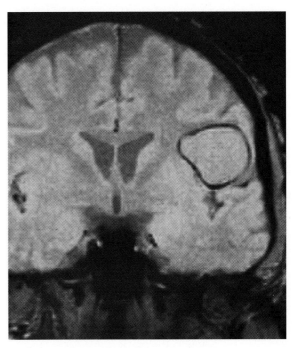

**Old Intracerebral Hematoma**

---

As discussed in Case 676, a characteristic MR feature of intracerebral hemorrhage is the signature of T2-shortening left at the site of bleeding. Breakdown products accumulated by macrophages at the perimeter of organized hematomas cause prominent low signal intensity on long TR spin echo images. Focal signal loss remains as a hallmark of prior hemorrhage even after the lesion has been completely resorbed. (This is strictly true only in areas of normal brain involved by hemorrhage; hemosiderin-laden macrophages within hemorrhagic neoplasms may gain abnormal vascular access and leave the region.)

In Case 679, T2-shortening causes low signal intensity along the margins of an old hematoma in the region of the left putamen *(arrows)*. This finding suggests a spontaneous hemorrhage that has been resorbed, leaving a hemosiderin-lined cleft (compare to Case 765). An appear-

ance similar to Case 679 would be the likely endpoint of the subacute hematoma illustrated in Cases 675 and 681.

Rarely, an old hematoma cavity persists and fills with fluid rather than collapsing. Case 680 illustrates such a "hematic cyst." The rim of low signal intensity identifies a period of hemorrhage in the history of the current lesion. The fluid within the cyst differs in signal intensity from CSF and is likely proteinaceous, but there is no evidence of mass effect or edema to suggest an inflammatory or malignant lesion.

As discussed in Case 678, gradient echo images are more sensitive than spin echo sequences to susceptibility effects caused by paramagnetic blood breakdown products. For this reason, GRE sequences are helpful in characterizing large hemorrhagic lesions and in screening for suspected small angiomas, hemorrhagic metastases, or shearing injuries (see Cases 693 and 694).

# DIFFERENTIAL DIAGNOSIS:
## HEMORRHAGIC MIDHEMISPHERE MASS

### Case 681

33-year-old hypertensive man, five days after a CVA. (axial, noncontrast T2-weighted SE scan)

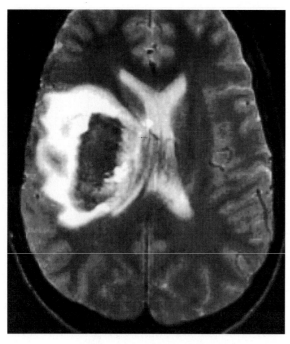

**Spontaneous Hematoma**
(same patient as Case 675)

### Case 682

89-year-old woman presenting with a two-day history of worsening confusion. (axial, noncontrast T2-weighed SE scan)

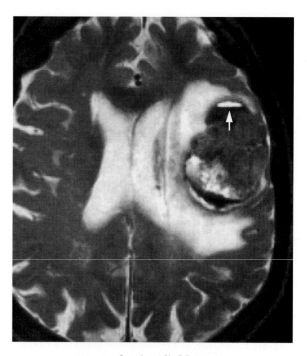

**Hemorrhagic Glioblastoma**

---

The discovery of an intracerebral hematoma should be followed by critical assessment of its location and morphology. The diagnosis of spontaneous hemorrage is reserved for hematomas occupying typical sites and demonstrating no unusual features.

Case 681 presents the characteristic appearance of an early subacute intracerebral hematoma. Although a core of homogenous T2-shortening remains, a broadening perimeter of the lesion evidences high signal intensity (compare to Case 674). After another week or two, the entire center of the lesion would be expected to demonstrate high intensity on a T2-weighted sequence (see Case 676).

Areas of T2-shortening due to hemorrhage are also present within the mass in Case 682. However, the internal architecture of this lesion is much more complex than the hematoma of Case 681. A sedimentation level is seen within a small cyst anteriorly *(arrow)*, but the midportion of the lesion appears to represent solid tissue. A cystic or necrotic zone of high signal intensity is present postero-

medially. This high degree of structure and heterogeneity strongly suggests an underlying mass with secondary hemorrhage.

The spontaneous hematoma in Case 681 is centered in the superior ganglionic region, whereas the lesion of Case 682 arises more peripherally. (Note that edema is predominantly lateral in Case 681 and predominantly medial in Case 682.) A superficial location of intracerebral hemorrhage should raise the suspicion of an underlying structural lesion, trauma, coagulopathy, or vasculopathy (such as amyloid angiopathy in older patients).

Cocaine use should be considered among the etiologies of spontaneous intracerebral hemorrhage in young patients. Such hematomas may originate from underlying vascular lesions (aneurysms or arteriovenous malformations) that bleed due to cocaine-induced hypertension.

Hemorrhage into a tumor is one mechanism by which mass lesions may present acutely, simulating a CVA (see also Case 10).

# DIFFERENTIAL DIAGNOSIS:
## MASS WITH A THIN, ENHANCING WALL

### Case 683

59-year-old woman presenting with
ataxia and left facial numbness.
(axial, postcontrast T1-weighted SE scan with MTS)

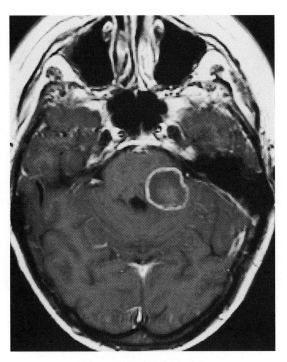

**Resolving Hematoma**
("spontaneous"/hypertensive)

### Case 684

74-year-old woman presenting with a seizure.
(axial, postcontrast T1-weighted SE scan with MTS)

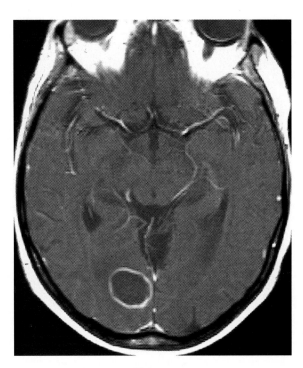

**Abscess**
(nocardia)

---

A uniform rim of contrast enhancement is often demonstrated at the margin of a resolving hematoma on CT or MR scans. Peripheral enhancement develops as the intrinsic T1-shortening of the lesion is fading due to the degradation of blood products. As a result, the rim-enhancing mass may come to resemble a tumor or abscess, like Case 684.

Clues to the correct diagnosis in such cases include: (1) a history of a recent CVA; (2) location at a common site of spontaneous hemorrhage; (3) a smooth, uniform rim *not* well seen on noncontrast scans; (4) faint residual T1-shortening near the center of the mass (as seen in Case 683); and (5) lack of adjacent edema. Enhancement surrounding an intracerebral hematoma has been noted within days of the hemorrhage and can persist for one or two months.

The hematoma in Case 683 is centered in the brachium pontis. The pons and cerebellum are among the common locations for "spontaneous" hemorrhages occurring in hypertensive patients, which was the clinical context in this case.

By itself, the abscess in Case 684 has no specific features. (Compare to the typical pyogenic abscesses in Cases 463-465.) Nocardia abscesses are often multiple and loculated, as was true of additional lesions at other sites in this patient. Cerebral infection by nocardia usually represents seeding from a pulmonary focus in an immunocompromised host.

Compare the above scans to Cases 100, 465, and 466.

## Case 685

3-year-old boy who fell through a
second story window screen.
(coronal, noncontrast T1-weighted SE scan)

## Case 686

23-year-old man admitted after
an automobile accident.
(axial, noncontrast T2-weighted SE scan)

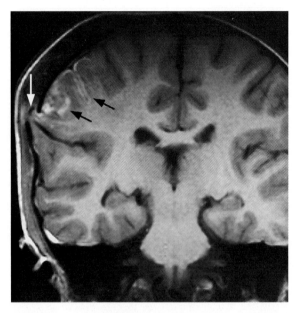

**Cerebral Contusion**
(and skull fracture)

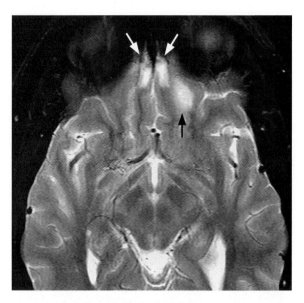

**Cerebral Contusion**

Posttraumatic intracerebral hemorrhages are often superficial lesions, reflecting bruising of the cortical surface against the adjacent calvarium. Common locations include the inferior frontal lobe, the anterior temporal lobe, the inferior surface of the temporal lobe, and the occipital pole. The mechanism of injury may involve direct impact or recoil. As a result, evidence of parenchymal damage should be sought both immediately beneath and directly opposite a skull fracture or scalp injury.

T1-shortening reflecting cortical hemorrhage in Case 685 *(black arrows)* includes both globular and laminar components. A ribbon-like distribution of subacute hemorrhage is commonly seen within zones of contusion, resembling the pattern of T1-shortening in laminar necrosis due to subacute infarction or anoxia (compare to Case 572).

Case 686 illustrates posttraumatic edema at the inferior surface of the frontal lobes, involving the gyrus rectus bilaterally *(white arrows)* and the supraorbital region on the left *(black arrow)*. Hemorrhagic contusions frequently occur in this location, sometimes associated with anosmia reflecting accompanying injury to the olfactory bulbs or tracts.

Cerebral contusions may be much more extensive than the focal lesions in the above cases. Scans may also demonstrate dramatic enlargement of posttraumatic intracerebral hemorrhages occurring hours or days after injury. This phenomenon should be suspected in any trauma patient whose condition deteriorates or fails to improve as expected.

"Posttraumatic" hemorrhages occurring in atypical locations must be carefully evaluated. Such hematomas may represent an initial cerebral event leading to trauma, or posttraumatic hemorrhage into a preexisting structural lesion.

Surprisingly minor head trauma may be associated with serious cerebral injury. For example, a simple fall from the standing position can cause extensive intracranial hemorrhage in elderly patients.

The small amount of brain tissue incarcerated within the skull fracture in Case 685 includes the flow void of an opercular branch of the middle cerebral artery *(white arrow)*. This finding was confirmed when the herniation was surgically reduced. Fortunately, the child recovered completely.

# DIFFERENTIAL DIAGNOSIS:
## FOCAL CORTICAL HEMORRHAGE AND EDEMA IN A CHILD

### Case 687

12-year-old boy presenting one day after a seizure, with a history of minor head trauma.
(axial, noncontrast T2-weighted SE scan)

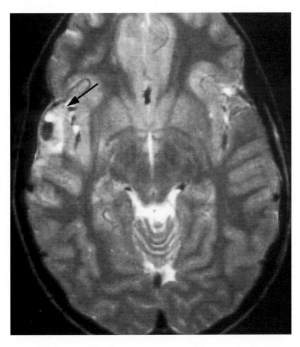

**Cerebral Contusion**

### Case 688

3-week-old girl presenting with decreased level of consciousness.
(coronal, noncontrast T2-weighted SE scan)

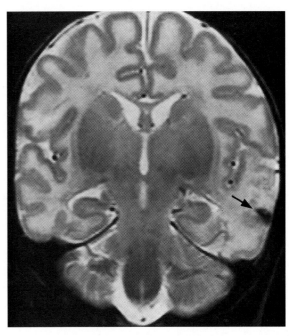

**Herpes Encephalitis**
(type 2)

The small lesion in Case 687 *(arrow)* represents localized contusion of the superior temporal gyrus. Central low signal intensity due to deoxyhemoglobin is surrounded by a rim of high intensity edema. A T1-weighted scan at this time showed only a small zone of mildly reduced signal intensity. This initial appearance is nonspecific; hemorrhage within a small neoplasm could not be excluded.

A follow-up scan in Case 687 demonstrated characteristic evolution and established the diagnosis of cerebral contusion. Edema and mass effect subsided. T1-shortening developed, with a gyriform contour following the cortical convolution (resembling Case 685).

Case 688 is an example of neonatal encephalitis due to herpes simplex virus type 2. Unlike encephalitis in older patients due to herpes simplex type 1 (see Cases 443-449),

neonatal cerebral infection by herpes often causes a devastating panencephalitis (see Case 451).

Involvement in Case 688 is unusually localized, affecting the lateral aspect of the left temporal lobe. Cortex in the region is edematous, so that it is poorly distinguished from unmyelinated subcortical white matter. (Compare to the reduced cortical definition of cerebral infarcts on T2-weighted scans in infants, illustrated in Case 555.) The small zone of low signal intensity near the center of the inflammatory region *(arrow)* represents focal hemorrhage, a common pathological feature of herpes encephalitis that may be demonstrated on MR images.

Case 836 documents the rapid evolution of subsequent parenchymal damage in Case 688.

### Case 689

4-year-old girl hit by a car.
(sagittal, noncontrast T1-weighted SE scan)

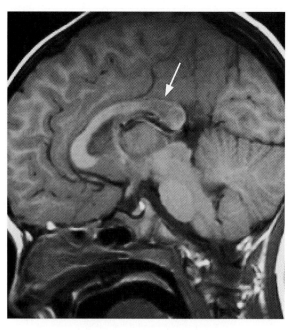

**Axonal (Shearing) Injury**

### Case 690

4-year-old boy admitted after
an automobile accident.
(axial, noncontrast T2-weighted SE scan)

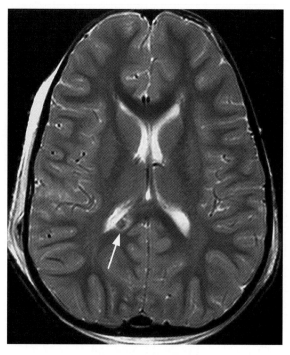

**Axonal (Shearing) Injury**

The superiority of MR over CT for defining white matter pathology as emphasized in Chapter 8 extends to the demonstration of shearing injuries. These foci of axonal disruption are usually inapparent on CT examinations; occasionally associated hemorrhages are noted. MR scans are much more sensitive to small sites of injury within white matter of the cerebral hemispheres and posterior fossa.

Shearing injuries occur in approximately 40% of patients with severe head trauma, most commonly in the frontal and temporal lobes. They may range from millimeters to centimeters in size. The majority are bland, but up to 25% are hemorrhagic.

The corpus callosum is a common location for shearing injury. The splenium is most frequently involved, as in the above patients.

Case 689 demonstrates patchy edema throughout the posterior body and splenium of the corpus callosum.

The lesion in the right major forceps of Case 690 *(arrow)* is much more discrete. It contains a small amount of hemorrhage, seen as a central zone of low intensity due to shortened T2 values. Diffuse scalp edema and hemorrhage are present extracranially.

Shearing injury to the corpus callosum is often associated with intraventricular hemorrhage, which can be a CT clue to the diagnosis.

### Case 691

4-year-old girl hit by a car.
(axial, noncontrast T2-weighted SE scan)

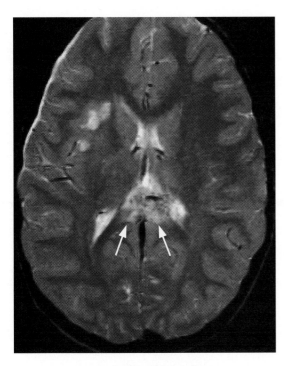

**Axonal (Shearing) Injury**
(same patient as Case 689)

### Case 692

36-year-old man, comatose after
an automobile accident.
(axial, noncontrast T2-weighted SE scan)

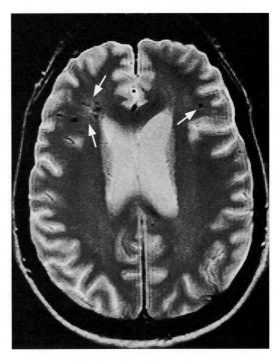

**Axonal (Shearing) Injury**

---

Axonal injury is common near interfaces between tissues of different consistency. Shearing forces develop in such locations when rotation/acceleration imparts different velocities and momentum to parenchyma on each side of the tissue boundary. The junction between gray and white matter of the cerebral convexity is a frequent site of "shear strain," as illustrated above.

Case 691 is a T2-weighted image of the patient in Case 689. The large area of axonal injury within the splenium is well demonstrated *(arrows)*. Several accompanying subcortical lesions are present in the right frontal lobe, with focal edema but no evidence of hemorrhage.

By contrast, the small foci of axonal injury in the frontal white matter of Case 692 *(arrows)* demonstrate signal loss from localized hemorrhage. There is little associated edema. Multiple additional sites of focal low signal intensity were present at other locations in this case, including lesions within the corpus callosum and the dorsolateral brainstem.

Cases 689 to 692 illustrate the variable MR appearance of supratentorial diffuse axonal injury (DAI). Lesions may be deep or subcortical, bland or hemorrhagic.

Diffusion-weighted images may demonstrate foci of posttraumatic edema that are inapparent on routine sequences. Both superficial injury and axonal damage may be much more impressive on diffusion-weighted scans than on standard images.

Similarly, reduced magnetization transfer ratios have been measured in areas of presumed axonal injury that appear normal on conventional MR images. Although MR is substantially more sensitive than CT for demonstrating shearing injuries, microscopically documented axonal damage is often undetected by either modality.

Callosal and hemispheric lesions of DAI correlate strongly with the presence of primary brainstem injury, which usually involves the posterolateral portions of the midbrain and pons. (Secondary brainstem injury after head trauma is often the result of transtentorial herniation, with caudal displacement of the brainstem stretching the penetrating branches of the basilar artery and leading to infarction and/or hemorrhage.)

A small subdural hematoma is present in the right frontal region of Case 691.

# DIFFERENTIAL DIAGNOSIS:
## MULTIPLE HEMORRHAGIC FOCI WITHIN THE CEREBRAL HEMISPHERES

### Case 693

13-year-old boy with decreased level of consciousness after an automobile accident. (axial, noncontrast T2*-weighted GRE scan)

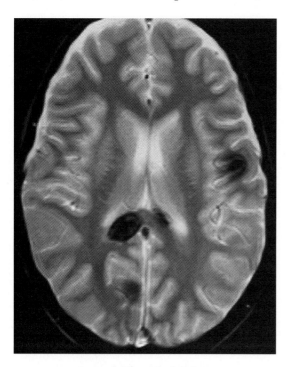

**Axonal (Shearing) Injury**

### Case 694

74-year-old man presenting with TIAs. (axial, noncontrast T2*-weighted GRE scan)

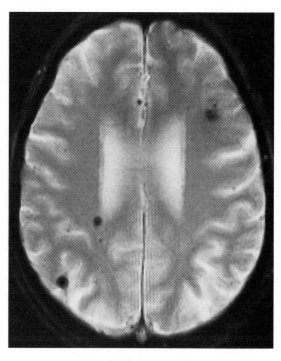

**Amyloid Angiopathy**

---

A number of pathologies can cause multiple small hemorrhages within cerebral parenchyma. As discussed on the previous pages, a substantial minority of shearing injuries are hemorrhagic. Case 693 is another example, demonstrating the characteristic combination of callosal and subcortical lesions.

The scattered hemorrhages in Case 694 are due to amyloid angiopathy. The deposition of amyloid weakens the walls of small arteries, often leading to focal or large hemorrhages at one or many sites. Other forms of vasculitis and hypertensive cerebrovascular disease may also cause multiple small intracerebral hemorrhages.

The differential diagnosis of multiple hemorrhagic cerebral lesions includes cerebral contusions, hemorrhagic metastases (see Cases 11 and 766), hemorrhage from cerebral emboli (see Case 678), dural sinus thrombosis with multifocal venous infarction, multiple cavernous angiomas, and hematomas due to coagulopathy.

Gradient echo sequences were used in both of the above cases to highlight magnetic susceptibility effects (see discussion of Case 678). Low signal intensity within hemorrhagic lesions on T2-weighted or T2*-weighted scans may reflect the presence of acute (deoxyhemoglobin) and/or chronic (hemosiderin) blood products.

# DIFFERENTIAL DIAGNOSIS:
## MULTIPLE FOCI OF SIGNAL ABNORMALITY IN PERIPHERAL WHITE MATTER

### Case 695

39-year-old woman presenting with
neuropsychological deficits nine months
after an automobile accident.
(axial, noncontrast T2-weighted SE scan)

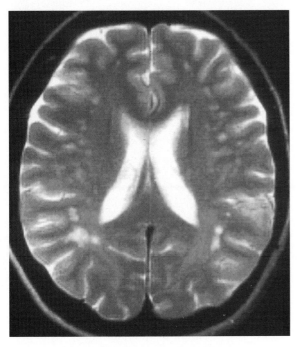

**Axonal (Shearing) Injuries**

### Case 696

56-year-old woman with a history
of hypertension and TIAs.
(axial, noncontrast T2-weighted SE scan)

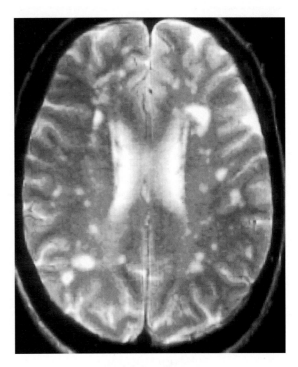

**Multiple Infarcts**

---

As discussed in Cases 691 and 692, subcortical white matter of the cerebral hemispheres is a common location of shear strain and axonal injury. Case 695 presents an additional example.

Shearing injury is often correlated with significant persistent neuropsychological deficits. MR scans can establish the diagnosis in such cases, whereas CT studies are usually negative.

The spectrum of multifocal infarction may include peripheral hemispheric lesions, as in Case 696. Close analysis usually demonstrates overall sparing of subcortical "U"

fibers (see discussion of Cases 608 and 609). In addition, deeper lesions in the centrum semiovale or corona radiata are almost always found in association with superficial ischemic foci.

A variety of inflammatory processes may also cause multiple small areas of signal abnormality within peripheral white matter of the cerebral hemispheres. Examples include demyelinating disease, collagen vascular disease, sarcoidosis, and Lyme disease (see Cases 495 and 496). Multiple sclerosis in particular may present with a combination of callosal and subcortical lesions that can resemble diffuse axonal injury.

### Case 697

9-year-old boy presenting with headaches,
three days after head trauma.
(axial, noncontrast T1-weighted SE scan)

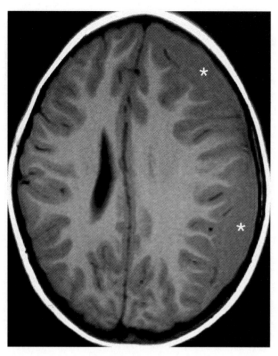

**Subdural Hematoma**
(acute)

### Case 698

10-month-old boy presenting with left hemiparesis.
(coronal, noncontrast T1-weighted SE scan)

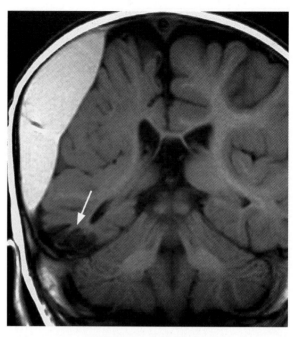

**Subdural Hematoma**
(subacute)

As discussed in Cases 673-676, the MR appearance of hemorrhage is a complex function of many variables. In general, acute intracerebral or extracerebral hematomas are isointense or slightly lower in signal intensity than cerebral parenchyma on T1-weighted images.

In Case 697, subdural collections overlie the left frontal and parietal lobes *(asterisks)*. The signal intensity of these acute hematomas is nearly equal to that of cerebral cortex.

The older subdural hematoma in Case 698 demonstrates homogeneously shortened T1 values. This appearance reflects the oxidation of deoxyhemoglobin to methemoglobin (compare to Case 675). Although blood products within extracerebral hematomas pass through the same degradation sequence as intracerebral hematomas, the rate of change is often slower and less predictable. Prominent T1-shortening due to the formation of methemoglobin may not be apparent until a week or more after injury.

CSF can mix with blood in the subdural space if the arachnoid membrane is torn (see discussion of subdural

hygromas in Cases 713 and 714). The signal changes caused by blood products in the collection are diluted in such cases.

The right cerebral hemisphere in Case 698 is small. A well-defined zone of encephalomalacia is present at the inferolateral margin of the right temporal lobe *(arrow)*, and other areas of focal parenchymal damage were noted on other sections. The subdural hematoma in this case may reflect subacute hemorrhage into a chronic collection, dating back to an injury weeks or months earlier.

The increase in signal intensity commonly seen on T1-weighted images of intracranial hemorrhages during the first week after bleeding contrasts with the CT pattern of immediate maximal attenuation. As a result, CT scans may be more characteristic than MR studies for diagnosis of acute intracranial hemorrhage, whereas MR scans are more specific than CT exams for the characterization of subacute or old hemorrhages.

### Case 699

77-year-old man whose family reported
him to be increasingly forgetful.
(axial, noncontrast T2-weighted SE scan)

### Case 700

10-year-old boy, after resection of a cerebellar
astrocytoma and shunt placement
for severe hydrocephalus.
(axial, noncontrast T2-weighted SE scan)

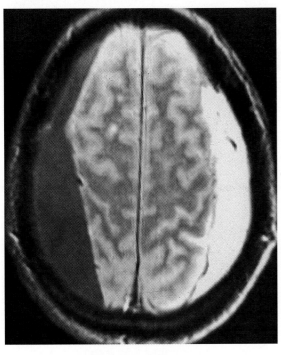

**Subdural Hematomas**
(acute and chronic)

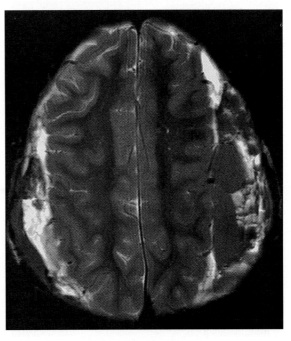

**Subdural Hematomas**
(subacute)

The appearance of subdural hematomas on long TR spin echo images depends on the age and compartmentalization of blood products within the lesion.

Case 699 illustrates the typical low signal intensity of an acute or early subacute subdural hematoma overlying the right hemisphere. A loculated chronic subdural hematoma is present on the left side. Comparison of the two collections demonstrates that lysis of cells, aqueous dilution, and removal of blood products from the extracerebral space convert the initially low intensity of fresh subdural hemorrhage on T2-weighted scans to the eventual high intensity appearance expected for a proteinaceous solution.

The subdural collections in Case 700 are much more complex. Heterogeneous signal intensity within subdural hematomas may be caused by old clots surrounded by fresh blood, loculated plasma separated from red cells, and/or encysted spinal fluid from an associated arachnoid tear.

Sedimentation levels of blood products are often noted after liquefaction of a subdural hematoma, which usually occurs by two to three weeks of age. A dependent zone of cellular material characteristically causes T2-shortening in such cases.

Approximately 25% of subacute and chronic subdural hematomas are bilateral, as in Cases 699 and 700. The above scans demonstrate bilateral compression of cerebral parenchyma, effacement of sulci, and medial displacement of cortical veins.

Subdural hematomas may become very large, particularly in elderly patients. The presence of pre-existing atrophy delays the onset of cerebral compression by an expanding collection. When the buffering capacity of enlarged CSF spaces has been exceeded, rapidly developing symptoms may lead to the discovery of a surprisingly thick hematoma.

The initial clinical presentation of patients with subdural hematomas can range from vague headaches to generalized disorientation and confusion (as in Case 699) to focal deficits mimicking an acute CVA (see Case 702). Hemiparesis may be contralateral or ipsilateral to the hematoma, with the latter occurrence reflecting brainstem displacement causing pressure on the contralateral cerebral peduncle. Elderly patients with subdural hematomas have a generally poorer prognosis than younger individuals.

### Case 701

53-year-old man presenting with headaches.
(sagittal, noncontrast T1-weighted SE scan)

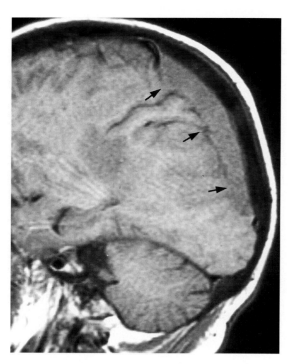

**Metastatic Carcinoma of the Prostate**

### Case 702

65-year-old man presenting with
rapidly developing hemiparesis.
(sagittal, noncontrast T1-weighted SE scan)

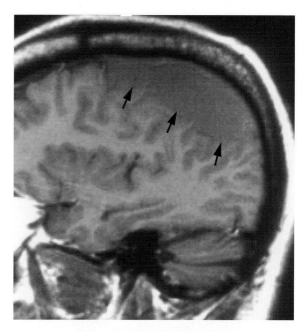

**Chronic Subdural Hematoma**

In Case 701, a homogeneous extracerebral "collection" causes displacement of the underlying hemisphere and cortical veins *(arrows)*. It is important to remember that epidural and/or subdural tumors can present in this manner, mimicking a subdural hematoma.

A clue to the diagnosis in Case 701 is abnormal signal intensity throughout the diploic space of the calvarium. Although dural-based metastases can occur without osseous involvement, associated skull lesions are often apparent (see Cases 25 and 28). The low signal intensity throughout the vault in Case 701 (compare to the normal diploic space in Case 702) may reflect cellular infiltration, reactive sclerosis, or both.

The greater sphenoid wing is another frequent location of dural-based metastatic disease, especially from carcinoma of the prostate (see Case 58). Breast carcinoma is the most common tumor to present in this manner in women. An appearance comparable to Case 701 may be seen in children due to neuroblastoma (see Case 27) or lymphoma.

Chronic subdural hematomas often demonstrate intermediate signal intensity on T1-weighted scans, as in Case 702. This appearance probably reflects the clearing of methemoglobin present during subacute stages, liquefaction, and aqueous dilution. Intermediate signal intensity may also represent an averaging of blood components of varying age. Rebleeding is common in subdural hematomas, contributing to their progressive enlargement. Recurrent hemorrhages may cause a layered or laminated appearance or simply add volume to a unilocular collection.

Postcontrast scans would clearly distinguish between the above lesions. Dural-based tumor typically demonstrates homogeneous enhancement (see Case 28 for a postcontrast scan of Case 701). The enhancement of subdural hematomas is usually limited to membranes that develop by about three weeks of age. Membrane enhancement is typically linear, adjacent to the cortical surface and along the inner table. Loculation of enhancing membranes occasionally presents a confusing appearance.

## Case 703

*82-year-old woman presenting after head trauma with seizures involving the left side of the body. (coronal, noncontrast T1-weighted SE scan)*

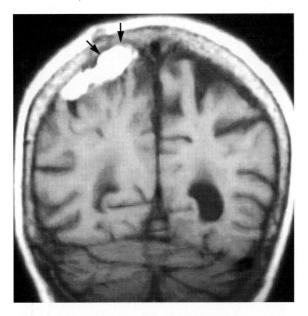

**Convexity Lipoma**

## Case 704

*80-year-old woman presenting with dementia. (coronal, noncontrast T1-weighted SE scan)*

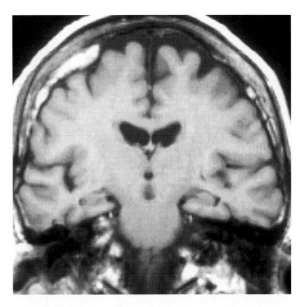

**Hyperostosis Frontalis Interna**

---

Subacute hemorrhage within the subdural space is the most common cause of a layered zone of short T1 values overlying the cerebral convexity. However, other conditions can mimic this appearance.

In Case 703, superficial high signal intensity is due to lipid protons within an unusual lipoma. Intracranial lipomas are more commonly encountered as midline lesions in the interhemispheric fissure or along the base of the brain (see Cases 276 and 859-862). The long-standing mass in Case 703 has caused remodeling of the calvarium *(arrows)* and depression of underlying cortex. (The small nodule within subcutaneous tissue of the scalp was unrelated to the intracranial mass.) The lipoma was removed, and seizures did not recur.

Case 704 presents a normal variant, which should not be mistaken for a layer of subdural hemorrhage. Prominent thickening of the inner aspect of the skull frequently occurs in elderly patients. This widened bone appears dense or "hyperostotic" on x-rays or CT scans, but its MR appearance may be dominated by short T1 values presumed to represent fatty marrow spaces. This finding is usually most prominent in the frontal region and is also characterized by a somewhat undulating inner margin. Bilaterality is usual, often with more symmetry than is seen above.

A similar pattern of layered high signal intensity may occur along the falx on T1-weighted scans of patients with calcified or ossified dural plaques. The short T1 values may reflect fatty marrow within bone or the effect of a calcium matrix on water protons. In any event, this normal variant frequently accounts for small or large areas of bright signal in the interhemispheric fissure on short TR scans. Such patches are characteristically very thin on coronal or axial images and are associated with calcification on CT scans or skull films.

Fat saturation pulse sequences would demonstrate reduced signal intensity of the "lesions" in each of the above cases, distinguishing them from subacute subdural hematomas. The presence of chemical shift artifact on long TR images can also help to identify lipomas (see Cases 276 and 861).

### Case 705

2-year-old boy presenting with irritability.
(axial, noncontrast T2-weighted SE scan)

### Case 706

71-year-old man presenting with right hemiparesis.
(axial, noncontrast T2-weighted SE scan)

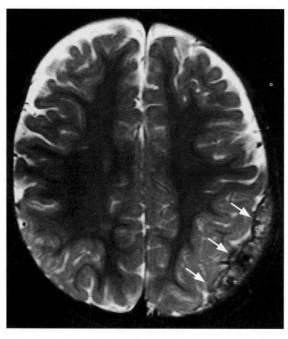

**Neuroblastoma**
(epidural)

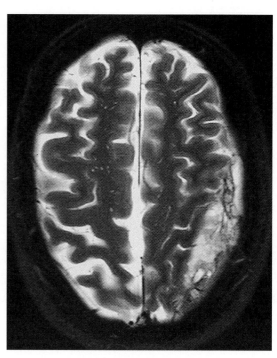

**Subdural Hematoma**
(subacute)

Case 705 is another reminder that a layer of dural-based tumor can mimic the appearance of an extracerebral hematoma. Like carcinomas of the prostate or breast in adults (see Case 701), neuroblastoma in children often involves the epidural space as an isolated process or in association with calvarial disease.

The heterogeneous signal intensity of the extracerebral tissue in Case 705 reflects small hemorrhages within the tumor. Epidural lymphoma or leukemia could present a similar appearance.

The subacute subdural hematoma in Case 706 demonstrated homogeneously high signal intensity on T1-weighted scans. T2-weighted images of subacute to chronic subdural collections often reveal more complexity and compartmentalization than is apparent on short TR scans. This heterogeneity is commonly observed in benign subdural hematomas and does not imply hemorrhage into pre-existing extracerebral pathology. On the other hand, dural metastases in adults (especially carcinomas of the breast or prostate) may be associated with subdural hemorrhage, so-called *pachymeningitis interna hemorrhagica*.

Postcontrast scans can distinguish between epidural neoplasms and extracerebral collections when noncontrast images are ambiguous. Enhancement is expected throughout the substance of tumor tissue, but only at the margins of a subdural hematoma.

Mass effect from the hematoma in Case 706 compresses sulci at the vertex of the left hemisphere and effaces the interhemispheric fissure on the left.

## Case 707

5-month-old boy.
(sagittal, noncontrast T1-weighted SE scan)

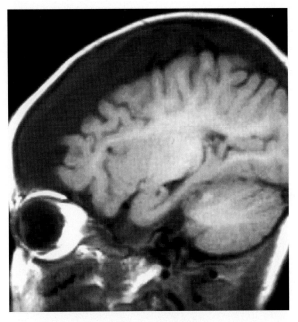

**Subdural Hygroma**

## Case 708

79-year-old man.
(sagittal, noncontrast T1-weighted SE scan)

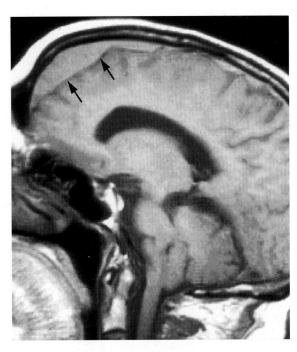

**Chronic Subdural Hematoma**

---

The distinction between a subdural hygroma (discussed in Cases 713 and 714) and a chronic subdural hematoma may be difficult on CT scans, since both lesions demonstrate uniformly low atttenuation. When this distinction is clinically or legally important, MR can provide useful characterization.

The large subdural collection in Case 707 contains signal intensity that is very close to that of spinal fluid. (Compare to the temporal horn or the vitreous humor of the globe.) This appearance favors a subdural hygroma rather than a chronic subdural hematoma, which usually contains fluid that is higher in intensity than CSF (as in Case 708; see also Case 702).

Some subdural hygromas are found to contain traces of hemorrhage or increased levels of protein at surgery. Such collections demonstrate signal intensities that are somewhat higher than CSF on all pulse sequences (see Cases 713 and 714). Even these complicated hygromas are rarely

as different from CSF signal intensity on T1-weighted images as the usual chronic subdural hematoma.

The signal intensity of the chronic hematoma in Case 708 has returned to a level intermediate between the acute and subacute stages illustrated in Case 699. Chronic subdural hematomas are often relatively isointense to cortex on T1-weighted scans. However, the interface between the extraaxial collection and the underlying brain is usually clearly defined by a combination of compressed subarachnoid space *(arrows)*, displaced cortical veins and/or subdural membranes.

The contrast between the signal intensity of the subdural collection in Case 708 and that of normal CSF would be less on T2-weighted scans, where both would appear bright. On the other hand, FLAIR images clearly distinguish simple CSF from other fluid collections with low attenuation values and long T1 and T2 relaxation times.

### Case 709

55-year-old woman presenting with
a ten-day history of headaches.
(coronal, noncontrast T1-weighted SE scan)

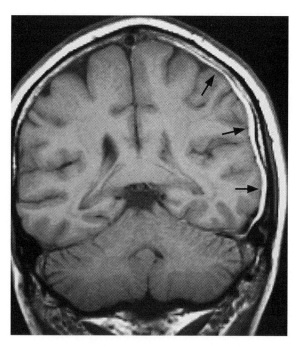

**Subdural Hematoma**

### Case 710

2-month-old girl presenting with a seizure.
(coronal, noncontrast T2-weighted SE scan)

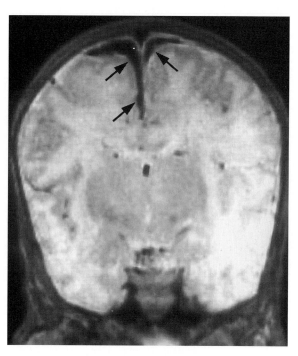

**Subdural Hematomas**

The increased attenuation of small acute or subacute subdural hematomas can be difficult to distinguish from the inner table on CT studies. MR offers two major advantages for detecting such lesions: (1) multiplanar display and (2) high contrast between subacute hematomas and adjacent bone.

The T1-shortening typically seen within subacute subdural hematomas makes these lesions conspicuous on T1-weighted images. In Case 709, a coronal scan clearly defines a thin hematoma overlying the convexity of the left cerebral hemisphere (*arrows;* compare Case 709 with Case 704).

In Case 710, a CT scan failed to demonstrate the acute subdural hematomas at the vertex due to partial volume artifact from the calvarium. The coronal projection and lack of bone artifact on the MR study clearly document the prognostically (and legally) important hemorrhages, which are seen as zones of low intensity reflecting the presence of deoxyhemoglobin.

Interhemispheric subdural hematomas characteristically demonstrate a flat medial margin along the falx and a variably thick lateral extension. (Compare to the subdural empyemas in Cases 436-439.)

## Case 711

6-month-old girl brought to the emergency
room because of lethargy.
(sagittal, noncontrast T1-weighted SE scan)

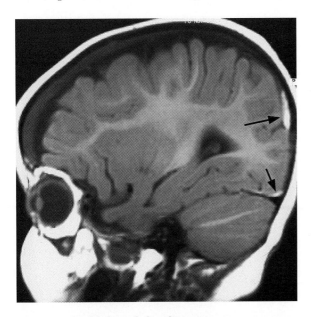

**Multiple Subdural Hematomas**

## Case 712

5-month-old boy presenting with lethargy.
(coronal, noncontrast T1-weighted SE scan)

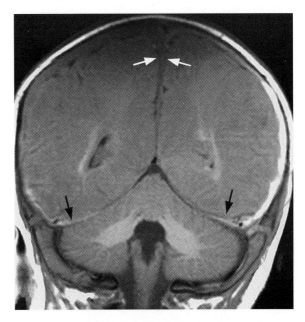

**Multiple Subdural Hematomas**

Subdural hematomas are common in children who have suffered physical abuse. The presence of one or more subdural collections is an important clue to the possibility of "nonaccidental trauma." MR can help to establish this diagnosis by: (1) documenting characteristic patterns of extracerebral hemorrhage and/or (2) demonstrating variable age of multiple intracranial hematomas, implying repetitive injury.

Posterior interhemispheric subdural hematomas often occur in children subjected to shaking and impact injuries and are a hallmark of the "battered child syndrome" or "shaken baby impact syndrome." Coronal MR scans can define the thin subdural hemorrhages adjacent to the posterior falx or tentorium that are typical of this disorder (see Case 710).

Multiple subdural hematomas of variable age are apparent in each of the above scans. In Case 711, small subacute hemorrhages are present at the occipital pole *(long arrow)* and along the superior surface of the tentorium *(short arrow)*. A larger subdural collection in the frontal region may represent an acute or chronic hematoma or a subdural hygroma with high protein or cell content. (The subarach-

noid space is seen as an underlying layer of lower signal intensity.)

Case 712 demonstrates thin layers of subdural hemorrhage surrounding both cerebral hemispheres, including components in the interhemispheric fissure *(white arrows)* and along the tentorium *(black arrows)*. The mixture of isointensity and short T1 values suggests hemorrhages of variable age.

The underlying cerebral parenchyma appears mildly atrophic in Case 711 and swollen in Case 712. These changes probably reflect remote trauma or hypoxic/ischemic injury in Case 711 and a recent cerebral insult in Case 712. Diffusion-weighted scans are more sensitive than routine MR images for demonstrating parenchymal injuries (usually cortical) that often accompany subdural hematomas in cases of child abuse.

Retinal hemorrhages are very common in infants or children who have experienced shaking/impact injury. The combination of this finding with the presence of an interhemispheric subdural hematoma strongly implies nonaccidental trauma.

### Case 713

2-year-old boy presenting with
bilateral sixth nerve palsies.
(coronal, noncontrast T1-weighted SE scan)

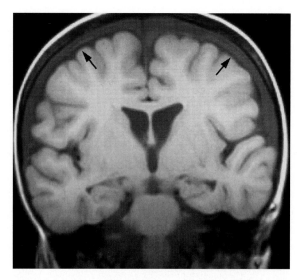

**Subdural Hygromas**

### Case 714

16-year-old girl presenting with headaches,
one week after head trauma.
(axial, noncontrast scan; SE 3000/30)

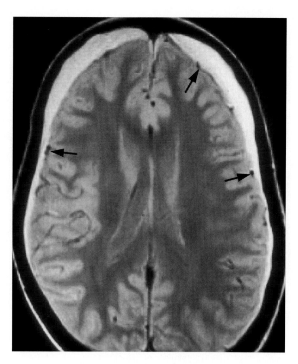

**Subdural Hygromas**

Some patients develop acute aqueous subdural collections after head trauma. These accumulations have been termed *subdural hygromas,* because they usually contain clear or lightly colored cerebrospinal fluid. The fluid apparently gains access to the subdural space through an arachnoid tear. Subdural hygromas are most often seen in elderly patients and young children. Most of these collections remain small and resolve spontaneously.

Subdural hygromas are sometimes confused with widened subarachnoid spaces due to cerebral atrophy. These two processes are usually distinguishable on the basis of (1) cortical contour and gyral position and (2) signal intensity, especially on FLAIR or long TR spin echo images. As seen in the above cases, the margin of compressed cortex beneath a subdural collection is abnormally smooth, contrasting with the irregular outline of atrophic cortex reflecting widened sulci. The tips of cortical gyri seldom retract significantly from the inner table even in the presence of marked atrophy (see Cases 534 and 535). By contrast, the cortical surface is unequivocally displaced from

the calvarium by subdural collections. Similarly, displacement of cortical veins from the inner table indicates subdural accumulation of fluid (*arrows* in Case 714).

The signal intensity of subdural hygromas is usually higher than that of subarachnoid or ventricular CSF due to the presence of increased protein content and/or cell count. Relative lack of signal loss from CSF pulsation may also contribute to this difference. The distinction between hygroma fluid and CSF is best appreciated on long TR, short TE images, such as Case 714, and on FLAIR sequences.

The child in Case 713 is unusual in that the subdural hygromas have grown sufficiently large to increase intracranial pressure and cause sixth nerve palsies. Drainage of the collections demonstrated clear, golden fluid. The mild ventricular prominence in this case may reflect impairment of CSF circulation through convexity subarachnoid spaces, which are faintly seen as a line of lower signal intensity at the medial margin of the hygromas *(arrows).*

### Case 715

1-month-old girl who suffered a parietal
skull fracture one week earlier.
(sagittal, noncontrast T1-weighted SE scan)

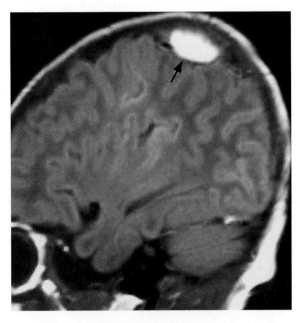

**Epidural Hematoma**
(subacute)

### Case 716

5-year-old girl presenting one
day after a bicycle accident.
(sagittal, postcontrast T1-weighted SE scan)

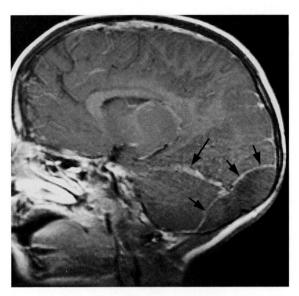

**Epidural Hematoma**
(acute)

---

The dura functions as periosteum for the inner table and is tightly adherent to the skull. For this reason, hemorrhage accumulating between the calvarium and the dura remains relatively confined. An epidural hematoma acquires substantial thickness and a convex margin before sufficient pressure develops to strip the dura for further expansion. This biconvex or lentiform shape, as illustrated in Case 715, contrasts with the thin, crescentic morphology of most acute subdural hematomas (compare to Case 709).

Subdural hematomas often widen with time. Subacute or chronic subdural collections may demonstrate a medial margin that is straight or even convex (see Cases 698-700), resembling an epidural hematoma. The dura is usually visible as a line of low signal intensity at the inner margin of an epidural collection; absence of this feature suggests a subdural process. Epidural hematomas are limited by the attachment of dura/periostem at suture lines, whereas subdural hematomas are not. Clinical context (e.g., association with skull fracture and rapidity of neurological deterioration) also helps to distinguish between the two lesions.

Most supratentorial epidural hematomas are due to lacerations of branches of the middle meningeal artery at the point of skull fracture. These hemorrhages may enlarge rapidly and warrant close observation in cases where emergency surgery is not performed. A "lucid interval" of several hours between trauma and the rapid onset of symptoms is a characteristic clinical feature. Small epidural hematomas in asymptomatic patients may resolve without surgery, as was true in Case 715.

Epidural hematomas in the posterior fossa are usually caused by venous bleeding from torn dural sinuses. As a result, they present less acutely and have less characteristic morphology than supratentorial epidural hemorrhages. Regardless of shape, an extracerebral hematoma is established as epidural if it crosses the plane of the tentorium or falx.

The acute epidural hematoma in Case 716 *(short arrows)* clearly crosses the plane of the tentorium *(long arrow)*. Linear enhancement at the anterior margin of the collection represents the displaced dura.

Mild T1-shortening within the cortex near the frontoparietal junction in Case 715 probably reflects contusion (see Case 685).

## Case 717

52-year-old woman, ten days
after collapsing at work.
(sagittal, noncontrast T1-weighted SE scan)

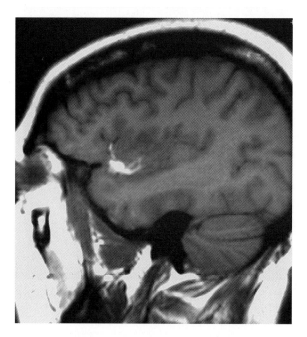

**Subarachnoid Hemorrhage**
(subacute)

## Case 718

45-year-old man being treated with
anticoagulants, now presenting with
decreased level of consciousness.
(axial, noncontrast FLAIR scan)

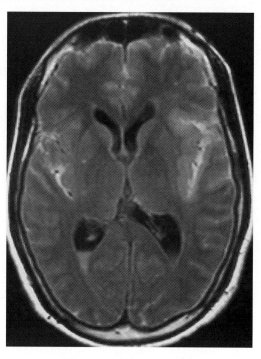

**Subarachnoid Hemorrhage**
(acute)

Acute subarachnoid hemorrhage may be inapparent on standard spin echo MR images. High oxygen tension within the CSF, spinal fluid pulsation, and averaging of subtle signal changes with the long T1 and T2 values of CSF have been suggested as reasons for this lack of sensitivity.

On the other hand, spin echo MR images can confirm the suspicion of subacute subarachnoid hemorrhage at a stage when the CT attenuation of cisterns has returned to near normal. In Case 717, focal T1-shortening due to methemoglobin is present within the sylvian cistern near the genu of the middle cerebral artery. A ruptured aneurysm at this site was demonstrated angiographically and surgically repaired. Mild edema thickens the adjacent insular cortex.

FLAIR pulse sequences substantially improve the MR detection of acute subarachnoid hemorrhage. By design, normal CSF is dark on FLAIR scans. The presence of cells or protein with sulci and cisterns causes a conspicuous increase in signal intensity.

Case 718 illustrates this appearance. Acute, diffuse subarachnoid hemorrhage fills all cisterns and sulci, contrast-ing with the low intensity of intraventricular CSF. (A small amount of hemorrhage is present in the trigone of the right lateral ventricle.)

Ruptured aneurysms account for about 80% of subarachnoid hemorrhages and should be sought in all cases. However, some patients present with hemorrhage centered in the prepontine and interpeduncular region and no evidence of an associated aneurysm. Such *benign perimesencephalic hemorrhage* or *pretruncal nonaneurysmal subarachnoid hemorrhage* may originate from small veins or perforating arteries and carries a good prognosis with rare recurrence.

Several complications of subarachnoid hemorrhage may be apparent on MR scans. Obstructive or communicating hydrocephalus may develop due to clot within the ventricular system or clogging of arachnoid granulations. Cerebral infarction may occur secondary to arterial spasm, which typically develops several days after hemorrhage and tends to be most severe in the areas of densest subarachnoid clot. Parenchymal hematomas associated with subarachnoid hemorrhage may provide clues to the location of a ruptured aneurysm.

## Case 719

86-year-old man presenting with left hemiparesis
two days after head trauma.
(axial, noncontrast FLAIR scan)

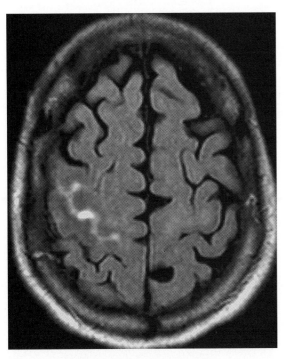

**Subarachnoid Hemorrhage**

## Case 720

34-year-old woman presenting with headaches.
(axial, noncontrast FLAIR scan)

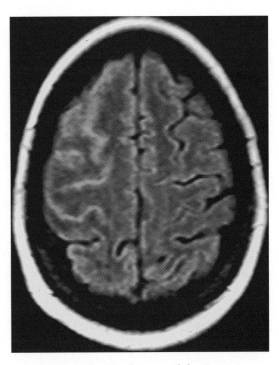

**Metastatic Carcinoma of the Breast**

---

As discussed on the previous page, subarachnoid hemorrhage is readily demonstrated on FLAIR images by increased signal intensity within sulci or cisterns. Hemorrhage in Case 719 is localized to the right central sulcus. Adjacent cortical edema is present.

In Case 720, CSF within sulci of the superior right frontal lobe is replaced by tissue that is nearly isointense to cortex. This finding proved to represent leptomeningeal metastasis from a previously unsuspected carcinoma of the breast. Metastatic disease should be included in the differential diagnosis of parenchymal or meningeal disease, even in young adults.

Meningitis is a third major category of pathology to be considered when MR scans demonstrate focal or diffuse abnormality of subarachnoid spaces (see Cases 424 and 425).

Congestion of the leptomeninges in an area of arterial or venous infarction is an additional potential etiology of abnormal signal intensity within sulci, most apparent on FLAIR images.

Finally, increased signal from subarachnoid CSF has been reported on FLAIR images of patients scanned during general anesthesia. This finding is believed to reflect the increased oxygen content of spinal fluid surrounding intracranial arteries when supplemental oxygen is administered.

See Cases 430 and 431 for discussion of the differential diagnosis of abnormal leptomeningeal enhancement.

### Case 721

65-year-old man with a history of multiple
subdural hematomas, now presenting with
bilateral hearing loss.
(axial, noncontrast T2-weighted SE scan)

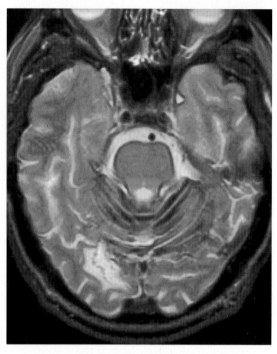

**Superficial Siderosis**

### Case 722

67-year-old man presenting with ataxia.
(axial, noncontrast T2-weighted SE scan)

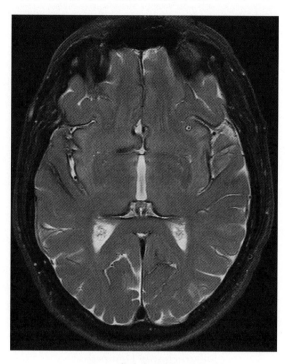

**Superficial Siderosis**

Case 721 demonstrates an unusual layer of low signal intensity along the surface of the cerebellum and brainstem. (Unrelated background findings include atrophy and a small area of encephalomalacia in the right occipital lobe.) A similar line of low intensity marginates the sylvian, interhemispheric, and pineal cisterns in Case 722. The strikingly uniform outline of parenchymal contours in these cases is caused by subpial accumulation of old blood products, mainly hemosiderin.

Such *superficial siderosis* is seen in situations of chronic or repetitive subarachnoid hemorrhage. The source of bleeding may be a leaking vascular lesion (e.g., aneurysm or vascular malformation), margins of a postoperative CSF space (e.g., pseudomeningocele or hemispherectomy), or a spinal or intracranial neoplasm. Hemorrhagic ependymomas of the spinal canal (see Cases 1082 and 1223) have been particularly frequently associated with intracranial siderosis.

Fragile vessels within the membranes of chronic subdural hematomas frequently bleed. This mechanism prob-

ably contributes to the growth of such lesions and is also a recognized cause of cerebral siderosis.

In 30% to 50% of cases the etiology of superficial siderosis cannot be established, even at autopsy. The source of the siderosis in Case 722 was unknown.

The meningeal surfaces of the posterior fossa are often most severely affected in cases of generalized siderosis. The superior aspect of the cerebellum is especially commonly involved. (Compare this localization to the preferential distribution of meningeal carcinomatosis, as discussed in Cases 165-167 and 627.)

Patients suffering from superficial siderosis frequently present with bilateral sensorineural hearing loss. The cisternal segments of the eighth cranial nerves are particularly susceptible to damage from the deposition of blood products on their surface. Cerebellar symptoms are usually absent, but ataxia has been noted in some cases.

Localized siderosis may occur anywhere over the cerebral convexity in proximity to a source of repeated subarachnoid hemorrhages. Examples include a long-standing neoplasm or an old operative site.

### Case 723

4-day-old girl, born at 36-weeks' gestation.
(sagittal, noncontrast T1-weighted SE scan)

### Case 724

5-day-old boy, born at 33-weeks' gestation.
(axial, noncontrast T2-weighted SE scan)

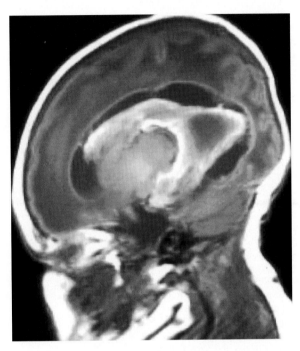

**Intraventricular Hemorrhage**

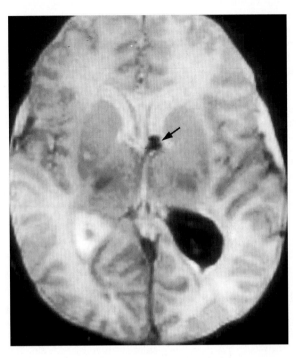

**Intraventricular Hemorrhage**

Hemorrhage commonly arises from fragile vessels in the periventricular germinal matrix of premature newborns. Hematomas may remain confined to the subependymal region or rupture into the ventricular system, often causing secondary hydrocephalus.

Cribside ultrasound (using the open fontanelles as acoustic windows) is the procedure of choice for following the initial course of such infants. CT or MR scans of neonatal intraventricular hemorrhage may be performed in ambiguous or complicated cases.

In Case 723, a hemorrhagic cast of the lateral ventricle was formed at the time it filled with blood. This clot now resides within a larger CSF space caused by consequent hydrocephalus. The predominant high signal intensity of the intraventricular thrombus indicates the presence of methemoglobin and suggests that the hemorrhagic event occurred several days earlier.

Case 724 illustrates prominent T2-shortening within intraventricular thrombus filling the trigone of the left lateral ventricle. Both deoxyhemoglobin and intracellular methemoglobin may cause this appearance. The former is associated with isointensity on T1-weighted scans (see Case 673), whereas the latter produces T1-shortening. In either case, the intraventricular hemorrhage is clearly recent and likely perinatal. A tiny clot at the foramen of Monro, as seen on the left in Case 724 *(arrow)*, is occasionally an isolated clue to recent intraventricular hemorrhage.

In adults, hematomas in the posterior fossa or basal ganglia may rupture into the fourth, third, or lateral ventricles. The ventricles may be grossly expanded by thrombus. Alternatively, the intraventricular hematoma may cause obstructive hydrocephalus.

# REFERENCES

Aoki N: Extracerebral fluid collections in infancy: role of magnetic resonance imaging in differentiation between subdural effusion and subarachnoid space enlargement. *J Neurosurg* 81:20-23, 1994.

Ashikaga R, Araki Y, Ishida O: MRI of head injury using FLAIR. *Neuroradiology* 39:239-242, 1997.

Atlas SW: MR imaging is highly sensitive for acute subarachnoid hemorrhage...Not! *Radiology* 186:319-322, 1993.

Atlas SW, DuBois P, Singer MB, Lu D: Diffusion measurements in intracranial hematomas: implications for MR imaging of acute stroke. *AJNR* 21:1190-1194, 2000.

Atlas SW, Mark AS, Grossman RI, Gomori JM: Intracranial hemorrhage: gradient-echo MR imaging at 1.5T. Comparisons with spin-echo imaging and clinical applications. *Radiology* 168:803-805, 1988.

Atlas SW, Thulborn KR: MR detection of hyperacute parenchymal hemorrhage of the brain. *AJNR* 19:1471-1478, 1998.

Bakshi R, Kamran S, Kinkel PR, et al: Fluid-attenuated inversion-recovery MR imaging in acute and subacute cerebral intraventricular hemorrhage. *AJNR* 20:629-636, 1999.

Bakshi R, Kamran S, Kinkel PR, et al: MRI in cerebral intraventricular hemorrhage: analysis of 50 consecutive cases. *Neuroradiology* 41:401-409, 1999.

Ball WS Jr: Nonaccidental craniocerebral trauma (child abuse): MR imaging. *Radiology* 173:609-610, 1989.

Barkovich AJ, Atlas SW: Magnetic resonance of intracranial hemorrhage. *Radiol Clin North Am* 26:801-820, 1988.

Bourgouin PM, Tampieri D, Melancon D, et al: Superficial siderosis of the brain following unexplained subarachnoid hemorrhage: MRI diagnosis and clinical significance. *Neuroradiology* 34:407-410, 1992.

Bracchi M, Savoiardo M, Triulzi F, et al: Superficial siderosis of the CNS: MR diagnosis and clinical findings. *AJNR* 14:227-236, 1993.

Bradley WG Jr: MR appearance of hemorrhage in the brain. *Radiology* 189:15-26, 1993.

Bradley WG Jr, Schmidt PG: Effect of methemoglobin formation of the MR appearance of subarachnoid hemorrhage. *Radiology* 156:99-103, 1985.

Brooks RA, Di Chiro G, Patronas N: MR imaging of cerebral hematomas as different field strengths: theory and applications. *J Comput Assist Tomogr* 13:194-206, 1989.

Brown E, Prager J, Lee H-Y, Ramsey RG: CNS complications of cocaine abuse: prevalence, pathophysiology and neuroradiology. *Am J Roentgenol* 159:137-147, 1992.

Chan S, Kartha K, Yoon SS, et al: Multifocal hypointense cerebral lesions on gradient-echo MR are associated with chronic hypertension. *AJNR* 17:1821-1827, 1996.

Clark RA, Watanabe AT, Bradley WG Jr, Roberts JD: Acute hematoma: effects of deoxygenation, hematocrit, and fibrin-clot formation and retraction on T2 shortening. *Radiology* 175:201-206, 1990.

Deliganis AV, Fisher DJ, Lam AM, Maravilla KR: Cerebrospinal fluid signal intensity increase on FLAIR MR images in patients under general anesthesia: the role of supplemental $O_2$. *Radiology* 218:152-156, 2001.

Dooms GC, Uske A, Brant-Zawadzki M, et al: Spin-echo MR imaging of intracranial hemorrhage. *Neuroradiology* 28:132-138, 1986.

Ebisu T, Naruse S, Horikawa Y, et al: Nonacute subdural hematoma: Fundamental interpretation of MR images based on biochemical and in vitro analysis. *Radiology* 171:449-454, 1989.

Fazekas F, Kleinert R, Roob G, et al: Histopathologic analysis of foci of signal loss on gradient-echo T2*-weighted MR images in patients with spontaneous intracerebral hemorrhage: evidence of microangiopathy-related microbleeds. *AJNR* 20:637-642, 1999.

Filippi CG, Ulug AM, Lin D, et al: Hyperintense signal abnormality in subarachnoid spaces and basal cisterns of children anesthetized with propofol: new fluid-attenuated inversion recovery findings. *AJNR* 22:394-399, 2001.

Fobben ES, Grossman RI, Atlas SW, et al: MR characteristics of subdural hematoma and hygromas at 1.5 T. *AJNR* 10:687-693, 1989.

Gentry LR: Imaging of closed head injury. *Radiology* 191:1-17, 1994.

Gentry LR: Primary neuronal injuries. *Neuroimaging Clin N Amer* 1:411-432, 1991.

Gentry LR, Gordersky JC, Thompson B: MR imaging of head trauma: review of the distribution and radiopathologic features of traumatic lesions. *AJNR* 9:101-110, 1988.

Gentry LR, Gordersky JC, Thompson BH: Traumatic brain stem injury: MR imaging. *Radiology* 171:177-187, 1989.

Gentry LR, Gordersky JC, Thompson B, Dunn VD: Prospective comparative study of intermediate-field MR and CT in the evaluation of closed head trauma. *AJNR* 9:91-100, 1988.

Gentry LR, Thompson B, Gordersky JC: Trauma to the corpus callosum: MR features. *AJNR* 9:1129-1138, 1988.

Ghazi-Birry HS, Brown WR, Moody DM, et al: Human germinal matrix: venous origin of hemorrhage and vascular characteristics. *AJNR* 18:219-229, 1997.

Gomori JM, Grossman RI: Mechanisms responsible for the MR appearance and evolution of intracranial hemorrhage. *Radiographics* 8:427-440, 1988.

Gomori JM, Grossman RI, Bilaniuk LT, et al: High field MR imaging of superficial siderosis of the central nervous system. *J Comput Assist Tomogr* 9:972-975, 1985.

Gomori JM, Grossman RI, Goldberg HI, et al: High-field spin-echo MR imaging of superficial and subependymal siderosis secondary to neonatal intraventricular hemorrhage. *Neuroradiology* 29:339, 1987.

Gomori JM, Grossman RI, Goldberg HI, et al: Intracranial hematoma: imaging by high-field MR. *Radiology* 157:87-93, 1985.

Gomori JM, Grossman RI, Hackney DB, et al: Variable appearances of subacute intracranial hematomas on high-field spin-echo MR. *AJNR* 8:1019-1026, 1987.

Good CD, Ng VWK, Clifton A, et al: Amyloid angiography causing widespread miliary haemorrhages within the brain evident on MRI. *Neuroradiology* 40:308-311, 1998.

Grossman RI, Gomori JM, Goldberg HI, et al: MR imaging of hemorrhagic conditions of the head and neck. *Radiographics* 8:441, 1988.

Groswasser Z, Reider-Groswasser I, Soroker N, Machtey Y: Magnetic resonance imaging in head injury patients with normal late computed tomography scans. *Surg Neurol* 27:331-337, 1987.

Hackney DB, Lesnick JE, Zimmerman RA, et al: MR identification of the bleeding site in subarachnoid hemorrhage with multiple intracranial aneurysms. *J Comput Assist Tomogr* 10:878-880, 1986.

Han JS, Kaufman B, Alfidi RJ, et al: Head trauma evaluated by magnetic resonance and computed tomography: a comparison. *Radiology* 150:71-77, 1984.

Harwood-Nash DC: Abuse to the pediatric central nervous system. *AJNR* 13:569-576, 1992.

Hasegawa M, Yamashima T, Yamashita J: Traumatic subdural hygroma: pathology and meningeal enhancement on magnetic resonance imaging. *Neurosurgery* 31:580-585, 1992.

Hayman LA, Taber KH, Ford JJ, Bryan RN: Mechanisms of MR signal alteration by acute intracerebral blood: old concepts and new theories. *AJNR* 12:899-907, 1991.

Hesselink JR, Dowd CF, Healy ME, et al: MR imaging of brain contusion: a comparative study with CT. *AJNR* 9:269-278, 1988.

Hosoda K, Tamaki N, Masumma M, et al: Magnetic resonance images of chronic subdural hematomas. *J Neurosurg* 67:677-683, 1987.

Hsu WC, Loevner LA, Forman MS, Thaler ER: Superficial siderosis of the CNS associated with multiple cavernous malformations. *AJNR* 20:1245-1248, 1999.

Janick PA, Hackney DB, Grossman RI, Asakura T: MR imaging of various oxidation of intracellular and extracellular hemoglobin. *AJNR* 12:891-897, 1991.

Janss AJ, Galetta SL, Freese A, et al: Superficial siderosis of the central nervous system: magnetic resonance imaging and pathologic correlation. Case report. *J Neurosurg* 79:756-760, 1993.

Jenkins A, Hadley D, Teasdale GM, et al: Magnetic resonance imaging of acute subarachnoid hemorrhage. *J Neurosurg* 68:731-736, 1988.

Jones KM, Mulkern RV, Mantell MT, et al: Brain hemorrhage: evaluation with fast spin-echo and conventional dural spin-echo images. *Radiology* 182:53-58, 1992.

Kaminogo M, Moroki J, Ochi A, et al: Characteristics of symptomatic chronic subdural haematomas on high-field MRI. *Neuroradiology* 41:109-116, 1999.

Kelly AB, Zimmerman RD, Snow RB, et al: Head trauma: comparison of MR and CT-experience in 100 patients. *AJNR* 9:699-708, 1988.

Landi JL, Spickler EM: Imaging of intracranial hemorrhage associated with drug abuse. *Neuroimaging Clin N Amer* 2:187-194, 1992.

Levin HS, Amparo EG, Eisenberg HM, et al: Magnetic resonance imaging after closed head injury in children. *Neurosurgery* 24:223-227, 1989.

Levin HS, Amparo EG, Eisenberg HM, et al: Magnetic resonance imaging and computerized tomography in relation to the neurobehavioral sequelae of mild and moderate head injuries. *J Neurosurg* 66:706-713, 1987.

Liang L, Korogi Y, Sugahara T, et al: Detection of intracranial hemorrhage with susceptibility-weighted MR sequences. *AJNR* 20:1527-1534, 1999.

Liu AY, Maldjian JA, Bagley LJ, et al: Traumatic brain injury: diffusion-weighted MR imaging findings. *AJNR* 20:1636-1641, 1999.

Mahallati H, Wallace CJ, Sevick RJ: Susceptibility artifact mimicking chemical shift artifact in acute and subacute hematoma. *Int J Neurorad* 5:22-26, 1999.

Marshall LF: Head injury: recent past, present and future. *Neurosurgery* 47:546-561, 2000.

McArdle CB, Richardson CJ, Hayden CK, et al: Abnormalities of the neonatal brain: MR imaging. Part I. Intracranial hemorrhage. *Radiology* 163:387-394, 1987.

McCluney KW, Yeakley JW, Fenstermache, MJ, et al: Subdural hygroma versus atrophy on MR brain scans: "The cortical vein sign." *AJNR* 13:1335-1339, 1992.

McGowan JC, Yang JH, Plotkin RC, et al: Magnetization transfer imaging in the detection of injury associated with mild head trauma. *AJNR* 21:875-880, 2000.

Melhem ER, Patel RT, Whitehead RE, et al: MR imaging of hemorrhagic brain lesions: a comparison of dual-echo gradient-and spin-echo and fast spin-echo techniques. *Am J Roentgenol* 171:797-802, 1998.

Mendelsohn DB, Levin HS, Harward H, Bruce D: Corpus callosum lesions after closed head-injury in children: MR clinical features and outcome. *Neuroradiology* 34:384-388, 1992.

Mittl RL Jr, Grossman RI, Hiehle JF Jr, et al: Prevalence of MR evidence of diffuse axonal injury in patients with mild head injury and normal head CT findings. *AJNR* 15:1583-1590, 1994.

Moon KL Jr, Brant-Zwadzki M, Pitts LH, Mills CM: Nuclear magnetic resonance imaging of CT-isodense subdural hematomas. *AJNR* 5:319-322, 1984.

Noguchi K, Ogawa T., Inugami A, et al: Acute subarachnoid hemorrhage: MR imaging with fluid-attenuated inversion recovery pulse sequences. *Radiology* 196:773-778, 1995.

Noguchi K, Ogawa T, Inugami A, et al: MR of acute subarachnoid hemorrhage: a preliminary report of fluid-attenuated inversion-recovery pulse sequences. *AJNR* 15,1940-1944, 1994.

Noguchi K, Ogawa T, Seto H, et al: Subacute and chronic subarachnoid hemorrhage diagnosis with fluid-attenuated inversion-recovery MR imaging. *Radiology* 203:257-262, 1997.

Noguchi K, Seto H, Kamisaki Y, et al: Comparison of fluid-attenuated inversion-recovery MR imaging with CT in a simulated model of subarachnoid hemorrhage. *AJNR* 21:923-927, 2000.

Offenbacher H. Fazekas F, Schmidt R, et al: MR of cerebral abnormalities concomitant with primary intracerebral hematomas. *AJNR* 17:573-578, 1996.

Offenbacher H, Fazekas F, Schmidt R, et al: Superficial siderosis of the central nervous system: MRI findings and clinical significance. *Neuroradiology* 38:S51-S56, 1996.

Ogawa T, Inugami A, Shimosegawa E, et al: Subarachnoid hemorrhage: evaluation with MR imaging. *Radiology* 186:345-351, 1993.

Orrison WW, Gentry LR, Stimac GK, et al: Blinded comparison of cranial CT and MR in closed head injury evaluation. *AJNR* 15:351-356, 1994.

Qureshi AI, Tuhrim S, Broderick JP, et al: Spontaneous intracerebral hemorrhage. *N Engl J Med* 344:1450-1460, 2001.

Pfleger MJ, Hardee EP, Contant CF Jr, Hayman LA: Sensitivity and specificity of fluid-blood levels for coagulopathy in acute intracerebral hematomas. *AJNR* 15:217-224, 1994.

Pyhtinen J, Paakko E, Ilkko E: Superficial siderosis in the central nervous system. *Neuroradiology* 37:127-128, 1995.

Rinkel GJE, Wijdicks EFM, Vermeulen M, et al: Nonaneurysmal perimesencephalic subarachnoid hemorrhage: CT and MR patterns that differ from aneurysmal rupture. *AJNR* 12:829-834, 1991.

Sato Y, Yuh WTC, Smith WL, et al: Head injury in child abuse: evaluation with MR imaging. *Radiology* 173:653-657, 1989.

Saton S, Kadoya S: Magnetic resonance imaging of subarachnoid hemorrhage. *Neuroradiology* 30:361, 1988.

Schwartz TH, Mayer SA: Quadrigeminal variant of perimesencephalic nonaneurysmal subarachnoid hemorrhage. *Neurosurgery* 46:584-588, 2000.

Schwartz TH, Solomon RA: Perimesencephalic nonaneurysmal subarachnoid hemorrhage: review of the literature. *Neurosurgery* 39:433-440, 1996.

Seidenwurm D, Meng T-K, Kowalski H, et al: Intracranial hemorrhage lesions: evaluation with spin-echo and gradient-refocused MR imaging at 0.5 and 1.5 T. *Radiology* 172:189-194, 1989.

Singer MB, Atlas SW, Drayer BP: Subarachnoid space disease: diagnosis with fluid-attenuated inversion-recovery MR imaging and comparison with Gadolinium-enhanced spin-echo MR imaging-blinded reader study. *Radiology* 208:417-422, 1998.

Sklar EML, Quencer RM, Bowen BC, et al: Magnetic resonance application in cerebral injury. *Radiol Clin North Am* 30:353-366, 1992.

Snow RB, Zimmerman RD, Gandy SE, Deck MDF: Comparison of magnetic resonance imaging and computed tomography in the evaluation of head injury. *Neurosurgery* 18:45-52, 1986.

Stein SC, Spettell C, Young C, Ross SE: Delayed and progressive brain injury in closed-head trauma: radiologic demonstration. *Neurosurgery* 32:25-31, 1993.

Taoka T, Yuh WTC, White ML, et al: Sulcal hyperintensity of fluid-attenuated inversion recovery MR images in patients without apparent cerebrospinal fluid abnormality. *Am J Roentgenol* 176: 519-524, 2001.

Walenga JM, Marmon JF: Coagulopathies associated with intracranial hemorrhage. *Neuroimaging Clin N Amer* 2:137-152, 1992.

Watanabe AT, Mackey JK, Lufkin RB: Imaging diagnosis and temporal appearance of subarachnoid hemorrhage. *Neuroimaging Clin N Amer* 2:53-59, 1992.

Wilberger JE Jr, Deeb Z, Rothfus W: Magnetic resonance imaging in cases of severe head injury. *Neurosurgery* 20:571-576, 1987.

Wilms G, Vanderschueren G, Demaerel PH, et al: CT and MR in infants with pericerebral collections and macrocephaly: benign enlargement of the subarachnoid spaces versus subdural collections. *AJNR* 14:855-860, 1993.

Yoon HC, Lufkin RB, Vinuela F, et al: MR of acute subarachnoid hemorrhage. *AJNR* 9:404-405, 1988.

Zimmerman RA, Bilaniuk LT: Pediatric head trauma. *Neuroimaging Clin North Am* 4:349-366, 1994.

Zimmerman RA, Bilaniuk LT Hackney DB, et al: Head injury: early results of comparing CT and high-field MR. *AJNR* 7:757-764, 1986.

Zimmerman RD, Heier LA, Snow RB, et al: Acute intracranial hemorrhage: intensity changes on sequential MR scans at 0.5 T. *AJNR* 9:47-58, 1988.

# CHAPTER 14

# Vascular Lesions

## Case 725

32-year-old woman presenting with headaches and
a family history of subarachnoid hemorrhage.
(axial, noncontrast scan; SE 2800/45)

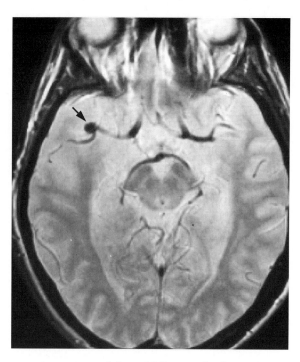

**Aneurysm of the Middle Cerebral Artery**

## Case 726

82-year-old man with a history of TIAs.
(axial, noncontrast T2-weighted FSE scan)

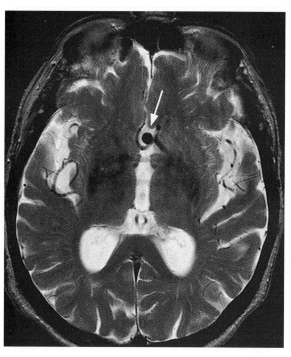

**Aneurysm of the Anterior Communicating Artery**

Small, patent aneurysms can be identified on spin echo MR studies as nodular expansions of flow void along the course of cerebral arteries. Such lesions are particularly well outlined by the high signal intensity of CSF on long TR sequences.

The genu or "trifurcation" region of the middle cerebral artery and the junction of the anterior cerebral and anterior communicating arteries are common sites for intracranial aneurysms, as illustrated above. Attention to these vessels is an appropriate component of interpreting MR scans (along with noting the presence or absence of flow void in major arteries at the base of the skull).

Larger patent aneurysms may present more complicated appearances. Zones of slow flow or stasis within giant aneurysms can generate regions of variable intensity that may be difficult to distinguish from thrombus. Gradient echo sequences emphasizing flow-related enhancement

help to separate these intraluminal components. Both slow flow and thrombus may be associated with enhancement on postcontrast MR scans.

Unruptured aneurysms can occasionally cause symptoms by embolization of thrombi formed within their lumens. It was not possible to clearly establish the source of the TIAs in Case 726.

Even "incidental" aneurysms in asymptomatic patients may be considered for surgery (or intraarterial occlusion with platinum coils), depending on the aneurysm size and patient age. Population studies have estimated the risk of bleeding from unruptured aneurysms to be about 1% to 2% per year.

MR angiography is an excellent tool for noninvasive screening of patients with an increased risk of or concern about intracranial aneurysms (see Case 729).

# DIFFERENTIAL DIAGNOSIS:
## FOCAL LOW SIGNAL INTENSITY ADJACENT TO AN ARTERY

### Case 727

23-year-old man presenting with headaches.
(axial, noncontrast scan; SE 2800/45)

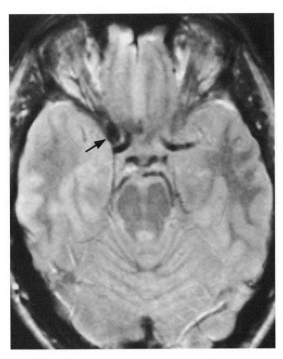

**Pneumatized Anterior Clinoid Process**

### Case 728

2-year-old girl studied for developmental delay.
(axial, noncontrast T2-weighted SE scan)

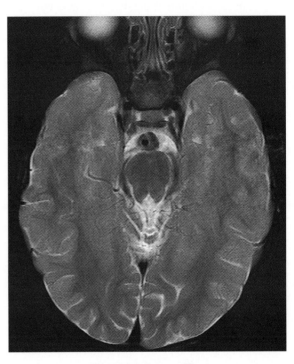

**CSF Pulsation Artifact**

---

The flow void within the lumen of a patent aneurysm on standard MR images can be mimicked by a number of anatomical or physiological findings. Two common examples are illustrated above.

A large pneumatized or sclerotic anterior clinoid process may cause a focal zone of low signal intensity adjacent to the lumen of the internal carotid artery, as in Case 727 *(arrow).* This appearance may be accentuated on axial scans by a small amount of head tilt causing right/left asymmetry. A similar "pseudoaneurysm" can occur in the region of the anterior communicating artery when partial volume of a prominent tuberculum sella is included on an axial scan.

Scans in the coronal plane will convincingly exclude or document an aneurysm in many cases. A flow-sensitive gra-

dient echo sequence should settle the question when necessary.

Signal loss due to CSF motion is common within the basal cisterns of children, who normally demonstrate dynamic pulsation of spinal fluid in the suprasellar and prepontine regions. In Case 728, a halo of reduced cisternal signal intensity surrounds the flow void of the rostral basilar artery, reflecting the pulsatility of the vessel and/or of the adjacent CSF circulation. This physiological variant should not be confused with vascular pathology.

Less prominent areas of reduced signal intensity parallel the perimesencephalic course of the posterior cerebral arteries in Case 728.

### Case 729A

38-year-old woman with a family
history of cerebral aneurysms.
(axial source image from a noncontrast, three-
dimensional, time-of-flight GRE sequence)

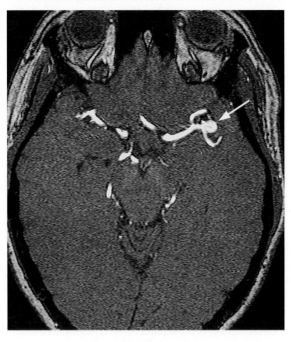

**Aneurysm of the Middle Cerebral Artery**

### Case 729B

Same patient.
(submentovertex view, maximal intensity projection
reconstruction, noncontrast, three-dimensional,
time-of-flight GRE sequence)

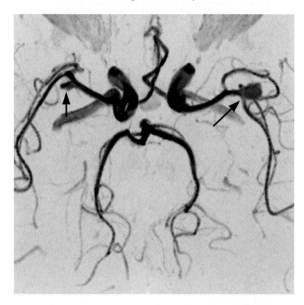

**Aneurysms of the Middle Cerebral Arteries**

---

MR angiography (MRA) and CT angiography can provide excellent demonstration of intracranial vascular pathology without the risk and cost of arterial catheterization. The noninvasive nature of MRA is particularly valuable for screening studies, as in this patient.

The source image in Case 729A demonstrates an aneurysm arising at the trifurcation or genu of the left middle cerebral artery *(arrow)*. The lumen is filled with the high signal intensity generated by unsaturated or "fresh" protons that have recently entered the plane of the image. Analysis of individual source images often clarifies details of aneurysmal morphology that may be ambiguous on three-dimensional reconstructions.

Case 729B is one of the multiple three-dimensional projections obtained by combining the data from a stack of source images. First and second order branches of major cerebral arteries are routinely defined on such reconstructions, covering the location of the great majority of spontaneous intracranial aneurysms.

The left MCA aneurysm is well displayed in Case 729B *(long arrow)*. In addition, a smaller "mirror" aneurysm is apparent at the right MCA trifurcation *(short arrow)*. Intracranial aneurysms are multiple in about 20% of cases, occurring more often in women.

The right-sided aneurysm in Case 729 was difficult to confidently distinguish from a branching vessel on individual source images. Source images and three-dimensional reconstructions are often complementary for detecting and defining vascular pathology.

Another clinical context in which screening for intracranial aneurysms by MRA has been utilized is polycystic kidney disease. Intracranial aneurysms are found in about 10% of patients with this disorder (compared with an incidence of 1% to 5% in the general population).

The annual risk of hemorrhage from an unruptured intracranial aneurysm depends on a number of factors and is a subject of controversy. Most overall estimates are in the range of 1%. Aneurysms that have bled have a high incidence of recurrent hemorrhage if untreated, approaching 50% in the six months following initial rupture.

## Case 730

41-year-old woman with a suprasellar
lesion discovered on a CT scan.
(axial, noncontrast scan; SE 2800/45)

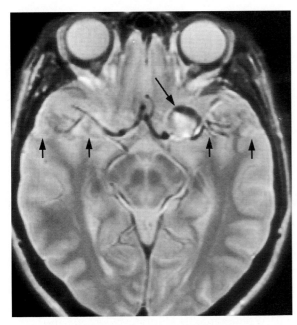

**Aneurysm of the Supraclinoid
Internal Carotid Artery**

## Case 731

53-year-old woman presenting with headaches.
(axial, noncontrast T2-weighted SE scan)

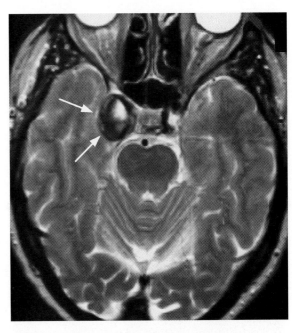

**Aneurysm of the Cavernous
Internal Carotid Artery**

---

The circulation of blood within medium- and large-sized aneurysms is often complex, with lower velocities and less turbulence than is typically present within the lumen of smaller lesions. As a result, large aneurysms may demonstrate mixed intraluminal signal intensity on noncontrast scans and prominent enhancement on postcontrast images.

It may be difficult to distinguish between slowly flowing but patent components of the aneurysm and intraluminal thrombus on standard spin echo scans. Gradient echo sequences emphasizing flow-related enhancement (as in Case 729A) are useful for demonstrating the patent portions of the lumen in such cases.

The paraclinoid mass in Case 730 (*long arrow*) had been interpreted as a parasellar meningioma on an outside CT scan, which demonstrated uniform high attenuation and intense contrast enhancement. The band of pulsation artifact passing through the lesion on the MR study (*short arrows;* see discussion below) favors the alternative diagnosis of a large aneurysm. The mixture of signal intensities within the lumen reflects typically complex and slow flow.

MR angiography and subsequent surgery demonstrated no intraluminal thrombus.

The content of the parasellar aneurysm in Case 731 is ambiguous on this routine image. Amorphous low signal intensity within the lesion could represent flow void or T2-shortening due to deoxyhemoglobin or hemosiderin within recent or old thrombus. An angiographic sequence is necessary to establish the degree of patency of such lesions.

Spatial mismapping of signal along the phase-encoding axis of the image may be caused by phase changes accumulated by protons in the blood as they flow across magnetic field gradients. Phase dispersion is increased by pulsation within an aneurysm and systolic/diastolic motion of its wall. The finding, illustrated in Case 730 (and also in Case 746), is most marked on long TR sequences without motion compensation. Pulsation artifact may be noted in association with both patent and thrombosed aneurysms. Its presence can be a useful clue to the vascular nature of an otherwise ambiguous mass.

## Case 732

59-year-old woman presenting with
a third nerve palsy.
(sagittal, noncontrast T1-weighted SE scan)

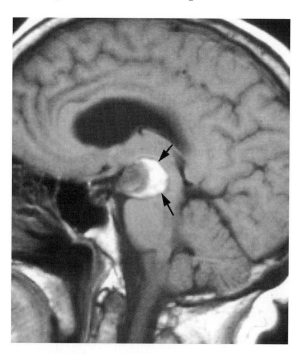

**Thrombosed Aneurysm of the Basilar Artery**

## Case 733

76-year-old man with progressive aphasia and
hemiparesis, referred for resection of a brain tumor.
(coronal, noncontrast T1-weighted SE scan)

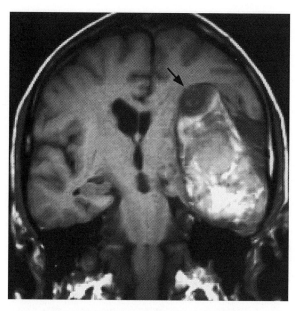

**Predominantly Thrombosed Aneurysm
of the Middle Cerebral Artery**

---

Thrombosed aneurysms present variable MR appearances, depending on the age of the intraluminal clot and the parameters of the pulse sequence. Thrombus may have an amorphous or coarsely heterogeneous appearance that is difficult to distinguish from eddies of slow flow within a patent lumen. Alternatively, well-defined components of T1- or T2-shortening may present characteristic morphologies that convincingly document thrombosis.

On T1-weighted images, thrombosed aneurysms often demonstrate a mixture of isointensity and high signal zones, as in Case 732. A craniopharyngioma might be considered in the differential diagnosis of this retrosellar lesion with T1-shortening (see Case 251), particularly since a CT scan of the mass demonstrated a peripheral shell of calcification (as is common in giant aneurysms). Characteristic morphology on long TR spin echo images (presented as Case 734) established the correct diagnosis.

The coronal scan in Case 733 indicates that the middle fossa "tumor" is an extraaxial mass, filled with subacute thrombus. The appearance suggests a giant aneurysm of the middle cerebral artery. At angiography the horizontal segment of the middle cerebral artery was draped over the top of the aneurysm. A small patent lumen was found, corresponding to the low-intensity zone at the dome of the lesion *(arrow)*.

Large aneurysms have been angiographically described as "giant" when their diameter reaches 2.5 centimeters. Giant aneurysms most commonly arise from the supraclinoid internal carotid artery or the middle cerebral artery. They often present as mass lesions, but hemorrhage is not as rare as previously believed.

The lumina of giant aneurysms are usually at least partially occupied by thrombus, which often has a lamellar or concentric appearance. The association of subarachnoid, subdural, or intracerebral hemorrhage with a large, marble-like mass near the skull base is highly characteristic of a ruptured giant aneurysm.

Case 733 demonstrates that giant aneurysms can reach remarkable size through slow expansion, gradually deforming the surrounding brain. The midline shift in this case is quite small for the size of the mass, attesting to its long-standing nature.

### Case 734

59-year-old woman presenting with diplopia.
(axial, noncontrast scan; SE 2500/28)

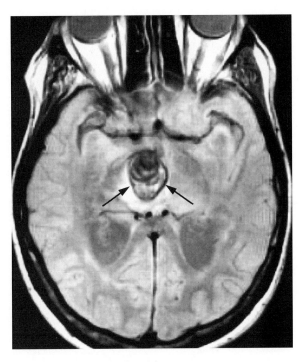

**Thrombosed Aneurysm**
(same patient as Case 732)

### Case 735

76-year-old man presenting with
aphasia and hemiparesis.
(axial, noncontrast scan; SE 3000/22)

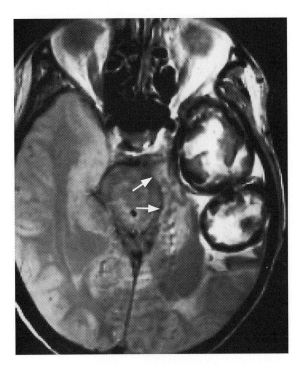

**Thrombosed Aneurysm**
(same patient as Case 733)

On long TR spin echo images, the presence of T2-shortening due to blood products helps to characterize thrombosed giant aneurysms. The pattern of such zones of low signal intensity is variable. They may be strikingly lamellar, as in Case 734, or peripherally clumped, as in Case 735. In some cases, T2-shortening due to deoxyhemoglobin and/or intracellular methemoglobin occupies most of the lumen of a thrombosed aneurysm, mimicking flow void.

The benefit of combining MR planes and sequence weightings in analysis of vascular masses is apparent when the above images are compared to the preceeding page. In Case 734, the layered morphology of blood products on the long TR image distinguishes the lesion from other suprasellar pathologies, while the T1-weighted scan (Case 732) is indeterminate. By contrast, the coronal T1-weighted scan in Case 733 is more definitive than the long TR axial image in Case 735. On the latter scan, the high signal intensity of distorted cisterns surrounding the mass could be

misinterpreted as edema, and blood products within the lesion could be attributed to intratumoral hemorrhage (compare to Case 682.)

The clinical presentation of patients with giant intracranial aneurysms often reflects the mass effect of the lesion, as in Cases 733 and 735. The bilobed mass in the left sylvian region has caused uncal herniation *(arrows)*.

Contrast enhancement of giant aneurysms may take several forms. Occasionally the lumen is entirely patent. Intense enhancement of slowly flowing blood within such lesions may mimic a meningioma. Completely thrombosed giant aneurysms typically demonstrate a thin rim of surrounding enhancement due to adventitia or a capsule. Finally, many lesions present a combination or target-like appearance. A small, often eccentric lumen (such as in Case 733) is surrounded by a large zone of nonenhancing thrombus, which is in turn bordered by a rim of peripheral enhancement.

451

### Case 736A

41-year-old woman admitted with subacute
bacterial endocarditis and confusion.
(axial, noncontrast T2-weighted SE scan)

### Case 736B

Same patient.
(axial, postcontrast T1-weighted SE scan with MTS)

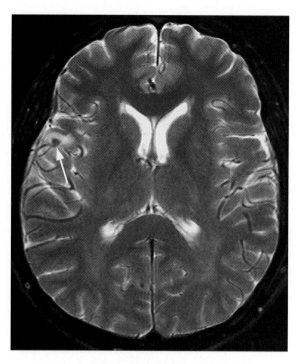

**Mycotic Aneurysm**

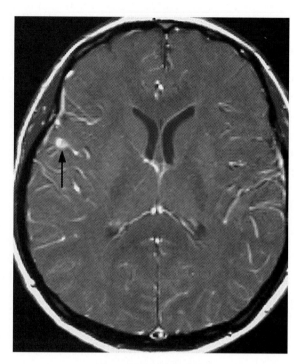

**Mycotic Aneurysm**

Aneurysms are occasionally found at sites distant from the circle of Willis. Peripheral aneurysms exhibit the same characteristics of extraaxial location and low signal intensity due to flow void as seen in more proximal lesions. When peripheral aneurysms are found, the possibility of mycotic, traumatic, neoplastic, or dysplastic origin should be considered.

Case 736A illustrates a small focus of low intensity adjacent to an opercular branch of the right middle cerebral artery *(arrow)*. This site is distal to the common location of spontaneous "berry" aneurysms involving the circle of Willis. The presence of adjacent edema outlining the lesion is also an atypical finding for an aneurysm of this size. The peripheral location and the adjacent inflammatory response combine with the history of the patient to suggest a mycotic aneurysm secondary to septic embolization. Case

736B demonstrates enhancement within the small aneurysm, which was confirmed angiographically.

Mycotic aneurysms are often multiple. They may form and rupture within days. Alternatively, they may continue to appear or enlarge for weeks during successful treatment of the underlying infectious process. For these reasons, follow-up angiography is indicated when a mycotic aneurysm is discovered.

Bleeding from a mycotic aneurysm is one of the causes of "spontaneous" subdural hematomas. (Others include coagulopathy and dural arteriovenous fistulae.) Rupture of a mycotic aneurysm is also among the etiologies of superficial intracerebral hemorrhage. The morphology in such cases often resembles the appearance of Case 750.

Multiple small peripheral aneurysms can additionally be seen in cases of vasculitis and in patients with cerebral emboli from an atrial myxoma.

# PSEUDOANEURYSMS

## Case 737A

28-year-old woman presenting with recurrent dizziness after chiropractic manipulation.
(AP view, maximal intensity projection reconstruction, noncontrast, three-dimensional, time-of-flight GRE sequence)

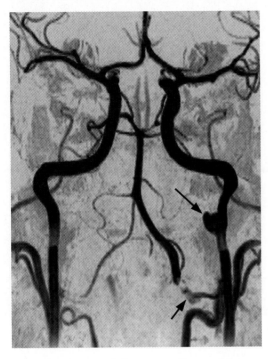

**Pseudoaneurysm of the Internal Carotid Artery**

## Case 737B

Same patient.
(targeted AP view, maximal intensity projection reconstruction, noncontrast, three-dimensional, time-of-flight GRE sequence)

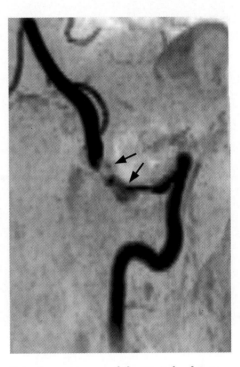

**Pseudoaneurysm of the Vertebral Artery**

---

Pseudoaneurysms are focal extensions of an arterial lumen through a defect in the inner layer of the wall (intima and media), contained by adventitia and/or surrounding fibrosis. They may develop after trauma or in the context of arterial dissection, posttraumatic or spontaneous. The cervical segments of the internal carotid and vertebral arteries are susceptible to dissection and the formation of pseudoaneurysms. Intracranial pseudoaneurysms are rare.

Case 737A illustrates a lobulated pseudoaneurysm arising from the distal cervical segment of the left internal carotid artery *(long arrow)*. This location is a common site for spontaneous or posttraumatic dissection (see Cases 632-635), which is the likely cause of the pseudoaneurysm in this case. The reduced intensity of flow signal within the artery immediately proximal to the pseudoaneurysm is an artifact at the junction of two imaging volumes.

Dissection of the distal left vertebral artery is also present in this case, visible in Case 737A *(short arrow)* but bet-

ter displayed by the targeted reconstruction in Case 737B. The dissection at this site narrows the lumen of the vessel. The associated pseudoaneurysm is smaller and more poorly defined than the accompanying carotid lesion.

Thrombi may form within or adjacent to a pseudoaneurysm of the internal carotid or vertebral artery, with subsequent intracranial embolization. This possibility should be considered among the etiologies of TIAs or CVAs in young patients.

Simultaneous or sequential dissection of more than one cervical artery is common, as discussed in Cases 632-635. Among the conditions predisposing to dissection of the carotid or vertebral arteries are fibromuscular dysplasia, Marfan syndrome, and Ehlers-Danlos syndrome. Cervical arteries with a prominent loop also seem prone to acquired dissection.

**Case 738**

34-year-old woman presenting with a seizure.
(axial, noncontrast T2-weighted SE scan)

**Case 739**

12-year-old boy presenting with a heart murmur.
(axial, noncontrast T2-weighted FSE scan)

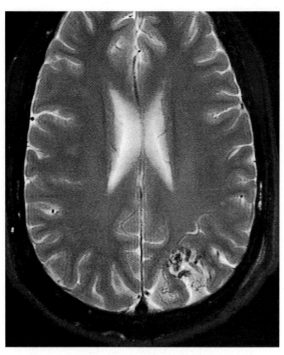

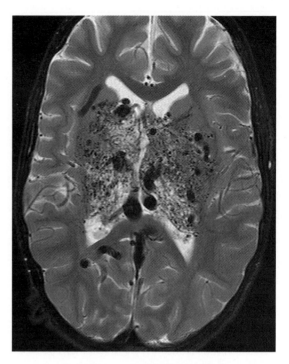

**Arteriovenous Malformation**

**Arteriovenous Malformation**

Uncomplicated arteriovenous malformations (AVMs) present on spin echo MR scans as tightly packed clusters of serpentine channels demonstrating flow void. The contour of the lesions varies from spherical to wedge-shaped, often based against the cerebral surface or the ventricular margin.

As illustrated by the above scans, AVMs may be superficial or deep, focal or extensive. The small cortical malformation in Case 738 is localized to a few gyri of the posterior parietal lobe. By contrast, the large malformation in Case 739 involves the basal ganglia, thalami, and lateral ventricles bilaterally. (Compare Case 739 to the appearance of moyamoya disease in Case 638.)

High intensity components interspersed with flow void in AVMs may represent zones of slow flow, hemorrhage, and/or intervening parenchyma or scar tissue. Mass effect is unusual in the absence of associated hemorrhage. How-

ever, some AVMs do contain sufficiently bulky vascular components to cause compression of the adjacent structures. Encephalomalacia may be present due to old hemorrhage or to parenchymal damage arising from the pulsations or "steal" of the malformation.

The high flow within the nidus, feeding arteries, and draining veins of arteriovenous malformations can be demonstrated on angiographic gradient echo scans (see Case 742). Phase contrast angiography with variable velocity encoding may be useful to separately image slow flow components of an AVM.

Patients with AVMs commonly experience seizures, as in Case 738. Other frequent symptoms include headache and focal hemispheric deficits. Hemorrhage is the initial manifestation of a cerebral AVM in about 50% of cases (see Case 752).

## Case 740

28-year-old man presenting with
left superior quadrantanopsia.
(axial, noncontrast scan; SE 2500/45)

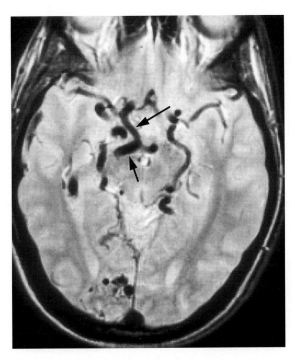

**Arteriovenous Malformation**

## Case 741

28-year-old woman presenting with numbness
and tingling on the right side of the body.
(coronal, noncontrast T2-weighted SE scan)

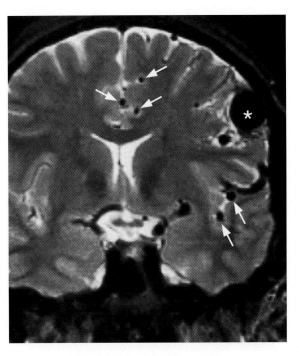

**Arteriovenous Malformation**

Ectatic feeding arteries or draining veins may be prominent components of high flow AVMs. Case 740 illustrates hypertrophy of multiple arteries that supplied an extensive right hemispheric AVM, predominantly involving the occipital lobe. For example, note the gross enlargement of the right posterior communicating artery *(long arrow)* and the proximal posterior cerebral artery *(short arrow)*.

Multiple hypertrophied branches of the anterior and middle cerebral arteries in Case 741 *(arrows)* supplied an AVM within the left cerebral hemisphere. The large superficial vascular channel *(asterisk)* in Case 741 proved to be a varix. Veins draining an AVM may be diffusely dilated or demonstrate localized ectasias called *venous aneurysms*.

One or more arterial aneurysms are frequently found along the course of vessels feeding an AVM. Their occurrence is likely flow related; they may thrombose spontaneously after the AVM is embolized or resected. Such prox-

imal aneurysms do not carry a significantly increased risk of hemorrhage, while intranidal aneurysms within the substance of an AVM are prone to rupture and should be treated.

Areas of low signal intensity within arteriovenous malformations on MR scans may alternatively be due to calcification, which is common within the walls of vascular channels or within dystrophic cerebral parenchyma. Zones of acute hemorrhage (containing deoxyhemoglobin) and/or hemosiderin accumulation from old hemorrhages may also contribute to low signal intensity on long TR spin echo images.

Structural features of AVMs associated with an increased risk of hemorrhage include periventricular location, central venous drainage, and the presence of an intranidal aneurysm.

### Case 742

23-year-old man presenting with headaches.
(axial source image from a noncontrast, three-dimensional, time-of-flight GRE sequence)

### Case 743

78-year-old woman presenting with headaches.
(axial, postcontrast T1-weighted SE scan with MTS)

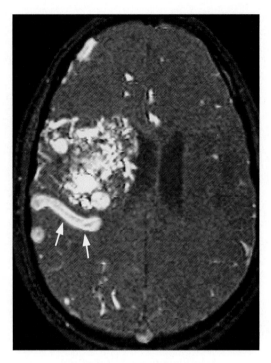

**Arteriovenous Malformation**

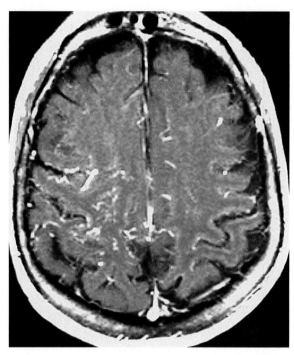

**Dilated Collateral Veins**
(due to thrombosis of the superior sagittal sinus)

Intracranial vessels may enlarge because they participate in an arteriovenous shunt or because they serve as collateral channels due to compromise of other arteries or veins.

Angiographic gradient echo scans such as Case 742 maximize the signal intensity of fresh spins entering the imaging volume while suppressing the surrounding signal through RF saturation of stationary tissue. As a result, flow appears bright against a dark background.

Case 742 demonstrates high flow within multiple vessels of variable size clustered in the right frontal lobe. The large channel at the posterior margin of the AVM *(arrows)* was angiographically proven to represent a varix draining the malformation.

The tortuously enlarged vessels in Case 743 are hypertrophied veins, which had developed secondary to long-standing occlusion of the superior sagittal sinus. The appearance superficially resembles an AVM, but the uniform size and relative separation of the involved channels are clues to an alternative diagnosis.

The pattern of enlarged intramedullary veins illustrated in Case 743 can also be seen in cases of dural arteriovenous fistulae. Increased flow and/or stenosis within major dural venous channels in such cases leads to congestion and hypertrophy of small parenchymal tributaries. This finding should prompt consideration of an AV fistula, which may be otherwise inapparent on standard MR images (see Cases 744 and 745).

Moyamoya disease (see Case 638) is an example of arterial hypertrophy providing collateral flow.

Prominent vessels also may be associated with intracranial tumors (see Cases 92 and 93), but the pattern is rarely as tightly interwoven as in AVMs or as uniformly dispersed as in situations of collateral hypertrophy.

### Case 744

41-year-old man presenting with
headaches and dizziness.
(axial, noncontrast scan; FSE 5033/14)

### Case 745

62-year-old man presenting with left-sided
tinnitus and mild ataxia.
(coronal, postcontrast T1-weighted SE scan)

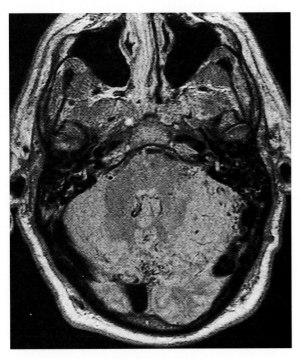

**Dural AV Fistula**

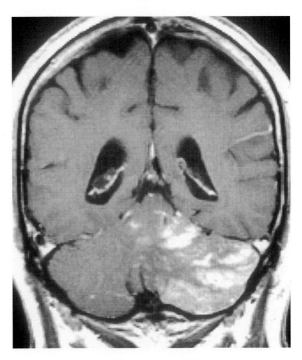

**Dural AV Fistula**

About 15% of intracranial vascular malformations are found within the dura. The most common locations for such lesions are the walls of major dural sinuses, especially the transverse sinus (as in the above examples) and the cavernous sinus. Many dural vascular malformations are true arteriovenous fistulae, with direct shunting of blood from dural arteries into a venous compartment.

If the outflow of a dural AVM is not compromised, symptoms are often nonspecific and standard MR scans may demonstrate no associated parenchymal changes. A negative MR scan does not exclude the diagnosis of a dural vascular malformation.

However, many dural AVMs are accompanied by partial or complete occlusion of the receiving venous sinus. There is evidence that primary sinus thrombosis leads to subsequent development of a dural AVM in some cases. In other patients, a flow-induced vasculopathy causes progressive constriction of the initially patent sinus draining a dural fistula.

Restriction of venous outflow may cause severe symptoms and characteristic parenchymal changes on MR images. These findings are due to cortical venous drainage that develops as a collateral system when the dural sinuses

are stenosed or occluded and to associated venous hypertension. Patients whose dural AVMs drain into cortical veins are at risk for venous infarction and/or intracranial hemorrhage.

Case 744 demonstrates typical findings of a dural AVM with restricted outflow. Multiple dilated, tortuous veins are seen as short, corkscrew-like flow voids within and near the surface of the left cerebellar hemisphere. Unlike the parenchymal AVMs in Cases 738-742, no hypertrophied feeding artery or parenchymal nidus is associated with the scattered venous ectasia. Dilated cortical veins in the absence of a pial AVM should suggest the diagnosis of a dural fistula.

Swelling of the left cerebellar hemisphere is apparent on the postcontrast scan in Case 745. Venous congestion and impaired parenchymal drainage are demonstrated by the diffuse tissue stain of abnormal enhancement.

Dural AVMs of the anterior cranial fossa are particularly prone to hemorrhage, which may be subdural, subarachnoid, or intracerebral (typically in the medial inferior frontal lobe). These fistulae are usually fed by ethmoidal branches of the ophthalmic artery and frequently drain into cortical veins along the base of the frontal lobes.

457

## Case 746

14-month-old girl with a history of borderline
heart failure since infancy.
(axial, noncontrast scan; SE 2800/45)

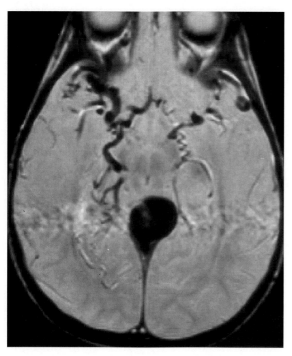

**Vein of Galen Malformation**

## Case 747

2-month-old girl presenting with a rapidly
enlarging head and a cranial bruit.
(axial, noncontrast T2-weighted SE scan)

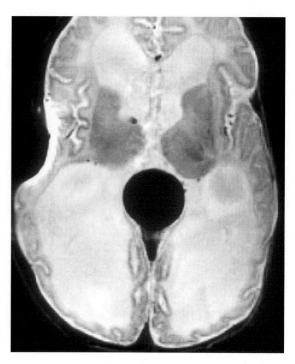

**Vein of Galen Malformation**

The vein of Galen develops from a fetal vessel called the *median vein of the prosencephalon.* Occasionally an arteriovenous fistula (or several) forms in the wall of this vein and leads to marked expansion, traditionally misnamed as a "vein of Galen aneurysm." The fistula may be a direct shunt from the pericallosal or posterior cerebral arteries ("mural" type) or be fed by smaller thalamoperforating or pial arteries ("choroidal" type). Vein of Galen malformations account for about one-third of intracranial vascular malformations in children and about 1% of all intracranial AVMs.

Rapid and turbulent flow through the arterialized veins of a vascular malformation exceeds the rephasing capability of most non-angiographic MR sequences. The signal void within such structures usually persists after the injection of contrast material. In the above cases, the dilated vein of Galen is strikingly defined as a midline zone of absent signal. Other possible sources of signal loss (e.g., dense calcification or marked T2-shortening) are rarely as uniform,

severe, and sharply marginated as seen here (but compare Case 747 to Case 771).

In Case 746, a transverse band of pulsation artifact passes through the varix, comparable to the appearance of an arterial aneurysm such as in Case 730. Multiple hypertrophied feeding arteries are apparent near the circle of Willis.

High flow through a vein of Galen malformation may cause congestive heart failure in the neonatal period. Infants and older children with less severe arteriovenous shunts often present with hydrocephalus, as in Case 747. Venous hypertension may impair resorption of CSF, leading to communicating hydrocephalus. Alternatively, the mass effect of the varix may cause obstructive hydrocephalus by compressing the posterior third ventricle and aqueduct.

Secondary development of distal stenoses along the path of drainage through dural veins and sinuses is a common feature of high flow vascular malformations. This process may play an important role in the morphological and symptomatic progression or regression of vein of Galen "aneurysms."

## Case 748

31-year-old man presenting with seizures
and right hand weakness.
(sagittal, noncontrast T1-weighted SE scan)

## Case 749

20-year-old man presenting with seizures.
(sagittal, noncontrast T1-weighted SE scan)

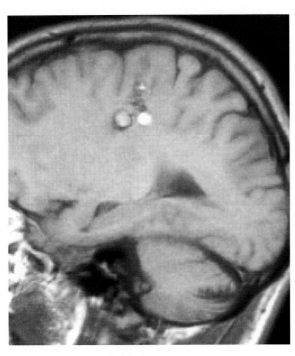

Thrombosed AVM

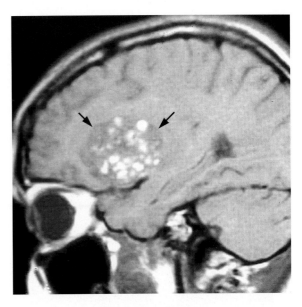

Thrombosed AVM

Thrombosed vascular malformations are often said to be "occult," meaning that they are not demonstrable by angiographic techniques. Such lesions are usually apparent on CT scans as small, high attenuation regions. Their CT density may be due to calcification, blood volume, and/or contrast enhancement.

Thrombosis of an AVM eliminates the characteristic flow patterns illustrated in Cases 738-742. However, the nidus of the malformation remains well defined on MR scans as a zone of mixed signal abnormality reflecting blood products and calcification within the lesion.

Case 748 illustrates the typical MR appearance of a thrombosed vascular malformation. A multinodular lesion contains prominent components of T1-shortening, suggesting the presence of methemoglobin. A T2-weighted scan demonstrated low signal intensity within and surrounding the lesion due to local accumulation of hemosiderin from old microhemorrhages.

Occasional thrombosed AVMs are sufficiently large and mass-like to mimic a cerebral neoplasm. The overall contour of the lesion in Case 749 is approximately spherical.

Multiple internal nodules of T1-shortening on the precontrast scan resemble the appearance of Case 748. However, their distribution throughout a larger mass raises the question of hemorrhagic loculations, proteinaceous cysts, or even lipid material within a complex tumor such as an oligodendroglioma or teratoma (see Cases 114 and 309-311).

On postcontrast scans in Case 749, tissue between the nodules enhanced intensely. The relative lack of mass effect for the size of the lesion is a clue to the correct diagnosis, but long-standing low grade tumors may also demonstrate this feature. The mass was resected and proved to be an entirely thrombosed AVM.

The lesion in Case 748 was known to represent an AVM from angiographic studies demonstrating patency on an earlier admission. However, the MR appearance is indistinguishable from that of a cavernous hemangioma (see Cases 761-768). For this reason, thrombosed AVMs and cavernous angiomas are sometimes discussed together as occult cerebrovascular malformations (OCVMs).

# DIFFERENTIAL DIAGNOSIS:
## COMPLEX INTRACEREBRAL HEMORRHAGE

### Case 750

53-year-old man presenting with
a cerebrovascular accident.
(axial, noncontrast T2-weighted FSE scan)

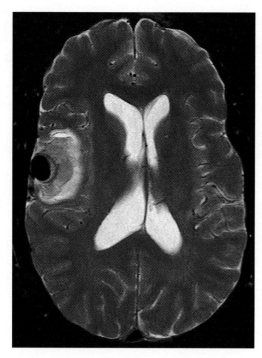

**Hemorrhage from an AVM**

### Case 751

58-year-old woman presenting with a seizure.
(sagittal, noncontrast T1-weighted SE scan)

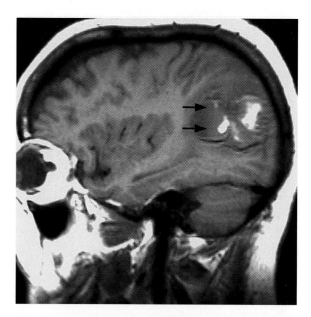

**Spontaneous Intracerebral Hemorrhage**
(with coagulopathy)

Complex morphology of an intracerebral hematoma raises the suspicion of an underlying structural lesion. AVMs are among the pathologies to be considered in such patients, as illustrated in Case 750 (and in Case 752).

The superficial hematoma in Case 750 forms a band of intermediate intensity separating a nodule of very low signal from a rim of edema. This concentric or layered morphology suggests hemorrhage originating from a vascular structure at the cerebral surface. A mycotic aneurysm would be among the potential etiologies for this composite lesion (see Case 736). The flow-containing nodule in Case 750 instead proved to be a localized varix ("venous aneurysm") draining a small AVM.

Thorough evaluation and follow-up studies in Case 751 demonstrated no evidence of other pathology at the site of the complex hematoma. (It is possible that a tiny vascular malformation was destroyed at the time of bleeding.) Benign or spontaneous intracerebral hemorrhages occasionally present with the multinodular morphology and heterogeneous intensity illustrated in this case, resembling the appearance of secondary bleeding into a preexisting mass.

(See Cases 673-676 for examples of the concentric zones of evolving signal intensity more typical of spontaneous hematomas.)

The small areas of short T1 values within the mass in Case 751 suggest methemoglobin and indicate the presence of blood products. The possibility that the *entire* mass represents a benign hematoma is raised by two additional features. Arcs of frequency misregistration artifact are present at the superior and inferior margins of the lesion (see discussion of Case 677). In addition, a sedimentation level ("hematocrit phenomenon") is faintly visible within the anterior lobulation of the mass *(arrows)*.

A sedimentation level can reflect hemorrhage into a preexisting cavity (see Case 95). However, a spontaneous hemorrhage may also present in this manner if impaired clotting mechanisms prevent coagulation. The presence of a sedimentation level within an intracerebral hematoma is therefore a clue to coagulopathy as the cause of bleeding. The patient in Case 751 was receiving coumadin and was found to have a significantly prolonged clotting time.

460

# DIFFERENTIAL DIAGNOSIS:
## MULTINODULAR HEMORRHAGIC MASS

### Case 752

7-year-old boy presenting with a seizure
and headaches after a fall.
(axial, noncontrast T2-weighted SE scan)

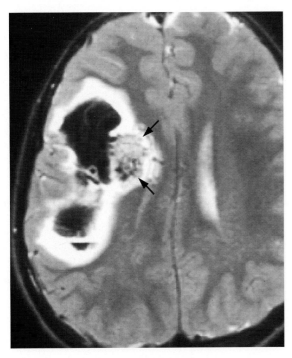

**AVM with Hemorrhage**

### Case 753

66-year-old man presenting with personality
change and right hemiparesis.
(axial, noncontrast T2-weighted SE scan)

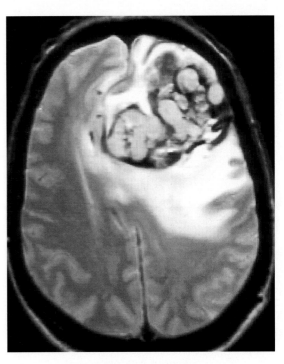

**Metastatic Carcinoma of the Lung**

---

Hemorrhage is the most common presentation of AVMs, occurring in one-third to two-thirds of patients in most series. The majority of these hemorrhages are intracerebral rather than subarachnoid.

The lateral component of the mass in Case 752 represents an acute intracerebral hematoma (compare to Case 674). Very low central signal intensity due to intracellular deoxyhemoglobin is surrounded by a thick collar of high intensity due to reactive edema.

An area of tissue with distinctly different architecture is apparent at the medial margin of the hemorrhage (*arrows, Case 752*). This feature strongly suggests a preexisting structural lesion as the source of bleeding. Although a neoplasm could be considered, the reticular or racemose morphology of the tissue nodule and the age of the patient favor the diagnosis of a vascular malformation.

In an older patient, the multinodular morphology of a vascular malformation with adjacent hemorrhage can resemble a tumor like Case 753. Several MR features help to distinguish these pathologies. Edema surrounding cerebral

tumors is often more extensive and irregular than the uniform rind encircling benign hematomas. (Compare the morphology of edema in the above cases.) More importantly, blood products are found within the substance of a hemorrhagic neoplasm, contrasting with the usual eccentricity of hematomas seen adjacent to the nidus of a vascular malformation.

The annual risk of bleeding from an unruptured AVM is estimated to be about 2% to 4% per year. For this reason, treatment by embolization, surgery, and/or radiation is recommended for most patients. The choice of modality is influenced by the size and location (i.e., resectability) of the malformation, as well as the age and symptoms of the patient.

Once an AVM has bled, the annual risk of new hemorrhage initially rises to 5% to 15% per year. Many surgeons choose to attempt resection of a malformation that has "declared itself" by an episode of hemorrhage. The space created by evacuation of an adjacent hematoma may aid excision.

**461**

## Case 754

28-year-old woman complaining of headaches.
(sagittal, noncontrast T1-weighted SE scan)

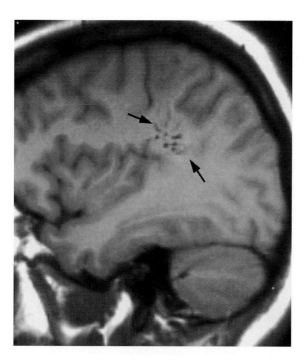

**Venous Angioma**

## Case 755

42-year-old woman presenting with dizziness.
(axial, noncontrast T2-weighted SE scan)

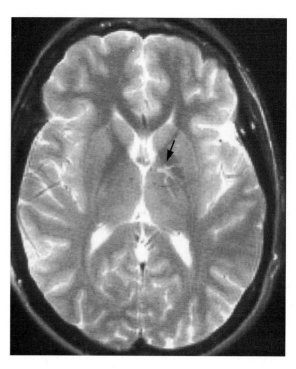

**Venous Angioma**

Venous angiomas (also called *venous malformations* or *developmental venous anomalies*) have a characteristic morphology that is often recognizable on CT and MR scans. The lesion has two components: (1) a group of radially oriented tributary veins converging like spokes of an umbrella to a central point and (2) a single, abnormally large draining vein formed at the confluence of the tributaries and following an aberrant route through cerebral parenchyma.

The above cases illustrate the appearance of the converging tributary channels, seen in cross section (Case 754) or parallel to the scan plane (Case 755).

Blood flow within venous angiomas is slow. As a result, these vascular anomalies usually demonstrate fluid-like signal intensity rather than flow void. For the same reason,

venous angiomas characteristically enhance with contrast material (see Cases 757 and 759). In fact, they may be visible only on postcontrast studies.

Venous angiomas are most often incidental anomalies rather than threatening "malformations." They are infrequently associated with seizures. Clinically significant bleeding is uncommon in the absence of outflow obstruction; a possibly increased incidence in cerebellar lesions is controversial.

Small hemorrhages localized to the vicinity of a venous angioma are probably more frequent. The common occurrence of cavernous angiomas adjacent to venous malformations has suggested that organization of small hemorrhages from a venous angioma may play a role in formation of some cavernous lesions.

### Case 756

6-year-old girl presenting with seizures.
(sagittal, noncontrast T1-weighted SE scan)

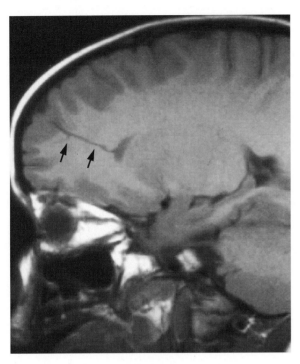

**Venous Angioma**

### Case 757

42-year-old woman presenting with headaches.
(coronal, postcontrast T1-weighted
SE scan with MTS)

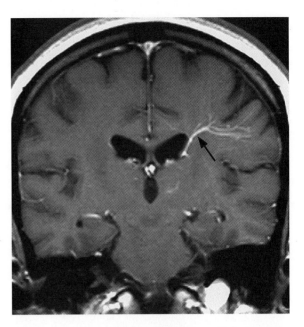

**Venous Angioma**

The typically aberrant, transparenchymal course of the major stem vein within a venous angioma is demonstrated in the above cases *(arrows)*. This channel emerges from the confluence of radially oriented tributary vessels and traverses broad regions of parenchyma to reach the cerebral surface or the ventricular margin. The central vein of the angioma usually terminates by merging with the normal venous system in one of these locations. Even when tributary veins are inconspicuous, the dilated and anomalously located stem of a venous angioma is highly characteristic.

In Cases 756 and 757, long segments of stem veins are visualized because they are parallel to the scan plane. The central channels of other venous angiomas may intersect the plane of the scan perpendicularly or at oblique angles, resulting in circular or elliptical cross-sections (see Case 760B).

As mentioned earlier, slow flow within venous angiomas results in obvious contrast enhancement, demonstrated in Case 757. Lack of enhancement within a vascular channel should raise doubt about the diagnosis of venous angioma.

Stenosis of the stem vein of a venous angioma may predispose to hemorrhage within its watershed. Such constriction typically occurs at the site where a stem vein penetrates the dura. A vague haze of contrast enhancement throughout the parenchyma drained by the angioma can be a clue to stasis caused by partial outflow obstruction. (A similar appearance may be produced by venous sinus occlusion in association with a dural arteriovenous fistula, often accompanied by a number of distended and tortuous parenchymal veins; see Case 745.)

Enhancement along the course of a prior shunt tube or ventriculostomy catheter can simulate the transcerebral stem vein of a venous angioma in patients with a recent history of hydrocephalus.

### Case 758

28-year-old man presenting with vague paresthesias.
(axial, noncontrast T2-weighted SE scan)

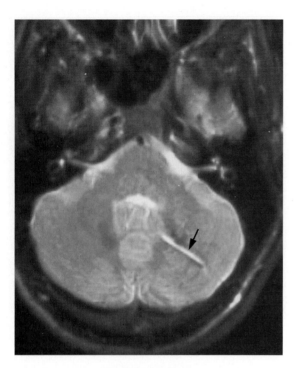

**Venous Angioma**

### Case 759

36-year-old man presenting with headaches.
(coronal, postcontrast T1-weighted
SE scan with MTS)

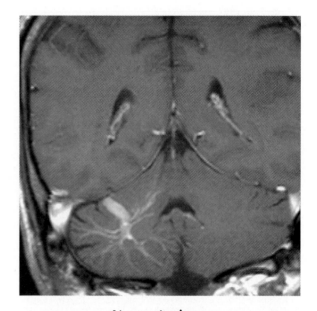

**Venous Angioma**

Venous angiomas may occur within the brainstem and are commonly encountered in the cerebellum. The majority of these anomalies are found incidentally, although the frequency of hemorrhage has been reported to exceed that of supratentorial angiomas.

Cases 758 and 759 demonstrate that the morphology of cerebellar venous angiomas is comparable to their cerebral counterparts. Large stem veins characteristically traverse the cerebellar hemispheres to reach the fourth ventricle or the pial surface. The direction of flow in such transcerebellar channels may be either centripetal or centrifugal.

In Case 758, a long segment of the central vein runs within the plane of the scan. High intensity within the large vein is due to successful rephasing of the signal from slowly flowing protons. This recovery of signal (i.e., avoidance of flow void) is mainly due to refocusing features of current spin echo pulse sequences, designed to reduce mismapping of CSF signal from pulsating cisterns. Rephasing can also be seen on even echoes of nonrefocused spin echo sequences.

The coronal scan in Case 759 demonstrates both the central channel and multiple tributaries of a large venous angioma. This anomalous system drains the entire right cerebellar hemisphere. Surgical interruption of the angioma would lead to extensive venous infarction, while stenosis of this stem vein at the tentorium could cause diffuse parenchymal edema and patchy enhancement (comparable to Case 745).

## Case 760A

16-year-old girl presenting with seizures.
(axial, postcontrast T1-weighted SE scan)

## Case 760B

Same patient.
(axial, postcontrast T1-weighted SE scan)

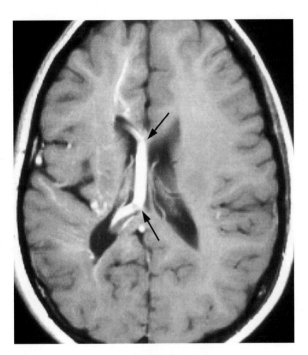

**Venous Malformation**

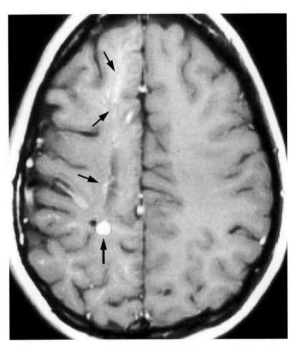

**Venous Malformation**

Occasional venous malformations are large and complex. The presence of two or three "heads" (i.e., systems of radial tributaries converging to a central stem) is relatively common. Anomalous venous drainage of an entire hemisphere, as in Case 760, is much rarer.

The above scans demonstrate abnormally large, contrast-filled veins throughout much of the white matter of the right cerebral hemisphere. These aberrant medullary channels receive flow from radially oriented tributaries (*thin arrows,* Case 760B) and drain centrally to a greatly enlarged ventricular vein (*arrows,* Case 760A). This vein subsequently courses superiorly through the parietal lobe (*thick arrow,* Case 760B) to reach the convexity.

Such cases emphasize that venous angiomas are best considered to represent anomalies of cerebral venous development. However aberrant their morphology, they provide functional venous drainage from major zones of cerebral parenchyma. Resection of these "lesions" may lead to venous infarction. In symptomatic cases with a history of hemorrhage, the size and location of a venous angioma must be considered to judge the advisability of resection.

## Case 761

43-year-old man with headaches and multiple high attenuation lesions discovered on a CT scan.
(sagittal, noncontrast T1-weighted SE scan)

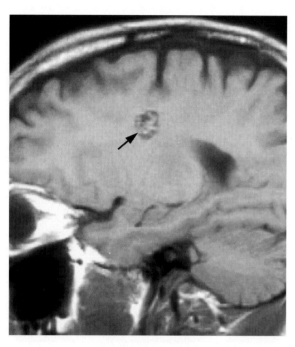

**Cavernous Angioma**

## Case 762

10-year-old boy presenting with a seizure and hemiparesis.
(sagittal, noncontrast T1-weighted SE scan)

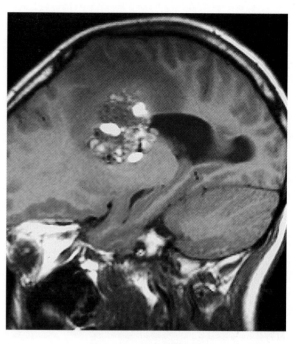

**Cavernous Angioma**

---

Cavernous hemangiomas or "angiomas" are collections of sinusoidal vascular spaces without intervening neuroglial tissue. Although well-recognized pathologically as one of the major categories of cerebrovascular malformations, these lesions have been difficult to diagnosis prior to CT scanning. Their frequent demonstration on CT and MR studies requires recognition and distinction from other masses. Cavernous angiomas are angiographically occult and account for the majority of so-called *cryptic* vascular malformations.

The MR appearance of cavernous angiomas is highly characteristic. An aggregate, multinodular, or "popcorn" morphology with prominent central zones of T1-shortening is surrounded by a rind of T2-shortening. Septations and focal areas of additional T2-shortening are often seen within the lesion.

Cavernous angiomas may range in size from a few millimeters to several centimeters in diameter. Any region of the brain may be affected. A diagnostically helpful feature of cavernous angiomas is frequent multiplicity, with occasional familial incidence. Ambiguous lesions are commonly accompanied by other more typical angiomas.

Case 761 illustrates the characteristic architecture of a small cavernous angioma. (Note that a hemorrhagic metastasis like Case 9 can present a similar appearance.)

The angioma in Case 762 is much larger but maintains the typical morphology of multinodularity and heterogeneous signal intensity. Acute hemorrhage at the lateral margin of the angioma accounted for the clinical presentation and the surrounding edema.

Thrombosed or low flow AVMs may have an appearance similar to cavernous angiomas (compare Case 761 to Case 748 and Case 762 to Case 749). Mixed vascular malformations containing several histological patterns are common, particularly the combination of venous angioma and cavernous angioma (see discussion of Cases 769 and 770).

Thrombosed aneurysms may present with a heterogeneous combination of signal intensities resembling that of cavernous angiomas. However, the morphology of such lesions is often laminar or concentric (see Case 734), in contrast to the "mulberry" or "honeycomb" architecture of most cavernous malformations.

# CAVERNOUS ANGIOMAS: T2-WEIGHTED IMAGES

## Case 763

38-year-old woman presenting with
a long history of seizures.
(coronal, noncontrast T2-weighted SE scan)

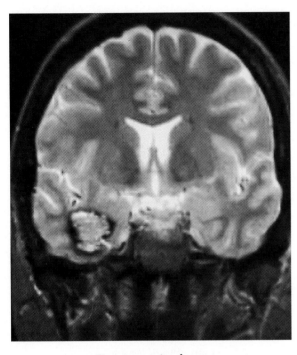

**Cavernous Angioma**

## Case 764

5-year-old boy with mild truncal ataxia.
(axial, noncontrast T2-weighted SE scan)

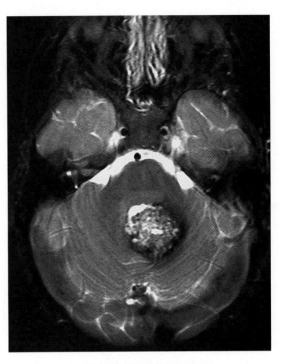

**Cavernous Angioma**

---

The perimeter of cavernous angiomas is usually outlined by a prominent zone of low signal intensity on T2-weighted images, as seen above. This rind of T2-shortening is attributable to an accumulation of hemosiderin from old hemorrhages.

Cavernous angiomas are commonly found in the temporal lobes, where they represent an important cause of seizures (as in Case 763). The absence of reactive edema and mass effect argues against neoplasm in such cases.

Case 764 illustrates that cavernous angiomas also occur below the tentorium. The cerebellar mass deforms the fourth ventricle and extends into the brachium pontis. The nodular texture of the lesion and the peripheral zone of short T2 values establish the diagnosis of a benign vascular malformation in this young patient. (See Cases 767 and 768 for a discussion of cavernous angiomas within the brainstem.)

Calcification may contribute to low signal intensity within and surrounding cavernous angiomas. (Calcification may cause localized signal loss by physical replacement of protons and/or by susceptibility effects that accelerate

proton relaxation.) The walls of cavernous channels within the malformations are often thickened, with secondary calcification or even ossification.

Serial scans have documented progressive enlargement of some cavernous angiomas, presumably due to recurrent small hemorrhages with subsequent organization and recanalization of thrombus. Such events are usually subclinical. Angiomas are occasionally implicated as the source of major parenchymal hematomas (as was true in Case 762; see also Cases 771 and 772).

Lesions resembling the MR appearance of cavernous angiomas may develop within the brain after radiation therapy. Such foci likely represent small, organizing hemorrhages secondary to radiation-induced vascular injury.

A focal, low grade glioma containing calcification may resemble a cavernous angioma. However, such tumors are usually surrounded by a perimeter of at least mildly prolonged T2 values, which differs from the rim of T2-shortening characteristically seen in cavernous malformations.

Case 770 presents a postcontrast scan of the lesion in Case 764.

# DIFFERENTIAL DIAGNOSIS:
## SMALL CEREBRAL LESIONS WITH RIMS OF LOW SIGNAL INTENSITY

### Case 765

56-year-old woman with a distant history of CVA.
(axial, noncontrast scan; SE 2500/45)

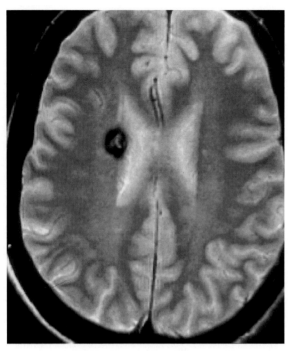

**Old Intracerebral Hematoma**

### Case 766

64-year-old woman with a known hypernephroma.
(axial, noncontrast scan; SE 2800/45)

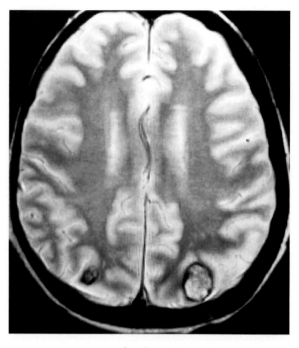

**Hemorrhagic Metastases**

---

The hemosiderin rim that is characteristic of cavernous angiomas is not specific for this diagnosis. As discussed previously, the organization of spontaneous parenchymal hematomas leads to a layer of hemosiderin-containing macrophages at the perimeter of the lesion. The stain persists indefinitely and may be demonstrated on subsequent MR studies or at autopsy.

Case 765 is an example of this occurrence. Since the region of the basal ganglia and corona radiata is a common location for both cavernous angiomas (see Case 761) and spontaneous intracerebral hemorrhage (see Case 675), a hemosiderin-lined lesion in this area may represent either pathology.

Case 766 illustrates that hemorrhage and/or calcification within primary or metastatic neoplasms may mimic the MR presentation of cavernous angiomas. Like angiomas, vascular metastases may contain blood products and demonstrate a rim of low signal intensity on T2-weighted scans.

As discussed in Chapter 1, metastases may incite little or no surrounding edema. Multiplicity is a common feature of both metastatic disease and cavernous angiomas. For these reasons, careful attention to clinical context and follow-up examinations are appropriate before the diagnosis of "multiple cavernous angiomas" is accepted. The lesions in Case 766 enlarged rapidly on subsequent scans.

## Case 767

45-year-old woman with a ten-year
history of "brainstem glioma."
(sagittal, noncontrast T1-weighted SE scan)

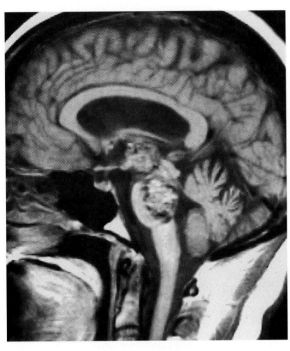

**Cavernous Angioma**

## Case 768

40-year-old man being evaluated for
suspected demyelinating disease.
(axial, noncontrast T2-weighted SE scan)

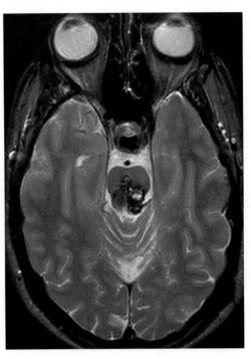

**Cavernous Angioma**

---

Cavernous angiomas commonly occur in the brainstem, where they may mimic primary or metastatic tumors. The gradual enlargement of an angioma can cause progressive symptoms suggesting an infiltrating neoplasm, as had been true in Case 767.

MR scans have now demonstrated that many patients previously assumed to have stable brainstem "tumors" have in fact harbored cavernous malformations. The characteristics of the lesion in Case 767 are highly suggestive of this diagnosis. Furthermore, the patient demonstrated accompanying cerebral lesions (one is apparent in the hypothalamic region on this scan) and had a sister whose subsequent MR evaluation for seizures disclosed multiple cavernous angiomas.

The repeated occurrence and organization of small hemorrhages within or adjacent to an angioma of the brainstem may alternatively lead to a relapsing/remitting course that resembles demyelinating disease, as in Case 768. The scan shows no evidence of edema to suggest recent hemorrhage outside the margin of the angioma. However, small changes in volume of such lesions due to internal hemorrhage can produce significant symptomatology because of the strategic position of the mass amid the nuclei and tracts of the brainstem.

Other varieties of vascular malformations may also involve the brainstem. Venous angiomas are occasionally found in this location. The pathologically common capillary telangiectasia (see Cases 773 and 774) is rarely evident on noncontrast MR scans but may cause pontine hemorrhage. True AVMs of the brainstem occur, often bordering the fourth ventricle. Bulky components of an AVM may fill the ventricle and simulate an intraventricular tumor (similar to Case 764).

**Case 769**

36-year-old man presenting with
headaches and a seizure.
(axial, postcontrast T1-weighted SE scan with MTS)

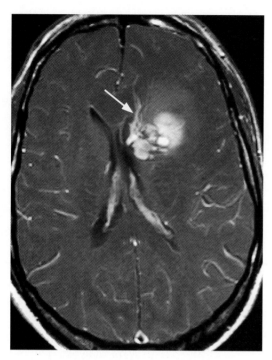

**Venous and Cavernous Angiomas**

**Case 770**

5-year-old boy presenting with mild truncal ataxia.
(sagittal, postcontrast T1-weighted
SE scan with MTS)

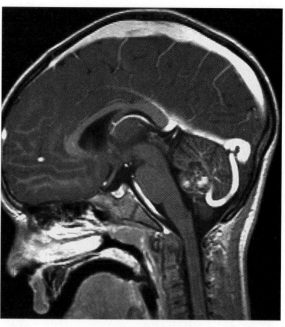

**Venous and Cavernous Angiomas**
(same patient as Case 764)

Vascular malformations of mixed classification are sometimes discovered at surgery or autopsy and on MR studies. A frequent combination is the association of a venous malformation with an adjacent mass demonstrating features of a cavernous angioma. With current imaging techniques, 5% to 10% of venous angiomas are found to be associated with cavernous malformations, while 20% to 30% of cavernous angiomas are located adjacent to a developmental venous anomaly.

In Case 769, tributary veins and a short stem channel of a venous angioma *(arrow)* are apparent at the anteromedial margin of the multinodular cavernous mass. Case 770 illustrates a large venous malformation that forms at the posterior-inferior margin of a cavernous angioma before coursing posteriorly and superiorly along the border of the inferior vermis. (Case 764 presents a clearer view of the cavernous malformation in this patient.)

The reason for the common association of venous and cavernous angiomas has been the subject of debate. In some cases, both malformations have been present and stable over long periods, suggesting coexisting developmental anomalies. In other patients, the cavernous component of the combined abnormality has developed or enlarged adjacent to a preexisting venous angioma, implying that occurrence and organization of hemorrhages in the territory drained by the venous malformation has led to formation of the cavernous mass.

Regardless of the etiological role of the venous angioma, its resection at the time of surgery for removal of a symptomatic cavernous lesion must be carefully considered to avoid the superimposed complication of venous infarction (see discussion in Cases 758-760). That is, it is important to define a developmental venous anomaly adjacent to a symptomatic cavernous angioma with the hope that the former can be preserved when the latter is resected.

### Case 771

43-year-old man presenting with the sudden
onset of right hemiparesis.
(axial, noncontrast scan; SE 2800/45)

### Case 772

36-year-old man presenting with
a seizure and headaches.
(coronal, postcontrast T1-weighted
SE scan with MTS)

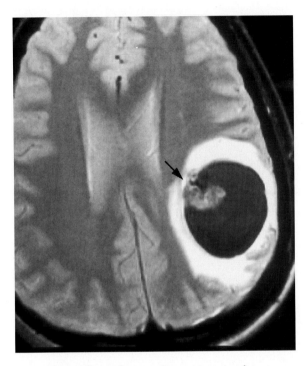

**Hemorrhage from a Cavernous Angioma**

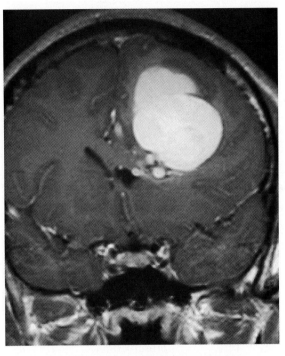

**Hemorrhage from a Cavernous Angioma**
(same patient as Case 769)

---

Small hemorrhages within or at the margins of cavernous angiomas occur with variable frequency. Many cavernous malformations are stable over years of follow-up. Others clearly enlarge with time. Recurrent hemorrhage and organization is presumed to be the mechanism for such growth, which is most common in deep hemispheric and infratentorial lesions.

Only rarely are cavernous angiomas associated with large intracerebral hematomas, as in the above cases. The acute hemorrhage in Case 771 is uniformly dark due to the presence of deoxyhemoglobin. A thick rim of surrounding edema accentuates the signal loss within the clot. A mildly

nodular mass at the anteromedial margin of the hemorrhage *(arrow)* proved to represent a cavernous angioma.

Case 772 presents another view of the patient in Case 769. A large hematoma containing methemoglobin is present at the lateral margin of the cavernous malformation, which was in turn adjacent to a venous angioma (see Case 769). Mass effect depresses the left lateral ventricle and causes subfalcial herniation.

The relationship of the hematoma to the periventricular angioma in Case 772 is nearly identical to the configuration in Case 762.

# CAPILLARY TELANGIECTASIAS

### Case 773

14-year-old boy presenting with headaches.
(axial, postcontrast T1-weighted SE scan )

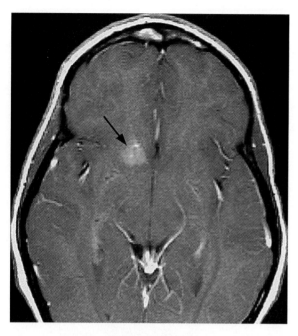

**Capillary Telangiectasia**
(presumed)

### Case 774

71-year-old woman presenting with dizziness.
(coronal, postcontrast T1-weighted SE scan)

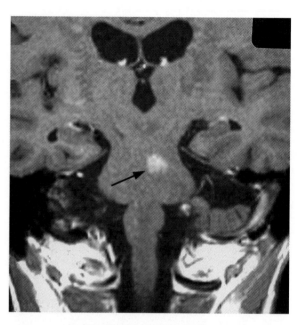

**Capillary Telangiectasia**
(presumed)

---

Capillary telangiectasias are vascular malformations comprised of dilated, thin-walled capillaries. These channels are separated by normal tissue, unlike the contiguous vascular spaces of cavernous angiomas. Capillary telangiectasias and cavernous angiomas may coexist at the same site or at different locations within the same patient. Like cavernous angiomas, capillary telangiectasias are often multiple.

Capillary telangiectasias may occur anywhere within the brain or spinal cord, but they are particularly common in the pons. These malformations are usually small (often less than one centimeter in diameter) and asymptomatic. Prior to CT and MR imaging, capillary telangiectasias were often discovered as incidental findings at autopsy.

Some capillary telangiectasias are associated with calcification and/or hemosiderin that results in increased attenuation on CT images and decreased signal intensity on T2- or T2*-weighted MR studies. More commonly, true telangiectasias (as distinct from cavernous malformations) are inapparent on standard noncontrast scans. The blood pool within the lesion does enhance on postcontrast studies, usually with a "soft" or "brush border" quality of relatively mild intensity and indistinct margins.

The lesions in Cases 773 and 774 match this appearance. Neither was visible on T1- or T2-weighted images. Both lesions have been stable over several years of follow-up, and neither has been biopsied.

Capillary telangiectasias may be detected as zones of low signal intensity on noncontrast sequences sensitive to magnetic susceptibility effects (e.g., T2*-weighted images). This characteristic likely reflects the slowly circulating blood volume within the lesions, containing a relatively high concentration of deoxyhemoglobin.

The differential diagnosis of small lesions with hazy enhancement in the brainstem (or elsewhere) includes many pathologies, such as demyelinating disease and subacute infarction (see Cases 775 and 776). However, most of these alternatives will be correlated with clinical clues and/or abnormalities on noncontrast scans. The lack of either should prompt consideration of a capillary telangiectasia.

Unlike cavernous angiomas of the brainstem, capillary telangiectasias usually do not progress or enlarge.

## Case 775

32-year-old man presenting with
left body numbness.
(axial, postcontrast T1-weighted SE scan)

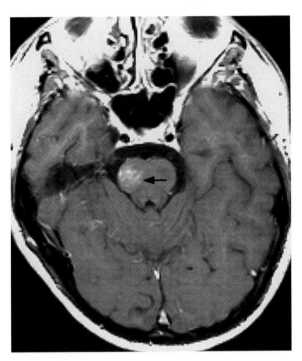

**Multiple Sclerosis**

## Case 776

72-year-old man presenting with diplopia.
(axial, postcontrast T1-weighted SE scan)

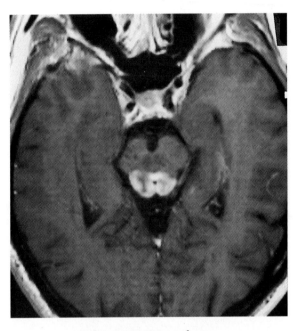

**Primary CNS Lymphoma**

---

Although the brainstem is a common location for vascular malformations such as capillary telangiectasias and cavernous angiomas, many other pathologies can cause focally enhancing lesions of the midbrain, pons, or medulla.

The "soft" character of enhancement within the demyelinating plaque in Case 775 resembles the quality of enhancement in a typical telangiectasia. Subacute infarction of the brainstem could present a similar appearance.

In Case 776, the bilateral enhancement of the tegmentum and tectum of the midbrain involves gray and white matter but does not follow a vascular distribution. The process is more infiltrative than mass-like, surrounding rather than displacing the aqueduct. These features argue against demyelinating disease, infarction, and metastasis. A rare metabolic disorder (e.g., Wernicke's encephalopathy) could be considered in the appropriate clinical context (see discussion of Cases 515 and 516).

The periaqueductal region is one of the sites frequently involved by CNS lymphoma, resembling the periventricular lesions commonly found in the supratentorial compartment (see Cases 347, 349, and 352). The patient in Case 776 had additional masses adjacent to the third ventricle. All of the lesions regressed rapidly after treatment with steroids but recurred within months.

## Case 777A

42-year-old man presenting with
left facial weakness.
(axial, noncontrast T2-weighted SE scan)

## Case 777B

Same patient.
(AP view, maximal intensity projection
reconstruction, noncontrast, three-dimensional,
time-of-flight GRE sequence)

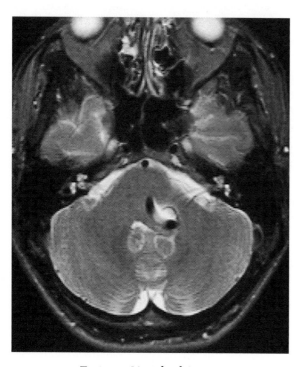

**Tortuous Vertebral Artery**

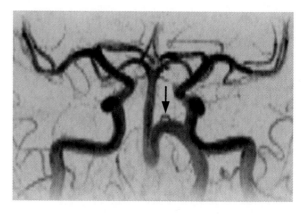

**Tortuous Vertebral Artery**

---

Some patients experience recurrent symptoms due to distortion of cranial nerves by adjacent vessels. Both tic douloureux (trigeminal nerve) and hemifacial spasm (facial nerve) may be caused by contact of an artery or vein with the nerve near its junction with the brainstem ("entry zone").

CT and MR scans rarely image the microvascular anatomy responsible for most cases of nerve irritation. Occasionally, symptomatic arterial loops can be identified.

In Case 777A, a large vascular channel appears to course through the dorsal brainstem, deforming the fourth ventricle. The small accompanying collection of cisternal CSF at the lateral aspect of the artery and the branch arising from the vessel (the PICA) indicate that the appearance is due to deep invagination of a loop of the distal left vertebral artery.

This tortuosity is impressively documented by the MR angiogram in Case 777B. The PICA originates at the apex of the loop *(arrow)*. Like other extraaxial masses, a tortuous artery can become deeply embedded within adjacent parenchyma over time (compare to the meningioma in Case 36 and the acoustic schwannoma in Case 194).

The precise vascular contact with a symptomatic cranial nerve is difficult to predict preoperatively even when an arterial anomaly is apparent. For example, the secondarily aberrant PICA could be the distorting vessel in Case 777 rather than the tortuous vertebral artery itself.

A combination of pulse sequences is helpful in screening for neurovascular compression. Thin, heavily T2-weighted axial and coronal scans define the cisternal segments of cranial nerves and their relationship to adjacent vessels (see Case 199). MR angiography documents the position of large arteries and their major branches but rarely demonstrates small neurovascular contacts.

## Case 778

49-year-old woman with a long history
of right hemifacial spasm.
(axial source image from a noncontrast, three-
dimensional, time-of-flight GRE sequence)

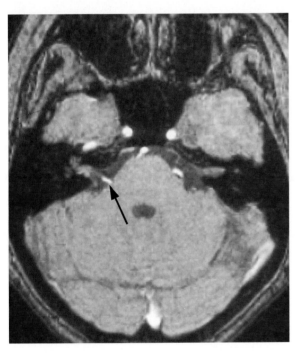

**AICA Loop Contacting the Facial Nerve**

## Case 779

6-year-old boy with "seizures" since infancy
manifested by facial twitching.
(mildly brow-up AP view, maximal intensity
projection reconstruction, noncontrast, three-
dimensional, time-of-flight GRE sequence)

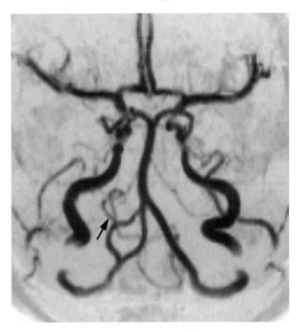

**Aberrant PICA**
(due to fenestration of the vertebral artery)

Case 777 on the preceding page is a rare example of a large vessel causing a cranial neuropathy. More commonly, screening MR studies in this context demonstrate localized tortuosity of a small artery (or are negative).

In Case 778, flow is demonstrated within a loop of the right AICA, which appears to be in direct contact with the facial nerve *(arrow)*. Surgery confirmed this finding. Facial spasm ceased after the artery was separated from the nerve.

Case 779 illustrates fenestration of the distal right vertebral artery. The right PICA *(arrow)* originates from the superior arm of this fenestration and courses further superiorly into the cerebellopontine angle. At surgery, this vessel was found to distort the cisternal portion of the facial nerve, accounting for the history of hemifacial spasm that had mimicked a seizure disorder.

Prominent arterial loops within the cerebellopontine angle are commonly seen in asymptomatic patients. The significance of such vascular tortuosity depends on correlation with symptoms and anticipated surgery. Even if a notable arterial loop is not directly responsible for distortion of the symptomatic cranial nerve, demonstration of the regional vascular anatomy is important preoperative information for a surgeon contemplating microvascular decompression.

Potentially symptomatic arterial loops are occasionally apparent on routine MR scans, particularly in the coronal plane. MR angiograms offer additional vascular evaluation in the setting of irritative cranial neuropathy. The above scans demonstrate that examination of both the individual partition images and the three-dimensional composite view is important for analysis of vascular detail.

### Case 780

77-year-old man presenting with brainstem TIAs.
(coronal, noncontrast T1-weighted SE scan)

### Case 781

76-year-old man presenting with
right trigeminal neuralgia.
(coronal, postcontrast T1-weighted
SE scan with MTS)

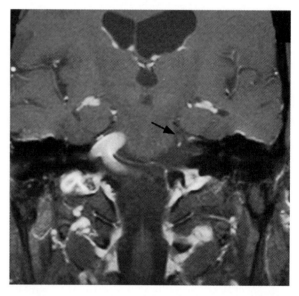

**Dolichoectasia of the Vertebrobasilar Junction**

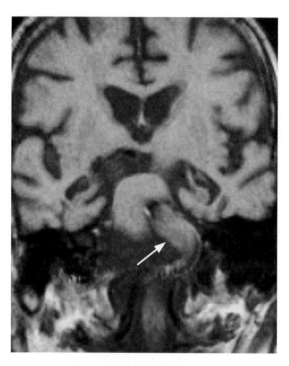

**Dolichoectasia of the Basilar Artery**

The basilar artery may undergo striking elongation and fusiform ectasia in elderly patients. This so-called *dolichoectasia* may cause the tip of the artery to rise as far superiorly as the foramen of Monro.

Case 780 demonstrates widening and tortuosity of the basilar artery *(arrow).* The vessel is filled with intraluminal signal intensity rather than flow void, suggesting slow flow and/or thrombus. The ectatic artery acts as a cerebellopontine angle mass, deforming the adjacent brainstem. In such cases, axial CT scans can be misinterpreted as demonstrating an enhancing extraaxial neoplasm.

Dolichoectatic basilar arteries rarely cause subarachnoid or parenchymal hemorrhage. Brainstem ischemia due to atherosclerotic disease affecting the origin of perforating vessels is a more common presentation, as in Case 780.

Mechanical distortion of cranial nerves is another mechanism by which dolichoectatic basilar arteries produce symptoms. Elongation of the artery may stretch the third cranial nerve by carrying it far superiorly, because the nerve is caught as it passes between the posterior cerebral and superior cerebellar arteries at the basilar tip. In Case 781, the tortuous and ectatic vertebrobasilar junction occupies the expected location of the cisternal segment of the trigeminal nerve. (Note the position of the normal left fifth nerve; *arrow.)* This case is a rare example of macrovascular compression causing trigeminal neuralgia.

Dolichoectasia of the supraclinoid internal carotid arteries or proximal middle cerebral arteries may also occur but is less common than basilar artery involvement.

An aneurysmal arteriopathy resembling adult dolichoectasia has been noted in children with AIDS. This ectasia of basal arteries correlates pathologically with destruction of the internal elastic lamina and thinning of the media.

### Case 782

4-year-old boy presenting with irritability.
(sagittal, noncontrast T1-weighted SE scan)

### Case 783

67-year-old woman presenting with headaches.
(axial, noncontrast T2-weighted FSE scan)

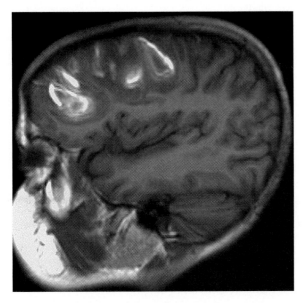

**Thrombosis of the Superior Sagittal Sinus**
(same patient as Case 677)

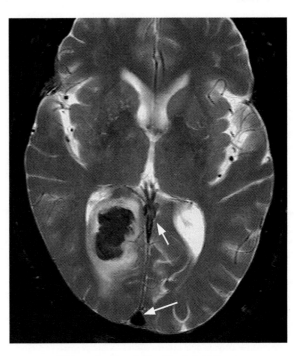

**Thrombosis of the Straight Sinus**

---

Among the vascular lesions to be considered as the source of intracerebral hemorrhage is thrombosis of a dural sinus. The general topic of dural sinus thrombosis has been discussed in Cases 647-660. The above patients illustrate the spectrum of parenchymal hemorrhages that can be associated with this condition.

In Case 782, gyriform T1-shortening is predominantly laminar and subcortical, paralleling the convolutions of the frontal lobe. Edema and hemorrhage due to venous infarction are often more apparent in subcortical white matter than in the overlying cortex. The hemorrhage in Case 782 is extensive; other venous infarcts contain smaller patches of blood products. (See Case 677 for an earlier scan of this patient and Case 650 for a T2-weighted image.)

The confluent hematoma at the temporal/occipital junction in Case 783 demonstrates prominent T2-shortening and a moderate rim of edema suggesting acute to early sub-acute age. Intermediate signal intensity within the nearby straight sinus *(short arrow)* contrasts with the normal flow void in the superior sagittal sinus *(long arrow)*. This finding suggests slow flow or thrombus within the straight sinus; thrombosis was confirmed by other images and an MR venogram.

Arterial infarction or laminar necrosis due to anoxia could be considered in the differential diagnosis of Case 782. Other potential etiologies for the hematoma in Case 783 include rupture of a vascular malformation (see Cases 750 and 752), hemorrhage into a primary or metastatic tumor (see Cases 9, 10, 96, and 97), amyloid angiopathy, coagulopathy (see Case 751) or spontaneous hemorrhage. Along with these conditions, dural sinus thrombosis should be remembered as a possible cause of laminar, patchy, or confluent intracerebral hemorrhage.

# REFERENCES

Abe T, Singer RJ, Marks MP, et al: Coexistence of occult vascular malformations and developmental venous anomalies in the central nervous system: MR evaluation. *AJNR* 19:51-58, 1998.

Adams WM, Laitt RD, Jackson A: The role of MR angiography in the pretreatment assessment of intracranial aneurysms: a comparative study. *AJNR* 21:1618-1628, 2000.

Aletich VA, Debrun GM, Monsein LH, et al: Giant serpentine aneurysms: a review and presentation of five cases. *AJNR* 16:1061-1072, 1995.

Atlas SW: Intracranial vascular malformations and aneurysms: current imaging applications. *Radiol Clin North Am* 26:821-837, 1988.

Atlas SW: Magnetic resonance imaging of intracranial aneurysms. *Neuroimaging Clin North Am* 7:709-720, 1997.

Atlas SW, Grossman RI, Goldberg HI, et al: Partially thrombosed giant intracranial aneurysms: correlation of MR and pathologic findings. *Radiology* 162:111-114, 1987.

Atlas SW, Mark AS, Fram EK, Grossman RI: Vascular intracranial lesions: applications of gradient-echo MR imaging. *Radiology* 169:455-462, 1988.

Atlas SW, Sheppard L, Goldberg HI, et al: Intracranial aneurysms: detection and characterization with MR angiography with use of an advanced postprocessing technique in a blinded-reader study. *Radiology* 203:807-814, 1997.

Augustyn GT, Scott JA, Olson E, et al: Cerebral venous angiomas: MR imaging. *Radiology* 156:391-396, 1985.

Award IA, Robinson JR Jr, Mohanty S, Estes ML: Mixed vascular malformations of the brain: clinical and pathogenetic considerations. *Neurosurgery* 33:179-188, 1993.

Awasthi D, Voorhies RM, Eick J, Mitchell WT: Cerebral amyloid angiopathy presenting as multiple intracranial lesions of magnetic resonance imaging. *J Neurosurg* 75:458-469, 1991.

Ballantyne ES, Page RD, Melaney JFM, et al: Coexistent trigeminal neuralgia, hemifacial spasm, and hypertension: preoperative imaging of neurovascular compression. Case report. *J Neurosurg* 80:559-563, 1994.

Barr RM, Dillon WP, Wilson CB: Slow-flow vascular malformations of the pons: capillary telangiectasias? *AJNR* 17:71-78, 1996.

Bellon RJ, Seeger JF: Cavernous angiomas: a radiologic review. *Int J Neurorad* 3:343-355, 1997.

Bernardi B, Zimmerman RA, Savino PJ, Adler C: Magnetic resonance tomographic angiography in the investigation of hemifacial spasm. *Neuroradiology* 35:606-611, 1993.

Biondi A, Scialfa G, Scotti G: Intracranial aneurysms: MR imaging. *Neuroradiology* 30:214-218, 1988.

Boecher-Schwarz HG, Bruehl K, Kessel G, et al: Sensitivity and specificity of MRA in the diagnosis of neurovascular compression in patients with trigeminal neuralgia. A correlation of MRA and surgical findings. *Neuroradiology* 40:88-95, 1998.

Bourgouin PM, Tampieri D, Johnston W, et al: Multiple occult vascular malformations of the brain and spinal cord: MRI diagnosis. *Neuroradiology* 34:110-111, 1992.

Bradley WG, Waluch V: Blood flow: magnetic resonance imaging. *Radiology* 154:443-450, 1985.

Brugieres P, Blustajn J, LeGuerinel C, et al: Magnetic resonance angiography of giant intracranial aneurysms. *Neuroradiology* 40:96-102, 1998.

Brunereau L, Labauge P, Tournier-Lasserve E, et al: Familial form of intracranial cavernous angioma: MR imaging findings in 51 families. *Radiology* 214:209-216, 2000.

Cammarata C, Han JS, Haaga JR, et al: Cerebral venous angiomas imaged by MR. *Radiology* 155:639-644, 1985.

Chung T-S, Joo J-Y, Lee S-K, et al: Evaluation of cerebral aneurysms with high-resolution MR angiography using a section-interpolation technique: correlation with digital subtraction angiography. *AJNR* 20:229-236, 1999.

Ciricillo SF, Dillon WP, Fink ME, Edwards MSB: Progression of multiple cryptic vascular malformations associated with anomalous venous drainage. *J Neurosurg* 81:477-481, 1994.

Clatterbuck RE, Elmaci I, Rigamonti D: The nature and fate of punctate (type IV) cavernous malformations. *Neurosurgery* 49:26-32, 2001.

Clatterbuck RE, Moriarity JL, Elmaci I, et al: Dynamic nature of cavernous malformations: a prospective magnetic resonance imaging study with volumetric analysis. *J Neurosurg* 93:981-986, 2000.

Cognard C, Gobin YP, Pierot L, et al: Cerebral dural arteriovenous fistulas; clinical and angiographic correlation with a revised classification of venous drainage. *Radiology* 194:671-680, 1995.

Corr P, Wright M, Handler LC: Endocarditis-related cerebral aneurysms: radiologic changes with treatment. *AJNR* 16:745-748, 1995.

Crecco M, Floris R, Vidiri A, et al: Venous angiomas: plain and contrast-enhanced MRI and MR angiography. *Neuroradiology* 37:20-24, 1995.

Curling OP, Kelly DI, Elster AD, Craven TE: An analysis of the natural history of cavernous hemangiomas. *J Neurosurg* 75:702-708, 1991.

Damiano TR, Truwit CL, Dowd CF, Symonds DL: Posterior fossa venous angiomas with drainage through the brain stem. *AJNR* 15:643-652, 1994.

DeMarco JK, Dillon WP, Halback VV, Tsuruda JS: Dural arteriovenous fistulas: evaluation with MR imaging. *Radiology* 175:193-199, 1990.

Dillon WP: Cryptic vascular malformations: controversies in terminology, diagnosis, pathophysiology, and treatment. *AJNR* 18:1839-1846, 1997.

Du C, Korogi Y, Nagahiro S, et al: Hemifacial spasm: three-dimensional MR images in the evaluation of neurovascular compression. *Radiology* 197:227-231, 1995.

Ebeling JD, Tranmer BI, Davis KA, et al: Thrombosed arteriovenous malformations: a type of occult vascular malformation. *Neurosurgery* 23:605-610, 1988.

Edelman RR, Wentz KU, Mattle HP, et al: Intracerebral arteriovenous malformation: evaluation with selective MR angiography and venography. *Radiology* 173:831, 1989.

Epstein MA, Packer RJ, Rorke LB, et al: Vascular malformations with radiation vasculopathy after treatment of chiasmatic/hypothalamic glioma. *Cancer* 70:887-893, 1992.

Field LR, Russell EJ: Spontaneous hemorrhage from a cerebral venous malformation related to thrombosis of the central draining vein: demonstration with angiography and serial MR. *AJNR* 16:1885-1888, 1995.

Fulbright RK, Chaloupka JC, Putman CM, et al: MR of hereditary hemorrhagic telangiectasia: prevalence and spectrum of cerebrovascular malformations. *AJNR* 19:477-484, 1998.

Gaen AD, Pile-Spellman J, Heros RC: A pneumatized anterior clinoid mimicking and aneurysm on MR imaging. Report of two cases. *J Neurosurg* 71:128-132, 1989.

Gaensler EHL, Dillon WP, Edwards MSB, et al: Radiation-induced telangiectasia in the brain simulates cryptic vascular malformations at MR imaging. *Radiology* 193:629-636, 1994.

Girard N, Poncet M, Caces F, et al: Three-dimensional MRI of hemifacial spasm with surgical correlation. *Neuroradiology* 39:46-51, 1997.

Gomori JM, Grossman RI, Goldberg HI, et al: Occult cerebral vascular malformations: high-field MR imaging. *Radiology* 158:707-713, 1986.

Graves VB, Duff TA: Intracranial arteriovenous malformations: current imaging and treatment. *Invest Radiol* 25:952-960, 1990.

Griffiths PD, Hoggard N, Warren DJ, et al: Brain arteriovenous malformations: assessment with dynamic MR digital subtraction angiography. *AJNR* 21:1892-1899, 2000.

Holtas S, Olsson M, Romner B, et al: Comparison of MR imaging and CT in patients with intracranial aneurysm clips. *AJNR* 9: 891-897, 1988.

Horowitz MB, Jungreis CA, Quisling RG, Pollack I: Vein of Galen aneurysms: a review and current perspective. *AJNR* 15:1486-1496, 1994.

Hosoya T, Watanabe N, Yamaguchi K, et al: Three-dimensional MRI of neurovascular compression in patients with hemifacial spasm. *Neuroradiology* 37:350-352, 1995.

Huddle DC, Chaloupka JC, Sehgal V: Clinically aggressive diffuse capillary telangiectasia of the brain stem: a clinical radiologic-pathologic case study. *AJNR* 20:1674-1677, 1999.

Hurst RW, Bagley LJ, Galetta S, et al: Dementia resulting from dural arteriovenous fistulas: the pathologic findings of venous hypertensive encephalopathy. *AJNR* 19:1267-1273, 1998.

Hurst RW, Judkins A, Bolger W, et al: Mycotic aneurysm and cerebral infarction resulting from fungal sinusitis: imaging and pathologic correlation. *AJNR* 22:858-863, 2001.

Huston J III, Nichols DA, Leutmer PH, et al: Blinded prospective evaluation of sensitivity of MR angiography to known intracranial aneurysms: importance of aneurysm size. *AJNR* 15:1607-1614, 1994.

Huston J III, Rufenacht DA, Ehman RL, Wiebers DO: Intracranial aneurysms and vascular malformations: comparison of time-of-flight and phase-contrast MR angiography. *Radiology* 181:721-730, 1991.

Ida M, Kurisu Y, Yamashita M: MR angiography of ruptured aneurysms in acute subarachnoid hemorrhage. *AJNR* 18:1025-1032, 1997.

Jager HR, Ellamushi H, Moore EA, et al: Contrast-enhanced MR angiography of intracranial giant aneurysms. *AJNR* 21:1900-1907, 2000.

Jaspan T, Wilson M, O'Donnell H, et al: Magnetic resonance imaging with even-echo rephasing sequences in assessment and management of giant intracranial aneurysm. *Br J Radiol* 61: 351, 1988.

Kallmes DF, Clark HP, Dix JE, et al: Ruptured vertebrobasilar aneurysms: frequency of the nonaneurysmal perimesencephalic pattern on CT scans. *Radiology* 201:657-660, 1996.

Kashiwagi S, Van Loueren HR, Tew JM Jr, et al: Diagnosis and treatment of vascular brain stem malformations. *J Neurosurg* 72:27-34, 1990.

Katayama Y, Tsubokawa T, Miyazaki S, et al: Magnetic resonance imaging of cavernous sinus cavernous hemangioma. *Neuroradiology* 33:118-122, 1991.

Konan AV, Raymond J, Bourgouin P, et al: Cerebellar infarct caused by spontaneous thrombosis of a developmental venous anomaly of the posterior fossa. *AJNR* 20:256-258, 1999.

Korogi Y, Takahashi M, Mabuchi N, et al: Intracranial aneurysms: diagnostic accuracy of MR angiography with evaluation of maximum intensity projection and source images. *Radiology* 199: 199-208, 1996.

Kucharczyk W, Kelly WM, Davis DO, et al: Intracranial lesions. Flow-related enhancement on MR images using time-of-flight effects. *Radiology* 161:767-772, 1986.

Kucharczyk W, Lemme-Pheghos L, Uske A, et al: Intracranial vascular malformations. MR and CT imaging. *Radiology* 156:383-389, 1985.

Labauge P, Brunereau L, Levy C, et al: The natural history of familial cerebral cavernomas: a retrospective MRI study of 40 patients. *Neuroradiology* 42:327-332, 2000.

Lasjaunias P, Burrows P, Planet C: Developmental venous anomalies (DVA): the so-called venous angioma. *Neurosurg Rev* 9: 233-244, 1986.

Latchaw RE, Truwit CL, Heros RC: Venous angioma, cavernous angioma, and hemorrhage. *AJNR* 15:1255-1258, 1994.

Leblanc R, Levesque M, Comair Y, Ethier, R: Magnetic resonance imaging of cerebral arteriovenous malformation. *Neurosurgery* 21:15-20, 1987.

Lee BCP, Herberg L, Zimmerman RD, Deck MDF: MR imaging of cerebral vascular malformations. *AJNR* 6:863-870, 1985.

Lee BCP, Vo KD, Kido DK, et al: MR high-resolution blood oxygenation level-dependent venography of occult (low-flow) vascular lesions. *AJNR* 20:1239-1242, 1999.

Lee C, Pennington MA, Kenney CM: MR evaluation of developmental venous anomalies: medullary venous anatomy of venous angiomas. *AJNR* 17:61-70, 1996.

Lee RR, Becher MW, Benson ML, Rigamonti D: Brain capillary telangiectasia: MR imaging appearance and clinicohistopathologic findings. *Radiology* 205:797-805, 1997

Lemme-Phaghos L, Kucharczyk W, Brant-Zawadzki M, et al: Mr imaging of angiographically occult vascular malformations. *AJNR* 7:217-222, 1986.

Majoie CBLM, Hulsmans F-JH, Verbeeten B Jr, et al: Trigeminal neuralgia: comparison of two MR imaging techniques in the demonstration of neurovascular contact. *Radiology* 204:455-460, 1997.

Mansmann U, Meisel J, Brock M, et al: Factors associated with intracranial hemorrhage in cases of cerebral arteriovenous malformation. *Neurosurgery* 46:272-281, 2000.

Marks MP, Lane B, Steinberg GK, Chang PJ: Hemorrhage in intracerebral aneurysms and arteriovenous malformations: frequency of intracranial hemorrhage and relationship of lesions. *J Neurosurg* 73:859-863, 1990.

Mawad ME, Klucznik RP: Giant serpentine aneurysms: radiographic features and endovascular treatment. *AJNR* 16:1053-1060, 1995.

Meisel HJ, Mansmann U, Alvarez H, et al: Cerebral arteriovenous malformations and associated aneurysms: analysis of 305 cases from a series of 662 patients. *Neurosurgery* 46:793-802, 2000.

Merten CL, Knitelius HO, Hedde JP, et al: Intracerebral haemorrhage from a venous angioma following thrombosis of a draining vein. *Neuroradiology* 40:15-18, 1998.

Metens T, Rio F, Baleriaux D, et al: Intracranial aneurysms: detection with gadolinium-enhanced dynamic three-dimensional MR angiography - initial results. *Radiology* 216:39-46, 2000.

Meyer FB, Huston J III, Riederer SS: Pulsatile increases in aneurysm size determined by cine phase-contrast MR angiography. *J Neurosurg* 78:879-883, 1993.

Mitsuoka H, Tsunoda A, Okuda O, et al: Delineation of small nerves and blood vessels with three-dimensional fast spin-echo MR imaging: comparison of presurgical and surgical findings in patients with hemifacial spasm. *AJNR* 19:1823-1830, 1998.

Momoshima S, Shiga H, Yuasa Y, et al: MR findings in extracerebral cavernous angiomas or the middle cranial fossa: Report of two cases and review of the literature. *AJNR* 12:756-760, 1991.

Nadel L, Braun IF, Kraft K, et al: Intracranial vascular abnormalities: value of MR phase imaging to distinguish thrombus from flowing blood. *AJNR* 11:1133-1140, 1990.

Naseem M, Leehey P, Russell E, et al: MR of basilar artery dolichoectasia. *AJNR* 9:391-392, 1988.

New PFJ, Ojemann RG, Davis KR, et al: MR and CT of occult vascular malformations of the brain. *AJNR* 7:771-780, 1986.

Noorbehesht B, Fabrikant JI, Enzmann DR, et al: Size determination of supratentorial arteriovenous malformations by MR, CT, and angio. *Neuroradiology* 29:512, 1987.

Olsen WL, Brant-Zawadzki M, Hodes J, et al: Giant intracranial aneurysms: MR imaging. *Radiology* 163:431-435, 1987.

Ostertun B, Solymosi L: Magnetic resonance angiography of cerebral developmental venous anomalies: its role in differential diagnosis. *Neuroradiology* 35:97-104, 1993.

Prayer L. Wimberger D, Stiglbauer R. et al: Haemorrhage in intracerebral arteriovenous malformations: detection with MRI and comparison with clinical history. *Neuroradiology* 35:424-427, 1993.

Putman CM, Chaloupka JC, Fulbright RK, et al: Exceptional multiplicity of cerebral arteriovenous malformations associated with hereditary hemorrhagic telangiectasia (Osler-Weber-Rendu syndrome). *AJNR* 17:1733-1742, 1996.

Rapacki TFX, Brantley MJ, Furlow TW, et al: Heterogeneity of cerebral cavernous hemangiomas diagnosed by MR imaging. *J Comput Assist Tomogr* 14:18-25, 1990.

Raybaud CA, Strother CM, Hald JK: Aneurysms of the vein of Galen: embryonic considerations and anatomical features relating to the pathogenesis of the malformations. *Neuroradiology* 31:109-128, 1989.

Rigamonti D, Hadley MN, Drayer BP, et al: Cerebral cavernous malformations: incidence and familial occurrence. *N Engl J Med* 319:343-347, 1988.

Rigamonti D, Johnson PC, Spetzler RF, et al: Cavernous malformations and capillary telangiectasia: a spectrum within a single pathological entity. *Neurosurgery* 28:60-64, 1991.

Rigamonti D, Spetzler D: The association of venous and cavenous malformations: report of four cases and discussions of the pathophysiological, diagnostic and therapeutic implications. *Acta Neurochir (Wien)* 92:100-105, 1988.

Rigamonti D, Spetzler RF, Medina M, et al: Cerebral venous malformations. *J Neurosurg* 73:560-564, 1998.

Rigamonti DE, Drayer BP, Johnson PC, et al: The MRI appearance of cavernous malformations (angiomas). *J Neurosurg* 67:518-524, 1987.

Robinson JR, Awad IA, Little JR: Natural history of the cavernous angioma. *J Neurosurg* 75:709-714, 1991.

Robinson JR Jr, Awad IA, Magdinec M, Paranandi L: Factors predisposing to clinical disability in patients with cavernous malformations of the brain. *Neurosurgery* 32:730-736, 1993.

Robinson JR Jr, Awad IA, Thomas J, et al: Pathological heterogeneity of angiographically occult-vascular malformations of the brain. *Neurosurgery* 33:547-555, 1993.

Rolen PB, Sze G: Small, patent cerebral aneurysms: atypical appearances at 1.5-T MR imaging. *Radiology* 208:129-136, 1998.

Ruggieri P, Poulos N, Masaryk T, et al: Occult intracranial aneurysms in polycystic kidney disease: screening with MR angiography. *Radiology* 191:33-40, 1994.

Sankhla SK, Gunawardena WJ, Coutinho CMA, et al: Magnetic resonance angiography in the management of aneurysmal subarachnoid haemorrhage: a study of 51 cases. *Neuroradiology* 38:724-729, 1996.

Sato N, Sze G, Awad IA, et al: Parenchymal perianeurysmal cystic changes in the brain: report of five cases. *Radiology* 215:229-234, 2000.

Schuierer G, Huk WJ, Laub G: Magnetic resonance angiography of intracranial aneurysms: comparison with intra-arterial digital subtraction angiography. *Neuroradiology* 35:50-54, 1993.

Seidenwurm D, Berenstein A: Vein of Galen malformation: clinical relevance of angiographic classification and utility of MRI in treatment planning. *Neuroradiology* 33(suppl):153-155, 1991.

Seidenwurm D, Berenstein A, Hyman A, Kowalsla H: Vein of Galen malformation: correlation of clinical presentation, arteriography, and MR imaging. *AJNR* 12:347-345, 1991.

Smith HJ, Strother CM, Kikuchi Y, et al: MR imaging in the management of supratentorial intracranial AVMs. *AJNR* 9:225-235, 1988.

Stone JL, Crowell RM, Grandhi YN, Jafar JJ: Multiple intracranial aneurysms: magnetic resonance imaging for determination of the site of rupture. *Neurosurgery* 23:97-100, 1988.

Strother CM, Eldevik P, Kikuchi Y, et al: Thrombus formation and structure and the evolution of mass effect in intracranial aneurysms treated by balloon embolization: Emphasis on MR findings. *AJNR* 10:787-796, 1989.

Sze G, Krol G, Olson WL, et al: Hemorrhagic neoplasms: MR mimics of occult vascular malformations. *AJNR* 8:795-802, 1987.

Tash R, DeMerritt J, Sze G, Leslie D: Hemifacial spasm: MR imaging features. *AJNR* 12:839-842, 1991.

Tash RE, Kier EL, Chyatte D: Hemifacial spasm caused by a tortuous vertebral artery: MR demonstration. *J Comput Assist Tomogr* 12:492-494, 1988.

Tech KE, Becker CJ, Lazo A, et al: Anomalous intracranial venous drainage mimicking orbital or cavernous arteriovenous fistula. *AJNR* 16:171-174, 1995.

Tein RD, Wilkins RH: MRA delineation of the vertebrovascular system in patients with hemifacial spasm and trigeminal neuralgia. *AJNR* 14:34-36, 1993.

Tomlinson FH, Houser OW, Scheithauer BW, et al: Angiographically occult vascular malformations: a corelative study of features on magnetic resonance imaging and histologic examination. *Neurosurgery* 34:792-800, 1994.

Toro VE, Gever CA, Sherman IL, et al: Cerebral venous angiomas: MR findings. *J Comput Assist Tomogr* 12:935-940, 1988.

Truwit CL: Venous angioma of the brain: history, significance and imaging findings. *Am J Roentgenol* 159:1299-1307, 1992.

Uchino a, Imador H, Ohno M: Magnetic resonance imaging of intracranial venous angioma. *Clinical Imaging* 14:309-314, 1990.

White PM, Wardlaw JM, Easton V: Can noninvasive imaging accurately depict intracranial aneurysms? A systemic review. *Radiology* 217:361-370, 2000.

Willinsky R, Goyal M, terBrugge K, Montanera W: Tortuous, engorged pial veins in intracranial dural arteriovenous fistulas: correlations with presentation, location, and MR findings in 122 patients. *AJNR* 20:1031-1036, 1999.

Willinsky R, Terbruge K, Montanera W, et al: Venous congestion: an MR finding in dural arteriovenous malformations with cortical venous drainage. *AJNR* 15:1501-1507, 1994.

Wilms G, Bleus E, Demaerel P, et al: Simultaneous occurrence of developmental venous anomalies and cavernous angiomas. *AJNR* 15:1247-1254, 1994.

Wilms G, Demaerel P, Marchal G, et al: Gadolinium-enhanced MR imaging of cerebral venous angiomas with emphasis on their drainage. *J Comput Assist Tomogr* 15:199-206, 1991.

Wilms G, Marchal G, Vas Hecke P, et al: Cerebral venous angioma: MR imaging at 1.5 Tesla. *Neuroradiology* 32:81-85, 1990.

Wilms G, Bleus E, Demaerel P, et al: Simultaneous occurrence of developmental venous anomalies and cavernous angiomas. *AJNR* 15:1247-1254, 1994.

Wilson CB: Cryptic vascular malformations. *Clin Neurosurg* 38:49-84, 1992.

Wong BW, Steinberg GK, Rosen L: Magnetic resonance imaging of vascular compression in trigeminal neuralgia: case report. *J Neurosurg* 70:132-134, 1989.

Worthington BS, Kean DM, Hawkes RC, et al: Nuclear magnetic resonance imaging in recognition of giant intracranial aneurysms. *AJNR* 4:835-836, 1983.

Yousem DM, Flamm ES, Grossman RI: Comparison of MR imaging with clinical history in the identification of hemorrhage in patients with cerebral arteriovenous malformations. *AJNR* 10:1151-1154, 1989.

Zimmerman RS, Spetzler RF, Lee KS, et al: Cavernous malformations of the brain stem. *J Neurosurg* 75:32-39, 1991.

# Chapter 15

# Hydrocephalus and Cysts

### Case 784

11-year-old boy presenting with headaches.
(axial, postcontrast T1-weighted SE scan)

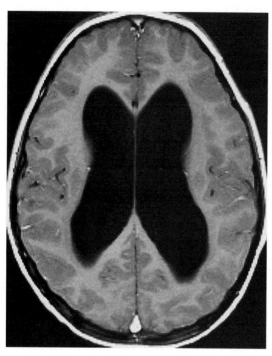

**Hydrocephalus**
(due to a midbrain glioma)

### Case 785

53-year-old woman presenting with
headaches and a large head.
(axial, noncontrast T2-weighted SE scan)

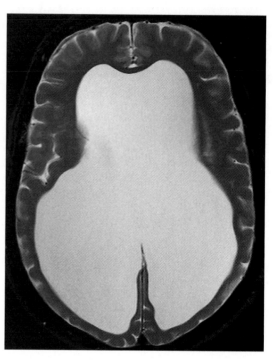

**Hydrocephalus**
(due to aqueductal stenosis)

Although the diagnosis of hydrocephalus is easily made by CT, MR is valuable for assessing etiology. Many cases of hydrocephalus are caused by obstruction at the level of the aqueduct or fourth ventricle. Sagittal and coronal MR views free from bone artifact provide much better visualization of the midbrain and posterior fossa than CT scans.

Cases 784 and 785 illustrate marked symmetrical enlargement of the lateral ventricular bodies. Hydrocephalic lateral ventricles may become hugely dilated, occupying most of the supratentorial compartment. Except in extreme cases, the thinness of the residual cortical mantle is an unreliable predictor of postshunt recovery.

The posterior bodies, atria, and occipital horns of hydrocephalic ventricles are often larger than the frontal horns. This disparity may increase after shunting, with the greatest reduction in ventricular size occurring anteriorly. Severe hydrocephalus may be associated with thinning or frank dehiscence of the septum pellucidum, as in Case 785.

Occasional intraventricular or periventricular masses obstruct one lateral ventricle without compromising the contralateral foramen of Monro. Potential causes of unilateral hydrocephalus include intraventricular meningiomas, subependymal giant cell astrocytomas in tuberous sclerosis (see Cases 896 and 897), ependymomas (see Case 123), subependymomas (see Cases 129 and 344), septal or intraventricular gliomas (see Cases 106, 107, 109, and 345), oligodendrogliomas, and central neurocytomas (see Cases 342 and 343).

Unilateral hydrocephalus may also result from benign strictures or adhesions at the foramen of Monro. Such septations are usually not definable on scans without intraventricular contrast material. The diagnosis is otherwise based on exclusion of an obstructing mass or cyst by careful examination of multiplanar, multisequence, precontrast and postcontrast MR images.

## Case 786

26-year-old woman presenting with
positional headaches.
(axial, noncontrast scan; SE 2500/28)

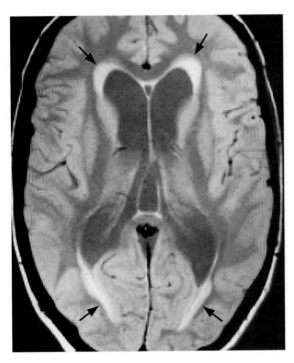

**Hydrocephalus**
(due to a colloid cyst of the third ventricle)

## Case 787

9-year-old boy presenting with ataxia.
(axial, noncontrast FLAIR scan)

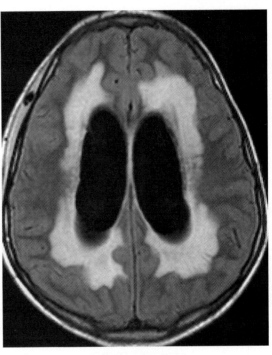

**Hydrocephalus**
(due to a cerebellar astrocytoma)

As the lateral ventricles enlarge in hydrocephalus, the tight junctions between ependymal cells are eventually disrupted. This discontinuity may allow cerebrospinal fluid under pressure to leak into the periventricular white matter. The normal centripetal movement of interstitial fluid from the brain through the subependymal region into the ventricles is also impaired by high intraventricular pressure. These factors cause a localized or diffuse layer of increased fluid around the ventricular margins.

Periventricular edema due to hydrocephalus is well demonstrated by MR, like other causes of increased water content in cerebral white matter. Cases with an equivocal CT appearance may be obvious on MR studies.

The zone of periventricular edema bordering hydrocephalic ventricles may be smooth and uniform, as in Case 786. Other cases present a broader and more irregular band of edema, as seen in Case 787. This shaggy morphology occurs with acute and/or severe elevation of in-

traventricular pressure. Regardless of severity, the fluid accumulation within periventricular white matter is usually most prominent near the frontal horns and trigones of the lateral ventricles.

Periventricular edema is best demonstrated on MR scans with "intermediate" weighting (long TR and short TE values) or on FLAIR images. On T2-weighted scans, the high signal intensity of ventricular CSF may merge with the high intensity of subependymal fluid.

Note that the dilated ventricles in Cases 784 and 785 on the previous page are not associated with increased periventricular fluid, even though they are larger than the ventricles in Cases 786 and 787. This discrepancy reflects the relative acuity and/or degree of raised intraventricular pressure. Chronic, mild impairment of CSF circulation may cause gradually progressive ventricular enlargement without accompanying edema in periventricular tissue.

### Case 788

2-day-old boy.
(coronal, noncontrast T1-weighted SE scan)

### Case 789

7-day-old girl.
(axial, noncontrast T2-weighted SE scan)

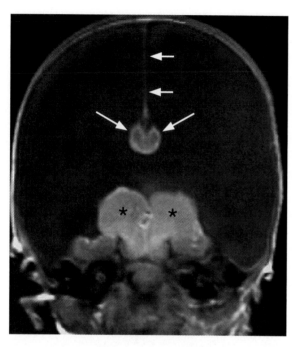

**Hydranencephaly**

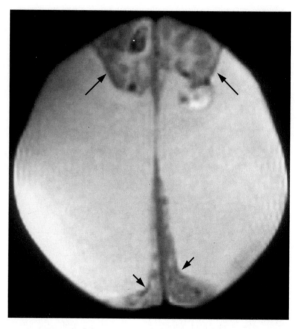

**Hydranencephaly**

Several congenital abnormalities are associated with large supratentorial CSF spaces that may resemble hydrocephalic ventricles.

Hydranencephaly represents loss of normal brain tissue due to an embryologic insult. Major portions of the cerebral hemispheres are absent, and the supratentorial region is filled with fluid. In most cases, the posterior fossa and diencephalon (*asterisks,* Case 788) are preserved. This finding suggests that the hemispheric deficiency is due to agenesis, hypoplasia, and/or occlusion of the supraclinoid internal carotid arteries.

The above scans illustrate a variant of hydranencephaly that may alternatively be considered to represent a severe form of bilateral schizencephaly (see discussion of Cases 884-888). Parasagittal parenchyma is spared in the distribution of the anterior cerebral arteries (*long arrows,* Cases 788 and 789) and in the distribution of the posterior cere-

bral arteries (*short arrows,* Case 789). That is, the absence of cerebral tissue approximates the distribution of the middle cerebral arteries, which presumably failed to develop or were occluded in utero.

Hydranencephaly may be mistaken for severe hydrocephalus. However, the scattered remnants of cortex in hydranencephaly do not form a complete rim around the hemisphere, as does the compressed cortical mantle of hydrocephalus. The presence of an intact falx cerebri, well seen in the above images (*short arrows,* Case 788), distinguishes hydranencephaly from alobar or semi-lobar holoprosencephaly.

A diffuse postnatal anoxic or inflammatory insult may resemble hydranencephaly when widespread damage to cerebral tissues spares the posterior fossa and diencephalon. A ghost of once-normal hemispheric structures is usually visible in such cases.

## Case 790A

2-month-old girl presenting with a large head.
(coronal, noncontrast T1-weighted SE scan)

## Case 790B

Same patient.
(axial, noncontrast T1-weighted SE scan)

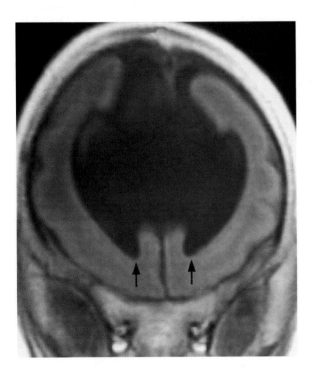

Holoprosencephaly

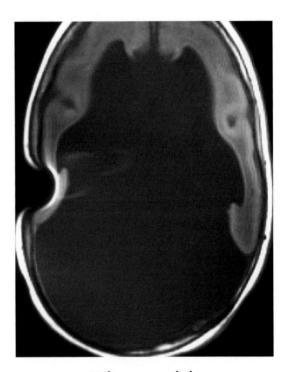

Holoprosencephaly

Holoprosencephaly is a developmental malformation characterized by absent or incomplete cerebral hemispherization. A horseshoe-shaped forebrain ("holoprosencephalon") surrounds a central monoventricle.

The typical batwing morphology of the single-chambered ventricle is seen anteriorly in Case 790. Inferior pointing of the frontal horns is prominent (*arrows,* Case 790A). This finding also occurs in less severe syndromes of midline dysgenesis (such as septooptic dysplasia; see Cases 863 and 864) and in some cases of Chiari II malformation.

A midline dorsal cyst is often found posterior and superior to cerebral tissue in cases of holoprosencephaly. The cyst may communicate broadly with the monoventricle, as seen above, or be an isolated, interhemispheric structure. Dorsal interhemispheric cysts can also accompany other congenital malformations of the brain, notably agenesis of the corpus callosum (see Cases 855-857).

Absence of the septum pellucidum does not by itself imply holoprosencephaly (or milder forms of midline cerebral dysgenesis). The septum may become markedly thinned or frankly dehiscent in severe hydrocephalus, with resulting communication between the lateral ventricles (see Case 785).

Cerebral cortex in Case 790 is abnormally smooth, demonstrating a lack of gyral development (see Cases 870-873). Metallic artifact in the right parietal region in Case 790B is due to a shunt valve.

Cases 865 and 866 provide further discussion of holoprosencephaly.

### Case 791

24-year-old man presenting with a seizure.
(axial, postcontrast T1-weighted SE scan)

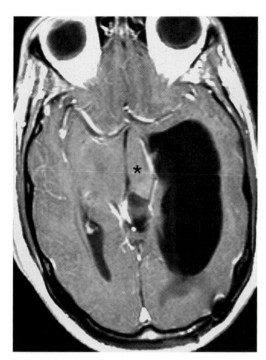

**Trapped Temporal Horn**

### Case 792

3-year-old girl with a history of communicating
hydrocephalus and recurrent shunt infection.
(sagittal, noncontrast T1-weighted SE scan)

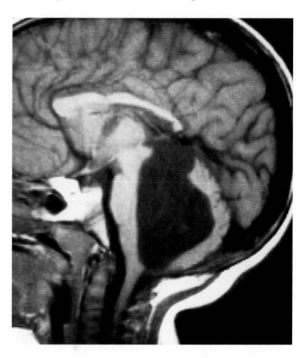

**Trapped Fourth Ventricle**

If a portion of the ventricular system containing choroid plexus becomes isolated from adjacent ventricular compartments, the trapped segment may enlarge due to continued production of CSF. Cases 791 and 792 present two examples of this situation.

In Case 791, higher scans demonstrated a cystic astrocytoma severely compressing the trigone of the left lateral ventricle. CSF formed within the temporal horn cannot circulate toward the foramen of Monro and accumulates locally. (The rate of CSF production by choroid plexus does not decrease until intraventricular pressure is substantially elevated.) The distended temporal horn acts as a cystic mass, causing medial herniation of the uncus and parahippocampal gyrus with flattening and compression of the midbrain at the level of the tentorial hiatus *(asterisk)*.

The lateral and third ventricles in Case 792 are well decompressed by a supratentorial shunt. The fourth ventricle is strikingly dilated, implying both functional inadequacy of the aqueduct (so that the fourth ventricle is isolated from drainage by the shunt) and obstruction of fourth ventricular outlet foramina. The degree of compression of the brainstem and cerebellum is comparable to that of a large fourth ventricular tumor (compare to Cases 150 and 158).

Trapping of the fourth ventricle is a potential complication of shunting in cases with obstruction of the fourth ventricular foramina. Reduction in the caliber of a previously distended aqueduct and/or reactive aqueductal gliosis may lead to functional disconnection of the fourth ventricle from the supratentorial ventricles. Continued formation of CSF within a trapped fourth ventricle leads to an expanding mass, which can cause life-threatening compression of the brainstem.

Small size of shunted ventricles (as is true of the lateral and third ventricles in Case 792) does not exclude the possibility of shunt malfunction. Chronic ventricular collapse may be associated with low compliance. Subsequent shunt obstruction can cause a rapid increase in pressure with little expansion of ventricular volume. This condition, the *slit-like ventricle syndrome* or *stiff ventricle syndrome,* is among the potential complications of ventricular shunts.

# DIFFERENTIAL DIAGNOSIS:
## SUPRASELLAR CYST ASSOCIATED WITH HYDROCEPHALUS

### Case 793

11-year-old boy presenting with headaches.
(axial, postcontrast T1-weighted SE scan)

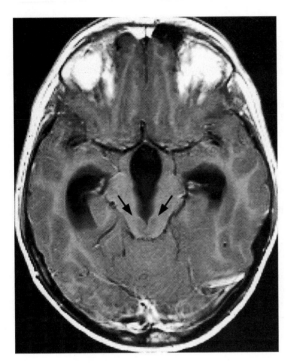

**Dilated Third Ventricle**

### Case 794

34-year-old man presenting with impaired vision.
(axial, noncontrast FLAIR scan)

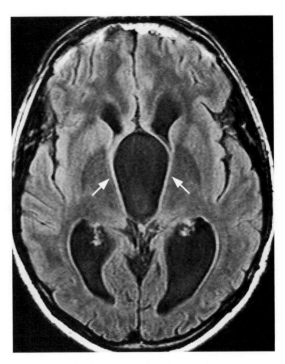

**Suprasellar Arachnoid Cyst**

---

As illustrated on the preceding page, hydrocephalic ventricles can resemble focal masses. Conversely, localized cysts or tumors can mimic dilated ventricular chambers.

A small glioma of the dorsal midbrain obstructs the aqueduct in Case 793 *(arrows)*, with secondary dilatation of the third ventricle and temporal horns. Even larger third ventricles can be encountered in cases of chronic aqueductal stenosis. These structures may act as suprasellar masses, causing erosion of the dorsum sella and expansion of the sella itself.

The suprasellar arachnoid cyst in Case 794 *(arrows)* mimicked an enlarged third ventricle on a preshunt CT study. The diagnosis of aqueductal stenosis was assumed. Subsequent evaluation demonstrated a suprasellar cyst that had compressed the third ventricle to cause obstructive hydrocephalus. An ependymal cyst or a cysticercosis cyst arising within the third ventricle could present similarly (see Cases 806 and 807).

The above cases emphasize that the diagnosis of benign aqueductal stenosis requires careful exclusion of other lesions. Small midbrain masses can obstruct the aqueduct while causing minimal abnormalities of CT density or contour. Alternatively, fluid-intensity lesions can be overlooked as they occupy or compress the third ventricle. Such lesions can be hidden within CSF or mistakenly interpreted as a dilated ventricle. (Cystic lesions can also enlarge the *fourth* ventricle and be initially masked by superimposed hydrocephalus; see Cases 806 and 807.)

Cases 816 and 817 discuss suprasellar arachnoid cysts. Other midline masses that may mimic third ventricular distension include hypothalamic gliomas (see Case 262), craniopharyngiomas (see Case 250), and occasional cysts of the septum pellucidum (see Case 845).

**Case 795A**

18-year-old man with a history of head trauma,
now presenting with headaches.
(axial, noncontrast T2-weighted SE scan)

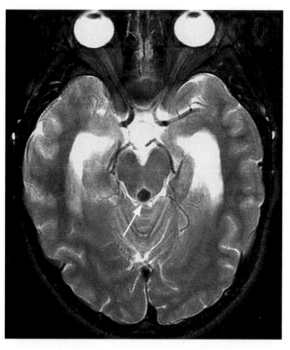

**Communicating Hydrocephalus**

**Case 795B**

Same patient.
(axial, noncontrast T2-weighted SE scan)

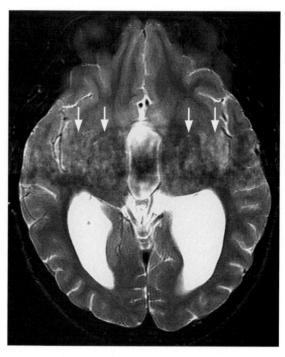

**Communicating Hydrocephalus**

The flow of CSF through the ventricular system is pulsatile, reflecting the transmission of cardiac systole and diastole to the cerebral hemispheres. CSF flow velocity is greatest where ventricular diameters are narrowest, notably at the aqueductal level. Normal aqueductal flow is bidirectional, with the magnitude of the caudal systolic component exceeding the rostral diastolic component.

In the presence of communicating hydrocephalus (or hydrocephalus due to fourth ventricular obstruction), CSF motion within the aqueduct may become hyperdynamic, with greater caudal and rostral excursions. The cause of this increased pulsatility has been suggested to be the reduced elasticity or compliance of the distended lateral ventricles and cerebral hemispheres. Greater velocity and turbulence of aqueductal flow in such cases may cause increased signal loss within the aqueduct.

Prominent aqueductal signal loss can therefore be a clue to abnormal CSF hydrodynamics. Although the finding is not specific and may be seen in some cases of atrophy, its presence should lead to consideration of hydrocephalus (and its absence argues against the diagnosis). The degree of aqueductal signal loss depends on the pulse sequence employed, especially the amount of motion compensation.

The aqueduct in Case 795 is abnormally large and black (*arrow*, Case 795A), reflecting signal loss due to flow void and/or turbulence. Low signal intensity is also apparent within the third ventricle, associated with a transverse band of artifact (*arrows*, Case 795B) due to mismapped phase information caused by exaggerated CSF pulsatility. (Compare this appearance to the phase artifact generated by the aneurysm in Case 730 and the dilated vein of Galen in Case 746.)

Low signal intensity due to exaggerated CSF flow is often most apparent on T2-weighted scans, when more static ventricular chambers are filled with high intensity values.

# THIRD VENTRICULOSTOMY

## Case 796A

22-year-old man treated for aqueductal stenosis.
(sagittal, noncontrast T2-weighted SE scan)

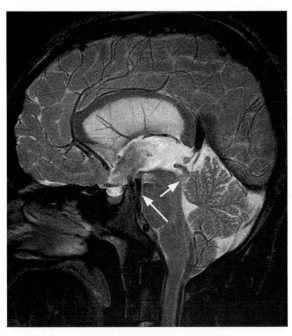

**Third Ventriculostomy**
(and aqueductal stenosis)

## Case 796B

Same patient.
(sagittal, noncontrast phase contrast scan)

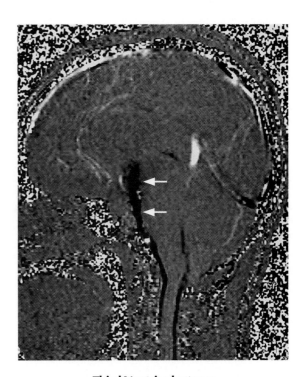

**Third Ventriculostomy**

Ventricular shunts are subject to a low but real risk of complications, including occlusion, infection, intracranial hemorrhage, and "slit ventricle syndrome" (see discussion of Case 792). For this reason, there has been increasing interest in alternative treatments for hydrocephalus.

One therapeutic option is third ventriculostomy, usually performed endoscopically via the foramen of Monro. A midline opening is made in the floor of the third ventricle, between the infundibular recess and the mammillary bodies. This aperture establishes communication between the ventricular system and the subarachnoid space of the interpeduncular and prepontine cisterns, bypassing obstruction to CSF circulation at the level of the aqueduct or fourth ventricle.

Sagittal MR scans can confirm the patency of a third ventriculostomy, as illustrated above. The T2-weighted image in Case 796A demonstrates aqueductal stenosis (*short arrow;* see discussion of Cases 800-803). The flow void of the basilar artery lies along the ventral margin of the pons *(long arrow)*. Anterior to the rostral basilar artery is another band of low intensity representing signal loss due to

exaggerated cisternal motion of CSF. This band extends superiorly across the floor of the third ventricle to blend with motion-induced signal loss in the anterior half of the ventricle. Thin, sagittal, heavily T2-weighted images from three-dimensional gradient echo sequences (e.g., "CISS" or "constructive interference in the steady state") may be used to visualize the margins of a ventriculostomy.

The phase contrast image in Case 796B confirms the continuity of a flow column from the third ventricle to the prepontine cistern *(arrows)*. This appearance establishes patency of the third ventriculostomy. If the ventriculostomy were significantly narrowed or occluded, the ventricular and cisternal phase information would be asynchronous.

Mid sagittal scans such as Case 796A are useful for demonstrating morphology of the third ventricle, aqueduct, and fourth ventricle in cases of hydrocephalus. The position of the tip of the basilar artery is important preoperative information in cases scheduled for third ventriculostomy.

**489**

### Case 797A

66-year-old woman presenting with
imbalance and vertigo.
(coronal, postcontrast T1-weighted SE scan)

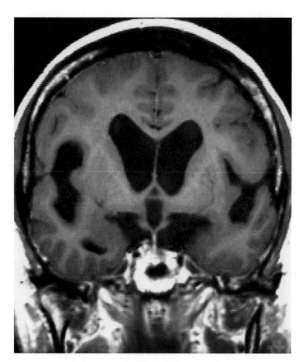

**Communicating Hydrocephalus**

### Case 797B

Same patient.
(axial, noncontrast T2-weighted SE scan)

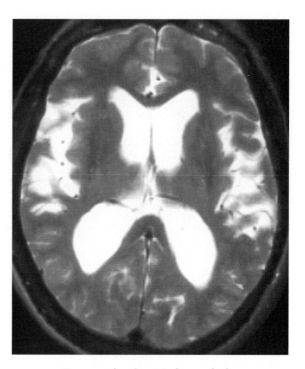

**Communicating Hydrocephalus**

Hydrocephalic expansion of all four ventricles suggests impairment of CSF flow or absorption along the surface pathways from the foramen magnum through the tentorial incisura to the parasagittal arachnoid granulations. This "communicating" pathophysiology contrasts with localized ventricular obstruction and is a common cause of infantile and adult hydrocephalus.

In infants, communicating hydrocephalus is frequently congenital and idiopathic but may also develop after meningitis or intracranial hemorrhage. Communicating hdyrocephalus in adults often follows an inflammatory meningeal process, either infectious (meningitis) or hemorrhagic (trauma or aneurysm rupture). Meningeal carcinomatosis may also present in this manner. Contrast-enhanced scans and CSF analysis to exclude meningeal pathology are important whenever ventricular enlargement is noted in the absence of an obstructing lesion.

Intracranial and spinal tumors may be associated with communicating hydrocephalus due to high CSF loads of cells, hemorrhage, and/or protein. Choroid plexus papillomas, ependymomas, and acoustic schwannomas are among the masses with this tendency. (A small acoustic schwannoma was present in Case 797.)

Multiplanar MR can support the diagnosis of communicating hydrocephalus by documenting widened superficial CSF pathways in addition to diffuse ventricular enlargement. In Case 797, the sylvian cisterns are prominently expanded with a tight contour that suggests active distention. The absence of atrophic sulci in other sites supports the interpretation of focal cisternal enlargement as a manifestation of communicating hydrocephalus.

Some adults develop low grade communicating hydrocephalus with no history of meningitis, subarachnoid hemorhage, or tumor. This "normal pressure hydrocephalus" may resemble atrophic enlargement of CSF spaces in an elderly patient.

Sagittal MR images can help to distinguish communicating hydrocephalus from atrophy. Superior bowing of the corpus callosum and inferior bulging of the third ventricular floor (causing partial effacement of the interpeduncular cistern) on such scans support the diagnosis of active ventricular distention. (See Cases 150, 294, 295, 326, 800, and 802 for examples of these findings.)

### Case 798

1-year-old boy with a large head since birth.
(coronal, noncontrast T1-weighted SE scan)

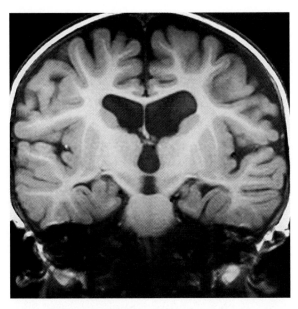

**Benign Enlargement of CSF Spaces**

### Case 799

5-month-old boy referred for
evaluation of a large head.
(axial, noncontrast T2-weighted SE scan)

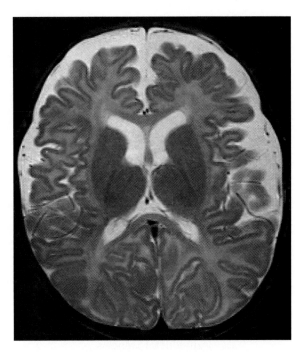

**Benign Enlargement of CSF Spaces**

Some infants who present with macrocephaly are found to have mildly enlarged ventricles in association with unusually wide subarachnoid spaces over the cerebral convexities. Cases 798 and 799 illustrate this appearance. The pattern is believed to represent a transient form of communicating hydrocephalus due to immaturity of arachnoid villi.

This condition has received many different labels, including *external hydrocephalus, benign macrocephaly of infancy,* and *benign extraaxial collections of infancy.* The head growth of affected infants usually stabilizes near the 95th percentile between ages 1 and 2. After age 2, the head size and scan appearance gradually return to normal.

It is important to recognize macrocephaly of infancy as a benign and self-limited process to be distinguished from progressive communicating hydrocephalus and from other causes of extracerebral fluid collections (subdural hygromas and hematomas). The clinical context is usually helpful: infants with benign macrocephaly are developmentally normal, with no signs of increased intracranial pressure.

MR scans establish that the convexity spaces in benign macrocephaly are subarachnoid and CSF-containing. Corti-cal vessels are usually apparent within the extracerebral fluid, which is typically symmetrical and most prominent in the frontal regions (as seen above). The cortical contour is loose, with exaggerated gyral convolutions. This appearance contrasts with the effaced sulcal markings usually seen at the vertex in cases of true hydrocephalus and underlying subdural hematomas or hygromas. (Compare the cerebral surface in the above scans to Cases 713 and 714.)

Children may alternatively have large heads because of increased intracranial tissue volume. Several pathological syndromes (e.g., mucopolysaccharidoses and gangliosidoses) are associated with megalencephaly, but many children with large brains are functionally normal. Clinical clues to benign megalencephaly include normal head shape, head growth curves parallel to standards, the absence of increased intracranial pressure, normal neurological development, and large head size of a parent.

Correlation with head size is necessary to interpret scans such as Cases 798 and 799. The same mild prominence of ventricles and subarachnoid spaces in an infant with a *small* head suggests reduced parenchymal volume due to malnutrition, dehydration, or atrophy.

## Case 800

38-year-old woman presenting with diplopia.
(sagittal, postcontrast T1-weighted SE scan)

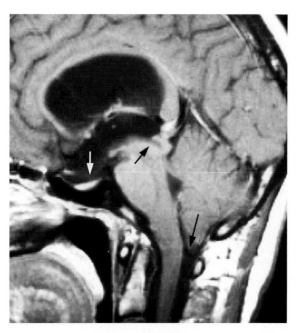

**Aqueductal Stenosis**

## Case 801

32-year-old woman presenting with
headaches and a large head.
(coronal, noncontrast T1-weighted SE scan)

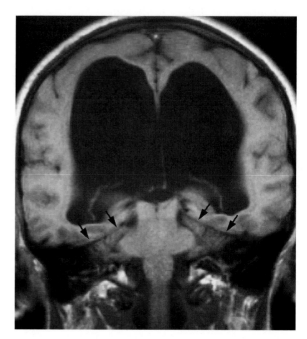

**Aqueductal Stenosis**

Aqueductal stenosis is a major cause of infantile hydrocephalus. Most cases are due to a congenital abnormality, usually "forking" or "gliosis." Infantile aqueductal stenosis may also follow ependymitis from infection or intraventricular hemorrhage. Cases of congenital origin often present in adulthood, when the borderline capacity of a narrowed aqueduct is further compromised or exceeded by some superimposed event.

The CT diagnosis of aqueductal stenosis has been based on (1) enlargement of the lateral and third ventricles without fourth ventricular expansion and (2) the absence of other lesions causing obstruction at the aqueductal level (see Cases 136 and 802). MR adds direct visualization of the aqueduct to these secondary observations. Multiplanar display and the absence of bone artifact in the posterior fossa contribute to an excellent view of midbrain anatomy on MR scans.

In Case 800, the lateral and third ventricles are distended (including inferior bowing of the third ventricular floor;

*white arrow)*, while the fourth ventricle is small. This disparity localizes obstruction to the aqueductal level. The proximal aqueduct is dilated *(short black arrow)* while the lumen of the distal aqueduct is not visualized, further defining the site of stenosis. (See Case 796A for a T2-weighted scan demonstrating similar morphology.)

The posterior fossa in Case 800 is crowded due to long-standing expansion of the supratentorial compartment. The brainstem is closely applied to clivus, and the cerebellar tonsils extend below the plane of the foramen magnum *(long black arrow)*.

Adults presenting with hydrocephalus due to aqueductal stenosis often demonstrate evidence of chronic ventricular enlargement. In Case 801, the markedly dilated lateral ventricles are associated with a small posterior fossa. (Arrows mark the low tentorium.) This finding suggests intrauterine or infantile onset of aqueductal compromise, with developmental expansion of the supratentorial compartment at the expense of the posterior fossa.

# DIFFERENTIAL DIAGNOSIS:
## HYDROCEPHALUS DUE TO AQUEDUCTAL OBSTRUCTION

### Case 802

15-year-old girl presenting with
headaches and papilledema.
(sagittal, noncontrast T1-weighted SE scan)

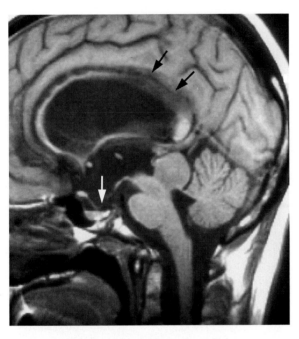

**Glioma of the Midbrain Tectum**

### Case 803

19-year-old woman presenting with blurred vision.
(sagittal, noncontrast T1-weighted SE scan)

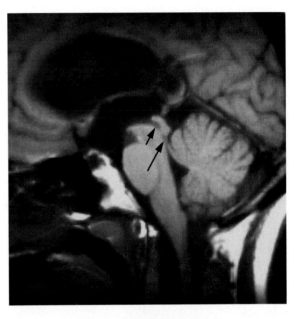

**Aqueductal Stenosis**

Case 802 demonstrates obstruction of the aqueduct due to the localized mass effect of a tectal glioma. The sagittal MR display clearly defines both the luminal compromise and the responsible tumor (compare to Case 136).

As discussed in Chapter 4, many midbrain gliomas are small, low grade lesions. The diagnosis of "benign aqueductal stenosis" on the basis of CT scans warrants an MR exam to exclude a subtle, obstructing glioma.

In Case 803, the proximal aqueduct is distended *(short arrow)*, while the lumen of the distal aqueduct is small *(long arrow)*. The junction between the segments represents the precise level of aqueductal compromise. Benign stenosis commonly occurs between the middle and distal thirds of the aqueduct, where an anatomical narrowing called the "inferior constriction" is normally located. Thin, saggittal, heavily T2-weighted CISS (constructive interference in the steady state) images are useful for defining a septum or focal narrowing within the aqueduct.

Both of the above cases demonstrate hydrocephalic stretching of the corpus callosum. In addition, callosal edema is present, particularly posteriorly in Case 802 *(black arrows)*. Edema between the transversely oriented axons of the corpus callosum often exhibits a striated appearance on sagittal or axial scans. Inferior bowing of the floor of the third ventricle is prominent in Case 802 *(white arrow)*.

In addition to small midbrain masses, another group of pathologies can mimic benign aqueductal stenosis. Cysts or tumors with fluid-like intensity values (e.g., cysticercosis, ependymal cyst, pilocytic astrocytoma, or epidermoid cyst) may obstruct the third ventricle while blending with the surrounding CSF. These masses can be easily overlooked, leading to the incorrect diagnosis of aqueductal stenosis.

Close attention to the intensity values of "CSF" within the enlarged third or fourth ventricles is warranted in all cases of hydrocephalus. "Intermediate" or "balanced" spin echo pulse sequences (long TR, short TE) and FLAIR images are particularly useful for demonstrating subtle intraventricular lesions.

## Case 804

1-year-old boy presenting with a large head.
(sagittal, noncontrast T1-weighted SE scan)

## Case 805

38-year-old woman presenting with depression.
(axial, noncontrast T2-weighted SE scan)

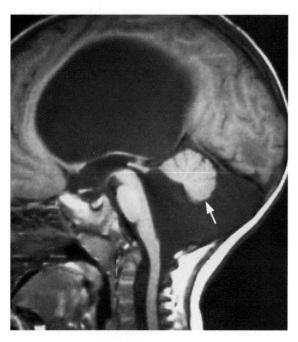

**Dandy-Walker Malformation**

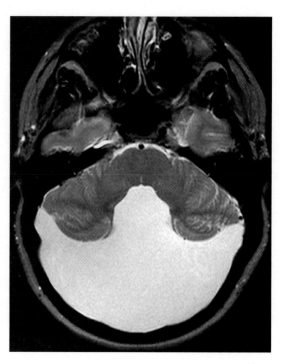

**Dandy-Walker Malformation**

The Dandy-Walker malformation consists of (1) hypoplasia and malrotation of the cerebellar vermis, and (2) a "roofless" fourth ventricle, which opens dorsally into a large posterior fossa cyst.

Associated hydrocephalus develops during the first year of life in more than three-fourths of infants born with this syndrome. The cause of ventricular enlargement is unclear, but hydrocephalus may be communicating rather than obstructive.

The sagittal MR plane has improved understanding of the Dandy-Walker malformation. As seen in Case 804, absence of the vermis on low axial sections through the posterior fossa is due more to superior rotation of this tissue than to complete aplasia. The broad communication between the fourth ventricle and the posterior fossa cyst lifts and rotates the vermis *(arrow)* superiorly against the tentorial apex. Although associated vermian hypoplasia is common, the amount of residual tissue demonstrated by MR is greater than previously appreciated on CT studies.

The cerebellar hemispheres are variably hypoplastic in patients with Dandy-Walker malformation. In Case 805, a broad communication is present between the fourth ventricle and the posterior fossa cyst. The cyst surrounds mildly compressed and hypoplastic hemispheres.

Posterior fossa arachnoid cysts (see Cases 820-823) and enlarged cisternae magnae may mimic the Dandy-Walker malformation. The integrity and position of the cerebellar vermis are keys to the differential diagnosis in such cases (see Cases 824 and 825).

Other congenital abnormalities frequently occur in association with the Dandy-Walker malformation, including hypogenesis or agenesis of the corpus callosum, heterotopic gray matter, schizencephaly, malformations of cortical development, and occipital encephaloceles.

Compare the hypogenesis of the vermis in the Dandy-Walker malformation to Joubert syndrome (Cases 867 and 868) and rhombencephalosynapsis (Case 869).

### Case 806

34-year-old man, three days after ventriculostomy
for hydrocephalus.
(axial, noncontrast T2-weighed FSE scan)

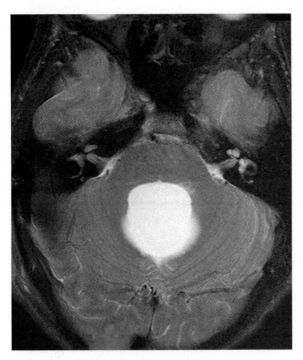

**Cysticercosis Cyst**

### Case 807

Same patient.
(sagittal, noncontrast T1-weighted SE scan)

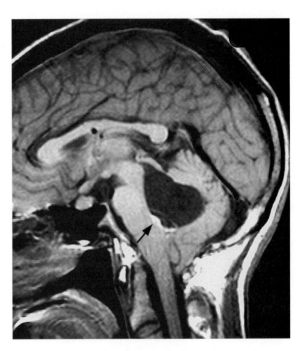

**Cysticercosis Cyst**

Expansion of the fourth ventricle may reflect distention by CSF (see Case 792) or enlargement due to an intraventricular cyst or mass, as above. A cyst obstructing the fourth ventricle and causing secondary enlargement of the lateral and third ventricles can mimic communicating hydrocephalus on initial scans.

The size and roundness of the fourth ventricle in Case 806 suggested localized pathology even before ventriculostomy was performed. Note that compressed vermian tissue clearly encloses the posterior portion of the expanded ventricle, distinguishing Case 806 from the Dandy-Walker malformations illustrated on the previous page.

An intraventricular cyst causing hydrocephalus becomes obvious when it fails to be decompressed by ventricular drainage. The lateral and third ventricles in Case 807 are small following ventriculostomy. The fourth ventricle remains prominently distended, causing ventral flattening of the pons and caudal herniation of the cerebellar tonsils.

The content of cysticercal cysts is often indistinguishable from CSF on non-contrast images, including FLAIR sequences.

Short T1 values at the inferior margin of the fourth ventricle in Case 807 *(arrow)* may represent calcification or hemorrhage at the site of the original larva.

Note the rostral extension of the cyst in Case 807, expanding the cerebral aqueduct. Compare the morphology of the aqueduct and fourth ventricle in this case to the trapped fourth ventricle in Case 792.

The fourth ventricle is the most common site for intraventricular cysticercosis. Case 525 illustrates a cysticercal cyst in the temporal horn of a lateral ventricle. Parenchymal cysticercosis is discussed in Case 469.

### Case 808

21-year-old woman presenting with seizures.
(sagittal, noncontrast T1-weighted SE scan)

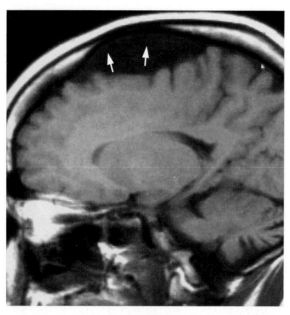

**Arachnoid Cyst**

### Case 809

16-year-old boy presenting with headaches.
(axial, noncontrast T2-weighted SE scan)

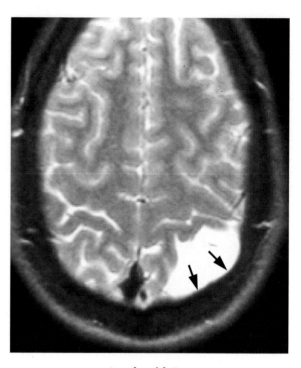

**Arachnoid Cyst**

---

Arachnoid cysts account for about 1% of intracranial masses. They are often discovered incidentally, presenting as fluid-intensity lesions in a number of characteristic locations. The cerebral convexity is a common site, as illustrated in these cases.

Convexity arachnoid cysts usually depress the underlying cerebral cortex (but see Case 810 on the next page). The interface between the cyst and the brain is often quite angular or linear. This characteristic feature may help to distinguish extensive arachnoid cysts from subdural hygromas or chronic hematomas on CT and MR studies.

Long-term pressure from arachnoid cysts frequently causes expansion or erosion of bone. This finding is well illustrated in the above cases, with scalloping of the inner table *(arrows)*. Bone remodeling establishes the chronicity of these low grade lesions, distinguishing them from subdural collections. (Compare to erosions of the inner table by low grade superficial tumors, as in Cases 73, 338, 340, and 660.)

Cortical deformity due to the arachnoid cyst in Case 808 is of questionable relevance to the patient's seizures. The cyst in Case 809 is probably incidental. Case 808 demonstrates cerebellar atrophy (possibly associated with dilantin therapy).

### Case 810

51-year-old woman presenting with
mild left hemiparesis.
(sagittal, noncontrast T1-weighted SE scan)

### Case 811

72-year-old woman presenting with ataxia.
(axial, noncontrast T2-weighted FSE scan)

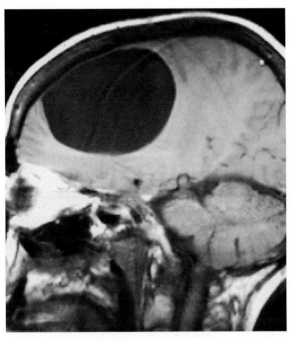

**Arachnoid Cyst**

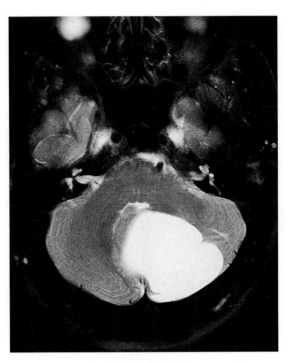

**Arachnoid Cyst**

Occasional arachnoid cysts invaginate into adjacent parenchyma, as in the above cases (see also Case 826). Such extension is relatively common with other long-standing extraaxial masses (e.g., meningiomas or schwannomas; see Cases 36 and 194) but is unusual for arachnoid cysts. As a result, an appearance such as Cases 810 and 811 may be misinterpreted as a cystic intraaxial lesion (e.g., ependymal cyst, neuroepithelial cyst, parasitic cyst, or cystic neoplasm).

Clues to the correct diagnosis in the above images include the meningeal base of the cyst, the simple character of the fluid, the absence of tissue nodules or irregularity along the margin, the lack of surrounding edema, and the morphology of compressed gyri and buckled white matter displaced by the lesion. (Compare this appearance in Case 810 to the similar ripples of compressed parenchyma adjacent to the meningioma in Case 46.)

Low attenuation CT lesions can be confirmed as CSF-containing cysts by magnetic resonance imaging. The signal intensity of such masses should match that of cisternal or ventricular fluid on all pulse sequences. FLAIR images are the most sensitive technique for demonstrating small amounts of protein or cellular debris within apparently simple fluid collections.

### Case 812

38-year-old man presenting with right orbital pain.
(coronal, noncontrast T1-weighted SE scan)

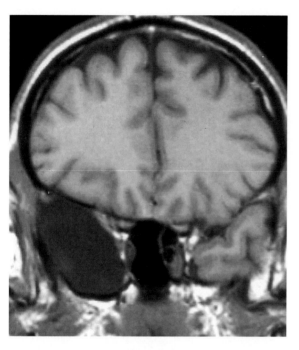

**Arachnoid Cyst**

### Case 813

19-year-old man complaining of headaches.
(axial, noncontrast T2-weighted SE scan)

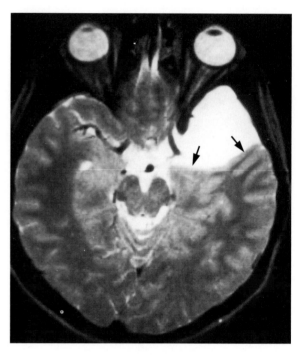

**Arachnoid Cyst**

---

Arachnoid cysts are most common near the skull base. The anterior portion of the middle cranial fossa is a particularly frequent location for these lesions, which are usually incidental findings.

In Case 812, an arachnoid cyst has caused expansion of the middle cranial fossa on the right (compare to the volume of the middle fossa on the left side). There is little midline shift because the slow growth of the cyst has been accommodated by calvarial expansion and parenchymal hypoplasia.

Case 813 presents a typical T2-weighted axial scan of another patient. Note the posterior flattening and compression of the hypoplastic left temporal lobe and the straight, somewhat angular margin between the cyst and the brain.

As illustrated above, there is usually no reactive edema surrounding arachnoid cysts. The walls of the cyst do not demonstrate abnormal contrast enhancement.

Hypoplasia of the ipsilateral temporal lobe is commonly associated with arachnoid cysts of the middle fossa. Debate

about whether this incomplete development is primary or secondary with respect to formation of the cyst does not reduce the diagnostic significance of the association.

A less frequent finding accompanying arachnoid cysts of the middle cranial fossa is hypertrophy and/or prominent pneumatization of the lesser wing of the sphenoid bone. Case 813 demonstrates enlargement of the anterior clinoid process on the side of the lesion. This appearance adjacent to a "mass" is somewhat paradoxical, resembling expansion of the sphenoid sinus beneath a meningioma of the planum sphenoidale (see Case 43). The mechanism causing this hypertrophy of bone/sinus has not been established. Speculation includes the possibilities of local meningeal traction by the cystic mass or primary parenchymal hypoplasia with secondary bone overgrowth and cyst formation.

An appearance similar to Case 812 is occasionally seen in children with chronic subdural hematomas of the middle cranial fossa. In adults, the major differential diagnosis on routine CT or MR images is an epidermoid cyst (see Cases 320-323).

### Case 814

5-month-old boy presenting with hydrocephalus.
(axial, noncontrast T2-weighted FSE scan)

### Case 815

9-year-old boy presenting with headaches.
(coronal, noncontrast T2-weighted FSE scan)

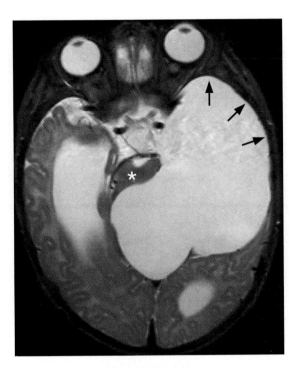

**Arachnoid Cyst**

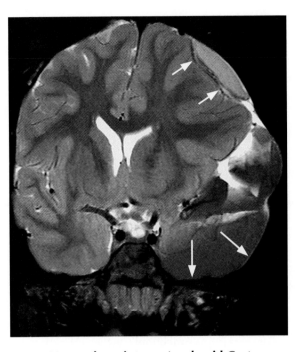

**Hemorrhage into an Arachnoid Cyst**

The characteristic extraaxial location and CSF content of typical arachnoid cysts establish the diagnosis in most cases. Occasional cysts cause confusion because of invagination (see Cases 810 and 811), large size (as in Case 814), or hemorrhage (illustrated by Case 815).

Arachnoid cysts are among the masses that may extend from one intracranial compartment to another. The cyst in Case 814 arose in the left middle cranial fossa, which is markedly enlarged *(arrows)*. Medial expansion of the cyst crosses the tentorial margin and extends inferiorly through the quadrigeminal cistern, displacing and compressing the midbrain *(asterisk)*.

The large areas of low signal intensity within the arachnoid cyst in Case 815 are due to recent hemorrhage (deoxyhemoglobin and/or intracellular methemoglobin). Bleeding within the cyst is accompanied by an adjacent subdural hematoma extending over the frontal convexity *(short arrows)*. Hemorrhage within or near an arachnoid

cyst may follow trauma (often mild) or be apparently spontaneous. Bleeding probably originates from stretched cortical veins near the perimeter of the cyst.

An appearance similar to Case 814 can be caused by a diverticulum ballooning medially from the atrium of a hydrocephalic lateral ventricle. (A coronal scan would distinguish such an intraaxial "cyst" from the extraaxial lesion illustrated above.) Like the arachnoid cyst in Case 814, medial atrial diverticula may extend inferiorly into the quadrigeminal cistern. The transtentorial morphology of the diverticulum can then be mistaken for a quadrigeminal arachnoid cyst *causing* the hydrocephalus by compressing the midbrain and aqueduct.

Note the expansion of the left middle cerebral fossa and the erosion of the inner table in Case 815 *(long arrows)*. The degree of midline shift is mild for the size of the extraaxial lesion. These findings indicate chronic mass effect that has clearly preceded the recent hemorrhage.

## Case 816

25-year-old man with a four-year
history of headaches.
(sagittal, noncontrast T1-weighted SE scan)

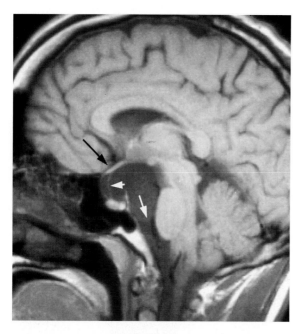

**Arachnoid Cyst**

## Case 817

34-year-old man presenting with a visual field cut.
(axial, noncontrast T2-weighted FSE scan)

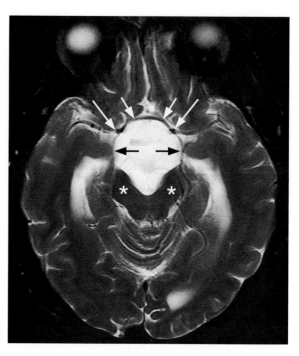

**Arachnoid Cyst**
(same patient as Case 794)

Arachnoid cysts may occur in the suprasellar region, mimicking other masses or a distended third ventricle (see Case 794). Cases 816 and 817 demonstrate the characteristic morphology of these lesions.

Suprasellar arachnoid cysts are usually associated with a prominent prepontine component. The interface between the cyst and the prepontine cistern is faintly visible in Case 816 *(long white arrow)* due to the slightly higher intensity of the cyst. This feature may reflect relatively less fluid movement within the enclosed cyst as compared to subarachnoid cisterns and/or slight elevation of protein content within the lesion.

Case 816 also documents superior displacement of the optic chiasm *(black arrow)* and anterior bowing of the pituitary infundibulum *(short white arrow)*. The floor of the third ventricle is elevated, and the basilar artery and pons are posteriorly displaced. Such evidence of mass effect distinguishes an arachnoid cyst from incidental widening of basal cisterns, which is common in children. The elevation of the optic chiasm and the posterior displacement

of the pons also distinguish a suprasellar arachnoid cyst from marked dilatation of the third ventricle.

The T2-weighted axial scan in Case 817 documents the displacements caused by the midline cyst. The A1 segments of the anterior cerebral arteries are stretched across the ventral margin of the lesion *(short white arrows)*, which spans the supraclinoid internal carotid arteries *(long white arrows)*, separates the medial temporal lobes *(black arrows)*, and splays the cerebral peduncles *(asterisks)*. Compression of the third ventricle has caused hydrocephalus, with dilatation of the temporal horns.

Epidermoid cysts should be included in the differential diagnosis of suprasellar masses with fluid-like intensity values on standard T1- and T2-weighted scans (see discussion of Cases 818, 819, 830, and 831).

Occasional suprasellar arachnoid cysts extend into the sella turcica, resembling the morphology of a cystic or necrotic pituitary adenoma or a craniopharyngioma like Case 250.

# DIFFERENTIAL DIAGNOSIS:
## MASS IN THE QUADRIGEMINAL CISTERN WITH FLUID-LIKE SIGNAL INTENSITY

### Case 818

1-year-old girl presenting with hydrocephalus.
(sagittal, noncontrast T1-weighted SE scan)

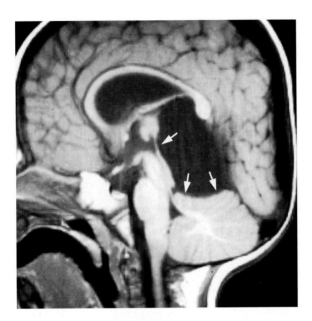

**Arachnoid Cyst**

### Case 819

36-year-old man presenting with papilledema.
(axial, postcontrast T1-weighted SE scan)

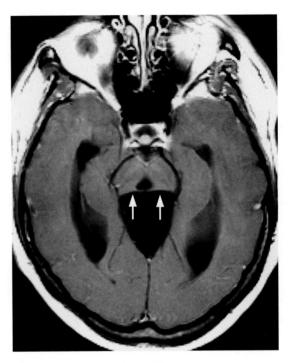

**Epidermoid Cyst**

---

The quadrigeminal cistern is a common location for both arachnoid cysts and epidermoid cysts. Small arachnoid cysts at this site resemble the pineal cysts discussed in Cases 290-293.

The large cyst in Case 818 causes marked inferior displacement of the cerebellum, anterior flattening of the midbrain and third ventricle, and elevation of the splenium of the corpus callosum. A scan at two months of age had demonstrated a cyst measuring one centimeter in diameter. The marked enlargement of an arachnoid cyst on follow-up studies is highly unusual but occasionally observed. Similarly, spontaneous decompression of arachnoid cysts has been noted (see Case 821).

The epidermoid cyst filling the tentorial apex and flattening the dorsal midbrain *(arrows)* in Case 819 resembles an arachnoid cyst due to long T1 values. The lesion would also mimic a CSF collection on T2-weighted scans (see Cases 322, 323, and 327).

The distinction between arachnoid and epidermoid cysts on standard spin echo images is based on the character of the margin and the pattern of growth. The borders of arachnoid cysts are usually smoothly rounded or angular, while the perimeter of epidermoid cysts is typically more irregular and scalloped. Arachnoid cysts displace nerves and vessels, while epidermoid cysts engulf them.

Newer MR techniques can separate these pathologies more easily. On FLAIR images, arachnoid cysts are characterized by low intensity while epidermoid cysts are not (see Case 324). Diffusion-weighted scans demonstrate facilitated diffusion (low signal intensity) in arachnoid cysts, versus restricted diffusion (high signal intensity) in epidermoid masses (see Case 325).

Compression of the aqueduct in Case 818 has caused obstructive hydrocephalus. In the presence of ventricular enlargement, the differential diagnosis of a transtentorial cyst includes a ventricular diverticulum. Such expansion of hydrocephalic ventricles may arise from the medial wall of the lateral ventricular trigone (see discussion of Case 814) or from the posterior portion of the third ventricle. Either type of diverticulum may expand to occupy the quadrigeminal cistern and/or extend infratentorially to deform the cerebellum in a manner similar to Case 818.

## Case 820

56-year-old woman presenting with
suboccipital pain.
(sagittal, noncontrast T1-weighted SE scan)

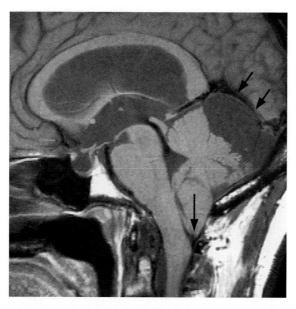

**Arachnoid Cyst**

## Case 821

1-year-old girl.
(sagittal, noncontrast T1-weighted SE scan)

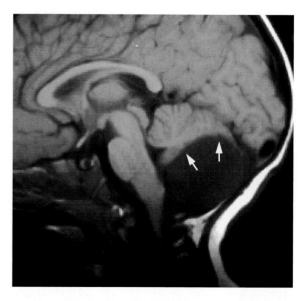

**Arachnoid Cyst**

Infratentorial arachnoid cysts occur in both retrocerebellar and anterolateral locations. The former cysts may be encountered superior or inferior to the cerebellar vermis and/or hemispheres, as seen in the above cases.

The cyst in Case 820 is marginated superiorly by the tentorium *(short arrows)*. Mass effect from the lesion has crowded the posterior fossa, with caudal herniation of the cerebellar tonsils *(long arrow)*. More anteriorly located supracerebellar arachnoid cysts may extend superiorly through the tentorial hiatus to resemble Case 818.

Case 821 demonstrates a midline cyst inferior to the cerebellum. Signal intensity within the cyst is slightly higher than cisternal or ventricular CSF (see discussion of Case 816). The morphology of displaced inferior cerebellar folia and the absence of enhancement on a postcontrast scan help to exclude the alternative diagnosis of a cystic cerebellar astrocytoma (compare to Case 142).

Posterior fossa arachnoid cysts should not be confused with the Dandy-Walker malformation, since they are not as-

sociated with defects or malrotation of the vermis. Compare the fourth ventricular morphology in the above cases to Case 804.

The child in Case 821 returned for a follow-up study three months later. The cyst was found to have spontaneously decompressed in the interval, leaving mild hypoplasia of the inferior cerebellum as the only apparent abnormality. Although most arachnoid cysts are stable lesions, occasional cysts may be observed to enlarge or shrink (see Case 818).

A partially "empty" sella and prominent CSF flow void within the aqueduct are seen in Case 820.

Low signal intensity within the basisphenoid in Case 821 suggests persistent hematopoietic marrow. This finding is common in infants and contrasts with the short T1 values of fatty marrow within the skull base in older children and adults. Fatty replacement of marrow within the clivus usually occurs by age six or seven.

**Case 822**

25-year-old woman presenting with numbness
of the arms and shoulders.
(axial, noncontrast T2-weighted SE scan)

**Case 823**

14-month-old boy.
(axial, noncontrast T2-weighted SE scan)

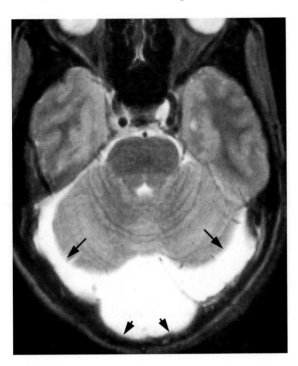

**Arachnoid Cyst**

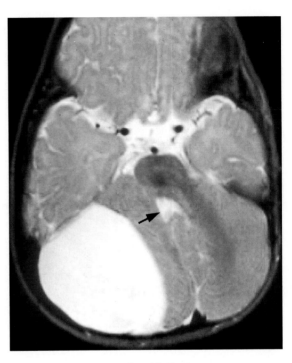

**Arachnoid Cyst**

The morphology and symmetry of retrocerebellar arachnoid cysts are variable. Case 822 demonstrates a midline lesion with symmetrical lateral extensions, while the cyst in Case 823 is more spherical and eccentric.

Arachnoid cysts near the occipital bone may overlap the spectrum of large cisternae magnae. Restricted communication between a large cisterna magna and other subarachnoid spaces may lead to evidence of mass effect, supporting the diagnosis of a functional "cyst."

In Case 822, the surface of the cerebellar hemispheres is abnormally smooth *(long arrows)* due to displacement by the lateral arms of the cyst. The midline component has caused erosion of the inner table *(short arrows)*, comparable to the supratentorial lesions in Cases 808 and 809.

The cyst is Case 823 clearly compresses underlying cerebellar tissue. The fourth ventricle *(arrow)* is displaced anteriorly and laterally.

Low signal intensity within the pons and middle cerebellar peduncles in Case 823 reflects the normal myelination of these structures in an infant. By contrast, the as yet unmyelinated white matter of the frontal and temporal lobes demonstrates high signal intensity reflecting higher water content. (Compare the relative intensity of gray and white matter within the temporal lobes in Case 823 to Case 822.)

# DIFFERENTIAL DIAGNOSIS:
## CYSTIC RETROCEREBELLAR LESION

### Case 824

25-year-old woman presenting with numbness
of the shoulders and arms.
(sagittal, noncontrast T1-weighted SE scan)

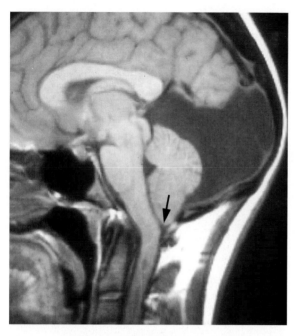

**Arachnoid Cyst**
(and hydromyelia; same patient as Case 822)

### Case 825

20-year-old woman with a history
of shunted hydrocephalus.
(sagittal, noncontrast T1-weighted SE scan)

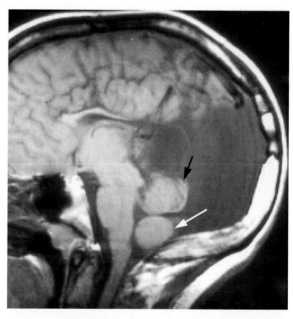

**Dandy-Walker Malformation**
(with tonsillar tissue as a pseudovermis)

---

The large arachnoid cyst in Case 824 surrounds the cerebellum posteriorly and superiorly, representing a combination of the locations in Cases 820 and 821. The cyst is clearly not an expansion of the fourth ventricle (compare to Case 804).

Mass effect is present with enlargement of the posterior fossa and erosion of the occipital bone. More importantly, the cerebellum has been displaced anteriorly and inferiorly into the foramen magnum *(arrow)*. The resulting crowding of cerebellar tissue dorsal to the cervicomedullary junction resembles a Chiari I malformation (see Cases 847 and 848) and is similarly associated with hydromyelia (faintly seen at the caudal margin of the scan).

In Case 825, the diagnosis of a Dandy-Walker malformation is confused by the presence of tissue in the expected location of vermian hypoplasia *(white arrow)*. Coronal scans demonstrated that this tissue represents medial extension of the cerebellar tonsils secondary to hypoplasia of

the inferior vermis. True vermian tissue in this case is limited to the more superior nodule of cerebellar parenchyma *(black arrow)*.

Both cases illustrate abnormally high position of the tentorium, reflecting congenital enlargement of the posterior fossa. The tentorium normally moves posteriorly and inferiorly as the cerebral hemispheres develop. Intrauterine presence of a cyst or mass within the posterior fossa prevents normal tentorial descent. (Compare to the appearance of exaggerated tentorial descent as in Cases 801, 849, and 850.)

The corpus callosum is markedly hypoplastic in Case 825. Agenesis or dysgenesis of the corpus callosum is present in about 20% of patients with the Dandy-Walker malformation. Less commonly associated congenital abnormalities include gray matter heterotopias, polymicrogyria, and occipital encephaloceles.

# DIFFERENTIAL DIAGNOSIS:
## CYSTIC CEREBELLAR MASS

### Case 826

*87-year-old woman presenting with headaches.*
*(coronal, noncontrast T1-weighted SE scan)*

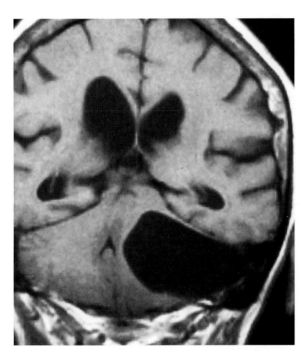

**Arachnoid Cyst**

### Case 827

*48-year-old woman presenting with ataxia.*
*(coronal, noncontrast T1-weighted SE scan)*

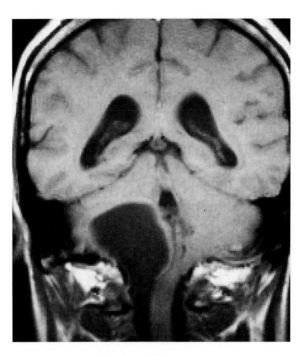

**Hemangioblastoma**

---

As discussed in Cases 810 and 811, occasional arachnoid cysts invaginate into underlying brain tissue rather than displacing it. The reasons for this unusual occurrence have not been established. Possible factors include early extension of the cyst into a sulcus or meningeal adhesions limiting convexity spread of the lesion.

The mass in Case 826 resembles a cystic cerebellar neoplasm. Clues to the correct diagnosis include the CSF-like content of the cyst, its base against the petrous bone, and the absence of a mural nodule. The relatively small shift of the fourth ventricle also favors a long-standing lesion. A postcontrast scan demonstrated no peripheral enhancement, supporting the diagnosis of a benign cyst. At surgery the lesion was documented to be extraaxial, originating from the meninges.

Case 827 is an example of a largely cystic hemangioblastoma. The signal intensity of the fluid is mildly but definitely higher than that of ventricular CSF. A small tissue nodule at the caudal pole of the cyst enhanced intensely after contrast injection, establishing the diagnosis of a cystic neoplasm. The differential diagnosis includes a cystic astrocytoma, which is rarer in adults (see Case 146).

**Case 828**

31-year-old man presenting with
a left sixth nerve palsy.
(axial, postcontrast T1-weighted SE scan)

**Case 829**

15-year-old girl presenting with
right-sided facial pain.
(axial, noncontrast T2-weighted SE scan)

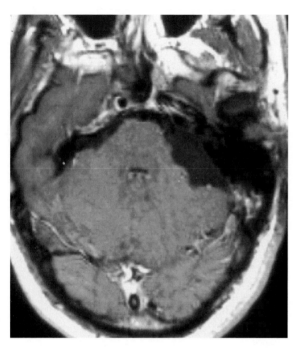

**Arachnoid Cyst**

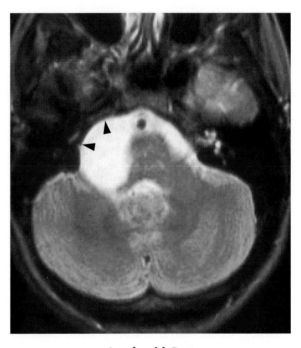

**Arachnoid Cyst**

The cerebellopontine angle is a common location for infratentorial arachnoid cysts. The lesions in Cases 828 and 829 are typical examples.

Signal intensity within the cysts is very close to cisternal or ventricular CSF on all pulse sequences. Margins are well defined. A smooth border (either linear or rounded) as in Case 829 is more characteristic than the mild irregularity of Case 828, which resembles the morphology of an epidermoid cyst (compare to Cases 320 and 322).

The cyst in Case 829 has caused erosion of the adjacent petrous bone *(arrowheads)*. This characteristic feature of arachnoid cysts helps to distinguish them from epidermoid tumors.

Masses within the cerebellopontine angle can account for a variety of cranial neuropathies. Syndromes caused by intermittent aberrant firing of sensory or motor neurons (e.g., trigeminal neuralgia and hemifacial spasm) and steadily progressive palsies (e.g., sixth nerve) may both be caused by cisternal tumors or cysts. Distortion of cranial nerves by adjacent vascular structures is another potential extraaxial etiology of cranial neuropathies (see Cases 778 and 779).

# DIFFERENTIAL DIAGNOSIS:
## CEREBELLOPONTINE ANGLE LESION WITH FLUID-LIKE SIGNAL INTENSITY

### Case 830

31-year-old man presenting with
a left sixth nerve palsy.
(axial, postcontrast T1-weighted SE scan)

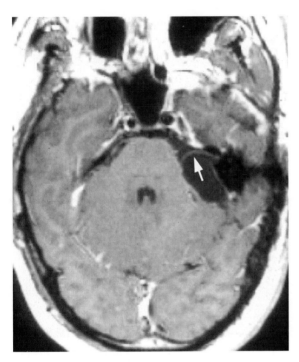

**Arachnoid Cyst**
(same patient as Case 828)

### Case 831

51-year-old man presenting with
right facial numbness.
(axial, postcontrast T1-weighted SE scan)

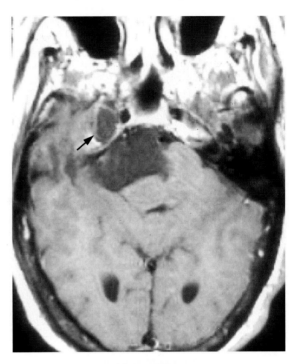

**Epidermoid Cyst**
(same patient as Case 320)

Magnetic resonance imaging can help to distinguish between arachnoid cysts and epidermoid cysts of the cerebellopontine angle. The signal intensity of these lesions is usually similar on standard spin echo images: long T1 and T2 values, with no contrast enhancement. However, their morphologies are typically characteristic.

Epidermoid cysts are soft, lobulated, infiltrating masses that tend to surround vessels and cranial nerves (see Cases 320 and 322). By contrast, arachnoid cysts are usually unilocular and smoothly marginated, stretching and displacing adjacent neurovascular structures. Bone erosion is commonly associated with arachnoid cysts and rarely seen with epidermoid masses.

Scalloped erosion of the petrous apex is suggested adjacent to the lesion in Case 830. The neurovascular bundle (seventh and eighth cranial nerves) crossing to the internal auditory canal is anteriorly displaced and bowed *(arrow).*

Neural structures can be seen *within* (i.e., surrounded by) the epidermoid mass in Case 831. The mass has extended ventrally into Meckel's cave *(arrow)*. The presenting symptom of facial numbness may reflect this component of the lesion or be due to distortion of the fifth nerve

more proximally, where it is surrounded by the cisternal portion of the mass. Arachnoid cysts rarely extend across the petrous apex in this manner.

As discussed in Cases 818 and 819, the MR distinction between arachnoid cysts and epidermoid cysts is aided by FLAIR and diffusion-weighted scans. The CSF within arachnoid cysts demonstrates uniformly low signal intensity on these images, whereas the keratinous semi-solid content of an epidermoid cyst is characterized by higher intensity on FLAIR studies and on diffusion-weighted images.

Occasional schwannomas within the cerebellopontine angle are cystic masses, as seen in Cases 192 and 196. Infrequently a cystic meningioma is encountered at this site. Coronal and sagittal MR scans help to establish the correct diagnosis in such cases by demonstrating the solid component of complex tumors, which usually enhances after contrast administration.

Racemose cysts of cysticercosis may involve the cerebellopontine angle. Another rare pathology in this differential diagnosis is a neurenteric cyst, more commonly encountered in the spinal canal (see Cases 1266 and 1267).

### Case 832

9-year-old girl with seizures and
a history of a stroke in infancy.
(coronal, noncontrast T1-weighted SE scan)

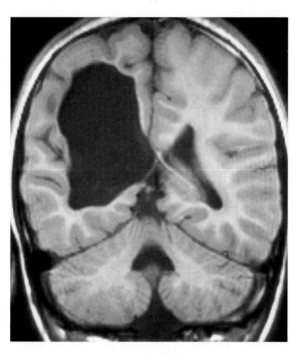

**Porencephalic Cyst**

### Case 833

27-year-old man presenting with seizures
and stable right hemiplegia.
(coronal, noncontrast T2-weighted SE scan)

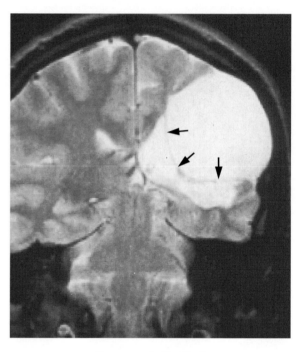

**Porencephalic Cyst**

---

The term *porencephalic cyst* is variously applied to cystic lesions that form in regions of cerebral encephalomalacia. The strict use of the phrase refers to localized expansion of the ventricular system into an area of parenchymal damage.

Case 832 is an example of this occurrence. Porencephalic expansion of the right ventricular trigone indicates the site of the childhood CVA.

Porencephalic cysts may grow and exert pressure, probably due to incomplete communication with the parent ventricle or subarachnoid pathways. Such lesions present a paradoxical appearance of mass effect in the midst of atrophy.

In Case 833, a large cyst of CSF-like intensity extends from the ventricular margin to the cortical surface of the left hemisphere. The overlying inner table is mildly eroded. A thin layer of tissue *(arrows)* separates the cyst from the ventricular chamber. Although the cyst itself is tightly rounded and associated with mass effect, ipsilateral ventricular enlargement suggests a porencephalic origin. The left hemicranium is slightly smaller than the right, supporting a history of parenchymal damage.

Compare the lack of tissue separating the intraaxial cyst from the adjacent ventricle in Case 833 to the appearance of an invaginating extraaxial arachnoid cyst in Case 826.

## DIFFERENTIAL DIAGNOSIS:
## CYST AT THE CEREBRAL SURFACE

### Case 834

48-year-old man presenting with headaches.
(coronal, noncontrast T1-weighted SE scan)

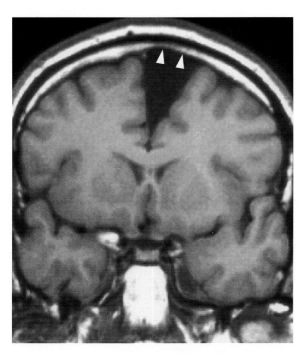

**Arachnoid Cyst**

### Case 835

22-year-old man with a history of
seizures and "cerebral palsy."
(coronal, noncontrast scan; SE 2500/28)

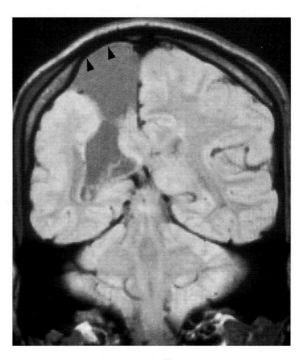

**Porencephalic Cyst**

---

Convexity arachnoid cysts occasionally involve the interhemispheric region, as in Case 834. The lateral margin of the lesion is quite linear. Mild erosion of the adjacent inner table is present superiorly *(arrowheads)*. The underlying cerebral cortex is intact although displaced. These features combine to indicate the correct diagnosis of a long-standing, extraaxial lesion.

In Case 835, a superficial cyst with CSF-like intensity values is seen at the right hemisphere vertex. The location and content of the lesion and the associated erosion of the overlying calvarium *(arrowheads)* might suggest an arachnoid cyst.

The key to the correct diagnosis in Case 835 is the status of the underlying cerebral parenchyma. The right hemisphere is small, with expansion of the right lateral ventricle. These features imply old volume loss and suggest that the superficial cyst has arisen in a region of encephalomalacia. Unlike Case 834, there is a gap between medial and lateral hemispheric cortex. Adjacent gliosis is not well seen on this scan but supports the MR diagnosis of porencephaly in other cases.

Fatty marrow within large anterior clinoid processes is present bilaterally in Case 834. This normal variant may be asymmetrical and can mimic a partially thrombosed aneurysm of the paraclinoid internal carotid artery.

## Case 836

4-week-old girl, eleven days after presenting with decreased level of consciousness.
(sagittal, noncontrast T1-weighted SE scan)

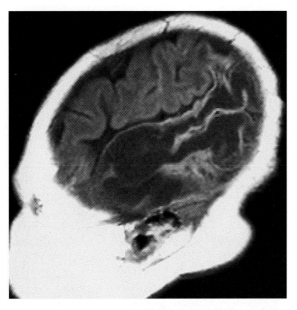

**Cystic Encephalomalacia**
(due to herpes encephalitis;
same patient as Case 688)

## Case 837

8-month-old boy with a history of perinatal anoxia.
(axial, noncontrast T2-weighted SE scan)

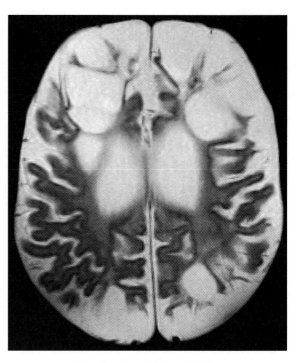

**Cystic Encephalomalacia**
(due to hypoxia/ischemia)

---

Areas of cystic encephalomalacia may occur as the result of ischemia, infection, or developmental insults. These regions may be relatively small and numerous *(multicystic encephalomalacia)* or large and unilocular *(porencephaly;* see Cases 832 and 833). The gliotic reaction that surrounds and contains zones of cystic encephalomalacia is a more mature response to cerebral injury than the generalized dissolution of tissue usually seen in cases of intrauterine or premature perinatal damage.

Neonatal herpes encephalitis is often diffuse and devastating (see Case 451). Infection in older infants may demonstrate a more multifocal pattern of hemorrhagic necrosis.

Case 836 illustrates severe parenchymal damage localized to the temporal lobe. (Scattered additional sites of encephalomalacia were present elsewhere.) A scan eleven days earlier had shown edema and mass effect in this region, with blurring of the interface between gray and white

matter and no evidence of volume loss (see Case 688). The rapid evolution to the appearance in Case 836 is typical of the progression of herpes encephalitis in infants.

As discussed in Chapter 11, diffuse ischemia or hypoxia late in gestation or in the perinatal period typically causes greatest damage to tissues at the intersection of the cortical watershed and intrahemispheric watershed zones. Case 837 demonstrates this pattern. Tissue loss is symmetrical and most severe in the border zone between the major arterial territories. Cavitation of necrotic parenchyma has resulted in large cysts in these regions. Overall reduction of cerebral volume is indicated by enlargement of the ventricles and sulci.

The multicystic nature of encephalomalacia is better demonstrated on MR scans than by CT studies, which may fail to define septations traversing and partitioning zones of low attenuation.

### Case 838A

58-year-old woman complaining of dizziness.
(coronal, postcontrast T1-weighted SE scan)

### Case 838B

Same patient.
(axial, noncontrast T2-weighted SE scan)

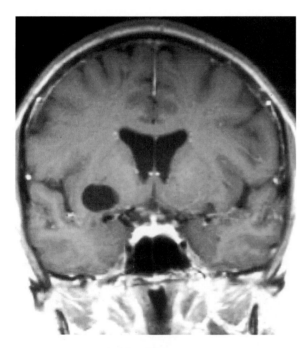

**Sublentiform Cyst**
(developmental variant)

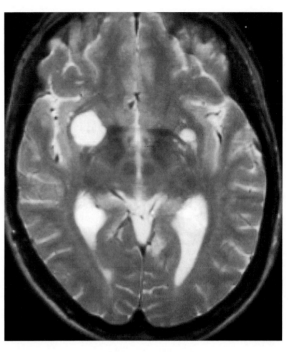

**Sublentiform Cysts**
(developmental variant)

Small developmental cysts occur in several characteristic locations within the cerebral hemispheres. A particularly common site is the sublentiform region, as illustrated above.

One or more cysts ranging in diameter from a few millimeters to several centimeters may be found unilaterally or bilaterally near the inferior margin of the putamen. The occurrence of cysts in this location usually represents localized exaggeration of prominent perivascular spaces accompanying lenticulostriate arteries into the basal ganglia.

Prominent perivascular spaces or "sublentiform cysts" are incidental and asymptomatic. They are distinguished from mass lesions by their characteristic location, sharply defined margins, round shape, lack of contrast enhancement, and absence of associated edema. The typical loca-

tion of sublentiform cysts is inferior to the site of most ganglionic infarctions. The common presence of bilateral (albeit asymmetrical) cysts helps to establish the diagnosis of a developmental variant in ambiguous cases.

Gelatinous pseudocysts within the basal ganglia due to cryptococcus could cause lesions similar in location to Case 838. Such "cysts" are typically round and nonenhancing, measuring five to ten millimeters in diameter. They are caused by fungal disease ascending from basal cisterns along perivascular spaces surrounding the lenticulostriate arteries. Cryptococcal pseudocysts are usually accompanied by clinical evidence of basal meningitis.

Compare the sublentiform location of the cysts in this case to the appearance of pallidal necrosis from carbon monoxide poisoning in Cases 671 and 672.

### Case 839

36-year-old woman presenting with dizziness.
(sagittal, noncontrast T1-weighted SE scan)

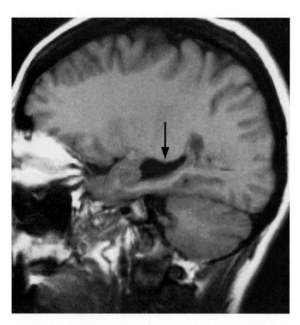

**Choroid Fissure Cyst**

### Case 840

10-year-old girl complaining of headaches.
(axial, noncontrast T2-weighted SE scan)

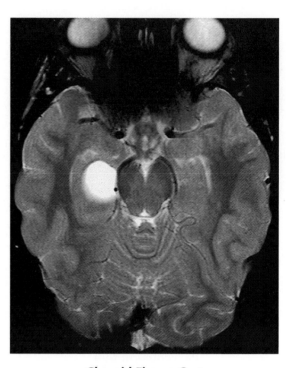

**Choroid Fissure Cyst**

---

Another common location of developmental cysts is in the choroid fissure. Such cysts may be either neuroepithelial or arachnoidal in origin.

Cases 839 and 840 present typical examples of this entity. The cysts are usually quite round on axial and coronal scans, with a characteristic spindle shape paralleling the long axis of the temporal lobe (and choroid fissure) on sagittal images. They are often about one centimeter in diameter but may be two or three times this size. Intensity values within choroid fissure cysts are close to those of CSF, and there is no associated contrast enhancement or reactive parenchymal edema.

As with the sublentiform cysts discussed on the preceding page, recognition of choroid fissure cysts as a developmental variant is important to avoid mistaking them for other lesions. The differential diagnosis of cystic masses in the medial temporal region is discussed in Cases 841 and 842.

Despite the proximity of choroid fissure cysts to the hippocampal formation, most patients with this finding do not experience seizures (or other referable symptoms).

Cysts measuring a few millimeters in diameter may be demonstrated within the hippocampal formation on high resolution scans. The small size and usual multiplicity of these incidental structures distinguish them from more medial cysts of the choroid fissure.

### Case 841

10-year-old girl presenting with headaches.
(coronal, noncontrast T1-weighted SE scan)

### Case 842

47-year-old man presenting with seizures.
(coronal, postcontrast T1-weighted GRE scan)

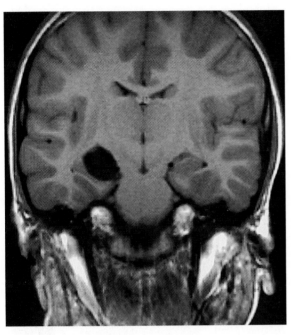

**Choroid Fissure Cyst**
(same patient as Case 840)

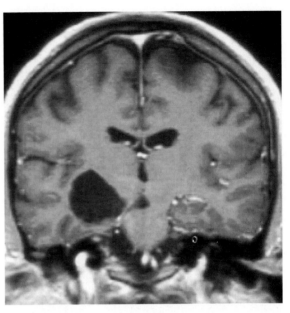

**Epidermoid Cyst**
(same patient as Case 321)

A variety of pathologies can cause a cyst-like mass in the medial temporal lobe. Potential fluid-containing lesions include a developmental cyst of the choroid fissure, as in Case 841, and a parasitic cyst within the temporal horn or adjacent tissue or sulci. (Compare the above images to the cysticercosis cyst in Case 525.)

Case 842 demonstrates that epidermoid cysts can invaginate into cerebral parenchyma to mimic an intraaxial lesion. (Compare to the dermoid cyst in Case 314.) The epidermoid mass in this case has developed within and widened the choroid fissure. The well-defined, homogeneous, non-enhancing appearance of the lesion closely resembles a simple fluid-containing cyst on routine spin echo images. (The epidermoid cyst would be brighter than CSF on FLAIR or diffusion-weighted scans.)

Low grade gliomas may involve the medial temporal lobe as well-defined, non-enhancing masses with long T1 and T2 values and should be included in this differential diagnosis (see Cases 81 and 526).

### Case 843

2-year-old boy with a "brain tumor"
reported on an outside CT scan.
(sagittal, noncontrast T1-weighted SE scan)

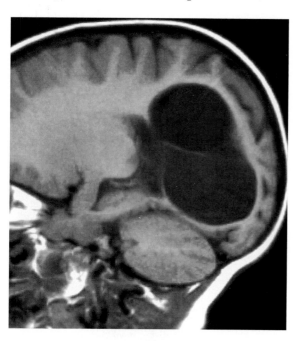

**Neuroepithelial Cyst**

### Case 844

2-year-old boy being evaluated for hypothyroidism.
(axial, postcontrast T1-weighted SE scan)

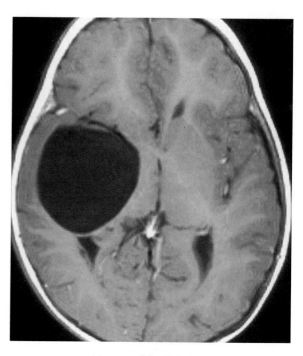

**Neuroepithelial Cyst**

When a cyst is encountered within the brain, diagnostic considerations include cystic neoplasm, abscess, parasitic cyst, cystic encephalomalacia or porencephaly, and dermoid or epidermoid cysts. The diagnosis of a benign developmental or "neuroepithelial" cyst is entertained when alternative etiologies have been excluded.

Sporadic cysts can occur anywhere within cerebral parenchyma and may be unrelated to fissures or ventricles. They likely arise from neuroepithelial or ependymal cell rests enclosed during embryogenesis. Although the above patients are children, neuroepithelial cysts may be incidentally discovered or present in adulthood.

The large cyst in Case 843 demonstrates at least one fold or septation. Location of the cyst adjacent to the ventricular margin suggests possible origin from aberrant ependymal development. Mass effect from the lesion causes ante-

rior displacement of the lateral ventricle, but there is no evidence of surrounding edema. Ependymal cysts may also arise within ventricular chambers, causing obstructive hydrocehalus while blending with surrounding CSF in a manner analogus to parasitic intraventricular lesions (see Cases 806 and 807).

The cyst in Case 844 had been observed to triple in size within one year. Despite this rapid growth, the cyst appears benign. Margins are smoothly rounded and well demarcated, demonstrating no abnormal contrast enhancement. Surgery disclosed a simple unilocular neuroepithelial cyst, with no communication to the subarachnoid space or ventricular system. The mechanism by which such cysts may enlarge has not been established. (Compare to the occasional dramatic growth of arachnoid cysts, as in Case 818.)

### Case 845

17-year-old boy with Down syndrome
and acute lymphocytic leukemia.
(axial, noncontrast T2-weighted SE scan)

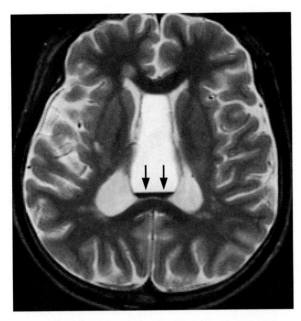

**Cavum Septi Pellucidi and Cavum Vergae**
(with hemorrhage)

### Case 846

10-year-old boy with macrocephaly and retardation.
(axial, postcontrast T1-weighted SE scan)

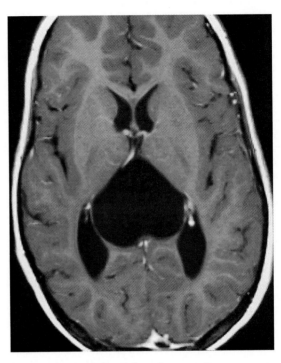

**Cyst of the Velum Interpositum**

---

A variety of CSF-containing midline cysts can occur as developmental variants. A fluid space enclosed by the leaves of the septum pellucidum is a normal feature of developing brains but is usually obliterated soon after birth. A persistent septal cyst between the frontal horns *(cavum septi pellucidi)* is demonstrated in about 5% to 10% of adults. The posterior extension of a cavum septi pellucidi beyond the columns of the fornix and foramina of Monro has been called a "cavum vergae," but this arbitrary distinction of nomenclature does not reflect anatomical partitioning of the single septal chamber.

Persistent cavi septi pellucidi are usually only a few millimeters in diameter. Larger septal cysts do occur, as illustrated in Case 845, but even these are rarely symptomatic. Occasionally a cavum within the anterior portion of the septum pellucidum obstructs the foramina of Monro like a colloid cyst and must be decompressed. There is no evidence of hydrocephalus in Case 845.

Cysts of the septum pellucidum normally contain simple CSF and demonstrate no enhancement. These features (and the truly midline location) distinguish cavi septi pellucidi from rare parasitic or neoplastic cysts within the lateral ventricles. The small sedimentation level of blood products within the dependent portion of the cyst in Case 845 *(arrows)* is unusual and may reflect coagulopathy related to the patient's leukemia.

The large midline cyst in Case 846 is CSF-filled and nonenhancing, but it is clearly not associated with persistence of a cavum within the septum pellucidum more anteriorly. The mass more likely represents a cyst arising in the velum interpositum, the normally narrow space between the roof of the third ventricle and the fornices at the inferior margin of the lateral ventricles. Such cysts may be arachnoidal or neuroepithelial in origin.

Small developmental cysts within the velum interpositum *(cavum veli interpositi)* typically have the shape of an elongated triangle pointing anteriorly. Larger cysts become more rounded and mass-like, as in Case 846. Large cysts of the velum interpositum can project posteroinferiorly to act as any other subsplenial mass (see Cases 295 and 296), potentially compressing the dorsal midbrain and aqueduct. The posterior portion of such lesions resembles a pineal cyst or an arachnoid cyst of the quadrigeminal cistern (see Case 818).

# REFERENCES

Aleman J, Jokura H, Higano S, et al: Value of constructive interference in steady state three-dimensional, fourier transformation magnetic resonance imaging for neuroendoscopic treatment of hydrocephalus and intracranial cysts. *Neurosurgery* 48:1291-1296, 2001.

Altman NR, Naidich TP, Braffman BH: Posterior fossa malformations. *AJNR* 13:691-724, 1992.

Aprile I, Iaiza F, Lavaroni A, et al: Analysis of cystic intracranial lesions performed with fluid-attenuated inversion recovery MR imaging. *AJNR* 20:1259-1267, 1999.

Aoki N: Extracerebral fluid collections in infancy: role of magnetic resonance imaging in differentiation between subdural effusion and subarachnoid space enlargement. *J Neurosurg* 81:20-23, 1994.

Atlas W, Mark AS, Fram EK: Aqueductal stenosis: evaluation with gradient echo imaging. *Radiology* 169:449-453, 1988.

Baker LL, Barkovich AJ: The large temporal horn: MR analysis in developmental brain anomalies versus hydrocephalus. *AJNR* 13:115-122, 1992.

Barkovich AJ, Kjos BO, Norman D, Edwards MS: Revised classification of posterior fossa cysts and cystlike malformations based on the results of multiplanar MR imaging. *AJNR* 10:977-988, 1989.

Barkovich AJ, Newton TH: MR of aqueductal stenosis. Evidence of a broad spectrum of tectal distortion. *AJNR* 10:471-476, 1989.

Boaz JC, Edwards-Brown MK: Hydrocephalus in children: neurosurgical and neuroimaging concerns. *Neuroimaging Clin North Am* 9:73-92, 1999.

Boockvar JA, Shafa R, Forman MS, O'Rourke DM: Symptomatic lateral ventricular ependymal cysts: criteria for distinguishing these rare cysts from other symptomatic cysts of the ventricles: case report. *Neurosurgery* 46:1229-1232, 2000.

Bourekas EC, Raji MR, Dastur KJ, et al: Retroclival arachnoid cyst. *AJNR* 13:353-354, 1992.

Bradley WG : Commentary—normal pressure hydrocephalus: new concepts on etiology and diagnosis. *AJNR* 21:1586-1590, 2000.

Bradley WG Jr: Commentary: MR prediction of shunt response to NPH: CSF morphology versus physiology. *AJNR* 19:1285-1286, 1998.

Bradley WG, Kortman KE, Burgoyne B: Flowing cerebrospinal fluid in normal and hydrocephalic states: appearance on MR image. *Radiology* 159:611-616, 1986.

Bradley WG Jr, Scalzo D, Queralt J, et al: Normal-pressure hydrocephalus: evaluation with cerebrospinal fluid flow measurements at MR imaging. *Radiology* 198:523-529, 1996.

Bradley WG Jr, Whittemore AR, Watanabe AS, et al: Association of deep white matter infarction with chronic communicating hydrocephalus: implications regarding the possible origin of normal-pressure hydrocephalus. *AJNR* 12:31-39, 1991.

Britton J, Marsh H, Kendall B, et al: MRI and hydrocephalus in childhood. *Neuroradiology* 30:310-314, 1988.

Chang K-H, Song IC, Kim SH, et al: In vivo single-voxel proton MR spectroscopy in intracranial cystic masses. *AJNR* 19:401-406, 1998.

Chaynes P, Thorn-Kany M, Sol JC, et al: Imaging in neurenteric cysts of the posterior cranial fossa. *Neuroradiology* 40:374-376, 1998.

Choi SK, Starshak RJ, Meyer GA, et al: Arachnoid cyst of the quadrigeminal plate cistern: report of two cases. *AJNR* 7:725-728, 1986.

Ciricillo SF, Cogen PH, Harsh GR, Edwards MSB: Intracranial arachnoid cysts in children. *J Neurosurg* 74:230-235, 1991.

Czervionke LF, Daniels DL, Meyer GA, et al: Neuroepithelial cyst of the lateral ventricles: MR appearance. *AJNR* 8:609-613, 1987.

Dross PE, Lally JF, Bonier B: Pneumosinus dilatans and arachnoid cyst: a unique association. *AJNR* 13:209-211, 1992.

El Gammal T, Allen MB Jr, Brooks BS, Mark EK: MR evaluation of hydrocephalus. *AJNR* 8:591-597 1987.

Elmadbouh H, Halpin SFS, Neal J, et al: Posterior fossa epithelial cyst: case report and review of the literature. *AJNR* 20:681-685, 1999.

Fitz CR: Disorders of ventricles and CSF spaces. *Semin US CT MR* 9:216-230, 1988.

Fukuhara T, Vorster SJ, Ruggieri P, Luciano MG: Third ventriculostomy patency: comparison of findings at cine phase-contrast MR imaging and at direct exploration. *AJNR* 20:1560-1566, 1999.

Gammal T, Allen M, Brooks B, et al: MR evaluation of hydrocephalus. *Am J Roentgenol* 149:807-813, 1987.

Gandy SE, Heier LA, Clinical and magnetic resonance features of primary intracranial arachnoid cysts. *Ann Neurol* 21:342-348, 1987.

Garcia Santos JM, Martinez-Lage J, Ubeda AG, et al: Arachnoid cysts of the middle fossa: a consideration of their origins based on imaging. *Neuroradiology* 39:395-358, 1993.

Gideon P, Stahlberg F, Thomsen C, et al: Cerebrospinal fluid flow and production in patients with normal pressure hydrocephalus studied by MRI. *Neuroradiology* 36:210-215, 1994.

Goeser CD, McLeary MS, Young LW: Diagnostic imaging of ventriculoperitoneal shunt malfunctions and complications. *Radiographics* 18:635-651, 1998.

Greitz D, Greitz T: The pathogenesis and hemodynamics of hydrocephalus: proposal for a new understanding. *Int J Neurorad* 3:367-375, 1997.

Hanigan WC, Wright R, Wright S: Magnetic resonance imaging of the Dandy-Walker malformations. *Pediatr Neurosci* 12:151-156, 1985-1986.

Ho SS, Kuzniecky RI, Gilliam F, et al: Congenital porencephaly: MR features and relationship to hippocampal sclerosis. *AJNR* 19:135-142, 1998.

Hoffmann KT, Hosten N, Meyer BU, et al: CSF flow studies of intracranial cysts and cyst-like lesions achieved using reversed fast imaging with steady-state precession MR sequences. *AJNR* 21:493-502, 2000.

Hofmann E, Becker T, Jackel M, et al: The corpus callosum in communicating and noncommunicating hydrocephalus. *Neuroradiology* 37:212-218, 1995.

Holodny AI, Waxman R, George AE, et al: MR differential diagnosis of normal-pressure hydrocephalus and Alzheimer disease: significance of perihippocampal fissures. *AJNR* 19:813-820, 1998.

Jack CR, Mokri B, Laws ER Jr, et al: MR findings in normal pressure hydrocephalus: significance and comparison to other forms of dementia. *J Comput Assist Tomogr* 11:923-931, 1987.

Jinkins JR: Clinical manifestations of hydrocephalus caused by impingement of the corpus callosum on the falx: an MR study in 40 patients. *AJNR* 12:331-340, 1991.

Jungreis CA, Kanal E, Hirsch WL, et al: Normal perivascular spaces mimicking lacunar infarction: MR imaging. *Radiology* 169:101-104, 1988.

Kalidasan V, Carroll T, Allcutt CT, Fitzgerald RJ: The Dandy-Walker syndrome—a 10-year experience of its management and outcome. *Eur J Pediatr Surg* 5:16-18, 1995.

Kemp SS, Zimmerman RA, Bilaniuk LT, et al: Magnetic resonance imaging of the cerebral aqueduct. *Neuroradiology* 29:430-436, 1987.

Kimura M, Tanaka A, Yoshinaga S: Significance of periventricular hemodynamics in normal pressure hydrocephalus. *Neurosurgery* 30:701-705, 1992.

Kitagaki H, Mori E, Ishii K, et al: CSF spaces in idiopathic normal pressure hydrocephalus: morphology and volumetry. *AJNR* 19:1277-1284, 1998.

Kjos BO, Brant-Zawadzki M, Kucharczyk W, et al: Cystic intracranial lesions: magnetic resonance imaging. *Radiology* 155:363-370, 1985.

Kollias SS, Ball WS Jr, Prenger EC: Cystic malformations of the posterior fossa: differential diagnosis clarified through embryologic analysis. *Radiographics* 13:1211-1232, 1993.

Kollias SS, Prenger EC, Becket WW Jr, et al: Posterior fossa cystic malformations: possible pitfalls in radiographics diagnosis. *Radiology* 185(suppl):403, 1992.

Kulkarni AV, Drake JM, Armstrong DC, Dirks PB: Imaging correlates of successful endoscopic third ventriculostomy. *J Neurosurg* 92:915-919, 2000.

Kulkarni V, Daniel RT, Haran RP: Extradural endodermal cyst of posterior fossa, review of the literature, and embryogenesis: *Neurosurgery* 47:764-767, 2000.

Kurihara N, Takahashi S, Tamura H, et al; Investigation of hydrocephalus with three-dimensional constructive interference in steady state MRI. *Neuroradiology* 42:634-638, 2000.

Lane JI, Luetmer PH, Atkinson JL: Corpus callosal signal changes in patients with obstructive hydrocephalus after ventriculoperitoneal shunting. *AJNR* 22:155-162, 2001.

Laitt RD, Mallucci CL, Jaspan T, et al: Constructive interference in steady-state 3D Fourier-transform MRI in management of hydrocephalus and third ventriculostomy. *Neuroradiology* 41:117-123, 1999.

LeBlang SD, Falcone S, Quencer RM: Enhancing meningeal blood vessels masquerading as leptomeningeal spread of tumor in obstructive hydrocephalus. *AJNR* 16:1742-1744, 1995.

Lev S, Bhadelia RA, Estin D, et al: Functional analysis of third ventriculostomy patency with phase-contrast MRI velocity measurements. *Neuroradiology* 39:175-179, 1997.

Machado MadC, Vieira NA, Matos PE, et al: External hydrocephalus: a review of 15 cases. *Int J Neurorad* 5:266-270, 1999.

Malcolm GP, Symon L, Kendall B, Pires M: Intracranial neurenteric cysts. *J Neurosurg* 75:115-120, 1991.

Miyajima M, Arai H, Okuda O, et al: Possible origin of suprasellar arachnoid cysts: neuroimaging and neurosurgical observations in nine cases. *J Neurosurg* 93:62-67, 2000.

Nakase H, Ishida Y, Tada T, et al: Neuroepithelial cysts of the lateral ventricle. *Surg Neurol* 37:94-100, 1992.

Prassopoulos P, Cavouras, Golfinopoulos S, Nezi M: The size of the intra- and extraventricular cerebrospinal fluid compartments in children with idiopathic benign widening of the frontal subarachnoid space. *Neuroradiology* 37:418-421, 1995.

Quencer RM: Intracranial CSF flow in pediatric hydrocephalus: evaluation with Cine-MR imaging. *AJNR* 13:601-608, 1992.

Quint DJ: Retroclival arachnoid cysts. *AJNR* 13:1503-1504, 1992.

Robertson SJ, Wolpert SM, Runge VM: MR imaging of middle cranial fossa arachnoid cysts: temporal lobe agenesis syndrome revisited. *AJNR* 10:1007-1010, 1989.

Rovira A, Capellades J, Grive E, et al: Spontaneous ventriculostomy: report of three cases revealed by flow-sensitive phase-contrast cine MR imaging. *AJNR* 20:1647-1652, 1999.

Sakamoto H, Fujitani K, Kitano S, et al: Cerebrospinal fluid edema associated with shunt obstruction. *J Neurosurg* 81:179-183, 1994.

Schumacher DJ, Tien RD, Friedman H: Gadolinium enhancement of the leptomeninges caused by hydrocephalus: a potential mimic of leptomeningeal metastasis. *AJNR* 15:639-641, 1994.

Sherman JL, Componovo E, Citrin CM: MR imaging of CSF-like choroidal fissure and parenchymal cysts of the brain. *AJNR* 11:939-945, 1990.

Silbert PL, Gubbay SS, Vaughan RJ: Cavum septum pellucidum and obstructive hydrocephalus. *J Neurol Neurosurg Psychiatry* 56:820-822, 1993.

Tsuchiya K, Hachiya J, Shiokawa Y, Saito I: Differentiating intracranial epidermoid tumors from arachnoid cysts by FLAIR magnetic resonance imaging. *Int J Neurorad* 3:376-380, 1997.

Tsuruda JS, Chew WM, Moseley ME, Norman D: Diffusion-weighted MR imaging of the brain: value of differentiating between extraaxial cysts and epidermoid tumors. *AJNR* 11:925-931, 1990.

Van Tassel P, Cure JK: Nonneoplastic intracranial cysts and cystic lesions. *Semin Ultrasound CT MRI* 16:186-211, 1995.

Weiner SN, Pearlstein AE, Eiber A: MR imaging of intracranial arachnoid cysts. *J Comput Assist Tomogr* 11:236-241, 1987.

Wester K: Gender distribution and sidedness of middle fossa arachnoid cysts: a review of cases diagnosed with computed imaging. *Neurosurgery* 31:940-944, 1992.

Wilms G, Venderschueren G, Demaerel PH, et al: CT and MR in infants with pericerebral collections and macrocephaly: benign enlargement of the subarachnoid spaces versus subdural collections. *AJNR* 14:855-860, 1993.

Yang D, Korogi Y, Ushio Y, Takahashi M: Increased conspicuity of intraventricular lesions revealed by three-dimensional constructive interference in steady state sequences. *AJNR* 21:1070-1072, 2000.

# CHAPTER 16

# Developmental Abnormalities

## Case 847

34-year-old man presenting with
bilateral arm numbness.
(sagittal, noncontrast T1-weighted SE scan)

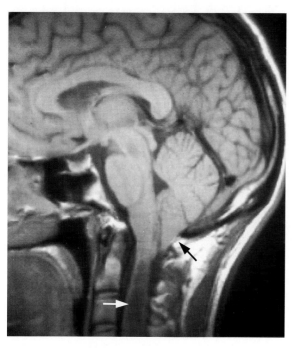

**Chiari I Malformation**

## Case 848

5-year-old boy presenting with occipital headaches.
(sagittal, noncontrast T1-weighted SE scan)

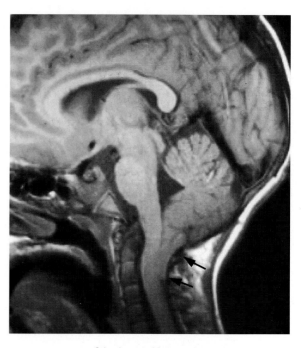

**Chiari I Malformation**

---

The Chiari I hindbrain malformation consists of abnormal inferior extension of the cerebellar tonsils through the plane of the foramen magnum. The low-lying tonsils tend to be peg-shaped or inferiorly pointed, as seen in the above cases *(black arrows)*.

This "malformation" probably represents secondary deformity caused by a small or crowded posterior fossa. The tonsils often become nearly normal in position and morphology when patients with Chiari I malformations are treated by decompression of the foramen magnum.

The caudal margin of normal tonsils may reside up to three or four millimeters below a line from the basion to the opisthion. Greater degrees of tonsillar ectopia suggest congenital malformation (or acquired herniation).

Chiari I malformations may be incidentally encountered in patients who have no related symptoms. Alternatively, crowding of tissue within the foramen magnum may compress the cervicomedullary junction, causing headaches (as in Case 848), neck pain, and/or lower cranial neuropathies.

Symptoms in other patients are due to hydromyelia, which develops in about 20% to 30% of cases. This association is believed to reflect abnormal hydrodynamics within the cervical spinal canal, with caudal systolic motion of the tonsils obstructing the foramen magnum and acting as a piston to increase cervical CSF pressure (see discussion of Cases 1228 and 1229). The frequent occurrence of syringomyelia warrants careful examination of the cervical spinal cord when a Chiari I hindbrain malformation is discovered. In Case 847, a cyst within the spinal cord is faintly seen at the inferior margin of the scan *(white arrow)*.

Intracranial hypotension (See Case 540) and secondary herniation (due to increased intracranial pressure or mass effect in the posterior fossa) should be considered along with Chiari I malformation in the differential diagnosis of low-lying cerebellar tonsils.

## Case 849

3-year-old girl with a history of myelomeningocele
repair at birth.
(sagittal, noncontrast T1-weighted SE scan)

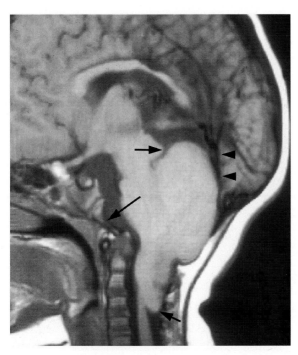

**Chiari II Malformation**

## Case 850

2-year-old girl with spina bifida.
(sagittal, noncontrast T1-weighted SE scan)

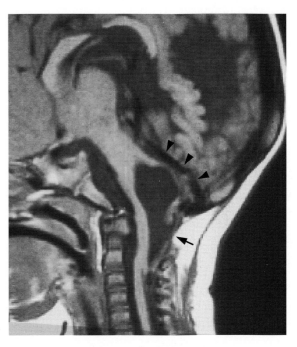

**Chiari II Malformation**

---

The Chiari II ("Arnold Chiari") hindbrain malformation is much more severe and complex than the Chiari I deformity. More extensive caudal herniation of the hindbrain into the cervical spinal canal is present, almost invariably associated with a lumbosacral myelomeningocele.

Case 849 illustrates a typical cascade of herniating tissue extending inferiorly from the small posterior fossa through the wide foramen magnum. Buckling of the caudally displaced medulla often forms a tissue layer between the herniated cerebellum and the spinal cord (*lowest arrow,* Case 849).

The fourth ventricle in Chiari II malformations is usually caudally elongated and slit-like due to tissue crowding. When a "normal"-sized or enlarged fourth ventricle is seen (as in Case 850), distention or trapping should be suspected (see discussion of Case 792).

The combination of herniating posterior fossa tissue and commonly associated supratentorial hydrocephalus results in a small posterior fossa. Accompanying cerebellar hypoplasia is variable. Very little cerebellar tissue is present in the tiny posterior fossa of Case 850.

Crowding of the hindbrain within the small posterior fossa causes characteristic patterns of bone erosion. Ventrally concave scalloping of the clivus (*long arrow,* Case 849) is typical and most apparent on sagittal MR scans after shunting has reduced intracranial pressure. Similar concave remodeling is often seen along the posterior margin of the petrous bones on axial scans.

The above cases illustrate additional abnormalities associated with the Chiari II hindbrain malformation. Hypoplasia of the corpus callosum (particularly posteriorly) is usually present, as is an abnormal gyral pattern most prominent in the medial occipital regions. "Beaking" of the midbrain tectum (*upper arrow,* Case 849) is characteristic, often reflecting both primary malformation (with fusion of colliculi into a single peak) and secondary deformity (due to long-standing lateral compression from hydrocephalic hemispheres). The straight sinus is abnormally low and vertical in both of these patients (*arrowheads*).

**Case 851**

18-year-old man with a history of
myelomeningocele repair at birth.
(axial, noncontrast T2-weighted SE scan)

**Case 852**

4-year-old girl, with a history of myelomeningocele
repair and shunted hydrocephalus.
(axial, noncontrast T2-weighted SE scan)

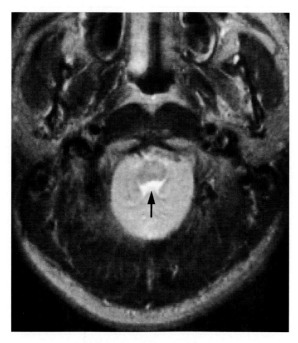

**Chiari II Malformation**

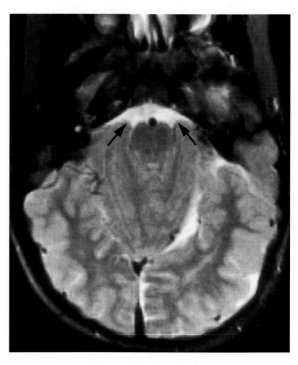

**Chiari II Malformation**

Axial scans document the crowding and deformity of infratentorial tissue in patients with Chiari II hindbrain malformations.

The abnormally large foramen magnum in Case 851 is filled by cerebellar parenchyma surrounding the lateral and posterior aspects of the medulla and low-lying fourth ventricle *(arrow).* A similar appearance is seen in Case 852, where the cerebellar hemispheres wrap ventrally around the pons to reach the prepontine cistern *(arrows).*

Case 852 illustrates a very narrow posterior fossa with a steeply sloping tentorium (see also Case 854). Mild concave erosion along the posterior surface of the petrous ridges is suggested medially. This remodeling of bone may be much more prominent in other cases.

The Chiari II malformation ranks with communicating hydrocephalus and aquedutal stenosis among the major causes of congenital hydrocephalus. If hydrocephalus is not present at birth, it usually develops rapidly following surgical closure of an associated myelomeningocele. Like aqueductal stenosis (see Case 801), the Chiari II malformation presents with overall cranial enlargement in the presence of a small posterior fossa.

The developmental sequence of events leading to the Chiari II malformation is believed to involve an abnormally small rhombencephalic ventricle due to patency or decompression of the intrathecal compartment at the site of the myelomeningocele. The volume enclosed by enchondral bone induced to surround the posterior fossa is therefore too small, leading to caudal herniation of the subsequently developing hindbrain parenchyma.

### Case 853

1-year-old girl with a history of myelomeningocele
repair and shunted hydrocephalus.
(axial, noncontrast T2-weighted SE scan)

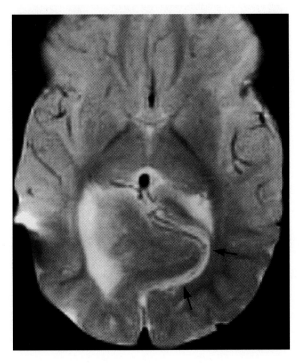

**Chiari II Malformation**

### Case 854

11-month-old boy with a history of
myelomeningocele repair and shunted
hydrocephalus.
(coronal, noncontrast T1-weighted SE scan)

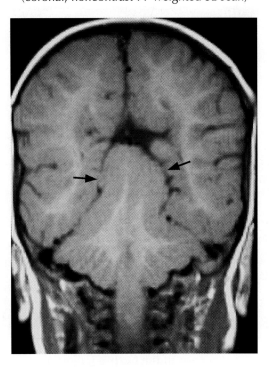

**Chiari II Malformation**

Several striking deformities of brain tissue may accompany Chiari II malformations at presentation or following treatment.

Hypoplasia and/or fenestration of the falx is common, often associated with interdigitation of gyri in the medial occipital regions. Case 853 presents a typical example of this deformity. The posterior interhemispheric fissure is bowed far to the left *(arrows)* as the right occipital lobe crosses midline.

Case 854 demonstrates the characteristically "towering" cerebellar vermis that often develops in patients with Chiari II malformations after shunting. Decompression of supratentorial mass effect allows the crowded cerebellum to expand superiorly, accentuated by the steeply sloping tentorium. This impressive rostral extension of bulky and dysmorphic tissue may be misinterpreted as a new midline mass, particularly on axial CT studies.

An abnormal gyral pattern on the medial surface of the cerebral hemispheres is again illustrated in Case 854.

Dysplasia of the hippocampus is common in association with other congenital malformations of the brain (see Case 866). The hippocampal formations may be abnormally vertical, globular, or noninverted in such cases.

The Chiari II malformation is occasionally accompanied by an occipital and/or cervical encephalocele containing herniated hindbrain tissue. See Cases 912 and 913 for discussion of this "Chiari III" deformity.

## Case 855

37-year-old woman being evaluated
for possible demyelinating disease.
(sagittal, noncontrast T1-weighted SE scan)

## Case 856

3-year-old boy presenting with developmental delay.
(coronal, noncontrast T1-weighted SE scan)

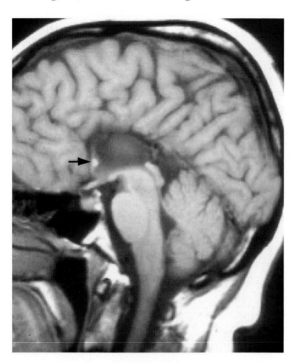

**Agenesis of the Corpus Callosum**

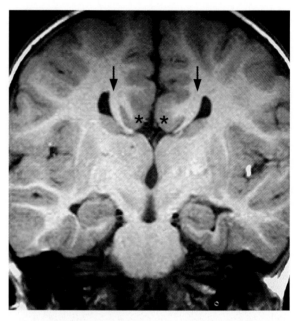

**Agenesis of the Corpus Callosum**

Callosal dysgenesis or agenesis is apparent on sagittal and coronal MR images. In Case 855, the expected structure of the corpus callosum is absent. Sulci on the medial surface of the hemisphere have an abnormal radial pattern, extending inferiorly to nearly reach the third ventricle and velum interpositum. The anterior commissure is hypertrophied *(arrow)*.

Case 856 demonstrates a "high-riding" third ventricle meeting the interhemispheric fissure, with no separation by crossing callosal tissue. Enlargement of the third ventricle in this position may form an interhemispheric cyst. (A separate and larger dorsal interhemispheric cyst may be seen in some cases of callosal agenesis, as in other congenital abnormalities; see Case 790.)

The lateral ventricles in Case 856 are widely separated, resembling the head of a longhorn steer when viewed coronally with the third ventricle. The narrow diameter and comma-shaped morphology of the lateral ventricles is due to indentation of their medial margin by the bundles of Probst *(arrows)*. These longitudinal fiber bands represent

axons that would normally cross in the corpus callosum but have instead formed parasagittal tracts (see Case 857). Malrotated cingulate gyri are present medial to the bundles of Probst *(asterisks)*; the gyri have not been normally inverted by development of a subjacent interhemispheric bridge of callosal tissue (compare to Case 863).

Dysgenesis of the corpus callosum may be incomplete. Most common is hypogenesis of the posterior portion, indicating arrest of callosal development. (Formation of the corpus callosum generally proceeds from anterior to posterior; development of the posterior portion of the genu is followed sequentially by the body, the anterior aspect of the genu, the splenium, and the rostrum.)

Agenesis or dysgenesis of the corpus callosum is frequently associated with other congenital abnormalities of the brain. Examples include the Dandy-Walker malformation, Chiari II malformation, encephaloceles, and neuronal migration abnormalities. Isolated callosal agenesis is often an incidental finding on scans obtained for unrelated complaints.

# DIFFERENTIAL DIAGNOSIS:
## DILATATION OF THE POSTERIOR PORTIONS OF THE LATERAL VENTRICLES

### Case 857

21-year-old man presenting with seizures.
(axial, noncontrast T2-weighted SE scan)

### Case 858

18-month-old girl with "cerebral palsy."
(axial, noncontrast T2-weighted SE scan)

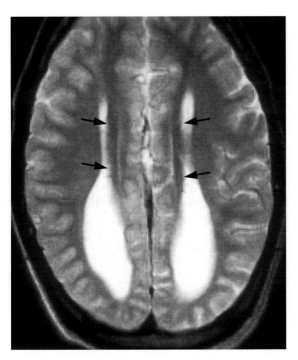

**Agenesis of the Corpus Callosum**

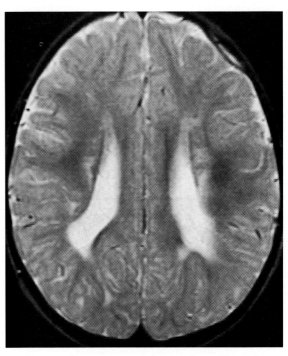

**Periventricular Leukomalacia**

---

"Colpocephaly," or dilatation of the posterior portion of the lateral ventricles, accompanies many congenital malformations. This feature may be especially prominent in agenesis of the corpus callosum, since the normal bulk and rigidity of the major forceps are missing from the posterior temporal and occipital lobes.

Case 857 presents a typical example of this finding. Also apparent is wide separation of the lateral ventricles, which are abnormally parallel. (This characteristic ventricular orientation is not present in all cases.) The parasagittally oriented bundles of Probst are well seen as longitudinal bands of white matter along the medial margin of the lateral ventricles *(arrows)*.

The posterior portions of the lateral ventricles are also enlarged in Case 858. However, the margins of the expanded ventricles are angular and irregular instead of smoothly rounded. The ventricular expansion is due to an acquired loss of periventricular white matter rather than to congenital malformation. Multiple foci of abnormal signal intensity in the periventricular regions corroborate a history of deep hemispheric insult (see discussion of Cases 592-595).

Seizures in patients with agenesis of the corpus callosum (as in Case 857) may be idiopathic or associated with recognizable accompanying abnormalities (e.g., neuronal migration disorders) or clinical syndromes. One of the latter is *Aicardi syndrome,* characterized by callosal agenesis, infantile spasms, chorioretinal lacunae, and mental retardation. This X-linked dominant disorder is observed only in girls, presumably because it is lethal in a male fetus. Multiple small or large interhemispheric cysts may be a prominent feature of MR scans in affected infants.

Children with periventricular leukomalacia often manifest spastic diplegia and are placed in the category of "cerebral palsy," as in Case 858.

## Case 859

36-year-old woman presenting with dizziness.
(sagittal, noncontrast T1-weighted SE scan)

## Case 860

10-year-old girl with a long history of seizures.
(sagittal, noncontrast T1-weighted SE scan)

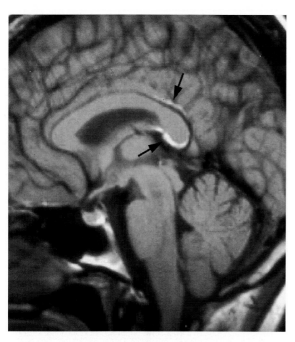

**Interhemispheric Lipoma**

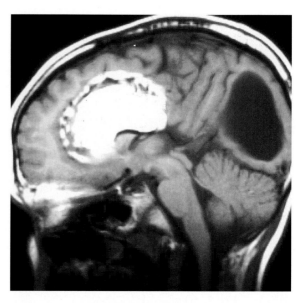

**Interhemispheric Lipoma**

"Lipomas of the corpus callosum" are better considered to be "interhemispheric lipomas with callosal dysgenesis." The lesions are believed to result from lipomatous mal-differentiation of primitive meningeal tissue in the interhemispheric fissure. The presence of an interhemispheric lipoma may secondarily impair callosal development, resulting in hypoplasia or agenesis.

The above scans demonstrate the variable size and morphology of interhemispheric lipomas. In Case 859, a thin layer of lipomatous tissue with short T1 values outlines the normally formed splenium of the corpus callosum *(arrows)*. By contrast, the large lipoma in Case 860 is a spherical mass, associated with severe dysgenesis of the corpus callosum. (Note the characteristic associated radial pattern of medial hemispheric gyri and accompanying colpocephaly.)

Foci of low signal intensity at the perimeter of an interhemispheric lipoma may represent calcification, commonly demonstrated on CT scans. Such calcification usually takes the form of a thin shell within cortex adjacent to the lipoma.

Flow voids of major arteries are another cause for low intensity areas within a lipoma. Such vessels are engulfed when the primitive tissue ("meninx") filling fetal cisterns differentiates into fat rather than involuting normally.

In cases of callosal agenesis, the proximal anterior cerebral arteries may follow an abnormally vertical and posterior course as they ascend along the anterior margin of the third ventricle. An azygous anterior cerebral artery is often seen in this context.

Calcification or ossification within the falx may be associated with T1-shortening due to paramagnetic effects or fatty marrow elements. Such thin dural plaques should not be mistaken for interhemispheric lipomas.

## Case 861

12-year-old boy with an abnormal
CT scan after head trauma.
(coronal, noncontrast scan; SE 2500/45)

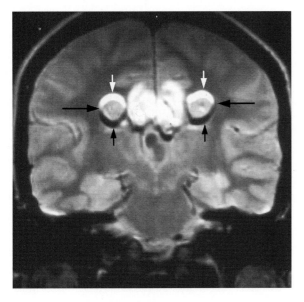

**Interhemispheric Lipoma**

## Case 862

15-year-old girl presenting with seizures.
(axial, noncontrast T2-weighted SE scan)

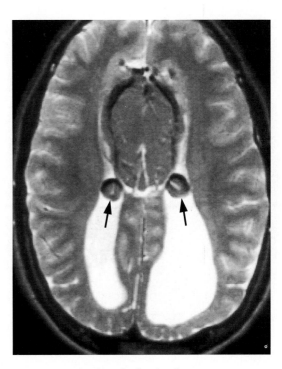

**Interhemispheric Lipoma**

---

Lipomas involving the choroid plexus of the lateral ventricles commonly accompany larger interhemispheric ("callosal") lipomas. The intraventricular lesions may be unilateral or bilateral and single or multinodular. They may be continuous with the interhemispheric mass or separate from it. Choroid plexus lipomas probably develop when maldifferentiating meningeal tissue invaginates through the choroid fissure.

In both of the above cases, the satellite lipomas are bilateral and symmetrical *(long arrows)*. Associated colpocephaly is present in Case 862.

Case 861 is a good example of chemical shift artifact at the interface between aqueous and fatty tissues. The naturally lower resonance frequency of lipid protons has caused the computer to plot their signal intensity a little closer to the low end of the frequency axis than is accurate. As a result, the lipoma is misregistered against the background of aqueous tissues, being artifactually shifted away from the inferior tissue (leaving a black gap; *short black arrows*) to overlap the superior tissue (causing a bright superimposition of signal; *white arrows*). This finding is a useful clue to the lipid nature of a mass on MR scans.

The expected short T2 values of fatty tissue are illustrated in Case 862. All three lipomas demonstrate uniformly low signal intensity, comparable to that of subcutaneous fat in the scalp. (Chemical shift artifact is present at the anterior and posterior margins of the lipomas in Case 862.)

Low signal intensity within the third ventricle in Case 861 is due to artifact from CSF pulsation.

### Case 863

2-year-old girl presenting with developmental delay.
(coronal, noncontrast T1-weighted SE scan)

### Case 864

10-year-old boy presenting with short stature.
(coronal, noncontrast T1-weighted SE scan)

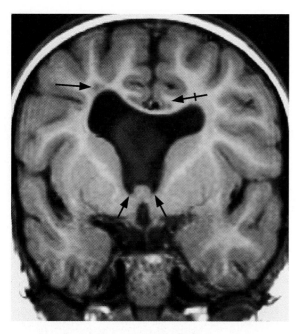

**Septooptic Dysplasia**

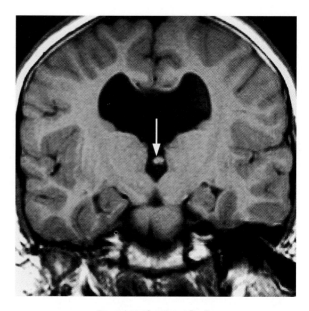

**Septooptic Dysplasia**

Several names have been applied to congenital malformations involving midline structures of the brain. Coexisting hypoplasia of the optic nerves and absence of the septum pellucidum has been called *septooptic dysplasia* or *de Morsier's syndrome*. The majority of such patients additionally demonstrate hypoplasia of the adenohypophysis, which may be the most important component of the complex clinically. Recently the generic nomenclature of "midline cerebral dysgenesis" has been proposed to include septooptic dysplasia and more complex malformations.

Absence of the septum pellucidum by itself has no functional significance. The finding is important only as a potential marker for associated hypoplasia of the optic nerves and/or pituitary gland. Patients with septooptic dysplasia may present with decreased visual acuity, nystagmus, or growth impairment secondary to insufficiency of the adenohypophysis.

MR scans clearly demonstrate absence of the septum pellucidum. The resulting fusion of the lateral ventricle superficially resembles the appearance of holoprosencephaly (compare the above scans to Case 865). Inferior

pointing of the frontal horns is usually prominent (*short arrows*, Case 863). This finding may also be noted in association with other congenital abnormalities, notably the Chiari II hindbrain malformation.

Because the septum pellucidum is absent, the columns of the fornix float characteristically within the third ventricle on coronal (or sagittal) images (*arrow*, Case 864).

Septooptic dysplasia may be accompanied by other developmental abnormalities, including schizencephaly (in up to 40% of cases), polymicrogyria, and heterotopic gray matter. A small nodule of neuronal tissue is present at the lateral margin of the right frontal horn in Case 863 *(long arrow)*, and additional subependymal heterotopias were noted elsewhere.

The corpus callosum is somewhat thin but is clearly present in the above images. As a result, the cingulate gyri have undergone normal inversion (*crossed arrow*, Case 863; compare to Case 856).

See Case 246 for an illustration of pituitary hypoplasia in septooptic dysplasia.

### Case 865

32-year-old woman with a history of
seizures and "mild cerebral palsy."
(coronal, noncontrast T1-weighted SE scan)

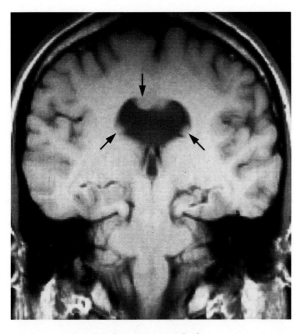

**Holoprosencephaly**

### Case 866

2-month-old girl presenting with a seizure.
(axial, noncontrast T1-weighted SE scan)

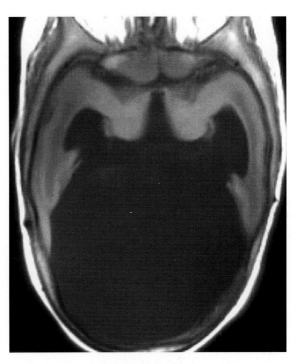

**Holoprosencephaly**

As discussed in Case 790, holoprosencephaly is a more severe midline malformation than septooptic dysplasia. Failure of normal hemisphere development results in a horseshoe-shaped forebrain ("holoprosencephalon") surrounding a central monoventricle.

Holoprosencephaly has traditionally been subdivided into lobar, semilobar, and alobar types. This somewhat artificial categorization refers to complete, partial, or absent separation of cerebral parenchyma into distinct hemispheres at the perimeter of the central ventricle. Hemispheric division (with presence of the falx) is often most complete posteriorly and least developed in the frontal region.

In Case 865, the interhemispheric fissure is bridged by tissue joining the frontal lobes (compare to the cases on the preceding page). The single-chambered ventricle resembles the morphology of septooptic dysplasia. (See Case 790 for an example of the classic "batwing" configuration often encountered in holoprosencephaly.) Nodules of heterotopic gray matter are present along the ventricular margins (*arrows;* see Cases 890 and 891).

Case 865 illustrates the variable severity of holoprosencephaly. The malformation demonstrated is intermediate between septooptic dysplasia and the more extensive abnormality in Case 866. Associated symptoms were correspondingly moderate.

Case 866 demonstrates partial hemispherization of the temporal lobes and thalami. However, all ventricular chambers join posteriorly to form a large cyst that occupies the posterior and superior portion of the cranium. Such a midline "dorsal cyst" is commonly found in association with cerebral malformations. The cyst may communicate with the ventricular system or be an isolated interhemispheric structure.

The hippocampal formations are severely hypoplastic in alobar and semilobar holoprosencephaly. As a result, the temporal horns in Case 866 are patulous, with a conspicuous lack of the normally complex tissue pattern along their medial margin. The visualized portions of the temporal lobes are lissencephalic (see Cases 870-873).

# JOUBERT'S SYNDROME

### Case 867

7-month-old girl presenting with
nystagmus and ataxia.
(axial, noncontrast T2-weighted SE scan)

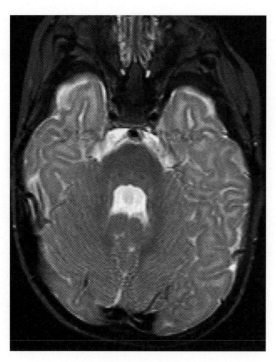

**Joubert's Syndrome**

### Case 868

7-week-old boy presenting with
periodic hyperpnea.
(axial, noncontrast T2-weighted SE scan)

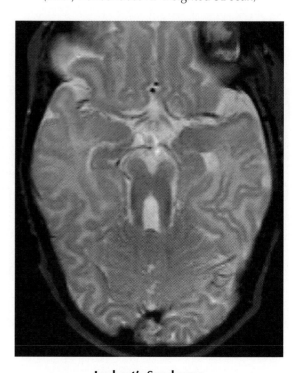

**Joubert's Syndrome**

---

Joubert's syndrome is an autosomal recessive disorder associated with a characteristic pattern of infratentorial midline dysgenesis. Affected infants present with episodic hyperpnea, nystagmus, ataxia, and psychomotor retardation. Imaging studies demonstrate failure of normal axonal decussation in the posterior fossa.

Disorganization and clefting of the superior cerebellar vermis is present with hypoplasia of the inferior vermis. The superior cerebellar peduncles are thick and parasagittally oriented, failing to decussate within the dorsal midbrain. The decussation of the pyramidal tracts is absent, and cerebellar nuclei, the olives, and dorsal column nuclei are often dysplastic. Retinal coloboma or dystrophy is a commonly associated finding.

The lack of vermian tissue at the posterior margin of the fourth ventricle causes it to appear abnormally triangular (with midline apex directed posteriorly) on low axial CT or MR scans. Axial images through the mid to superior fourth ventricle demonstrate a "batwing" morphology, as in Case 867, with the normal midline dorsal indentation of the vermis replaced by paired parasagittal convexities of hemispheric tissue. (Compare Case 867 to the normal ventricular configuration in Cases 193 and 199.)

The thick, parasagittally oriented superior cerebellar peduncles combine with the small midbrain (which lacks the normal volume of their decussation) to form a "molar tooth" configuration on axial scans, illustrated by case 868.

Patients may demonstrate the developmental abnormalities ("rhombencephaloschisis") associated with Joubert's syndrome without manifesting the characteristic infantile hyperpnea. That is, the clinical syndrome described by Joubert is only one possible presentation of this malformation.

**Case 869A**

4-year-old girl presenting with developmental delay.
(coronal, noncontrast T1-weighted SE scan)

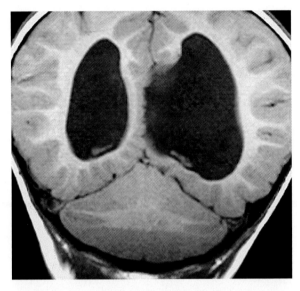

**Rhombencephalosynapsis**

**Case 869B**

Same patient.
(axial, noncontrast T2-weighted SE scan)

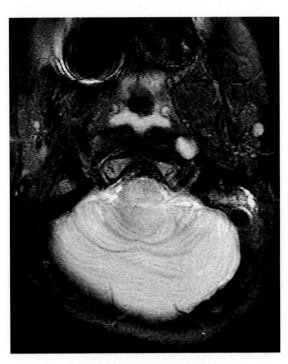

**Rhombencephalosynapsis**

Hypoplasia or absence of the cerebellar vermis is often associated with close apposition of the cerebellar hemispheres (see Cases 825 and 867). Alternatively, vermian agenesis may be accompanied by fusion of the hemispheres, a condition called *rhombencephalosynapsis.*

Case 869 is a typical example. Cerebellar folia and white matter are continuous across the midline, with no intervening vermis. In most cases, the dentate nuclei and superior cerebellar peduncles are also fused.

Axial CT or MR scans of patients with rhombencephalosynapsis may demonstrate posterior pointing of the fourth ventricle in the midline, reflecting the absence of

vermian tissue and resembling the morphology seen in Joubert's syndrome as discussed on the preceding page.

The clinical presentation of patients with rhombencephalosynapsis reflects the nature and severity of accompanying supratentorial abnormalities. Frequently associated anomalies include absence of the septum pellucidum, agenesis of the corpus callosum, fusion of the thalami, and malformations of cortical development. Hypogenesis of the corpus callosum was demonstrated on other scans in Case 869. Hydrocephalus is a common association, as seen in Case 869A.

### Case 870

3-month-old girl presenting with infantile spasms.
(axial, noncontrast scan; SE 3000/30)

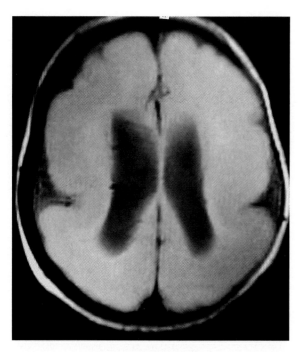

**Lissencephaly (Type I)**

### Case 871

21-year-old man presenting with seizures.
(coronal, noncontrast T1-weighted GRE scan)

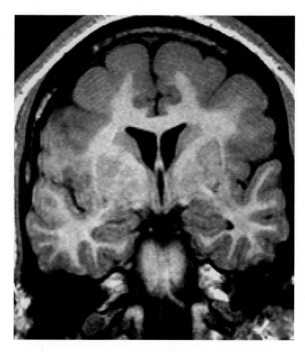

**Pachygyria**

---

Abnormalities of neuronal proliferation, migration, and organization lead to a variety of recognizable developmental malformations. These conditions have traditionally been called *neuronal migration disorders*. A more generic label of *malformations of cortical development* has recently been proposed to more accurately encompass the disordered proliferation and organization of neurons that frequently accompany aberrant migration.

Among these developmental anomalies is lissencephaly, or "smooth brain." Lissencephaly is characterized by lack of normal cortical gyration, as seen in the above cases.

Case 870 demonstrates several associated features. Poor opercularization is present in the sylvian region, with the shallow sylvian grooves giving the brain a "figure of eight" appearance on axial images. Hypoplasia of white matter accompanies the abnormal cortical mantle. (White matter in Case 870 is represented by the thin band of relatively high signal intensity in the periventricular region.) Ventricles are typically enlarged and dysmorphic.

When smooth and thick cerebral cortex is localized rather than generalized, the condition is termed *pachy-*

*gyria*. Case 871 demonstrates pachygyria over the frontal convexity bilaterally. The temporal lobes have a more normal gyral pattern.

Cases 870 to 873 illustrate "classical," or Type I lissencephaly. This disorder has been associated with abnormal genes on chromosome 17 and the X chromosome. Histology of the thick cortical mantle demonstrates four distinct layers, including a "cell sparse zone" between the wide "inner cellular" layer and the thinner "outer cellular" layer (see Case 873). The interface between malformed cortex and underlying white matter is smooth, lacking normal interdigitations.

Type II or "cobblestone" lissencephaly demonstrates an irregular interface between gray and white matter. This disorder is associated with congenital muscular dystrophies such as Walker-Warburg syndrome, Fukuyama muscular dystrophy, and muscle-eye-brain disease.

Lissencephaly with *thin* cerebral cortex may be seen in cases of congenital CMV infection, often in association with delayed myelination and cerebellar hypoplasia.

## Case 872

9-year-old girl presenting with seizures.
(axial, noncontrast scan; SE 3000/45)

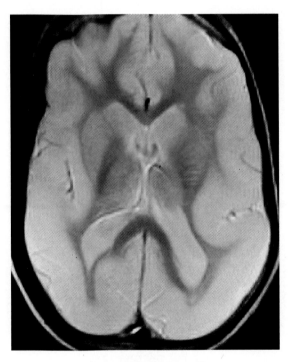

**Lissencephaly (Type I)**

## Case 873

3-month-old boy presenting with infantile spasms.
(coronal, noncontrast T2-weighted SE scan)

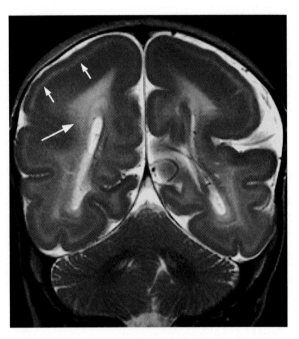

**Lissencephaly (Type I)**

Case 872 demonstrates symmetrical lissencephaly localized to the posterior portion of the cerebral hemispheres. Hypoplasia of underlying white matter and dilatation of the adjacent ventricular system accompany the marked cortical thickening. (Compare the thickness and complexity of parietal white matter to that in the frontal lobes.)

In Case 873, greatly thickened cortex occupies most of the cerebral mantle. A band of dysplastic white matter is seen as a zone of high signal intensity in the periventricular region *(long arrow)*. A stripe of signal abnormality near the cortical periphery *(short arrows)* probably represents the "cell sparse zone" typically found between the inner and outer cellular layers of the cortex in classical or Type I lissencephaly.

Cases 870 to 873 illustrate that lissencephaly can remain strikingly symmetrical while demonstrating variable hemispheric extent. In other cases, pachygyria is entirely unilateral, with widespread or focal involvement (see Cases 879 and 881).

Focal, unilateral pachygyria can be misinterpreted as an infiltrating mass lesion (see Case 879 and compare it to Case 77). Correct interpretation in such cases is based on recognizing that the signal intensity of the questioned area matches that of gray matter on all pulse sequences.

Abnormalities of neuronal migration are commonly associated with seizures, as in the above cases.

## Case 874A

9-month-old boy presenting with seizures.
(sagittal, noncontrast T1-weighted SE scan)

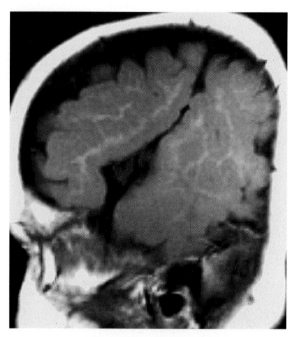

**Polymicrogyria**

## Case 874B

Same patient.
(coronal, noncontrast T1-weighted SE scan)

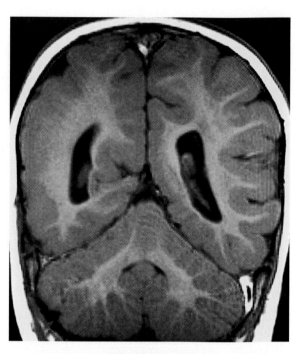

**Polymicrogyria**

---

Another pattern of abnormal neuronal migration and cortical development is polymicrogyria. As the name implies, this malformation is characterized by multiple tiny secondary gyri on the cortical surface. These shallow irregularities are often crowded together and not clearly separated by intervening CSF spaces. As a result, the involved cortex may appear abnormally smooth, resembling pachygyria.

Case 874A demonstrates abnormal morphology of the sylvian fissure, with an anomalous superior extension at its posterior margin. Fine nodularity is superimposed on the laminar morphology of cortex in the frontal and temporal regions, reflecting the close spacing of secondary gyri.

Involved cortex of the right parietal lobe in Case 874B appears mildly thickened, mimicking pachygyria. The blurred interface between gray and white matter in the affected region is probably due to the presence of scattered neurons throughout subcortical tissue, a common finding in areas of abnormal neuronal migration. White matter fronds often do not arborize normally into areas of polymi-

crogyria, as is apparent comparing the right and left hemispheres in Case 874B (but see Case 875).

Polymicrogyria may be localized or diffuse, symmetrical (see Case 875) or asymmetrical, as above. Cortex surrounding the sylvian fissure is commonly involved. Bilateral perisylvian polymicrogyria has been associated with a congenital syndrome characterized by pseudobulbar palsy including oropharyngeal dysfunction and dysarthria ("bilateral perisylvian syndrome").

Both genetic and acquired disorders are associated with polymicrogyria. Intrauterine infection with cyomegalovirus is among the latter.

Focal areas of intrauterine or perinatal infarction may present as localized regions in which the volume of individual cerebral gyri is markedly reduced. Subsequent development of the remainder of the brain may crowd the shrunken gyri, creating an appearance of secondary polymicrogyria.

## Case 875

45-year-old woman presenting with seizures.
(coronal, noncontrast T2-weighted FSE scan)

## Case 876

45-year-old man presenting with a seizure.
(axial, noncontrast T2-weighted FSE scan)

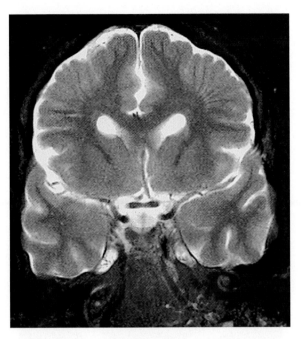

**Polymicrogyria**

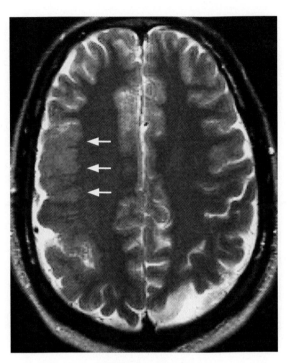

**Polymicrogyria**

High resolution T2-weighted scans may highlight the fine irregularity of the cortical surface in patients with polymicrogyria, helping to distinguish these cases from pachygyria. Intrinsic cortical morphology may also be better resolved on T2-weighted scans than on T1-weighted images, aiding diagnosis.

In Case 875, the pattern of gray and white matter within frontal cortex clearly suggests the crowding of multiple small gyri and is distinct from the coarsely laminar appearance of lissencephaly (compare to Case 873). Sulci between the small gyri are inapparent and have probably been obliterated. A lower resolution scan could give the impression of vague, generalized cortical thickening in such a case.

It is not possible to distinguish superficial gyral contours or white matter arborization within the zone of thickened cortex involving the posterior right frontal lobe in Case 876. However, the interface between gray and white matter in the affected region is irregularly nodular or serrated *(arrows)*. This bumpy *inner* cortical margin often helps to establish the diagnosis of polymicrogyria.

The orientation of the scan plane with respect to the axis of secondary gyri can make a substantial difference in the degree to which they are individually resolved (compare Cases 874A and 874B).

## Case 877

2-year-old girl presenting with developmental delay.
(axial, noncontrast T2-weighted SE scan)

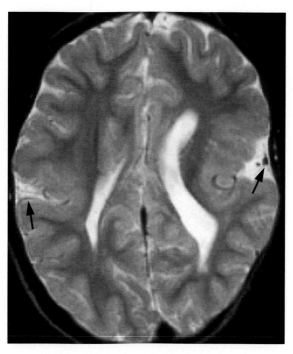

**Perisylvian Cortical Dysplasia**

## Case 878

38-year-old woman presenting with a
grand mal seizure involving the right arm.
(axial, noncontrast FLAIR scan)

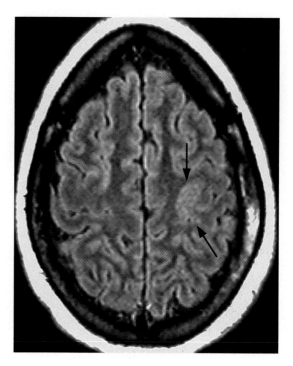

**Focal Cortical Dysplasia**

The sylvian and rolandic regions are commonly affected by localized cortical dysplasia, as seen bilaterally in Case 877. The mid hemispheric cortex is abnormally thick, suggesting pachygyria and/or polymicrogyria. Involved gray matter also invaginates abnormally toward the ventricular system. Such cortical infolding commonly accompanies focal pachygyria or polymicrogyria and can mimic schizencephaly (compare to Case 885).

Localized widening of CSF spaces often overlies focal cortical dysplasia and can be a helpful clue in distinguishing neuronal migration disorders from superficial mass lesions. Prominent anomalous superficial vessels (usually veins) are frequently present in these distorted subarachnoid spaces, as seen bilaterally in Case 877 *(arrows)*.

Cortical dysplasia may be very focal and subtle. Case 878 illustrates a small island of thickened cortex in the superior left frontal lobe *(arrows)*. Isointensity of this "mass" with adjacent gray matter and the absence of reactive edema identify the lesion as a cortical malformation rather than acquired pathology.

Aberrant giant cells ("balloon cells") may be found in areas of focal cortical dysplasia (FCD) and are a histologic marker for this diagnosis. Similar cells occur in the cortical hamartomas of tuberous sclerosis. Like the peripheral lesions of tuberous sclerosis, superficial FCD may be associated with a linear or wedge-shaped track of signal abnormality leading back to the periventricular region and implying a transmantle dysplasia (see Cases 898 and 899).

High resolution scans with good contrast between gray and white matter are necessary to define localized cortical malformations. Fine nodularity of cortical margins and/or localized decrease in definition of the junction between gray and white matter support the diagnosis.

Focal cortical dysplasia is often intrinsically epileptogenic and accounts for up to 25% of the lesions demonstrated by MRI in children with seizures.

# DIFFERENTIAL DIAGNOSIS:
## FOCAL SUBCORTICAL SIGNAL ABNORMALITY IN A YOUNG PATIENT WITH SEIZURES

### Case 879

5-year-old girl presenting with a seizure.
(axial, noncontrast T2-weighted SE scan)

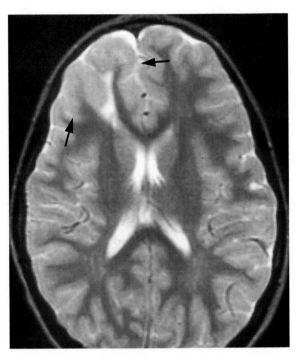

**Focal Cortical Dysplasia**

### Case 880

29-year-old woman with a history of seizures.
(coronal, noncontrast T2-weighted FSE scan)

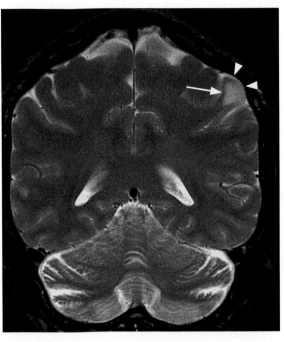

**Dysembryoplastic Neuroepithelial Tumor**

---

Abnormal signal intensity (usually T2 prolongation) is commonly seen within white matter adjacent to an area of cortical dysplasia. This finding likely represents lack of normal myelination and/or mild gliosis. Subcortical signal abnormality may call attention to an otherwise inconspicuous cortical malformation or mimic edema bordering a mass lesion.

In Case 879, the zone of high signal intensity within white matter of the right frontal lobe outlines the medial margin of a thickened gyrus. Signal intensity within the cortex itself is normal, and cortical thickening extends anteriorly for a short distance. The inward buckling of the malformed gray matter in this area is a common feature of cortical dysplasia.

The superficial lesion in Case 880 *(arrow)* differs from cortical dysplasia in several ways. Subcortical signal abnormality outlines cortex that is *not* thickened. A small area of T2 prolongation is present *within* the cortex itself. Most important, there is adjacent localized erosion of the inner table *(arrowheads)*, implying the presence of long-

standing mass effect. These features suggest a low grade mass and are typical of a dysembryoplastic neuroepithelial tumor (see Cases 338-341).

Tuberous sclerosis should also be considered in the differential diagnosis of a focal superficial lesion in a young patient with seizures (see Cases 900 and 901). Like low grade gliomas, hamartomas of tuberous sclerosis may involve cortex and subcortical white matter with prolonged T1 and T2 values and no abnormal contrast enhancement.

When a mass such as Case 880 is discovered, a search for potential corollary findings of tuberous sclerosis is indicated. These include subependymal nodules, other hemispheric tubers, and lines or wedges of abnormal signal intensity extending radially from the ventricular wall to the cerebral surface (see Cases 898 and 899). The clinical context (e.g., duration of seizures and presence or absence of associated retardation) may help to categorize cases with ambiguous scan findings.

Cerebellar atrophy in Case 880 is probably related to the history of seizures and Dilantin therapy.

537

### Case 881A

5-year-old girl with seizures since birth.
(coronal, noncontrast T1-weighted SE scan)

### Case 881B

Same patient.
(axial, noncontrast T2-weighted SE scan)

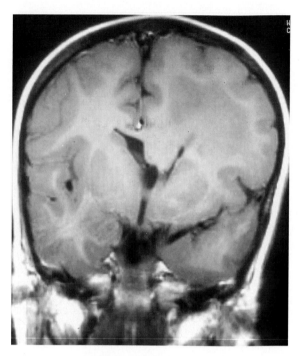

**Unilateral Megalencephaly**

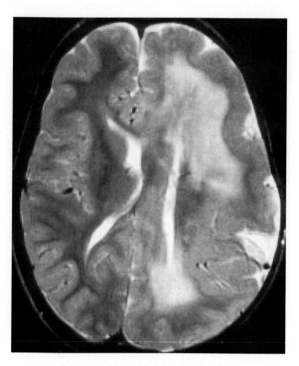

**Unilateral Megalencephaly**

Unilateral megalencephaly is an uncommon neuronal migration abnormality extensively involving one hemisphere. The affected half of the cerebrum is enlarged, with widespread cortical thickening and hypertophied white matter. The cortical thickening may reflect pachygyria and/or polymicrogyria. White matter may be of normal signal intensity or variably dysplastic, demonstrating high intensity on T2-weighted images.

An important clue to the diagnosis in many cases is dilatation of the ipsilateral ventricle. Such ventricular enlargement is commonly associated with other neuronal migration disorders, as seen in the preceding pages. However, Case 881 demonstrates that ventricular expansion is not invariable in unilateral megalencephaly. The hemispheric enlargement and abnormal signal intensity within white matter may then suggest an infiltrating mass.

The coronal scan of Case 881A documents asymmetry in the volume of the hemispheres. Bulky mass effect de-

forms the left frontal horn. Abnormal signal intensity is present in the left centrum semiovale.

The T2-weighted image in Case 881B provides key information by highlighting the abnormal thickness and contour of cortex over the left hemisphere. The pattern resembles the more common cortical dysplasias previously illustrated. Signal intensity within the dysmorphic cortical ribbon is normal. (Cortical calcification causes reduced signal intensity in occasional patients with unilateral megalencephaly.) However, the signal intensity of underlying white matter is distinctly abnormal, another common observation in cases of neuronal migration disorders (compare to Case 879).

Rare cases of tuberous sclerosis uniformly involving one cerebral hemisphere can demonstrate thick cortex, abnormal signal intensity of underlying white matter, and enlargement of the ipsilateral ventricle, resembling unilateral megalencephaly. Associated subependymal nodules usually establish the correct diagnosis in such patients.

## Case 882

22-year-old woman presenting with seizures.
(coronal, noncontrast T1-weighted GRE scan)

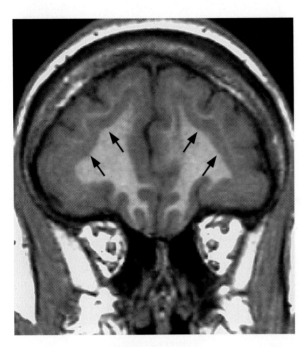

**Band Heterotopia**

## Case 883

15-year-old girl presenting with seizures.
(axial, noncontrast T2-weighted SE scan)

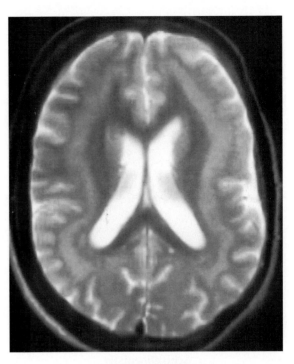

**Band Heterotopia**

Disorders of the embryologic migration of neurons from the germinal matrix to the cerebral cortex may take many forms. If neurons fail to leave the periventricular region, subependymal heterotopias are found (see Cases 890 and 891). If neurons fail to organize normally on reaching the surface of the brain, pachygyria or polymicrogyria result (see Cases 870-876).

Band heterotopias represent a geographically intermediate form of neuronal migration abnormality. In these cases, waves of migrating neurons move outward from their periventricular origin but fail to reach the cerebral convexity. Instead, their migration is arrested at a location part way through the cerebral mantle. There they reside as islands or "bands," surrounded by midhemispheric white matter.

Like other disorders of neuronal migration, band heterotopias may be (1) unilateral or bilateral and (2) holohemispheric or localized. They may be centimeters thick or as thin as a millimeter. The thickness of overlying cortex may be normal, increased (i.e., pachygyria), or decreased; sulcation is often shallow.

Symmetrical band heterotopia is demonstrated within the frontal lobes in Case 882. Uniform layers of ectopic

neurons *(arrows)* are separated from the thin overlying cortex by a band of white matter. The result is a laminated or "double cortex" morphology.

Case 883 illustrates bilateral, symmetrically thick bands of heterotopic gray matter. These broad zones of neuronal tissue are separated from the cerebral cortex by a narrow strip of subcortical white matter and from the lateral ventricles by a broader layer of myelinated parenchyma. Note that the bands of abnormal tissue in Cases 882 and 883 are isointense to gray matter, the hallmark of heterotopic neurons.

Heterotopic gray matter within the centrum semiovale often has a more irregular and nodular morphology than the uniform bands in Case 883. Such islands are frequently round or amorphous in contour and markedly asymmetrical or unilateral.

Uniform and symmetrical band heterotopia (like Case 883) may be misinterpreted as a leukodystrophy, since diffusely abnormal signal intensity extends throughout large regions of cerebral white matter.

About 90% of reported patients with bilateral band heterotopia have been women. These patients are often carriers of X-linked lissencephaly.

539

**Case 884**

8-year-old boy with a history of seizures
and "unilateral cerebral palsy."
(sagittal, noncontrast T1-weighted SE scan)

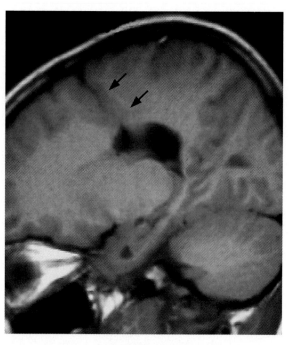

**Schizencephaly**

**Case 885**

4-year-old girl presenting with seizures
and right hemiparesis.
(axial, noncontrast T2-weighted SE scan)

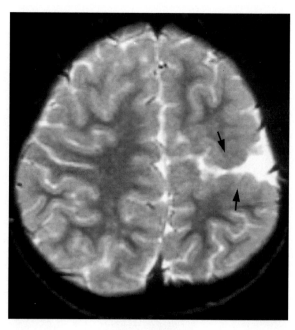

**Schizencephaly**

Schizencephaly is a malformation of cortical development characterized by a transcerebral cleft, usually extending from the lateral ventricle to the cerebral surface. Unlike encephaloclastic clefts from damage to normally formed parenchyma, schizencephalic clefts are lined by gray matter. This margin of transparenchymal cortex is clearly seen in the above cases *(arrows)*.

The clefts of schizencephaly may be unilateral or bilateral. They most frequently involve the midhemispheric region, near the central sulcus. Gray matter at the margins of schizencephalic clefts usually demonstrates abnormal thickness and morphology. Polymicrogyria is common in these areas.

Schizencephalic clefts vary considerably in width. Many are broader than the examples above. The apparent width of a parenchymal defect in schizencephaly also depends on the angulation of the cleft with respect to the plane of imaging. In some cases, the margins of the clefts are closely apposed ("closed lip" schizencephaly; see Cases 886 and 887).

Even narrow clefts are typically associated with small, CSF-containing diverticula at the ventricular and superficial limits of the lesion. These focal deformities of the subarachnoid space or the ventricular contour can be a clue to the presence of a largely closed cleft traversing the intervening cerebral tissue.

## Case 886

9-month-old girl with mild right hemiparesis.
(coronal, noncontrast T1-weighted SE scan)

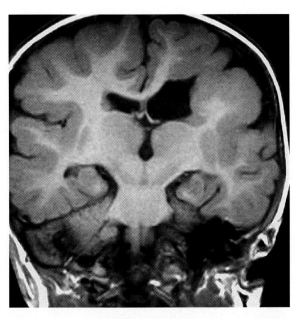

**Schizencephaly**

## Case 887

18-year-old man with a history of seizures.
(coronal, noncontrast scan; SE 2500/28)

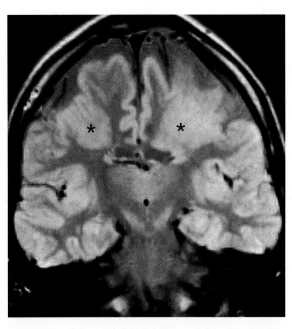

**Schizencephaly**

Schizencephalic clefts may be completely closed, with fusion of gray matter along the zone of disordered migration. Like localized cortical dysplasia (see Cases 878 and 879), these intraparenchymal "masses" may mimic a cerebral neoplasm. In such cases, the gray/white matter differentiation on MR scans helps to identify abnormalities of neuronal migration.

A zone of bulky gray matter extends from the cerebral surface to the ventricular margin in the left frontal lobe of Case 886. Typical expansion of the overlying subarachnoid space and the underlying ventricle distinguishes this developmental anomaly from a mass lesion. The diverticulum at the ventricular end of the fused cleft is particularly characteristic. Cortical thickening continues inferiorly from the area of schizencephaly to involve the sylvian region.

Case 887 demonstrates transcerebral columns of gray matter extending from the cerebral surface to the ventricular margin in the posterior frontal regions bilaterally *(as-*

*terisks)*. There is mild deformity of overlying subarachnoid spaces but no associated ventricular diverticula. Tissue along the bands demonstrates the same signal intensity as cortical gray matter in other locations, suggesting heterotopic neurons.

A narrow schizencephalic cleft may be obscured on scans that are parallel or oblique to its plane. Multiplanar MR is more effective than CT for documenting schizencephaly by means of images that are perpendicular to the cleft.

Patients with schizencephaly often present with seizures. Focal neurological deficits may also occur (as in Case 886), reflecting the location and size of the cleft.

Schizencephaly is accompanied by septooptic dysplasia in a large minority of cases. Evidence of one of these congenital malformations should prompt a search for the other.

### Case 888

8-year-old boy presenting with
seizures and hemiparesis.
(axial, noncontrast T2-weighted SE scan)

### Case 889

3-year-old boy presenting with
developmental delay.
(axial, noncontrast T2-weighted SE scan)

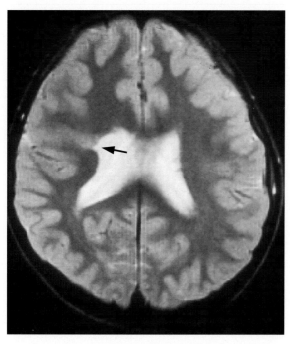

**Schizencephaly**
(same patient as Case 884)

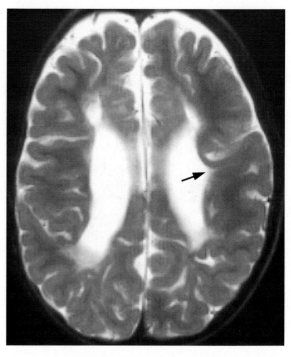

**Periventricular Leukomalacia**

As discussed in Cases 884-887, schizencephaly is frequently associated with a diverticular deformity at the ventricular end of the transparenchymal cleft. This focal irregularity is usually recognizable, even when the cleft itself has largely closed.

Case 888 illustrates this appearance. The localized outpouching along the lateral wall of the right lateral ventricle *(arrow)* is positioned at the base of a transhemispheric column of gray matter. (See Case 884 for better demonstration of the thin residual cleft in this patient.)

In Case 889, the focal irregularity of ventricular contours reflects localized damage to periventricular white matter.

As discussed in Cases 592-595, zones of necrosis and cavitation in periventricular leukomalacia may persist as independent cysts or coalesce with the ventricular chamber. In the latter circumstance, the lateral wall of the lateral ventricle becomes characteristically irregular and angular (see Cases 594 and 595 for other examples).

In both of the above cases, the lateral ventricles are abnormally large. Dysmorphic dilatation of ventricles commonly accompanies congenital malformations of the brain, and parenchymal loss regularly causes secondary ventricular expansion in periventricular leukeomalacia. Hydrocephalus is not a consideration in either case.

## Case 890

25-year-old woman with intractable seizures.
(coronal, noncontrast T1-weighted GRE scan)

## Case 891

4-year-old girl presenting with
gross motor incoordination.
(axial, noncontrast T2-weighted SE scan)

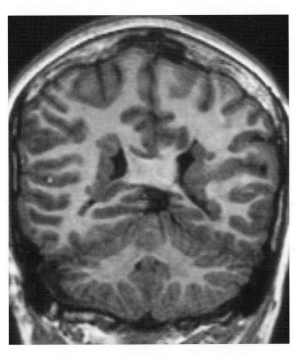

**Subependymal Nodular Heterotopia**

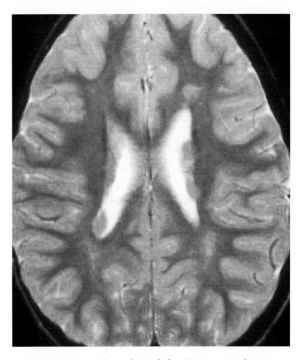

**Subependymal Nodular Heterotopia**

---

Nodules of heterotopic gray matter are commonly found along the margins of the lateral ventricles. Such "subependymal nodular heterotopias" result from an embryological failure of neurons to migrate away from the periventricular germinal matrix. The extent of involvement may vary from a few isolated nodules, as in Case 891, to a diffuse cobblestone pattern lining the ventricular wall, illustrated by Case 890. The findings may be bilaterally symmetrical or strikingly unilateral. An X-linked form of bilateral periventricular nodular heterotopia has been identified, but most cases are sporadic.

Isolated periventricular heterotopias are often discovered incidentally in patients with no associated symptoms. More extensive cases are usually correlated with seizures. Accompanying callosal or cerebellar hypoplasia is present in some patients.

The key to correct identification of subependymal nodules as heterotopias is the signal intensity of the masses. They should match the intensity of normal gray matter on all pulse sequences, with no abnormal contrast enhancement. Cases 890 and 891 demonstrate this concordance.

Heavily T1-weighted gradient echo sequences with an initial inverting pulse or "magnetization preparation" accentuate the contrast between gray and white matter. Such techniques are useful for examining patients with seizures, since (1) the hippocampal formation is well-defined (see discussion of mesial temporal sclerosis in Cases 523 and 524) and (2) gray matter heterotopias are sharply marginated, as in Case 890.

The reason for failure of normal neuronal migration has not been established. Possibilities include damage to the guiding radial glial fibers and/or lack of normal surface receptor recognition between these astrocytes and the migrating neurons.

### Case 892

2-day-old girl with several cardiac masses
demonstrated by ultrasound.
(sagittal, noncontrast T1-weighted SE scan)

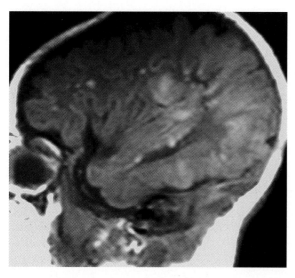

**Tuberous Sclerosis**

### Case 893

2-year-old boy presenting with myoclonic seizures.
(axial, postcontrast T1-weighted SE scan)

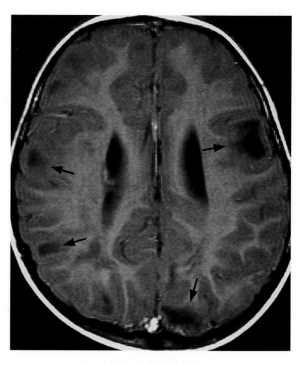

**Tuberous Sclerosis**

Tuberous sclerosis is one of the neurocutaneous syndromes or "neurophakomatoses," along with neurofibromatosis, Sturge-Weber syndrome, von Hippel-Lindau disease, and ataxia telangiectasia. The disorder is inherited as an autosomal dominant trait with frequent sporadic cases. Mutations of genes on chromosomes 9, 11, and 16 have been identified in affected patients. Clinical features include seizures, mental retardation, and a papular facial rash ("adenoma sebaceum").

Affected individuals have nodules of disorganized tissue (containing large cells with variable neuronal or astrocytic differentiation) along ventricular margins and/or within cerebral parenchyma. In infants, both the subependymal and the parenchymal nodules of tuberous sclerosis typically demonstrate T1-shortening, as in Case 892. The etiology of this high intensity on T1-weighted scans is not established; disordered accumulation of myelin-like lipids may play a role.

Subependymal nodules in older children and adults are often isointense on T1-weighted MR scans. In some cases, the characteristic calcification of periventricular tubers causes focally low intensity.

Parenchymal hamartomas in tuberous sclerosis are usually larger than the subependymal nodules and are often located in subcortical white matter. Case 893 illustrates several typical lesions *(arrows),* demonstrating that the malformations may be clearly defined by long T1 values. More commonly, hemispheric lesions in tuberous sclerosis are relatively inapparent on T1-weighted scans (and on CT studies), with much greater conspicuity on T2-weighted images (see Cases 900 and 901).

Tuberous sclerosis is a common cause of "infantile spasms" (myoclonic seizures) and should be considered in this clinical context. Characteristic periventricular and parenchymal lesions on MR scans usually enable diagnosis well before specific clinical findings or CT calcifications are apparent.

Cardiac rhabdomyomas may be present at birth in children with tuberous sclerosis, as in Case 892. These benign masses typically involute with age but can cause congestive heart failure in the neonatal period.

### Case 894

2-year-old boy presenting with seizures.
(sagittal, noncontrast T1-weighted SE scan)

### Case 895

4-year-old girl presenting with seizures.
(sagittal, noncontrast T1-weighted SE scan)

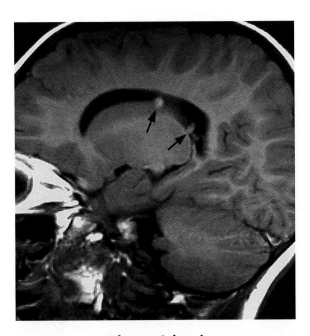

**Tuberous Sclerosis**

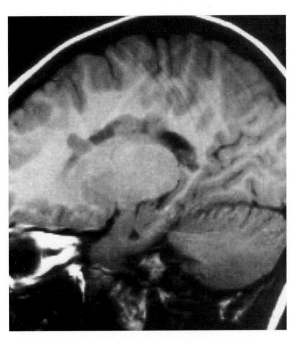

**Heterotopic Gray Matter**

Both heterotopic gray matter and tuberous sclerosis may cause small periventricular masses in patients with seizures. The characteristic subependymal nodules of tuberous sclerosis are well seen as focal irregularities along the ventricular margins on MR examinations such as in Case 894. Periventricular islands of heterotopic gray matter are usually larger and more amorphous than uncomplicated subependymal tubers, as demonstrated in Case 895.

More importantly, the signal intensity of heterotopic gray matter matches that of cerebral cortex, while the subependymal lesions of tuberous sclerosis do not. (As discussed on the preceding page, subependymal tubers may demonstrate short, long, or intermediate T1 values.) This distinction is apparent in the above examples.

Associated developmental anomalies (e.g., agenesis of the corpus callosum or absence of the septum pellucidum) may accompany heterotopic gray matter, confirming the diagnosis of congenital malformation.

Calcification is common within subependymal lesions on CT scans of older children and adults with tuberous sclerosis. This finding is not seen in nodules of heterotopic gray matter.

Subependymal calcifications can also result from prior cerebral inflammation (e.g., congenital infection with CMV or toxoplasmosis). Calcified tubers are usually larger and fewer than the periventricular calcifications of inflammatory disease. Congenital inflammatory disorders are also usually associated with parenchymal damage (e.g., microcephaly in CMV) and/or hydrocephalus (commonly occurring in toxoplasmosis), which would be unusual in cases of tuberous sclerosis.

If periventricular nodules are accompanied by an intracranial mass, the possibility of ependymal seeding from CSF dissemination of tumor should be considered (see Cases 110 and 111).

## Case 896

2-day-old girl presenting with cardiac masses.
(coronal, noncontrast T1-weighted SE scan)

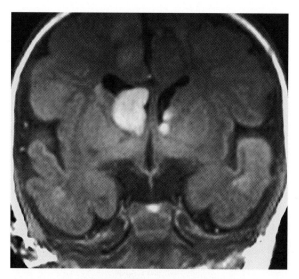

**Giant Cell Astrocytoma**
(same patient as Case 892)

## Case 897

8-year-old girl presenting with seizures.
(axial, postcontrast T1-weighted SE scan)

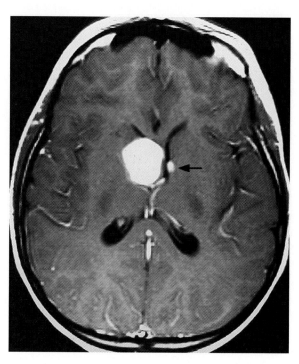

**Giant Cell Astrocytoma**

---

Subependymal nodules in tuberous sclerosis commonly occur near the foramen of Monro. Tubers in this location are prone to develop into subependymal giant cell astrocytomas, as illustrated above.

These low grade gliomas are often large, fleshy, lobulated masses. They demonstrate benign behavior but may cause obstructive hydrocephalus because of their strategic location. Recurrence is rare, and prognosis is good after surgical resection.

The short T1 values within the right frontal mass in Case 896 match the intensity of other tubers in this newborn (see Case 892). Subependymal giant cell astrocytomas are typically more isointense on T1-weighted scans in older children and adults.

Transformation of a subependymal nodule into a giant cell astrocytoma is suggested by increasing diameter and contrast enhancement. The right-sided mass in Case 897 had been identical in size to the small left frontal nodule *(arrow)* on a scan four years earlier.

Many static subependymal nodules enhance on MR studies. That is, the presence of enhancement does not by itself imply astrocytic transformation.

The differential diagnosis of a mass near the foramen of Monro includes several other lesions. Colloid cysts of the third ventricle can be identified by their origin from the third ventricular roof and their midline location. The usual lack of abnormal contrast enhancement also distinguishes colloid cysts from most other neoplasms.

Diffuse astrocytomas or lymphoma may infiltrate and thicken the septum pellucidum. Such midline masses contrast with the typical origin of subependymal tubers and giant cell astrocytomas from the *lateral* margin of the foramen of Monro.

Subependymal giant cell astrocytomas are classified as "circumscribed," "grade I" gliomas by the World Health Organization (along with pilocytic astrocytomas and pleomorphic xanthoastrocytomas). These tumors can occur as isolated lesions, unaccompanied by other findings of tuberous sclerosis.

## Case 898

12-year-old girl presenting with seizures.
(axial, noncontrast scan; SE 2500/30)

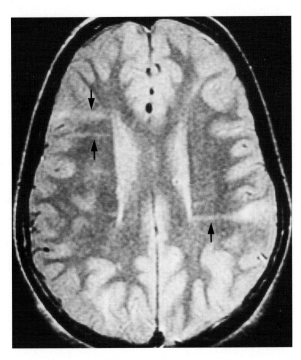

**Tuberous Sclerosis**

## Case 899

2-year-old boy presenting with seizures.
(coronal, noncontrast T1-weighted
SE scan with MTS)

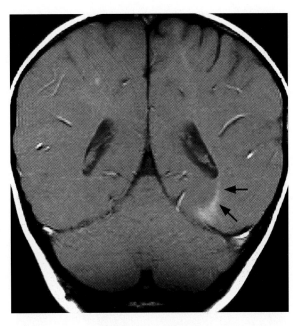

**Tuberous Sclerosis**
(same patient as Case 893)

The above cases illustrate bands of high signal intensity extending from the ventricular margin to the cortical surface *(arrows)*. These striations or wedges are oriented along the direction of neuronal migration and have been termed "migration lines" or "linear transmantle hyperintensities." Some of these rays lead to cortical/subcortical hamartomas.

The findings suggest that tuberous sclerosis involves disorganization and dysplasia of stem cells migrating from the periventricular germinal zone. The rays of abnormal signal intensity likely represent a combination of neuronal heterotopia and disordered myelination.

The presence of one or more radial migration lines or wedges is highly suggestive of tuberous sclerosis. A similar transmantle striation may be seen underlying focal cortical dysplasias, as discussed in Cases 877 and 878.

Images obtained with FLAIR or magnetization transfer suppression (MTS) techniques accentuate the contrast between the abnormal tissue within migration lines and surrounding parenchyma. In Case 899, the subcortical signal abnormality at the inferior margin of the posterior left temporal lobe was ambiguous on routine T1- and T2-weighted scans. The MTS image demonstrates a narrowing wedge-shaped track or tail *(arrows)* leading from the lesion to the periventricular region and suggesting a developmental disorder.

A few smaller lesions are also highlighted as foci of high signal intensity elsewhere within the cerebral hemispheres in Case 899.

## Case 900

17-year-old boy presenting with a seizure.
(axial, noncontrast T2-weighted FSE scan)

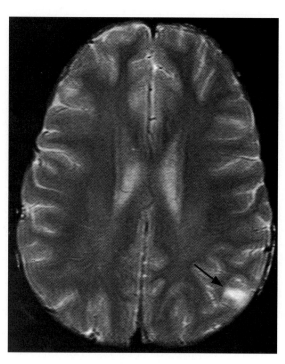

**Tuberous Sclerosis**

## Case 901

5-month-old girl presenting with infantile spasms.
(axial, noncontrast T2-weighted SE scan)

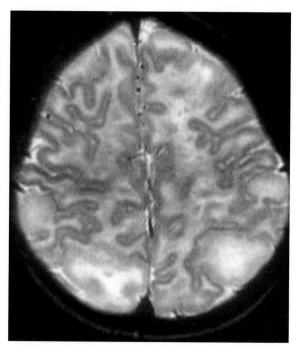

**Tuberous Sclerosis**

Parenchymal lesions in tuberous sclerosis represent heterotopic islands of abnormal neurons associated with disordered myelination and fibrillary gliosis. They are typically one or two centimeters in diameter, considerably larger than accompanying subependymal nodules. These focal areas of disorganized and dysplastic tissue are usually more apparent on T2-weighted MR scans than on T1-weighted images or CT studies. Although parenchymal nodules tend to be centered in subcortical white matter, they may vary greatly in size and number.

The small left parietal lesion in Case 900 is nonspecific (compare to Cases 879 and 880). Associated subependymal nodules, migration lines, and/or clinical stigmata would be necessary to establish the diagnosis of tuberous sclerosis in this patient.

Case 901 illustrates multiple superficial tubers that are truly "potato-like," with expansion of gyri. Although the signal intensity of the lesions is only slightly higher than adjacent unmyelinated white matter, they are identifiable because of anatomical distortion. Subcortical tubers in older children and adults are typically more sharply marginated (see Case 902).

Calcification may occur within small or large parenchymal nodules in children or adults with tuberous sclerosis. Low signal intensity within such lesions on T2- or T2*-weighted scans often contrasts with the more common T2 prolongation of adjacent foci. Parenchymal tubers rarely enhance.

Subependymal and cortical hamartomas with short T1 values in infants (see Cases 892 and 896) usually demonstrate low signal intensity on T2-weighted images.

# DIFFERENTIAL DIAGNOSIS:
## MULTIPLE PATCHY SUBCORTICAL LESIONS

### Case 902

3-year-old boy presenting with seizures.
(axial, noncontrast T2-weighted FSE scan)

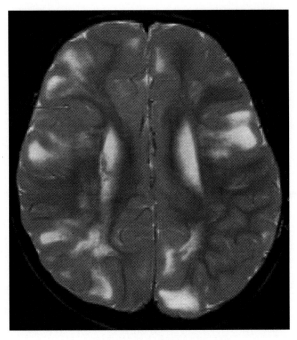

**Tuberous Sclerosis**

### Case 903

14-year-old boy presenting with decreasing
level of consciousness.
(axial, noncontrast T2-weighted SE scan)

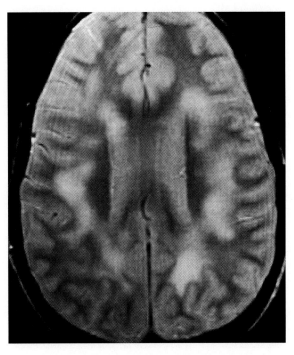

**Acute Disseminated Encephalomyelitis**

---

The white matter lesions in tuberous sclerosis often have an irregular, angular, or stellate morphology. The patchy morphology and multiplicity of such foci may resemble an inflammatory process or demyelinating disease.

It is important to realize that the shaggy subcortical abnormalities in Case 902 fall within the spectrum of tuberous sclerosis. Attention to possible associated findings (e.g., subependymal nodules or migration lines) and clinical context can prevent unwarranted evaluation for leukoencephalopathy or systemic disease.

The superficial lesions of tuberous sclerosis are often more peripheral (with more cortical involvement) than demyelinating or dysmyelinating foci. In Case 903, patchy areas of signal abnormality are concentrated in central white matter, with relative sparing of subarcuate fibers.

Cerebral vasculitis (see Cases 641 and 642), mitochondrial encephalomyopathies (see Case 510), or systemic lupus erythematosus (see Cases 481 and 483) could cause multifocal lesions with combined cortical and subcortical involvement similar to Case 902. Acuity of symptoms and systemic manifestations usually distinguish these entities from tuberous sclerosis.

**Case 904**

5-year-old girl being followed for an optic glioma.
(axial, noncontrast T2-weighted FSE scan)

**Case 905**

14-year-old boy with multiple café-au-lait spots.
(axial, noncontrast T2-weighted FSE scan)

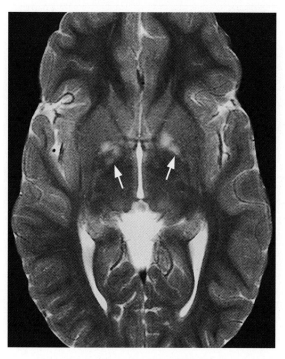

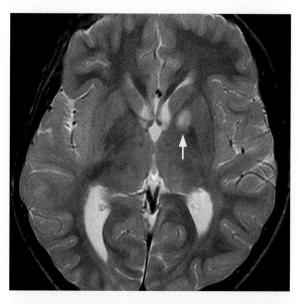

**Neurofibromatosis (Type 1)**

**Neurofibromatosis (Type 1)**

The intracranial and spinal tumors frequently associated with neurofibromatosis are discussed in Chapters 3, 4, 6, and 19. Non-neoplastic abnormalities may also be encountered on MR scans of patients with this diagnosis.

Zones of high signal intensity on long TR images are common deep within the cerebral hemispheres in children with type 1 neurofibromatosis. The basal ganglia (particularly the globus pallidus) and internal capsule are frequent sites of such "regional signal hyperintensities."

These areas most often represent disordered or retarded myelination and/or maldevelopment, analogous to the parenchymal abnormalities of tuberous sclerosis. Most such lesions are not neoplastic and do not enlarge over time. In fact, many disappear during years of follow-up.

However, the possibility of a developing astrocytoma warrants close observation of any patient with neurofibromatosis whose MR scan demonstrates areas of abnormal signal intensity. Increasing size and contrast enhancement

of a lesion suggest neoplasia rather than malformation. (Compare to the assessment of subependymal nodules in tuberous sclerosis, as discussed in Cases 896 and 897.)

The benign deep hemispheric zones of T2 prolongation common in neurofibromatosis type 1 demonstrate variable size, multiplicity, and symmetry. In Case 904, small areas of patchy signal abnormality are present within the globus pallidus bilaterally *(arrows)*. A unilateral focus is present in a similar location in Case 905 *(arrow)*. Much larger ganglionic "lesions" may occur in neurofibromatosis and still represent dysplastic, disorganized, and/or immature tissue rather than neoplasms.

As evidenced by the scans above, neurofibromatosis should be considered among the etiologies of unilateral or bilateral ganglionic pathology (together with various anoxic, toxic, and metabolic disorders; see Cases 505-508, 511-514, 671, and 672).

### Case 906

8-year-old girl presenting with optic gliomas.
(axial, noncontrast T2-weighted SE scan)

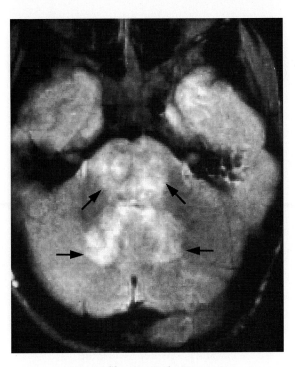

**Neurofibromatosis (Type 1)**

### Case 907

5-year-old girl being followed for an optic glioma.
(axial, noncontrast T2-weighted FSE scan)

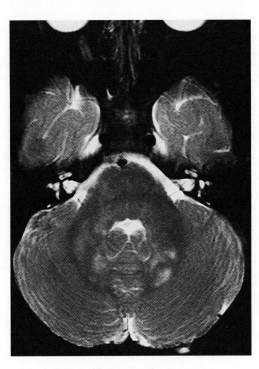

**Neurofibromatosis (Type 1)**
(same patient as Case 904)

---

The brainstem, cerebellar peduncles, and cerebellum are other locations where non-neoplastic zones of signal abnormality commonly occur in type 1 neurofibromatosis.

The scan in Case 906 is degraded by patient motion, but extensive areas of high intensity are apparent throughout the pons and posterolateral to the fourth ventricle *(arrows)*. There was no associated mass effect or abnormal contrast enhancement. The abnormalities became progressively less conspicuous on follow-up scans over a four-year period. This course indicates that the widespread prolongation of T2 in Case 906 likely represents disordered development or immaturity of tissue that becomes more normal with age. However, the possibility of a low grade brainstem glioma must be considered when such a scan is first encountered.

Case 907 demonstrates smaller patches of signal abnormality within the dorsal pons and medial cerebellum, which are characteristic sites for neurofibromatosis-related "lesions." In an ambiguous clinical context, this appearance could be mistaken for multifocal inflammatory disease (e.g., acute disseminated encephalomyelitis).

Associated findings may help to establish the diagnosis in such cases. Symmetrical widening of the internal auditory canals (with no evidence of acoustic schwannomas), as seen in Case 907, is a common incidental finding in neurofibromatosis type 1.

Focal or patchy areas of signal abnormality on long TR spin echo images like the lesions in Cases 904 through 907 may also be seen in the thalamus, corpus callosum, and centrum semiovale of patients with neurofibromatosis type 1.

### Case 908

29-year-old man with a long history of seizures.
(axial, noncontrast T1-weighted SE scan)

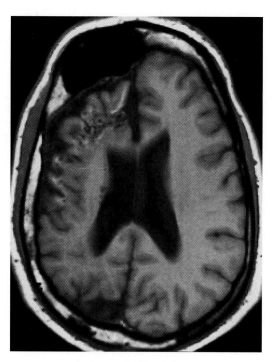

**Sturge-Weber Syndrome**

### Case 909

19-year-old man presenting with seizures.
(coronal, noncontrast T2-weighted SE scan)

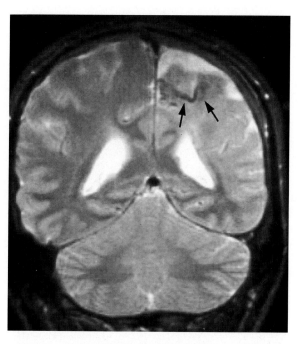

**Sturge-Weber Syndrome**

---

Sturge-Weber syndrome is one of the neurophako-matoses combining cutaneous and intracranial abnormalities. The external manifestation of the syndrome is a unilateral facial angioma or "port-wine stain" in the distribution of a division of the trigeminal nerve. This hallmark is associated with an ipsilateral venous angioma of the meninges, most common in the parietooccipital region. (An alternative name for this syndrome is "encephalotrigeminal angiomatosis.")

Cerebral cortex underlying the meningeal angioma of Sturge-Weber syndrome exhibits a characteristic "tram-track" pattern of dystrophic calcification, easily appreciated on skull films or CT scans. The calcification may be observed to develop in an infant or toddler over a period of weeks or months.

On noncontrast MR scans there may be little or no evidence of the meningeal angioma. Cortical calcification may cause T1-shortening or focal low signal intensity on short TR scans; both are seen in the right frontal lobe of Case 908. Calcification of cortex (and/or associated iron

deposition) is usually apparent as discrete or hazy regions of low intensity on T2-weighted images, illustrated by Case 909 *(arrows).* Vague low signal intensity may also be present within white matter in affected areas on T2-weighted scans.

Cerebral atrophy is commonly associated with Sturge-Weber syndrome and may be focal or hemispheric. Both of the above cases demonstrate this finding.

The right cerebral hemisphere is small in Case 908, with particular volume loss of the frontal lobe. Associated expansion of the right frontal sinus and asymmetrical thickening of the calvarium on the right indicate that the reduced cerebral volume dates back to early childhood (or before).

In Case 909, the volume of the left hemicranium is smaller than the right, with eccentric position of the falx. The interface between gray and white matter is abnormal over a large region of the left hemisphere, extending well beyond the zone of calcification.

### Case 910

29-year-old man with a long history of seizures.
(axial, postcontrast T1-weighted SE scan with MTS)

### Case 911

40-year-old man with seizures since childhood.
(coronal, postcontrast T1-weighted SE scan)

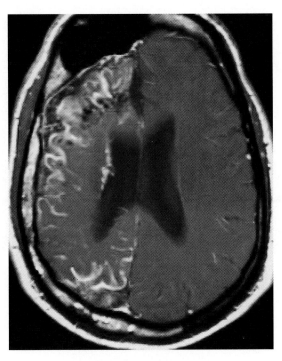

**Sturge-Weber Syndrome**
(same patient as Case 908)

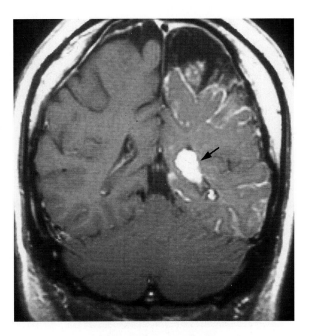

**Sturge-Weber Syndrome**

A number of abnormalities may be demonstrated on postcontrast MR scans in patients with Sturge-Weber syndrome.

The meningeal angioma covering the surface of the small right hemisphere in Case 910 is seen as a superficial layer of enhancement. Abnormal leptomeningeal enhancement often extends beyond the area of cortical calcification and parenchymal atrophy, as demonstrated in this case (compare Case 910 to Case 908). Vascular congestion within the meninges reflecting the commonly associated abnormality of cortical venous drainage probably contributes to this diffuse involvement. In any event, Sturge-Weber syndrome should be included in the differential diagnosis of leptomeningeal enhancement (along with meningeal inflammation, neoplasm, and hyperemia).

Intense, confluent enhancement is present within choroid plexus of the left lateral ventricle in Case 911 *(arrow)*. An angioma of the ipsilateral choroid plexus is commonly associated with other findings of the Sturge-Weber syndrome.

Large superficial and deep veins are often seen in the region involved by Sturge-Weber syndrome. (Note the prominent subependymal veins along the margin of the right lateral ventricle in Case 910.) These hypertrophied and/or aberrant channels reflect abnormal cortical venous drainage, with collateral flow away from the superior sagittal sinus.

Seizures are almost always a dominant feature in the clinical presentation of patients with Sturge-Weber syndrome, often beginning at age one or two.

Case 910 is an example of the Dyke-Davidoff-Masson syndrome of cerebral hemiatrophy with hemicranial hypertrophy. The reduced volume of the right cerebral hemisphere has led to ipsilateral changes in calvarial morphology, demonstrating the interrelationship of brain growth and skull contour. The involved hemicranium is small, with eccentric falx position. The skull is thickened on the side of cerebral atrophy, and there is asymmetrical enlargement of ipsilateral sinuses.

# OCCIPITAL ENCEPHALOCELES

## Case 912

1-day-old boy.
(sagittal, noncontrast T1-weighted SE scan)

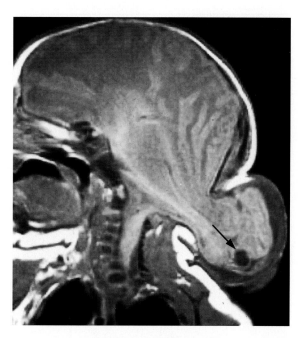

**Occipital Encephalocele**

## Case 913

1-day-old girl.
(sagittal, noncontrast T1-weighted SE scan)

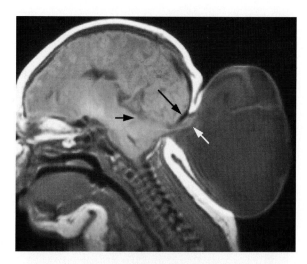

**Occipital Encephalocele**

Encephaloceles are extracranial extensions of brain tissue, most commonly encountered along the skull base. Potential locations include the nose, sphenoid sinus, petrous bones, occipital region, and parietal bones. Frontonasal, parietal, and occipital meningoceles or encephaloceles are usually apparent at birth. Cephaloceles in the sphenoid or temporal region of the skull base are much more occult, often not presenting or detected until adulthood (see Cases 914 and 915).

MR is the modality of choice for noninvasive evaluation of congenital cephaloceles. Scans clearly document whether the extracranial sac is filled with brain tissue, as in Case 912, or largely contains CSF, as in Case 913.

A small amount of cerebellar parenchyma enters the superior margin of the encephalocele in Case 913 *(white arrow)*. The more amorphous zones of intermediate signal intensity in the superior portion of the encephalocele sac are artifactual.

MR scans can also demonstrate the presence of flow void indicating major vascular structures within cephalocele sacs. This is particularly relevant to the evaluation of occipital encephaloceles, which develop near major dural sinuses. In Case 912, a large vessel is imaged in cross section at the posteroinferior margin of the herniation *(arrow)*. A venous sinus is present immediately superior to the herniating cerebellar tissue in Case 913 *(long black arrow)*.

Both of the above cases demonstrate distorted morphology of intracranial parenchyma as it is pulled in the direction of the encephalocele. This traction pattern remains as evidence of the congenital malformation even after a cephalocele has been repaired.

Associated hindbrain malformations are present in the above patients. Deformed cerebellar tissue extends into the cervical spinal canal in Case 912. "Beaking" of the midbrain tectum is seen in Case 913 *(short black arrow)*. This combination of Chiari type II hindbrain deformities with an occipital and/or high cervical encephalocele is often referred to as a "Chiari III" malformation.

### Case 914

48-year-old woman presenting with CSF rhinorrhea.
(coronal, noncontrast T1-weighted SE scan)

### Case 915

45-year-old woman presenting with seizures.
(coronal, postcontrast T1-weighted SE scan)

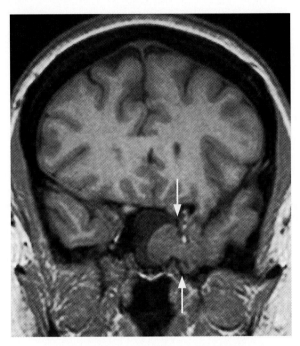

**Lateral Sphenoidal Encephalocele**

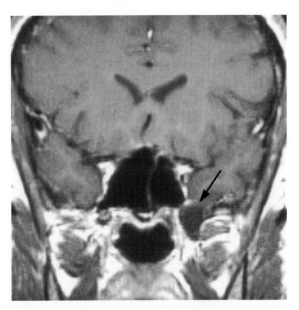

**Lateral Sphenoidal Encephalocele**

Transphenoidal meningoceles or encephaloceles are often initially occult. Midline sphenoidal encephaloceles may present in adolescence or childhood with nasopharyngeal obstruction, impaired vision, or reduced endocrine function. The latter symptoms are due to dysfunction of the optic apparatus and/or hypothalamic/pituitary axis caused by inferior displacement or traction of these structures. Parasagittal sphenoidal cephaloceles are more likely to present with meningitis, CSF rhinorrhea, or seizures, as in the above cases.

The scan in Case 914 demonstrates medial temporal gyri extending into the left side of the sphenoid sinus through a deficient lateral wall *(arrows)*. The remainder of the sinus is filled with CSF. Communication of the sphenoid sinus with the nose provides a route for CSF rhinorrhea and potential meningitis.

The cephalocele sac in Case 915 is more subtle, occurring in the left pterygoid region *(arrow)*. Meningoceles or encephaloceles involving the medial portion of the middle cranial fossa are often associated with distortion and scarring of the adjacent temporal lobe. This parenchymal abnormality may present clinically as seizures. As a result, small lateral sphenoidal or petrous cephaloceles are among the lesions to be sought on coronal scans of epileptic patients.

The cephalocele sac in Case 915 is filled with CSF and demonstrated high signal intensity on a T2-weighted scan. This appearance had initially been interpreted as a schwannoma near the foramen ovale. Although uniform prolongation of T2 is common in schwannomas, the alternative possibility of a CSF-containing sac should be considered when such a lesion is encountered along the skull base. The lack of contrast enhancement within a cephalocele can distinguish it from a solid mass in otherwise ambiguous cases.

### Case 916A

64-year-old man with a long history of
nasal obstruction on the right.
(axial, noncontrast T2-weighted SE scan)

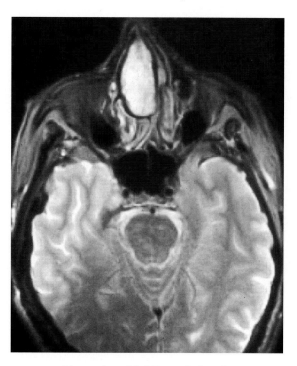

**Nasoethmoidal Encephalocele**

### Case 916B

Same patient.
(sagittal, noncontrast T1-weighted SE scan)

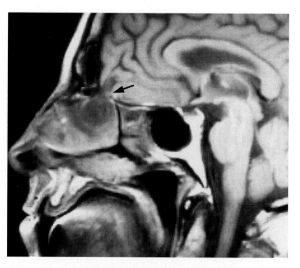

**Nasoethmoidal Encephalocele**

The smoothly rounded mass within the right nasal cavity in Case 916A seems to be long-standing. There is associated deviation of the nasal septum and deformity of the ipsilateral turbinates.

This appearance should raise the possibility of a nasoethmoidal encephalocele. Biopsy or removal of such masses carries the risk of CSF leak and meningitis. Important vessels or functional neural tissue may extend into the encephalocele and be vulnerable to surgical injury.

Discovery of a soft tissue mass beneath the skull base warrants a careful search for bone defects or anatomical distortions linking the lesion with the intracranial compartment. In Case 916B, a defect along the floor of the anterior cranial fossa is apparent in the cribform region *(arrow)*. The crista galli is poorly seen and presumably dis-

placed and/or eroded. There is continuity of soft tissue between a small intracranial component and the larger intranasal mass. Note that gyri and sulci of the frontal lobe are not pulled toward the encephalocele in this case (compare to Cases 912 and 913). Surgery confirmed an encephalocele containing dysplastic glial tissue.

Occasionally the stalk connecting a nasal encephalocele with its origin in the anterior cranial fossa is obliterated. The resulting island of glial tissue within the nose is often called a *nasal glioma.*

Dermal sinus tracts may also span the skull base with nasal and intracranial components (see Case 917). Both encephaloceles and dermal sinuses involving the nasoethmoid region may predispose to isolated or recurrent meningitis.

## Case 917A

16-month-old boy presenting with a small mass
and a dimple on the bridge of the nose.
(sagittal, postcontrast T1-weighted GRE scan)

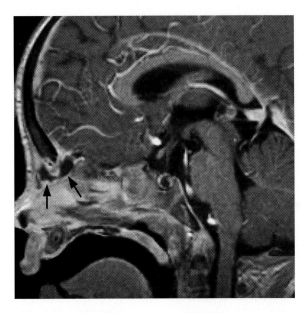

**Frontonasal Dermoid Cyst**

## Case 917B

Same patient.
(coronal, postcontrast T1-weighted GRE scan)

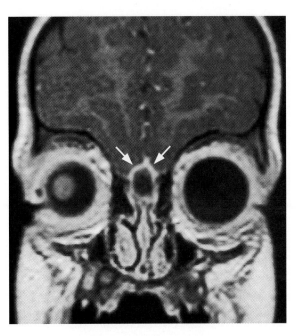

**Frontonasal Dermoid Cyst**

Failure of dysjunction of cutaneous and neuroectoderm leads to a dermal sinus tract from the skin surface to (or through) the dura. The spinal form of this embryological malformation is relatively common; see Cases 1264 and 1265 for discussion of the "dorsal dermal sinus syndrome."

Transcranial dermal sinuses also occur, typically in the midline. Common locations include the frontonasal region, the vertex, and the occipital area. Such sinuses may be associated with epidermoid or dermoid cysts in the epidural or intradural spaces.

Case 917A demonstrates a bilobed midline mass extending from the anterior-inferior corner of the anterior cranial fossa to the base of the nose *(arrows)*. The center of the lesion demonstrates uniformly long T1 values, outlined by a thin layer of contrast enhancement. The midline location and peripheral enhancement of the frontonasal mass are confirmed in the coronal projection *(arrows, Case 917B)*.

This appearance is typical for a nasal dermoid sinus/cyst. Such congenital tracts traverse the foramen cecum, following the same route as nasoethmoidal encephaloceles (see Case 916). This common pathway reflects the normal embryological projection of dura that extends from the ante-

rior fossa through the foramen cecum and between the nasal bone and nasal cartilage to contact the skin surface at the glabella. If this normally transient dural extension fails to involute, brain tissue can follow the channel into the ethmoid sinuses and nose, leading to a fronto-ethmoidal ("sincipital") encephalocele or a "nasal glioma." Alternatively, if the dural projection retracts while retaining contact with the skin, a dermal sinus tract is created along the same pathway. Subsequent proliferation of cutaneous ectoderm can lead to dermoid or epidermoid cysts at any point along the route from the nose through the foramen cecum to the intracranial compartment.

As discussed in Chapter 7, the signal intensity within dermoid cysts is variable. Distinction between an inclusion cyst and a cephalocele in the frontonasal region is more reliably based on the morphology of adjacent brain tissue than on specific signal characteristics. When frontonasal dermoid or epidermoid cysts project into the anterior cranial fossa, they displace CSF and cerebral parenchyma. Conversely, these structures are usually drawn toward or into the foramen cecum in cases of nasoethmoidal encephaloceles (but see Case 916).

**Case 918A**

6-month-old girl with a soft lump
on the back of the head.
(sagittal, noncontrast T1-weighted SE scan)

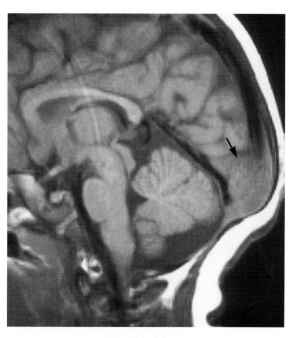

**Dermoid Cyst**

**Case 918B**

Same patient.
(axial, noncontrast T2-weighted SE scan)

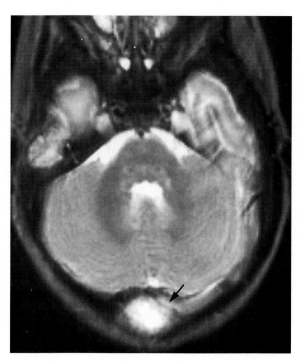

**Dermoid Cyst**

Intracranial dermoid masses may develop as isolated inclusion cysts or in association with a dermal sinus (as in Case 917). Intradural dermoid cysts have been discussed in Cases 312-315. Case 918 demonstrates an epidural cyst, presenting as a homogeneous midline lesion posterior to the torcular herophili. The occipital bone overlying the mass is markedly thinned or absent. (CT would offer a better assessment of osseous deformity.)

The signal intensity of the lesion (intermediate T1 values, long T2 values) is nonspecific. Epidermoid cysts usually demonstrate lower intensity on T1-weighted scans than seen in Case 918A. However, superimposed inflammatory changes due to an associated sinus tract may modify the classic appearance.

As discussed in Cases 312-315, the signal intensity of dermoid cysts is variable. Relevant factors include (1) the proportion of proteinaceous content versus lipid material, (2) the presence or absence of simple fluid (see Case 919), and (3) the presence or absence of superimposed infection.

It is important to consider dermal sinus tracts and associated dermoid or epidermoid cysts along with cephaloceles in the differential diagnosis of small, midline transcranial lesions. Both pathologies commonly involve the frontonasal and occipital regions. Traction of intracranial parenchyma toward the calvarial defect favors a cephalocele. Conversely, dermal sinuses often lead to epidural or intradural masses that displace cerebral tissue away from the skull, as seen in this case.

**Case 919A**

9-month-old girl with a progressively
enlarging lump on the head.
(coronal, postcontrast T1-weighted SE scan)

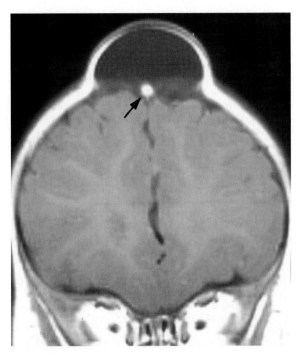

**Dermoid Cyst**

**Case 919B**

Same patient.
(axial, noncontrast T2-weighted SE scan)

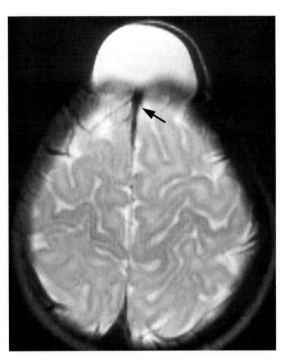

**Dermoid Cyst**

---

Dermoid cysts are the most common cause of a scalp mass in an infant. They are particularly frequent near the anterior fontanelle and along the course of cranial sutures. Associated dermal sinuses and intracranial extension commonly accompany lesions near the nasion and torcular (see Cases 917 and 918) but rarely occur with dermoid cysts overlying the sagittal suture.

The extracranial mass in Case 919 had been observed to enlarge steadily since the newborn period. Such rapid growth would be unusual for the slow accumulation of semisolid material within a dermoid or epidermoid cyst. However, the coronal scan in Case 919A clearly indicates that the lesion is superficial to the normally formed dura and superior sagittal sinus *(arrow)*, excluding a meningocele.

At surgery, the mass proved to be a fluid-filled dermoid cyst within the scalp. A small amount of granular, greasy material was also present within the cyst.

This case demonstrates that dermoid cysts occasionally accumulate aqueous fluid. Together, Cases 918 and 919 illustrate that dermoid or epidermoid cysts may cause midline extracranial or transcranial masses clinically resembling cephaloceles.

In addition to dermoid cysts and encephaloceles, the differential diagnosis of a lump on the head of a child includes cephalohematoma, subgaleal hematoma, hemangioma, lymphangioma, neurofibroma, eosinophilic granuloma, osteoma, and sinus pericranii.

# REFERENCES

Aboulezz AO, Sartor K, Geyer CA, et al: Position of cerebellar tonsils in the normal population and in patients with Chiari malformation: a quantitative approach with MR imaging. *J Comput Assist Tomogr* 1033-1036, 1985.

Aida N, Tamagawa K, Takada K, et al: Brain MR in Fukuyama congenital muscular dystrophy. *AJNR* 17:605-614, 1996.

Aida N, Yagishita A, Takada K, Katsumata Y: Cerebellar MR in Fukuyama congenital muscular dystrophy: polymicrogyria with cystic lesions. *AJNR* 15:1755-1760, 1994.

Altman NR, Purser RK, Post MJD: Tuberous sclerosis: characteristics at CT and MR imaging. *Radiology* 167:527-532, 1988.

Aoki S, Barkovich AJ, Nishimura K, et al: Neurofibromatosis types 1 and 2: cranial MR findings. *Radiology* 172:527-534, 1989.

Arbelaez A, Castillo M: Magnetic resonance imaging of cerebellar lesions in patients with tuberous sclerosis. *Int J Neurorad* 4: 412-416, 1998.

Armonda RA, Citrin CM, Foley KT, Ellenbogen RG: Quantitative cine-mode magnetic resonance imaging of Chiari I malformations: an analysis of cerebrospinal fluid dynamics. *Neurosurgery* 35:214-224, 1994.

Atlas SW, Zimmerman RA, Bilaniuk LT, et al: Corpus callosum and limbic system: Neuroanatmic MR evaluation of developmental anomalies. *Radiology* 160:355-362, 1986.

Ball WS, Crone KR: Chiari I malformation: from Dr. Chiari to MR imaging. *Radiology* 195:602-604, 1995.

Barkovich AJ: Analyzing the corpus callosum. *AJNR* 17:1643-1645, 1996.

Barkovich AJ: Apparent atypical callosal dysgenesis: analysis of MR findings in six cases and their relationship to holoprosencephaly. *AJNR* 11:333-339, 1990.

Barkovich AJ: Imaging of the cobblestone lissencephalies. *AJNR* 17:615-618, 1996.

Barkovich AJ: Morphologic characteristics of subcortical heterotopia: MR imaging study. *AJNR* 21:290-295, 2000.

Barkovich AJ: Neuroimaging manifestations and classification of congenital muscular dystrophies. *AJNR* 19:1389-1396, 1998.

Barkovich AJ: Subcortical heterotopia: a distinct clinicoradiologic entity. *AJNR* 17:1315-1322, 1996.

Barkovich AJ, Chuang SH: Unilateral megalencephaly: correlation of MR imaging and pathologic characteristics. *AJNR* 11:523-531, 1990.

Barkovich AJ, Chuang SH, Norman D: MR of neuronal migration anomalies. *AJNR* 8:1009-1017, 1987.

Barkovich AJ, Fram EK, Norman D: Septo-optic dysplasia: MR imaging. *Radiology* 171:189-192, 1989.

Barkovich AJ, Frieden IJ, Williams ML: MR of neurocutaneous melanosis. *AJNR* 15:859-860, 1994.

Barkovich AJ, Gressens P, Evrard P: Formation, maturation, and disorders of brain neocortex. *AJNR* 13:423-446, 1992.

Barkovich AJ, Guerrini R, Battaglia G, et al: Band heterotopia: correlation of outcome with magnetic resonance imaging parameters. *Ann Neurol* 36:609-617, 1994.

Barkovich AJ, Hevner R, Guerrini R: Syndromes of bilateral symmetrical polymicrogyria. *AJNR* 20:1814-1821, 1999.

Barkovich AJ, Jackson DE Jr, Boyer RS: Band heterotopias: a newly recognized neuronal migration anomaly. *Radiology* 171:455-458, 1989.

Barkovich AJ, Kjos BO: Gray matter heterotopias: MR characteristics and correlation with developmental and neurologic manifestations. *Radiology* 182:493-499, 1992.

Barkovich AJ, Kjos BO: Nonlissencephalic cortical dysplasias: correlation of imaging findings with clinical deficits. *AJNR* 13:95-103, 1992.

Barkovich AJ, Kjos BO: Schizencephaly: correlation of clinical findings with MR characteristics. *AJNR* 13:85-94, 1992.

Barkovich AJ, Kuzniecky RI, Bollen AW, Grant PE: Focal transmantle dysplasia: a specific malformation of cortical development. *Neurology* 49:1148-1152, 1997.

Barkovich AJ, Kuzniecky RI, Dobyns WB, et al: A classification scheme for malformations of cortical development. *Neuropediatrics* 27:59-63, 1996.

Barkovich AJ, Norman D: Absence of the septum pellucidum: a useful sign in the diagnosis of congenital brain malformations. *AJNR* 9:1107-1114, 1988.

Barkovich AJ, Norman D: Anomalies of the corpus callosum: correlation with further anomalies of the brain. *AJNR* 9:493-501, 1988.

Barkovich AJ, Norman D: MR imaging of schizencephaly. *AJNR* 9:297-302, 1988.

Barkovich AJ, Quint DJ: Middle interhemispheric fusion: an unusual variant of holoprosencephaly. *AJNR* 14:431-440, 1993.

Barkovich AJ, Rowley HA, Andermann F: MR in partial epilepsy: value of high-resolution volumetric techniques. *AJNR* 16:339-344, 1995.

Barkovich AJ, Rowley H, Bollen A: Correlation of prenatal events with the development of polymicrogyria. *AJNR* 16:822-827. 1995.

Barkovich AJ, Vandermarck P, Edwards MSB, Cagen PH: Congenital nasal masses: CT and imaging features in 16 cases. *AJNR* 12: 105-116, 1991.

Barkovich AJ, Wippold FJ, Sherman JL, et al: Significance of cerebellar tonsillar position on MR. *AJNR* 7:795-799, 1986.

Baron Y, Barkovich AJ: MR imaging of tuberous sclerosis in neonates and young infants. *AJNR* 20:907-916, 1999.

Benedikt RA, Brown DC, Ghaed VN, et al: Sturge-Weber syndrome: cranial MR imaging with Gd-DTPA. *AJNR* 14:409-415, 1993.

Berns DH, Masaryk TJ, Weisman B, et al: Tuberous sclerosis: increased MR detection using gradient echo techniques. *J Comput Assist Tomogr* 13:896-898, 1989.

Bilaniuk L, Zimmerman R, Hochman M, et al: MR of the Sturge-Weber syndrome. *AJNR* 8:945, 1987.

Blaser SI, Jay V: Disorders of cortical formation: radiologic-pathologic correlation. *Neuroimaging Clin North Am* 9:53-72, 1999.

Bognanno JR, Edwards MK, Lee TA, et al: Cranial MR imaging in neurofibromatosis. *AJNR* 9:461-468, 1988.

Bonawitz C, Castillo M, Chin CT, et al: Usefulness of contrast material in MR of patients with neurofibromatosis type 1. *AJNR* 19:541-546, 1998.

Braffman BH, Bilaniuk LT, Naidich TP, et al: MR imaging of tuberous sclerosis: pathogenesis of this phakomatosis. Use of gadopentetate dimeglumine, and literature review. *Radiology* 183: 227-238, 1992.

Braffman BH, Bilaniuk LT, Zimmerman RA: The central nervous system manifestation of the phakomatoses on MR. *Radiology* 26:773-800, 1988.

Braffman BH, Bilaniuk CT, Zimmerman RA: MR of central nervous system neoplasia of the phakomatoses. *Sem Roentgenol* 25:198-217, 1990.

Braffman B, Naidich TP: The phakomatoses: part II. Von Hippel-Lindau disease, Sturge-Weber syndrome, and less common conditions. *Neuroimaging Clin North Am* 4:325-348, 1994.

Bronen RA, Spencer DD, Fulbright RK: Cerebrospinal fluid cleft with cortical dimple: MR imaging marker for focal cortical dysgenesis. *Radiology* 214:657-664, 2000.

Bronen RA, Vives KP, Kim JH, et al: Focal cortical dysplasia of Taylor, balloon cell subtype: MR differentiation from low-grade tumors. *AJNR* 18:1141-1152, 1997.

Byrd SE, Bohan TP, Osborn RE, Naidich TP: The CT and MR evaluation of lissencephaly. *AJNR* 9:923-927, 1988.

Byrd SE, Naidich TP: Common congenital brain anomalies. *Radiol Clin North Am* 26:755-772, 1988.

Byrd SE, Osborn RE, Bohan TP, et al: CT and MR evaluation of migrational disorders of the brain. Part I. Lissencephaly and pachygyria. *Pediatr Radiol* 19:151, 1989.

Byrd SE, Osborn RE, Bohan TP, et al: CT and MR evaluation of migrational disorders of the brain. Part II. Schizencephaly, heterotopia, and polymicrogyria. *Pediatr Radiol* 19:219, 1989.

Byrd SE, Osborn RE, Radkowski MA, et al: Disorders of midline structures: holoprosencephaly, absence of corpus callosum and Chiari malformations. *Semin US CT MR* 9:201-215, 1988.

Cai C, Oakes WJ: Hindbrain herniation syndromes: the Chiari malformation (I and II). *Semin Pediatr Neurol* 4:179-191, 1997.

Castillo M: Congenital abnormalities of the nose: CT and MR findings. *Am J Roentgenol* 162:1211-1217, 1994.

Castillo M, Bouldin TW, Scatliff JH, Suzuki K: Radiologic-pathologic correlation. Alobar holoprosencephaly. *AJNR* 14:1151-1156, 1993.

Castillo M, Wilson JD: Spontaneous resolution of a Chiari I malformation: MR demonstration. *AJNR* 16:1158-1160, 1995.

Chamberlain M, Press G, Hesselink J: MR imaging and CT in Sturge-Weber syndrome. *AJNR* 10:491, 1989.

Cho WH, Seidenwurm D, Barkovich AJ: Adult-onset neurologic dysfunction associated with cortical malformations. *AJNR* 20:1037-1043, 1999.

Cure JK, Holden KR, Van Tassel P: Progressive venous occlusion in a neonate with Sturge-Weber syndrome: demonstration with MR venography. *AJNR* 16:1539-1542, 1995.

Curnes JT, Laster DW, Koubek TD, et al: MRI of corpus callosal syndromes. *AJNR* 7:617-622, 1986.

Curnes JT, Oakes W, Boyko OB: MR imaging of hindbrain deformity in patients with and without symptoms of brain stem compression. *AJNR* 10:293-302, 1989.

Dean B, Drayer BP, Berisini DC, Bird CR: MR imaging of pericallosal lipoma. *AJNR* 9:929-931, 1988.

Deasy NP, Jarosz JM, Al Sarraj S, Cox TCS: Intrasphenoid cephalocele: MRI in two cases. *Neuroradiology* 41:497-500, 1999.

Demaerel P, Van de Gaer P, Wilms G, et al: Interhemispheric lipoma with variable callosal dysgenesis: relationship between embryology, morphology, and symptomatology. *Eur Radiol* 6:904-909, 1996.

Demirci A, Kawamura Y, Sze G, Duncan C: MR of parenchymal neurocutaneous melanosis. *AJNR* 16:603-608, 1995.

Dietrich RB, Kocit DD, et al: Lissencephaly: MR and CT appearances with different subtypes. *Radiology* 185(suppl):123, 1992.

DiPaolo D, Zimmerman RA: Solitary cortical tubers. *AJNR* 16:1360-1364, 1995.

DiPaolo DP, Zimmerman RA, Rorke LB, et al: Neurofibromatosis type I: pathologic substrate of high-signal intensity foci in the brain. *Radiology* 195:721-724, 1995.

Dubeau F, Tampieri D, Lee N, et al: Periventricular and subcortical nodular heterotopia: a study of 33 patients. *Brain* 118:1273-1287, 1995.

Dunn V, Mock T, Bell WE, et al: Detection of heterotopic gray matter in children by magnetic resonance imaging. *Magn Reson Imaging* 4:33-39, 1986.

El Gammal T, Mark EK, Brooks BS: MR imaging of Chiari II malformation. *AJNR* 8:1037-1044, 1987.

Elster AD: Radiologic screening in the neurocutaneous syndromes: strategies and controversies. *AJNR* 13:1078-1082, 1992.

Elster AD, Chen MYM: Chiari I malformations: clinical and radiologic reappraisal. *Radiology* 183:347-353, 1992.

Elster AD, Chen MYM: MR imaging of Sturge-Weber syndrome: role of gadopentetate dimeglumine and gradient echo techniques. *AJNR* 11:685-689, 1990.

Fitz CR: Holoprosencephaly and septo-optic dysplasia. *Neuroimaging Clin North Am* 4:263-281, 1994.

Gallucci M, Bozzao A, Curatolo P, et al: MR imaging of incomplete band heterotopia. *AJNR* 12:701-702, 1991.

Georgy BA, Hesselink JR, Jernigan TL: MR imaging of the corpus callosum. *Am J Roentgenol* 160:949-955, 1993.

Girard N, Zimmerman RA, Schnur RE, et al: Magnetization transfer in the investigation of patients with tuberous sclerosis. *Neuroradiology* 39:523-528, 1997.

Gomez-Anson B, Thom M, Moran N, et al: Imaging and radiological-pathological correlation in histologically proven cases of focal cortical dysplasia and other glial and neuronoglial malformative lesions in adults. *Neuroradiology* 42:157-167, 2000.

Grant PE, Barkovich AJ, Wald LL, et al: High-resolution surface-coil MR of cortical lesions in medically-refractory epilepsy: a prospective study. *AJNR* 18:291-301, 1997.

Griffiths PD, Blaser S, Boodram MB, et al: Choroid plexus size in young children with Sturge-Weber syndrome. *AJNR* 17:175-180, 1996.

Guyot LL, Kazmierczak CD, Michael DB: Adult rhombencephalosynapsis. Case report. *J Neurosurg* 93:323-325, 2000.

Hurst R, Newman S, Cail W: Multifocal intracranial MR abnormalities in neurofibromatosis. *AJNR* 9:293, 1988.

Inoue Y, Nakajima S, Fukuda T, et al: Magnetic resonance imaging of tuberous sclerosis: further observations and clinical correlations. *Neuroradiology* 30:379, 1988.

Itoh T, Magnaldi S, White RM, et al: Neurofibromatosis type I: the evolution of deep gray and white matter MR abnormalities. *AJNR* 15:1513-1520, 1994.

Iwasaki S, Nakagawa H, Kichikawa K, et al: MR and CT of tuberous sclerosis: linear abnormalities in the cerebral white matter. *AJNR* 11:1029-1034, 1990.

Jinkins JR, Whittemore AR, Bradley WG: MR imaging of callosal and corticocallosal dysgenesis. *AJNR* 10:339-344, 1989.

Kash F, Brown G, Smirniotopoulos JA, et al: Intracranial lipomas: pathology and imaging spectrum. *Int J Neurorad* 2:109-116, 1996.

Kato T, Yamanouchi H, Sugai K, Takashima S: Improved detection of cortical and subcortical tubers in tuberous sclerosis by fluid-attenuated inversion recovery MRI. *Neuroradiology* 39:378-380, 1997.

Kier EL, Truwit CL: The normal and abnormal genu of the corpus callosum: an evolutionary, embryologic, anatomic, and MR analysis. *AJNR* 17:1631-1641, 1996.

Kingsley D, Kendall B, Fitz C: Tuberous sclerosis: a clinicoradiological evaluation of 110 cases with particular reference to atypical presentation. *Neuroradiology* 28:171-190, 1986.

Kuzniecky R, Andermann F: The congenital bilateral perisylvian syndrome: imaging findings in a multicenter study. *AJNR* 15:139-144, 1994.

Landrieu P, Husson B, Pariente D, Lacroix C: MRI-neuropathological correlations in type 1 lissencephaly. *Neuroradiology* 40:173-176, 1998.

Lee BCP, Engle M: MR of lissencephaly. *AJNR* 9:804, 1988.

Lee BCP, Schmidt RE, Hatfield GA, et al: MRI of focal cortical dysplasia. *Neuroradiology* 40:675-683, 1998.

Lehericy S, Dormont D, Semah F, et al: Developmental abnormalities of the medial temporal lobe in patients with temporal lobe epilepsy. *AJNR* 16:617-626, 1995.

Levine D, Barnes PD, Madsen JR, et al: Fetal central nervous system anomalies: MR imaging augments sonographic diagnosis. *Radiology* 204:635-642, 1997.

Levine D, Barnes PD, Madsen JR, et al: Fetal CNS anomalies revealed on ultrafast MR imaging. *Am J Roentgenol* 172:813-818, 1999.

Lindbichler F, Braun H, Raith J, et al: Nasal dermoid cyst with a sinus tract extending to the frontal dura mater: MRI. *Neuroradiology* 39:529-531, 1997.

Lipski S, Brunelle F, Aicardi J, et al: Gd-DTPA-enhanced MR imaging in two cases of Sturge-Weber syndrome. *AJNR* 11:690-692, 1990.

Marti-Bonmati L, Menor F, Dosda R: Tuberous sclerosis: differences between cerebral and cerebellar cortical tubers in a pediatric population. *AJNR* 21:557-560, 2000.

Martinez-Lage JF, Poza M, Sola J, et al: The child with a cephalocele: etiology, neuroimaging, and outcome. *Childs Nerv Syst* 12:540-550, 1996.

Martinez-Lage JF, Sola J, Casas C, et al: Atretic cephalocele: the tip of the iceberg. *J Neurosurg* 77:230-235, 1992.

Mautner VF, Lindenau M, Baser ME, et al: The neuroimaging and clinical spectrum of neurofibromatosis 2. *Neurosurgery* 38:880-886, 1996.

McLone DG, Naidich TP: Developmental morphology of the subarachnoid space, brain vasculature, and contiguous structures, and the cause of the Chiari II malformation. *AJNR* 13:463-482, 1992.

McMurdo SK Jr, Moore SG, Brant-Zawadzki M, et al: MR imaging of intracranial tuberous sclerosis. *AJNR* 8:77-82, 1987.

Meadows J, Kraut M, Guarnieri M, et al: Asymptomatic Chiari type I malformations identified on magnetic resonance imaging. *J Neurosurg* 92:920-926, 2000.

Menkes JH, Curran J: Clinical and MR correlates in children with extra-pyramidal cerebral palsy. *AJNR* 15:451-458, 1994.

Menor F, Marti-Bonmati L: CT detection of basal ganglia lesions in neurofibromatosis type1: correlation with MRI. *Neuroradiology* 34:305-307, 1992.

Menor F, Marti-Bonmati L, Mulas F, et al: Imaging considerations of central nervous system manifestations in pediatric patients with neurofibromatosis type 1. *Pediatr Radiol* 21:389-394, 1991.

Menor F, Marti-Bonmati L, Mulas F, et al: Neuroimaging in tuberous sclerosis: a clinicoradiological evaluation in pediatric patients. *Pediatr Radiol* 22:485-489, 1992.

Mirowitz SA, Sarton K, Gado M: High-intensity basal ganglia lesions on T1-weighted MR images in neurofibromatosis. *AJNR* 10:1159-1163, 1989.

Mori K: Giant interhemispheric cysts associated with agenesis of the corpus callosum. *J Neurosurg* 76:224-230, 1992.

Naidich TP, Altman NR, Braffman BH, et al: Cephaloceles and related malformations. *AJNR* 13:655-690, 1992.

Nixon JR, Houser OW, Gomez MR, Okazaki H: Cerebral tuberous sclerosis: MR imaging. *Radiology* 170:869-874, 1989.

Noorani PA, Bodensteiner JB, Barnes PD: Colpocephaly: frequency and associated findings. *J Child Neurol* 3:100, 1988.

Oba H, Barkovich AJ: Holoprosencephaly: analysis of callosal formation and its relation to development of the interhemispheric fissure. *AJNR* 16:453-460, 1995.

Osborn RE, Byrd SE, Naidich TP, et al: MR imaging of neuronal migrational disorders. *AJNR* 9:1101-1106, 1988.

Packard AM, Miller VS, Delgado MR: Schizencephaly: correlations of clinical and radiologic features. *Neurology* 48:1527-1434, 1997.

Payner TD, Prenger E, Berger TS, Crone KR: Acquired Chiari malformations: incidence, diagnosis, and management. *Neurosurgery* 34:429-434, 1994.

Pillay PK, Awad IA, Little JR, Hahn JF: Symptomatic Chiari malformation in adults: a new classification based on magnetic resonance imaging with clinical and prognostic significance. *Neurosurgery* 28:639-645, 1991.

Poe LB, Coleman LL, Mahmud F: Congenital central nervous system abnormalities. *Radiographics* 9:801-826, 1989.

Pont MS, Elster AD: Lesions of skin and brain. Modern imaging of the neurocutaneous syndrome. *Am J Roentgenol* 158:1193-1201, 1992.

Raffel C, McComb JG, Bodner S, Gilles FE: Benign brain stem lesions in pediatric patients with neurofibromatosis: case reports. *Neurosurgery* 25:959-964, 1989.

Raybaud C, Canto-Moreira N, Girard N, Poncet M: Polymicrogyria: MR appearance and its relationship to the fetal development of the cortex and its microvasculature. *Int J Neurorad* 1:161-170, 1995.

Reinarz SJ, Coffman CE, Smoker WRK et al: MR imaging of the corpus callosum. Normal and pathologic findings and correlation with CT. *AJNR* 9:649-656, 1988.

Rice JF, Eggers DM: Basal transsphenoidal encephalocele: MR findings. *AJNR* 10:579-580, 1989.

Roach ES, Williams DP, Laster DW: Magnetic resonance imaging in tuberous sclerosis. *Arch Neurol* 44:301-303, 1987.

Rubinstein D, Youngman V, Hise JH, Damiano TR: Partial development of the corpus callosum. *AJNR* 15:869-875, 1994.

Ruge JR, Tomitashita T, Naidich TP, et al: Scalp and calvarial mass of infants and children. *Neurosurgery* 22:1037-1042, 1988.

Sato N, Hatakeyama S, Shimizu N, et al: MR evaluation of the hippocampus in patients with congenital malformations of the brain. *AJNR* 22:389-393, 2001.

Sato Y, Kao SCS, Smith WL: Radiographic manifestations of anomalies of the brain. *Radiol Clin North Am* 29:179-194, 1991.

Sevick RJ, Barkovich AJ, Edwards MSB, et al: Evolution of white matter lesions in neurofibromatosis type 1: MR findings. *Am J Roentgenol* 159:171-175, 1992.

Shepherd CW, Houser OW, Gomez MR: MR findings in tuberous sclerosis complex and correlation with seizure development and mental impairment. *AJNR* 16:149-155, 1995.

Simon EM, Goldstein RB, Coakley FV, et al: Fast MR imaging of fetal CNS anomalies in utero. *AJNR* 21:1688-1698, 2000.

Simon EM, Hevner R, Pinter JD, et al: Assessment of the deep gray nuclei in holoprosencephaly. *AJNR* 21:1955-1961, 2000.

Smirniotopoulos JG, Murphy FM: The phakomatoses. *AJNR* 13:725-746, 1992.

Smith AS, Blaser SI, Ross JS, Weinstein MA: Magnetic resonance imaging of disturbances in neuronal migration: illustration of an embryologic process. *Radiographics* 9:509-523, 1989.

Smith A, Weinstein M, Quencer R, et al: Association of heterotopic gray matter with seizures: MR imaging. *Radiology* 168-195, 1988.

Stark JE, Glasier CM: MR demonstration of ectopic fourth ventricular choroid plexus I Chiara II malformation. *AJNR* 14:618-621, 1993.

Steen RG, Taylor JS, Langston JW, et al: Prospective evaluation of the brain in asymptomatic children with neurofibromatosis type 1: relationship of macrocephaly to T1 relaxation changes and structural brain abnormalities. *AJNR* 22:810-817, 2001.

Takanashi J-I, Sugita K, Fujii K, Niimi H: MR evaluation of tuberous sclerosis: increased sensitivity with fluid-attenuated inversion recovery and relation to severity of seizures and mental retardation. *AJNR* 16:1923-1928, 1995.

Tart RP, Quisling RG: Curvilinear and tubulonodular varieties of lipoma of the corpus callosum: an MR and CT study. *J Comput Assist Tomogr* 15:805-810, 1991.

Terada H, Barkovich AJ, Edwards MSB, Ciricillo SF: Evolution of high-intensity basal ganglia lesions on T1-weighted MR in neurofibromatosis type I. *AJNR* 17:755-760, 1996.

Terwey B, Doose H: Tuberous sclerosis: magnetic resonance imaging of the brain. *Neuropediatrics* 18:67-69, 1987.

Thompson JE, Castillo M, Thomas D, et al: Radiologic-pathologic correlation: polymicrogyria. *AJNR* 18:307-312, 1997.

Titelbaum DS, Haward JC, Zimmerman RA: Pachygyriclike changes: topographic appearance at MR imaging and CT and correlation with neurologic status. *Radiology* 173:663-668, 1989.

Truwit CL, Barkovich AJ: Pathogenesis of intracranial lipoma: an MR study in 42 patients. *AJNR* 11:665-674, 1990.

Truwit CL, Barkovich AJ, Koch TK, Ferriero DM: Cerebral palsy: MR findings in 40 patients. *AJNR* 13:67-78, 1992.

Truwit CL, Barkovich AJ, Shanahan R, Maroldo TV: MR imaging of rhombencephalosynapsis: report of three cases. *AJNR* 12:957-965, 1991.

Truwit C, Williams RG, Armstrong EA, Marlin AE: MR imaging of choroid plexus lipomas. *AJNR* 11:202-204, 1990.

Uchino A, Hasuo K, Matsumoto S, Masuda K: Solitary choroid plexus lipomas: CT and MR appearance. *AJNR* 14:116-118, 1993.

Utsunomiya H, Ogasawara T, Hayashi T, et al: Dysgenesis of the corpus callosum and associated telencephalic anomalies: MRI. *Neuroradiology* 39:302-310, 1997.

Utsunomiya H, Takano K, Ogasawara T, et al: Rhombencephalosynapsis: cerebellar embryogenesis. *AJNR* 19:547-549, 1998.

Van Bogaert P, Baleriaux D, Christope C, Szliwowski HB: MRI of patients with cerebral palsy and normal CT scan. *Neuroradiology* 34:52-56, 1992.

van beck EJR, Majoie CBLM: Joubert syndrome. *Radiology* 216:379-382, 2000.

Van Tassel P, Cure JK, Holden KR: Cystlike white matter lesions in tuberous sclerosis. *AJNR* 18:1367-1374, 1997.

Vogl TJ, Stemmler J, Bergman C, et al: MR and MR angiography of Sturge-Weber syndrome. *AJNR* 14:417-425, 1993.

Volpe JJ: Value of MR in definition of the neuropathology of cerebral palsy in vivo. *AJNR* 13:79-83, 1992.

Wasenko JJ, Rosenbloom SA, Duchesneau PM, et al: The Sturge-Weber syndrome: comparison of MR and CT characteristics. *AJNR* 11:131-134, 1990.

Wilms G, Van Wijck E, Dermaerel PH, et al: Gyriform calcifications in tuberous sclerosis simulating the appearance of Sturge-Weber disease. *AJNR* 13:295-298, 1992.

Wippold FJ II, Baber WW, Gado M, et al: Pre- and post-contrast MR studies in tuberous sclerosis. *J Comput Assist Tomogr* 16:69-72, 1992.

Wolpert SM, Anderson M, Scott RM, et al: The Chiari II malformation: MR imaging evaluation. *AJNR* 8:783-792, 1987.

Wolpert SM, Cohen A, Libenson MH: Hemimegalencephaly: a longitudinal MR study. *AJNR* 15:1479-1482, 1994.

Wolpert SM, Scott RM, Platenberg C, Runge VM: The clinical significance of hindbrain herniation and deformity as shown on MR images of patients with Chiari II malformation. *AJNR* 9:1075-1078, 1988.

Yagishita A, Arai N: Cortical tubers without other stigmata of tuberous sclerosis: imaging and pathological findings. *Neuroradiology* 41:428-432, 1999.

Yagishita A, Arai N, Taketoshi M, et al: Focal cortical dysplasia: appearance on MR images. *Radiology* 203:553-560, 1997.

Yagishita A, Arai N, Tamagawa K, Oda M: Hemimegalencephaly: signal changes suggesting abnormal myelination on MRI. *Neuroradiology* 40:734-738, 1998.

Yasumoro K, Hasuo K, Nagata S, et al: Neuronal migration anomalies causing extensive ventricular indentation. *Neurosurgery* 26:504-506, 1990.

Young JN, Oakes WJ, Hatten HP Jr: Dorsal third ventricular cyst: an entity distinct from holoprosencephaly. *J Neurosurg* 77:556-561, 1992.

Zimmerman RA, Yachnis AT, Rorke CT, et al: Pathology of findings of cerebral high signal intensity in two patients with type I neurofibromatosis. *Radiology* 185(suppl):123, 1992.

# CHAPTER 17

# Disc Disease and Spondylosis

### Case 920

78-year-old woman presenting with
pseudoclaudication.
(sagittal, noncontrast T1-weighted SE scan)

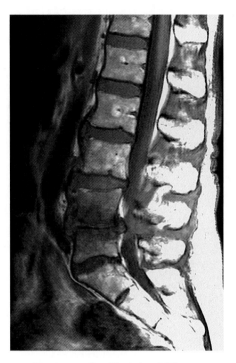

**Degenerative Vertebral Edema**

### Case 921

57-year-old woman presenting with back pain.
(sagittal, noncontrast T2-weighted FSE scan)

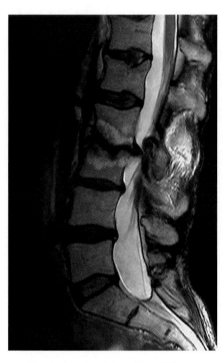

**Degenerative Vertebral Edema**

Sagittal or coronal MR scans may demonstrate reactive changes in the vertebral bodies adjacent to degenerating discs. Subchondral zones of long T1 and long T2 values are often seen, representing edema, vascularization, and cellular infiltration within the marrow. At a later stage, fatty atrophy of the marrow may cause the opposite pattern of signal changes: bright on T1-weighted images, with reduced signal intensity on T2-weighted scans (see Cases 922 and 923).

Severe disc space narrowing is present at the L4-5 level in Case 920, accompanied by anterior and posterior disc bulging. Poorly defined areas of low signal intensity occupy the subchondral regions of the adjacent vertebral bodies.

Case 921 demonstrates narrowing, reduced hydration signal and a Schmorl's node at the L2-3 disc level (as well as a herniated disc compressing the thecal sac). Prominent bands of T2 prolongation in subchondral regions of the L2 and L3 vertebral bodies correlated with low signal intensity on T1-weighted scans. This increase in water content suggests reactive inflammation.

Prolongation of T1 and T2 values within subchondral bone is also seen in patients with discitis and osteomyelitis (see Cases 1107-1110). Several features help to distinguish degenerative bone changes from osseous infection: (1) cortical end plates are preserved in degenerative disease (except for well-defined Schmorl's nodes) and irregularly eroded by infection; (2) the adjacent disc space usually demonstrates little or no hydration signal in degenerative disease but is commonly bright on T2-weighted scans when inflamed by discitis; (3) associated epidural or paraspinal masses are rarely seen in degenerative disease (unless there is superimposed disc herniation) but are often present with discitis; (4) contrast enhancement of affected vertebral bodies is moderate and uniform in degenerative disease, whereas enhancement in discitis/osteomyelitis is more irregular and intense.

The clinical context is also helpful in assessing the significance of signal abnormalities within vertebral bodies. Patients with discitis/osteomyelitis are usually in severe pain. The diagnosis is unlikely in the absence of significant discomfort.

High grade stenosis of the central canal in Case 920 explains the patient's pseudoclaudication (see Cases 956-959). Large anterior disc bulges elevate the anterior longitudinal ligament at L2-3, L3-4, and L4-5.

# BONE CHANGES ACCOMPANYING DISC DEGENERATION: FATTY ATROPHY

## Case 922

48-year-old man with a long history of back pain.
(sagittal, noncontrast T1-weighted SE scan)

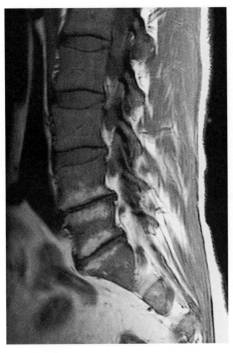

**Degenerative Marrow Atrophy**
(with otherwise increased cellularity)

## Case 923

49-year-old man presenting with back and leg pain.
(sagittal, noncontrast T2-weighted FSE scan)

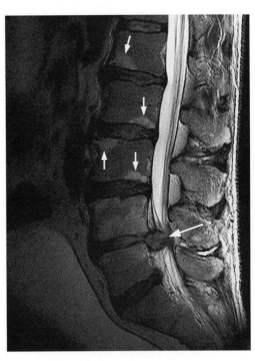

**Degenerative Marrow Atrophy**
(and disc herniation)

---

Chronic degenerative disc disease may be associated with atrophic changes in adjacent vertebral bodies. Marrow cellularity is decreased, with a corresponding increase in the proportion of fat. This altered water/lipid ratio causes shortening of T1 values in the affected regions, as illustrated at the L4-5 and L5-S1 levels in Case 922. (The subchondral fatty atrophy in this case is accentuated by a background of otherwise increased marrow cellularity due to chronic anemia.)

Relatively high signal intensity may also be noted in subchondral zones of marrow atrophy on T2-weighted scans performed with fast spin echo techniques, as seen at multiple levels *(short arrows)* in Case 923. The retention of high signal intensity within fatty tissue on T2-weighted FSE images (as compared to decreased signal intensity on conventional T2-weighted spin echo scans) is attributed to reduced spin-spin coupling ("J modulation"). This phase modulation causing destructive interference on late echoes of a standard spin echo sequence is suppressed by the close echo spacing used for an FSE sequence.

Subchondral marrow atrophy is often not as bright as subchondral edema on T2-weighted images. Correlation with a T1-weighted scan will eliminate potential confusion between fatty atrophy and increased water content on a T2-weighted FSE image. Sequences with fat-saturation technique can also clarify cases in which the etiology of the high intensity in subchondral regions on a T2-weighted FSE study is unclear.

The scattered, well-defined subchondral zones of relatively high signal intensity in Case 923 lie adjacent to discs with reduced height and/or hydration signal indicating degeneration. The most extensive marrow atrophy, within the L4 and L5 vertebral bodies, adjoins the level of herniation *(long arrow)* and greatest narrowing of the disc space. Cortical margins of the affected bodies remain well defined, unlike the usual appearance of discitis (see Cases 1107-1110).

## Case 924

45-year-old man presenting with low back pain.
(sagittal, noncontrast T1-weighted SE scan)

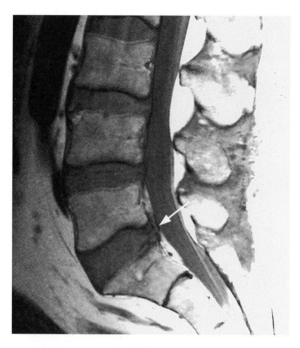

**Annular Tear**

## Case 925

36-year-old man presenting with back stiffness.
(sagittal, noncontrast T2-weighted FSE scan)

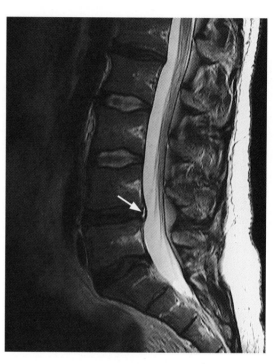

**Annular Tear**

Normal intervertebral discs demonstrate generally high signal intensity on long TR spin echo images. This appearance reflects the high water content of the nucleus pulposus and the integrity of the complex polysaccharides within the nuclear matrix.

Degeneration of a disc is accompanied by progressive loss of long T2 values, as seen at the L1-2, L4-5, and L5-S1 levels in Case 925. This change probably represents both a decrease in water content and an alteration of the macromolecular matrix of the disc (with increased binding of water molecules shortening relaxation times).

Disc degeneration is often associated with one or more tears of the annulus. These disruptions may play a role in causing or exacerbating "dehydration" or other components of the degenerative process.

The outer annular fibers form a dense zone at the perimeter of a normal disc. This band of collagenous tissue contains little water and is normally seen as a thick line of low signal intensity separating nuclear material from epidural fat and the thecal sac. Disruption of the outer annulus is imaged as discontinuity along the normally dark perimeter of a disc.

In Case 924, a gap is demonstrated near the middle of the annulus at the posterior margin of the L5-S1 disc (*arrow;* compare to the intact annulus at L4-5). Such transverse tears are more common at the junction of the annulus with the ring apophysis of one of the vertebral end plates, probably representing an avulsion. Granulation tissue within these disruptions causes a small zone of high signal intensity at the inferior or superior insertion of the normally dark outer annulus on T2-weighted scans (see Case 931).

Case 925 demonstrates a thin, vertically oriented layer of abnormal T2 prolongation within the posterior annulus at L4-5 *(arrow)*. This cleft likely reflects a concentric tear separating annular lamellae.

A radial tear is a third type of annular disruption, crossing multiple annular lamellae with greater vertical dimension but more limited horizontal extent than a transverse tear. These tears (in combination with concentric tears) account for the majority of the high intensity zones demonstrated near the center of the annulus on T2-weighted MR images. Radial tears are better correlated with other degenerative changes of the disc space than concentric or transverse tears.

## Case 926

54-year-old woman complaining of back pain.
(axial, noncontrast T2-weighted
FSE scan; L4-5 level)

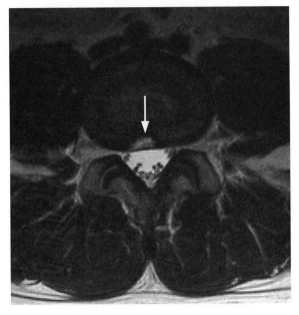

**Annular Tear**

## Case 927

45-year-old man presenting with low back pain.
(axial, postcontrast T1-weighted
SE scan; L5-S1 level)

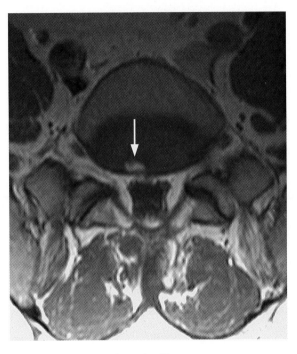

**Annular Tear**
(same patient as Case 924)

Granulation tissue within annular tears typically demonstrates high water content and contrast enhancement. These features increase the conspicuity of the tears on T2-weighted and postcontrast images.

The focal tear within the posterior annulus in Case 926 *(arrow)* is bright because of prolonged T2 values of the contained reparative tissue. Similarly, focal enhancement within the posterior annulus of the disc in Case 927 *(arrow)* reflects localized hyperemia of the inflammatory/healing response. Comparable findings occur at a site of surgical interruption of the annulus (see Case 949).

Disruption of the annulus fibrosus is necessary for herniation of the nucleus pulposus. However, an annular tear does not necessarily imply the presence of disc herniation. Granulation tissue and edema within a disruption of the annulus may expand the defect and be incorrectly interpreted as herniated nuclear material.

Many authors have suspected that annular tears may be associated with discogenic pain in the absence of accompanying herniation. Suggested mechanisms include: (1) leakage of irritating substances from the disc into the epidural space with subsequent inflammation; (2) growth of innervated granulation tissue into the annular defect, establishing a zone of pain receptors; and (3) mechanical destabilization of the disc level.

## Case 928

32-year-old woman complaining
of chronic back pain.
(axial, noncontrast T1-weighted SE scan; L4-5 level)

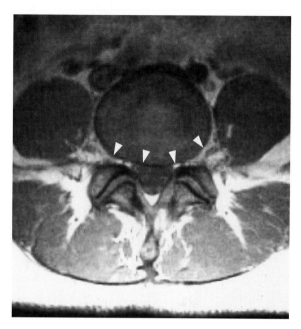

**Bulging Disc**

## Case 929

39-year-old man presenting with left leg
pain and diminished ankle reflex.
(axial, noncontrast T1-weighted SE scan; L5-S1 level)

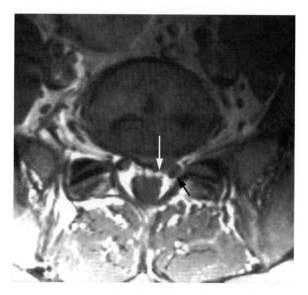

**Herniated Disc**

The MR demonstration of lumbar disc abnormalities is based on the differential signal intensity of bone, disc, spinal fluid, and epidural fat. In Case 928, the posterior margin of the bulging disc *(arrowheads)* is defined by the slightly lower intensity of spinal fluid within the dural sac and the higher signal intensity of epidural fat within the nerve root canals.

The posterior margin of lumbar discs is normally slightly concave at the L1 through L5 levels and nearly straight at L5-S1. Bulging discs demonstrate a uniform, symmetrical convexity. This broad curve contrasts with the focal asymmetry of disc herniation, as seen in Case 929.

The false appearance of a posterior disc bulge may be caused by oblique angulation of axial scans with respect to the disc level, most commonly seen at L5-S1. Spondylolisthesis may also cause a prominent disc shelf resembling a diffuse bulge (see Case 967).

The focal protrusion of disc material in Case 929 *(white arrow)* has a small radius of curvature and a relatively abrupt angle of origin from the parent disc. This localized change in contour contrasts with the diffuse bulge in Case 928. A discontinuity in the dark line of posterior annular fibers is apparent at the base of the herniation.

Disc herniations involving the central canal are often asymmetrical. Eccentric herniations may severely distort individual nerve roots without compressing the dural sac. The disc in Case 929 displaces and compresses the proximal left S1 nerve root *(black arrow)* within the lateral recess.

Some cases present features intermediate between Cases 928 and 929, so that distinguishing between an asymmetrical disc bulge and a frank disc herniation is difficult. MR scans have demonstrated evidence of annular tears and extruded disc material in cases where the overall contour of the disc remains generally symmetrical or "bulge-like." Sagittal views are particularly useful for assessing the integrity of the annulus fibrosis.

Disc herniations are most common in a posterolateral direction, as in Case 929. However, midline herniations also occur (see Case 935).

## Case 930

55-year-old man presenting with back pain.
(sagittal, noncontrast T1-weighted SE scan)

## Case 931

33-year-old man presenting with back and leg pain.
(sagittal, noncontrast T2-weighted FSE scan)

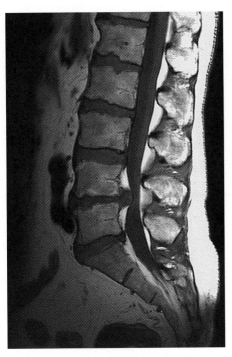

**Herniated Disc**

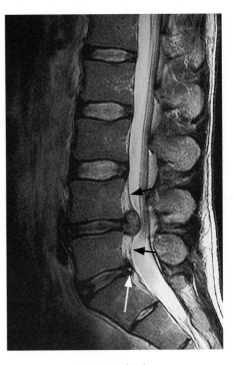

**Herniated Disc**

Centrally herniated discs are outlined on T1-weighted images by the slightly lower intensity of CSF within the subarachnoid space and/or by the higher signal intensity of ventral epidural fat. In Case 930, an anterior epidural mass is centered at the L4-5 disc level, suggesting discogenic origin. The ventral margin of the thecal sac is posteriorly displaced and compressed, with widening of the epidural space superior and inferior to the herniation. Associated edema, venous congestion, granulation tissue, and/or localized epidural hemorrhage may contribute to prominent extradural deformities at the site of a disc herniation (see Cases 942 and 943).

The signal intensity of herniated discs is variable on long TR spin echo images. Many herniated discs demonstrate intermediate to high intensity values on such scans (see Case 971). This apparent high water content may reflect the hydrophilic nature of herniated nuclear material and/or the presence of reactive granulation tissue.

In other cases, the signal intensity of disc herniations is relatively low, and they are well outlined by bright CSF on

T2-weighted studies. Case 931 illustrates this appearance (see also Case 923). The posterior longitudinal ligament and dura are tented above and below the level of the L4-5 disc herniation *(black arrows)*. Relatively high signal intensity within the anterior epidural space superior and inferior to the herniation may simply represent epidural fat (see discussion of FSE images in Case 923), although congested anterior epidural veins may also contribute. Disc space narrowing and reduced hydration signal are present at L4-5 and at L5-S1, where a small annular tear is noted *(white arrow)*.

On sagittal scans, the roots of the cauda equina may appear to form a dorsal band within the thecal sac in the superior lumbar region. This normal appearance should not be mistaken for thickening of the filum terminale or an abnormally low-lying spinal cord (see Cases 1236, 1237, 1242, and 1244). Axial images will resolve confusion in most cases.

Small Schmorl's nodes are present within multiple vertebral end plates in Case 930.

## Case 932

36-year-old man presenting with leg pain.
(sagittal, noncontrast T1-weighted SE scan)

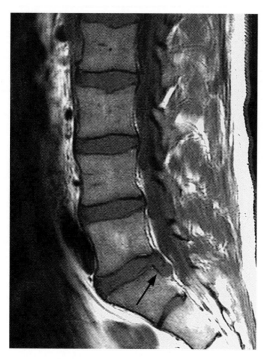

**Herniated Disc with Migration**

## Case 933

45-year-old woman presenting with leg pain.
(sagittal, noncontrast T1-weighted SE scan)

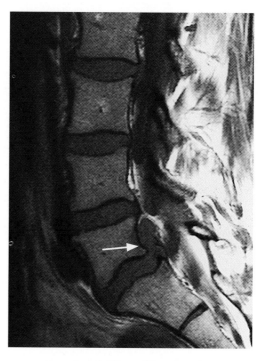

**Herniated Disc with Migration**

Many herniations remain centered at the level of the parent disc space, as illustrated on the previous page. In other cases, herniated discs extend caudally or cephalically from the level of origin. Superior or inferior projections of disc material may retain continuity with the parent disc or become isolated fragments (see Cases 934 and 935).

The L5-S1 disc herniation in Case 932 extends caudally through a disruption in the inferior portion of the posterior annulus *(arrow)*. The bulk of the herniation lies posterior to the S1 vertebral body, rather than at the L5-S1 disc level.

In Case 933, the herniated disc at L5-S1 projects superiorly, lying along the posterior cortex of the L5 vertebral body and reaching the inferior margin of the L4-5 disc level *(arrow)*. The herniation has passed through a gap within the superior portion of the posterior annulus.

Migration of a herniated disc has implications for the level of associated nerve compression. Although each of the above herniations originates at L5-S1, the disc in Case 932 will most likely distort the ipsilateral S1 root, whereas the disc in Case 933 will predominantly compress the ipsilateral L5 root.

## Case 934

28-year-old woman presenting with
S1 radiculopathy.
(sagittal, noncontrast T1-weighted SE scan)

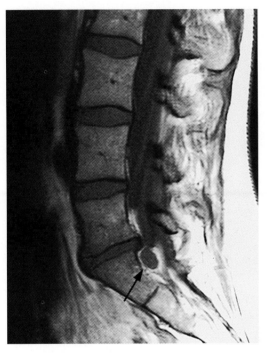

**Free Fragment Herniated Disc**

## Case 935

32-year-old man presenting with low back pain.
(axial, noncontrast T2-weighted
FSE scan; L5-S1 level)

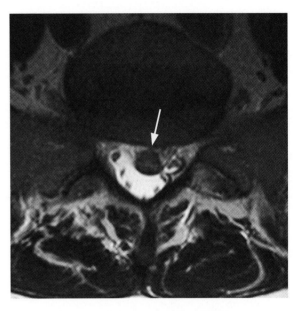

**Free Fragment Herniated Disc**

---

Herniated nuclear material (which is often accompanied by fragments of annulus and/or cartilage from the vertebral end plate) may become separated from the parent disc. Such "free fragments" may remain at the level of the disc space or migrate cephalically or caudally as isolated masses.

Case 934 illustrates an island of herniated disc material surrounded by epidural fat at the S1 level *(arrow)*. This fragment has migrated caudally from its origin and is separated from the posterior margin of the L5-S1 disc (compare to Case 932). The herniation is positioned to interrupt the course of the S1 nerve root, which can be faintly seen within the subarachnoid space superior to the fragment.

The herniated disc in Case 935 *(arrow)* has also migrated caudally from the L5-S1 disc level to lie posterior to S1. This fragment is more central, causing mild deformity of the thecal sac and the proximal left S1 root.

Note that the signal intensity of the disc herniation in Case 935 is a little lower than the herniation in Case 931. The apparent hydration of a herniated disc is widely variable on T2-weighted scans. (See Case 937 and 939 for herniations demonstrating even lower signal intensity.) Depending upon their size and position, herniated discs with low signal intensity can be difficult to distinguish from potential accompanying osteophytes on long TR spin echo images.

### Case 936

27-year-old man presenting with
pain in the back and right leg.
(axial, noncontrast T1-weighted SE scan; L5-S1 level)

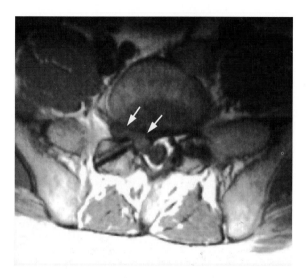

**Herniated Disc**

### Case 937

48-year-old man presenting with
left leg pain and foot drop.
(axial, noncontrast T2-weighted FSE scan; L4-5 level)

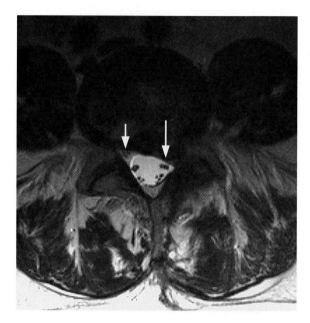

**Herniated Disc**

Herniated discs may compress nerve roots by distorting the dural sac, by narrowing the lateral recess, or by restricting the intervertebral foramen.

The lateral recess is formed at the anterolateral corner of the spinal canal by the junction of the vertebral body and pedicle. A lumbar nerve occupies this angle as it prepares to exit beneath the pedicle through the superior portion of the intervertebral foramen.

Posterolateral disc herniations commonly involve the region of the lateral recess, as in the above cases (see Cases 951 and 953 for additional examples). Case 936 demonstrates the amorphous, homogeneous signal intensity of herniated nuclear material replacing epidural fat within the right lateral recess (nerve root canal). The proximal right S1 nerve root, which would normally reside in this location, is severely compressed. (Note the position of the normal left S1 nerve root.)

In Case 937, a lateral disc herniation with low signal intensity occupies the left anterolateral recess *(long arrow)*. The thecal sac is only mildly deformed, but the exiting left L5 root is severely compressed prior to its entry into the nerve root canal. (Note the position of the normal right L5 root at this level; *short arrow.*)

Adjacent lumbar roots may share a common sleeve. A "conjoined" or "compound" sleeve is larger than an individual nerve and is located between the levels of the contributing roots. This normal variant presents as an asymmetrical structure occupying the lateral recess and may be misinterpreted as a herniated disc. However, the CSF-like signal intensity within a compound sleeve on all pulse sequences contrasts with the soft tissue values expected of disc material. In addition, the involved lateral recess is often large, suggesting a congenital variation. A compound sleeve can also be identified by more caudal sections demonstrating the emergence of two separate roots.

**Case 938**

43-year-old woman presenting with
S1 radiculopathy.
(sagittal, noncontrast T1-weighted SE scan)

**Case 939**

32-year-old woman presenting with right leg pain.
(coronal, noncontrast T2-weighted FSE scan)

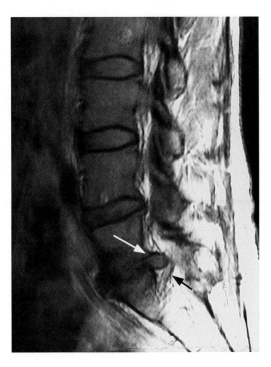

**Herniated Disc**
(recurrent)

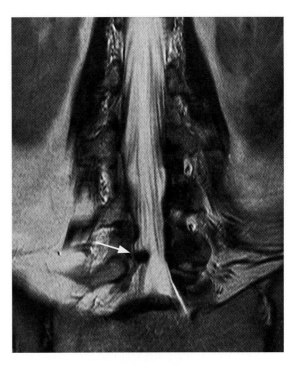

**Herniated Disc**

---

The above scans illustrate the position of herniated discs involving the anterolateral recess as displayed in the sagittal and coronal planes.

The image in Case 938 is parasagittal, located lateral to the thecal sac but just medial to the nerve root canals. A moderately large posterolateral disc herniation at L5-S1 is well defined by surrounding epidural fat *(white arrow)*. The disc displaces and distorts the S1 nerve root *(black arrow)* as it traverses the anterolateral recess to reach the intervertebral foramen.

The right-sided posterolateral disc herniation at L4-5 in Case 939 is conspicuous because of very low signal intensity. It clearly compresses the traversing right L5 root (and also deforms the more medial S1 root). Coronal scans are useful for demonstrating the exact relationship of herniated discs or other masses (e.g., schwannomas) to the margins of the nerve root canal.

The disc herniation in Case 939 *(arrow)* is surrounded by the bright signal of CSF. This appearance implies that the disc has focally invaginated the thecal sac. Occasional herniations erode through the dura and present as intradural masses.

### Case 940

58-year-old man complaining of left leg pain.
(axial, noncontrast T1-weighted SE scan; L4-5 level)

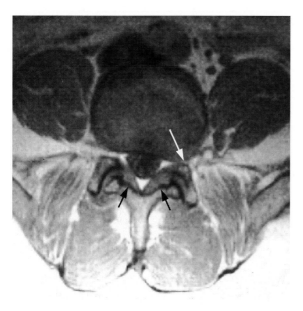

**Herniated Disc**

### Case 941

50-year-old man presenting with leg pain.
(sagittal, noncontrast T1-weighted SE scan)

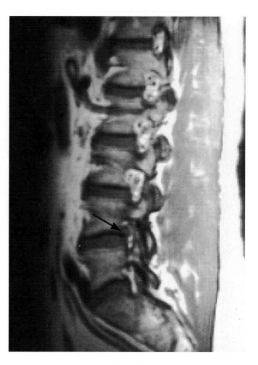

**Herniated Disc**

Lateral disc herniations may cause radiculopathy by compressing nerve roots as they leave the spinal canal. Disc material may extend into an intervertebral foramen and/or distort a nerve root distal to the neural canal.

In Case 940, a left lateral disc herniation *(white arrow)* occupies the inferior portion of the L4-5 nerve root canal. Compare the diameter of the right intervertebral foramen in Case 940 to the affected side.

The cephalocaudal dimension of intervertebral foramina can be difficult to judge on axial CT or MR scans. Sagittal views are helpful in this assessment. Since the orientation of lumbar nerve root canals is close to the coronal plane, sagittal MR scans provide cross-sectional views of foraminal margins and contents.

On T1-weighted images, the intervertebral foramina are normally filled with high intensity fat surrounding a nerve root of intermediate intensity. (In the lumbar region the root exits close to the superior pedicle; in the cervical spine, the nerve root exits closer to the inferior pedicle.) Disc material or osteophyte is well defined when encroaching into the zone of high contrast.

Case 941 demonstrates a lobulated disc herniation extending into the L4-5 nerve root canal *(arrow;* compare to foramina at the higher levels). The L4 root is mildly compressed between the disc margin and the overlying pedicle.

Disc herniations may occur even further laterally, distorting nerve roots as they exit from the intervertebral foramen. It is important to follow all roots through their foramina when reviewing CT and MR studies, so that foraminal or extraforaminal impingement is recognized. The surgical approach to "far lateral" root compression is a lateral exposure; traditional laminectomy will fail to identify the source of symptoms.

The symmetrical areas of tissue with intermediate signal intensity along the posterolateral margins of the spinal canal in Case 940 *(black arrows)* are the ligamenta flava. Thickening of these ligaments often accompanies degenerative disc disease and contributes to narrowing of the spinal canal or intervertebral foramina (see Cases 958 and 959).

### Case 942

59-year-old man presenting with bilateral leg pain, worse with walking. A prior CT scan was read as negative.
(sagittal, noncontrast T1-weighted SE scan)

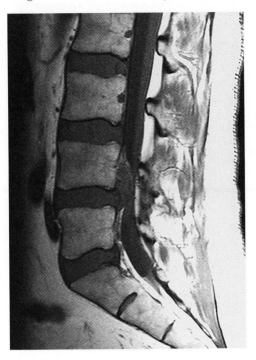

**Herniated Disc**

### Case 943

49-year-old man presenting with severe back pain.
(axial, noncontrast T1-weighted SE scan; L4-5 level)

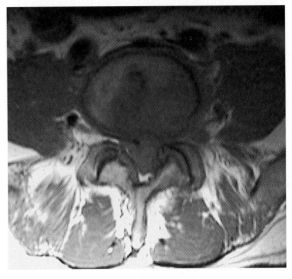

**Herniated Disc**

---

Lumbar disc herniations occasionally cause very large anterior epidural masses. Absorption of water, reactive edema, congestion of epidural veins, and epidural hemorrhage may all contribute to bulky mass effect.

The anterior epidural mass in Case 942 effaces the subarachnoid space, compressing the nerve roots of the cauda equina. The extradural deformity extends superiorly from the L4-5 disc level, suggesting migration of herniated nucleus pulposus (compare to Case 933).

Giant disc herniations are occasionally overlooked on axial CT scans, as had occurred in Case 942. If abnormal soft tissue fills the spinal canal, there may be no recognizable interface between the herniation and the compressed dural sac.

Case 943 illustrates this potential pitfall. A mild circumferential disc bulge is apparent. Diagnosis of the very large superimposed central herniation is less obvious and depends on recognizing that the homogeneous signal intensity within the spinal canal is higher than expected for intrathecal CSF. Correlation with sagittal and T2-weighted images makes misinterpretation of this appearance less likely on MR scans than on CT studies.

As mentioned above, epidural hemorrhage may contribute to the symptomatology and appearance of lumbar disc herniations. Disruption of an anterior epidural vein by a herniating disc can lead to localized bleeding that accentuates the mass effect of the herniation. The signal intensity of such lesions is often intermediate and nonspecific. This is particularly true on T1-weighted scans, where T1-shortening attributable to methemoglobin is rarely observed. (The intensity of epidural hemorrhage on long TR images may be low, intermediate or high.)

Epidural hematomas accompanying disc herniations usually regress spontaneously over a period of weeks to months. The resorption of such hemorrhages (together with reduction in epidural edema and venous congestion) may account for some of the spontaneously resolving disc herniations previously reported on myelographic and CT studies.

## Case 944

43-year-old man presenting with a three-month
history of back pain (no prior surgery).
(axial, postcontrast T1-weighted SE scan; L4-5 level)

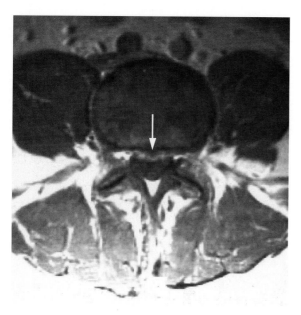

**Central Herniated Disc**

## Case 945

38-year-old man presenting with severe
right leg pain (no prior surgery).
(axial, postcontrast T1-weighted SE scan; L4 level)

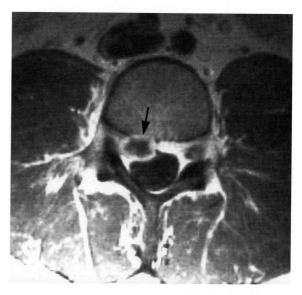

**Lateral Herniated Disc**
(free fragment)

The margin of herniated discs is usually outlined by a rim of enhancement on postcontrast scans. This enhancing border has been correlated histologically with a layer of vascular granulation tissue. Marginal enhancement can help to distinguish herniated discs from other epidural masses (e.g., lymphoma or metastasis) or from postoperative epidural fibrosis (see Cases 952 and 953).

The above cases demonstrate that peripheral enhancement may outline disc herniations prior to surgical intervention. (See Case 953 for discussion of postoperative disc enhancement.) The small central herniation in Case 944 is defined by the thin layer of adjacent enhancement; the herniation might otherwise be undetected on a T1-weighted scan.

In Case 945, peripheral contrast enhancement helps to characterize the large mass occupying the right lateral re-

cess. This lesion is not a solidly enhancing lymphoma or schwannoma but a fragment of disc material that has migrated rostrally to reside posterior to the vertebral body of L4. The dural sac is deformed, and both the exiting right L4 nerve root and the traversing right L5 nerve root are likely distorted.

Epidural abscesses and epidural hematomas may also present the appearance of marginal enhancement surrounding a nonenhancing center (see Cases 1190 and 1191). These pathologies should be considered in the appropriate clinical context.

Contrast material may diffuse from the perimeter of a herniated disc into the center on delayed scans. This gradual accumulation of contrast over a period of minutes to hours may obscure the initially characteristic morphology and reduce diagnostic specificity (see Case 1061).

# DISCOGENIC ENHANCEMENT OF INTRADURAL NERVE ROOTS

## Case 946

32-year-old man presenting with
leg pain and numbness.
(sagittal, postcontrast T1-weighted SE scan)

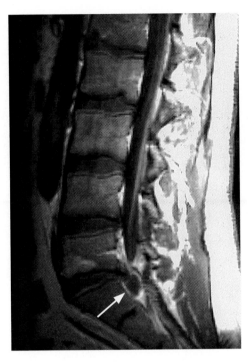

**Enhancing Root Due to Disc Herniation**

## Case 947

30-year-old man presenting with back pain.
(axial, postcontrast T1-weighted SE scan; L2-3 level)

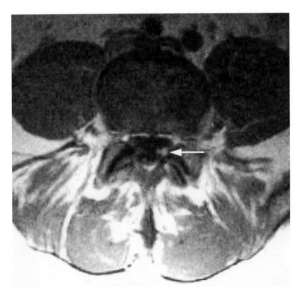

**Enhancing Root Due to Disc Herniation**

---

Postcontrast scans in cases of disc herniation may demonstrate intrathecal enhancement of compressed nerve roots. This enhancement can extend for several centimeters proximal to the site of herniation.

Case 946 is a typical example. A free fragment herniation is present within the anterolateral recess caudal to the L5-S1 level (*arrow;* compare to Case 934). The disc material is well defined as a low intensity mass surrounded by the short T1 values of peripheral enhancement and epidural fat. More superiorly, a prominently enhancing nerve root is demonstrated within the thecal sac from L3 through L5. The course of this nerve suggests that it represents the S1 root proximal to the site of compression by the L5-S1 herniation.

Axial images such as Case 947 can confirm that abnormal intrathecal enhancement is confined to a specific root, which can be followed distally to a point of compression by a herniated disc. In this case, the left L5 root was deformed by a large herniation at L4-5.

Disc-related enhancement of intrathecal nerve roots is more isolated and more prominent than the normal mildly increased intensity of all intradural roots on postcontrast scans. The affected root remains smoothly uniform in caliber, without the nodularity commonly noted in leptomeningeal carcinomatosis or drop metastases (see Cases 1042-1047).

Inflammatory disorders (e.g., meningitis, sarcoidosis, tuberculosis, herpes zoster, cytomegalovirus, arachnoiditis, and Guillain-Barré syndrome) occasionally cause focal enhancement of isolated roots. It is important to recognize that irritation of a root by extradural disc disease can be associated with abnormal intrathecal enhancement mimicking these other pathologies.

Prominent, asymmetrical contrast enhancement of an intradural nerve root is occasionally seen as a normal variant due to a large accompanying radicular vein. (The largest vein of the cauda equina usually courses along the filum terminale, at least proximally.)

### Case 948

43-year-old woman several years
after right-sided laminectomy.
(axial, noncontrast T1-weighted SE scan; L4 level)

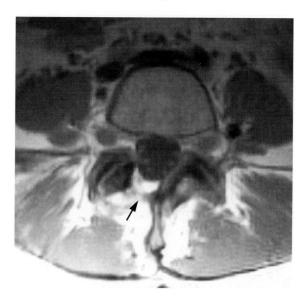

**Postoperative Change**

### Case 949

39-year-old man four months
after microdiscectomy.
(axial, postcontrast T1-weighted SE scan; L4-5 level)

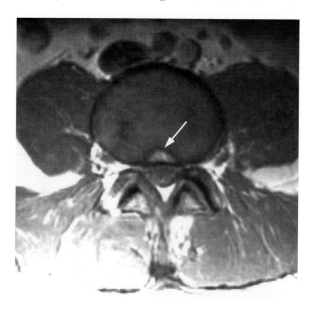

**Postoperative Change**

Lumbar laminectomy and discectomy lead to character-istic postoperative MR findings. A laminectomy defect is usually well defined as a gap in the vertebral arch posterior to the facet joint. The ligamentum flavum is absent on the side of surgery.

Case 945 illustrates that both the lamina and the liga-mentum flavum have been removed on the right side *(arrow)*. The dural sac bulges dorsally toward the operative defect. Epidural fibrosis is minimal in this case, and there is no evidence of recurrent disc herniation. Nerve roots are well visualized within the intervertebral foramina and within the thecal sac.

Focal contrast enhancement normally occurs along the posterior margin of intervertebral discs at the site of prior herniation and surgery. This localized finding probably reflects the presence of granulation tissue within the heal-ing annulus. Case 949 illustrates such enhancement in the midline *(arrow)* after resection of a central herniation.

More extensive enhancement involving central portions of the disc space is unusual after uncomplicated discec-tomy. The possibility of infection should be considered in such cases (see Cases 1119, 1120, and 1122).

Note that a laminectomy defect is not apparent in Case 949. Microdiscectomy techniques involving little or no bone removal are increasingly common. As a result, the ab-sence of an obvious laminectomy does not preclude post-operative changes as a potential etiology for abnormal find-ings on CT or MR scans.

Postoperative MR studies performed in the first several months after surgery often demonstrate a soft tissue "mass" at the site of the original herniation. This appearance probably reflects granulation tissue and edema filling the bed of the former herniated disc. The frequent occurrence of such pseudoherniations limits the value of early postop-erative scans.

# DIFFERENTIAL DIAGNOSIS:
## ABNORMAL EPIDURAL TISSUE WITHIN THE LATERAL RECESS

### Case 950

42-year-old woman with persistent left
leg pain six months after laminectomy.
(axial, noncontrast T1-weighted SE scan; L4-5 level)

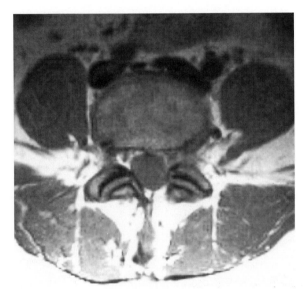

**Epidural Fibrosis**

### Case 951

58-year-old man presenting with left leg pain.
(axial, noncontrast T1-weighted SE scan; L4-5 level)

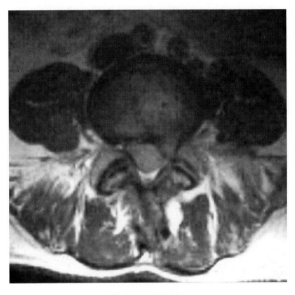

**Herniated Disc**

---

Residual or recurrent symptoms after lumbar discectomy may have many sources other than persistent or recurrent herniation at the operated level. The main purpose of scans performed in this context is to establish the presence or absence of disc herniation to help determine whether further surgery is warranted.

Following discectomy, epidural fat is often replaced or infiltrated by tissue with longer T1 values. This postoperative scarring or "epidural fibrosis" is an expected consequence of surgery and by itself is rarely significant. However, epidural fibrosis reduces or obliterates the natural contrast between a disc and epidural tissue. Amorphous, intermediate signal intensity in the region of surgery may make it difficult to diagnose or exclude disc herniation. Prominent epidural fibrosis can itself appear mass-like and simulate disc material.

In Case 950, a left-sided laminectomy defect is present. Abnormal low signal intensity surrounds the proximal left L5 nerve root within the lateral recess. (Compare to the normal L5 root on the right side.) The fact that the root can be faintly seen in approximately normal position within the postoperative change argues against recurrent disc herniation.

The small disc herniation in Case 951 has a more mass-like contour, with better defined margins than the postoperative fibrosis of Case 950. Adjacent deformity of the dural sac is present. This finding is uncommon in cases of simple epidural fibrosis and should suggest the presence of herniated nuclear material. More importantly, the left L5 nerve root cannot be identified within the lateral recess in Case 951. This lack of visualization suggests displacement or compression of the root and contrasts with Case 950.

Long TR spin echo scans can be helpful in distinguishing between recurrent disc herniation and epidural fibrosis. Herniated discs may demonstrate either higher or lower signal intensity than surrounding postoperative changes on "intermediate" or T2-weighted images. A low intensity fibrous capsule is frequently seen at the margin of a recurrent herniation, separating it from epidural fibrosis of nearly equal intensity.

### Case 952A

47-year-old man complaining of persistent right
leg pain nine months after L4-5 discectomy.
(axial, noncontrast T1-weighted SE scan; L4-5 level)

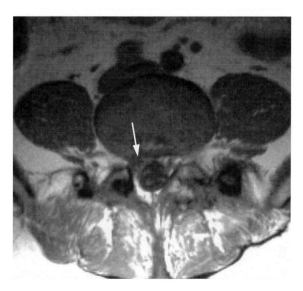

**Epidural Fibrosis**
(postoperative)

### Case 952B

Same patient.
(axial, postcontrast T1-weighted SE scan; same level)

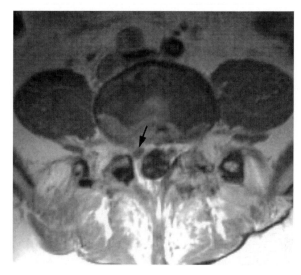

**Epidural Fibrosis**
(postoperative)

Abnormal soft tissue with a mass-like contour is present in the right anterolateral recess of Case 952A *(arrow)*. The ipsilateral L5 nerve root is not defined, and the overall appearance resembles the herniated disc in Case 951.

Contrast enhancement is useful for distinguishing residual or recurrent disc herniation from epidural fibrosis in such situations. As discussed in Cases 944 and 945, scans performed soon after the injection of contrast material usually demonstrate marginal enhancement at the perimeter of a herniated disc. The vascular granulation and scar tissue within zones of epidural fibrosis generally enhances more

homogeneously. That is, the early presence of contrast enhancement *within* the area of precontrast abnormality favors the diagnosis of epidural fibrosis over that of disc herniation.

In Case 952B, the majority of the "mass" within the right lateral recess demonstrates enhancement. Enhancing scar tissue defines the nondisplaced L5 nerve root *(arrow)*, which was not clearly identified on the precontrast scan. Such epidural enhancement simultaneously excludes recurrent herniation and establishes the position of symptomatic nerve roots.

## Case 953A

48-year-old man with worsening left
leg pain two months after surgery.
(axial, noncontrast T1-weighted SE scan; L4-5 level)

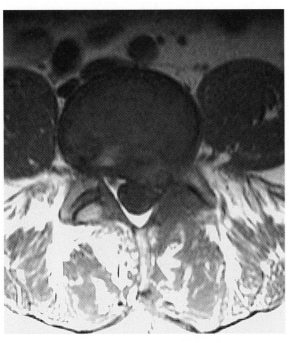

**Recurrent Herniated Disc**

## Case 953B

Same patient.
(axial, postcontrast T1-weighted SE scan; same level)

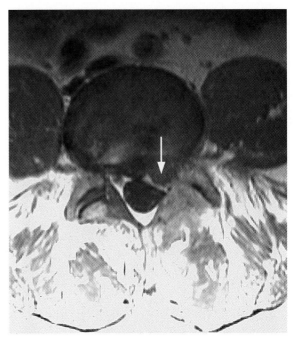

**Recurrent Herniated Disc**

---

The left-sided anterior epidural mass in Case 953A suggests recurrent herniation. There is mild compression of the thecal sac, and the proximal left L5 root cannot be identified. The overall appearance resembles Case 951 more than Case 950.

However, the margin of the mass is poorly defined. It is difficult to estimate the relative contribution of nuclear material and postoperative changes to the appearance at the site of surgery.

The postcontrast scan in Case 953B clarifies the situation. Enhancing granulation tissue (fibrosis) defines the margin of the nonenhancing recurrent herniation *(arrow)*. The left L5 root remains effaced (compare to the right L5 root in Case 952B).

Scans performed immediately after contrast injection are most helpful in making the distinction between recurrent disc herniation and epidural fibrosis. Contrast material may penetrate into the center of herniated discs on delayed images (see Case 1061).

Uniform enhancement of postoperative tissue in the region of the left facetectomy in Case 953B is an expected finding and does not imply (or exclude) infection.

### Case 954A

48-year-old man with increasing back pain one week after laminectomy and discectomy at L4-5. (sagittal, noncontrast T1-weighted SE scan)

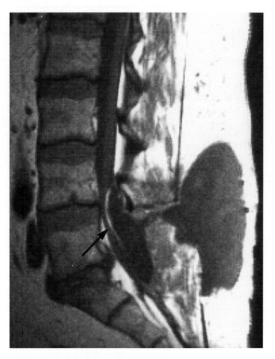

**Pseudomeningocele**

### Case 954B

Same patient.
(sagittal, noncontrast T2-weighted SE scan)

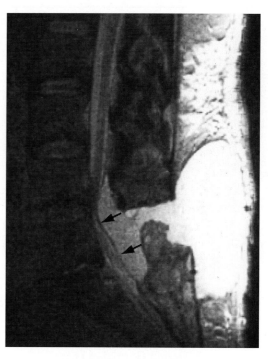

**Pseudomeningocele**

---

An uncommon cause of recurrent symptoms following surgery to remove a herniated disc is the development of a pseudomeningocele. These cystic collections of CSF may accumulate within epidural and paraspinal tissues when a tear of the dura occurs during surgery and is not completely repaired. Persistent communication with the thecal sac may cause pseudomeningoceles to enlarge, with increasing compression of adjacent nerve roots.

In Case 954A a large, fluid-filled sac is present within subcutaneous fat posterior to the lumbar spine. The appearance superficially resembles the congenital meningoceles discussed in Chapter 22. The relationship of the dorsal cyst to the dural sac is difficult to define on this T1-weighted scan. A curvilinear strand of high signal intensity within the anterior portion of the spinal canal at L4-5 *(arrow)* in fact represents a stripe of doral epidural fat, displaced ventrally by an epidural loculation of the cyst.

Case 954B documents the dumbbell morphology of the pseudomeningocele. A broad communication through the area of surgery connects the subcutaneous cyst with a dorsal epidural component. The epidural mass causes severe compression of the dural sac and cauda equina *(arrows)*.

Epidural or paraspinal abscesses may also cause localized fluid collections following surgery. Paraspinal abscesses are usually associated with systemic evidence of infection and severe local pain and tenderness (see Chapter 20). However, more indolent abscesses could be considered in the differential diagnosis of a pseudomeningocele, particularly if communication between the fluid collection and the dural sac is not convincingly demonstrated.

Epidural hematomas may also develop in the postoperative period to cause localized mass effect and recurrent or worsening symptoms (see Case 1186).

### Case 955A

46-year-old man with a history of spinal trauma and lumbar fusion twenty years earlier, now presenting with bladder and bowel dysfunction.
(sagittal, noncontrast T2-weighted SE scan)

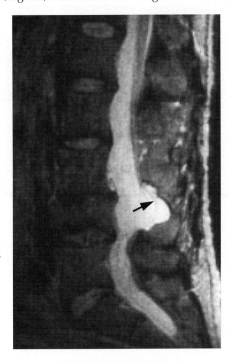

**Dural Diverticulae**

### Case 955B

Same patient.
(axial, noncontrast T1-weighted SE scan; L4 level)

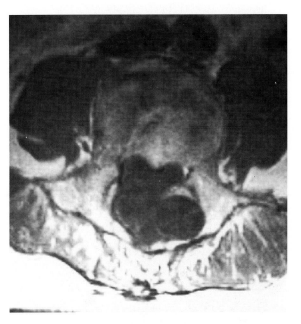

**Dural Diverticulae**

Lobulated ectasia of the dura ("dural diverticulae") may develop in patients with ankylosing spondylitis. The basis for this outpouching is not established but may include a component of chronic meningeal inflammation.

The patient in Case 955 did not have true ankylosing spondylitis. However, the lumbar fusion performed two decades earlier has apparently simulated the pathophysiology of the spondylitic disorder. The impressive lobulated dural ectasia seen above is very comparable to the pattern observed in patients with a long history of ankylosing disease.

Case 955 is distinct from Case 954 in several respects. The CSF-containing sac seen here reflects localized enlargement of the intradural compartment rather than the accumulation of extradural fluid. The ectasia in this case had developed gradually over many years, whereas a pseudomeningocele typically manifests within days or weeks of surgery or trauma. Finally, the morphology of the cystic CSF collection in Case 955 is characteristically lobulated, whereas pseudomeningoceles tend to be unilocular or dumbbell-shaped, as in Case 954.

The appearance in this case should not be confused with the dural ectasia seen in some patients with neurofibromatosis or connective tissue disorders (e.g., Marfan's syndrome or Ehlers-Danlos syndrome). In the latter conditions, dural expansion is more generalized, with smooth, concave erosion along the posterior margins of vertebral bodies. Such morphology contrasts with more focal scalloping, dorsal predominance, and limited extent of dural diverticulae in spondylitic syndromes.

The cause of the cauda equina syndrome in patients with ankylosing spondylitis and dorsal dural ectasia is probably an associated arachnoiditis. Nerve roots may become adherent or tethered to the inflamed meninges, with consequent distortion and traction. In Case 955A, the roots of the cauda equina are positioned along the posterior margin of the spinal canal at the L2-3 level. At least one root *(arrow)* follows an aberrant course into the dural diverticulae. The axial scan in Case 955B documents both the lobulated dural expansion (and bone erosion) and the distorted morphology of intrathecal nerve roots.

585

### Case 956

56-year-old man presenting with
pseudoclaudication.
(sagittal, noncontrast T1-weighted SE scan)

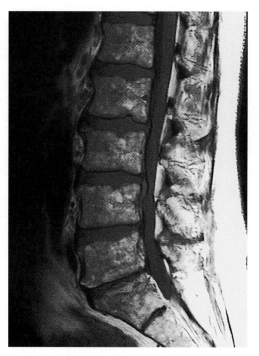

**Central Canal Stenosis**

### Case 957

77-year-old woman presenting with
severe back and leg pain.
(sagittal, noncontrast T2-weighted FSE scan)

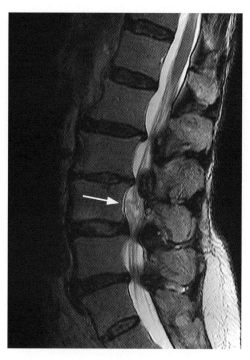

**Central Canal Stenosis**

---

A variety of congenital and acquired factors may cause narrowing of the spinal canal at any level. Central stenosis due to degenerative changes is most common in the lumbar region. Disc bulges and osteophytes cause spondylotic ridges indenting the anterior aspect of the spinal canal. Accompanying hypertrophy of the facet joints and thickening of the ligamenta flava encroach on the posterolateral portion of the canal. The combination of these features produces a circumferential or "napkin-ring" narrowing that encircles and constricts the dural sac. Superimposed static or dynamic subluxations exacerbate the crowding and compression of the nerve roots of the cauda equina.

Sagittal MR scans effectively demonstrate narrowing of the spinal canal. In Case 956, the anteroposterior diameter of the lumbar spinal canal is developmentally small. Superimposed on this congenital narrowing are acquired disc bulges at each level from L1 to L4. The combination of these features causes high grade stenosis of the central canal, most severe at L3-4. The normal low signal intensity of CSF within the thecal sac is replaced by amorphous intermediate signal intensity of compressed tissue in the region from L2 to the sacrum.

T2-weighted sagittal scans such as Case 957 often define the posterior components of degenerative spinal stenosis more clearly than T1-weighted images. In this case, large dorsal extradural deformities due to posterior element hypertrophy combine with a "washboard" of ventral spondylotic ridges to cause a series of napkin-ring constrictions.

Redundancy of intradural roots, as seen at the L3 level in Case 957 *(arrow)*, is often noted in cases of severe central lumbar stenosis. This tortuosity probably reflects elongation of the roots due to repeated stretching, with localized slack between points of current constriction. The finding confirms the significance and chronicity of spinal stenosis. Tortuous intrathecal nerve roots should not be confused with hypertrophied vessels (see Cases 1209, 1211, and 1215).

Case 956 demonstrates the substantial heterogeneity of signal intensity that normally can occur within vertebral bodies (see Cases 992 and 993). Severe disc space narrowing is present at L5-S1.

## Case 958

82-year-old man presenting with
back and leg pain.
(axial, noncontrast T1-weighted SE scan; L3-4 level)

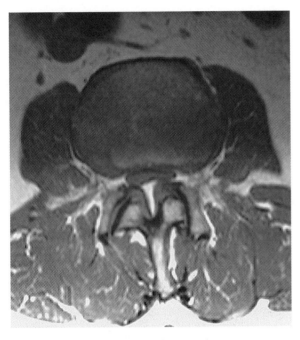

**Central Canal Stenosis**

## Case 959

78-year-old woman presenting with
pseudoclaudication.
(axial, noncontrast T1-weighted SE scan; L4-5 level)

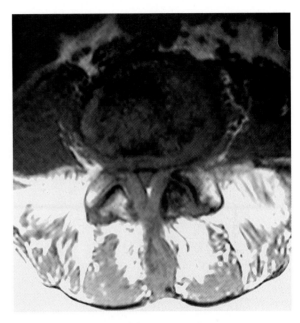

**Central Canal Stenosis**

---

Axial scans define the cross-sectional morphology and severity of spinal stenosis. Central canal compromise is often caused by the superimposition of acquired pathology on congenitally narrowed dimensions. The acquired factors may be specific processes (e.g., Paget's disease or ossification of the posterior longitudinal ligament) or simple degenerative changes.

In Case 958, congenitally small canal dimensions have been further narrowed by hypertrophy of the facets and thickening of the ligamentum flavum/facet capsule. The thecal sac is flattened anteriorly.

Case 959 demonstrates a combination of disc bulge, facet hypertrophy, and prominent thickening of the ligamentum flavum causing circumferential constriction of the lumbar canal. (Compare the size of the dural sac in these images to the more normal dimensions in Cases 948 and 950). The thecal sac and nerve roots of the cauda equina are severely compressed into a small central triangle of isointense tissue. A T2-weighted axial image at this level would demonstrate no residual CSF within the subarachnoid space. A complete block would be expected if myelography were performed.

## Case 960A

18-year-old man presenting with leg spasticity.
(sagittal, noncontrast T2-weighted SE scan)

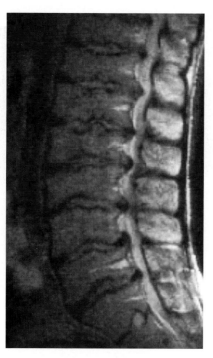

**Achondroplasia**

## Case 960B

Same patient.
(axial, noncontrast T1-weighted SE scan; L3-4 level)

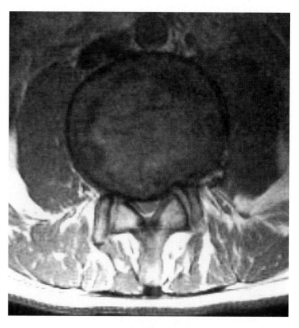

**Achondroplasia**

Achondroplasia is among the congenital causes of spinal stenosis. This autosomal dominant disorder results in dwarfism, with abnormal formation of enchondral bone. The head and spine are prominently affected.

Calvarial involvement characteristically results in a hypoplastic skull base. The foramen magnum is typically very small, with constriction of the cervicomedullary junction. Shelf-like hypertrophy of the posterior lip of the foramen magnum often contributes to the narrow bony dimensions.

Spinal manifestations of achondroplasia include abnormally formed vertebral bodies and high grade central canal stenosis. Case 960A demonstrates a congenitally narrow AP diameter of the lumbar canal, which is due predominantly to short pedicles. Superimposed disc bulges at all levels further constrict the canal. The axial scan of Case 960B confirms that the combination of a small bony canal and prominent disc bulging results in severe compression of the thecal sac.

Axial scans of congenitally stenotic canals often demonstrate a triangular or "trefoil" morphology, with short pedicles and medially bowing laminae. Such congenital deformity is frequently most prominent in the lumbar region.

Other systemic bone disorders that may cause multi-level spinal stenosis include Paget's disease, rickets, and diffuse idiopathic skeletal hyperostosis.

### Case 961A

62-year-old man presenting with back and
leg pain. The patient was otherwise
well and taking no medications.
(sagittal, noncontrast T1-weighted SE scan)

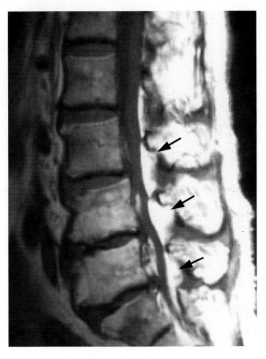

**Epidural Lipomatosis**

### Case 961B

Same patient.
(axial, noncontrast T1-weighted
SE scan; L4 level)

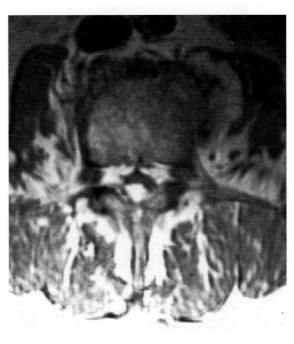

**Epidural Lipomatosis**

Abnormal accumulation of epidural fat is a rare cause of central canal stenosis. Symptomatic epidural lipomatosis is most common in the thoracic region (see Case 1192) but may also involve the lumbar canal, as in this case. Excessive exogenous or endogenous glucocorticoids (i.e., steroid therapy or Cushing's disease) is the usual clinical setting for this disorder. Uncomplicated obesity may occasionally be associated with symptomatic thickening of epidural fat.

In Case 961A, a prominent layer of epidural fat occupies the dorsal portion of the lumbar canal from L2 to S1 *(arrows)*. Ventral deposits of epidural fat are seen posterior to several vertebral bodies. The dural sac is reduced to a ribbon-like band passing between these accumulations of lipid material. The axial plane (Case 961B) confirms compression and deformity of the thecal sac due to dorsal and ventral layers of epidural fat.

When the dural sac is deformed by epidural tissue demonstrating short T1 values, the possibility of hematoma should be considered along with lipomatosis. Subacute blood products (i.e., methemoglobin) may cause a subdural or epidural hemorrhage to appear bright on T1-weighted scans (see Cases 1185-1187). A scan performed with fat suppression techniques will establish the etiology of epidural T1-shortening in questionable cases.

Occasional angiolipomas and hemangiomas occur in the spinal epidural space, particularly in the thoracic region (see Cases 995 and 996). Such tumors should be considered among the causes of T1-shortening in this location.

Cases 1192 and 1193 present additional examples of epidural lipomatosis.

## Case 962

80-year-old woman presenting with
bilateral leg pain.
(axial, noncontrast T1-weighted SE scan; L4 level)

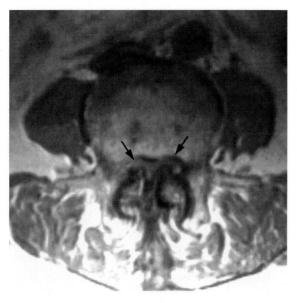

**Lateral Recess Stenosis**

## Case 963

77-year-old man with severe back pain.
(axial, noncontrast T1-weighted SE scan; L4-5 level)

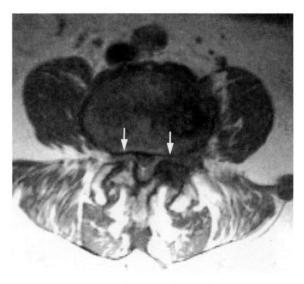

**Lateral Recess Stenosis**

The lateral recess of the spinal canal is formed by the junction of the vertebral body and pedicle. A lumbar nerve root occupies this angle as it prepares to pass beneath the pedicle through the superior portion of the intervertebral foramen. The root may be compressed in this location by a posterolateral disc herniation, as discussed in Cases 936 and 937. Alternatively, bony narrowing of the lateral recess can severely distort the contained nerve.

The base of the superior articular facet of a lumbar vertebra forms the posterolateral margin of the lateral recess. Hypertrophy of the facet (and/or related osteophytes) may significantly narrow the recess, either alone or in combination with disc pathology.

In Case 962, hypertrophy and spurring of the facet joints encroach on the posterior portion of the lateral recesses bilaterally. The proximal L4 nerve roots are flattened anteroposteriorly *(arrows)*. High grade central canal stenosis commonly accompanies bony narrowing of the lateral recesses, as in this case.

The axial scan of Case 963 is at a slightly lower level than Case 962, passing through the junction of the lateral recesses and the intervertebral foramina. Bone overgrowth and associated spondylotic thickening of soft tissue obliterate normal epidural fat in this region. Exiting nerve roots are distorted as they traverse the constricted lateral recess and enter the nerve root canals. Moderate central canal stenosis is also present in Case 963 due to the combination of facet hypertrophy and thickening of the ligamenta flava.

## Case 964

50-year-old woman presenting with
back and leg pain.
(sagittal, noncontrast T1-weighted SE scan)

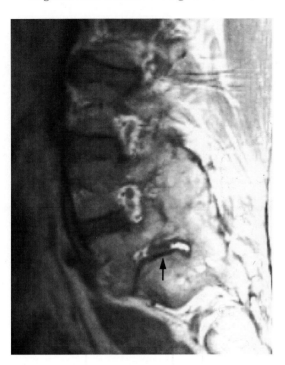

**Lateral (Foraminal) Stenosis**

## Case 965

60-year-old woman presenting with
leg pain and numbness.
(sagittal, noncontrast T1-weighted SE scan)

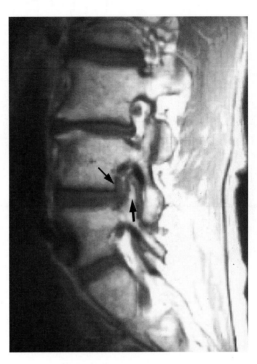

**Lateral (Foraminal) Stenosis**

---

Lateral disc herniation causing foraminal compression of lumbar nerve roots has been illustrated in Cases 940 and 941. An equally important cause of foraminal compromise is bony stenosis.

Bony narrowing of a nerve root canal may develop as a consequence of disc space narrowing. Case 964 presents a typical example. Severe narrowing of the disc space (and mild spondylolisthesis) were noted at the L5-S1 level on more medial images. Associated cephalocaudal narrowing of the nerve root canal flattens the exiting L5 root *(arrow)*.

Case 965 illustrates another form of bony foraminal compromise. No significant disc space narrowing or subluxation is present. Instead, the L4-5 intervertebral foramen is constricted by hypertrophy of the superior articular facet of L5 *(thick arrow)*. A superimposed disc bulge *(thin arrow)* adds to the crowding that compresses the L4 nerve root against the overlying pedicle.

Parasagittal scans are very useful for demonstrating the relative contributions of disc and bone to compromise of an intervertebral foramen (compare Case 965 to Case 941).

### Case 966A

71-year-old man presenting with L4 radiculopathy.
(sagittal, noncontrast T1-weighted SE scan)

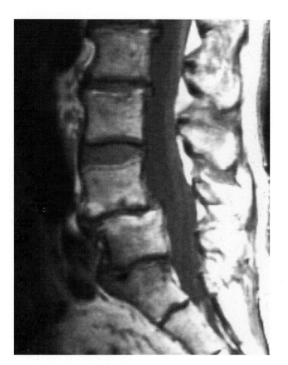

**Spondylolisthesis**

### Case 966B

Same patient.
(axial, noncontrast T1-weighted SE scan; L4 level)

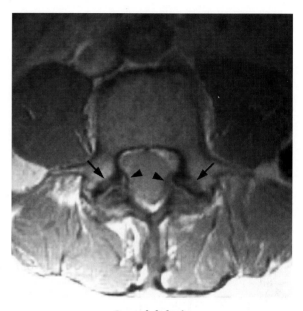

**Spondylolysis**

Ventral subluxation of one vertebral body on another may occur in the presence of intact vertebral arches when degenerative changes cause disc space narrowing and ligamentous laxity. Spondylolisthesis may alternatively reflect defects in the pars interarticularis of the forward-slipping vertebra. Such discontinuity of the posterior arch allows the body and superior articular facet to slide anteriorly, unrestrained by linkage to the inferior articular facet (which maintains its articulation to the next inferior vertebra).

Often spondylolysis and degenerative changes are both present at the level of subluxation, as in Case 966. The sagittal scan demonstrates severe narrowing of the L4-5 disc space and reactive marrow changes (compare to Case 922), whereas the axial view documents narrow bilateral defects of spondylolysis *(arrows)*. Reactive sclerosis and/or callus frequently accompany a thin tissue line traversing the pars interarticularis, as seen in this case. AP elongation of

the spinal canal due to the mild subluxation is well demonstrated in both projections.

When present, the bone defect of spondylolysis resembles an extra facet joint crossing anterior to the normal articulation. Spondylolysis is best seen at the midvertebral level, whereas the facet joint is best seen at the disc level. The plane of a spondylolitic defect is typically more coronal than that of the facet joints.

Case 966B demonstrates mild soft tissue thickening at the medial margin of the spondylolitic defects *(arrowheads)*. More prominent callus formation, bone fragmentation, and granulation tissue at the site of spondylolysis may form a composite mass that encroaches on the spinal canal. Alternatively, nerve roots may be tethered within the fibrotic reaction adjacent to a pars defect.

Spondylolysis is more common at L5 than at any other lumbar level. Cervical spondylolysis occurs but is rare.

# NERVE ROOT COMPRESSION DUE TO SPONDYLOLISTHESIS

## Case 967

35-year-old woman presenting with
bilateral leg pain.
(axial, noncontrast T1-weighted SE scan; L5-S1 level)

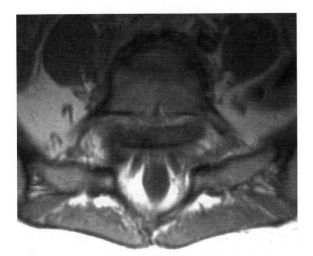

**Spondylolisthesis**

## Case 968

49-year-old man presenting with
bilateral L5 radiculopathy.
(sagittal, noncontrast T2-weighted FSE scan)

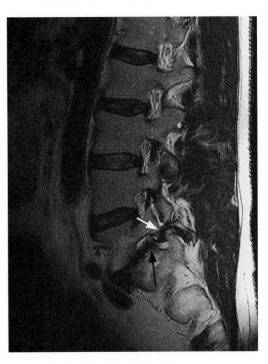

**Spondylolisthesis**

---

Axial CT or MR images in cases of spondylolysis with spondylolisthesis demonstrate typical morphological features. Anterior movement of the rostral body away from its posterior arch causes the spinal canal to become elongated in anteroposterior diameter and elliptical in configuration. Since the intervertebral disc usually maintains its relationship to the caudal vertebral body, the ledge or step-off from the rostral body to disc resembles a disc bulge. Case 967 illustrates these characteristic findings.

The central canal is usually not compromised by spondylolisthesis due to spondylolysis. However, the nerve roots exiting beneath the pedicles of the forward-slipping vertebra are often distorted. Displacement of the rostral vertebra carries the lateral recesses anteriorly, so that they come to lie above the nondisplaced disc. This malalignment narrows the cephalocaudal dimension of the intervertebral foramina, with consequent flattening of the exiting nerve roots.

An analysis of Case 967 presents the problem. The L5 nerve roots must pass beneath the pedicles of L5 but above the L5-S1 disc. However, both structures are imaged at the same axial level, indicating that there is little space remaining between them.

This foraminal distortion is more easily appreciated on sagittal scans such as Case 968. The L5 nerve root is mildly flattened between the overlying pedicle and the underlying disc (*black arrow;* compare to the normally rounded root morphology and abundant epidural fat in higher foramina). Severe narrowing of the disc space contributes to reduced cephalocaudal dimension of the nerve root canal. The spondylolysis defect is well seen crossing the pars interarticularis of L5 *(white arrow)*.

Spondylolisthesis due to spondylolysis can be distinguished from degenerative spondylolisthesis on midsagittal MR scans by the position of the posterior arch of the forward-slipping vertebra. The disconnected spinous process is *not* anteriorly displaced in cases of spondylolysis, whereas it necessarily moves anteriorly along with the vertebral body in degenerative spondylolisthesis.

## Case 969

56-year-old woman presenting with back pain.
(sagittal, noncontrast T2-weighted SE scan)

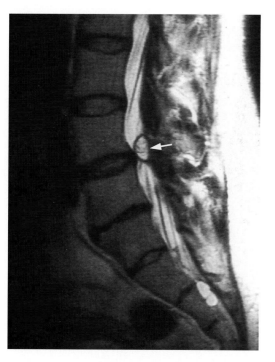

**Synovial Cyst**

## Case 970

63-year-old woman presenting with right leg pain.
(axial, postcontrast T1-weighted SE scan; L4-5 level)

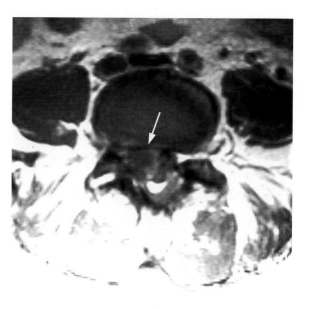

**Synovial Cyst**

Degenerative changes of the lumbar facet joints may be associated with the development of a synovial cyst. These structures represent expansion or herniation of synovial membranes beneath or through the facet capsule/ligamentum flavum.

Synovial cysts are characteristically found at the medial margin of the facet joint. The resulting extradural deformity along the posterolateral border of the spinal canal can usually be distinguished from more anteriorly based disc herniations.

Case 969 illustrates the typical appearance of synovial cysts on sagittal studies. A round mass measuring approximately one centimeter in diameter is present within the spinal canal at the L4-5 level. The lesion is defined by a thin, uniform rim of low signal intensity on a long TR spin echo image. This rim correlates with the dense perimeter of synovial cysts usually seen on CT scans and reflects calcification and/or old blood products. The center of the cyst may be heterogeneous or homogeneously bright on T2-weighted images.

In Case 970, the cyst is located medial to the right facet joint. The dural sac is compressed and displaced contralaterally. Enhancement is present along the margins of the cyst, most apparent medially. (See Case 1063 for a sagittal view of this lesion.) Some synovial cysts demonstrate central high signal intensity on precontrast T1-weighted scans, reflecting subacute blood produces within the lesion.

The great majority of synovial cysts are found at L4-5, possibly relating to the relatively large amount of motion and facet stress occurring at this level. (As discussed in Case 966, spondylolysis is also most common at L5.)

Synovial cysts may fluctuate in size on follow-up studies, suggesting variable distention by joint effusion or fluid. Occasional cysts cause persistent compression of nerve roots and require aspiration or surgery.

# DIFFERENTIAL DIAGNOSIS:
## SMALL, ROUND INTRASPINAL MASS WITH A RIM OF LOW INTENSITY

### Case 971

55-year-old woman presenting with back pain.
(sagittal, noncontrast scan; SE 2500/45)

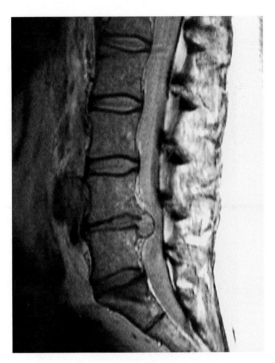

**Herniated Disc**

### Case 972

49-year-old woman presenting with leg pain.
(sagittal, noncontrast scan; SE 2700/45)

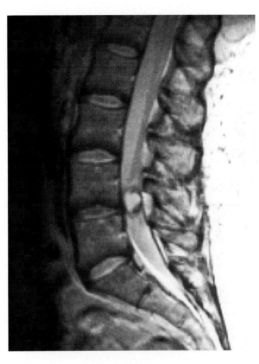

**Synovial Cyst**

---

In each of these cases, a small mass with round contours is present within the spinal canal at the L4-5 level. Both masses demonstrate intermediate to high signal intensity surrounded by a rim of low intensity. There is narrowing of the adjacent L4-5 disc in both cases.

Case 971 is an example of the long T2 values often seen within a herniated disc, even when the parent disc appears "dehydrated." The lesion is based against the posterior margin of the disc space. The band of low signal intensity enclosing the mass posteriorly represents residual fibers of the outer annulus and posterior longitudinal ligament partially containing the focal herniation.

The synovial cyst in Case 972 is more central with respect to the anteroposterior diameter of the spinal canal (because it arises laterally rather than ventrally). The characteristic rim of low signal intensity is somewhat more irregular in this case than in Case 969. This feature combines with the size and shape of the mass, its midcanal position, and is occurrence at the L4-5 level to suggest the correct diagnosis.

Both of the above lesions would be expected to demonstrate peripheral enhancement on postcontrast scans (compare to Cases 1190 and 1191).

### Case 973

42-year-old man presenting with
bladder dysfunction.
(sagittal, noncontrast T1-weighted SE scan)

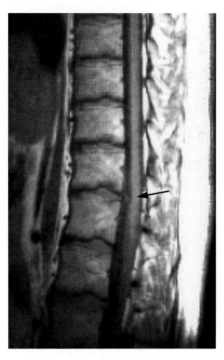

**Herniated Disc**

### Case 974

37-year-old woman presenting with "shooting"
midthoracic pain on coughing or sneezing
and vague numbness below the waist.
(sagittal, noncontrast T2-weighted FSE scan)

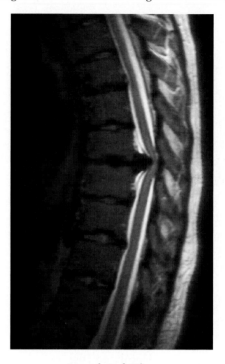

**Herniated Disc**

---

Magnetic resonance imaging has demonstrated that herniated thoracic discs are much more common than had been previously appreciated. Many such lesions are asymptomatic and clinically incidental. However, the small diameter of the thoracic spinal canal and its kyphotic curvature predispose to neurological impairment from even small anterior extradural deformities. About two thirds of patients with symptomatic thoracic disc herniations present with motor and sensory complaints, whereas one third experience bowel or bladder dysfunction.

In Case 973, a small herniated disc is seen at T11-12 as an indentation along the dark line of ventral subarachnoid space, dura, and posterior longitudinal ligament *(arrow)*. Slight ventral flattening of the conus medullaris confirms the presence of an extradural lesion.

Case 974 illustrates the opposite extreme in the spectrum of herniated thoracic discs. A very large epidural mass is based against the anterior margin of the spinal canal and centered at a disc level. The low signal intensity of the lesion correlated with dense calcification on x-ray and CT studies and matches the appearance of the adjacent disc. The spinal cord is severely displaced and compressed.

In some cases, the volume of a herniated thoracic disc seems to exceed the volume of a normal intervertebral disc space. It is likely that hydration of extruded nuclear material, reactive edema, granulation tissue, focal hemorrhage, and calcification contribute to the epidural mass in such cases. (See the discussion of giant lumbar disc herniations in Cases 942 and 943.)

Large herniated thoracic discs are often more rounded or hemispheral in morphology than in Case 974 (see Case 977). The size and calcification of the lesion may then resemble the appearance of a spinal meningioma or schwannoma. The relationship of such herniations to a parent disc is the key feature enabling correct diagnosis.

## Case 975

69-year-old woman presenting with
midthoracic pain.
(axial, noncontrast T1-weighted
SE scan; T7-8 level)

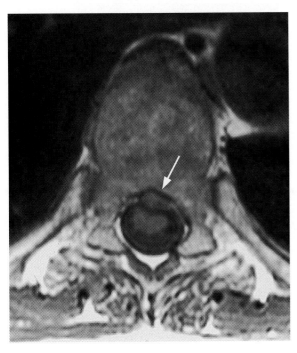

**Herniated Disc**

## Case 976

50-year-old man complaining of sudden
severe back and right flank pain.
(axial, noncontrast T1-weighted
SE scan; T10-11 level)

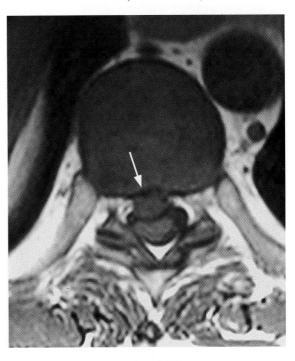

**Herniated Disc**

Herniated thoracic discs cause radicular pain more frequently than symptoms of cord compression. The pain may be bilateral in the presence of large or central herniations or unilateral in association with more eccentric herniation.

The ventral margin of the spinal cord is mildly indented by the small disc herniation in Case 975. The larger herniation in Case 976 displaces the spinal cord dorsally and flattens its anterior margin.

As mentioned on the preceding page, herniated discs are a common incidental finding on MR scans of the thoracic spinal canal. However, even herniations as small as Case 975 can cause severe local or long tract symptoms and signs. Clinical correlation is necessary to determine the significance of small thoracic herniations.

Localized epidural hemorrhage may accompany herniated thoracic discs, as is true in the lumbar region. The presence of blood products within the epidural space may cause heterogeneous and confusing patterns of signal abnormality. An anterior epidural mass centered at a disc level should raise the question of disc herniation, regardless of the size, morphology, and signal intensity of the lesion.

# DIFFERENTIAL DIAGNOSIS:
## ANTERIOR EXTRAMEDULLARY MASS IN THE THORACIC SPINAL CANAL

### Case 977

19-year-old man presenting with
worsening paraparesis.
(sagittal, noncontrast T1-weighted SE scan)

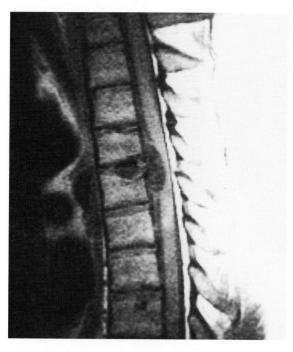

**Herniated Disc**

### Case 978

43-year-old woman presenting with
difficulty walking.
(sagittal, noncontrast T1-weighted SE scan)

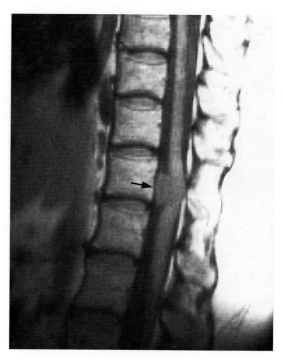

**Schwannoma**

As discussed in Case 974, occasional herniated thoracic discs are large lesions that can resemble intraspinal neoplasms. The herniation in Case 977 is at least as large as the tumor in Case 978 and causes substanial deformity of the spinal cord. Low signal intensity within the lesion and the parent disc space is due to calcification, which was documented on routine x-rays. The hemispheral morphology and calcification of the mass mimic a meningioma (see Cases 1050 and 1051).

Spinal schwannomas may be indistinguishable from meningiomas on preconstrast or postcontrast MR studies. (Potential differentiating features are discussed in Cases 1050-1059.) Both types of tumors are commonly intra-

dural, causing widening of the adjacent subarachnoid space. This finding is illustrated by Case 978 and contrasts with the epidural mass effect effacing the subarachnoid space adjacent to the mass in Case 977.

A vague zone of high signal intensity within the signal cord slightly inferior to the herniation in Case 977 may reflect subacute hemorrhage or contusion (see Case 1177). It is possible that superimposed trauma, albeit minor, exacerbated the neurological deficit caused by long-standing cord compression in this patient.

The ventral location of the tumor in Case 978 is typical of spinal schwannomas (see also Cases 1054, 1066, and 1067).

## Case 979

50-year-old woman complaining of back pain.
(axial, noncontrast T1-weighted SE scan; T7-8 level)

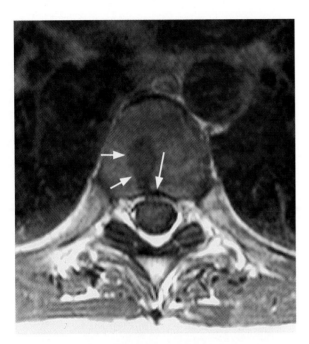

**End Plate Trail**
(adjacent to a herniated disc)

## Case 980

47-year-old man presenting with right
radicular midthoracic pain.
(axial, noncontrast T1-weighted SE scan; T6-7 level)

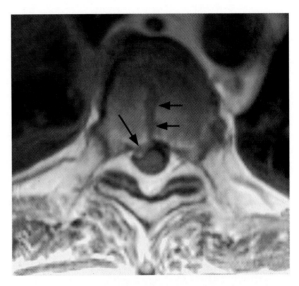

**End Plate Trail**
(adjacent to a herniated disc)

Herniated thoracic discs are sometimes associated with a characteristic trail or track within one of the adjacent end plates. This finding represents a groove and/or a band of sclerosis with a sagittal or mildly oblique orientation that may be midline or paramedian. The appearance suggests a furrow of reactive changes created by gradual migration of a Schmorl's node toward the posterior margin of the disc space. Such end plate trails or tracks often lead to a herniated disc, which may be best seen on an adjacent image. The finding is most apparent on CT scans, where it has been reported to accompany more than 40% of herniated thoracic discs. End plate tracks are not common in the cervical or lumbar region.

Case 979 illustrates a relatively broad parasagittal groove in the inferior end plate of T7 *(short arrows)*. A small por-

tion of the disc herniation at T7-8 replaces ventral epidural fat near the midline *(long arrow);* the majority of the herniated disc was demonstrated on the next inferior scan.

In Case 980, a narrow nuclear trail is seen as a sagittal groove of decreased signal intensity traversing the cortex of the inferior end plate of T6 *(small arrows)*. The shallow furrow leads posteriorly to a small, right-sided disc herniation that focally deforms the anterior margin of the spinal cord *(long arrow)*.

End plate tracks can help to identify an otherwise ambiguous anterior epidural mass. Nuclear trails also serve as a reminder that herniation of the nucleus pulposus is often accompanied by posterior displacement of annular fragments and pieces of cartilage from the end plate.

## Case 981

77-year-old man presenting with
mild spastic quadriparesis.
(sagittal, noncontrast T1-weighted SE scan)

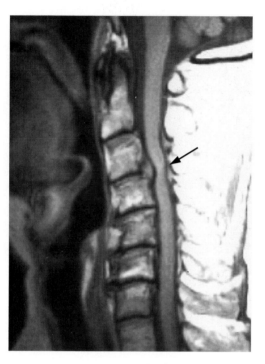

**Herniated Disc**

## Case 982

34-year-old man presenting with bilateral arm
pain and weakness and difficulty walking.
(sagittal, noncontrast T2-weighted FSE scan)

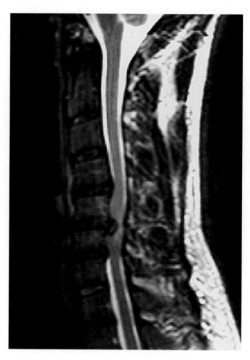

**Herniated Disc**

Herniated cervical discs present in a variety of clinical contexts and with a spectrum of MR appearances. The most common associated symptoms are neck and arm pain due to small or lateral herniations. Symptoms of cord compression, as in the above cases, are seen with larger herniations and/or in a setting of spinal stenosis. (Case 981 illustrates the combination of both factors.)

The signal intensity within herniated cervical discs is variable, resembling the range of appearances previously illustrated in the lumbar and thoracic regions. Most cervical herniations are relatively isointense to the parent disc and to cord parenchyma on T1-weighted scans, as seen in Case 981. On T2-weighted images, herniated cervical discs may demonstrate low intensity, intermediate values, or high intensity.

The subarachnoid space is completely effaced at the level of herniation in each of the above cases. Cord compression is present in both patients. The T2-weighted scan in Case 980 demonstrates associated intramedullary edema.

A small disc herniation or bulge may be difficult to appreciate on T1-weighted scans, since the low signal intensity of the annulus blends with that of the posterior longitudinal ligament, dura, and ventral subarachnoid space. Techniques with bright CSF (i.e., spin echo sequences with long TR values or gradient echo sequences with low flip angles) demonstrate more clearly the interface between the disc margin and the dural sac.

Large herniated cervical discs may elevate or tent the posterior longitudinal ligament away from the adjacent vertebral bodies. Soft tissue with long T1 and T2 values then imaged between the bodies and the posteriorly displaced ligament usually represents prominent epidural veins rather than rostral or caudal migration of disc fragments.

Artifact from the thick tissue and bone of the shoulders often compromises CT scans at inferior cervical levels. Sagittal MR images provide an alternative, artifact-free means of evaluating the cervicothoracic junction.

### Case 983

26-year-old woman presenting with neck pain.
(axial, noncontrast T1-weighted SE scan; C3-4 level)

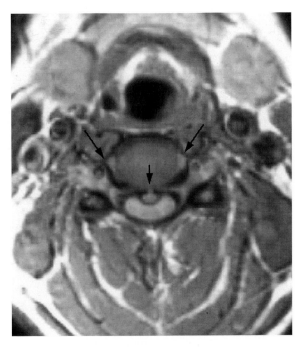

**Herniated Disc**

### Case 984

29-year-old man presenting with right arm pain.
(axial, noncontrast T2*-weighted
GRE scan; C4-5 level)

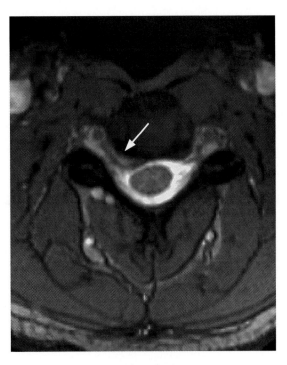

**Herniated Disc**

The axial perspective is as useful in the cervical spine as in the lumbar or thoracic region. However, the small size of cervical vertebrae and discs requires close placement of thin sections for adequate definition of anatomical and pathological features. Even with good technique, the relative lack of epidural fat in the cervical region and the reduced contrast resolution of thin sections may make diagnosis difficult.

A small central disc herniation *(short arrow)* is well seen on the T1-weighted image in Case 983, indenting the ventral margin of the dural sac and spinal cord. A black line between the disc and the cord probably represents a combination of outer annulus, posterior longitudinal ligament, and dura. The marrow-containing uncinate processes *(long arrows)* are of higher signal intensity than the disc they enclose.

Axial scans performed with low flip angle gradient echo technique, such as Case 984, provide a myelographic effect that is useful in evaluating herniated cervical discs. Such sequences also produce high signal intensity within epidural veins of the cervical canal and neural foramina, in-creasing the contrast with disc material or osteophytes in both locations.

In Case 984, the spinal cord is well defined, with intramedullary discrimination of gray and white matter. A lateral disc herniation occupies the right anterolateral recess of the spinal canal and extends into the neural foramen *(arrow)*. The ventral subarachnoid space is effaced with mild flattening of the anterior margin of the spinal cord, and the right nerve root canal is narrowed.

The signal intensity of herniated discs on low flip angle gradient echo images varies from low to intermediate to bright. High intensity in the region of herniation, as in Case 984, may include partial volume contributions from prominent epidural veins immediately superior or inferior to the herniated disc itself.

Enlarged epidural veins can be an independent occurrence, causing masses that mimic herniated discs. Distention of veins due to recent suboccipital surgery or in association with spontaneous intracranial hypotension (see Case 540) are two such circumstances.

## Case 985

81-year-old woman presenting with
cervical myelopathy.
(sagittal, noncontrast T2-weighted SE scan)

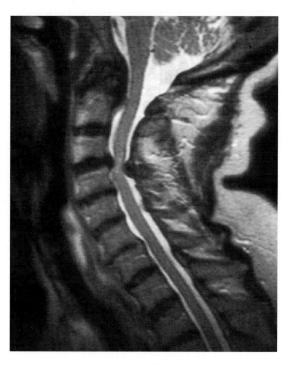

**Central Canal Stenosis**

## Case 986

91-year-old woman presenting with
arm and leg weakness.
(sagittal, noncontrast T2-weighted FSE scan)

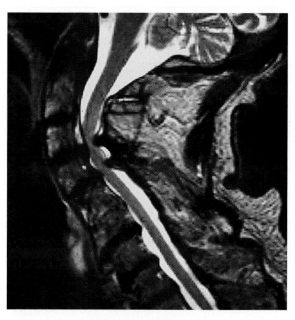

**Central Canal Stenosis**

---

Central canal stenosis in the cervical region is often due to disc-based ridges accompanied by thickening and buckling of dorsal ligaments. Case 985 illustrates this combination of ventral and dorsal extradural deformities. A disc bulge or herniation indents the anterior margin of the dural sac at C3-4, while thickening of posterior elements causes a dorsal impression.

The spinal cord in Case 985 is pinched between the focal extradural masses. A small area of high signal intensity is present within the mildly flattened cord, characteristic of compressive myelopathy. Both reversible edema and irreversible myelomalacia may contribute to this appearance, which may be correlated with limited postoperative improvement. Remarkable flattening of the spinal cord can be asymptomatic if epidural compression develops slowly (see Cases 990 and 1168).

Central canal stenosis at C3-4 and C4-5 in Case 986 is due predominantly to hypertrophy of dorsal elements.

Disc bulges are also present at the anterior margin of the spinal canal. Although the spinal cord is severely compressed at C3-4, there is little evidence of associated edema or myelomalacia.

The C5-6 disc space is obliterated in Case 986 with probable fusion at this level. Disc levels superior to spontaneous or operative fusion experience increased motion and stress, which may exacerbate the development of degenerative changes.

The small anterior extradural deformities at disc levels from C6 to T2 in Case 986 probably represent both bulging discs and accompanying osteophytes. It is often difficult to distinguish between these two potential components; the generic phrase "spondylotic ridge" may be the most appropriate description in such cases.

See Case 1041 for another example of central cervical stenosis.

## Case 987

26-year-old man presenting with right arm pain.
(axial, noncontrast T2*-weighted
GRE scan; C5-6 level)

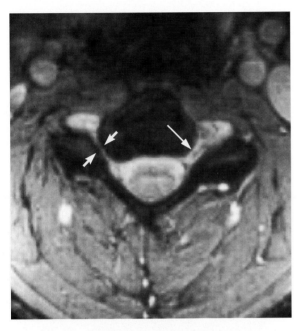

**Lateral (Foraminal) Stenosis**

## Case 988

41-year-old woman presenting with
arm pain and numbness.
(oblique coronal, noncontrast T1-weighted SE scan)

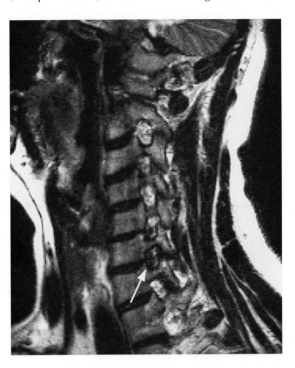

**Lateral (Foraminal) Stenosis**

In Case 987, the left nerve root canal *(long arrow)* is seen as a band of high signal intensity reflecting its content of epidural veins and CSF-containing root sleeve. (Compare to the T1-weighted appearance of the foramina in Case 983.) By contrast, the right intervertebral foramen is severely narrowed due to hypertrophy of the uncinate process and facet joint *(short arrows)*.

A small amount of cervical scoliosis or tilt will cause asymmetrical visualization of the right and left intervertebral foramina on any one axial scan. Care should be taken to evaluate adjacent sections before foraminal asymmetry is judged to represent stenosis.

Case 987 demonstrates that nerve root canals in the cervical region are aligned at about a 45-degree angle to the sagittal or coronal planes. For this reason, cervical intervertebral foramina are sectioned obliquely by sagittal or coronal scans. A true cross-sectional view of cervical nerve root canals requires an oblique acquisition (or reconstruction), as in Case 988. This projection displays the column of foramina in a manner comparable to parasagittal scans in the lumbar region.

Osteophyte extends into the anterior-inferior corner of the C5-6 nerve root canal in Case 988. A disc herniation significantly compromises the canal at C6-7 *(arrow)*, with probable compression of the exiting C7 root. (Compare to the morphology of the widely patent canals at C4-5 and C7-T1.)

Discrimination between osteophyte and dehydrated disc material can be difficult on cervical MR scans, since both present as low intensity extradural deformities. This distinction is more easily made on CT studies.

### Case 989A

52-year-old man presenting with neck
and arm pain and leg weakness.
(sagittal, noncontrast T1-weighted SE scan)

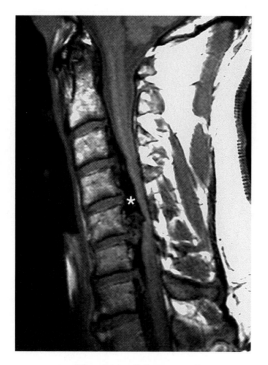

**Ossification of the Posterior
Longitudinal Ligament**

### Case 989B

Same patient.
(sagittal, noncontrast T2-weighted FSE scan)

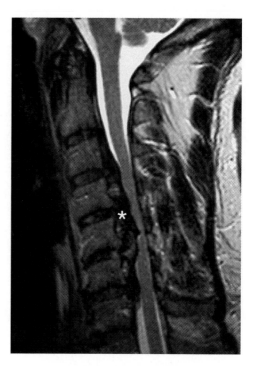

**Ossification of the Posterior
Longitudinal Ligament**

Stenosis of the cervical canal and compressive myelopathy may be caused by ossification of the posterior longitudinal ligament (OPLL). This bone formation along the posterior margin of cervical vertebral bodies may be segmental or diffuse. In either case, progressive thickening of the layer of epidural ossification causes gradual flattening of the thecal sac.

OPLL may demonstrate high or low signal intensity on T1-weighted scans, depending on the presence or absence of lipid-containing marrow elements. In Case 989A, a thick layer of predominantly low signal intensity *(asterisk)* is apparent along the posterior margin of vertebral bodies from C3 to C7. The ossified tissue is mildly heterogeneous and irregular, with variable diameter.

In other cases, OPLL may be smoother in contour and more uniform in signal intensity (usually low) and dimension. The low intensity of the ossified ligament may then be poorly defined on T1-weighted images, due to the adjacent low intensity of the ventral subarachnoid space.

The T2-weighted scan in Case 989B documents complete effacement of CSF spaces in the mid cervical region. The spinal cord is posteriorly displaced and severely compressed, but there is little intramedullary edema.

# OSSEOUS DEFORMITY OF THE CERVICAL CANAL

### Case 990

61-year-old man presenting with abnormal posture and quadriparesis.
(sagittal, noncontrast T2-weighted SE scan)

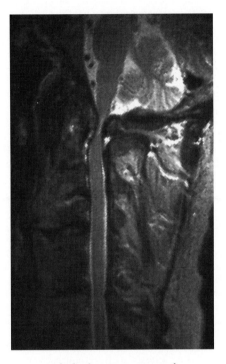

**Ankylosing Hyperostosis**

### Case 991

2-year-old boy with spinal deformity incidentally noted on x-rays of the pharynx.
(sagittal, noncontrast T2-weighted SE scan)

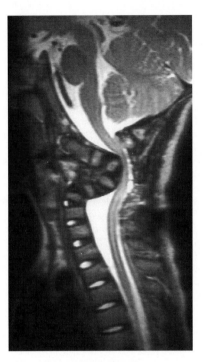

**Idiopathic Kyphosis**

---

The ability of MR scans to display long segments of the spinal canal while demonstrating the intradural consequences of vertebral abnormalities is useful for evaluation of spinal deformities. A common application of MR in this regard is the assessment of thoracic scoliosis, checking for potentially associated intradural or extradural malformations or masses and/or secondary cord compression (see Cases 1072, 1079, and 1256).

The above cases illustrate more unusual examples of osseous deformity involving the cervical canal. The patient in Case 990 suffers from severe constriction of the neural canal at the craniocervical junction. This stenosis is caused by subluxation and degenerative changes at the C1 level due to long-standing immobility of the remainder of the

cervical spine. The thick, hyperostotic bone fusing the anterior margins of cervical vertebrae is faintly visualized.

High signal intensity within the compressed cervicomedullary junction in Case 990 may represent reversible edema and/or irreversible myelomalacia (compare to Case 985). See Cases 1167, 1168, and 1273-1276 for additional examples of canal stenosis at the craniocervical junction.

The cause of the severe cervical kyphosis in Case 991 has not been determined. No other skeletal abnormalities have been demonstrated in this patient. The sagittal MR scan clearly documents cord deformity, with abnormal intramedullary signal. This unusual cervical gibbus was resected by an anterior approach and replaced by bone struts to reconstitute reasonable alignment of the cervical canal.

# REFERENCES

Ackerman SJ, Steinberg EP, Bryan RN, et al: Persistent low back pain in patients suspected of having herniated nucleus pulposus: radiologic predictors of functional outcome—implications for treatment selection. *Radiology* 203:815-822, 1997.

Ackerman SJ, Steinberg EP, Bryan RN, et al: Trends in diagnostic imaging for low back pain: has MR imaging been a substitute or add-on? *Radiology* 203:533-538, 1997.

Agula LA, Piraino DW, Modie MT: The intranuclear cleft of the intervertebral disk: magnetic resonance imaging. *Radiology* 155:155, 1985.

Al-Mefty O, Harkey LH, Middleton TH, et al: Myelopathic cervical spondylitic lesions demonstrated by magnetic resonance imaging. *J Neurosurg* 68:217-222, 1988.

Amunosen T, Weber H, Lilleas F, et al: Lumbar spinal stenosis: clinical and radiologic features. *Spine* 20:1178-1186, 1995.

Annertz M , Jonsson B, Stromqvist B, Holtas S: Serial MRI in the early postoperative period after lumbar discectomy. *Neuroradiology* 37:177-182, 1995.

Awwad EE, Martin DS, Smith KR: The nuclear trial sign in thoracic herniated disks. *AJNR* 13:137-143, 1992.

Awwad EE, Martin DS, Smith KR Jr, Buchotz RD: MR imaging of lumbar juxtaarticular cysts. *J Comput Assist Tomogr* 14:415-417, 1990.

Barnett GH, Hardy RW Jr, Little JR, et al: Thoracic spinal canal stenosis. *J Neurosurg* 66:338-344, 1987.

Benitah S, Raftopoulos C, Baleriaux D, et al: Upper cervical spinal cord compression due to bony stenosis of the spinal canal. *Neuroradiology* 36:231-233, 1994.

Berger PE, Atkinson D, Wilson WJ, Wiltse L: High resolution surface coil magnetic resonance imaging of the spine: normal and pathologic anatomy. *Radiographics* 6:573-602, 1986.

Bergleit R, Gebarski SS, Brunberg JA, et al: Lumbar synovial cysts: correlation of myelographic MR and pathologic findings. *AJNR* 11:777-779, 1990.

Blumenkoph B: Thoracic intervertebral disc herniations: diagnostic value of magnetic resonance imaging. *Neurosurgery* 23:36-40, 1988.

Boden SD, Davis DO, Dina TS, et al: Abnormal magnetic resonance scans of the lumbar spine in asymptomatic patients. *J Bone Joint Surg* 72:403-408, 1990.

Boden SD, Davis DO, Dina TS, et al: Contrast-enhanced MR imaging performed after successful lumbar disk surgery: prospective study. *Radiology* 182:59-64, 1992.

Boden SD, Davis DO, Dina TS, et al: Postoperative diskitis: distinguishing early MR imaging findings from normal postoperative disk space changes. *Radiology* 184:765-771, 1992.

Borm W, Bohnstedt T: Intradural cervical disc herniation. Case report and review of the literature. *J Neurosurg Spine* 92:221-224, 2000.

Bozzao A, Gallucci M, Masciocchi C, et al: Lumbar disk herniation: MR imaging assessment of natural history in patients treated without surgery. *Radiology* 185:135-142, 1992.

Brown BM, Schwartz RH, Frank E, Blank NK: Preoperative evaluation of cervical radiculopathy and myelopathy by surface-coil MR imaging. *AJNR* 9:859-866, 1988.

Bundschuh CV, Modic MT, Ross JS, et al: Epidural fibrosis and recurrent disk herniation in lumbar spine: MR imaging assessment. *AJNR* 9:169-178, 1988.

Bundschuh CV, Stein L, Slusser JH, et al: Distinguishing between scar and recurrent herniated disk in postoperative patients: value of contrast-enhanced CT and MR imaging. *AJNR* 11:949-958, 1990.

Castillo M: Neural foramen remodeling caused by a sequestered disk fragment. *AJNR* 12:566-567, 1991.

Charest DR, Kenny BG: Radicular pain caused by synovial cyst: an underdiagnosed entity in the elderly? *J Neurosurg Spine* 92:57-60, 2000.

Clatterbuck RE, Belzberg AJ, Ducker TB: Intradural cervical disc herniation and Brown-Sequard's syndrome. Report of three cases and review of the literature. *J Neurosurg Spine* 92:236-240, 2000.

Crisi G, Carpeggiani P, Trevisan C: Gadolinium-enhanced nerve roots in lumbar disk herniation. *AJNR* 14:1379-1392, 1993.

Czervionke LF: Lumbar intervertebral disc disease. *Neuroimaging Clin N Amer* 3:465-486, 1993.

Czervionke LF, Daniels DL, Ho PSP, et al: The cervical neural foramina: a correlative anatomic and MR study. *Radiology* 1:753-759, 1988.

DeRoos A, Kressel H, Spritzer C, Dalinka M: MR imaging of marrow changes adjacent to end-plates in degenerative lumbar disk disease. *Am J Roentgenol* 149:531-534, 1987.

Devor M, Rappaport ZH: Relation of foraminal (lateral) stenosis to radicular pain. *AJNR* 17:1615-1618, 1996.

Dina TS, Boden SD, Davis DO: Lumbar spine after surgery of herniated disk: imaging findings in the early postoperative period. *Am J Roentgenol* 164:665-672, 1995.

El Gammal TAM, Crews CE: MR myelography of the cervical spine. *Radiographics* 16:77-88, 1996.

Emamian SA, Skriver EB, Henriksen L, Cortsen ME: Lumbar herniated disk mimicking neuroma. *Acta Radiol* 34,fasc.2:127-129, 1993.

Enzmann DR, Rubin JB: Cervical spine: MR imaging with a partial flip angle, gradient-refocused pulse sequence. Part I. General considerations and disk disease. *Radiology* 166:467-472, 1988.

Erkintalo MO, Salminen JJ, Alanen AM, et al: Development of degenerative changes in the lumbar intervertebral disk: results of a prospective MR imaging study in adolescents with and without low-back pain. *Radiology* 196:529-534, 1995.

Fletcher G, Haughton VM, Ho K-C, Yu S: Age-related changes in cervical facet joints: studies with cryomicrotomy, MR and CT. *AJNR* 11:27-30, 1990.

Fox MW, Onofrio BM, Kilgore JE: Neurological complications of ankylosing spondylitis. *J Neurosurg* 78:871-878, 1993.

Friedberg SR, Fellows T, Thomas CB, et al: Experience with symptomatic spinal epidural cysts. *Neurosurgery* 34:989-993, 1994.

Gaskill MF, Lukin R, Wiot JG: Lumbar disc disease and stenosis. *Radiol Clin North Am* 29:753-764, 1991.

Georgy BA, Hesselink JR: MR imaging of the spine: recent advances in pulse sequences and special techniques. *Am J Roentgenol* 162:923-934, 1994.

Georgy BA, Hesselink JR, Middleton MS: Fat suppression contrast-enhanced MRI in the failed back surgery syndrome: a prospective study. *Neuroradiology* 37:51-57, 1995.

Georgy BA, Snow RD, Hesselink JR: MR imaging of the spinal nerve roots: techniques, enhancement patterns, and imaging findings. *Am J Roentgenol* 166:173-180, 1996.

Glickstein MF, Sussman SK: Time-dependent scar enhancement in magnetic resonance imaging of the postoperative lumbar spine. *Skeletal Radiol* 20:333-337, 1991.

Gorey MT, Hyman RA, Black KS, et al: Lumbar synovial cysts eroding bone. *AJNR* 13:161-163, 1992.

Grand CM, Bank WO, Baleriaux D, et al: Gadolinium enhancement of vertebral endplates following lumbar disc surgery. *Neuroradiology* 35:503-505, 1993.

Grenier N, Greselle JF, Douws C, et al: MR imaging of foraminal and extraforaminal lumbar disk herniations. *J Comput Assist Tomogr* 14:243-249, 1990.

Grenier N, Greselle J, Vital J, et al: Normal and disrupted lumbar longitudinal ligaments: correlative MR and anatomic study. *Radiology* 171:197-205, 1989.

Grenier N, Kressel HY, Schiebler MI, et al: Normal and degenerative posterior spinal structures: MR imaging. *Radiology* 165:517-525, 1987.

Gundry CR, Heithoff KB: Epidural hematoma of the lumbar spine: 18 surgically confirmed cases. *Radiology* 187:427-432, 1993.

Haughton VM: MR imaging of the spine. *Radiology* 166:297-301, 1988.

Hedberg MC, Drayer BP, Flom RA, et al: Gradient echo (GRASS) MR imaging in cervical radiculopathy. *AJNR* 150:683-689, 1988.

Hierholzer J, Benndorf G, Lehmann T, et al: Epidural lipomatosis: case report and literature review. *Neuroradiology* 38:343-348, 1996.

Ho PSP, Yu S, Sether LA, et al: Ligamentum flavum: appearance on sagittal and coronal MR images. *Radiology* 168:469-472, 1988.

Ho PSP, Yu S, Sether LA, et al: Progressive and regressive changes in the nucleus pulposus: part I. The neonate. *Radiology* 169:87-91, 1988.

Howington JU, Connolly ES, Voorhies RM: Intraspinal synovial cysts; 10-year experience at the Ochsner Clinic. *J Neurosurg Spine* 91:193-199, 1999.

Hueftle M, Modic MT, Ross JS, et al: Lumbar spine: postoperative MR imaging with Gd-DTPA. *Radiology* 167:817-824, 1988.

Ibrahim MA, Jesmanowicz A, Hyde JS, et al: Contrast enhancement of normal intervertebral disks: time and dose dependent. *AJNR* 15:419-424, 1994.

Itoh R, Murata K, Kamata M, et al: Lumbosacral nerve root enhancement with disk herniation on contrast-enhanced MR. *AJNR* 17:1619-1625, 1996.

Jackson DE, Atlas SW, Mani JR, Norman D: Intraspinal synovial cysts: MR imaging. *Radiology* 170:527-530, 1989.

Jahnke RW, Hart BL: Cervical stenosis, spondylosis, and herniated disc disease. *Radiol Clin North Am* 29:777-792, 1991.

Jarvik JG, Deyo RA: Imaging of lumbar intervertebral disk degeneration and aging, excluding disk herniations. *Radiol Clin North Am* 38:1255-1266, 2000.

Jarvik JG, Maravilla KR, Haynor DR, et al: Rapid MR imaging versus plain radiography in patients with low back pain: initial results of a randomized study. *Radiology* 204:447-454, 1997.

Jinkins JR: Gd-DTPA enhanced MR of the lumbar spinal canal in patients with claudication. *J Comput Assist Tomogr* 17:555-561, 1993.

Jinkins JR: MR of enhancing nerve roots in the unoperated lumbosacral spine. *AJNR* 14:193-202, 1993.

Jinkins JR, Matthes JC, Sener RN, et al: Spondylolysis, spondylolisthesis, and associated nerve root entrapment in the lumbosacral spine: MR evaluation. *Am J Roentgenol* 159:799-803, 1992.

Jinkins JR, Osborn AG, Garrett D, et al: Spinal nerve enhancement with Gd-DTPA: MR correlation with the postoperative lumbosacral spine. *AJNR* 14:383-394, 1993.

Jinkins JR, Van Goethem JWM: The postsurgical lumbar spine: magnetic resonance imaging evluation following intervertebral disk surgery, surgical decompression, intervertebral bony fusion, and spinal instrumentation. *Radiol Clin North Am* 39:1-29, 2001.

Johnson DW, Farnum GN, Latchaw RE, et al: MR imaging of the pars interarticularis in patients with spondylolisthesis. *AJNR* 9:1215-1220, 1988.

Kent DL, Haynor DR, Larson EB, Deyo RA: Diagnosis of lumbar spinal stenosis in adults: a metaanalysis of the accuracy of CT, MR and myelography. *Am J Roentgenol* 158:1135-1144, 1992.

Kim FM, Poussaint TY, Barnes PD: Neuroimaging of scoliosis in childhood. *Neuroimaging Clin North Am* 9:195-222, 1999.

Kostelic J, Haughton MV, Sether L: Proximal lumbar spinal nerves in axial MR imaging, CT, and anatomic sections. *Radiology* 183:239, 1992.

Krauss WE, Atkinson JLD, Miller GM: Juxtafacet cysts of the cervical spine. *Neurosurgery* 43:1363-1368, 1998.

Lane JI, Koeller KK, Atkinson JLD: Contrast-enhanced radicular veins on MR of the lumbar spine in an asymptomatic study group. *AJNR* 16:269-274, 1995.

Lane JI, Koeller KK, Atkinson JLD: Enhanced lumbar nerve roots in the spine without prior surgery: radiculitis or radicular veins? *AJNR* 15:1317-1325, 1994.

Lee SH, Coleman PE, Hahn FJ: Magnetic resonance imaging of degenerative disk disease of the spine. *Radiol Clin North Am* 26:949-964, 1988.

Liu SS, Williams KD, Drayer BP, et al: Synovial cysts of the lumbosacral spine: diagnosis by MR imaging. *AJNR* 10:1239-1242, 1989.

Luetkehans TJ, Coughlin BF, Weinstein MA: Ossification of the posterior longitudinal ligament by MR. *AJNR* 8:924-925, 1987.

Lyons MK, Atkinson JLD, Wharen RE, et al: Surgical evaluation and management of lumbar synovial cysts: the Mayo Clinic experience. *J Neurosurg Spine* 93:53-57, 2000.

Mahallati H, Wallace CJ, Hunter KM, et al: MR imaging of a hemorrhagic and granulomatous cyst of the ligamentum flavum with pathologic correlation. *AJNR* 20:1166-1168, 1999.

Masaryk TJ, Ross TS, Modic MT, et al: High-resolution MR imaging of sequestered lumbar intervertebral disks. *AJNR* 9:351-358, 1988.

Matsubara Y, Kato F, Mimatsu K, et al: Serial changes on MRI in lumbar disc herniations treated conservatively. *Neuroradiology* 37:378-383, 1995.

McCall IW: Lumbar herniated disks. *Radiol Clin North Am* 38:1293-1309, 2000.

Mehalic TF, Pezzuti RT, Applebaum BI: Magnetic resonance imaging and cervical spondylitic myelography. *Neurosurgery* 26:216-227, 1990.

Melhem ER, Benson ML, Beauchamp NJ, Lee RR: Cervical spondylosis: three-dimensional gradient-echo MR with magnetization transfer. *AJNR* 17:705-712, 1996.

Milette PC: Classification, diagnostic imaging, and imaging characterization of lumbar herniated disk. *Radiol Clin North Am* 38:1267-1292, 2000.

Mirowitz SA, Shady KL: Gadopentetate dimeglumine-enhanced MR imaging of the postoperative lumbar spine: comparison of fat-suppressed and conventional T1-weighted MR scans. *Am J Roentgenol* 159:385-389, 1992.

Modic MT, Herfkens RJ: Intervertebral disk: normal age-related changes in MR signal intensity. *Radiology* 166:332-334, 1990.

Modic MT, Masaryk TJ, Boumphrey F, et al: Lumbar herniated disk disease and canal stenosis: prospective evaluation by surface coil MR, CT, and myelography. *AJNR* 7:709-717, 1986.

Modic MT, Masaryk TJ, Mulopulos GP, et al: Cervical radiculopathy: prospective evaluation with surface coil MR imaging, CT with metrizamide, and metrizamide myelopgraphy. *Radiology* 161:753-760, 1986.

Modic MT, Masaryk T, Paushter D: Magnetic resonance imaging of the spine. *Radiol Clin North Am* 24:229-245, 1986.

Modic MT, Masaryk TJ, Ross JS, et al: Cervical radiculopathy: value of oblique MR imaging. *Radiology* 163:227-232, 1987.

Modic MT, Masaryk RJ, Ross JS, Carter JR: Imaging of degenerative disk disease. *Radiology* 168:177-186, 1988.

Modic MT, Ross JS, Obuchowski NA, et al: Contrast-enhanced MR imaging in acute lumbar radiculopathy: a pilot study of the natural history. *Radiology* 195:429-435, 1995.

Modic MT, Steinberg PM, Ross JS, et al: Degenerative disk disease assessment of changes in vertebral body marrow with MR imaging. *Radiology* 166:193-199, 1988.

Muhle C, Metzner J, Weinert D, et al: Classification system based on kinematic MR imaging in cervical spondylitic myelopathy. *AJNR* 19:1763-1772, 1998.

Murayama S, Numaguchi Y, Robinson AE: The diagnosis of herniated intervertebral disks with MR imaging: a comparison of gradient-refocused-echo and spin-echo pulse sequences. *AJNR* 11:17-22, 1990.

Nguyen C, An H, Ho K-C, et al: Utility of high-dose contrast enhancement for detecting recurrent herniated intervertebral disks. *AJNR* 15:1291-1298, 1994.

Nguyen CM, Ho K-C, An H, et al: Ionic versus nonionic paramagnetic contrast media in differentiating between scar and herniated disk. *AJNR* 17:501-506, 1996.

Nguyen-minh C, Hughton VM, An HS, et al: Contrast media of high and low molecular weights in the detection of recurrent herniated disks. *AJNR* 19:889-893, 1998.

Nizara RS, Wybier M, Laredo J-D: Radiologic assessment of lumbar intervertebral instability and degenerative spondylolisthesis. *Radiol Clin North Am* 39:55-71, 2001.

Nowicki BH, Haughton VM: Neural foraminal ligaments of the lumbar spine: appearance at CT and MR imaging. *Radiology* 183:257-264, 1992.

Nowicki BH, Haughton VM, Schmidt TA, et al: Occult lumbar lateral spinal stenosis in neural foramina subjected to physiologic loading. *AJNR* 17:1605-1614, 1996.

Nowicki BH, Haughton VM, Yu S, An HS: Radial tears of the intervertebral disc: anatomic appearance, biomechanics, and clinical effects. *Int J Neurorad* 3:270-284, 1997.

Osborn AG, Hood RS, Sherry RG, et al: CT/MR spectrum of far lateral and anterior lumbosacral disk herniations. *AJNR* 9:775-778, 1988.

Otake S, Matsuo M, Nishizawa S, et al: Ossification of the posterior longitudinal ligament: MR evaluation. *AJNR* 13:1059-1067, 1992.

Pech P, Haughton VM: Lumbar intervertebral disk: correlative MR and anatomic study. *Radiology* 156:699-701, 1985.

Pfirrmann CWA, Resnick D: Schmorl nodes of the thoracic and lumbar spine: radiographic-pathologic study of prevalence, characterization, and correlation with degenerative changes of 1,650 spinal levels in 100 cadavers. *Radiology* 219:368-374, 2001.

Ramanauskas WL, Wilner HI, Metes JJ, et al: MR imaging of compressive myelomalacia. *J Comput Assist Tomogr* 13:399-404, 1989.

Resnick D: Degenerative diseases of the vertebral column. *Radiology* 156:3-14, 1985.

Robertson WD, Jarvik JG, Tsuruda JS, et al: The comparison of a rapid screening MR protocol with a conventional MR protocol for lumbar spondylosis. *Am J Roentgenol* 166:909-916, 1996.

Rosenbloom SA: Thoracic disc disease and stenosis. *Radiol Clin North Am* 29:765-776, 1991,

Rosenbloom J, Mojtahedi S, Foust RJ: Synovial cysts in the lumbar spine: MR characteristics. *AJNR* 10:S94, 1989.

Ross JS: Magnetic resonance assessment of the postoperative spine: degenerative disc disease. *Radiol Clin North Am* 29:793-809, 1991.

Ross JS: The postoperative lumbar spine. *Semin Spine Surg* 9:28-37, 1997.

Ross JS, Frederickson RCA, Petrie JL, et al: Association between peridural scar and recurrent radicular pain after lumbar discectomy: MR evaluation. *Neurosurgery* 38:855-863, 1996.

Ross JS, Masaryk TJ, Modic MT, et al: Lumbar spine: postoperative assessment with surface-coil MR imaging. *Radiology* 164:851-860, 1987.

Ross JS, Masaryk TJ, Modic MT: Postoperative cervical spine: MR assessment. *J Comput Assist Tomogr* 11:955-962, 1987.

Ross JS, Masaryk TJ, Schrader M, et al: MR imaging of the postoperative lumbar spine: assessment with gadopentetate dimegluine. *AJNR* 11:771-776, 1990.

Ross JS, Modic MT, Masaryk TJ, et al: Assessment of extradural degenerative disease with Gd-DTPA-enhanced MR imaging: correlation with surgical and pathologic findings. *AJNR* 10:1243-1249, 1989.

Ross JS, Modic MT, Masaryk TJ: Tears of the anulus fibrosus: assessment with Gd-DTPA-enhanced MR imaging. *AJNR* 10:1251-1254, 1989.

Ross JS, Modic MT, Masaryk TJ, et al: The postoperative lumbar spine. *Semin Roentgenol* 23:125-136, 1988.

Ross JS, Obuchowski N, Zepp R: The postoperative lumbar spine: evaluation of epidural scar over a 1-year period. *AJNR* 19:183-186, 1998.

Ross JS, Perez-Reyes N, Masaryk TJ, et al: Thoracic disk herniation: MR imaging. *Radiology* 165:511-516, 1987.

Ross JS, Ruggieri PM, Tkach JA, et al: Gd-DTPA-enhanced 3D MR imaging of cervical degenerative disk disease: initial experience. *AJNR* 13:127-136, 1992.

Ross JS, Ruggieri P, Tkach J, et al: Lumbar degenerative disk disease: prospective comparison of conventional T2-weighted spin-echo imaging and T2-weighted rapid acquisition relaxation enhanced imaging. *AJNR* 14:1215-1224, 1993.

Ross JS, Zepp R, Modic MT: The postoperative lumbar spine: enhanced MR evaluation of the intervertebral disk. *AJNR* 17:323-331, 1996.

Rubenstein DJ, Alvarez O, Ghelman B, Marchisello P: Cauda equina syndrome complicating ankylosing spondylitis: MR features. *J Comput Assist Tomogr* 13:511-513, 1989.

Russell EG: Cervical disk disease. *Radiology* 177:313-325, 1990.

Ryken TC, Menezes AH: Cervicomedullary compression in achondroplasia. *J Neurosurg* 81:43-48, 1994.

Schellinger D, Manz HJ, Vidic B, et al: Disk fragment migration. *Radiology* 175:831-836, 1990.

Schiebler ML, Grenier N, Fallon M, et al: Normal and degenerated intervertebral disk: in vivo and in vitro MR imaging with histopathologic correlation. *Am J Roentgenol* 157:93-97, 1991.

Schmid MR, Stucki G, Duewell S, et al: Changes in cross-sectional measurements of the spinal canal and intervertebral foramina as a function of body position: in vivo studies on an open-configuration MR system. *Am J Roentgenol* 172:1095-1102, 1999.

Schönström N, Willen J: Imaging lumbar spinal stenosis. *Radiol Clin North Am* 39:31-53, 2001.

Sether LA, Yu S, Haughton VM, Fischer ME: Intervertebral disk: normal age-related changes in MR signal intensity. *Radiology* 177:385-388, 1990.

Silbergleit R, Gebarski SS, Brunberg JA, et al: Lumbar synovial cysts: correlation of myelographic, CT, MR, and pathological findings. *AJNR* 11:777-779, 1990.

Silverman CS, Lenchik L, Shimkin PM, et al: The value of MR in differentiating subligamentous from supraligamentous lumbar disk herniations. *AJNR* 16:571-579, 1995.

Smith KA, Rekate HL: Delayed postoperative tethering of the cervical spinal cord. *J Neurosurg* 81:196-201, 1994.

Sobel DF, Zyroll J, Thorne RP: Discogenic vertebral sclerosis: MR imaging. *J Comput Assist Tomogr* 11:855-858, 1987.

Sotiropoulos S, Chafetz NI, Lang P, et al: Differentiation between postoperative scar and recurrent disk herniation: prospective comparison of MR, CT, and contrast-enhanced CT. *AJNR* 10:639-643, 1989.

Stabler A, Bellan M, Weiss M, et al: MR imaging of enhancing intraosseous disk herniation (Schmorl's nodes). *Am J Roentgenol* 168:933-938, 1997.

Stadnik TW, Lee RR, Coen HL, et al: Annular tears and disk herniation: prevalence and contrast enhancement on MR images in the absence of low back pain or sciatica. *Radiology* 206:49-56, 1998.

Stollman A, Pinto R, Benjamin V, et al: Radiologic imaging of symptomatic ligamentum flavum thickening with and without ossification. *AJNR* 8:991-994, 1987.

Sze G, Kawamura Y, Neaishi C, et al: Fast spin-echo MR imaging of the cervical spine: influence of echo train length and echo spacing on image contrast and quality. *AJNR* 14:1203-1214, 1993.

Takahashi M, Yamashita T, Sakamoto Y, Kojima R: Chronic cervical cord compression: clinical significance of increased signal intensity on MR imaging. *Radiology* 173:219-224, 1989.

Tartaglino LM, Flanders AE, Vinitski S, Fiedman DP: Metallic artifacts on MR images of the postoperative spine: reduction with fast spin echo techniques. *Radiology* 190:565-572, 1994.

Tehranzadeh J, Andrews C, Wong E: Lumbar spine imaging: normal variants, imaging pitfalls, and artifacts. *Radiol Clin North Am* 38:1207-1253, 2000.

Teresi LM, Lufkin RB, Reicher MA, et al: Asymptomatic degenerative disk disease and spondylosis of the cervical spine: MR imaging. *Radiology* 164:83-88, 1997.

Thornbury JR, Fryback DG, Turski PA, et al: Disk-caused nerve compression in patients with acute low back pain: diagnosis with MR, CT myelography, and plain CT. *Radiology* 186:731-738, 1993.

Toyone T, Takahashi K, Kitahara H, et al: Visualization of symptomatic nerve roots. *J Bone Joint Surg* (Br) 75-B:529-533, 1993.

Tsuruda JS, Norman D, Dillown W, et al: Three-dimensional gradient-recalled MR imaging as a screening tool for the diagnosis of cervical radiculopathy. *AJNR* 10:1263-1271, 1989.

Ulmer JL, Elster AD, Matthews VP, et al: Distinction between degenerative and isthmic spondylolisthesis on sagittal MR images: importance of increased anteroposterior diameter of the spinal canal ("wide canal sigh"). *Am J Roentgenol* 163:411-416, 1994.

Ulmer JL, Mathews VP, Elster AD, et al: MR imaging of lumbar spondylolysis: the importance of ancillary observations. *Am J Roentgenol* 169:233-239, 1997.

Ulmer JL, Mathews VP, Elster AD, King JC: Lumbar spondylolysis without spondylolisthesis: recognition of isolated posterior element subluxation on sagittal MR. *AJNR* 16:1393-1398, 1995.

VanDyke C, Ross JS, Tkach J, et al: Gradient-echo MR imaging of the cervical spine: evaluation of extradural disease. *AJNR* 10:627-632, 1989.

Vroomen PCAJ, Van Hapert SJM, Van Acker REH, et al: The clinical significance of gadolinium enhancement of lumbar disc herniation and nerve roots on preoperative MRI. *Neuroradiology* 40:800-806, 1998.

Wagner AL, Murtagh FR, Arrington JA, Stallworth D: Relationship of Schmorl's nodes to vertebral body endplate fractures and acute endplate disk extrusions. *AJNR* 21:276-281, 2000.

Wagner M, Sether LA, Yu S, et al: Age changes in the lumbar intervertebral disc studied with magnetic resonance and cryomicrotomy. *Clin Anat* 1:93-103, 1988.

Walker HS, Dietrich RB, Flannigan DB, et al: Magnetic resonance imaging of the pediatric spine. *Radiographics* 7:1129, 1987.

Wasserstrom R, Mamouian AC, Black JF, Lehman RAW: Intradural lumbar disk fragment with ring enhancement on MR. *AJNR* 14:401-404, 1993.

Weishaupt D, Schmid MR, Zanetti M, et al: Positional MR imaging of the lumbar spine: does it demonstrate nerve root compromise not visible at conventional MR imaging? *Radiology* 215:247-253, 2000.

Weishaupt D, Zanetti M, Hodler J, Boos N: MR imaging of the lumbar spine: prevalence of intervertebral disk extrusion and sequestration, nerve root compression, end plate abnormalities, and osteoarthritis of the facet joints in asymptomatic volunteers. *Radiology* 209:661-666, 1998.

Weishaupt D, Zanetti M, Hodler J, et al: Painful lumbar disk derangement: relevance of endplate abnormalities at MR imaging. *Radiology* 218:420-427, 2001.

Widder DJ: MR imaging of ossification of the posterior longitudinal ligament. *AJNR* 153:194-195, 1989.

Wildermuth S, Zanetti M, Duewell S, et al: Lumbar spine: quantitative and qualitative assessment of positional (upright flexion and extension) MR imaging and myelography. *Radiology* 207:391-398, 1998.

Williams MP, Cherryman GR, Husband JE: Significance of thoracic disc herniation demonstrated by MR imaging. *J Comput Assist Tomogr* 13:211-214, 1989.

Wilmink JT, Hofman PAM: MRI of the postoperative lumbar spine: triple-dose gadodiamide and fat suppression. *Neuroradiology* 39:589-592, 1997.

Wybier M: Imaging of lumbar degenerative changes involving structures other than the disk space. *Radiol Clin North Am* 39:101-114, 2001.

Yousem DM, Atlas SW, Goldberg HI, Grossman RI: Degenerative narrowing of the cervical spine neural foramina: evaluation with high-resolution 3DFT gradient-echo MR imaging. *AJNR* 12:228-236, 1991.

Yu S, Haughton VM, Ho PSP, et al: Progressive and regressive changes in the nucleus pulposus: part II. The adult. *Radiology* 169:93-97, 1988.

Yu S, Haughton VM, Lynch KL, et al: Fibrous structure in the intervertebral disk: correlation of MR appearance with anatomic sections. *AJNR* 10:1105-1110, 1989.

Yu S, Haughton VM, Sether LA, et al: Criteria for classifying normal and degenerated intervertebral disks. *Radiology* 170:523-526, 1989.

Yu S, Haughton VM, Sether LA, Wagner M: Comparison of MR and diskography in detecting radial tears of the annulus: a post-mortem study. *AJNR* 10:1077-1082, 1989.

Yu S, Sether LA, Ho PSP, et al: Tears of the anulus fibrosus: correlation between MR and pathologic findings in cadavers. *AJNR* 9:367-370, 1988.

Yuh WTC, Dres JM, Weinstein JN, et al: Intraspinal synovial cysts: magnetic resonance evaluation. *Spine* 16:740-745, 1991.

# CHAPTER 18

# Vertebral and Epidural Tumors

**Case 992**

74-year-old woman presenting with back pain.
(sagittal, noncontrast T1-weighted SE scan)

**Case 993**

39-year-old woman complaining of leg pain.
(sagittal, noncontrast T1-weighted SE scan)

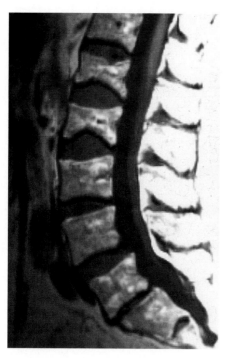

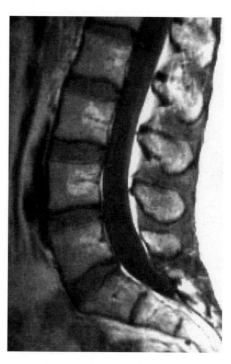

**Normal Variation in Vertebral Intensity**

**Normal Variation in Vertebral Intensity**

The vertebral marrow of most adults demonstrates uniformly high intensity on T1-weighted scans. However, a number of normal variations may produce a more heterogeneous appearance, which can be mistaken for multifocal metastatic disease.

Diffuse, mottled irregularity in the signal intensity of vertebral marrow is common in elderly patients, as illustrated in Case 992. This heterogeneity may reflect scattered fatty atrophy of the marrow alternating with zones of residual hematopoiesis. The dark areas within such spines on T1-weighted scans are not as well defined as focal metastases, such as those in Cases 1000 and 1004, or as pervasive as the diffuse marrow infiltration in Case 1005. Clinical correlation is necessary when an appearance like Case 992 is encountered (see Case 1007), but it is important to recognize this pattern as a potential normal variant.

Younger patients may have zones of signal abnormality within the midposterior portion of one or more vertebral bodies. Such areas can demonstrate T1 values that are shorter (as in Case 993; see also Case 1233) or longer than adjacent marrow. They differ in size and prominence from patient to patient and from one vertebra to the next.

These normal pseudolesions reflect localized anatomical variation surrounding the basivertebral veins. The basivertebral vein drains the posterior half of the vertebral body, exiting through the midposterior cortex to join the anterior epidural plexus. The characteristic location of signal changes surrounding this vessel help to establish the incidental nature of the finding.

Benign compression fractures of the L1 and L2 vertebral bodies are present in Case 992. There is mild ventral subluxation of L4 on L5 and severe disc space narrowing at L5-S1.

# VERTEBRAL HEMANGIOMAS

## Case 994A

49-year-old man complaining of back pain.
(axial, noncontrast T1-weighted SE scan; L1 level)

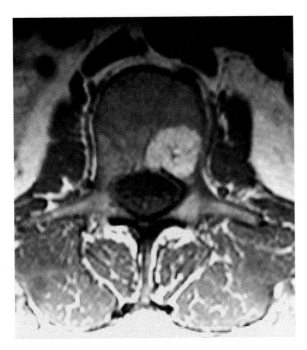

**Hemangioma**

## Case 994B

Same patient.
(sagittal, noncontrast T2-weighted FSE scan)

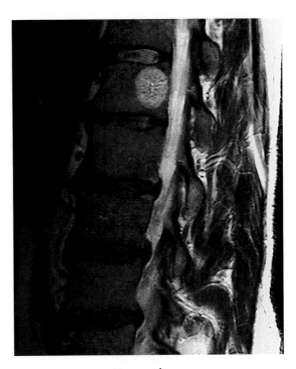

**Hemangioma**

---

Hemangiomas are among the most common benign vertebral pathologies. These lesions consist of dilated vascular spaces replacing portions of the marrow and cancellous bone. They may occur anywhere within the vertebral body and/or posterior arch. As osseous lesions, hemangiomas must be distinguished from metastatic deposits.

The characteristic features of vertebral hemangiomas on CT scans are well recognized. A small number of vertically oriented trabeculae remain within the overall lucency caused by the hemangioma. The residual weight-bearing trabeculae are typically thickened, resulting in a coarse "honeycomb" or "polka-dot" pattern on axial scans and a striated texture on sagittal or coronal reconstructions.

Hemangiomas present a more variable appearance on MR studies. The lesions may have predominantly low or predominantly high signal intensity relative to surrounding marrow on T1-weighted scans. This range of T1 values probably reflects variable amounts of accompanying fat as well as potential components of thrombus.

Case 994A demonstrates a lumbar hemangioma with uniformly high signal intensity on a short TR image. Hemangiomas with longer T1 values than adjacent marrow can more closely resemble isolated vertebral metastases. (See the lesion within T3 in Case 996 for an example.)

High signal intensity is usually present within vertebral hemangiomas on T2-weighted images, as in Case 994B. Long T2 values of blood pools within the lesion contribute to this finding, as does accompanying fat that retains significant signal intensity on T2-weighted fast spin echo scans. (Note the intensity of subcutaneous fat in Case 994B and see discussion of Case 923.)

Margins of a hemangioma may be indistinct or sharply defined. A reticulated (as in Case 994B) or striated (see Case 995) texture may be appreciable within the lesion, although this feature is less prominent than on CT studies.

The parasagittal scan in Case 994B demonstrates reduced hydration signal at all disc levels from L1 to L5.

### Case 995

65-year-old woman presenting with
difficulty walking.
(sagittal, postcontrast T1-weighted SE scan)

### Case 996

29-year-old man presenting with
back pain and myelopathy.
(sagittal, noncontrast T1-weighted SE scan)

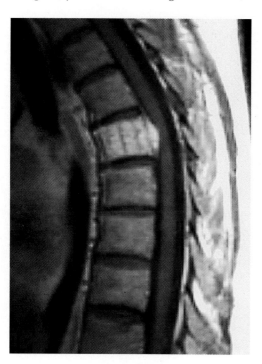

**Hemangioma**

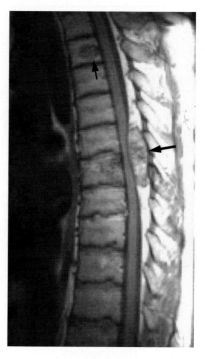

**Hemangioma**

Vertebral hemangiomas are a common incidental finding on MR scans of the spine. These lesions are rarely symptomatic. Occasional hemangiomas cause expansion of bone or give rise to bulky paraspinal or intraspinal masses.

In Case 995, the entire vertebral body of T7 has been replaced by enhancing tissue traversed by vertically oriented striations. Although the body is only mildly compressed, there is a contiguous anterior epidural mass effacing the ventral subarachnoid space and deforming the spinal cord. At surgery, the mass proved to be an epidural component of a hemangioma arising from the adjacent vertebral body.

Case 996 illustrates epidural extension of a hemangioma involving the body and posterior arch of T7 *(large arrow)*. A smaller hemangioma is present within the body of T3 *(small arrow)*. The epidural mass compresses the spinal cord and is responsible for the patient's myelopathy. The hemangiomas at T3 and T7 enhanced to become isointense with surrounding vertebral marrow and epidural fat on postcontrast scans. However, they were well defined by high signal intensity on T2-weighted images.

The mixed signal intensity of the process at T7 and the low intensity of the lesion at T3 in Case 996 (together with the predominantly short T1 values of the mass in Case 994) illustrate the spectrum of potential signal intensities within spinal hemangiomas.

Aneurysmal bone cysts (see Cases 1037 and 1038) and osteoblastomas are other benign vertebral masses that can cause expansion of bone and secondary compromise of the spinal canal.

### Case 997

6-year-old girl presenting with a
stiff back and difficulty walking.
(axial, noncontrast T2-weighted FSE scan; L1-2 level)

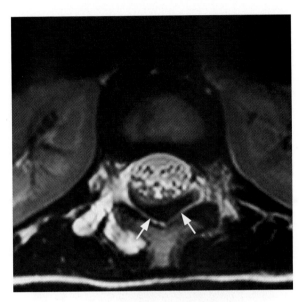

**Paraspinal Hemangioma**
(and epidural hematoma)

### Case 998

3-year-old girl presenting with leg weakness.
(axial, noncontrast T2-weighted SE scan; L1 level)

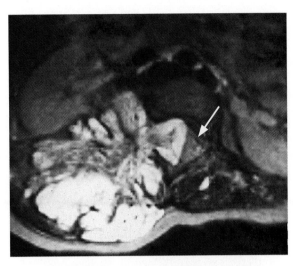

**Paraspinal and Epidural Hemangioma**

---

Hemangiomas can occur in paraspinal tissue with potential epidural involvement, as illustrated in the above children.

The right-sided paraspinal mass in Case 997 is more lobulated and higher in signal intensity that would be expected for malignant paraspinal lesions in a pediatric patient (see discussion of "small blue cell" tumors, Cases 1022-1025). These features and the apparent extension through an intervertebral foramen could suggest a nerve sheath tumor (see Chapter 19), but are also characteristic of soft tissue hemangiomas. The association of an acute dorsal epidural hematoma *(arrows)* favors the latter diagnosis, which was confirmed at surgery.

The paraspinal hemangioma in Case 998 is much larger. It extends medially through a widened intervertebral foramen, with an epidural component causing displacement and compression of the conus medullaris *(arrow)*. At surgery, the mass was firm to palpation, correlating with the fibrous stroma apparent within the vascular spaces of the lesion. The differential diagnosis of this appearance would include a plexiform neurofibroma (see Case 1071), but presentation of the latter would be unusual at this age.

## Case 999

69-year-old man presenting with back pain.
(sagittal, noncontrast T1-weighted SE scan)

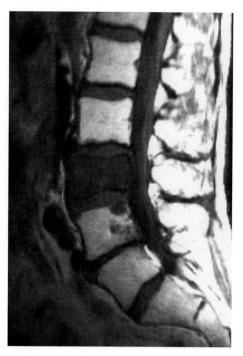

**Metastatic Small Cell Carcinoma of the Lung**

## Case 1000

70-year-old man presenting with a stumbling gait.
(sagittal, noncontrast T1-weighted SE scan)

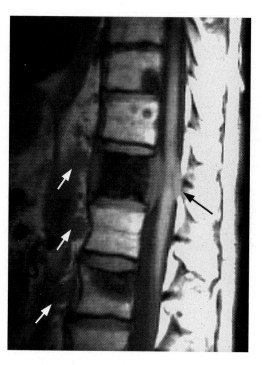

**Metastatic Carcinoma of the Prostate**

Vertebral and epidural metastases are usually well defined on T1-weighted MR studies. Fat within vertebral marrow and the epidural space provides a normal background of high signal intensity. Marrow replacement by cellular infiltration (malignant or benign; see Cases 1107 and 1108) causes a conspicuous reduction in intensity. In Case 999, the entire vertebral body of L3 is filled with "watery" metastatic tissue. Reactive sclerosis contributes to the dark spots of metastatic disease within thoracic and lumbar vertebrae in Case 1000.

T1-weighted images also demonstrate the contours of the spinal cord as outlined by CSF. Cord compression by epidural components of metastatic tumor can be readily assessed. In Case 1000, an epidural mass at the T12 level effaces the subarachnoid space and deforms the cord (*black arrow;* compare to Case 1175). The other vertebral lesions are not associated with epidural masses.

Contrast-enhanced T1-weighted scans may be less effective than noncontrast studies for detecting vertebral and epidural metastases (unless fat-saturation techniques are superimposed). Metastatic lesions may enhance to a level isointense with marrow or epidural fat, masking their presence (see Case 1046 and compare Cases 1014 and 1016 and Cases 1112 and 1119).

Inflammatory etiologies should also be considered in the differential diagnosis of multiple vertebral lesions. Tuberculosis and coccidioidomycosis can cause destruction at several vertebral levels due to subligamentous extension, often with sparing of the intervening disc spaces. Pyogenic vertebral osteomyelitis is usually associated with characteristic features of discitis, as discussed in Chapter 20.

Mildly enlarged retroperitoneal lymph nodes are present in Case 1000 *(white arrows).* Whenever the question of vertebral metastases is raised, a search for associated paraspinal adenopathy or masses is warranted.

### Case 1001

48-year-old woman presenting with
back pain and leg numbness.
(sagittal, noncontrast T2-weighted FSE scan)

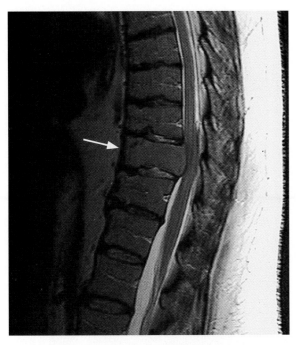

**Metastatic Small Cell Carcinoma of the Lung**

### Case 1002

48-year-old man presenting with back pain.
(sagittal, noncontrast T2*-weighted GRE scan)

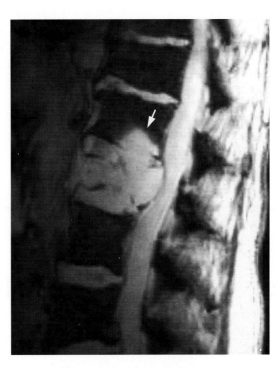

**Metastatic Hypernephroma**

Vertebral metastases demonstrate variable signal intensity on pulse sequences that emphasize T2 relaxation times. Some lesions are nearly isointense to surrounding marrow on T2-weighted spin echo scans, as seen in Case 1001 *(arrow)*. The relative lack of T2 prolongation probably reflects a densely cellular tumor with a high nuclear to cytoplasmic ratio. (Compare to the appearance of cerebral germinomas and lymphomas, as in Cases 294 and 348.)

The affected vertebral body in Case 1001 was uniformly low in signal intensity on T1-weighted scans, resembling Cases 999 and 1000. Detectability on the above T2-weighted image depends more on associated mass effect than on signal abnormality: the ventral subarachnoid space is effaced, and the spinal cord is posteriorly displaced.

By contrast, the vertebral lesion in Case 1002 demonstrates very high signal intensity on a "myelographic" gradient echo sequence. A compression fracture of the involved body is apparent, with mild compromise of the spinal canal (see Cases 1174 and 1175).

Metastatic tissue has crossed the superior disc space in Case 1002 to involve the adjacent vertebra *(arrow)*. This contiguous extension to an adjoining level is more characteristic of inflammatory disease but does not exclude vertebral metastasis (see Cases 1113 and 1114).

Rare vertebral chordomas (usually involving the C2 to C4 levels) may also extend across disc spaces. This feature can combine with characteristically long T2 values to produce an appearance similar to Case 1002.

### Case 1003

68-year-old man.
(axial, noncontrast T1-weighted SE scan; L3 level)

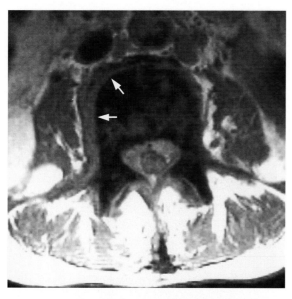

**Metastatic Carcinoma of the Prostate**

### Case 1004

59-year-old woman.
(sagittal, noncontrast T1-weighted SE scan)

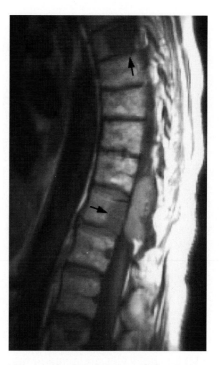

**Metastatic Carcinoma of the Breast**

---

Vertebral metastases are commonly accompanied by epidural extension of tumor. These masses may compromise the spinal canal and compress neural tissue, causing local symptoms and/or long tract findings.

The lumbar vertebral body in Case 1003 is diffusely sclerotic. The epidural space is filled with soft tissue of intermediate signal intensity, replacing epidural fat and encircling the thecal sac. The proximal L3 nerve roots are surrounded by tumor in the lateral recesses. A layer of paraspinal tumor is present along the vertebral margins anteriorly and on the right *(arrows)*.

Case 1004 demonstrates a more mass-like epidural metastasis. The tumor within the spinal canal differs in signal intensity from the vertebral body of origin. By itself, the epidural mass resembles a spinal meningioma (compare to

Case 1050). Associated bone lesions both adjacent to and removed from the mass *(arrows)* establish the diagnosis.

The anterior epidural space is divided in the midline by a sagittally oriented band of tissue extending from the ventral surface of the dural sac to the posterior longitudinal ligament. This "ligament of Trolard" may influence the shape of slowly growing epidural masses, causing them to initially accumulate in the lateral portions of the anterior epidural compartment (with relative sparing of the midline). Epidural metastases may demonstrate this "theater curtain" morphology.

See Cases 1174 and 1175 for discussion of pathological fractures, another cause of epidural deformity due to vertebral metastases.

# DIFFERENTIAL DIAGNOSIS:
## DIFFUSELY ABNORMAL SIGNAL INTENSITY OF THE SPINE

### Case 1005

70-year-old man presenting with fatigue.
(sagittal, noncontrast T1-weighted SE scan)

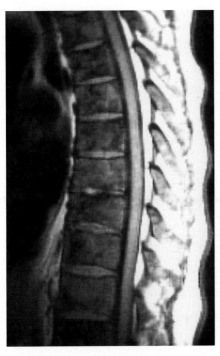

**Metastatic Carcinoma of the Prostate**

### Case 1006

78-year-old woman presenting with paraplegia.
(sagittal, noncontrast T1-weighted SE scan)

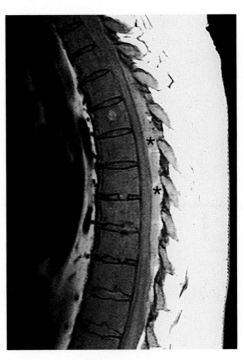

**Myelofibrosis**
(with extramedullary hematopoiesis)

---

Metastatic infiltration of vertebral bodies can be extensive, with uniform involvement of all visualized levels. Diffuse prolongation of T1 values throughout the spine may cause disc spaces to appear brighter than the adjacent vertebrae on short TR spin echo images. Case 1005 illustrates this pattern, which is the reverse of the normal relationship of signal intensities in adults. No epidural mass is apparent.

Prolongation of T1 values throughout all vertebral bodies in Case 1006 is as extensive as in Case 1005 but even more uniform. This pattern suggests a hematological malignancy (leukemia or lymphoma; see Case 1014) or myelofibrosis. The accompanying dorsal epidural mass *(asterisks)* could represent a chloroma, epidural involvement by lymphoma (compare to Cases 1014-1016), or an epidural hematoma secondary to associated coagulopathy (see Cases 1185 and

1186). Surgery in this patient documented dorsal epidural extramedullary hematopoiesis due to severe obliteration of normal marrow by myelofibrosis.

Abnormal low signal intensity may also be seen throughout the spine in hematological conditions leading to accumulation of iron within the marrow. Among these is "anemia of chronic disease," which can be observed in patients with AIDS (see Case 1103).

Dorsal epidural fat is prominent in Case 1005. (See the discussion of epidural lipomatosis in Cases 691, 1192, and 1193.)

The small area of relatively high signal intensity within a superior thoracic vertebral body in Case 1006 probably represents an incidental hemangioma.

### Case 1007

44-year-old man presenting with back pain.
(sagittal, noncontrast T1-weighted SE scan)

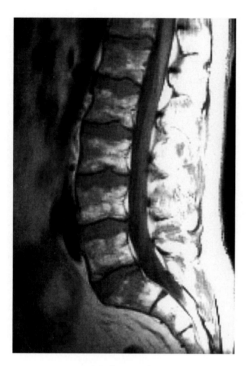

**Multiple Myeloma**

### Case 1008

50-year-old man presenting with back
pain and mild gait abnormality.
(sagittal, noncontrast T1-weighted SE scan)

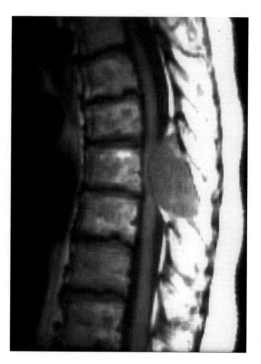

**Multiple Myeloma**

The extent and pattern of findings on MR scans of the spine in patients with multiple myeloma are widely variable. Multifocal infiltration of spinal marrow may be encountered, as in Case 1007. The heterogeneous appearance in this example resembles the potential normal variant in older patients illustrated in Case 992. More uniform marrow replacement in myeloma can resemble Cases 1005 and 1006.

In other patients with multiple myeloma, focal vertebral lesions predominate at one or several levels. Case 1008 demonstrates a large mass that has expanded from the posterior arch of a midthoracic vertebra (compare to Case 1004). The spinal cord is severely compressed. A back-

ground of mottled signal intensity within all thoracic vertebral bodies is nonspecific but may reflect more generalized and subtle disease. Focal lesions within vertebral bodies (comparable to the metastases in Cases 1000 and 1004) are also seen within the spectrum of myeloma.

Pain may be the only symptom of patients with early cord compression by epidural metastasis or multiple myeloma. A high index of suspicion is warranted in cancer patients with new or worsening back pain, and prompt evaluation is indicated. Magnetic resonance imaging has replaced emergency myelography as the procedure of choice for this purpose.

# DIFFERENTIAL DIAGNOSIS:
## MASS EXPANDING THE POSTERIOR ARCH OF A VERTEBRA

### Case 1009

52-year-old man presenting with
radicular flank pain.
(axial, noncontrast T1-weighted SE scan; L3 level)

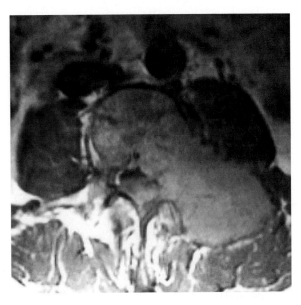

**Multiple Myeloma**

### Case 1010

62-year-old man complaining of
radicular midthoracic pain.
(axial, noncontrast T1-weighted SE scan; T6 level)

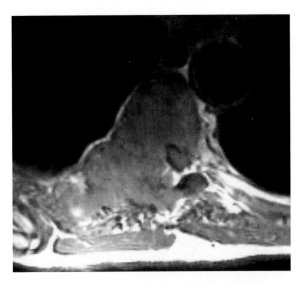

**Metastatic Carcinoma of the Colon**

---

Multiple myeloma (or solitary plasmocytoma) is a leading consideration when an expansile tumor is discovered arising from posterior elements of the spine in adults, as illustrated in Case 1009. Case 1010 demonstrates that metastatic disease can also produce an expansile mass with bulky paraspinal and epidural components.

For practical purposes, metastasis and multiple myeloma should both be considered whenever either pathology is entertained as the etiology of a spinal lesion. Both tumors can involve the vertebral body and/or the posterior arch.

In younger patients, benign bone tumors such as osteoblastomas and aneurysmal bone cysts may cause expansile lesions of the pedicle or lamina. Many aneurysmal bone cysts are multiloculated, demonstrating one or more sedimentation levels of blood products within cystic components of the mass (see Case 1038). In other cases, aneurysmal bone cysts present as solid tissue surrounded by characteristic "egg shells" of expanded cortex (see Case 1037).

Osteomyelitis (e.g., coccidioidomycosis) and chondrosarcomas (see Cases 1039 and 1040) are additional rare causes of expansile lesions arising from a vertebral body or posterior arch.

## Case 1011A

50-year-old man presenting with
sacral pain and weight loss.
(sagittal, noncontrast T1-weighted SE scan)

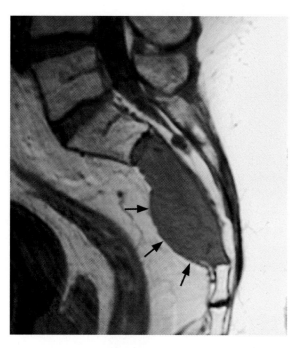

**Plasmacytoma**

## Case 1011B

Same patient.
(axial, postcontrast T1-weighted
SE scan with fat saturation)

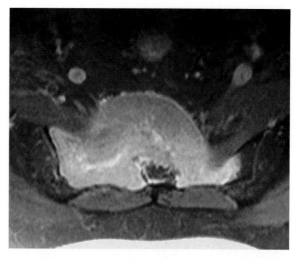

**Plasmacytoma**

Malignant proliferation of plasma cells may be localized to a single vertebra. Like multiple myeloma, such solitary plasmacytomas are most common in adults between ages 50 and 70. Thoracic vertebrae are most frequently involved, but any level of the spine can be affected.

Plasmacytomas often arise in the vertebral body and progress to completely replace and expand it. Case 1011 is a good example: the S2 and S3 segments are nearly filled by cellular tissue. (There is a small amount of residual normal marrow near the left sacroiliac joint in Case 1011B.) The anterior sacral cortex has been destroyed, with a convex margin of tissue bulging into presacral fat (*arrows,* Case 1011A).

The homogeneous appearance of the above lesion on both precontrast and postcontrast images is characteristic of plasmacytomas. Signal intensity on T2-weighted images can vary from relatively low to moderately increased.

Solitary plasmacytomas at higher spinal levels may be associated with pathological fractures and/or epidural masses causing compression of the spinal cord (see Case 1013).

Cases of solitary plasmacytoma frequently progress to multiple myeloma within three to ten years.

# DIFFERENTIAL DIAGNOSIS:
## PATHOLOGY INVOLVING ADJACENT VERTEBRAL BODIES

### Case 1012

81-year-old man presenting with leg weakness.
(sagittal, noncontrast T1-weighted SE scan)

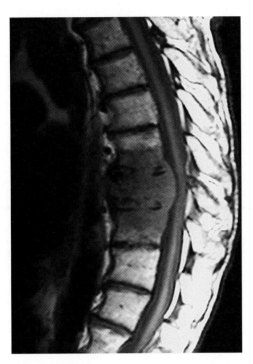

**Metastatic Hypernephroma**

### Case 1013

79-year-old man presenting with neck and arm pain.
(sagittal, postcontrast T1-weighted SE scan)

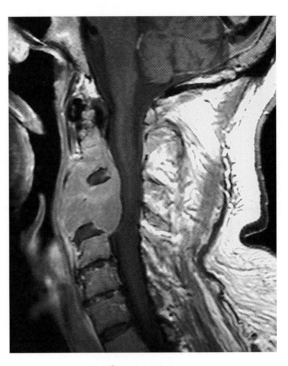

**Plasmacytoma**

---

Involvement of contiguous vertebral bodies is a well-known characteristic of discitis/osteomyelitis (see Chapter 20). However, several neoplasms can also extend across disc spaces, as illustrated above.

The metastasis in Case 1012 is centered at T8 but has grown into the inferior aspect of T7 and the superior portion of T9. Associated prevertebral and anterior epidural masses are present. The latter causes posterior displacement and compression of the spinal cord.

Case 1013 illustrates a plasmacytoma arising from the vertebral body of C3 and extending superiorly to involve C2. The expansile nature and homogeneous enhancement of the lesion are comparable to Case 1011. Prevertebral and anterior epidural masses are present, resembling Case 1012.

Chordomas can also extend from one vertebral body to the next. Nonsacral chordomas of the spine are most common in the superior cervical region.

## Case 1014

62-year-old woman presenting with
anemia and back pain.
(sagittal, noncontrast T1-weighted SE scan)

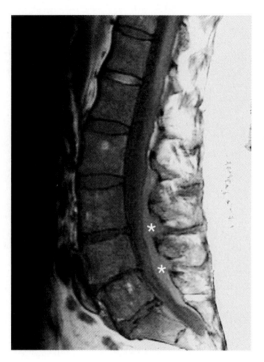

**Lymphoma**

## Case 1015

65-year-old woman presenting with
progressive paraparesis.
(sagittal, noncontrast T2-weighted FSE scan)

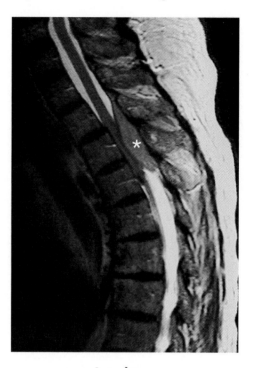

**Lymphoma**

Although less common than metastasis or multiple myeloma, lymphoma should be included in the differential diagnosis of epidural masses in adults (and in children). Like metastasis and myeloma, lymphoma may cause destructive and/or expansile lesions of vertebral bodies or posterior arches at one or more levels. However, lymphomatous epidural masses may also occur in the absence of adjacent osseous lesions. (Compare to primary epidural involvement by neuroblastoma in children; see Cases 1018 and 1019.)

Case 1014 illustrates abnormally low signal intensity throughout all visualized vertebrae, resembling Cases 1005 and 1006. In addition, a homogeneous layer of dorsal epidural tumor is present from L2 to S1 *(asterisks)*, de-

forming the thecal sac. This tissue enhanced intensely following contrast injection (see Case 1016).

The dorsal epidural mass compressing the spinal cord in Case 1015 *(asterisk)* was not associated with vertebral pathology. The tumor demonstrates homogeneously low signal intensity on this T2-weighted scan, suggesting dense cellularity. Lymphoma should be considered whenever an epidural mass with these features is discovered, whether or not there is adjacent vertebral abnormality.

Non-neoplastic epidural masses (e.g., abscess or hematoma; see Cases 1124, 1126, 1185, and 1186) could be included in the differential diagnosis of the above cases. The more rapid development of symptoms usually helps to distinguish an epidural hematoma or abscess from neoplasms.

### Case 1016

62-year-old woman presenting with
anemia and back pain.
(sagittal, postcontrast T1-weighted SE scan)

### Case 1017

78-year-old woman presenting with paraplegia.
(sagittal, postcontrast T1-weighted SE scan)

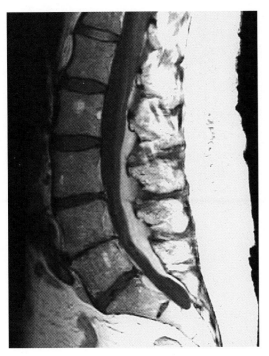

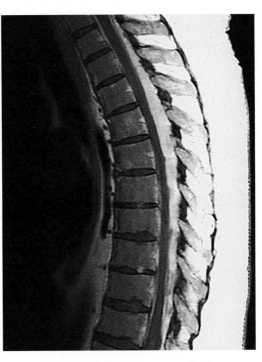

**Lymphoma**
(same patient as Case 1014)

**Extramedullary Hematopoiesis**
(due to myelofibrosis;
same patient as Case 1006)

Several pathologies can cause epidural masses that extend over many vertebral levels. Lymphoma is a primary consideration when a long epidural process is encountered, as in Case 1016.

The dorsal epidural mass in Case 1017 is typical for the rare occurrence of extramedullary hematopoiesis within the spinal canal. Severe myelofibrosis in this patient has led to proliferation of hematopoietic tissue in auxiliary locations, including the epidural space. This possibility should be considered (along with leukemia and lymphoma) in patients who demonstrate extensive epidural masses in association with diffusely abnormal vertebral marrow.

Epidural metastases in adults are usually more focal and mass-like than the layers of abnormal tissue in the above cases. Epidural involvement by neuroblastoma or other "small blue cell" tumors in children can be indistinguishable from spinal lymphoma.

Spinal epidural phlegmons or abscesses typically involve multiple vertebral levels (see Case 1124) and would be considered in the differential diagnosis of the above scans in an appropriate clinical context. Epidural hematomas can demonstrate precontrast T1-shortening, but do not enhance centrally like cellular masses.

Note that enhancement of the vertebral bodies in Case 1016 has made them appear more normal than their precontrast pattern in Case 1014. Focal or diffuse pathology of the spine may be obscured by enhancement to isointensity on postcontrast images without fat saturation. (Compare Cases 1112 and 1119 for another example.)

The lack of significant enhancement within vertebral bodies in Case 1017 reflects the fibrous replacement of the marrow space.

## Case 1018

7-year-old girl complaining of intermittent
back pain and mild gait abnormality.
(sagittal, noncontrast T1-weighted SE scan)

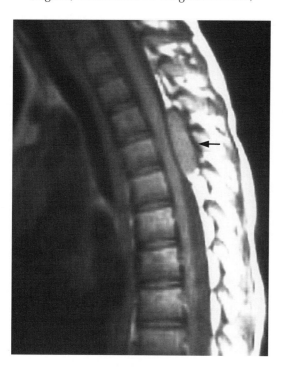

**Neuroblastoma**

## Case 1019

2-month-old girl presenting with
an abdominal mass.
(coronal, noncontrast T1-weighted SE scan)

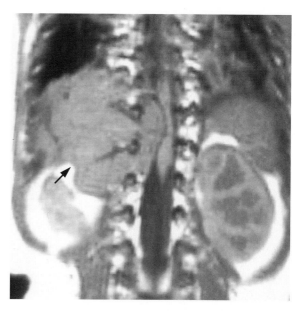

**Neuroblastoma**

Epidural neuroblastoma is often primary, with no associated vertebral lesions. Case 1018 demonstrates a smoothly marginated mass within dorsal epidural fat in the superior thoracic region *(arrow)*. The lesion extends across three vertebral levels, compressing the dural sac and spinal cord. There is no evidence of osseous infiltration or destruction.

Epidural masses in the pediatric population are frequently of paraspinal origin. In Case 1019, a coronal scan establishes continuity between the paraspinal and epidural components of a large tumor. The mass extends from the right suprarenal area through two intervertebral foramina to displace the spinal cord and conus medullaris. The le-

sion is homogeneous in signal intensity. Calcification, which is characteristic of abdominal neuroblastoma on CT scans, is rarely appreciated on MR studies.

The differential diagnosis of an epidural and/or paraspinal mass in a child includes leukemia, lymphoma, Ewing's sarcoma, and rhabdomyosarcoma in addition to neuroblastoma. Occasional benign hemangiomas present in the paraspinal region (see Case 998).

Cases 1020 and 1021 illustrate examples of neuroblastoma involving the lumbosacral spinal canal.

Compare Case 1018 to the adult with lymphoma in Case 1015.

## Case 1020

4-year-old girl presenting with constipation.
(sagittal, noncontrast T1-weighted SE scan)

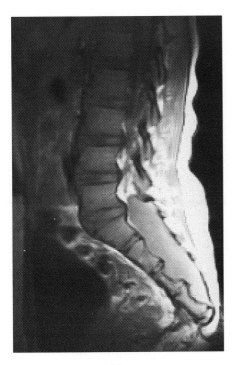

**Neuroblastoma**

## Case 1021

9-year-old boy presenting with
clumsiness of the left leg.
(coronal, postcontrast T1-weighted SE scan)

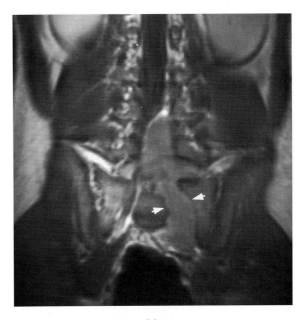

**Neuroblastoma**

As discussed on the previous page, neuroblastoma commonly involves the spinal canal in the thoracolumbar region, either as a primary epidural process or by extension from a paraspinal origin.

Cases 1020 and 1021 illustrate a somewhat different presentation of spinal neuroblastoma in the lumbosacral area. The long-standing, slowly growing intraspinal masses in these patients have caused expansion of the spinal canal and contiguous intervertebral foramina. In Case 1020, posterior scalloping of sacral vertebral bodies is apparent. In Case 1021, tongues of tumor flow through widened lumbar and sacral foramina on the left side *(arrows)*. The adjacent left sacral ala is sclerotic and probably permeated by neoplasm.

Pathological examination of tumor tissue in the above cases demonstrated mature neuroblastoma, containing ar-

eas better classified as ganglioneuroma. Neuroblastomas characteristically stabilize or involute after infancy, so that older children may present with low grade, long-standing versions of this tumor.

The appearance of a lobulated intraspinal mass causing scalloped bone erosion and foraminal widening may suggest the diagnosis of neurofibroma, schwannoma, or myxopapillary ependymoma. Neuroblastoma/ganglioneuroma should be considered among diagnostic possibilities in such cases.

Other long-standing, low grade masses (e.g., epidermoid cysts) may cause expansion of the sacral canal comparable to the scalloping in Case 1020. A similar morphology may also be associated with dural ectasia (as in neurofibromatosis or Marfan's syndrome) or cysts of the sacral canal (see Cases 1202 and 1203).

### Case 1022

2-year-old boy presenting with difficulty walking.
(axial, noncontrast T1-weighted SE scan; T10 level)

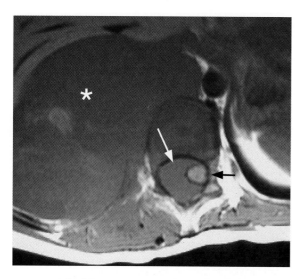

**Primitive Neuroectodermal Tumor**

### Case 1023

6-year-old boy presenting with leg weakness.
(sagittal, noncontrast T2-weighted FSE scan)

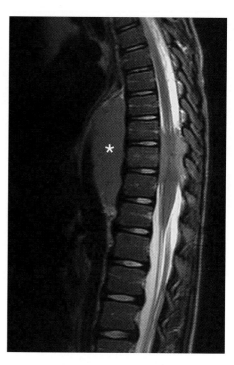

**Rhabdomyosarcoma**

---

A number of childhood malignancies are characterized histologically by small round cells with little cytoplasm. The closely spaced, blue-staining nuclei in such lesions have caused them to be known as "small blue cell" tumors. Included in this category are neuroblastoma, more undifferentiated primitive neuroectodermal tumors (PNET), lymphoma, rhabdomyosarcoma, and extraosseous Ewing's sarcoma. Pathological distinction among these lesions often requires special histochemical stains, electron microscopy, and/or correlation with increased levels of specific metabolites in the blood or urine.

Any of the "small blue cell" neoplasms can arise in a paraspinal location with intraspinal extension. The tumor in Case 1022 has accumulated as a large abdominal mass *(asterisk)*. The lesion traversed several intervertebral foramina, with a major epidural component *(white arrow)* displacing the dural sac and spinal cord *(black arrow)*. Compare this morphology to Case 1019.

Case 1023 demonstrates an encircling rind of epidural tumor effacing the subarachnoid space from T9 to T11. A large accompanying prevertebral mass is present *(asterisk)*.

The epidural component of pediatric paraspinal masses as illustrated above is comparable to the adult intraspinal masses arising from vertebral metastases (compare to Cases 1000 and 1003).

## Case 1024

2-year-old boy presenting with difficulty walking.
(axial, postcontrast T1-weighted SE scan; T11 level)

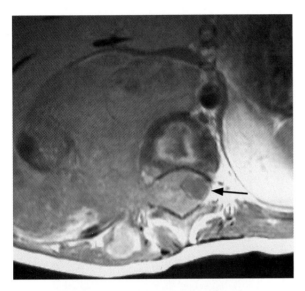

**Primitive Neuroectodermal Tumor**
(same patient as Case 1022)

## Case 1025

2-year-old girl presenting with abdominal pain.
(axial, postcontrast T1-weighted SE scan; L1-2 level)

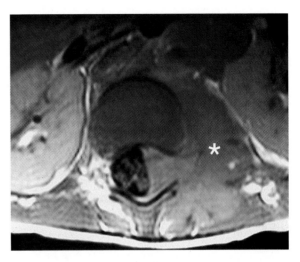

**Lymphoma**

---

Each of the above cases illustrates the extension of a paraspinal tumor through an intervertebral foramen to cause epidural mass effect.

Case 1024 presents a postcontrast scan of the lesion in Case 1022. The large tumor enhances quite homogeneously. The epidural component surrounds the right side of the thecal sac and spinal cord, which are displaced to the left *(arrow)*. An irregular ring of enhancement within the vertebral body suggests osseous involvement by the neoplasm.

The paraspinal lymphoma in Case 1025 *(asterisk)* is moderately lobulated. Intraspinal extension deforms the thecal sac but does not significantly compress the roots of the cauda equina. The overall morphology of the lesion resembles the hemangioma in Case 998, but the latter is much more heterogenous (and would enhance more intensely).

Nerve sheath tumors can also present as masses spanning an intervertebral foramen with both epidural and paraspinal components (see Cases 1056, 1058, and 1060). However, such lesions are rare in toddlers, and their characteristically long T2 values differ from the usually isointense appearance of "blue cell" tumors on T2-weighted images (as illustrated in Case 1023).

## Case 1026A

5-year-old girl with a posterior mediastinal mass discovered on a chest x-ray.
(coronal, noncontrast T1-weighted SE scan)

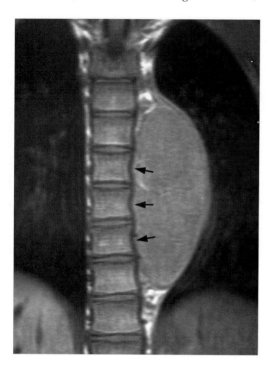

**Ganglioneuroma**

## Case 1026B

Same patient.
(sagittal, noncontrast T2-weighted SE scan)

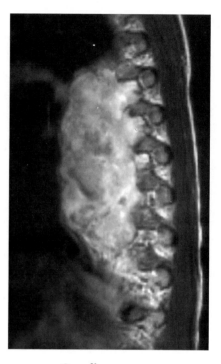

**Ganglioneuroma**

---

Ganglioneuromas are well-differentiated neoplasms comprised primarily of mature ganglion cells. These tumors tend to occur in older children and young adults. In some cases, they represent maturation of an earlier neuroblastoma. Ganglioneuromas frequently arise from the sympathetic chain in a paraspinal location.

The tumor in Case 1026 is typical, presenting as a large mediastinal mass. The size of the well-defined lesion and the mild scalloping of adjacent vertebral bodies *(arrows)* suggest a slow-growing neoplasm. Note, however, that the internal architecture of the tumor appears much more complex on the T2-weighted scan in Case 1026B than on the T1-weighted image in Case 1026A. This heterogeneous texture might suggest an aggressive paraspinal neoplasm, but the prolonged T2 values would be unusual in a malignant "blue cell" tumor.

The mass in this case did not traverse intervertebral foramina to involve the spinal canal. Mature ganglioneuromas may do so, resembling the appearance of the neuroblastoma in Case 1019.

## Case 1027A

10-year-old boy presenting with constipation.
(sagittal, noncontrast T1-weighted SE scan)

## Case 1027B

Same patient.
(axial, noncontrast T2-weighted SE scan)

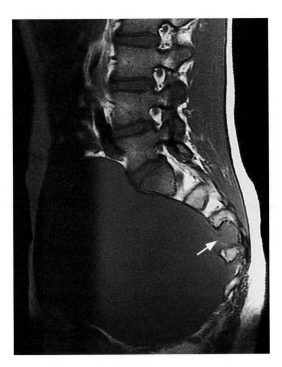

**Ganglioneuroma**

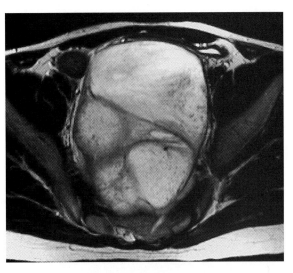

**Ganglioneuroma**

Ganglioneuromas should be included in the differential diagnosis of pelvic masses in children and young adults. Like lumbosacral neuroblastomas (see Cases 1020 and 1021), ganglioneuromas may cause expansion of sacral foramina (*arrow,* Case 1027A). This feature and the frequently large size of the lesion suggest a slow-growing mass of potentially neurogenic origin.

The lobulated morphology demonstrated in Case 1027B is common in ganglioneuromas, but not specific (see Cases 1029, 1033, and 1071). Prolonged T2 values within the mass resemble Case 1026B.

The differential diagnosis of a large, lobulated paraspinal mass with foraminal expansion and prolonged T2 values includes a nerve sheath tumor (neurofibroma or schwannoma; see Case 1071) and extension of a myxopapillary ependymoma (see Cases 1092-1094).

## Case 1028

72-year-old man presenting with sacral pain
and difficulty with bowel movements.
(sagittal, noncontrast T1-weighted SE scan)

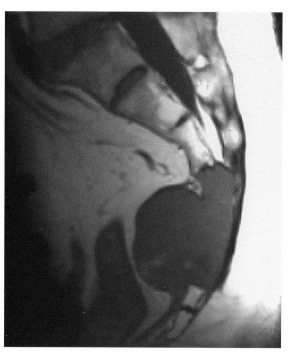

**Chordoma**

## Case 1029

29-year-old man presenting with leg weakness.
(axial, noncontrast T2-weighted FSE scan)

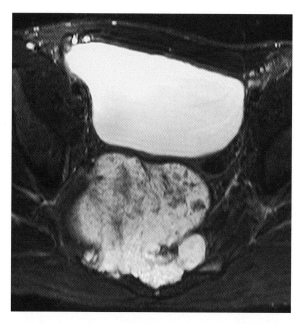

**Chordoma**

About 50% of chordomas arise from the sacrum, most presenting in adults over age 60. These lobulated masses are typically expansile and should be included in the differential diagnosis of "bubbly" sacral lesions (see discussion of Case 1038). Although sacral chordomas are slow-growing tumors, they recur and progress if incompletely resected.

The mass in Case 1028 has destroyed the S4 and S5 segments, expanding ventrally into the presacral space. A thin layer of tumor extends caudally along the anterior surface of the coccyx. Many chordomas demonstrate greater heterogeneity than this lesion, including cysts and areas of hemorrhage.

Case 1029 illustrates the typical lobulation and T2 prolongation of sacral chordomas. This appearance correlates with the histopathologic presence of large, vacuolated "physaliferous" cells. Involved bone is typically both expanded and destroyed.

The islands of low signal intensity within the bright tumor in Case 1029 corresponded pathologically with multifocal hemorrhage. The same foci were apparent as bright spots within an otherwise dark tumor on T1-weighted scans.

Myxopapillary ependymomas (see Cases 1092-1094) occasionally arise within the sacrum or immediately dorsal to it in a "subcutaneous" location. Such tumors could cause sacral erosion resembling a chordoma.

The sacrum is intact most cases of sacrococcygeal teratoma (see Cases 1031-1033). These tumors usually originate near the coccyx and present in early childhood, but sporadic cases are reported in adults.

Metastasis or myeloma should also be considered in the differential diagnosis of a mass arising from the sacrum (see Case 1011).

Compare the characteristics of the above tumors to the clival chordomas in Cases 168-170.

## Case 1030A

27-year-old man presenting with a four-year history of increasing back pain.
(sagittal, noncontrast T1-weighted SE scan)

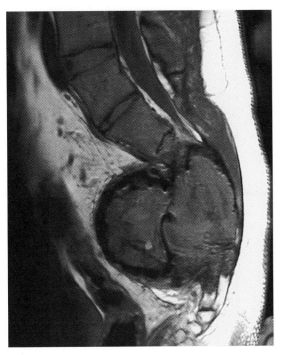

**Giant Cell Tumor**

## Case 1030B

Same patient.
(sagittal, noncontrast T2-weighted SE scan)

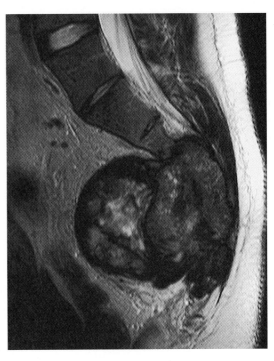

**Giant Cell Tumor**

Giant cell tumors are primary neoplasms of bone that are rarely malignant but often locally aggressive. Young adults are most commonly affected. Few than 10% of giant cell tumors involve the spine, most frequently at sacral levels. A giant cell tumor should be considered when a destructive sacral mass is discovered in patient between ages 20 and 40; chordomas and plasmacytomas are less common in this group (but see Case 1029).

The morphology of the mass in Case 1030 resembles the tumors in Cases 1011 and 1028. However, the pattern of signal intensity within the lesion is very different. Giant cell tumors are typically heterogeneous masses, often containing extensive hemorrhage related to their characteristic hypervascularity. The complex texture and overall short T2 values demonstrated in Case 1030B contrast with the homogeneous character of a plasmacytoma (see Case 1011) and the usually prominent T2 prolongation within a chordoma (compare Case 1030B to Case 1029).

## Case 1031

2-year-old girl being evaluated for constipation.
(sagittal, noncontrast T1-weighted SE scan)

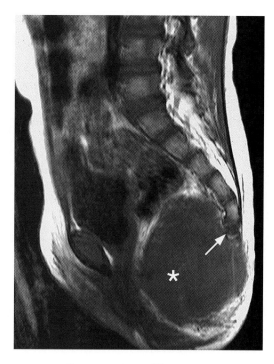

**Sacrococcygeal Teratoma**

## Case 1032

11-month-old girl with reduced
leg motion.
(sagittal, postcontrast T1-weighted SE scan)

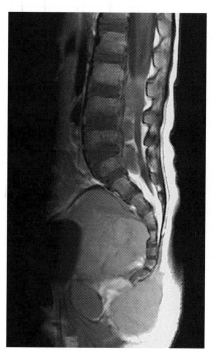

**Sacrococcygeal Teratoma**

Sacrococcygeal teratomas present as masses in the sacral region of infants or young children, with a female to male ratio of 4 to 1. These tumors originate near the coccyx and grow inferior, anterior, or posterior to the sacrum, which is often intact. Sacrococcygeal teratomas are typically lobulated and heterogeneous, usually containing a cystic component. The degree of anaplasia or maturity within a particular tumor is difficult to predict from its MR characteristics.

The large teratoma in Case 1031 *(asterisk)* is associated with focal signal abnormality in a segment of the coccyx *(arrow)*. Compare the level of the center of this mass to the sacral lesions in Case 1028 and 1030. T2-weighted scans demonstrated uniformly high signal intensity throughout the tumor and in the affected coccygeal segment.

The sacrum appears intact in Case 1032. However, noncontrast T1-weighted scans demonstrated abnormally low signal intensity throughout vertebral bodies from L3 through S1. Intraspinal extension of the tumor is apparent, with several epidural lobulations compressing the thecal sac in the lumbar region. A T2-weighted scan disclosed substantial heterogeneity within the pelvic tumor and the epidural masses, with mixed high and intermediate signal intensity (see Case 1033).

Subcutaneous myxopapillary ependymomas may arise in the sacrococcygeal region and present as a mass with minimal bone destruction or erosion. However, these tumors are rare in infants or children and typically involve the dorsal surface of the sacrum, features that distinguish them from the usual presentation of sacrococcygeal teratomas.

# DIFFERENTIAL DIAGNOSIS:
## LOBULATED PRESACRAL MASS IN A CHILD

### Case 1033

11-month-old girl presenting with
reduced leg motion.
(sagittal, noncontrast T2-weighted FSE scan)

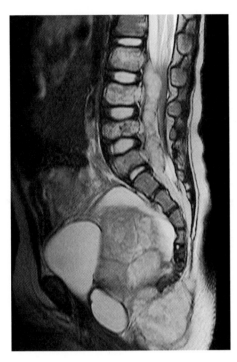

**Sacrococcygeal Teratoma**
(same patient as Case 1032)

### Case 1034

10-year-old boy presenting with constipation.
(sagittal, noncontrast T2-weighted FSE scan)

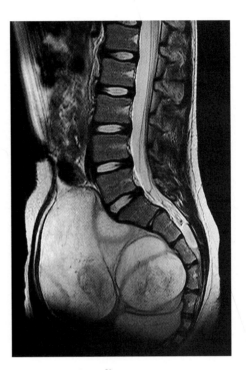

**Ganglioneuroma**
(same patient as Case 1027)

---

Large, lobulated pelvic masses in infants and children are often of developmental or neurogenic origin.

The heterogenous tumor surrounding the inferior and anterior aspect of the sacrum in Case 1033 is typical for a sacrococcygeal teratoma in an infant. The vertebral and epidural involvement in this case is unusual; in most children the teratoma is largely extraspinal (see Case 1031).

Case 1034 is an additional scan of the patient presented in Case 1027. The lobulation, heterogeneity, and prolonged T2 values of this mature neuronal tumor closely resemble the teratoma in Case 1033. The older age of the patient and the associated widening of a sacral foramen (see Case 1027A) are clues to the correct diagnosis.

A large plexiform neurofibroma of the pelvis could be included in the differential diagnosis (see Case 1071), although such tumors are rare in children. Extraspinal myxopapillary ependymomas can also present as pelvic masses (or as "subcutaneous" lesions posterior to the sacrum).

## Case 1035

9-year-old boy presenting with back pain.
(sagittal, noncontrast T1-weighted SE scan)

## Case 1036

4-year-old boy presenting with back pain.
(sagittal, noncontrast T2-weighted FSE scan)

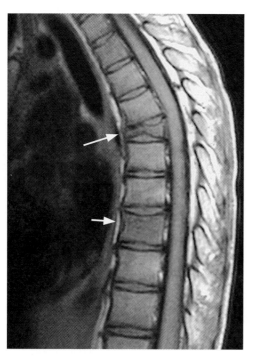

**Langerhans Cell Histiocytosis**

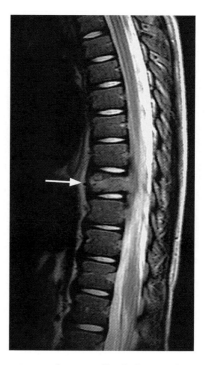

**Langerhans Cell Histiocytosis**

Langerhans cell histiocytosis is an idiopathic proliferation of large mononuclear cells, probably representing a disordered immune response rather than a neoplasm. Intracranial manifestations have been discussed in Cases 270-272.

Spinal involvement in histiocytosis may be an isolated finding or accompanied by systemic disease. Vertebral lesions typically affect the body and may be solitary or multiple. Both lytic foci and compression fractures are common. Near complete collapse of an affected vertebral body ("vertebra plana") is frequent and should suggest the diagnosis.

Case 1035 illustrates severe compression of the T6 vertebral body *(long arrow)* and depression of the superior end plate of T9 *(short arrow)*. Mild T1 prolongation is present at both levels. Both lesions demonstrated high signal intensity on T2-weighted scans. Neither is associated with significant compromise of the spinal canal.

Partial collapse of the T9 vertebral body in Case 1036 *(arrow)* is accompanied by a shallow anterior epidural mass. Mild T2 prolongation is present within the vertebra.

Postcontrast scans in histiocytosis usually demonstrate uniform enhancement of the involved body and any accompanying prevertebral or epidural masses.

The differential diagnosis of a collapsed vertebral body in a child includes leukemia, metastatic neuroblastoma, and Ewing's sarcoma as well as primary bone tumors.

### Case 1037

15-year-old girl presenting with
back pain and leg weakness.
(axial, noncontrast T1-weighted SE scan; T8 level)

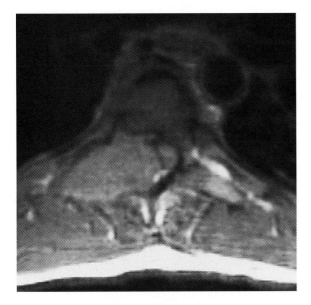

**Aneurysmal Bone Cyst**

### Case 1038

10-year-old girl presenting with a stiff
back and mild difficulty walking.
(sagittal, noncontrast T2-weighted SE scan)

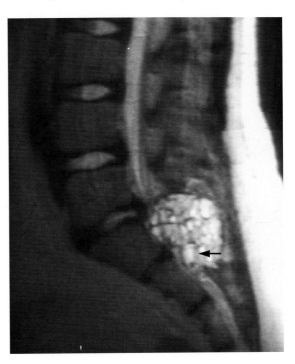

**Aneurysmal Bone Cyst**

---

Primary vertebral tumors are an unusual cause of epidural masses and neurological symptoms. Benign lesions such as osteoblastomas and aneurysmal bone cysts may be encountered in young patients, as illustrated above.

Aneurysmal bone cysts are osteolytic masses, typically comprised of lobulated compartments containing blood. The origin of these lesions is not well established. In many cases they seem to represent a reactive process incited by a primary pathology such as fibrous dysplasia, nonossifying fibroma, osteoblastoma, or giant cell tumor. Aneurysmal bone cysts themselves are not neoplastic. About 20% of aneurysmal bone cysts occur in the spine, frequently arising from posterior elements as in these cases.

The mass in Case 1037 has expanded from the vertebral pedicle and transverse process to involve the spinal canal. The appearance represents a pediatric analogy to the adult lesions in Cases 1009 and 1010. Characteristic "egg shells" of displaced cortex are often demonstrated at the perimeter of aneurysmal bone cysts on CT scans.

Case 1037 is unusual because the mass appears homogeneous and the lesion was predominantly solid at surgery. The more typical architecture of aneurysmal bone cysts is the multicystic pattern illustrated in Case 1038. Several of the small loculations contain sedimentation levels *(arrow)*, suggesting the presence of blood products.

Other potential "bubbly" lesions of the sacrum in children include giant cell tumors (see Case 1030), histiocytosis, chondrosarcomas, and hemophiliac pseudotumors. In adults, myeloma, metastases (e.g., from hypernephroma and thyroid carcinoma), and hyperparathyroidism may cause multiloculated sacral expansion. (Also see the discussion of sacral chordomas in Cases 1028 and 1029.)

### Case 1039

52-year-old man presenting with arm
weakness and difficulty walking.
(sagittal, noncontrast T2-weighted FSE scan)

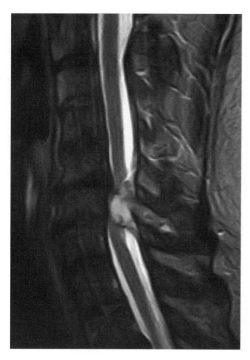

**Chondrosarcoma**

### Case 1040

34-year-old woman presenting with
back pain and paraparesis.
(axial, postcontrast T1-weighted SE scan; T4 level)

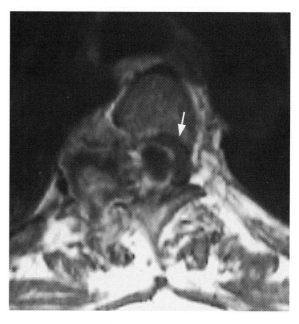

**Chondrosarcoma**

---

Malignant primary vertebral tumors may also cause epidural masses and compression of the spinal cord. Chondrosarcomas are the most common lesions to do so in adults, usually affecting patients from 30 to 60 years of age. Other rare primary malignant bone tumors that occasionally involve the spinal canal include osteosarcomas (most common at ages 10 to 20), primary Ewing's sarcomas (most common at ages 15 to 25), and fibrosarcomas.

Both of the tumors illustrated above arise from the posterior arch of the involved vertebra, and both demonstrate lobulated morphology. These features are typical for vertebral chondrosarcomas. The high signal intensity of the mass in Case 1039 suggests high water content within the tumor matrix, another characteristic feature of chondroid neoplasms. Scattered areas of low signal intensity may also be seen within chondrosarcomas on T2-weighted images due to calcification and/or hemorrhage.

The heterogeneous enhancement pattern in Case 1040 includes both solid and peripheral components, with an overall multinodular structure. This pattern correlates with histology demonstrating a mixture of cellular tumor regions and areas that primarily contain matrix. The mass expands from its vertebral origin to produce bulky paraspinal and epidural components.

The spinal cord in Case 1039 is well defined and clearly compressed. The cord in Case 1040 is less well demarcated but appears to be displaced and flattened against the left side of the spinal canal *(arrow)*.

## Case 1041A

68-year-old woman presenting with quadriparesis
and hyperreflexia of the legs.
(sagittal, noncontrast T1-weighted SE scan)

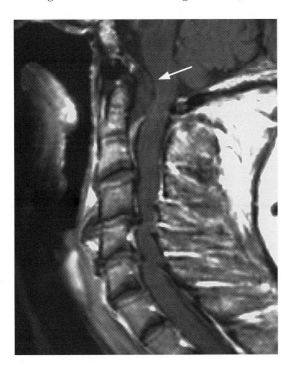

**Fibrous Pseudotumor at C1-2**
(and central canal stenosis)

## Case 1041B

Same patient.
(sagittal, noncontrast T2-weighted FSE scan)

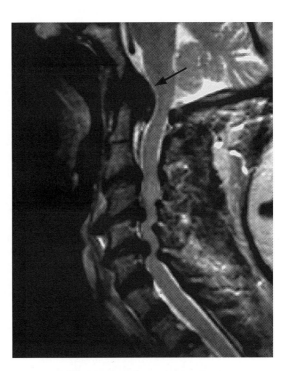

**Fibrous Pseudotumor at C1-2**
(and central canal stenosis)

---

Fibrous pseudotumors may develop along the anterior margin of the foramen magnum, often associated with chronic instability or abnormal stress at the C1-2 articulation. Soft tissue thickening posterior to the odontoid process may reflect old trauma or ligamentous laxity leading to excessive motion and secondary degenerative change.

In Case 1041, congenital abnormality including atlantooccipital assimilation and fusion of the C2 and C3 vertebral bodies has probably caused an abnormal distribution of forces at C1-2. Tissue at the level of the transverse ligament of the atlas is markedly thickened *(arrows)*. The very low signal intensity of this anterior epidural mass on the T2-weighted scan in Case 1041B is characteristic of dense fibrosis and distinct from the watery granulation tissue of rheumatoid arthritis (compare to Cases 1165 and 1166).

The low intensity of the lesion in Case 1041B combines with its epidural location to largely exclude a schwannoma

or meningioma, both of which can occur at the ventral margin of the foramen magnum (see Cases 1053 and 1054). Contrast enhancement within fibrous pseudotumors at C1-2 is usually minimal, unlike the expected intense enhancement of a schwannoma or a meningioma.

Although the C1-2 pseudolesion in Case 1041 does compromise the foramen magnum, the patient's symptoms are more likely due to the stenosis of the central canal from C3 to C6. Anterior extradural ridges from bulging discs combine with hypertrophy of dorsal ligaments (and congenitally small canal dimensions) to severely deform and compress the spinal cord. A haze of prolonged T2 values within the cord in Case 1041B may reflect edema, ischemia, and/or myelomalacia.

The differential diagnosis of a ventral epidural mass at C1-2 includes rheumatoid arthritis and calcium pyrophosphate dihydrate deposition disease (see Cases 1163-1166).

# REFERENCES

Algra PR, Bloem JL, Tissing H, et al: Detection of vertebral metastases: comparison between MR imaging and bone scintigraphy. *Radiology* 11:219-232, 1991.

Avrahami E, Tadmor R, Dally O, Hadar H: Earl MR demonstration of spinal metastases in patients with normal radiographs and CT and radionuclide bone scans. *J Comput Assist Tomogr* 13:598-602, 1989.

Aydingoz U, Oto A, Cila A: Spinal cord compression due to epidural extramedullary haematopoiesis in thalassaemia: MRI. *Neuroradiology* 39:870-872, 1997.

Baker LL, Goodman SB, Perkash I, et al: Benign versus pathological compression fractures of vertebral bodies: assessment with conventional spin echo, chemical-shift, and STIR MR imaging. *Radiology* 174:495-502, 1990.

Beltram J, Noto AM, Chakeres DW, Christoforidis AJ: Tumors of the osseous spine: staging with MR imaging versus CT. *Radiology* 162:565-569, 1987.

Beltram J, Simon DC, Levy M, et al: Aneurysmal bone cysts: MR imaging at 1.5 T. *Radiology* 158:689-690, 1986.

Boukobza M, Mazel C, Touboul E: Primary vertebral and spinal epidural non-Hodgkin's lymphoma with spinal cord compression. *Neuroradiology* 38:333-337, 1996.

Carmody RF, Yang PJ, Seeley GM, et al: Spinal cord compression due to metastatic disease: diagnosis with MR imaging versus myelography. *Radiology* 173:225-229, 1989.

Castillo M, Arbelaez A, Smith JK, Fisher LL: Diffusion-weighted MR imaging offers no advantage over routine noncontrast MR imaging in the detection of vertebral metastases. *AJNR* 21:948-953, 2000.

Cory DA, Fritsch SA, Cohen MD, et al: Aneurysmal bone cysts: imaging findings and embolotherapy. *Am J Roentgenol* 153:369-373, 1989.

Daffner RH, Lupetin AR, Dash N, et al: MRI in the detection of malignant infiltration of bone marrow. *Am J Roentgenol* 146:353-358, 1986.

De Schepper AMA, Ramon F, Van Marck E: MR imaging of eosinophilic granuloma: report of 11 cases. *Skeletal Radiol* 22:163-166, 1993.

Dietrich RB, Kangarloo H, Lenarsky C, Feig SA: Neuroblastoma: the role of MR imaging. *Am J Roentgenol* 148:937-942, 1987.

Disler DG, Miklic D: Imaging findings in tumors of the sacrum. *Am J Roentgenol* 173:1699-1706, 1999.

Fox MW, Onofrio BM: The natural history of management of symptomatic and asymptomatic vertebral hemangiomas. *J Neurosurg* 78:36-45, 1993.

Friedman DP: Symptomatic vertebral hemangiomas: MR findings. *Am J Roentgenol* 167:359-364, 1996.

Ginsberg LE, Williams DW, Stanton C: Intrasacral myxopapillary ependymoma. *Neuroradiology* 36:56-58, 1994.

Godersky JC, Smoker WRK, Knutzon R: Use of magnetic resonance imaging in the evaluation of metastatic spine disease. *Neurosurg* 21:676-680, 1987.

Guermazi A, Miaux Y, Chiras J: Imaging of spinal cord compression due to thoracic extramedullary haematopoiesis in myelofibrosis. *Neuroradiology* 39:733-736, 1997.

Hajek PC, Baker LL, Goobar JE, et al: Focal fat deposition in axial bone marrow: MR characteristics. *Radiology* 162:245, 1987.

Hayes CW, Jensen ME, Conway WF: Non-neoplastic lesions of vertebral bodies. Findings in magnetic resonance imaging. *Radiographics* 9:883-904, 1989.

Jones KM, Schwartz RB, Mantello MT, et al: Fast spin-echo MR in the detection of vertebral metastases: comparison of three sequences. *AJNR* 15:401-408, 1994.

Kamholtz R, Sze G: Current imaging in spinal metastatic disease. *Semin Oncol* 18:158-169, 1991.

Keslar PJ, Buck JL, Suarez ES: Germ cell tumors of the sacrococcy geal region: radiologic-pathologic correlation. *Radiographics* 14:607-620, 1994.

Klein SL, Sanford RA, Muhlbauer MS: Pediatric spinal epidural metastases. *J Neurosurg* 74:70-75, 1991.

Lanir A, Aghai E, Simon JR, et al: MR imaging in myelofibrosis. *J Comput Assist Tomogr* 10:634, 1986.

Laredo JD, Assouline E, Gelbert F, et al: Vertebral hemangioma—fat content as a sign of aggressiveness. *Radiology* 177:467, 1990.

Laredo J-D, Quessar AE, Bossard P, Vuillemin-Bodaghi V: Veretebral tumors and pseudotumors. *Radiol Clin North Am* 39:137-163, 2001.

Libshitz HI, Malthouse SR, Cunningham D, et al: Multiple myeloma: appearance at MR imaging. *Radiology* 182:833-837, 1992.

Llauger J, Palmer J, Amores S, et al: Primary tumors of the sacrum: diagnostic imaging. *Am J Roentgenol* 174:417-424, 2000.

Lyons MK, O'Neill BP, March WR, Kurtin DJ: Primary spinal epidural non-Hodgkin's lymphoma: report of eight patients and review of the literature. *Neurosurgery* 30:675-680, 1992.

Mascalchi M, Arnetoli G, Pozzo G, et al: Spinal epidural angiolipoma: MR findings. *AJNR* 12:744-745, 1991.

Mehta RC, Marks MP, Hinks RS, et al: MR evaluation of vertebral metastases: T1-weighted, short-inversion-time in-version recovery, fast spin-echo, and inversion-recovery fast spin-echo sequences. *AJNR* 16:281-288, 1995.

Meyers SP, Yaw K, Devaney K: Giant cell tumor of the thoracic spine: MR appearance. *AJNR* 15:962-964, 1994.

Moulopoulos LA, Varma DGK, Dimopoulos MA, et al: Multiple myeloma: spinal MR imaging in patients with untreated newly diagnosed. *Radiology* 185:833-840, 1992.

Munday TL, Johnson MH, Hayes CW, et al: Musculoskeletal causes of spinal axis compromise. *Radiographics* 14:1225-1245, 1994.

Munk PL, Helms CA, Holt RG, et al: MR imaging of aneurysmal bone cysts. *Am J Roentgenol* 153:99-101, 1989.

Murphey MD, Andrews CL, Flemming DJ, et al: Primary tumors of the spine: radiologic-pathologic correlation. *Radiographics* 16:1131-1158, 1996.

Olson DO, Shields AF, Sheunch CJ, et al: Magnetic resonance imaging of the bone marrow in patients with leukemia, aplastic anemia, and lymphoma. *Invest Radiol* 21:540, 1986.

Perry JR, Deodhare SS, Bilbao JM, et al: The significance of spinal cord compression as the initial manifestation of lymphoma. *Neurosurgery* 32:157-162, 1993.

Preul MC, Leblanc R, Tampieri D: Spinal angiolipomas: report of three cases. *J Neurosurg* 78:280-286, 1993.

Provenzale JM, McLendon RE: Spinal angiolipomas: MR features. *AJNR* 17:713-720, 1996.

Quirini GE, Meyer JR, Herman M, Russell EJ: Osteochondroma of the thoracic spine: an unusual cause of spinal cord compression. *AJNR* 17:961-964, 1996.

Ragland RL, Knorr JR, Kamath SV, et al: Magnetic resonance patterns of epidural impression from spinal metastases: review of 200 cases. *Int J Neurorad* 2:69-72, 1996.

Rahmouni A, Divine M, Mathieu D, et al: Detection of multiple myeloma involving the spine: efficiency of fat-suppression and contrast-enchanced MR imaging. *Am J Roentgenol* 160:1049-1052, 1993.

Rosenthal DI, Scott JA, Mankin HJ, et al: Sacrococcygeal chrodoma: magnetic resonance imaging and computed tomography. *Am J Roentgenol* 145-143, 1985.

Rovira A, Rovira A, Capellades J, et all: Lumbar extradural hemangiomas: report of three cases. *AJNR* 20:27-32, 1999.

Ross JS, Masaryk TJ, Modic MT et al: Vertebral hemangiomas: MR imaging. *Radiology* 165:165-169, 1987.

Schellinger D: Patterns of anterior spinal canal involvement by neoplasms and infections. *AJNR* 17:953-960, 1996.

Siegel MJ, Jamroz GA, Glazer HS, Abramson CL: MR imaging of intraspinal extension of neuroblastoma. *J Comput Assist Tomogr* 10:593-595, 1986.

Syklawer R, Osborn RE, Kerber CW, Glass RF: Magnetic resonance imaging of vertebral osteoblastome: a report of two cases. *Surg Neurol* 34:421-426, 1990.

Smoker WRK, Godersky JC, Knutzon RK, et al: The role of MR imaging in evaluation of metastatic spinal disease. *AJNR* 8:901-908, 1987.

Sze G, Krol G, Zimmerman RD, Deck MDF: Malignant extradural spinal tumors: MR imaging with Gd-DTPA. *Radiology* 167:217-223, 1988.

Weaver GR, Sandler MP: Increased sensitivity of magnetic resonance imaging compared to radionuclide bone scintigraphy in the detection of lymphoma of the spine. *Clin Nucl Med* 12:333-334, 1987.

Wippold FJ II, Koeller KK, Smirniotopoulos JG: Clinical and imaging features of cervical chordoma. *Am J Roentgenol* 172:1423-1426, 1999.

Yochum TR, Lile RL, Schultz GD, et al: Acquired spinal stenosis secondary to an expanding thoracic vertebral hemangioma. *Spine* 18:299-305, 1993.

York JE, Berk RH, Fuller GN, et al: Chondrosarcoma of the spine: 1954 to 1997. *J Neurosurg Spine* 90:73-78, 1999.

Yuh WTC, Zachar CK, Barloon TJ, et al: Vertebral compression fractures: distinction between benign and malignant causes with MR imaging. *Radiology* 172:215-218, 1989.

# CHAPTER 19

# Intradural and
# Nerve Sheath Tumors

## Case 1042

64-year-old man presenting with
lumbar radiculopathy.
(sagittal, noncontrast T2-weighted FSE scan)

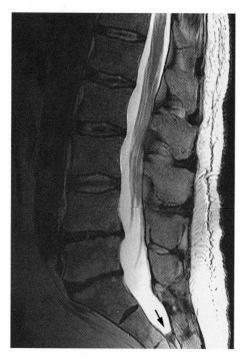

**Leptomeningeal Metastases from
Carcinoma of the Lung**

## Case 1043

11-year-old girl with extensive intracranial
recurrence of a primitive neuroectodermal tumor.
(sagittal, postcontrast T1-weighted SE scan)

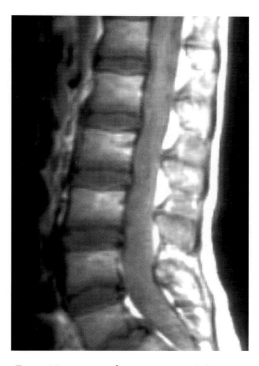

**Drop Metastases from Intracranial PNET**

Hematogenous metastases to the spinal canal most frequently involve the vertebral bodies and/or the epidural space, as illustrated in Chapter 18. However, intradural metastases are more common than previously appreciated.

Intramedullary metastases may occur at any level of the spinal cord (see Cases 1105 and 1106). The conus medullaris is a particularly common site and should be carefully examined on all lumbar scans.

Alternatively, intradural metastases may involve the cauda equina, causing nodularity (see Case 1046) and/or thickening of the nerve roots. In Case 1042, intrathecal roots are diffusely enlarged due to metastatic carcinoma of the lung. (Compare to the normal appearance of the cauda equina in Cases 923 and 925.) Carcinoma of the breast and melanoma are other tumors that commonly metastasize to the intrathecal compartment.

Case 1043 demonstrates a second form of intradural metastasis: CSF-borne dissemination of intracranial tumors to the spinal canal. Such "drop" metastases may present as uniform coating and/or nodularity (see Case 1047) of the

spinal cord or cauda equina or as one or more discrete masses.

In Case 1043, the pathology is poorly defined because it is so extensive. The entire thecal sac is abnormal, with signal intensity greater than that expected for CSF. The amorphous or featureless appearance of the intradural compartment is due to the presence of cells, protein, and contrast material within the spinal fluid. This suspension surrounds the cauda equina and eliminates the normal definition of intradural anatomy. A similar appearance is occasionally seen with hematogenous metastases of systemic origin, (e.g., breast carcinoma) filling the subarachnoid space.

Primary intradural or epidural tumors may also cause a featureless lumbar canal by filling or effacing the thecal sac. Examples include intradural epidermoid masses, large intradural ependymomas (see Case 1094), and epidural neuroblastomas (see Case 1020).

Blunting of the caudal end of the thecal sac in Case 1042 *(arrow)* probably represents cellular debris and/or blood products related to the intradural metastases (compare to Case 1093).

# DIFFERENTIAL DIAGNOSIS:
## THICKENED INTRADURAL NERVE ROOTS

### Case 1044

64-year-old man presenting with
lumbar radiculopathy.
(axial, noncontrast T2-weighted FSE scan; L3 level)

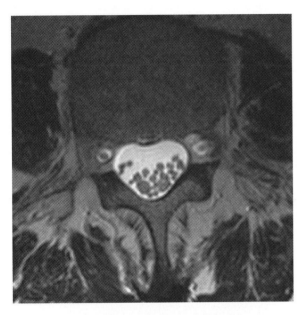

**Metastatic Carcinoma of the Lung**
(same patient as Case 1042)

### Case 1045

68-year-old man presenting with
progressive leg weakness.
(axial, noncontrast T1-weighted SE scan; L4-5 level)

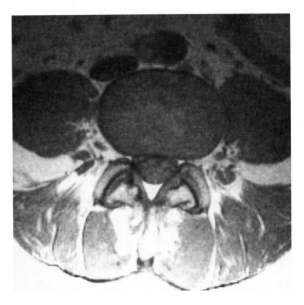

**Lymphomatous Meningitis**

---

Intrathecal nerve roots are abnormally thickened in each of the above cases. Intradural metastases should be a leading consideration when this appearance is encountered.

Case 1044 presents an axial scan of the patient in Case 1042. Most of the roots of the cauda equina are enlarged, some more than others.

Case 1045 illustrates that systemic lymphoma may coat the surface of intradural tissues in a manner analogous to leptomeningeal carcinomatosis. Thickening of nerve roots is often more uniform in lymphomatous meningitis than in cases of intradural metastases from carcinomas.

"Drop" metastases from cranial (or other spinal) masses may cause an appearance very comparable to the above images (see Case 1162).

Nerve roots of the cauda equina normally appear more prominent on postcontrast scans (particularly in the axial plane) than on precontrast studies. This mild, uniform enhancement can raise the question of carcinomatous meningitis, as discussed in Case 1121.

Non-neoplastic etiologies of thickened intradural nerve roots include edema caused by mechanical compression (e.g., in cases of disc herniation or spinal stenosis), inflammation and/or adhesions secondary to arachnoiditis (see Cases 1157-1159), and rare primary hypertrophic neuropathies (e.g., Charcot-Marie-Tooth disease and Dejerine-Sottas disease).

Intradural metastases should be remembered as an occasional cause of radiculopathy, cauda equina symptoms, or conus dysfunction in patients with no preceding evidence of neoplasm or a distant history of malignancy. In particular, it is not uncommon to discover cerebral or spinal metastases from breast carcinoma developing a decade or more after treatment of the primary tumor.

# DIFFERENTIAL DIAGNOSIS:
## ENHANCING INTRADURAL NODULES

### Case 1046

90-year-old woman presenting with leg pain.
(sagittal, postcontrast T1-weighted SE scan)

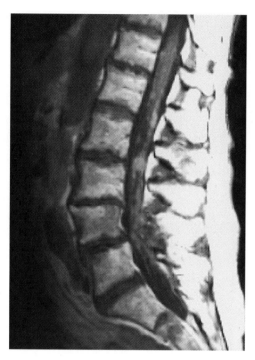

**Metastatic Carcinoma of the Breast**

### Case 1047

40-year-old man complaining of
headaches and low back pain.
(sagittal, postcontrast T1-weighted SE scan)

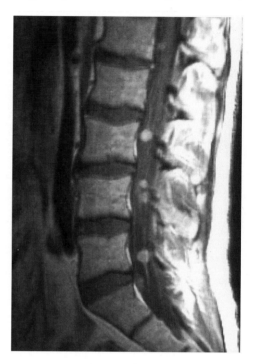

**Drop Metastases from a Cerebral
Glioblastoma Multiforme**

Intradural metastases can arise from hematogenous dissemination of systemic neoplasms or from CSF spread of primary CNS tumors. Cases 1046 and 1047 illustrate the potential similarity of these two pathologies.

In Case 1046, a precontrast scan showed nodularity along intradural nerve roots. The scan also demonstrated multiple, low intensity vertebral metastases. Most of the osseous lesions have enhanced to isointensity and are poorly seen on the above scan (see discussion of Cases 999 and 1000).

The enhancing tumor nodules along the roots of the cauda equina in Case 1047 are nonspecific and could easily represent metastases from a systemic source. Instead, they were due to CSF seeding of a malignant glioma. "Drop" metastases from gliomas are less frequent than spinal dissemination of germinomas, medulloblastomas, ependymomas and pineal cell tumors.

Multiple enhancing nerve root tumors (neurofibromas or schwannomas) in a patient with neurofibromatosis type 1 or 2 could result in a pattern very similar to the above images.

Case 1217 presents another example of nodular metastases involving nerve roots of the cauda equina.

# DIFFERENTIAL DIAGNOSIS:
## UNIFORM ENHANCEMENT COATING THE SPINAL CORD

### Case 1048

46-year-old man presenting with mild leg weakness.
(sagittal, postcontrast T1-weighted SE scan)

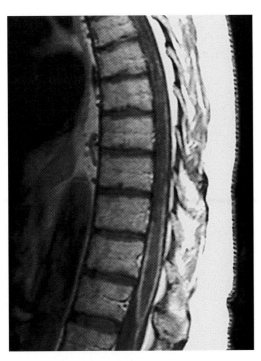

**Leptomeningeal Metastases**
(from carcinoma of the lung)

### Case 1049

48-year-old man presenting with back
pain and cauda equina syndrome.
(sagittal, postcontrast T1-weighted SE scan)

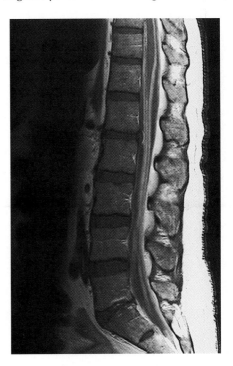

**Bacterial Meningitis**
(*Streptococcus pneumoniae*)

---

Hematogenous and CSF-borne metastases within the thecal sac are often nodular, as illustrated on the preceding page. Dissemination of tumor by either route may alternatively cause a uniform layer of enhancing tissue along the surface of the spinal cord and/or cauda equina.

Case 1048 is an example of such pial coating or "frosting," most apparent at the margins of the conus medullaris. Pial-based metastatic disease may be more subtle, discontinuous, asymmetric, and/or nodular, as seen in the mid thoracic region in Case 1048.

Superficial enhancement along cord margins is not specific for malignant disease, as emphasized by Case 1049. The diffuse pial and radicular enhancement in this patient was due to pneumococcal meningitis.

In addition to meningitis, inflammatory disorders such as sarcoidosis, CMV myelitis/radiculitis (see Case 1148), and Guillain-Barré syndrome (see Cases 1151-1153) can cause pial enhancement of the spinal cord and/or uniform enhancement of intrathecal nerve roots.

In both the neoplastic and inflammatory categories, subpial spread of disease can be associated with enhancing nodules of tissue extending into the cord from the surface (see Cases 1143-1146).

### Case 1050

53-year-old woman with a six-month history of "rubbery" legs and diminished sacral sensation.
(sagittal, noncontrast T1-weighted SE scan)

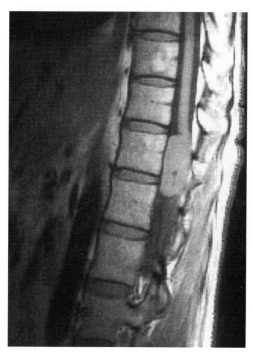

**Meningioma**

### Case 1051

67-year-old woman presenting with back and bilateral leg pain.
(sagittal, noncontrast T2-weighted FSE scan)

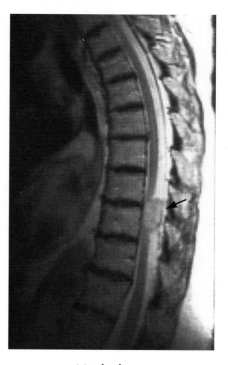

**Meningioma**

Meningiomas and schwannomas are the most common primary intradural tumors of the spinal canal. Although the masses may be nearly isointense to the spinal cord on noncontrast images, distortion of anatomy and capping of the tumors by spinal fluid establish their presence.

The large, homogeneous intradural meningioma in Case 1050 fills the spinal canal at the level of the conus medullaris and proximal cauda equina. Cord margins are obscured and the subarachnoid space is effaced. The differential diagnosis of this intradural mass includes ependymoma and schwannoma (see Cases 1062 and 1092).

Spinal meningiomas may demonstrate a range of signal intensities on T2-weighted scans, comparable to cerebral lesions (see Cases 35 and 36). Case 1051 demonstrates a tumor of intermediate intensity and homogeneous texture.

The spinal cord is anteriorly displaced and compressed. The dorsal subarachnoid space is widened at the margins of the mass, the hallmark of an intradural extramedullary process.

Spinal meningiomas are most common in the thoracic canal, often arising laterally (as in Case 1050) or dorsolaterally (as in Case 1051). They occur much more frequently in women than in men: the male to female ratio is about 1:4.

Ventral location within the spinal canal is common for cervical meningiomas. In the thoracic canal, ventral location of an intradural extramedullary mass is more typical of schwannomas (see Cases 978, 1066, and 1067). Meningiomas rarely occur in the lumbar region.

## Case 1052

67-year-old woman presenting with
back and bilateral leg pain.
(coronal, postcontrast T1-weighted SE scan)

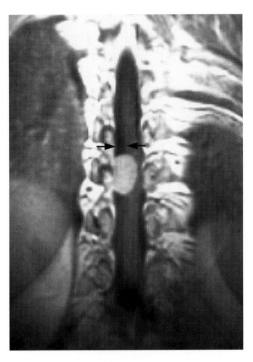

**Meningioma**
(same patient as Case 1051)

## Case 1053

48-year-old woman presenting with abnormal gait.
(coronal, postcontrast T1-weighted SE scan)

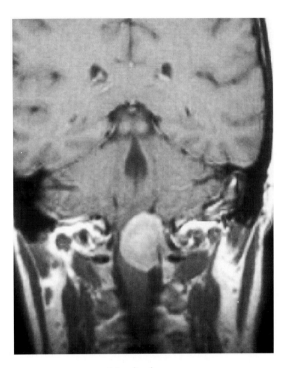

**Meningioma**

Like their intracranial counterparts, spinal meningiomas usually enhance intensely and uniformly.

In Case 1052, a meningioma arises from the dorsolateral margin of the dural sac and compresses the spinal cord contralaterally and anteriorly (see Case 1051). Note the widening of the subarachnoid space above *(arrows)* and below the tumor, documenting its location as intradural but extramedullary.

The meningioma in Case 1053 is centered at the C1 level. The mass occupies most of the spinal canal and distorts the cervicomedullary junction. Within the lesion a faint circular or target-like architecture can be seen. This occasional finding is highly suggestive of a meningioma.

The presence and uniformity of contrast enhancement within an intradural lesion are nonspecific. Intense, ho-

mogeneous enhancement as seen above is compatible with meningioma, but schwannomas, ependymomas, and intradural metastases may have a similar appearance. On the other hand, many spinal schwannomas and ependymomas contain cystic or necrotic areas that cause an inhomogeneous pattern of enhancement (see Case 1062).

The lesion in Case 1052 was apparent on noncontrast scans. Contrast was given to (1) more clearly demonstrate the interface between the tumor and the spinal cord (particularly on axial images) and (2) detect possible additional intradural masses.

The great majority of spinal meningiomas are entirely intradural. Approximately 5% are extradural lesions, whereas another 5% have both intradural and extradural components.

### Case 1054

26-year-old woman presenting with
arm paresthesias.
(sagittal, noncontrast T1-weighted SE scan)

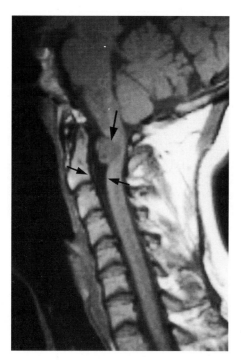

**Schwannoma**

### Case 1055

5-year-old girl presenting with paraparesis.
(sagittal, noncontrast T1-weighted SE scan)

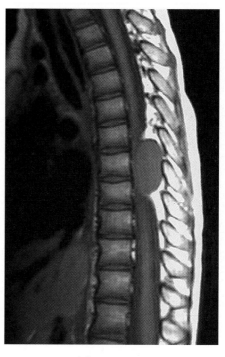

**Schwannoma**

Most spinal schwannomas are homogeneous and nearly isointense to neural tissue on T1-weighted scans. A minority of these tumors demonstrate prolonged T1 values, and T1-shortening due to subacute hemorrhage is occasionally seen in large lesions.

The intradural schwannoma in Case 1054 *(upper arrow)* displaces and compresses the cervicomedullary junction with widening of the ventral subarachnoid space *(lower arrows)*. A meningioma along the ventral margin of the foramen magnum could cause an identical appearance.

Case 1055 demonstrates that spinal schwannomas are occasionally extradural. The subarachnoid space at the level of the tumor is compressed rather than widened, as in Case 1054. Dorsal epidural fat caps the rostral and caudal poles of the mass.

In addition to intraspinal origin in either the intradural or extradural compartment, schwannomas may arise within an intervertebral foramen (see Cases 1056, 1058, and 1060). A combination of these components is often present. The schwannoma in Case 1055 extended laterally through an expanded nerve root canal to form a small paraspinal mass.

Masses at the foramen magnum may cause a variety of nonspecific symptoms. Demyelinating disease was suspected in Case 1053 on the previous page and in Case 1054 above. Attention to the foramen magnum (and the visible segment of the cervical spinal cord) is important during review of all cranial scans, especially those obtained for "possible multiple sclerosis."

Another clinical syndrome associated with compromise of the foramen magnum is spastic diplegia, often categorized in children as "cerebral palsy." Spinal masses at the craniocervical junction or within the cervical canal should be considered in patients with such histories.

## Case 1056

24-year-old man with an apical mass
discovered on a chest x-ray.
(axial, noncontrast T2*-weighted GRE scan; T1 level)

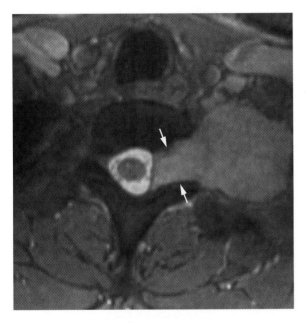

**Schwannoma**

## Case 1057

36-year-old man presenting with left arm numbness
and incoordination of the left leg.
(sagittal, noncontrast T2-weighted SE scan)

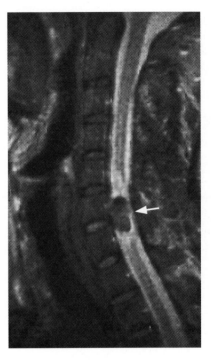

**Schwannoma**

The signal intensity of spinal schwannomas on T2-weighted scans is widely variable. (Compare to the appearance of acoustic schwannomas, discussed in Cases 193 and 194.)

Many of these tumors demonstrate moderate to marked prolongation of T2 values. The large mass expanding the left intervertebral foramen *(arrows)* and extending into paraspinal tissue in Case 1056 is homogeneously higher in signal intensity than surrounding muscle. T2 prolongation in other schwannomas may be more pronounced and more heterogeneous (see Case 1058).

Prolonged T2 values within schwannomas may arise from a watery tissue matrix, reflecting the predominance of Antoni "B" zones with a relatively loose arrangement of cells. Alternatively, high signal intensity within schwannomas on long TR spin echo images may be caused by cystic or necrotic degeneration, which often occurs as these tumors enlarge.

Other spinal schwannomas are characterized by low signal intensity on T2-weighted scans, as in Case 1057. This finding often correlates with the presence of old blood products. Small or large areas of hemorrhage are commonly noted within schwannomas at surgery or on histological examination.

The appearance in Case 1057 is nonspecific. Low signal intensity may occur within meningiomas due to dense fibrous tissue or calcification. Calcified or ossified extradural lesions (e.g., osteochondromas) could also present with morphology and signal intensity resembling Case 1057. Occasional cavernous angiomas of the spinal canal occur as small intradural or extradural masses with short T1 and T2 values due to the presence of subacute and chronic hemorrhage (see Cases 1220-1222).

Like the cases on the preceding page, the above scans demonstrate that spinal schwannomas may be extradural and/or intradural, paraspinal and/or intraspinal.

# DIFFERENTIAL DIAGNOSIS:
## FORAMINAL MASS WITH PROLONGED T2 VALUES

### Case 1058

42-year-old man presenting with L2 radiculopathy.
(sagittal, noncontrast T2-weighted FSE scan)

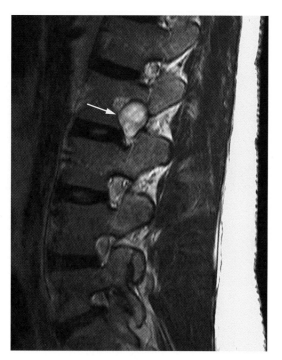

**Schwannoma**

### Case 1059

69-year-old woman presenting with back pain.
(axial, noncontrast T2-weighted FSE scan; T9 level)

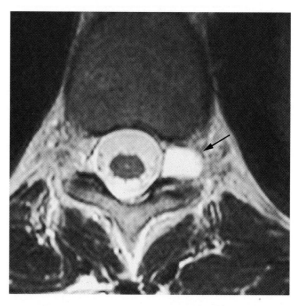

**Root Sleeve Cyst**
(normal variant)

---

Case 1058 demonstrates enlargement of the L2 nerve root within the nerve root canal *(arrow)*. The intervertebral foramen is itself expanded (compare to the foramen at L1-2). This bone remodeling suggests a long-standing, slow-growing tumor. The mottled prolongation of T2 within the lesion is among the common presentations of spinal schwannomas.

The high intensity "mass" within the left intervertebral foramen in Case 1059 *(arrow)* is a cyst of the root sleeve. This developmental variant may be solitary or multiple and can occur at any level of the spine. Root sleeve cysts are rarely symptomatic. An exception is the occasional cyst

that leaks CSF, causing the syndrome of spontaneous intracranial hypotension (see Case 540). In most cases, recognition of a root sleeve cyst is important only to avoid confusion with a tumor arising from a spinal nerve.

Like schwannomas, neurofibromas often demonstrate high signal intensity on T2-weighted scans (see Case 1068B). The distinction between these two root sheath tumors often depends on clinical context (and subsequent pathology) rather than on MR characteristics.

Parasagittal scans such as Case 1058 provide an excellent cross-sectional display of nerve root canals in the thoracic or lumbar regions.

# DIFFERENTIAL DIAGNOSIS:
## ENHANCING MASS WITHIN AN INTERVERTEBRAL FORAMEN

### Case 1060

42-year-old man presenting with
hearing loss and right leg pain.
(axial, postcontrast T1-weighted SE scan; L2-3 level)

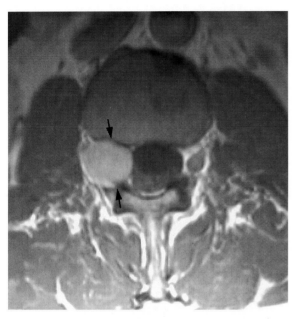

**Schwannoma**
(in type 2 neurofibromatosis)

### Case 1061

69-year-old woman presenting with left leg pain.
(axial, postcontrast T1-weighted SE scan; L3 level)

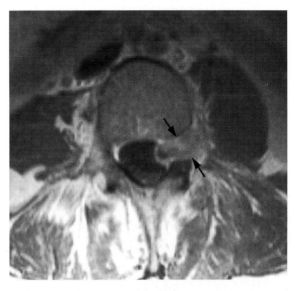

**Herniated Disc**

---

Masses within the intervertebral foramen may be neoplastic or discogenic in origin. The most common benign tumor in this location is a schwannoma, as in Case 1060.

The majority of spinal schwannomas are solitary lesions. Multiple intradural and extradural schwannomas occur in patients with type 2 neurofibromatosis. Sagittal scans in Case 1060 demonstrated several intensely enhancing masses within the thecal sac, resembling Cases 1046 and 1047.

Schwannomas often have CT attenuation values and MR intensity values resembling an enlarged root sleeve on noncontrast scans. Associated expansion of the intervertebral foramen *(arrows)* is a clue to the long-standing presence of a benign mass. Contrast enhancement confirms the solid nature of the lesion; uniform enhancement as in Case 1060 is characteristic of small and medium-sized schwannomas.

Forminal disc herniations may resemble schwannomas on both CT and MR studies. Occasional herniated discs are accompanied by erosive changes or remodeling of bone mimicking a nerve root tumor. MR scans with contrast enhancement will usually distinguish between these entities, demonstrating peripheral enhancement at the margins of disc fragments (see Cases 945 and 953B) and more solid enhancement within neoplasms.

The enhancement pattern in Case 1061 is a mixture of a peripheral component medially and a more solid and amorphous component laterally. As discussed in Chapter 17, central enhancement within disc herniations increases with time. On delayed scans, disc fragments may simulate enhancing tumors.

Lymphoma and epidural metastasis should also be included in the differential diagnosis of a foraminal mass. These pathologies are suggested when poorly defined tissue fills an intervertebral foramen without adjacent bone remodeling. Paraspinal "small blue cell" tumors can involve one or more intervertebral foramina in children (see Cases 1019, 1024, and 1025).

Finally, occasional vascular lesions can fill and expand an intervertebral foramen. Hemangiomas (see Case 998) and epidural cavernous angiomas may extend through a nerve root canal. A spinal dural arteriovenous fistula with predominant epidural rather than intradural drainage could also present in this manner.

### Case 1062

44-year-old woman presenting with a three-month history of increasing back pain and a negative lumbar CT scan.
(sagittal, postcontrast T1-weighted SE scan)

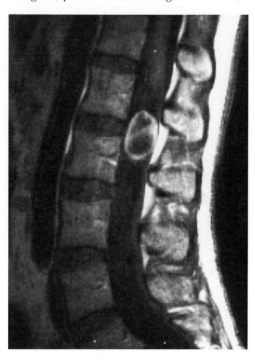

**Schwannoma**

### Case 1063

63-year-old woman presenting with leg pain.
(sagittal, postcontrast T1-weighted SE scan)

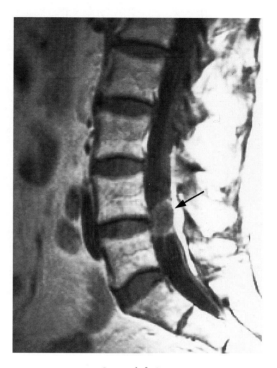

**Synovial Cyst**

---

Spinal schwannomas often contain nonenhancing areas of necrosis, hemorrhage, or cystic degeneration. Such tumors demonstrate heterogeneous contrast enhancement, illustrated by Case 1062. At surgery, this mass was found to be both hemorrhagic and necrotic.

Peripheral contrast enhancement is also characteristic of synovial cysts, discussed in Cases 969 and 970. The typical size and shape of the lesion in Case 1063 and its location at the L4-5 level are clues to the correct diagnosis. Axial scans would distinguish the epidural location of this synovial cyst from an intradural mass like Case 1062.

Herniated disc fragments should be included in the differential diagnosis. They are the most common epidural masses, and they are typically outlined by enhancement on early postcontrast scans (see Cases 945 and 953B).

Ependymomas of the filum terminale may be partially cystic or necrotic, resembling the above lesions. Rare cavernous angiomas within the spinal canal can also present a complex, lobulated appearance with rims of contrast enhancement.

Intrathecal masses may be missed on screening CT examinations of the lumar spine (as in Case 1062), either because they are located outside of the CT imaging volume or because their attenuation values do not differ significantly from CSF within the dural sac.

# DIFFERENTIAL DIAGNOSIS:
## ROUND, HETEROGENEOUSLY ENHANCING PARASPINAL MASS

### Case 1064

36-year-old woman presenting with left leg pain.
(coronal, postcontrast T1-weighted SE scan)

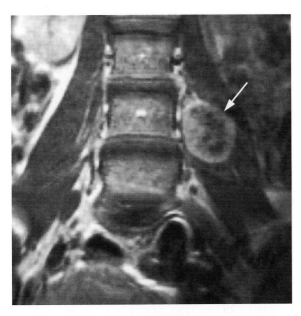

**Schwannoma**

### Case 1065

37-year-old woman presenting with right leg pain.
(axial, postcontrast T1-weighted SE scan; T12 level)

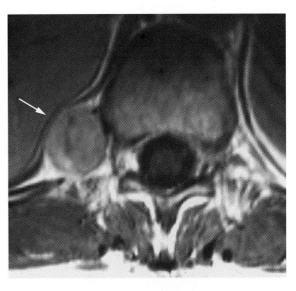

**Metastatic Adenopathy**
(from a fibrosarcoma)

Schwannomas and neurofibromas may be completely extraspinal, as illustrated in Case 1064. The mass in this case is centered along the axis of a single lumbar root. Peripheral enhancement surrounds a nonenhancing center, which may reflect cystic or necrotic components of the tumor (compare to Case 1062).

Case 1065 is a reminder that not all paraspinal masses are neurogenic. Adenopathy is always in the differential diagnosis of paraspinal pathology. A search for enlarged prevertebral or paraspinal nodes should be a routine component of spinal MR interpretations.

Solitary or plexiform neurofibromas may occur in the paraspinal region. When large, these tumors often present a characteristic appearance on noncontrast T2-weighted

scans, with a low intensity core surrounded by a perimeter of long T2 values (see Case 1071).

Ganglioneuromas should also be considered in the differential diagnosis of slow-growing paraspinal lesions (see Cases 1026 and 1027). Paraspinal ganglioneuromas most commonly arise from the sympathetic chain and are often discovered incidentally.

Lateral meningoceles may cause a paraspinal mass in patients with neurofibromatosis type 1, particularly in the thoracic region. These fluid-containing sacs can mimic solid paraspinal tumors on radiographic studies. MR scans establish the diagnosis in such cases by demonstrating CSF-like signal intensity (and lack of contrast enhancement) within the lesions.

### Case 1066

34-year-old woman presenting with clumsy arms.
(sagittal, noncontrast T1-weighted SE scan)

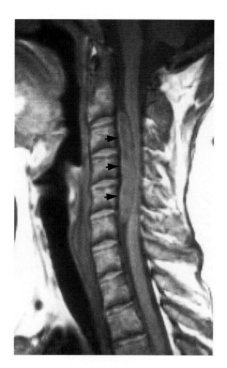

**Schwannoma**

### Case 1067

54-year-old woman presenting with
back pain and leg weakness.
(sagittal, postcontrast T1-weighted SE scan)

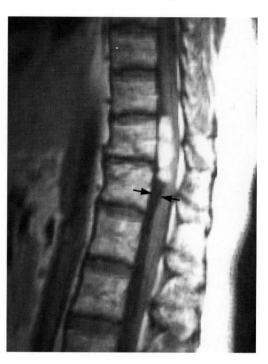

**Schwannoma**

---

Most schwannomas of the spinal canal are round or lobulated masses, as illustrated on the preceding pages. In some cases, spinal schwannomas assume an unusually flat, plaque-like morphology. Such lesions may extend along the spine for several segments.

Case 1066 demonstrates a thick layer of abnormal tissue occupying the anterior portion of the spinal canal from C2 to C6 *(arrows)*. The length of the lesion might raise the question of an epidural process such as lymphoma or metastasis. However, the subarachnoid space is widened at the rostral and caudal margins of the tumor, indicating intradural location of the mass. At surgery, the lesion proved to be a schwannoma attached to a single cervical root.

The intensely enhancing mass in Case 1067 has a similar plaque-like morphology, with mild superimposed lobula-

tions. As in Case 1066, the spinal cord is severely compressed, and caps of widened subarachnoid space are present at the poles of the mass *(arrows)*.

A meningioma should be considered in the differential diagnosis of Case 1067. "En plaque" meningiomas do occur in the spinal canal but are relatively less common than intracranial tumors with this morphology.

Examination of the remainder of the spinal canal on postcontrast images is indicated when one intradural mass is discovered. The presence of additional lesions raises the possibilities of multiple nerve root tumors (e.g., schwannomas in neurofibromatosis type 2 or neurofibromas in neurofibromatosis type 1) or intradural metastases of systemic or CNS origin (see Cases 1046 and 1047).

## Case 1068A

28-year-old woman presenting with neck pain, left arm weakness, and spasticity of the left leg. (sagittal, noncontrast T1-weighted SE scan)

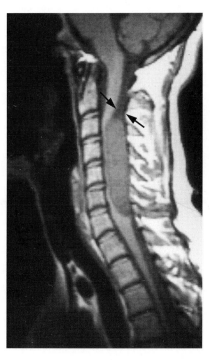

**Neurofibroma**

## Case 1068B

Same patient.
(axial, nonconstrast T2*-weighted GRE scan; C5-6 level)

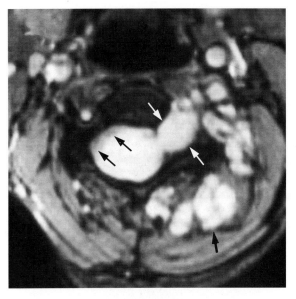

**Neurofibroma**

The MR characteristics of schwannomas and neurofibromas are largely indistinguishable. For this reason, they are often discussed together as "nerve sheath tumors" or "nerve root tumors." Both schwannomas and neurofibromas commonly arise from the dorsal sensory root of a spinal nerve.

Clinically and pathologically the lesions are distinct. Schwannomas occur sporadically. They originate from proliferation of schwann cells at one location on the perimeter of a nerve, leading to an eccentric mass that compresses and displaces the otherwise uninvolved axons. Neurofibromas are essentially limited to and specific for neurofibromatosis type 1. They arise from proliferation of both the internal fibroblastic and external schwann cell components of the nerve, resulting in symmetrical enlargement that surrounds individual axons. Neurofibromas are usually multiple, whereas schwannomas are usually solitary. (Multiple schwannomas are seen in neurofibromatosis type 2.)

The majority of nerve root tumors are entirely intradural, as illustrated by the schwannomas on the previous pages.

About 40% of nerve root tumors are extradural or demonstrate both intradural and extradural components.

Such dumbbell-shaped tumors typically involve and expand intervertebral foramina, as seen in Case 1068B. The large intradural component of this tumor (which causes widening of the dorsal subarachnoid space outlined by arrows in Case 1068A) flattens the spinal cord (*thin black arrows*, Case 1068B) contralaterally. The adjacent extradural portion of the neurofibroma extends into the left intervertebral foramen, which has been widened by chronic mass effect *(white arrows)*. A plexiform neurofibroma within dorsal soft tissues of the neck *(thick black arrow)* establishes the underlying diagnosis of type 1 neurofibromatosis.

The high signal intensity of neurofibromas on T2-weighted pulse sequences is indistinguishable from the appearance of many schwannomas (see Case 1058). Central zones of low signal intensity within an otherwise bright tumor on T2-weighted scans is a characteristic feature seen in plexiform neurofibromas (see Case 1071).

### Case 1069

10-year-old boy with neurofibromatosis type 1.
(sagittal, noncontrast T1-weighted SE scan)

### Case 1070

59-year-old man presenting with neck pain.
(sagittal, noncontrast T1-weighted SE scan)

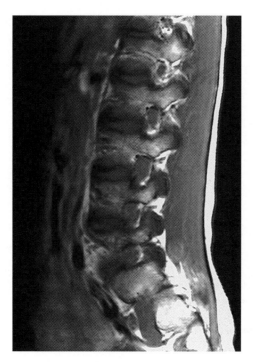

**Multiple Individual Neurofibromas**

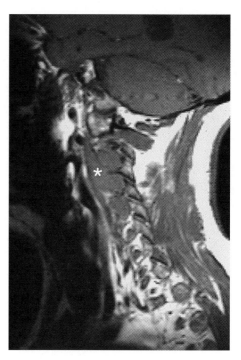

**Plexiform Neurofibroma**

The presence of multiple nerve root tumors suggests the diagnosis of neurofibromatosis. Neurofibromatosis type 1 may be associated with multiple individual neurofibromas, as in Case 1069, or with plexiform neurofibromas contiguously involving several adjacent roots, as in Case 1070. Multiple individual schwannomas may be encountered in patients with neurofibromatosis type 2.

All exiting lumbar roots are enlarged in Case 1069 (compare to Case 1058). The nerves nearly fill their intervertebral foramina, which have not yet been significantly expanded. The differential diagnosis for this appearance would include multiple root sleeve cysts (which could be excluded on postcontrast images) or a rare hypertrophic neuropathy (e.g., Dejerine Sottas disease or Charcot-Marie-Tooth disease).

The enlarged superior cervical roots in Case 1070 have eroded the margins of the associated intervertebral foramina. Unlike Case 1069, these nerves blend together to form a composite mass as they exit from the root canals *(asterisk).* The presence of such a plexiform neurofibroma is considered to be diagnostic of neurofibromatosis type 1, which had not been previously suspected in this patient. Plexiform neurofibromas can become much bulkier than the lesion illustrated above (see Case 1071).

## Case 1071A

26-year-old woman presenting with
back and leg pain.
(sagittal, noncontrast T1-weighted SE scan)

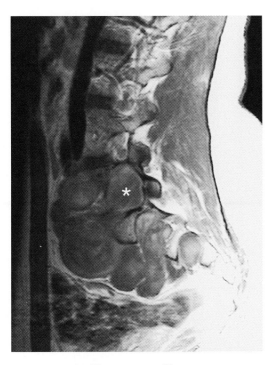

**Plexiform Neurofibroma**

## Case 1071B

Same patient.
(sagittal, noncontrast T2-weighted FSE scan)

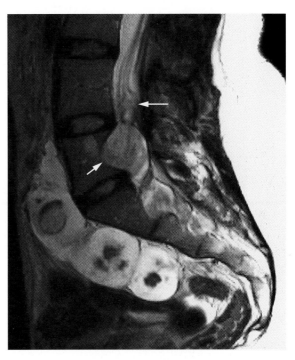

**Plexiform Neurofibroma**

Plexiform neurofibromas are a distinct type of nerve sheath tumor occurring exclusively in patients with neurofibromatosis type 1. The masses consist of fusiform expansion of contiguous nerves or branches of a nerve. Growth of the lesion can extensively infiltrate tissue planes and/or cause bulky, multinodular masses, illustrated by Case 1071.

The scan in Case 1071A demonstrates expansion of multiple lumbar and sacral roots in continuity with a lobulated presacral mass. Note the marked enlargement of the intervertebral foramen at L5-S1 *(asterisk)*.

Plexiform neurofibromas often have a characteristic appearance on T2-weighted images. The majority of each lobulation demonstrates high signal intensity, correlating with

the mucoid matrix common in these lesions. Near the center of each nodule is a contrasting zone of low signal intensity, representing a core of dense fibrocollagenous tissue. The combination of these features produces a target-like morphology that is demonstrated in Case 1071B and is highly suggestive of the diagnosis (see also Case 1205).

A large intraspinal component of the tumor is apparent in Case 1071B, causing erosion of the posterior cortices of the L5 vertebral body and the sacrum *(short arrow)*. Nerve roots of the cauda equina are compressed and distorted *(long arrow)*.

Contrast enhancement in plexiform neurofibromas may be moderate or intense, with variable heterogeneity.

### Case 1072

11-month-old boy presenting with decreased
crawling and mild scoliosis.
(sagittal, noncontrast T1-weighted SE scan)

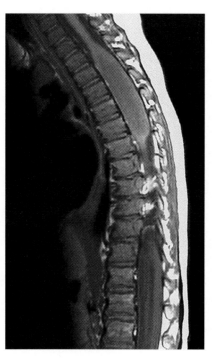

**Astrocytoma**

### Case 1073

3-year-old boy presenting with back pain.
(coronal, noncontrast T1-weighted SE scan)

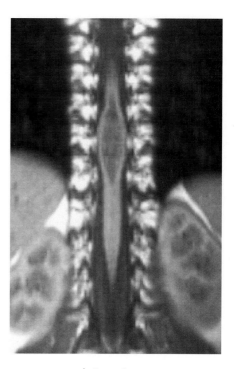

**Astrocytoma**

Magnetic resonance imaging far exceeds the capability of CT scanning to demonstrate intramedullary pathology. Contour abnormalities of the spinal cord are apparent on MR studies without intrathecal injection of contrast material. More importantly, MR can detect intramedullary lesions that are unaccompanied by cord expansion.

The differential diagnosis of intramedullary masses includes tumors, cysts, inflammatory processes, and vascular lesions. Within the tumor category, astrocytomas and ependymomas are the most common lesions. Of these two pathologies, astrocytomas are more frequently seen in children and in the thoracic region, as illustrated above.

Astrocytomas of the spinal cord may be histologically pilocytic or diffuse/infiltrating. The latter are usually lower grade tumors than intracranial masses of the same type.

On T1-weighted scans, intramedullary astrocytomas may be defined by abnormal signal intensity and/or cord expansion. Many of these lesions are relatively isointense. Others demonstrate mild or moderate prolongation of T1 values, as seen respectively in the superior thoracic cord in Case 1072 and in the midthoracic region in Case 1073.

Intramedullary astrocytomas vary considerably in texture and architecture. Some tumors are homogeneously solid lesions like the above masses. Other cases demonstrate heterogeneous signal intensity and/or a mixed solid/cystic morphology (see Case 1076).

Thoracic scoliosis is apparent in Case 1072. Intraspinal or paraspinal tumors are a potential cause of pediatric spinal deformity. Screening MR studies of such patients are warranted, particularly if scoliosis is progressive. Back pain (especially nocturnal) is another frequent complaint of children with intramedullary neoplasms.

## Case 1074

11-month-old boy presenting with decreased
crawling and mild scoliosis.
(sagittal, noncontrast T2-weighted FSE scan)

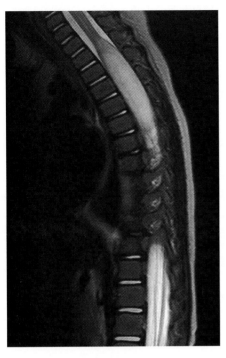

**Astrocytoma**
(same patient as Case 1072)

## Case 1075

55-year-old man presenting with
bilateral arm numbness.
(sagittal, noncontrast T2-weighted FSE scan)

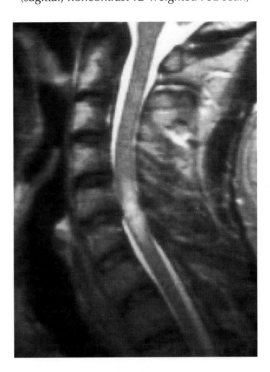

**Astrocytoma**

Astrocytomas usually demonstrate high signal intensity on T2-weighted scans. The region of abnormality may include components of neoplasm, adjacent gliosis, and reactive edema. Intramedullary cysts commonly accompany spinal cord tumors (see Cases 1076, 1077, and 1079) and may contribute to both mass effect and T2 prolongation.

Case 1074 presents a T2-weighted image of the astrocytoma in Case 1072. Prolonged T2 values within this lesion are homogeneous, with no evidence of focal cyst, hemorrhage, necrosis, or varying cellularity. The frequently uniform texture of astrocytomas contrasts with the typical heterogeneity of ependymomas (compare Case 1074 to Case 1082).

Small tumors of the spinal cord may be limited to one or two vertebral levels, with minimal mass effect. Case 1075 illustrates a very focal astrocytoma. The appearance of this lesion is nonspecific, and the differential diagnosis would include myelitis (see Cases 1133 and 1134).

The myelographic effect of the T2-weighted scan in Case 1074 clearly outlines the fusiform expansion of the superior thoracic spinal cord. The spinal cord in Case 1075 is mildly enlarged, occupying the entire anteroposterior diameter of the spinal canal. Subtle expansion of the cord can be difficult to judge in the inferior cervical region, where mildly increased diameter is normally found at the level of the lower motor neurons for the upper extremities.

### Case 1076

4-year-old boy presenting with abnormal gait.
(sagittal, noncontrast T1-weighted SE scan)

### Case 1077

16-year-old boy presenting with neck pain.
(sagittal, noncontrast T2-weighted SE scan)

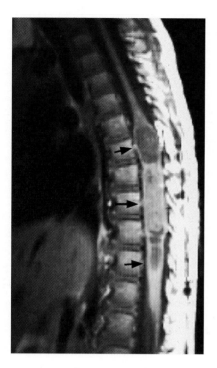

**Astrocytoma**

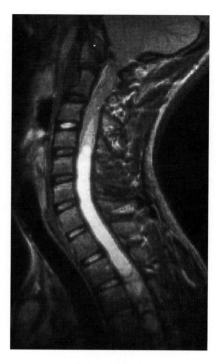

**Astrocytoma**

Cysts are commonly found within or adjacent to intramedullary tumors. Both astrocytomas and ependymomas may contain cystic cavities lined by tumor cells and/or may be bordered by benign, reactive intramedullary cysts. The distinction between primary tumor cysts and secondary syrinxes is usually best made on postcontrast scans (see Cases 1079 and 1085).

In Case 1076, a central mass of isointense tumor tissue *(thick arrow)* is located between rostral and caudal cysts *(thin arrows)*. The solid mass enhanced uniformly, whereas the cyst margins did not. At surgery, neoplastic tissue was limited to the solid nodule, and the polar cysts were found to be reactive.

The majority of the intramedullary expansion in Case 1077 is due to a long cyst containing uniformly high signal intensity on this T2-weighted scan. Surgery demonstrated a low grade astrocytoma at the T3 to T5 level. The cervical cyst contained simple fluid and was not lined by tumor.

Cases 1079 and 1097 present additional examples of spinal astrocytomas with adjacent cysts.

Syringomyelia frequently develops secondarily when mass lesions obstruct the spinal canal, altering normal hydrodynamics. For example, spinal meningiomas or schwannomas may be associated with intramedullary cysts. A fluid loculation within the spinal cord does not necessarily imply that an accompanying mass is intramedullary.

## Case 1078

11-month-old boy presenting with decreased
crawling and mild scoliosis.
(sagittal, postcontrast T1-weighted SE scan)

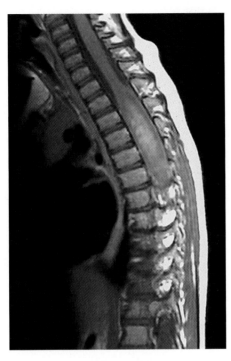

**Astrocytoma**
(same patient as Case 1072)

## Case 1079

13-year-old boy presenting with
back pain and scoliosis.
(coronal, postcontrast T1-weighted SE scan)

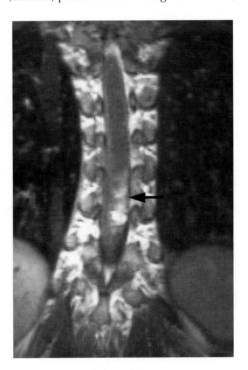

**Astrocytoma**

---

Although the majority of spinal astrocytomas are low grade lesions, these tumors characteristically enhance with contrast material. The absence of enhancement argues against neoplasm as the etiology of an intramedullary mass.

The pattern of contrast enhancement within spinal astrocytomas is highly variable. Many cases demonstrate shaggy or patchy enhancement mixed with nonenhancing portions of the tumor. The modest, predominantly central enhancement of the mass in Case 1078 is typical. (Compare to the precontrast scan of this tumor in Case 1072.)

In Case 1079, more intense, multinodular enhancement is present at the caudal margin of a large intramedullary cyst. There is no enhancement along the superior borders of the fluid collection. Surgery demonstrated an astrocytoma limited to the area of enhancement; the rostral cyst represented benign secondary syringomyelia.

See Case 1097 for an additional example of enhancement within a spinal astrocytoma.

## Case 1080

31-year-old man presenting with
neck pain and intermittent paresthesias.
(sagittal, noncontrast T1-weighted SE scan)

## Case 1081

21-year-old man presenting with
progressive cervical myelopathy.
(sagittal, noncontrast T1-weighted SE scan)

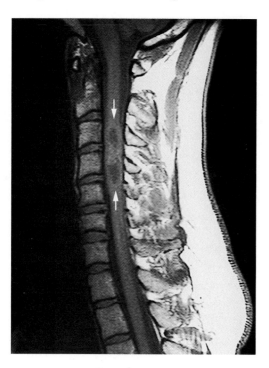

**Ependymoma**

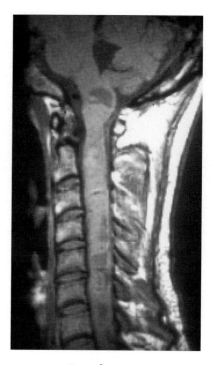

**Ependymoma**

Ependymomas are the most common intramedullary tumors in adults. The average age of patients with spinal ependymomas is about 15 years older than the population presenting with astrocytomas of the cord (early 40s versus mid 20s). Nevertheless, the above cases indicate that young adults may develop tumors of ependymal histology.

Ependymomas are commonly heterogeneous, often containing cysts and hemorrhage. The small tumor in Case 1080 *(arrows)* consists of a central nodule of tissue bordered by rostral and caudal cysts.

Case 1081 presents a larger and more complex ependymoma. The heterogeneous tumor expands the entire cervical spinal cord and extends into the medulla. Scattered areas of high and low signal intensity within the mass probably reflect components of hemorrhage, cystic change, and

calcification. (Correlate with the T2-weighted scan of this patient in Case 1082 and compare to Case 1100.)

At surgery, spinal ependymomas are usually more clearly demarcated from surrounding normal tissue than are intramedullary astrocytomas. However, the sharpness of the tumor margin is not a useful discriminating feature in the MR differential diagnosis between these pathologies.

Intramedullary ependymomas and astrocytomas both occur most commonly in the cervical spinal cord, but the predominance of this location is higher among ependymomas.

The patient in Case 1081 was known to have bilateral acoustic schwannomas. Ependymomas of the spinal cord are among the neoplasms associated with neurofibromatosis type 2, whereas neurofibromatosis type 1 is associated with an increased risk of intramedullary astrocytomas.

### Case 1082

21-year-old man presenting with
cervical myelopathy.
(sagittal, noncontrast T2-weighted SE scan)

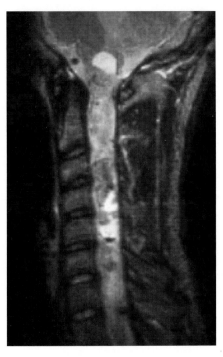

**Ependymoma**
(same patient as Case 1081)

### Case 1083

47-year-old woman presenting with
neck and back pain.
(sagittal, noncontrast T2-weighted SE scan)

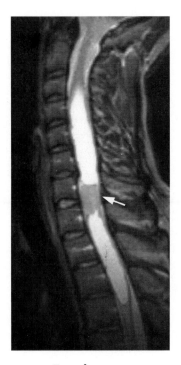

**Ependymoma**

Spinal ependymomas are often strikingly complex on T2-weighted scans. Cyst formation commonly causes small or large areas of high signal intensity on long TR images, seen in Cases 1082 and 1083 respectively.

In addition, blood products are frequently present within or adjacent to spinal ependymomas, contributing zones of low signal intensity to their heterogeneous appearance. In Case 1082, areas of T2-shortening are interspersed throughout the tumor. In other cases, caps of low signal intensity reflecting old blood products are seen at the rostral and/or caudal margins of an intramedullary ependymoma.

Case 1083 presents a simpler appearance. At surgery, tumor was limited to the homogeneous solid tissue in the middle of the lesion *(arrow)*. Benign rostral and caudal cysts were drained and have not recurred on follow-up studies.

Unlike astrocytomas, ependymomas are usually well encapsulated with good demarcation from surrounding parenchyma. As a result, even extensive tumors can often be completely removed with good preservation of function and excellent prognosis.

## Case 1084

27-year-old man presenting with
arm weakness and spastic gait.
(sagittal, postcontrast T1-weighted SE scan)

## Case 1085

47-year-old woman presenting with neck pain.
(sagittal, postcontrast T1-weighted SE scan)

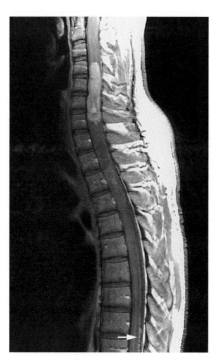

**Ependymoma**

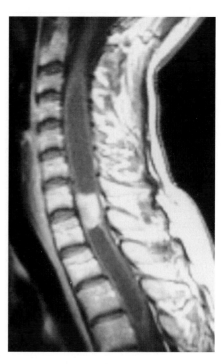

**Ependymoma**
(same patient as Case 1083)

Intense, homogeneous contrast enhancement is usually present within solid components of spinal ependymomas. Uniform enhancement can also be seen within astrocytomas (see Case 1097), but poorly enhancing tumors are more likely to be of astrocytic origin.

The enhancing cervical segment of the intramedullary mass in Case 1084 identifies the region most probably representing cellular neoplasm and most appropriate for biopsy or initial surgical exploration. The nonenhancing expansion of the thoracic spinal cord is of unknown etiology; it is difficult to distinguish poorly enhancing tumor from reactive edema (see Case 1100).

Case 1085 demonstrates enhancement throughout the central mass of Case 1083. No enhancement is present along the margin of the adjacent cysts, suggesting their benign nature.

Enhancement along the dorsal surface of the inferior thoracic spinal cord in Case 1084 is unusually prominent *(arrow)*. Although this finding could reflect venous engorgement due to obstruction of normal drainage patterns, the alternative possibility of pial metastases would have to be considered.

## Case 1086

17-year-old girl presenting with
cranial nerve deficits.
(coronal, postcontrast T1-weighted SE scan)

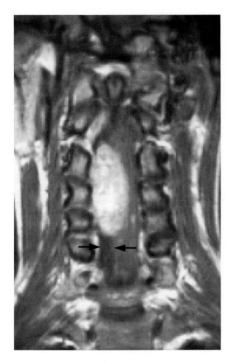

**Ependymoma**

## Case 1087

19-year-old man presenting with back
pain after a volleyball game.
(coronal, postcontrast T1-weighted SE scan)

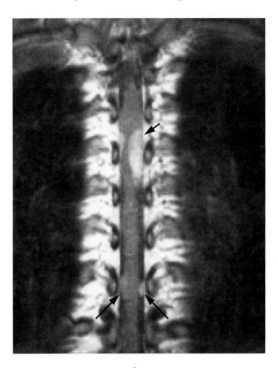

**Ependymoma**

---

Astrocytomas and ependymomas of the spinal canal are occasionally eccentric masses. Ependymomas are particularly prone to exophytic growth, which can be associated with CSF seeding.

The patient in Case 1086 was referred for a cerebral MR scan because of several cranial neuropathies. The study demonstrated leptomeningeal tumors within the posterior fossa, with no apparent intracranial source. The possibility of a disseminating spinal neoplasm was considered, and the cervical tumor was discovered.

Note that the exophytic ependymoma in Case 1086 has displaced the spinal cord in a manner resembling an intradural, extramedullary mass (*arrows;* compare to Cases

1052 and 1096). Together with uniform contrast enhancement, this morphology mimics a meningioma or schwannoma. The rare possibility of an exophytic ependymoma should be included in the differential diagnosis of intradural, extramedullary neoplasms.

Case 1087 illustrates a similar lesion. The primary ependymoma exophytically encircles the spinal cord in the superior thoracic region *(short arrow).* CSF spread of the tumor has occurred, with several distant nodules enhancing along the surface of the thoracic cord more inferiorly *(long arrows).*

Case 1090 presents a smaller exophytic ependymoma of the spinal cord.

# DIFFERENTIAL DIAGNOSIS:
## FOCAL, EXOPHYTIC INTRAMEDULLARY MASS

### Case 1088

37-year-old woman presenting with
clumsiness of the hands.
(sagittal, noncontrast T2-weighted FSE scan)

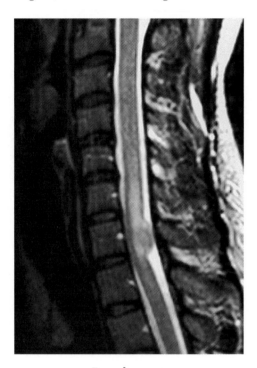

**Ependymoma**

### Case 1089

35-year-old woman presenting with a two-
year history of mild leg weakness.
(sagittal, noncontrast T2-weighted FSE scan)

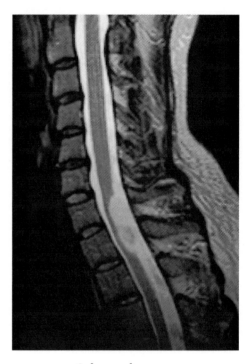

**Subependymoma**

As discussed on the preceding page, ependymomas of the spinal cord are occasionally eccentric and/or exophytic. Case 1088 presents another example. A relatively isointense nodule projects posteriorly from the dorsal surface of the cord, displacing the remainder of the cord anteriorly and widening the dorsal subarachnoid space. Adjacent intramedullary edema is present.

The tumor in Case 1089 is also eccentric and dorsally exophytic. At surgery, this mass proved to be a subependymoma. The MR features of the lesion do not distinguish it from an ependymoma (or an astrocytoma). However, contrast enhancement of the tumor in Case 1089 was minimal,

which would be unusual for even a low grade astrocytoma or ependymoma of the spinal cord but is typical for subependymomas. (Enhancement of the ependymoma in Case 1088 was focal and intense; see Case 1090.)

Intracranial subependymomas have been discussed in Case 129. Spinal forms of this tumor are similarly rare, slow-growing, and poorly enhancing.

The differential diagnosis in the above cases would include a pial-based lesion such as CSF-borne "drop" metastases or sarcoidosis (see Case 1146). Intradural extramedullary tumors could also be considered, as discussed on the next page.

### Case 1090

37-year-old woman presenting with
clumsiness of the hands.
(sagittal, postcontrast T1-weighted SE scan)

### Case 1091

54-year-old woman presenting with leg weakness.
(axial, postcontrast T1-weighted
SE scan; T10-11 level)

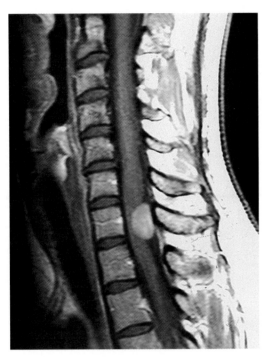

**Ependymoma**
(same patient as Case 1088)

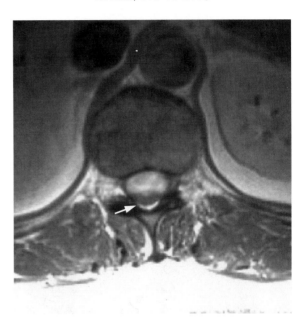

**Schwannoma**
(same patient as Case 1067)

Uniform and intense contrast enhancement within an exophytic ependymoma of the spinal cord may mimic a benign, intradural extramedullary mass, as illustrated above.

Case 1090 presents a postcontrast image of the patient in Case 1088. Enhancement is limited to the dorsal nodule; the surrounding zone of nonenhancing T2 prolongation likely represents edema. The sharp definition of the margin of enhancement in this case (and in Cases 1084 to 1087) contrasts with the usually less well-demarcated margin of enhancement in intramedullary astrocytomas.

The ventral schwannoma in Case 1091 occupies most of the dural sac. The spinal cord is severely displaced and compressed dorsally (*arrow;* see Case 1067 for a sagittal view). Uniform contrast enhancement within the lesion is typical but nonspecific. A meningioma or an intradural metastasis (of systemic or CNS origin) would be included in the differential diagnosis.

Ventral location (as in Case 1091) is relatively uncommon for meningiomas below the foramen magnum. These tumors more typically arise dorsally or laterally (see Cases 1051, 1052, and 1096).

Occasional intradural hemangiomas are extramedullary and intensely enhancing, resembling the above lesions.

### Case 1092

9-year-old boy presenting with low back pain.
(sagittal, noncontrast T1-weighted SE scan)

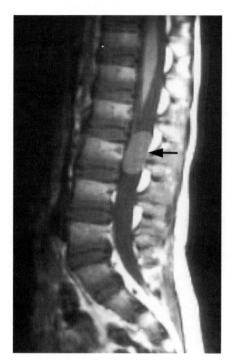

**Myxopapillary Ependymoma**

### Case 1093

55-year-old woman referred by a chiropractor
because of increasing leg weakness.
(sagittal, noncontrast T2-weighted FSE scan)

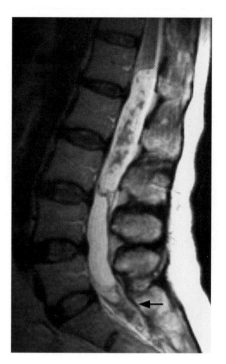

**Myxopapillary Ependymoma**

---

Myxopapillary ependymomas arise from the conus medullaris or filum terminale and are histologically distinct from intramedullary ependymomas of the cervical or thoracic region. The myxopapillary tumors contain a mucoid matrix surrounding cellular regions with papillary morphology and moderate vascularity. These masses grow slowly and can eventually fill the lumbosacral canal with scalloping of vertebral bodies and enlargement of intervertebral foramina.

The lumbar tumor in Case 1092 is homogeneous. (A T2-weighted scan demonstrated uniformly high signal intensity.) The morphology of this intradural lesion suggests a meningioma (compare to Case 1050), but meningiomas are rarely encountered in the lumbar region, particularly in a child. A schwannoma would be another diagnostic possibility (compare the character of the mass to Case 1055), although schwannomas this large are often cystic or hemorrhagic. Surgery demonstrated a myxopapillary ependymoma arising from the filum terminale.

The neoplasm in Case 1093 is more heterogeneous. Overall prolonged T2 values surround multiple areas of lower signal intensity, correlating with both the myxoid matrix and the presence of small hemorrhages within the tumor. The mass occupies the entire anteroposterior diameter of the spinal canal, displacing and compressing the nerve roots of the cauda equina.

Note the cellular debris and/or blood products filling the caudal end of the thecal sac in Case 1093 *(arrow)*. Subtle deposits of tissue in this gravitationally dependent location can be an early clue to the presence of CSF-borne metastases. (See Case 1042 for another example.)

As illustrated above, myxopapillary ependymomas of the conus medullaris or cauda equina can present in childhood or in adult patients. These tumors are substantially more common in males than in females.

Because the filum terminale (with associated rests of ependymal cells) extends caudally as far as the second sacral vertebra, myxopapillary ependymomas may arise in the sacral region. Occasional presacral ependymomas present as lobulated pelvic masses. Alternatively, "subcutaneous" myxopapillary ependymomas may be encountered posterior to the sacrum.

### Case 1094A

7-year-old girl presenting with back pain, leg stiffness, and urinary urgency. (sagittal, noncontrast T2-weighted SE scan)

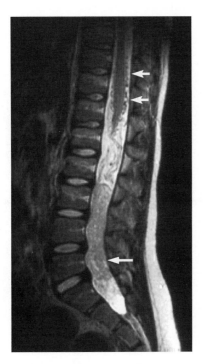

**Myxopapillary Ependymoma**

### Case 1094B

Same patient. (sagittal, postconstrast T1-weighted SE scan)

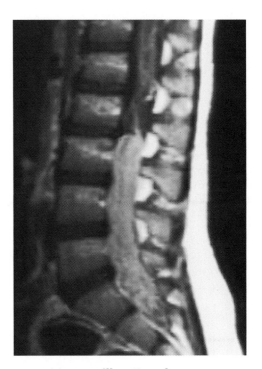

**Myxopapillary Ependymoma**

Low grade myxopapillary ependymomas of the filum terminale may enlarge to fill and expand the lumbar spinal canal. Further growth may extend through intervertebral foramina into the paraspinal region. Such bulky tumors may resemble a lobulated schwannoma or neurofibroma (or the occasional intraspinal neuroblastoma, as in Cases 1020 and 1021).

The signal intensity of the large intradural mass in Case 1094A *(long arrow)* is intermediate and homogeneous. The long-standing mass has caused mild scalloping of the posterior margin of the L4 and L5 vertebral bodies (compare to Case 1020). Tortuous intrathecal nerve roots are seen above the tumor, reflecting a long history of traction and displacement.

Prominent vessels are present on the surface of the conus medullaris in Case 1094A *(short arrows).* Distention of intrathecal veins near an ependymoma has been well recognized myelographically and should be considered in the differential diagnosis of spinal vascular malformations.

The finding may reflect congestion due to the obstructing mass effect of the tumor and/or hypervascularity of the mass itself. Spinal ependymomas are among the potential causes of intracranial superficial siderosis (see Cases 721 and 722) due to recurrent small subarachnoid hemorrhages.

The postcontrast scan in Case 1094B is blurred by patient motion. However, uniform enhancement is apparent throughout the tumor. Enhancement along the surface of the conus medullaris may represent the prominent vessels noted on the noncontrast scan or pial extension of tumor. A large schwannoma or ganglioneuroma could fill the lumbar canal and resemble Case 1094B.

The potential variation in size and morphology of myxopapillary ependymomas (as illustrated by Cases 1092-1094) means that these tumors should be considered in the differential diagnosis of most intrathecal masses in the lumbar region.

## Case 1095

9-year-old boy presenting with low back pain.
(sagittal, postcontrast T1-weighted SE scan)

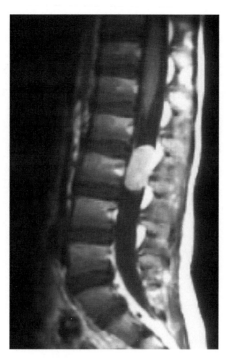

**Myxopapillary Ependymoma**
(same patient as Case 1092)

## Case 1096

41-year-old woman with increasing
difficulty walking.
(sagittal, postcontrast T1-weighted SE scan)

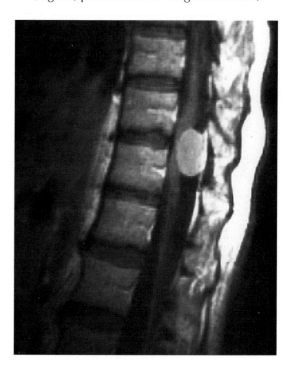

**Meningioma**

---

Myxopapillary ependymomas of the conus medullaris and cauda equina are often more homogeneous than ependymomas within the cervical or thoracic spinal cord. Case 1095 is a postcontrast image of the myxopapillary tumor presented in Case 1092. The morphology, homogeneity, and uniformly intense enhancement of the lesion resemble the meningioma in Case 1096. However, a meningioma would be extremely rare in the lumbar region of a 9-year-old boy. (The "clear cell" variant of meningiomas occasionally occurs in the lumbar canal of children.)

Meningiomas typically demonstrate homogeneous and intense enhancement, as in Case 1096. Dorsolateral location in the thoracic region of women from 40 to 70 years of age is a characteristic setting for these lesions (see Cases 1050-1052).

A schwannoma would also be considered in each of the above cases. However, schwannomas as large as these lesions often demonstrate more heterogeneous contrast enhancement (see Case 1062).

Hematogenous or "drop" metastases should be included in the differential diagnosis of a uniformly enhancing intradural mass. The gravitationally dependent caudal end of the thecal sac is commonly involved by settling of metastatic cells. Subtle amputation of the terminal sac by accumulation of soft tissue may help to characterize nodular or spherical masses at higher levels.

Intradural extramedullary hemangiomas occur rarely and can mimic the MR appearance of the cellular tumors discussed above.

# DIFFERENTIAL DIAGNOSIS:
## TUMOR INVOLVING THE CONUS MEDULLARIS IN A CHILD

### Case 1097

9-year-old girl presenting with a several-year history of itching on the dorsum of the feet. (coronal, postcontrast T1-weighted SE scan)

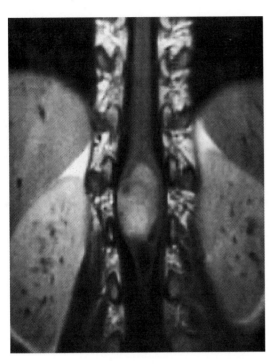

**Astrocytoma**

### Case 1098

8-year-old boy presenting with severe back pain. (sagittal, postcontrast T1-weighted SE scan)

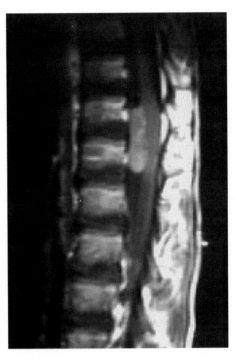

**Primitive Neuroectodermal Tumor**

---

Myxopapillary ependymomas are the most common primary neoplasms of the conus medullaris and cauda equina, but many other tumors can occur in this region.

Astrocytomas may involve any portion of the spinal cord, including the conus medullaris. The mass in Case 1097 demonstrates predominantly uniform enhancement. Small cysts are seen at the caudal pole of the tumor. Although the interface between the enhancing lesion and adjacent parenchyma appears well defined, astrocytomas are usually poorly encapsulated.

Primitive neuroectodermal tumors are among the rarer malignancies encountered in the region of the conus medullaris. The intensely enhancing exophytic mass in Case 1098 resembles the ependymomas in Cases 1086 and 1087.

Paragangliomas occasionally arise in the intradural compartment, usually near the thoracolumbar junction. Although a characteristic microscopic pattern of compact cell nests or "Zellballen" has been described in paragangliomas, special immunohistochemical stains may be necessary to distinguish these neuroendocrine tumors from lumbar ependymomas. Paragangliomas are highly vascular, and marked enlargement of pial veins is an imaging clue that should lead to their consideration.

Hemangioblastomas are sometimes discovered at the level of the conus medullaris (see Case 1099), but pediatric presentation would be rare.

The intensely enhancing astrocytoma in Case 1097 proved to be a low grade lesion. The presence and degree of contrast enhancement within spinal gliomas do not correlate with the grade of malignancy as closely as in intracranial tumors.

### Case 1099

77-year-old woman presenting with
back pain and leg numbness.
(sagittal, postcontrast T1-weighted SE scan)

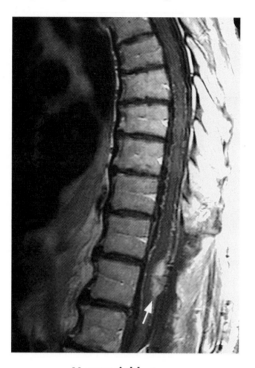

**Hemangioblastoma**

### Case 1100

37-year-old man presenting with progressive
spastic quadriparesis.
(sagittal, postcontrast T1-weighted SE scan)

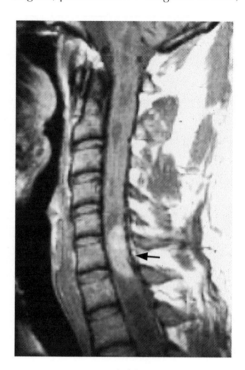

**Hemangioblastoma**

Hemangioblastomas are the third most common primary tumor of the spinal cord but account for less than 5% of intramedullary neoplasms. They involve the cervical and thoracic regions with nearly equal frequency. Affected patients typically present around the age of 40 years.

Most spinal hemangioblastomas are solitary lesions. About a third of patients with spinal hemangioblastomas have von Hippel-Lindau syndrome, with associated retinal and cerebellar tumors.

The MR characteristics of spinal hemangioblastomas resemble the intracranial lesions described in Cases 183-187. Solid tumor tissue is usually well defined by intense enhancement and abuts the pial surface of the cord. Prominent vessels may be apparent. Although hemangioblastomas of the spinal cord are usually small lesions, they often incite extensive edema and/or cyst formation within adjacent parenchyma. About 30% of spinal hemangioblastomas are partially or entirely extramedullary.

In Case 1099, surgery had been performed with partial resection of the intensely enhancing mass at the dorsal margin of the conus medullaris. The pial base of the residual tumor *(arrow)* and the very prominent vessels surrounding the spinal cord are typical features of spinal he-

mangioblastomas. No intramedullary cyst is present in this case.

Noncontrast scans in Case 1100 demonstrated mottled signal intensity throughout the cervical cord. A focal mass was not defined. Intense contrast enhancement of the tumor nodule *(arrow)* established the appropriate site for biopsy. At surgery, a hemangioblastoma was found to precisely conform to the margins of enhancement. The more rostral and caudal expansion of the cord was due to swampy edema, with a chain of small cysts that drained clear fluid when the tumor was removed.

The above cases illustrate that the extent of abnormal vascularity adjacent to spinal hemangioblastomas is variable. The enlarged pial vessels in Case 1099 resemble the appearance of a vascular malformation (compare to Cases 1209, 1211, and 1215), while no abnormal vessels are apparent in Case 1100.

Large vascular channels within or adjacent to a spinal mass can support the diagnosis of hemangioblastoma, but it should be remembered that prominent superficial vessels may also be associated with other intramedullary tumors (see Case 1094).

# DIFFERENTIAL DIAGNOSIS:
## INTRAMEDULLARY TUMOR WITH ADJACENT CYSTS

### Case 1101

31-year-old man presenting with
neck pain and intermittent paresthesias.
(sagittal, postcontrast T1-weighted SE scan)

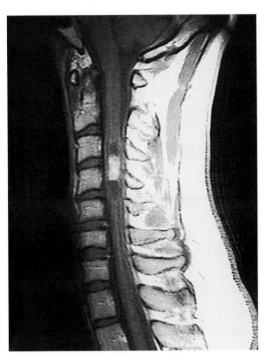

**Ependymoma**
(same patient as Case 1080)

### Case 1102

34-year-old man presenting with
neck pain and arm weakness.
(sagittal, postcontrast T1-weighted SE scan)

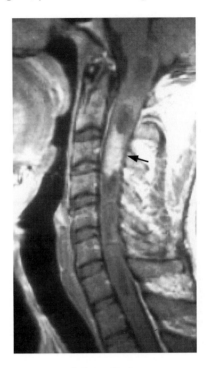

**Astrocytoma**

---

Glial tumors can present with a combination of enhancing nodules and adjacent cysts resembling hemangioblastomas.

Case 1101 is a postcontrast view of the small cervical ependymoma in Case 1080. The intensely enhancing central tumor is bordered by nonenhancing cysts that proved to be non-neoplastic. Note that the enhancing nodule does not contact the pial surface of the cord. If confirmed in all projections, this feature decreases the likelihood of hemangioblastoma in the differential diagnosis.

The astrocytoma in Case 1102 mimics the heman-

gioblastoma in Case 1100: a limited area of contrast enhancement *(arrow)* is seen within a larger lesion. However, additional subtle areas of enhancement are present both rostral and caudal to the main nodule. These more infiltrating components of enhancement are typical of astrocytomas and are distinct from the usual solitary enhancing focus of a hemangioblastoma.

Cases 1101 and 1102 again demonstrate that both astrocytomas and ependymomas are commonly associated with intramedullary cysts. Confident MR distinction between these pathologies is often difficult.

### Case 1103

28-year-old man with AIDS.
(sagittal, noncontrast T1-weighted SE scan)

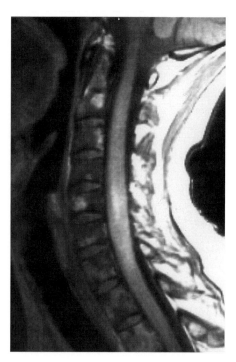

**Primary CNS Lymphoma**

### Case 1104

2-year-old girl with a history of surgery
for a spinal cord tumor.
(sagittal, noncontrast T1-weighted SE scan)

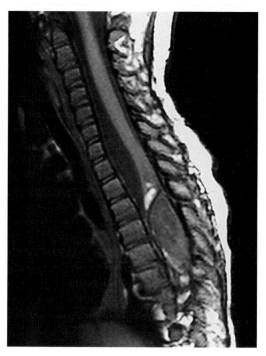

**Teratoma**

A number of rare primary tumors may involve the spinal cord and conus medullaris. Oligodendrogliomas occasionally arise within the spinal cord, as do gangliogliomas and primitive neuroectodermal tumors (see Case 1098). Intramedullary schwannomas and paragangliomas have been reported; the latter are most common near the conus medullaris.

The expansion of the cervical spinal cord in Case 1103 is nonspecific. The patient had known intracerebral lymphoma. Spinal cord involvement in such cases may include CSF seeding of the central canal, which is occasionally also seen in patients with medulloblastoma.

Abnormally low signal intensity within the marrow of cervical vertebrae provides a diagnostic clue in Case 1103. This finding is frequent in AIDS patients, reflecting increased iron stores due to "anemia of chronic disease."

Teratomas are rare tumors within the spinal canal, representing about 0.1% of all intraspinal neoplasms. They may be intramedullary or extramedullary, solid or cystic, simple or complex.

The mass in Case 1104 has previously expanded the spinal canal at the cervicothoracic junction and is associated with scoliosis. The central component of the tumor is homogeneous. The regions of short T1 values at the poles of the lesion demonstrated low signal intensity on fast spin echo images (see Case 1268), suggesting blood products or thickly proteinaceous material.

The alternative possibility of a neurenteric cyst would be considered in the differential diagnosis of Case 1104 (see Cases 1266 and 1267), although no associated vertebral anomaly is apparent.

676

### Case 1105

55-year-old woman presenting with
gait abnormality.
(sagittal, noncontrast T1-weighted SE scan)

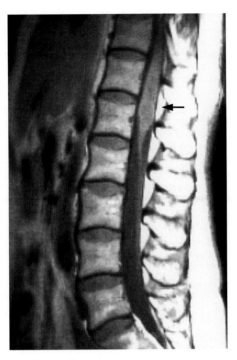

**Metastatic Carcinoma of the Breast**

### Case 1106

53-year-old woman presenting with
dysfunction of the conus medullaris.
(sagittal, postcontrast T1-weighted SE scan)

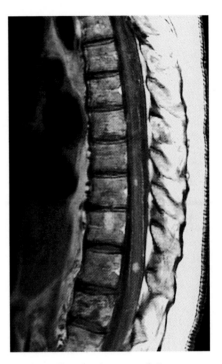

**Metastatic Carcinoma of the Breast**

Metastases to the spinal cord from systemic carcinomas are much less common than vertebral and epidural implants. However, intramedullary metastases should be considered in any patient presenting with myelopathy and a history of cancer. Carcinoma of the lung is the most frequent cause of intramedullary metastases, followed by carcinoma of the breast, melanoma, and hypernephroma.

The conus medullaris is a common site for metastatic involvement of the spinal cord, as illustrated in Case 1105 (see also Case 1214). Expansion and low signal intensity of the conus on this scan are nonspecific (compare to Cases 1150 and 1206), but a postcontrast scan demonstrated a central enhancing nodule. No accompanying vertebral or intradural extramedullary metastases were noted.

Case 1106 demonstrates several enhancing intramedullary masses. Nodules in the inferior thoracic spinal cord and the conus medullaris are well defined, with more patchy intramedullary enhancement in the superior thoracic region.

In some patients, intramedullary metastases incite edema extending several segments beyond the tumor, causing expansion of the spinal cord with prolonged T1 and T2 values. The appearance in such cases can resemble Cases 1100 and 1102.

Extensive enhancement is present at the surface of the spinal cord in Case 1106, raising the question of meningeal carcinomatosis (versus unusually prominent pial vessels). Some of the heterogeneous signal intensity within vertebral bodies on this scan may be benign (see Cases 992 and 993), but osseous metastases are probably present.

The patient in Case 1106 had undergone mastectomy and radiation for carcinoma of the breast ten years earlier. It is not uncommon to discover cerebral or spinal metastases from breast carcinoma developing a decade or more after treatment of the primary tumor.

Compare Case 1106 to the examples of pial and intramedullary sarcoidosis in Cases 1143 and 1144.

# REFERENCES

Aggarwal S, Deck JHN, Kucharczyk W: Neuroendocrine tumor (paraganglioma) of the cauda equina: MR and pathologic findings. *AJNR* 14:1003-1007, 1993.

Araki Y, Ishida T, Ootani M, et al: MRI of paraganglioma of the cauda equina. *Neuroradiology* 35:232-233, 1993.

Arnautovic KI, Al-Mefty O, Husain M: Ventral foramen magnum meningioma. *J Neurosurg Spine* 92:71-80, 2000.

Ashkenazi E, Onesti ST, Kader A, et al: Paraganglioma of the filum terminale: case report and literature review. *J Spinal Disord* 11:540-542, 1998.

Baker KB, Moran CJ, Wippold FJ II, et al: MR imaging of spinal hemangioblastoma. *Am J Roentgenol* 174:377-382, 2000.

Barloon TJ, Yuh WTC, Yang CJC, Schultz DH: Spinal subarachnoid tumor seeding from intracranial metastases: MR findings. *J Comput Assist Tomogr* 11:242-244, 1987.

Bazan C III: Imaging of lumbosacral spine neoplasms. *Neuroimaging Clin N Amer* 3:591-608, 1993.

Berns DH, Blaser S, Ross JS, et al: MR imaging with Gd-DTPA in leptomeningeal spread of lymphoma. *J Comput Assist Tomogr* 12:499-500, 1988.

Boncoeur-Martel MP, Lesort A, Moreau JJ, et al: MRI of paraganglioma of the filum terminale. *J Comput Assist Tomog* 20:162-165, 1996.

Bouffet E, Pierre-Kahn A, Marchal JC, et al: Prognostic factors in pediatric spinal cord astrocytoma. *Cancer* 83:2391-2399, 1998.

Bourgouin PM, Lesage J, Fontaine S, et al: A pattern approach to the differential diagnosis of intramedullary spinal cord lesions on MR imaging. *Am J Roentgenol* 170:1645-1649, 1998.

Brunberg JA, DiPietro MA, Venes JL, et al: Intramedullary lesions of the pediatric spinal cord: correlation of findings from MR imaging, intraoperative sonography, surgery, and histologic study. *Radiology* 181:573-579, 1991.

Burk D, Brunberg J, Kanal E, et al: Spinal and paraspinal neurofibromatosis: MR imaging. *Radiology* 162:797, 1987.

Cellerini M, Salti S, Desideri V, Marconi G: MR imaging of the cauda equina in hereditary motor sensory neuropathies: correlations with sural nerve biopsy. *AJNR* 21:1793-1798, 2000.

Chamberlain MC, Sandy AD, Press GA: Spinal tumors: gadolinium-DTPA-enhanced MR imaging. *Neuroradiology* 33:469-474, 1991.

Choi SK, Bowers RP, Buckthal PE: MR imaging in hypertrophic neuropathy: a case of hereditary motor and sensory neuropathy, type I (Charcot-Marie-Tooth). *Clin Imaging* 14:204-207, 1990.

Chung JY, Lee SK, Yang KH, Song MK: Subcutaneous sacrococcygeal myxopapillary ependymoma. *AJNR* 20:344-347, 1999.

Chu B-C, Terae S, Hida K, et al: MR findings in spinal hemangioblastoma: correlation with symptoms and with angiographic and surgical findings. *AJNR* 22:206-217, 2001.

Conway JE, Chou D, Clatterbuck RE, et al: Hemangioblastomas of the central nervous system in von Hippel-Lindau syndrome and sporadic disease. *Neurosurgery* 48:55-63, 2001.

Corr P, Dicker T, Wright M: Exophytic intramedullary hemangioblastoma presenting as an extramedullary mass on myelography. *AJNR* 16:883-884, 1995.

Davis PC, Friedman NC, Fry SM, et al: Leptomeningeal metastasis: MR imaging. *Radiology* 163:449-454, 1987.

DeAngelis LM: Current diagnosis and treatment of leptomeningeal metastasis. *J Neurooncol* 38:245-252, 1998.

Demachi H, Takashima T, Kadoya M, et al: MR imaging of spinal neurinomas with pathological correlation. *J Comput Assist Tomogr* 14:250-254, 1992.

Dillon WP, Norman D, Newton TH, et al: Intradural spinal cord lesions: Gd-DTPA-enhanced MR imaging. *Radiology* 170:229-232, 1989.

Domingues RC, Mikulis D, Swearingen B, et al: Subcutaneous sacrococcygeal myxopapillary ependymona: CT and MR findings. *AJNR* 12:171-172, 1991.

Egelhoff JC, Bates DJ, Ross JS, et al: Spinal MR findings in neurofibromatosis types 1 and 2. *AJNR* 13:1071-1077, 1990.

Epstein FJ, Farmer J-P, Freed D: Adult intramedullary astrocytomas of the spinal cord. *J Neurosurg* 77:355-359, 1992.

Faro SH, Turtz AR, Koenigsberg, RA, et al: Paraganglioma of the cauda equina with associated intramedullary cysts: MR findings. *AJNR* 18:1588-1590, 1997.

Fine MJ, Kricheff II, Freed D, Epstein FJ: Spinal cord ependymomas: MR imaging features. *Radiology* 197:655-658, 1995.

Friedman DP, Flanders AE, Tartaglino LM: Vascular neoplasms and malformations, ischemia, and hemorrhage affecting the spinal cord: MR imaging findings. *Am J Roentgenol* 162:685-692, 1994.

Friedman DP, Tartaglino LM, Flanders AE: Intradural schwannomas of the spine: MR findings with emphasis on contrast-enhancement characteristics. *Am J Roentgenol* 158:1347-1350, 1992.

Ginsberg LE, Williams DW, Stanton C: Intrasacral myxopapillary ependymoma. *Neuroradiology* 36:56-58, 1994.

Goy AMC, Pinto RS, Raghavendra BN, et al: Intramedullary spinal-cord tumors: MR imaging with emphasis on associated cysts. *Radiology* 161:381-386, 1986.

Halliday AL, Sobel RA, Martuza RL: Benign spinal nerve sheath tumors: their occurrence sporadically and in neurofibromatosis type 1 and 2. *J Neurosurg* 74:248-253, 1991.

Heinz R, Wiener D, Friedman H, Tien R: Detection of cerebrospinal fluid metastasis: CT myelography or MR? *AJNR* 16:1147-1151, 1995.

Hu HP, Huang QL: Signal intensity correlation of MRI with pathological findings in spinal neurinomas. *Neuroradiology* 34:98-102, 1992.

Ishii N, Matsuzaswa H, Houkin K, et al: An evaluation of 70 spinal schwannomas using conventional computed tomography and magnetic resonance imaging. *Neuroradiology* 33:542, 1991.

Kaffenberger DA, Shah CP, Murtagh FR, et al: MR imaging of spinal cord hemangioblastoma associated with syringomyelia. *J Comput Assist Tomogr* 12:495-498, 1988.

Kahan H, Sklar EM, Post MJD, Bruce JH: MR characteristics of histopathologic subtypes of spinal ependymomas. *AJNR* 17:143-150, 1996.

Knopp EA, Chynn KY, Hughes J: Primary lymphoma of the cauda equina: myelographic, CT myelographic, and MR appearance. *AJNR* 15:1187-1189, 1994.

Koeller KK, Rosenblum RS, Morrison AL: Neoplasms of the spinal cord and filum terminale: radiologic-pathologic correlation. *Radiographics* 20:1721-1749, 2000.

Krol G, Sze G, Malkin M, Walker R: MR of cranial and spinal meningeal carcinomatosis, comparison with CT and myelography. *AJNR* 9:709-714, 1988.

Lefton DR, Pinto RS, Martin SW: MRI features of intracranial and spinal ependymomas. *Pediatr Neurosurg* 28:97-105, 1998.

Levy RA: Paraganglioma of the filum terminale: MR findings. *Am J Roentgenol* 160:851-852, 1993.

Li MH, Holtas S: MR imaging of spinal neurofibromatosis. *Acta Radiol* 32, fasc 4:279-285, 1991.

Li MH, Holtas S. Larsson E-M: MR imaging of intradural extramedullary tumors. *Acta Radiol* 33:207-212, 1992.

Lim V, Sobel DF, Zyroff J: Spinal cord pial metastases: MR imaging with gadopentetate dimeglumine. *AJNR* 11:975-982, 1990.

Maki DD, Yousem DM, Corcoran C, Galetta SL: MR imaging of Dejerine-Sottas disease. *AJNR* 20:378-380, 1999.

Masaryk TJ: Neoplastic disease of the spine. *Radiol Clin North Am* 29:829-846, 1991.

Masuda N, Hayashi H, Tanebe H: Nerve root and sciatic trunk enlargement in Dejerine-Sottas disease: MRI appearances. *Neuroradiology* 35:36-37, 1992.

Matsumoto S, Hasu K, Uchino A, et al: MRI of intradural-extramedullary spinal neurinomas and meningiomas. *Clinical Imaging* 17:46-52, 1993.

Mautner VF, Tatagiba M, Lindenau M, et al: Spinal tumors in patients with neurofibromatosis type 2: MR imaging study of frequency, multiplicity, and variety. *Am J Roentgenol* 165:951-958, 1995.

McCormick PC, Torres R, Post KD, Stein BM: Intramedullary ependymoma of the spinal cord. *J Neurosurg* 62:523-532, 1990.

Meyers SP, Wildenhain SL, Chang J-K, et al: Postoperative evaluation for disseminated medulloblastoma involving the spine: contrast-enhanced MR findings, CSF cytologic analysis, timing of disease occurrence, and patient outcomes. *AJNR* 21:1757-1766, 2000.

Murota T, Symon L: Surgical management of hemangioblastoma of the spinal cord: a report of 18 cases. *Neurosurgery* 25:699-708, 1989.

Murphey MD, Smith WS, Smith SE, et al: Imaging of musculoskeletal neurogenic tumors: radiologic-pathologic correlation. *Radiographics* 19:1253-1280, 1999.

Nakasu Y, Minouchi K, Hatsuda N, et al: Thoracic meningiocele vs neurofibromatosis: CT and MR findings. *J Comput Assist Tomogr* 15:1062-1064, 1991.

Nemoto Y, Inoue Y, Tashiro T, et al: Intramedullary spinal cord tumors: significance of associated hemorrhage at MR imaging. *Radiology* 182:793-796, 1992.

Nokes SR, Murtagh FR, Jones JD, et al: Childhood scoliosis: MR imaging. *Radiology* 164:791, 1987.

Packer RJ, Zimmerman RA, Sutton LN, et al: Magnetic resonance imaging of spinal cord disease in childhood. *Pediatrics* 78:251, 1986.

Papadatos D, Albrecht S, Mohr G, del Carpio-O'Donovan R: Exophytic primitive neuroectodermal tumor of the spinal cord. *AJNR* 19:787-790, 1998.

Parizel PM, Baleriaux D, Rodesch G, et al: Gd-DTPA-enhanced MR imaging of spinal tumors. *AJNR* 10:249-258, 1989.

Patel U, Pinto RS, Miller DC, et al: MR of spinal cord ganglioglioma. *AJNR* 19:879-888, 1998.

Post MJD, Quencer RM, Green BA, et al: Intramedullary spinal cord metastases, mainly of nonneurogenic origin. *AJNR* 8:339-346, 1987.

Patronas NJ, Courcoutsakis N, Bromley C, et al: Intramedullary and spinal canal tumors in patients with neurofibromatosis 2: MR imaging fiindings and correlation with genotype. *Radiology* 218:434-442, 2001.

Rees JH, Smirniotopoulos JG, Moran C, Mena H: Paragangliomas of the cauda equina: imaging features with radiologic-pathologic correlation. *Int J Neurorad* 2:242-250, 1996.

Roux FX, Nataf F, Pinaudeau M, et al: Intraspinal meningiomas: review of 54 cases with discussion of poor prognosis factors and modern therapeutic management. *Surg Neurol* 46:458-463, 1996.

Rubin JM, Aisen AM, DiPietro MA: Ambiguities of MR imaging of tumoral cysts in the spinal cord. *J Comput Assist Tomogr* 10:395-398, 1986.

Schroth G, Thron A, Guhl L, et al: Magnetic resonance imaging of spinal meningiomas and neurinomas: improvement of imaging by paramagnetic contrast enhancement. *J Neurosurg* 66:695-700, 1987.

Schuknecht B, Huber P, Buller B, Nadjimi M: Spinal leptomeningeal neoplastic disease. *Eur Neurol* 32:11-16, 1992.

Schweitzer JS, Batzdorf U: Ependymomas of the cauda equina region: diagnosis, treatment, and outcome in 15 patients. *Neurosurgery* 30:202-207, 1992.

Scotti G, Scialfa G, Columbo N, et al: Magnetic resonance diagnosis of intramedullary tumors of the spinal cord. *Neuroradiology* 29:130-135, 1987.

Sevick RJ: Cervical spine tumors. *Neuroimaging Clin North Am* 5:385-400, 1995.

Shen W, Ho Y, Lee S, Lee K: Ependymoma of the cauda equina presenting with subarachnoid hemorrhage. *AJNR* 14:399-400, 1993.

Shen WC, Lee SK, Chang CY, Ho WL: Cystic spinal neurilemmoma on magnetic resonance imaging. *Neuroradiology* 34:447-448, 1992.

Silbergeld J, Cohen WA, Maravilla KR, et al: Supratentorial and spinal cord hemangioblastomas: gadolinium-enhanced MR appearance with pathologic correlation. *J Comput Assist Tomogr* 13:1048-1051, 1989.

Slasky BS, Bydder GM, Niendorf HP, Young IR: MR imaging with gadolinium-DTPA in the differentiation of tumor, syrinz, and cyst of the spinal cord. *J Comput Assist Tomogr* 11:845-850, 1987.

Smyth MD, Pitts L, Jackler RK, Aldape KD: Metastatic spinal ependymoma presenting as a vestibular schwannoma. Case illustration. *J Neurosurg:Spine* 92:247, 2000.

Solero CL, Fornari M, Giombini S, et al: Spinal meningiomas: review of 174 operated cases. *Neurosurgery* 25:153-160, 1989.

Stimac GK, Porter BA, Olson DO, et al: Gadolinium-DTPA-enhanced MR imaging of spinal neoplasms: preliminary investigation and comparison with unenhanced spin echo and STIR sequences. *AJNR* 9:839-846, 1988.

Sugahara T, Korogi Y, Hirai T, et al: Contrast-enhanced T1-weighted three-dimensional gradient-echo imaging of the whole spine for intradural tumor dissemination. *AJNR* 19:1773-1779, 1998.

Sze G: Magnetic resonance imaging in the evaluation of spinal tumors. *Cancer* 67:1229-1241, 1991.

Sze G, Abramson A, Krol G, et al: Gadolinium-DTPA/dimeglumine in the MR evaluation of intradural extramedullary spinal disease. *AJNR* 9:153-163, 1988.

Sze, G, Krol G, Zimmerman RD, Deck DMF: Intramedullary disease of the spine: diagnosis of using gadolinium-DPTA-enhanced MR imaging. *AJNR* 9:847-858, 1988.

Sze G, Merriam M, Oshio K, Jolez FA: Fast spin-echo imaging in the evaluation of intradural disease of the spine. *AJNR* 13:1383-1393, 1992.

Sze G, Stimac GK, Barlett C, et al: Multicenter study or gadopentetate dimeglumine as an MR contrast agent: evaluation in patients with spinal cord tumors. *AJNR* 11:967-974, 1990.

Thakkar SD, Feigen U, Mautner V-F: Spinal tumours in neurofibromatosis type 1: an MRI study of frequency, multiplicity and variety. *Neuroradiology* 41:625-629, 1999.

Weber AL, Montandon C, Robson C: Neurogenic tumors of the neck. *Radiol Clin North Am* 38:1077-1090, 2000.

Williams AL, Haughton VM, Pojunas KW, et al: Differentiation of intramedullary neoplasms and cysts by MR. *AJNR* 8:527-532, 1987.

Yousem DM, Patrone PM, Grossman RI: Leptomeningeal metastases: MR evaluation. *J Comput Assist Tomog* 14:255-261, 1990.

Zimmerman RA, Bilaniuk LT: Imaging of tumors of the spinal canal and cord. *Radiol Clin North Am* 26:965-1007, 1988.

# CHAPTER 20

# Inflammatory Disorders
# of the Spinal Canal

### Case 1107

73-year-old man presenting with arm and leg
weakness and staphylococcal septicemia.
(sagittal, noncontrast T1-weighted SE scan)

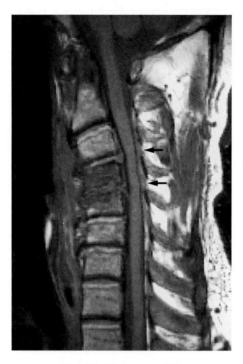

**Discitis/Osteomyelitis**

### Case 1108

79-year-old woman presenting with
severe back pain.
(sagittal, noncontrast T1-weighted SE scan)

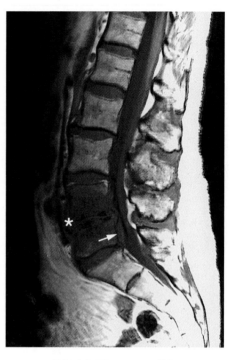

**Discitis/Osteomyelitis**

Infection of an intervertebral disc and adjacent vertebrae may occur in adults or children at any level of the spinal column. The majority of such infections are hematogenous, originating in the subchondral portion of a vertebral body and spreading to involve the neighboring disc. In young children the reverse sequence may occur: hematogenous infection may initially seed the disc before extending to subchondral bone. Direct infection of the disc space may follow surgery or instrumentation at any age.

The radiographic hallmark of discitis is involvement of the subchondral regions of adjacent vertebral bodies. This finding is well displayed on sagittal or coronal MR studies. Infiltration of marrow by edema and inflammatory cells causes a water-like signal pattern, with reduced intensity on T1-weighted images.

In Case 1107, the normally bright signal of marrow fat has been replaced throughout most of the C4 and C5 vertebral bodies. The inferior end plate of C4 and the supe-

rior end plate of C5 are demineralized and eroded. A shallow anterior epidural mass is present along the ventral margin of the spinal canal, and dorsal epidural fat is replaced by thickened tissue of intermediate signal intensity *(arrows)*. The thecal sac is compressed, and mild kyphosis is present.

Case 1108 demonstrates low signal intensity occupying most of the L4 and L5 vertebral bodies. The intervening disc space is barely discernible, since cortical bone along its margins has been destroyed. Prevertebral *(asterisk)* and anterior epidural *(arrow)* masses are present.

It is important to note that vertebral changes may be late to develop (and to resolve) during the course of discitis in some patients (see Case 1125 for an example). Abnormalities of the disc space (and possible adjacent soft tissue masses) may be the only manifestation of discitis in occasional cases.

## Case 1109

79-year-old woman presenting with
severe back pain.
(sagittal, noncontrast T2-weighted FSE scan)

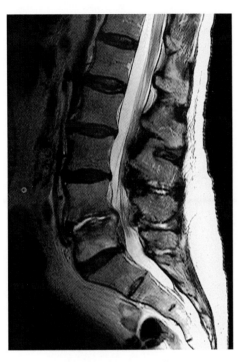

**Discitis/Osteomyelitis**
(same patient as Case 1108)

## Case 1110

35-year-old woman complaining
of worsening back pain.
(sagittal, noncontrast T2-weighted SE scan)

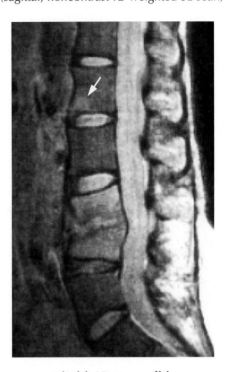

**Discitis/Osteomyelitis**

---

The cellular infiltration and edema accompanying discitis and osteomyelitis usually cause increased signal intensity on long TR spin echo images.

T2 prolongation within the L4 and L5 vertebral bodies in Case 1109 is subtle (compare to the more obvious prolongation of T1 values within the same vertebrae in Case 1108). However, the high signal intensity of the L4-5 disc space is strikingly abnormal for a narrowed lumbar disc in an elderly patient. (Compare to the "normal" dehydration at other levels.) Even if accompanying vertebral changes are not impressive, such high water content within a degenerated disc space raises the question of discitis. A small anterior epidural mass in Case 1109 causes moderate compression of the thecal sac.

In Case 1110, abnormally high intensity is seen throughout the L3 and L4 vertebral bodies. Adjacent portions of the bodies have been destroyed. The intervening disc space is narrow and irregular. Signal intensity within the disc is comparable to that of the infected vertebrae. (Low intensity would be expected in a degenerated disc that has caused sterile reactive changes of neighboring bodies; see Cases 920 and 921.)

Compare the sharp definition of uninvolved vertebral margins in Case 1110 to the poor visualization of cortex bordering the infected disc. Erosion and fragmentation of adjacent vertebral end plates are hallmarks of discitis. Inflammatory erosions are usually more numerous and irregular than the depressions caused by intravertebral disc herniations ("Schmorl's nodes"; see Case 1171).

The smaller lesion within the anterior inferior corner of the L1 vertebral body in Case 1110 *(arrow)* illustrates that hematogenous disc space infection usually originates from seeding of subchondral bone. The term "spondylitis" may be better than "discitis" to accurately represent the vertebral component of these combined infections.

# DIFFERENTIAL DIAGNOSIS:
## NARROWED, IRREGULAR DISC SPACE WITH ADJACENT SUBCHONDRAL REACTION

### Case 1111

57-year-old woman presenting with
chronic back pain.
(sagittal, noncontrast T1-weighted SE scan)

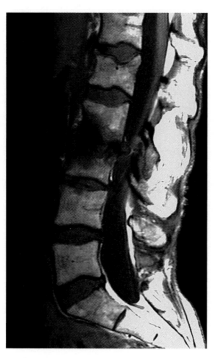

**Sterile Degenerative Changes**

### Case 1112

73-year-old man presenting with increasing back
pain after lumbar decompression for spinal stenosis.
(sagittal, noncontrast T1-weighted SE scan)

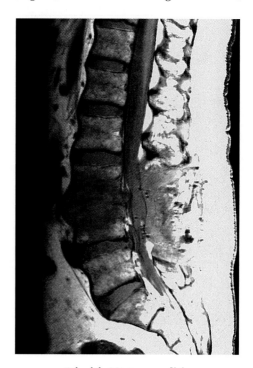

**Discitis/Osteomyelitis**

As discussed in Chapter 17 (see Cases 920 and 921), degenerative disc disease is frequently associated with reactive changes in subchondral bone. Prolonged T1 and T2 values within neighboring vertebral bodies may border a disc narrowed by degeneration and resemble the appearance of disc space infection.

Case 1111 illustrates this pattern. Stable degenerative changes at L2-3 had been noted on multiple previous studies, and there was no clinical evidence of infection. Low signal intensity within subchondral portions of the L2 and L3 bodies probably includes a component of sclerosis as well as reactive inflammation. An associated disc herniation and stenosis of the central canal are present.

Similar features of subchondral edema and diminished visualization of the disc space are seen at L3-4 in Case 1112. However, the loss of definition of the vertebral end plates is more extensive than in most cases of sterile degenerative disease. Associated focal prevertebral and intraspinal masses favor an inflammatory process (but can accompany

degenerative disease, as in Case 1111). Postlaminectomy changes are present in dorsal soft tissues.

A spondyloarthropathy resembling discitis/osteomyelitis may develop in patients with chronic renal failure undergoing dialysis. This disorder is believed to be caused by the accumulation and deposition of a low molecular weight protein ("beta-2-microglobulin") that is not removed by dialysis.

Neuropathic arthropathy ("Charcot spine") can cause destruction of a disc space resembling discitis. Clues to the former diagnosis include prominent degenerative erosion of the facet joints, the presence of gas within the disc space ("vacuum disc"), and extensive osseous debris.

The clinical condition of the patient is helpful in assessing scans demonstrating abnormal disc spaces. Discitis/osteomyelitis is severely painful. The diagnosis should be suggested even if MR findings are subtle when back pain is intense. Conversely, disc space changes are less likely to represent infection if associated pain is not significant and worsening.

# DIFFERENTIAL DIAGNOSIS:
## INFILTRATION AND DESTRUCTION OF ADJACENT VERTEBRAL BODIES

### Case 1113

70-year-old man presenting with severe back pain.
(sagittal, noncontrast T1-weighted SE scan)

### Case 1114

81-year-old man presenting with leg weakness.
(sagittal, noncontrast T1-weighted SE scan)

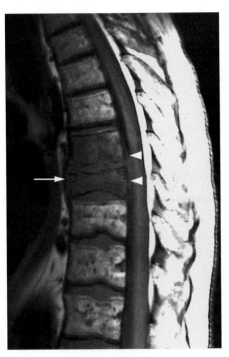

**Discitis/Osteomyelitis**

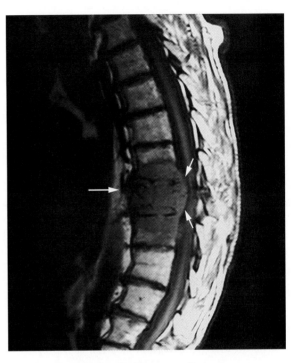

**Metastatic Hypernephroma**

Infiltration and destruction of adjacent vertebral bodies is a common presentation of discitis/osteomyelitis, as illustrated on the previous pages. Case 1113 presents an additional example involving the T6 and T7 vertebrae. The inflammatory process in this patient probably began at the T6-7 level but has now extended through the entire vertebral body of T7, with erosion of the inferior end plate and pathological fracture. Small associated prevertebral *(arrow)* and anterior epidural *(arrowheads)* masses are present.

Case 1114 demonstrates that neoplasms can also cross a disc space to involve contiguous vertebrae. A metastasis to the body of T8 has grown both superiorly and inferiorly into T7 and T9. The overall appearance resembles Case 1113, with erosion of end plates and accompanying pre-

vertebral *(long arrow)* and anterior epidural *(short arrows)* masses.

Clinical context helps to distinguish between these pathologies. Evidence of systemic infection is usual in patients with discitis. In addition, infectious spondylitis is typically associated with severe back pain, which is often a more impressive component of the initial presentation than in patients with vertebral metastases.

Tuberculosis or fungal (e.g., coccidioidomycosis) spondylitis frequently involves contiguous vertebral bodies by means of subligamentous extension. Intervening disc spaces may be relatively preserved in such cases.

Other spinal tumors that may extend from one vertebral body to the next include multiple myeloma (see Case 1013) and chordoma.

### Case 1115

34-year-old woman presenting with hand numbness and mildly spastic gait six months after admission for pneumonia and a mediastinal abscess.
(sagittal, noncontrast T1-weighted SE scan)

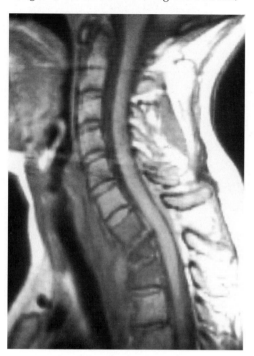

**Discitis/Osteomyelitis**

### Case 1116

83-year-old woman presenting with back pain and acute paraplegia.
(sagittal, noncontrast T1-weighted SE scan)

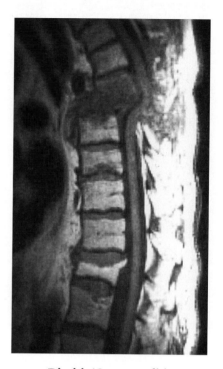

**Discitis/Osteomyelitis**

As seen on the preceding pages, discitis and osteomyelitis may cause extensive bone destruction. Cases 1115 and 1116 demonstrate that this loss of vertebral body height and stability may in turn lead to spinal deformity and cord compression.

In Case 1115, osteomyelitis involves the C7 through T2 levels, spanning two disc spaces. Anterior wedging of the T1 vertebral body is associated with kyphotic angulation and subluxation that is beginning to compromise the spinal canal. The subarachnoid space is partially effaced at the cervicothoracic junction.

The subluxation in Case 1116 is more extreme, with a bayonet-like deformity of the thoracic spinal canal. Cord compression in cases of discitis/osteomyelitis may be caused by such abnormalities of alignment and/or by associated epidural inflammatory masses. (The posterior arches in the involved region of Case 1115 had been resected in an attempt to decompress the spinal canal.)

### Case 1117

2-year-old boy with apparent back pain.
(sagittal, noncontrast T2-weighted SE scan)

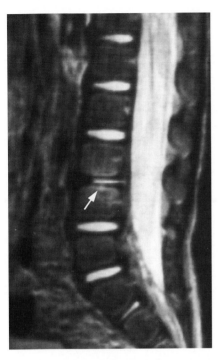

**Discitis**

### Case 1118

8-month-old boy presenting with
fever and irritability.
(sagittal, noncontrast T2-weighted SE scan)

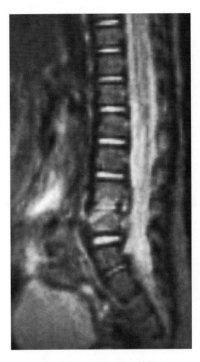

**Discitis/Osteomyelitis**

Pediatric discitis may be a low grade and self-limited inflammation, typically involving a single lumbar level. In many cases no causative organism is established. The clinical presentation is often nonspecific and may initially suggest hip pathology or appendicitis.

Case 1117 demonstrates narrowing of the L3-4 disc, with mild reduction of signal intensity. A faint haze of inflammatory edema is present within the adjacent vertebral bodies, but cortical end-plates are intact. The appearance is compatible with idiopathic nonsuppurative primary discitis.

More bone destruction is apparent at the L4-5 level in Case 1118. Adjacent cortices have been eroded, and there is more prominent signal abnormality within the involved vertebral bodies. These findings suggest pyogenic infection and would support early antibiotic therapy.

A syndrome of "benign calcification of an intervertebral disc" has been recognized in older children as an idiopathic, noninfectious, inflammatory condition. The process typically involves one or several adjacent discs in a child of age 5 to 12 years who complains of neck or back pain. Fever and leukocytosis may be present, mimicking infectious discitis. The affected disc space may be widened or narrowed but is characteristically calcified. There may be associated disc herniation or loss of vertebral height. Both the calcification and the symptoms usually resolve spontaneously over a period of weeks to months.

## Case 1119

73-year-old man presenting with increasing
back and leg pain after lumbar surgery.
(sagittal, postcontrast T1-weighted SE scan)

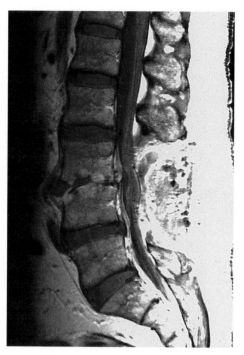

**Discitis/Osteomyelitis**
(same patient as Case 1112)

## Case 1120

64-year-old woman presenting with back pain.
(sagittal, postcontrast T1-weighted SE scan)

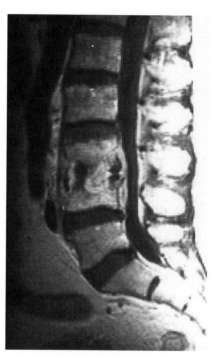

**Discitis/Osteomyelitis**

Contrast enhancement in discitis/osteomyelitis is usually intense, with variable morphology. Homogeneous enhancement within portions of affected vertebrae is frequently combined with very irregular enhancement of the disc space, subchondral bone, and/or paraspinal tissues.

Case 1119 is a postcontrast scan of the patient presented in Case 1112. Enhancement within the L3 and L4 vertebral bodies has caused them to become nearly isointense to normal marrow. Comparison of Cases 1112 and 1119 (or of Cases 1014 and 1016) demonstrates that enhancement may obscure the definition of vertebral (or epidural) pathology on T1-weighted scans. This possibility is frequently of concern in the evaluation of metastatic disease to the spinal canal. Scans in such cases should not be limited to postcontrast T1-weighted images without fat suppression.

The marked disc space narrowing, erosions of cortical end plates, and irregular enhancement of subchondral bone in Case 1119 suggest discitis as the source of the adjacent vertebral infiltration. Nonenhancing prevertebral and anterior epidural masses at the L3-4 disc level likely represent small abscesses rather than disc material.

In Case 1120, a central area of intense enhancement straddles the disc space and extends into the center of the involved vertebrae. This zone represents the core of the infection, with aggressive bone destruction comparable to Cases 1110 and 1116. Surrounding reactive inflammation enhances with a more uniform pattern, resembling Case 1119 and appearing isointense to adjacent normal vertebrae. An associated anterior epidural mass enhances intensely, representing an epidural phlegmon.

# DIFFERENTIAL DIAGNOSIS:
## IRREGULAR CONTRAST ENHANCEMENT WITHIN A VERTEBRAL BODY

### Case 1121

66-year-old woman presenting with back pain.
(axial, postcontrast T1-weighted SE scan; L2 level)

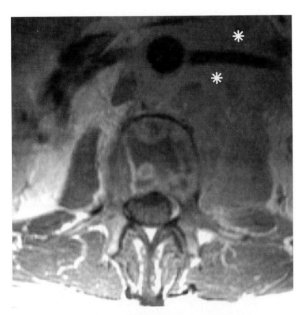

**Metastatic Carcinoma of the Breast**

### Case 1122

64-year-old woman presenting with back pain.
(axial, postcontrast T1-weighted SE scan; L4 level)

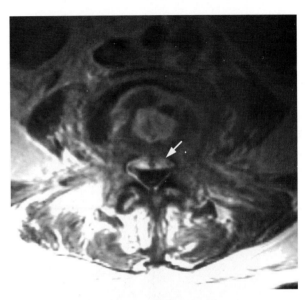

**Discitis/Osteomyelitis**
(same patient as Case 1120)

---

Metastatic disease and discitis/osteomyelitis must often be considered together in the differential diagnosis of vertebral lesions (see Cases 1113 and 1114). Both pathologies can cause irregular enhancement within involved bodies, as illustrated above. The clinical context and pattern of spinal disease (i.e., multiplicity and continuity of affected levels) will usually differentiate between these lesions.

Both infection and metastatic disease of the spine may cause associated paraspinal and epidural masses. A large left-sided paraspinal mass in Case 1121 involves the psoas region. An anterior epidural mass enhances intensely in Case 1122 (*arrow;* compare to the sagittal scan in Case 1120).

Retroperitoneal adenopathy, as seen in Case 1121 (*asterisks*), strongly suggests the context of systemic metastases. (See Case 1000 for another example.)

Intrathecal nerve roots of the cauda equina are somewhat prominent in Case 1121. This can be a normal postcontrast appearance due to mild diffuse enhancement. Pathologically enlarged or inflamed roots usually demonstrate more striking and asymmetrical enhancement, often in association with unequivocal precontrast abnormality of size and/or morphology (see Cases 1042-1045, 1151-1154, and 1162).

## Case 1123

63-year-old woman presenting with severe back pain two weeks after implantation of fusion cages. (sagittal, noncontrast T1-weighted SE scan)

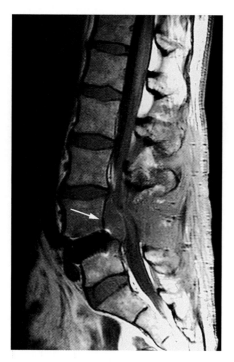

**Epidural Abscess**

## Case 1124

15-year-old boy presenting with back pain, leg numbness, and leg weakness. (sagittal, noncontrast T1-weighted SE scan)

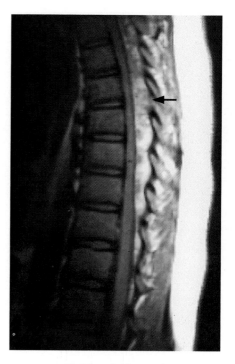

**Epidural Abscess**

Abscesses may develop in the epidural space by direct extension of spinal infection, by hematogenous seeding from distant sources, or by iatrogenic inoculation. Once established, epidural abscesses often involve long segments of the spinal canal (e.g., 10 or 20 vertebral levels). Initial symptoms may be mild or nondescript. Rapid loss of neurological function occurs with the onset of septic thrombophlebitis extending to the spinal cord.

In Case 1123, metallic fusion cages had been placed at the L4-5 level to treat instability and spondylolisthesis. The homogeneous anterior epidural mass at the surgical level *(arrow)* demonstrated uniformly high signal intensity on T2-weighted scans and peripheral contrast enhancement. Re-exploration disclosed a drainable abscess.

The long dorsal epidural mass in Case 1124 contains a mixture of signal intensities. The long T1 regions probably represent purulent loculations surrounded by residual dorsal epidural fat. (See Case 1188 for another example of a lobulated epidural abscess outlined by fat within the posterior portion of the spinal canal.) Hemorrhage is commonly found within epidural abscesses, and subacute blood products may also contribute to T1-shortening in the involved region.

There was no history of lumbar puncture or surgery in Case 1124, and there is no evidence of discitis/osteomyelitis. Instead, the dorsal epidural abscess represents hematogenous dissemination of infection, comparable to the occurrence of isolated epidural metastases. The dorsal portion of the thoracic spinal canal is a common location for such hematogenous lesions, and *Staphylococcus aureus* is the pathogen most frequently cultured.

The differential diagnosis in Case 1124 includes epidural hematoma (see Cases 1185 and 1186) and epidural metastasis. Rare epidural angiolipomas and hemangiomas (see Case 996) could cause a similar appearance.

## Case 1125

75-year-old woman presenting with a one-week history of neck pain and progressive quadriparesis.
(sagittal, noncontrast T2-weighted FSE scan)

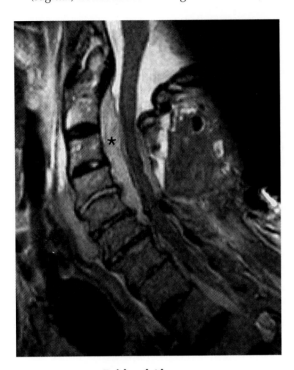

**Epidural Abscess**

## Case 1126

38-year-old man presenting with a four-day history of worsening back pain.
(sagittal, noncontrast T2-weighted FSE scan)

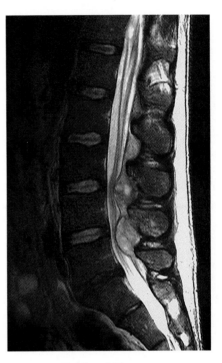

**Epidural Abscess**

Spinal epidural abscesses may present as thin layers of fluid or as thick and/or lobulated masses. Their signal intensity on T2-weighted images is variable; some lesions demonstrate longer T2 values than Cases 1125 and 1126.

The predominantly anterior epidural mass in Case 1125 *(asterisk)* is associated with discitis. Abnormally high signal intensity is present within several mid cervical discs. (Dehydration of these discs would be expected in view of their severe degenerative narrowing.) However, no vertebral destruction is seen, demonstrating that the extent of osseous erosion in discitis is variable and independent of the presence or size of epidural masses. A decompressive laminectomy had been performed in this case; re-operation drained a large collection of epidural pus encircling the thecal sac and effacing the subarachnoid space.

The dorsal epidural abscess in Case 1126 differs from Case 1125 in several respects. There is no evidence of associated discitis or osteomyelitis (and there was no history of lumbar puncture), so the source of the infection was probably hematogenous. The morphology of the collection is distinctly lobulated rather than laminar. Finally, the signal intensity within the abscess is heterogeneous, with average values slightly less than CSF. This feature likely reflects the presence of hemorrhage and/or thickly proteinaceous material.

A scan performed three days earlier in Case 1126 had been nearly normal, illustrating that epidural abscesses can progress rapidly to compromise the spinal canal. Worsening myelopathy in patients with even small epidural abscesses may alternatively reflect septic thrombophlebitis causing impaired venous drainage and infarction of the spinal cord.

It is often difficult to distinguish between epidural and subdural localization of spinal empyemas. Involvement of either compartment causes compression of the dural sac. Subdural and epidural abscesses should be considered in the differential diagnosis of a featureless spinal canal with obliteration of normal cord/CSF interfaces.

**Case 1127**

32-year-old man presenting with back pain.
(sagittal, noncontrast T1-weighted SE scan)

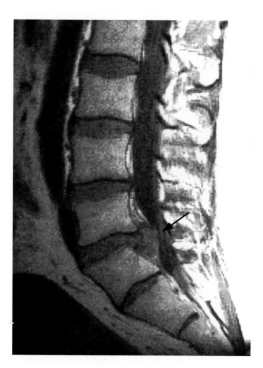

**Herniated Disc**

**Case 1128**

44-year-old man presenting with rapidly increasing back pain two weeks after lumbar discectomy.
(sagittal, noncontrast T1-weighted SE scan)

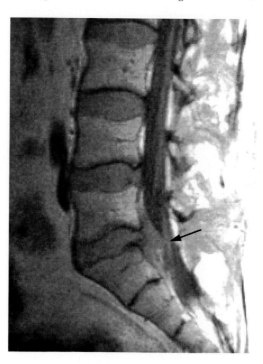

**Epidural Phlegmon**

An anterior epidural mass at the level of an intervertebral disc is a common manifestation of disc hernation, as in Case 1127. Associated edema, granulation tissue, venous congestion, and epidural hemorrhage may contribute to the bulk of such masses (see Cases 942 and 943).

Case 1128 illustrates that epidural infection should also be considered in this differential diagnosis. In some patients the disc space changes of infection are less impressive (or later to develop) than the epidural or paraspinal soft tissue components. The resulting appearance may simulate a herniated disc.

An epidural mass at the level of an infected disc may represent either a true abscess or a mound of edematous tissue referred to as a *phlegmon.* An epidural phlegmon often contains small loculations of pus.

It is very difficult to distinguish between a drainable abscess cavity and a boggy, semisolid phlegmon on MR scans. Both processes typically demonstrate intermediate to low signal intensity on T1-weighted scans and high intensity on T2-weighted studies. Contrast enhancement may be more clearly peripheral in frank abscesses (see Cases 1129 and 1130), but even this appearance is not a reliable distinguishing criterion.

### Case 1129

57-year-old woman presenting with a two-week
history of fever and increasing back pain.
(axial, postcontrast T1-weighted SE scan; L2 level)

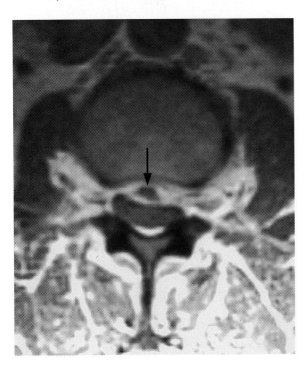

**Epidural Abscess**

### Case 1130

38-year-old man presenting with
rapidly worsening back pain.
(sagittal, postcontrast T1-weighted SE scan)

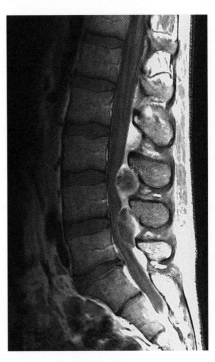

**Epidural Abscess**
(same patient as Case 1126)

---

Most epidural abscesses demonstrate peripheral enhancement that highlights central collections of pus. Both the small anterior epidural abscess in Case 1129 *(arrow)* and the larger dorsal epidural abscess in Case 1130 illustrate this pattern.

Occasionally epidural abscesses enhance more uniformly. Such homogeneity probably reflects leakage and accumulation of contrast material within the purulent loculations of the infected tissue.

Conversely, poorly enhancing areas within an inflammatory mass may represent microabscesses and induration rather than a macroscopic fluid compartment. Neither peripheral nor solid enhancement patterns guarantee or exclude the presence of a drainable cavity.

The differential diagnosis of a peripherally enhancing anterior epidural mass includes a herniated disc surrounded by granulation tissue (see Case 945). Epidural hematomas can occur ventral or dorsal to the thecal sac, with a pattern of surrounding enhancement potentially resembling the above scans (see Case 1190).

### Case 1131

36-year-old man presenting with
numbness of the hands and feet.
(sagittal, noncontrast T1-weighted SE scan)

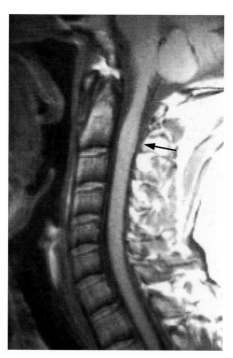

**Multiple Sclerosis**

### Case 1132

55-year-old woman presenting with unsteady gait.
(axial, noncontrast T2*-weighted
GRE scan; C2-3 level)

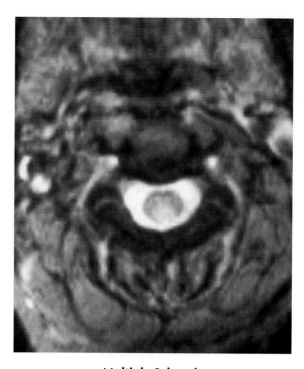

**Multiple Sclerosis**

Myelitis may be caused by a variety of agents and conditions. Demyelinating disease is a leading diagnostic possibility in young and middle-aged adults. Involvement of the spinal cord in multiple sclerosis may be focal, multifocal, or diffuse.

The T1-weighted scan in Case 1131 shows mild, isointense swelling of the cord at the C2-3 level *(arrow)*. This localized expansion is nonspecific; a small primary or metastatic tumor could cause a similar appearance. However, it is important to realize that such focal swelling does occur within the spectrum of demyelinating disease. The location of this lesion (i.e., the C2-3 level) and its size

(about one vertebral body in length) are both typical of multiple sclerosis within the cervical cord.

Case 1132 illustrates another small demyelinating plaque within the spinal cord at the C2-3 level. The edema associated with cord lesions in multiple sclerosis usually causes prominent prolongation of T2. High signal intensity on T2-weighted scans may be sharply defined, as in Case 1132 (see also Case 1133), or quite hazy and indistinct (see Case 1135).

The dorsal eccentricity of the lesion in Case 1132 is a common feature of intramedullary demyelinating disease.

# DIFFERENTIAL DIAGNOSIS:
## FOCAL INTRAMEDULLARY LESION

### Case 1133

20-year-old woman presenting with
arm and leg numbness.
(sagittal, noncontrast T2-weighted SE scan)

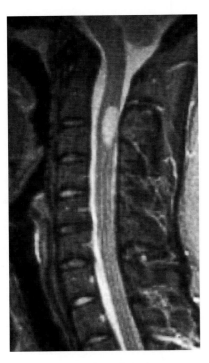

**Multiple Sclerosis**

### Case 1134

55-year-old man presenting with
arm numbness and weakness.
(sagittal, noncontrast T2-weighted SE scan)

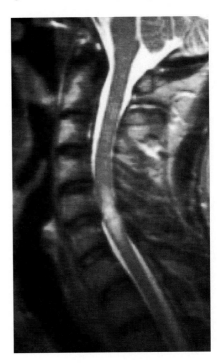

**Astrocytoma**

The very well-defined lesion in Case 1133 is another example of focal demyelination due to multiple sclerosis. The location of the plaque within the dorsal portion of the cord at the C2-3 level and its size (approximately one vertebral body in length) are characteristic findings in this disorder.

Case 1134 demonstrates that cord tumors may present a similar appearance. The astrocytoma in this case is somewhat more localized and homogeneous than usual. However, it is important to realize the potential overlap in appearance between inflammatory and neoplastic involvement of the spinal cord. (This overlap extends to contrast-enhanced images; see Cases 1140 and 1141.)

Edema and enhancement within demyelinating plaques of the spinal cord can be surprisingly stable over weeks or months of follow-up, further confusing the imaging distinction from neoplasms.

A cerebral scan may document intracranial demyelinating foci associated with an ambiguous cord lesion. In other cases, clinical and radiographic evidence of multiple sclerosis is limited to the spinal cord.

### Case 1135

27-year-old woman presenting with
paresthesias of the arms and legs.
(sagittal, noncontrast T2-weighted FSE scan)

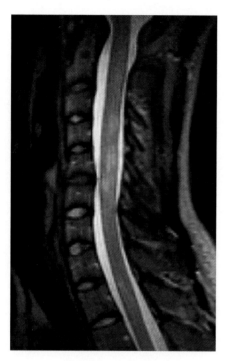

**Multiple Sclerosis**

### Case 1136

33-year-old woman presenting with
diplopia and incoordination.
(sagittal, noncontrast T2-weighted SE scan)

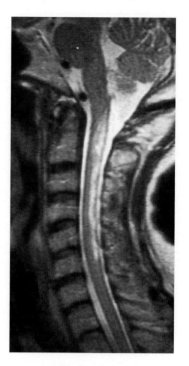

**Multiple Sclerosis**

---

Myelitis due to multiple sclerosis may present as multifocal or diffuse disease involving long segments of the spinal cord. Such lesions are often patchy and poorly defined, unlike the focal plaques in Cases 1131 and 1133.

Several hazy areas of mildly prolonged T2 values are present within the cervical cord (and also at the T2 level) in Case 1135. The partial coalescence of the plaques at the C4 to C6 levels causes mild expansion of the spinal cord. In other cases, greater confluence of lesions leads to diffuse intramedullary edema and swelling, resembling transverse myelitis.

The long column of abnormal signal intensity paralleling the posterior margin of the spinal cord in Case 1136 represents a series of multiple small areas of demyelination. Dorsal eccentricity is a common feature of intramedullary

plaques in the cervical region. The lesions in this case are more clearly defined than the plaques in Case 1135, illustrating the potential variation in conspicuity of demyelinating foci.

STIR images (inversion recovery sequences with short inversion times) may be helpful for accentuating intramedullary lesions with mildly prolonged T1 and T2 values. FLAIR images (inversion recovery sequences with long repetition and inversion times) have not proved useful for this purpose.

Systemic lupus erythematosus and sarcoidosis are additional potential inflammatory etiologies of multifocal or diffuse cord edema and mass effect in young or middle-aged adults (see Cases 1143, 1144, and 1149).

## Case 1137

2-year-old girl presenting with
progressive myelopathy.
(sagittal, noncontrast T1-weighted SE scan)

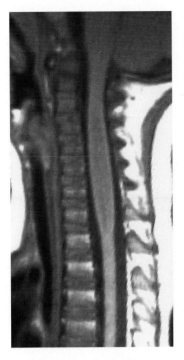

**Transverse Myelitis**

## Case 1138

3-year-old girl presenting with
quadriparesis and confusion.
(sagittal, noncontrast T2-weighted FSE scan)

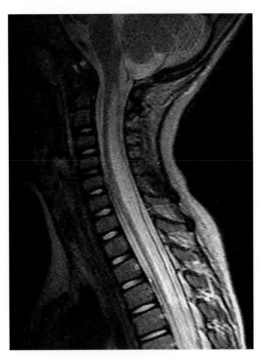

**Transverse Myelitis**

---

Inflammatory myelopathy with no identifiable cause is frequently called *transverse myelitis*. Many such cases probably represent an autoimmune response to an antigenic challenge, analogous to acute disseminated encephalomyelitis (see Cases 388-397). Transverse myelitis ranks with multiple sclerosis as the leading causes of spinal cord inflammation in adults.

Transverse myelitis is also seen in children, as illustrated above. In both adults and children, the cord swelling and dysfunction caused by transverse myelitis may mimic an intramedullary neoplasm. Expansion of the spinal cord by central edema in Case 1137 resembles the astrocytoma in Case 1074.

The above cases emphasize that the name "transverse" myelitis is somewhat misleading. Cord involvement is usually quite *longitudinal*, extending over many levels. In fact, transverse myelitis typically involves longer segments of the spinal cord than multiple sclerosis.

The spectrum of intramedullary edema in transverse myelitis overlaps that of multiple sclerosis. Clinical context (e.g., a history of optic neuritis) may help to distinguish between these inflammatory myelopathies. Alternatively, MR scans of the brain may demonstrate characteristic findings of multiple sclerosis (or of ADEM) when the pattern of spinal cord involvement is ambiguous.

Contrast enhancement usually does not separate myelitis due to multiple sclerosis from transverse myelitis. Both pathologies may demonstrate minimal or patchy enhancement. Discrete nodular enhancement favors multiple sclerosis (or another pathology) over idiopathic myelitis.

Transverse myelitis often responds dramatically to treatment with steroids. The diagnosis should be considered and a therapeutic trial entertained prior to biopsy for presumed neoplasm. A follow-up scan in Case 1137 was normal after ten days of steroid administration.

An MR scan of the head in Case 1138 revealed multiple cerebral and cerebellar lesions compatible with acute disseminated encephalitis.

### Case 1139

27-year-old woman presenting with
paresthesias of the arms and legs.
(sagittal, postcontrast T1-weighted SE scan)

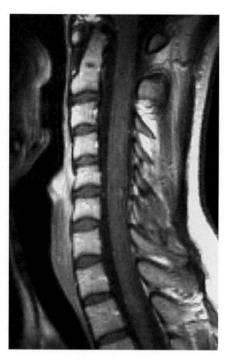

**Multiple Sclerosis**
(same patient as Case 1135)

### Case 1140

24-year-old man presenting with numbness
and paresthesias of the legs and feet.
(sagittal, postcontrast T1-weighted SE scan)

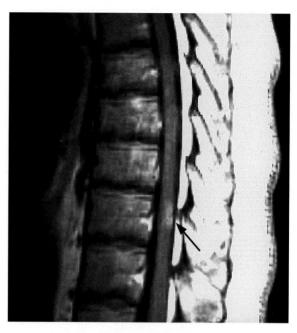

**Multiple Sclerosis**

---

Contrast enhancement is often demonstrated at sites of active demyelination within the spinal cord. The above cases illustrate that this enhancement may be subtle or intense, hazy or nodular.

Case 1139 is a postcontrast scan of the patient presented as Case 1135. A background of mild, diffuse intramedullary enhancement is suggested in the region from C4 through C6, where plaques were most prominent on the T2-weighted image. Small areas of more focally intense enhancement are poorly defined at C4, C5-6, and T2.

The localized intramedullary enhancement in Case 1140 *(arrow)* correlated with the new onset of lower extremity symptoms in a patient with known multiple sclerosis. The appearance is nonspecific. In an ambiguous clinical context, the possibility of neoplasm, infection, or vascular insult (arterial or venous) would have to be considered (see the next page and compare to Case 1206B).

The absence of demonstrable cord lesions on precontrast and postcontrast MR scans does not exclude the diagnosis of myelitis due to multiple sclerosis. Some intramedullary plaques are small and/or poorly defined from surrounding parenchyma. Together with the variability introduced by slice placement and partial volume effects, these factors may limit the detection of localized pathology.

# DIFFERENTIAL DIAGNOSIS:
## FOCAL INTRAMEDULLARY ENHANCEMENT

### Case 1141

55-year-old man presenting with
arm numbness and weakness.
(sagittal, postcontrast T1-weighted SE scan)

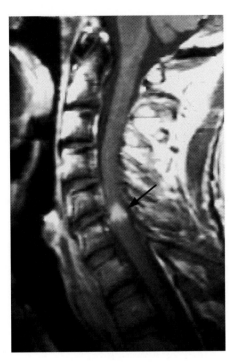

**Astrocytoma**
(same patient as Case 1134)

### Case 1142

49-year-old woman presenting with abnormal gait.
(sagittal, postcontrast T1-weighted SE scan)

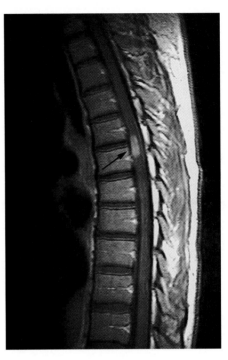

**Sarcoidosis**

---

Multiple sclerosis is one of several pathologies that may cause focal or multifocal enhancement within the spinal cord.

Primary or metastatic tumors should be included in the differential diagnosis. Astrocytomas (as in Case 1141), ependymomas, and hemangioblastomas may be discovered when they are quite small. Such neoplasms may be unassociated with the characteristic cysts or hemorrhages expected of larger lesions. Metastases to the spinal cord must also be considered whenever a focal intramedullary lesion is found (see Cases 1105 and 1106).

Granulomatous inflammatory processes can present with focal intramedullary enhancement, as seen in Case 1142

*(arrow)*. Sarcoidosis frequently involves the pial surface of the spinal cord, with variable intramedullary extension (see Cases 1143 and 1144). Tuberculosis is also among the potential etiologies of a localized intramedullary mass.

Finally, a number of vascular pathologies can cause focal cord enhancement. Arterial and venous infarction may be extensive or limited to small regions of the spinal cord (see Case 1206B). Vascular malformations (e.g., cavernous hemangiomas) within the cord may demonstrate enhancement, often in association with surrounding blood products indicating previous hemorrhage (see Cases 1220-1224).

### Case 1143

42-year-old man presenting with
cervical myelopathy.
(sagittal, postcontrast T1-weighted SE scan)

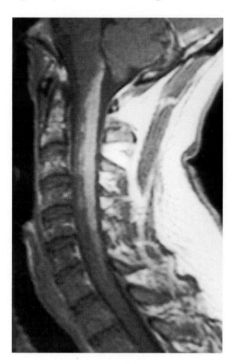

**Sarcoidosis**

### Case 1144

27-year-old woman presenting with paraparesis.
(sagittal, postcontrast T1-weighted SE scan)

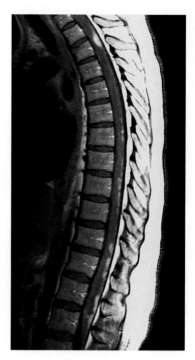

**Sarcoidosis**

The solitary intramedullary mass in Case 1142 is an unusual presentation of intrathecal sarcoidosis. Extensive or multifocal pial-based disease is more common in this disorder, as illustrated in the above cases.

A thick layer of abnormal contrast enhancement is present along the dorsal surface of the spinal cord in Case 1143. Projections of abnormal enhancement extend ventrally from this base into cord parenchyma. The affected portion of the spinal cord is widened, and T2-weighted scans demonstrated intramedullary edema.

The pial-based enhancement in Case 1144 is more scattered and nodular. This appearance closely resembles intradural metastatic disease coating the surface of the spinal cord (compare to Cases 1048 and 1106).

Associated intracranial disease should be sought when spinal sarcoidosis is suspected (see Cases 487-489).

# DIFFERENTIAL DIAGNOSIS:
## DORSALLY BASED INTRAMEDULLARY ENHANCEMENT

### Case 1145

54-year-old woman presenting with
gait abnormality.
(sagittal, postcontrast T1-weighted SE scan)

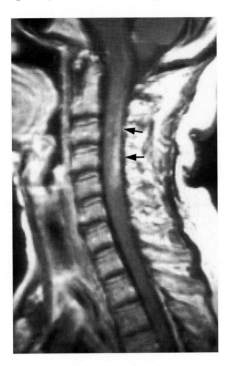

**Multiple Sclerosis**

### Case 1146

17-year-old girl presenting with
cranial neuropathies.
(sagittal, postcontrast T1-weighted SE scan)

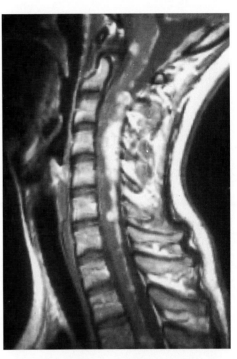

**CSF Seeding from an Exophytic Ependymoma**
(same patient as Case 1086)

A pial-based pattern of cord enhancement is not specific for sarcoidosis. Several other inflammatory diseases can cause a similar appearance. Case 1145 demonstrates that intramedullary contrast enhancement in multiple sclerosis may be eccentric (especially dorsally) and appear pial-based. Bacterial or fungal meningitis may cause a thick layer of pial enhancement coating the cord (see Case 1049). Leptomeningeal enhancement along the margins of the spinal cord has been reported in Lyme disease. Thin, superficial enhancement can be seen along the surface of the thoracic cord and conus medullaris in AIDS patients with CMV myelitis (see Case 1148).

Meningeal carcinomatosis may also coat the spinal cord with a layer of tumor, which can become thick and nodular. Case 1146 illustrates this pattern; see also Cases 1048 and 1106. Several small hemangioblastomas arising at the pial surface in a patient with Von Hippel-Lindau disease could present a similar morphology. Primary leptomeningeal melanoma or melanomatosis is an additional neoplastic etiology of abnormal superficial enhancement of the spinal cord (or brain).

Finally, arterial or venous infarcts of the spinal cord may demonstrate peripheral enhancement surrounding central edema.

## Case 1147

27-year-old man presenting with arm and back pain and cervical myelopathy.
(sagittal, noncontrast T2-weighted SE scan)

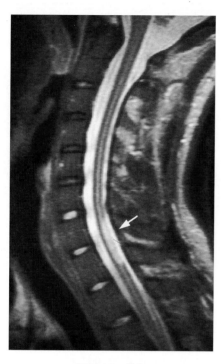

**HIV Myelitis**

## Case 1148

31-year-old man presenting with leg numbness and paresthesias, and bowel and bladder dysfunction.
(axial, postcontrast T1-weighted SE scan; T12-L1 level)

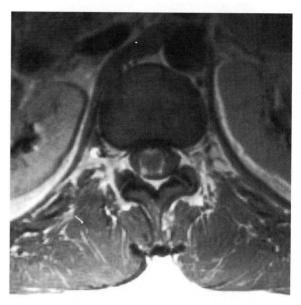

**CMV Myelitis and Radiculitis**

Patients with AIDS may develop meningitis, myelitis, and/or polyradiculitis due to a variety of inflammatory agents. Viruses (HIV, herpes simplex, varicella-zoster, and CMV) cause the majority of such cases.

Infection of the spinal cord by HIV can result in focal, multifocal, patchy, or diffuse intramedullary edema. This range of appearances resembles the spectrum of myelitis in multiple sclerosis.

The lesion in Case 1147 is better defined than in most cases of HIV myelopathy. Dorsally eccentric vacuolization and demyelination involving the posterior and lateral columns of the spinal cord have been pathologically correlated with HIV myelitis, but MR scans in AIDS patients with proven vacuolar myelopathy are often normal.

CMV is a frequent cause of polyradiculitis and myelitis involving the cauda equina and conus medullaris in AIDS patients. The pial enhancement demonstrated in Case 1148 is a characteristic feature of this condition. Enhancement of individual roots within the cauda equina may also be noted.

Myelopathy in a patient with AIDS may reflect neoplastic rather than inflammatory disease (see Case 1103). Likewise, pial enhancement similar to Case 1148 may be caused by meningeal tumor coating the surface of the spinal cord (see Case 1048).

### Case 1149

11-year-old girl presenting with
back pain and paraparesis.
(sagittal, noncontrast T2-weighted FSE scan)

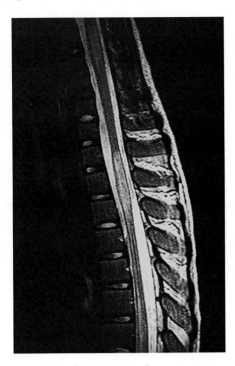

**Systemic Lupus Erythematosus**

### Case 1150

28-year-old man presenting with leg weakness
and bowel and bladder dysfunction.
(sagittal, postcontrast T1-weighted SE scan)

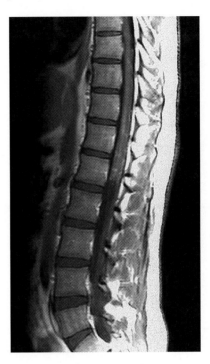

**Schistosomiasis**

Inflammation of the spinal cord may occur in a wide variety of noninfectious and infectious conditions.

Systemic lupus erythematosus (SLE) may affect children younger than ten years old, but the majority of pediatric cases occur between the ages of ten and fifteen years. Involvement of the spinal cord may be isolated or accompanied by cerebral disease. Like the cerebritis discussed in Cases 481, 483, and 485, myelitis in SLE may reflect autoimmune demyelination and/or vasculitis with associated ischemia.

The appearance of swelling and edema illustrated in Case 1149 is typical but nonspecific. A small amount of peripheral contrast enhancement has been noted in some cases of SLE myelitis; none was seen in this patient.

Myelitis involving the conus medullaris in Case 1150 proved to be caused by schistosomiasis, which the patient contracted while working in Africa. The conus and the adjacent spinal cord are expanded. Abnormal contrast enhancement is present both within the substance of the cord and at the pial surface. These findings are compatible with myelitis but nonspecific, requiring clinical correlation.

Radiation should be considered as a potential cause of myelitis in patients who have been treated for a malignancy. Radiation damage to the spinal cord may present subacutely or years after a course of therapy. The clinical syndrome of myelopathy in such cases is usually correlated with intramedullary edema causing long T1 and T2 values. Such changes often extend over several vertebral levels and are associated with expansion of the spinal cord. Nodular or patchy contrast enhancement may be present. The combination of findings may mimic inflammatory myelitis or intramedullary metastasis from the originally treated tumor. Fatty atrophy within adjacent vertebral marrow is a useful clue to a history of spinal radiation.

Deficiency of vitamin $B_{12}$ may cause myelopathy with edema localized to the posterior columns or diffusely involving a segment of the spinal cord. The clinical and MR presentation of such "subacute combined degeneration" can resemble inflammatory myelitis.

Similarly, primary angiitis of the central nervous system (see Cases 641 and 642) may cause multifocal intramedullary edema and enhancement, mimicking infectious or immune-mediated myelitis.

703

### Case 1151

11-year-old boy presenting with
progressive paraparesis.
(sagittal, postcontrast T1-weighted SE scan)

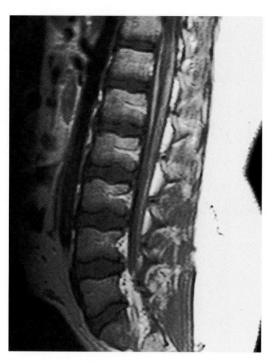

**Guillain-Barré Syndrome**

### Case 1152

6-year-old boy presenting with polyradiculopathy.
(axial, postcontrast T1-weighted
SE scan; T12-L1 level)

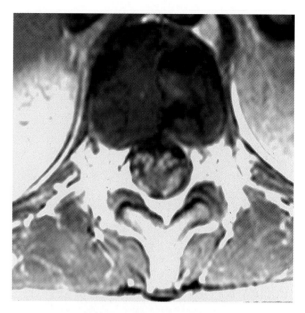

**Guillain-Barré Syndrome**

Guillain-Barré syndrome is an immune-mediated demyelinating polyradiculopathy presenting clinically with rapidly progressive weakness and hyporeflexia. The legs are usually affected first, with subsequent ascending involvement of the arms and face. Autonomic and cranial nerve dysfunction develops in some cases. The disorder occurs in both adults and children, with pathophysiology resembling a neuropathic form of acute disseminated encephalomyelitis.

MR scans of the spine in patients with Guillain-Barré syndrome may be normal. However, many cases demonstrate thickening and enhancement of the nerve roots of the cauda equina, as seen above. Case 1151 illustrates intense enhancement along ventral and dorsal nerve roots throughout the length of the lumbar canal; the conus medullaris itself is nonenhancing. Case 1152 demonstrates a nonen-

hancing conus surrounded by abnormally enhancing roots of normal size.

Mild enhancement of intrathecal nerves is a normal finding on postcontrast scans (see Case 1121). The degree of enhancement demonstrated in the above scans is pathological, although nonspecific (compare to Cases 1048, 1049, 1162, 1216, and 1217).

A brief clinical note is worth adding to this discussion. Children with rapidly progressive ascending paralysis may be misdiagnosed with Guillain-Barré syndrome when they are in fact suffering from tick paralysis. Tick paralysis is caused by a very potent neurotoxin produced by an engorged tick attached to the patient. A careful physical examination (particularly of the scalp) is important in children with worsening paresis; removal of the tick cures tick paralysis, which can otherwise be fatal.

# DIFFERENTIAL DIAGNOSIS:
## ENHANCING INTRADURAL NERVE ROOTS

### Case 1153

11-year-old boy presenting with
progressive paraparesis.
(axial, postcontrast T1-weighted SE scan; L1 level)

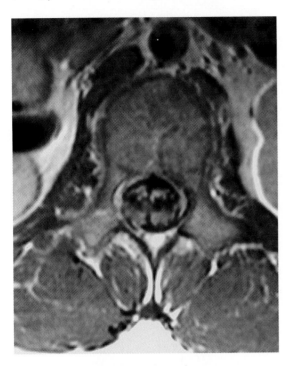

**Guillain-Barré Syndrome**
(same patient as Case 1151)

### Case 1154

48-year-old man presenting with
back pain and leg weakness.
(axial, postcontrast T1-weighted SE scan; T12 level)

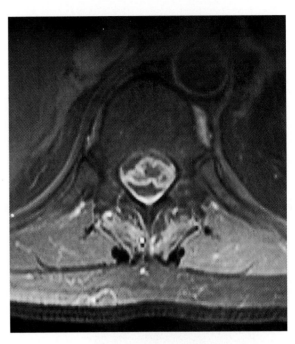

**Bacterial Meningitis**

---

As discussed with respect to cranial nerves in Chapter 5, abnormal enhancement of spinal nerves may be caused by inflammatory or neoplastic processes involving the nerve itself or its meningeal surface.

Case 1153 is an axial scan of the patient presented in Case 1151 and is comparable to Case 1152. Abnormally enhancing roots of the cauda equina surround the nonenhancing tip of the conus medullaris (which serves as a reference for the expected signal intensity of normal neural tissue).

The enhancement pattern in Case 1154 is subtly different. T1-shortening coats the surface of the conus medul-

laris and the aggregated nerve roots of the cauda equina. The neural structures themselves do not demonstrate central enhancement. This appearance suggests meningeal disease surrounding the intrathecal roots and narrows the differential diagnosis to meningitis versus meningeal carcinomatosis (see Case 1048). *Streptococcus pneumoniae* was cultured from the CSF in this case.

Abnormally enhancing ventral roots of the cauda equina (unilateral or bilateral) have been reported in a syndrome of acute flaccid paralysis associated with systemic infection by enterovirus 71. Affected patients present clinically as hand-foot-and-mouth disease or herpangina.

### Case 1155

40-year-old woman with a history of multiple myelograms and lumbar operations.
(sagittal, noncontrast T1-weighted SE scan)

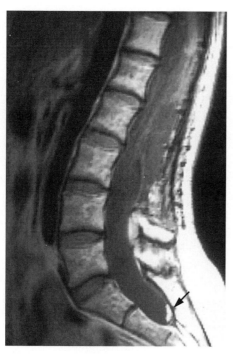

**Arachnoiditis**

### Case 1156

56-year-old woman two years after an automobile accident.
(sagittal, noncontrast T1-weighted SE scan)

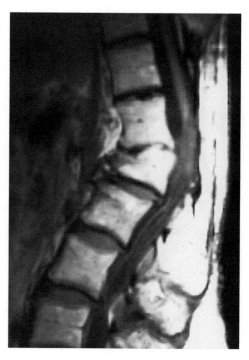

**Arachnoiditis**

Spinal arachnoiditis may be idiopathic or secondary to inflammation caused by subarachnoid hemorrhage, meningitis, surgery, or trauma. The MR hallmark of arachnoiditis is the presence of adhesions distorting intrathecal nerve roots. The intradural course of the roots may be abnormally angled or displaced by traction from scar tissue. Alternatively, roots may be clumped together or scarred to the margins of the dural sac.

Case 1155 illustrates a wide dural sac at the thoracolumbar junction, reflecting previous laminectomies. Residual intrathecal Pantopaque is seen as small foci of T1-shortening within the caudal sac *(arrow)* and along the dorsal surface of the spinal canal in the region of surgery. The latter

droplets of contrast material are likely encysted or scarred in place.

Within the dural sac, the morphology of the conus medullaris and cauda equina is severely distorted. Intradural nerve roots are thick and abnormally positioned, with abrupt angulation suggesting tethering by fibrous bands.

Case 1156 demonstrates more localized arachnoiditis adjacent to a vertebral fracture. Amorphous scarring obliterates the normal contour of the conus medullaris. This fibrosis probably reflects the organization of previous hemorrhage at the level of trauma. A decompressive laminectomy is present dorsally.

# DIFFERENTIAL DIAGNOSIS:
## THICKENED INTRADURAL NERVE ROOTS

### Case 1157

56-year-old woman with recurrent back and leg pain after several lumbar laminectomies.
(sagittal, noncontrast T1-weighted SE scan)

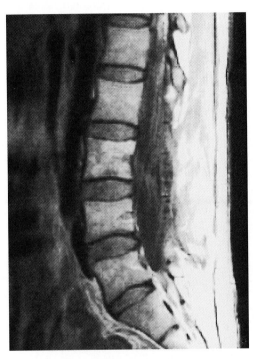

**Arachnoiditis**

### Case 1158

68-year-old man presenting with
leg pain and weakness.
(sagittal, noncontrast T1-weighted SE scan)

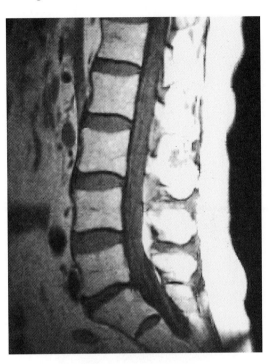

**Lymphomatous Meningitis**
(same patient as in Case 1045)

As illustrated on the preceding page, arachnoiditis may cause extensive thickening, clumping, and distortion of intrathecal nerve roots. Case 1157 is another example of this appearance in a patient who has undergone multiple back operations. The recognition of arachnoiditis in such cases is an important factor in judging the likelihood of symptomatic improvement from additional surgery.

In Case 1158, the thickening of intradural roots is due to a coating of neoplastic cells. (Case 1045 presents an axial view of this patient.) Meningeal carcinomatosis may reflect hematogenous metastases from systemic carcinomas or CSF seeding by primary intrathecal tumors. (See Cases 1042 to 1048 for additional examples.)

Neoplastic thickening of nerve roots often demonstrates contrast enhancement. Radicular enhancement is less prominent in most cases of arachnoiditis.

Arachnoiditis and meningeal carcinomatosis are among the potential etiologies of a featureless lumbar sac lacking normal definition of the conus medullaris and cauda equina (see Case 1043). High CSF levels of cells or protein (making spinal fluid nearly isointense to neural parenchyma) may also cause this appearance. Large intradural or epidural tumors (e.g., ependymoma, as in Case 1094, and neuroblastoma, as in Case 1020) may fill or compress the thecal sac, obscuring intraspinal anatomy. Finally, epidural or subdural empyemas may fill the spinal canal and efface the subarachnoid space, causing an amorphous lack of intraspinal detail.

Hypertrophic neuropathies such as Charcot-Marie-Tooth disease and Déjérine-Sottas disease are a rare cause of nerve root thickening similar to the above cases.

## Case 1159

39-year-old woman complaining of persistent
back pain after prior lumbar surgery.
(sagittal, noncontrast T2-weighted FSE scan)

## Case 1160

44-year-old woman with a history of multiple
lumbar operations and myelograms, now
presenting with bilateral lumbar radiculopathy.
(sagittal, noncontrast T2-weighted FSE scan)

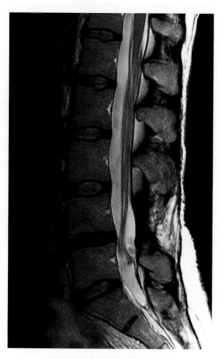

**Arachnoiditis**

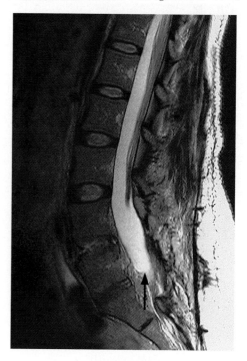

**Arachnoiditis**

Intrathecal adhesions caused by arachnoiditis may tether nerve roots to each other or to the margins of the dural sac.

In Case 1159, nerve roots of the cauda equina are thickened and aggregated. The band of clumped roots is focally distorted at L4-5, tethered ventrally at the disc level and dorsally at the L5 level. Dense scar tissue is present within the laminectomy defect at L4.

Case 1160 illustrates a different pattern of arachnoiditis. The subarachnoid space at L4-5 appears empty because nerve roots are scarred to the perimeter of the dural sac (see Case 1161). The thecal sac terminates abnormally at the L5 level *(arrow)*, with the more inferior portion obliterated by scar tissue.

A central intrathecal band of aggregated nerve roots extending caudally from the conus medullaris may be misin-

terpreted as a tethered spinal cord or thickened filum terminale. (Compare Case 1159 to Cases 1236 and 1237.)

The differential diagnosis in Case 1160 would include an intradural mass with long T1 and T2 values causing displacement of nerve roots. Epidermoid or parasitic cysts could be considered in this category.

Postoperative changes are apparent in dorsal soft tissues from L4 to S1 in Case 1160. The L4-5 and L5-S1 disc spaces are severely narrowed and may be at least partially fused.

In addition to tethering of nerve roots, adhesions due to arachnoiditis may cause loculation of the subarachnoid space, forming secondary arachnoid cysts. Another potential complication of arachnoiditis is syringomyelia, which can develop whenever CSF circulation within the thecal sac is impaired.

# DIFFERENTIAL DIAGNOSIS:
## CLUMPING OF INTRADURAL NERVE ROOTS

### Case 1161

44-year-old woman presenting with
bilateral lumbar radiculopathy.
(axial, noncontrast T2-weighted FSE scan; L3-4 level)

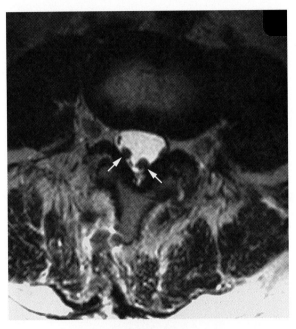

**Arachnoiditis**
(same patient as Case 1160)

### Case 1162

17-year-old girl presenting with back
pain and cranial nerve deficits.
(axial, postcontrast T1-weighted SE scan; L4-5 level)

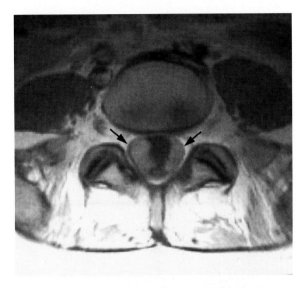

**Drop Metastases from a Cervical Ependymoma**
(same patient as Case 1086)

---

The aggregation of intrathecal nerve roots may reflect either inflammatory or neoplastic disease.

Case 1161 is an axial scan of the patient presented in Case 1160. The empty thecal sac on the sagittal view is explained on axial images by adhesion of clumped lumbar nerve roots to the dura bilaterally *(arrows)*.

Neoplastic coating of the cauda equina in Case 1162 is approximately symmetrical, as is often true in the inferior lumbar region. The aggregated nerve roots have greater volume than the clumped roots of arachnoiditis in Case 1161.

Gravitational settling of intrathecal cells makes the caudal sac a frequent location of meningeal carcinomatosis. This area should be carefully examined whenever meningeal tumor is considered clinically (see Cases 1042 and 1093).

### Case 1163

49-year-old woman complaining
of intermittent stumbling.
(sagittal, noncontrast T1-weighted SE scan)

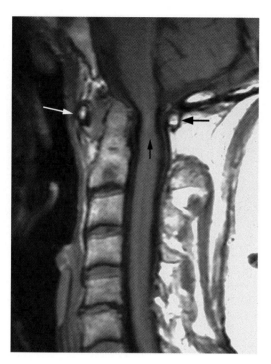

**Rheumatoid Arthritis**

### Case 1164

52-year-old woman presenting with
neck pain and scattered paresthesias.
(sagittal, noncontrast T1-weighted SE scan)

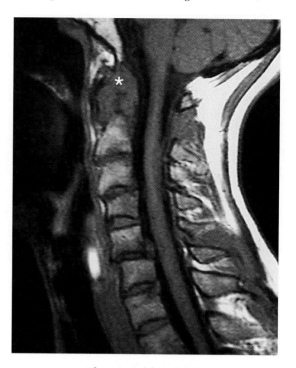

**Rheumatoid Arthritis**

Synovial inflammation in rheumatoid arthritis may involve the articulation of the odontoid process with the anterior arch of C1 and the transverse ligament of the atlas. Bone erosion and soft tissue inflammation at C1-2 often lead to ligamentous laxity and subluxation. The head and C1 can then move ventrally with respect to the odontoid process and the remainder of the cervical spine, widening the atlanto-dental interval and narrowing the spinal canal at C1-2.

Case 1163 illustrates these features. There is anterior displacement of C1 with respect to C2, with abnormal separation between the anterior arch of the atlas *(white arrow)* and the odontoid process. Anterior subluxation of the posterior arch of C1 indents the dorsal subarachnoid space *(long black arrow)*. Focal flattening of the cervicomedullary junction *(short black arrow)* suggests that subluxa-

tion at C1-2 is sometimes more severe than is demonstrated in the neutral position at the time of the scan. (Sagittal images can be obtained in flexion and extension to better estimate the range of subluxation in such cases.)

Although the odontoid process in Case 1163 is largely intact, erosion of the odontoid is a common feature of rheumatoid disease. A surrounding pannus of thickened soft tissue usually develops. Both of these findings are apparent in Case 1164. The odontoid process is reduced to a thin, irregular spicule of bone enveloped by an amorphous mass *(asterisk)*.

There is moderate ventral subluxation of C5 on C6 in Case 1164, with mild subluxation of C3 on C4. A superimposed disc herniation is present at C5-6 with a smaller herniation at C6-7.

### Case 1165

49-year-old woman complaining of
intermittent stumbling.
(axial, noncontrast T2*-weighted GRE scan; C1-2 level)

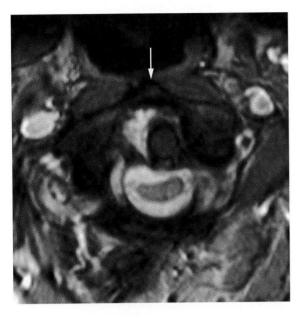

**Rheumatoid Arthritis**
(same patient as Case 1163)

### Case 1166

52-year-old woman presenting with
neck pain and scattered paresthesias.
(axial, noncontrast T2*-weighted GRE scan; C1-2 level)

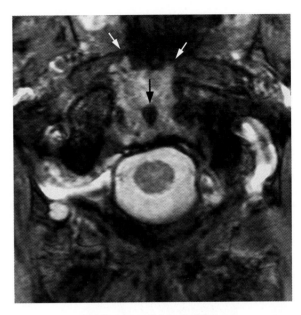

**Rheumatoid Arthritis**
(same patient as Case 1164)

---

The above scans present axial views of the patients illustrated on the preceding page.

Case 1165 emphasizes the laxity and subluxation at C1-2. The odontoid process is laterally and posteriorly positioned with respect to the anterior arch of C1 *(arrow.)* Although patent subarachnoid spaces surround the spinal cord on this image, the flattened contour of the cord attests to previous anteroposterior compression from greater degrees of subluxation.

The most impressive finding in Case 1166 is the striking penciling or whittling of the odontoid process, which has been reduced to a thin peg *(black arrow)*. The remnant of the odontoid is surrounded by a sea of granulation tissue demonstrating high water content. The anterior margins of this tissue erode the anterior arch of C1 *(white arrows)*.

Chronic instability at C1-2 can result in the development of a fibrous mass along the ventral margin of the foramen magnum (see Case 1041). Such pseudotumors may themselves cause compressive myelopathy. Unlike most cases of active rheumatoid pannus and granulation tissue, C1-2 pseudotumors usually demonstrate low signal intensity on T2-weighted scans and little contrast enhancement. How-

ever, fibrosis secondary to instability may be superimposed on the findings of rheumatoid disease at C1-2.

Calcium pyrophosphate dihydrate deposition disease (CPPD or "tophaceous pseudogout") may also involve the C1-2 articulation, producing an anterior epidural mass that compromises the foramen magnum. These pseudotumors often demonstrate small calcifications on CT scans and are typically heterogeneous on T2-weighted MR images. The incidence of CPPD increases with age, and the diagnosis should be considered in elderly patients with arthritic changes at C1-2, whether or not other joints are involved.

High signal intensity is present surrounding the distal vertebral arteries at the level of the posterior arch of C1 in both of the above cases. The arteries are normally surrounded by a venous plexus at C1-2, and these channels of slowly flowing blood can be prominent on T2-weighted or T2*-weighted scans. The finding, which has been compared to the anatomy of the internal carotid arteries surrounded by the cavernous sinus, is a normal variant which should not be confused with dissection or thrombosis of the vertebral arteries themselves.

### Case 1167

53-year-old woman presenting with neck pain.
(sagittal, noncontrast T1-weighted SE scan)

### Case 1168

10-year-old boy presenting with quadriparesis.
(sagittal, noncontrast T1-weighted SE scan)

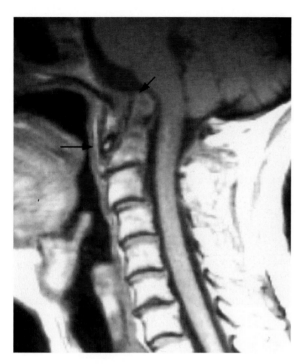

**Rheumatoid Arthritis**

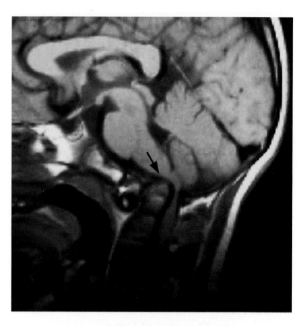

**Congenital Subluxation at C1-2**

A number of conditions may involve subluxation at C1-2, allowing the odontoid process to ascend into the foramen magnum. The most common cause of a high-riding odontoid process in adults is rheumatoid arthritis, as illustrated in Case 1167. In this patient, the dens *(short arrow)* has risen through the ring of C1 *(long arrow)* to present as a premedullary mass.

Superior displacement of the odontoid process in rheumatoid arthritis is aggravated by "cranial settling" due to erosion and reduced height of the lateral masses of C1. Resultant distortion of the medulla or cervicomedullary junction may be much more severe than demonstrated in Case 1167.

The deformity of the craniocervical junction in Case 1168 was congenital and idiopathic. Many patients with abnormal flattening of the skull base ("platybasia") suffer from compromise of the foramen magnum due to associated basilar invagination with encroachment of the dens (see Cases 1273 and 1274). The displaced odontoid process in Case 1168 has caused severe distortion and compression of the cervicomedullary junction. Transoral resection of the odontoid was performed to relieve the brainstem deformity in this case.

Compare the degree of compression of the cervicomedullary junction in Case 1168 to the adult patient in Case 990. Remarkable thinning of the medulla or spinal cord may be surprisingly well tolerated if the deformity progresses gradually. Eventual symptoms may then lead to the discovery of a ribbon-like band of flattened parenchyma.

# ANKYLOSING SPONDYLITIS

## Case 1169A

71-year-old man presenting with dysfunction of the cauda equina.
(sagittal, noncontrast T2-weighted FSE scan)

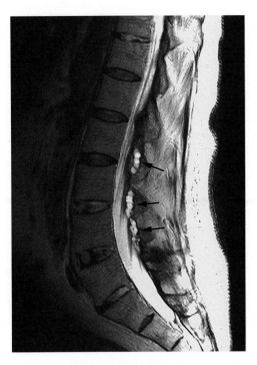

**Ankylosing Spondylitis**

## Case 1169B

Same patient.
(axial, noncontrast T2-weighted FSE scan)

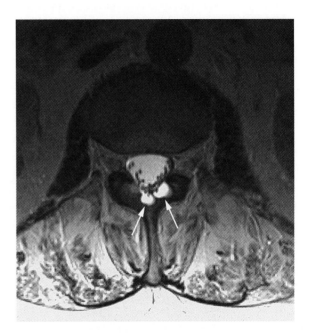

**Ankylosing Spondylitis**

---

Ankylosing spondylitis is an inflammatory spondyloarthropathy involving the insertion of ligaments into bone. The sacroiliac joints and the spine are most commonly and severely affected. The disorder is more frequent in men than in women and is associated with a specific histocompatibility antigen (B27).

Case 1169A illustrates smoothing and squaring of the anterior margins of lumbar vertebral bodies, a characteristic feature in ankylosing spondylitis. Bridging syndesmophytes cross the anterior aspect of disc spaces at L3-4 and L4-5. Other cases of ankylosing spondylitis demonstrate a more prominent "bamboo spine" with fusion of multiple vertebral segments.

Small erosions of the laminae and spinous process, as seen in Case 1169 *(arrows)*, are a characteristic MR feature of ankylosing spondylitis. These erosions presumably relate to the underlying inflammation of ligamentous insertions. As they enlarge, the erosions are occupied by dorsal diverticula of the thecal sac, which can become grossly expanded (see Case 955).

Patients with ankylosing spondylitis often present with a cauda equina syndrome. The etiology of this polyradiculopathy is not established but likely includes arachnoiditis related to inflammation of the posterior spinal ligaments and dura. Note that several nerve roots are prolapsed into and/or adhesed to the anterior margin of the laminar erosions in Case 1169B.

# REFERENCES

Ahmadi J, Bajaj A, Destian S, et al: Spinal tuberculosis: atypical observations at MR imaging. *Radiology* 189:489-493, 1993.

Austin SG, Zee C-S, Waters C: The role of magnetic resonance imaging in acute transverse myelitis. *Can J Neurol Sci* 19:508-511, 1992.

Barakos JA, Mark AS, Dillon WP, et al: MR imaging of acute transverse myelitis and AIDS myelopathy. *J Comput Assist Tomogr* 14:45-50, 1990.

Bassi SS, Bulundwe KK, Greeff GP, et al: MRI of the spinal cord in myelopathy complicating vitamin B12 deficiency: two additional cases and a review of the literature. *Neuroradiology* 41:271-274, 1999.

Berger JR, Quencer R: Reversible myelopathy with pernicious anemia: clinical/MR correlation. *Neurology* 41:947-948, 1991.

Bilgen IG, Yunten N, Ustun EE, et al: Adhesive arachnoiditis causing cauda equina syndrome in ankylosing spondylitis: CT and MRI demonstration of dural calcification and a dorsal dural diverticulum. *Neuroradiology* 41:508-511, 1999.

Boden SD, Davis DO, Dina TS, et al: Postoperative diskitis. Distinguishing early MR imaging findings from normal postoperative disk space changes. *Radiology* 184:765-771, 1992.

Byun WM, Park WK, Park BH, et al: Guillain-Barré syndrome: MR imaging findings of the spine in eight patients. *Radiology* 208:137-141, 1998.

Campi A, Benndorf G, Martinelli V, et al: Spinal cord involvement in primary angiitis of the central nervous system. *AJNR* 22:577-582, 2001.

Campi A, Filippi M, Comi G, et al: Acute transverse myelopathy: spinal and cranial MR study with clinical follow-up. *AJNR* 16:115-124, 1995.

Campi A, Pontesilli S, Gerevini S, Scotti G: Comparison of MRI pulse sequences for investigation of lesions of the cervical spinal cord. *Neuroradiology* 42:669-675, 2000.

Chan CT, Gold WL: Intramedullary abscess of the spinal cord in the antibiotic era: clinical features, microbial etiologies, trends in pathogenesis, and outcomes. *Clin Infect Dis* 27:619-626, 1998.

Chang KH, Han MH, Choi YW, et al: Tuberculous arachnoiditis of the spine: findings on myelography, CT, and MR findings. *AJNR* 10:1255-1262, 1989.

Chang K, Han M, Roh J, et al: Gd-DTPA-enhanced MR imaging in patients with meningitis. *AJNR* 11:69-76, 1990.

Charlesworth CH, Savy LE, Stevens J, et al: MRI demon of arachnoiditis in cauda equina syndrome of ankylosing spondylitis. *Neuroradiology* 38:462-465, 1996.

Chen C-Y, Chang Y-C, Huang C-C, et al: Acute flaccid paralysis in infants and young children with enterovirus 71 infection: MR imaging findings and clinical correlates. *AJNR* 22:200-205, 2001.

Choi KH, Lee KS, Chung So, et al: Idiopathic transverse myelitis: MR characteristics. *AJNR* 17:1151-1160, 1996.

Chong J, Di Rocco A, Tagliati M, et al: MR findings in AIDS-associated myelopathy. *AJNR* 20:1412-1416, 1999.

Coffe MJ, Hadley MN, Herrera GA, Morawetz RB: Dialysis-associated spondyloarthropathy. *J Neurosurg* 80:694-700, 1994.

Dagirmanjian A, Schils J, McHenry M, et al: MR imaging of vertebral osteomyelitis revisited. *Am J Roentgenol* 167:1539-1543, 1996.

Del COJ, Gower DJ, McWhorter JM: Changing concepts in spinal epidural abscess: a report of 29 cases. *Neurosurgery* 27:185-192, 1990.

Demaerel P, Wilms G, Van Lierde S, et al: Lyme disease in childhood presenting as primary leptomeningeal enhancement without parenchymal findings on MR. *AJNR* 15:302-304, 1994.

Duprez TP, Malghem J, Vande Berg BC, et al: Gout in the cervical spine: MR pattern mimicking diskovertebral infection. *AJNR* 17:151-153, 1996.

Edwards MK, Farlow MR, Stevens JC: Cranial MR in spinal cord MS: diagnosing patients with isolated spinal cord symptoms. *AJNR* 7:1003-1005, 1986.

Filippi M, Campi A, Martinelli, et al: Brain and spinal cord MR in benign multiple sclerosis: a follow-up study. *J Neurol Sci* 143:143-149, 1996.

Filippi M, Yousry TA, Alkadhi H, et al: Spinal cord MRI in multiple sclerosis with multicoil arrays: a comparison between fast spin echo and fast FLAIR. *J Neurol Neurosurg Psychiatry* 61:632-635, 1996.

Fitt GJ, Stevens JM: Postoperative arachnoiditis diagnosed by high resolution fast spin-echo MRI of the lumbar spine. *Neuroradiology* 37:139-144, 1995.

Friedman DP: Herpes zoster myelitis: MR appearance. *AJNR* 13:1404-1406, 1992.

Georgy BA, Chong B, Chamberlain M, et al: MR of the spine in Guillain-Barré syndrome. *AJNR* 15:300-301, 1994.

Gero B, Sze G, Sharif H: MR imaging of intradural inflammatory diseases of the spine. *AJNR* 12:1009-1019, 1991.

Gillams AR, Chaddha B, Carter AP: MR appearances of the temporal evolution and resolution of infectious spondylitis. *Am J Roentgenol* 166:903-908, 1996.

Gorson KC, Ropper AH, Muriello MA, et al: Prospective evaluation of MRI lumbosacral nerve root enhancement in acute Guillain-Barré syndrome. *Neurology* 47:813-817, 1996.

Gupta RK, Gupta S, Kumar S, et al: MRI in intraspinal tuberculosis. *Neuroradiology* 36:39-43, 1994.

Hackney DB: MR studies of the spinal cord in patients with multiple sclerosis: what should we do? *AJNR* 20:1581-1583, 1999.

Heller RM, Szalay EA, Green HE, et al: Disc space infection in children: magnetic resonance imaging. *Radiol Clin North Am* 26:207-210, 1988.

Hemmer B, Glocker FX, Schumacher M, et al: Subacute combined degeneration: clinical, electrophysiological, and magnetic resonance imaging findings. *J Neurol Neurosurg Psychiatry* 65:822-827, 1998.

Hickman SJ, Miller DH: Imaging of the spine in multiple sclerosis. *Neuroimaging Clin North Am* 10:689-704, 2000.

Hittmair K, Mallek R, Prayer D, et al: Spinal cord lesions in patients with multiple sclerosis: comparison of MR pulse sequences. *AJNR* 17:1555-1565, 1996.

Hlavin ML, Kaminski HJ, Ross JS, et al: Spinal epidural abscess: a ten-year perspective. *Neurosurgery* 27:177-184, 1990.

Holtas S, Basibuyuk N, Frederiksson K: MRI in acute transverse myelopathy. *Neuroradiology* 35:221-226, 1993.

Iwata F, Utsumi Y: MR imaging in Guillain-Barré syndrome. *Pediatr Radiol* 27:36-38, 1997.

Johnson CE, Sze G: Benign lumbar arachnoidisis: MR imaging with gadopentetate dimeglumine. *AJNR* 11:763-770, 1990.

Kakitsubata Y, Boutin RD, Theodorou DJ, et al: Calcium pyrophosphate dihydrate crystal deposition in and around the atlantoaxial joint: association with type 2 odontoid fractures in nine patients. *Radiology* 216:213-219, 2000.

Katsaros VK, Glocker FX, Hemmer B, et al: MRI of spinal cord and brain lesions in subacute combined degeneration. *Neuroradiology* 40:716-719, 1998.

Keiper MD, Grossman RI, Brunson JC, et al: The low sensitivity of fluid-attenuated inversion-recovery MR in the detection of multiple sclerosis of the spinal cord. *AJNR* 18:1035-1039, 1997.

Kelly RB, Mahoney PD, Cawley KM: MR demonstration of spinal cord sarcoidosis: report of a case. *AJNR* 9:197-199, 1988.

Kricun R, Shoemaker EL, Chovanes GI, Stephens HW: Epidural abscess of the cervical spine: MR findings in five cases. *Am J Roentgenol* 158:1145-1149, 1992.

Larsson E-M, Holtas S, Nilsson O: Gd-DTPA-enhanced MR of suspected spinal multiple sclerosis. *AJNR* 10:1071-1076, 1989.

Leite CC, Jinkins JR, Escobar BE, et al: MR imaging of intramedullary and intradural extramedullary spinal cysticercosis. *Am J Roentgenol* 169:1713-1718, 1997.

Levy ML, Wieder BH, Schneider J, et al: Subdural empyema of the cervical spine: clinicopathological correlates and magnetic resonance imaging. Report of three cases. *J Neurosurg* 79:929-935, 1993.

Lexa FJ, Grossman RI: MR of sarcoidosis of the head and spine: spectrum of manifestations and radiographic response to steroid therapy. *AJNR* 15:973-982, 1994.

Lycklama a Nijeholt GJ, Barkhof F, Castelijns JA, et al: Comparison of two MR sequences for detection of multiple sclerosis lesions in the spinal cord. *AJNR* 17:1533-1538, 1996.

Lycklama a Nijeholt GJ, Barkhoff F, Scheltens P, et al: MR of the spinal cord in multiple sclerosis: relation to clinical subtype and disability. *AJNR* 18:1041-1048, 1997.

Lycklama A Nijeholt GJ, Castelijns JA, Weerts J, et al: Sagittal MR of multiple sclerosis in the spinal cord: fast versus conventional spin-echo imaging. *AJNR* 19:355-360, 1998.

Malzberg MS, Rogg JM, Tate CA, et al: Poliomyelitis: hyperintensity of the anterior horn cells on MR images of the spinal cord. *Am J Roentgenol* 161:863-865, 1993.

Maravilla KR: Weinreb JC, Suss R, Nunnally RL: Magnetic resonance demonstration of multiple sclerosis plaques in the cervical cord. *AJNR* 5:685-689, 1984.

Matsui H, Tsuji H, Kanamori M, et al: Laminectomy-induced arachnoradiculitis: a postoperative serial MRI study. *Neuroradiology* 37:660-666, 1995.

Merine D, Wang H, Kumar AJ, et al: CT myelography and MR imaging of acute transverse myelitis. *J Comput Assist Tomogr* 11:606-608, 1987.

Meurice A, Flandroy P, Dondelinger RF, Reznik M: A single focus of probable multiple sclerosis in the cervical spinal cord mimicking a tumour. *Neuroradiology* 36:234-235, 1994.

Michikawa M, Wada Y, Sano M, et al: Radiation myelopathy: significance of gadolinium-DTPA enhancement in the diagnosis. *Neuroradiology* 33:286-289, 1991.

Miller GM, Baker HL Jr, et al: Spinal cord sarcoidosis: a new finding at MR imaging with Gd-DTPA enhancement. *Radiology* 173:839-843, 1989.

Modic MT, Feiglin DH, Piraino DW, et al: Vertebral osteomyelitis: assessment using MR. *Radiology* 157:157-166, 1985.

Mohanty A: Spinal intramedullary cysticercosis. *Neurosurgery* 40(1):82-87, 1997.

Murphy KJ, Brunberg JA, Kazanjian PH: Spinal cord infection: myelitis and abscess formation. *AJNR* 19:341-348, 1998.

Nesbit GM, Miller GM, Baker HL Jr, et al: Spinal cord sarcoidosis: a new finding at MR imaging with Gd-DTPA enhancement. *Radiology* 173:839-843, 1989.

Numaguchi Y, Rigamonti D, Rothman MI, et al: Spinal epidural abscess: evaluation with gadolinium-enhanced MR imaging. *Radiographics* 13:545-559, 1993.

Nussbaum ES, Rigamonti D, Standiford H, et al: Spinal epidural abscess: a report of 40 cases and review. *Surg Neurol* 38:225-231, 1992.

Olson EM, Duberg AC, Herron LD, et al: Coccidioidal spondylitis: MR findings in 15 patients. *Am J Roentgenol* 176:85-790, 1998.

Papadopoulos A, Garzonis S, Gouliamos A, et al: Correlation between spinal cord MRI and clinical features in patients with demyelinating disease. *Neuroradiology* 36:130-133, 1994.

Perry JR, Fung A, Poon P, Bayer N: Magnetic resonance imaging of nerve root inflammation in the Guillain-Barré syndrome. *Neuroradiology* 36:139-140, 1994.

Post MJD, Sze G, Quencer RM, et al: Gadolinium-enhanced MR in spinal infection. *J Comput Assist Tomogr* 14:721-729, 1990.

Post MJD, Quencer RM, Montalvo BM, et al: Spinal infections: evaluation with MR imaging and intraoperative US. *Radiology* 169:765-771, 1988.

Provenzale JM, Barboriak DP, Gaensler EHL, et al: Lupus-related myelitis: serial MR findings. *AJNR* 15:1911-1917, 1994.

Quencer RM: AIDS-associated myelopathy: clinical severity, MR findings, and underlying etiologies. *AJNR* 20:1387-1385, 1999.

Ratliff JK, Connolly ES: Intramedullary tuberculoma of the spinal cord. Case report and review of the literature. *J Neurosurg Spine* 90:125-128, 1999.

Reda MI, Bakr II: Tuberculous spondylitis: the role of magnetic resonance imaging in Pott's disease of the spine. *Int J Neurorad* 3:470-481, 1997.

Ross JS: Myelopathy. *Neuroimaging Clin North Am* 5:367-384, 1995.

Ross JS, Masaryk TJ, Modic MT, et al: Magnetic resonance imaging of lumbar arachnoiditis. *AJNR* 8:885-892, 1987.

Sadato N, Numaguchi Y, Rigamonti D, et al: Spinal epidural abscess with gadolinium-enhanced MRI: serial follow-up studies and clinical correlation. *Neuroradiology* 36:44-48, 1994.

Sandhu FS, Dillon WP: Spinal epidural abscess: evaluation with contrast-enhanced MR imaging. *AJNR* 12:1087-1093.

Santosh CG, Bell JE, Best JJK: Spinal tract pathology in AIDS: postmortem MRI correlation with neuropathology. *Neuroradiology* 37:134-138, 1995.

Sartoretti Schefer S, Blattler T, Wichmann W: Spinal MRI in vacuolar myelopathy, and correlation with histopathological findings. *Neuroradiology* 39:865-869, 1997.

Schultheiss TE, Stephens LC: Radiation myelopathy. *AJNR* 13:1056-1058, 1992.

Sharif HS: Role of MR imaging in the management of spinal infections. *Am J Roentgenol* 158:1333-1345, 1992.

Sharif HS, Aideyan OA, Clark DC, et al: Brucellar and tuberculosis spondylitis: comparative imaging features. *Radiology* 171:419-425, 1989.

Sharif HS, Morgan JL, Al Shahed MS, Al Thagafi MYA: Role of CT and MR imaging in the management of tuberculous spondylitis. *Radiol Clin North Am* 33:787-804, 1995.

Sharma S, Khilnani GC, Berry M: Megaloblastic anemia with subacute combined degeneration (SCD) of the spinal cord. *Semin Roentgenol* 34:2-4, 1999.

Sheth RD, Riggs JE, Schochet SS Jr: Demyelinating lesions mimicking spinal cord neoplasms. *Int J Neurorad* 3:496-502, 1997.

Sklar EML, Post MJD, Lebwohl NH: Imaging of infection of the lumbo-sacral spine. *Neuroimaging* 3:577-590, 1993.

Smith AS, Blaser SI: Infections and inflammatory processes of the spine. *Radiol Clin North Am* 29:809-828, 1991.

Smith AS, Weinstein MA, Mizushima A, et al: MR imaging of characteristics of tuberculosis spondylitis vs. vertebral osteomyelitis. *AJNR* 10:619-625, 1989.

Stäbler A, Reiser MF: Imaging of spinal infection. *Radiol Clin North Am* 39:1115-135, 2001.

Synder RD, King JN, Keck GM, Orrison WW: MR imaging of the spinal cord in 23 subjects with ALD-AMN complex. *AJNR* 12:1095-1098, 1991.

Talpos D, Tien RD, Hesselink JR: Magnetic resonance imaging of AIDS related polyradiculopathy. *Neurology* 41:1996-1998, 1991.

Tartaglino LM, Croul SE, Flanders AE, et al: Idiopathic acute transverse myelitis: MR imaging findings. *Radiology* 201:661-670, 1996.

Tartaglino LM, Friedman DP, Flanders AE, et al: Multiple sclerosis in the spinal cord: MR appearance and correlation with clinical parameters. *Radiology* 195:725-732, 1995.

Thorpe JW, Kidd D, Moseley IF, et al: Spinal MRI in patients with suspected multiple sclerosis and negative brain MRI. *Brain* 119: 709-714, 1996.

Thrush A, Enzmann D: MR imaging of infectious spondylitis. *AJNR* 11:1171-1180. 1990.

Thurnher MM, Post MJD, Jinkins JR: MRI of infections and neoplasms of the spine and spinal cord in 55 patients with AIDS. *Neuroradiology* 42:551-563, 2000.

Timms SR, Cure JK, Kurent JE: Subacute combined degeneration of the spinal cord: MR findings. *AJNR* 14:1224-1228, 1993.

Trop I, Bourgouin PM, Lapierre Y, et al: Multiple sclerosis of the spinal cord: diagnosis and follow-up with contrast-enhanced MR and correlation with clinical activity. *AJNR* 19:1025-1033, 1998.

Tung GA, Yim JWK, Mermel LA, et al: Spinal epidural abscess: correlation between MRI findings and outcome. *Neuroradiology* 41:904-909, 1999.

Unger E, Moldofsky P, Gatenby R, et al: Diagnosis of osteomyelitis by MR imaging. *Am J Roentgenol* 150:605-610, 1988.

Ursekar MA, Shetty PG, Dastur DK, Manghani DK: Tuberculous spinal meningitides and myeloradiculitis: imaging features with radiologic-pathologic correlation. *Int J Neurorad* 5:192-199, 1999.

Van Goethem JWM, Parizel PM, van den Hauwe L, et al: The value of MRI in the diagnosis of postoperative spondylodiscitis. *Neuroradiology* 42:580-585, 2000.

Varma R, Lander P, Assaf A: Imaging of pyogenic infectious spondylodiskitis. *Radiol Clin North Am* 39:203-213, 2001.

Wagner SC, Schweitzer ME, Morrison WB, et al: Can imaging findings help differentiate spinal neuropathic arthropathy from disk space infection? Initial experience. *Radiology* 214:693-699, 2000.

Wang PY, Shen WC, Jan JS: MR imaging in radiation myelopathy. *AJNR* 13:1049-1055, 1992.

Wang PY, Shen WC, Jan JS: Serial MRI changes in radiation myelopathy. *Neuroradiology* 37:374-377, 1995.

Welk LA, Wuint DJ: Amyloidosis of the spine in a patient on long-term hemodialysis. *Neuroradiology* 32:334-336, 1990.

Williams RL, Fukui MB, Meltzer CC, et al: Fungal spinal osteomyelitis in the immunocompromised patient: MR findings in three cases. *AJNR* 20:381-385. 1999.

Yasui T, Yagura H, Komiyama M, et al: Significance of gadolinium-enhanced magnetic resonance imaging of differentiating spinal cord radiation myelopathy from tumor. Case report. *J Neurosurg* 77:628-631, 1992.

Zweig G, Russell EJ: Radiation myelopathy of the cervical spinal cord: MR findings. *AJNR* 11:1188-1190, 1990.

# CHAPTER 21

# Spinal Trauma, Cysts, and Vascular Lesions

## Case 1170

77-year-old-man presenting with persistent
back pain two weeks after a fall.
(sagittal, noncontrast T1-weighted SE scan)

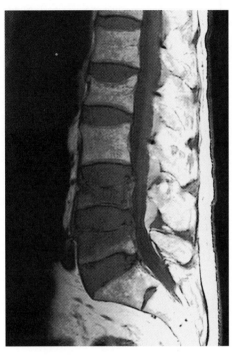

**Benign Compression Fractures**
(subacute)

## Case 1171

76-year-old woman presenting with back pain.
(sagittal, noncontrast T1-weighted SE scan)

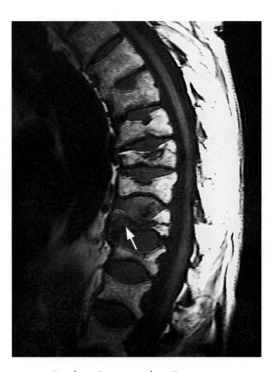

**Benign Compression Fractures**
(chronic)

Recent compression fractures of vertebral bodies typically demonstrate altered signal intensity. The normally short T1 and T2 values of fatty marrow are replaced by water-like signal characteristics due to hemorrhage, reactive edema and cellular infiltration.

In Case 1170, the superior end plates of the L4 and L5 vertebral bodies have been fractured and depressed. Subjacent edema occupies the majority of the L4 body and the superior two-thirds of the L5 body. Posterior displacement of bone and localized epidural hemorrhage cause mild anterior extradural deformity at both levels.

The reactive marrow edema associated with recent benign vertebral fractures may persist for weeks to months. Eventually, the appearance of the compressed vertebra returns to the baseline of short T1 values.

Case 1171 illustrates multiple old compression fractures of the thoracic spine. Focal Schmorl's nodes are superimposed on generalized depression of end plates at several levels. The one area of prolonged T1 values within vertebral marrow at the T11 level *(arrow)* probably indicates the site of a more recent fracture. There is overall exaggeration of thoracic kyphosis, but the spinal canal is not compromised.

Old depression of the superior end plate of the L2 vertebral body is present in Case 1170.

Low signal intensity within the disc at T10-11 in Case 1171 could represent either calcification or gas.

### Case 1172

65-year-old man presenting with cauda equina
syndrome after an automobile accident.
(sagittal, noncontrast T1-weighted SE scan)

### Case 1173

15-year-old boy injured in a
three-wheeler accident.
(sagittal, noncontrast T1-weighted SE scan)

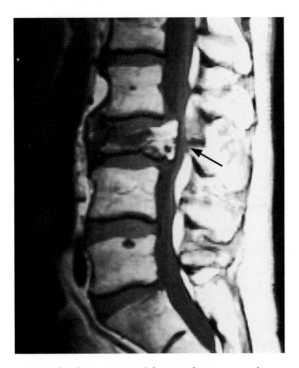

**Vertebral Fracture with Canal Compromise**

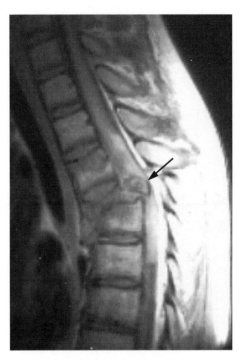

**Vertebral Fracture/Dislocation
with Canal Compromise**

---

MR effectively demonstrates compromise of the spinal canal and injury to the spinal cord in trauma cases. Sagittal T1-weighted scans provide a rapid survey of vertebral alignment. Epidural soft tissue masses are defined, and cord compression is quantified.

Posttraumatic narrowing of the spinal canal may be due to displacement of fracture fragments, associated hematomas, acute disc herniation, and/or frank dislocation. In Case 1172, posterior displacement of the fractured L3 vertebral body occupies the majority of the lumbar canal. Nerve roots of the cauda equina are dorsally displaced and compressed *(arrow)*. A small prevertebral mass at the L3 level probably represents recent hemorrhage superimposed on old degenerative changes.

Case 1173 demonstrates severe compression of the T4 vertebral body with associated dislocation. A fragment of the fractured vertebra has been displaced into the spinal canal *(arrow)*. Epidural (and possibly intradural) hemorrhage fills the canal from T2 to T6, obscuring the thecal sac and spinal cord. A localized prevertebral hematoma is present at the T5 level.

### Case 1174

77-year-old woman presenting with back pain.
(sagittal, noncontrast T1-weighted SE scan)

### Case 1175

48-year-old woman presenting with
back pain and bladder dysfunction.
(sagittal, noncontrast T1-weighted SE scan)

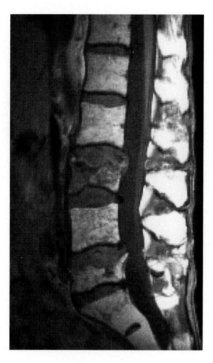

**Benign Fractures**

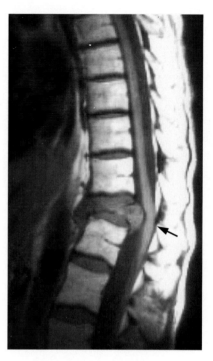

**Pathological Fracture**
(metastatic hypernephroma)

---

The distinction between benign and pathological fractures of vertebral bodies is a frequent clinical problem. MR scans can be helpful in this context.

Benign compression fractures that are subacute to chronic usually demonstrate residual high signal intensity due to marrow fat on T1-weighted scans. The L5 vertebral body in Case 1174 is a typical example: despite the obvious loss of height, the body is normally bright. This appearance contrasts with replacement of marrow signal by more water-like intensity in pathological fractures, as in Case 1175.

More recent benign vertebral fractures can be problematic. Hemorrhage and edema within a newly compressed vertebral body usually result in prolonged T1 and variable T2 values that may mimic primary vertebral disease with secondary pathological fracture. The L3 vertebra in Case 1174 demonstrates this appearance, which is more prominent in other cases (see Case 1170).

In such circumstances, secondary findings (e.g., the amount of cortical destruction, the presence of smaller le-

sions at other vertebral levels, or associated retroperitoneal or mediastinal adenopathy) may provide useful clues. STIR (Short Tau Inversion Recovery) sequences often help to detect subtle vertebral metastases at other levels. Postcontrast scans with fat-suppression techniques may define enhancing tumor, both within the compressed body and at possible additional sites.

Compressed vertebral bodies containing some residual normal marrow signal likely represent benign fractures; most pathological vertebral fractures are associated with complete replacement of normal marrow. Diffusion-weighted images have recently been suggested as a means of separating pathologic vertebral fractures (which demonstrate restricted diffusion) from benign lesions (which are often characterized by facilitated diffusion).

The pathological fracture in Case 1175 compresses the conus medullaris. Symptoms of conus dysfunction in cancer patients may also be caused by intramedullary metastases (see Case 1105).

## Case 1176A

85-year-old man being treated with corticosteroids,
now presenting with back pain.
(sagittal, noncontrast T1-weighted SE scan)

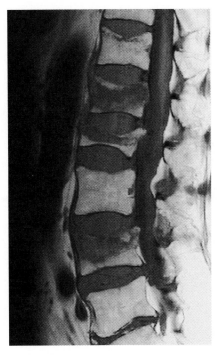

**Vertebral Osteonecrosis**

## Case 1176B

Same patient.
(sagittal, noncontrast T2-weighted FSE scan)

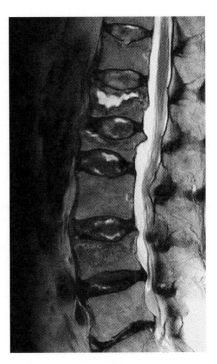

**Vertebral Osteonecrosis**

Avascular necrosis of a vertebral body typically occurs in association with a compression fracture. Primary ischemic necrosis may weaken the bone and predispose to fracture, or a benign compression fracture may compromise vertebral blood supply with subsequent osseous infarction.

Most patients with vertebral osteonecrosis are elderly individuals with osteoporosis. Corticosteroid therapy is a common component of the history. The osteonecrotic vertebra is often accompanied by simple compression fractures at other levels of the spine.

A characteristic imaging feature of vertebral osteonecrosis is the formation of a transverse or horizontal cleft within the ischemic body. When filled with gas, the clefts can be appreciated on standard radiographs ("intravertebral vacuum sign").

Alternatively, the clefts may be fluid-filled, as in Case 1176. The T1-weighted scan in Case 1176A demonstrates prolonged T1 values in several vertebral bodies with varying degrees of compression. (Note the preservation of normal marrow signal in portions of each compressed vertebrae, as is usually the case in benign fractures.) The T2-weighted image in Case 1176B defines a large, fluid-filled cleft within the L1 vertebra. A much smaller cleft is seen anteriorly at the L2 level, and there is a subtle suggestion of early cleft formation within the superior anterior portion of the L4 body. (Fissures containing watery granulation tissue or fluid are also present in several intervertebral discs.)

Ischemic necrosis and cleft formation within vertebral bodies are most common at levels from T8 to L2, with the highest incidence at T12 and L1. The demonstration of a cleft within a compressed vertebra strongly supports benignancy of the fracture and suggests avascular necrosis as a contributing factor.

Compare the localized, sharply defined fluid-filled cleft in Case 1176B to the less intense and more diffuse subchondral edema typically seen in discitis/osteomyelitis, as in Cases 1109 and 1110.

### Case 1177

6-year-old girl, paraplegic after an automobile
accident, with normal spine x-rays.
(sagittal, noncontrast T1-weighted SE scan)

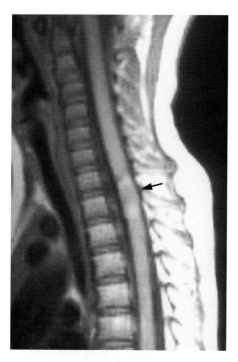

**Spinal Cord Contusion**

### Case 1178

8-month-old girl, paraplegic after an automobile
accident, with normal spine x-rays.
(sagittal, noncontrast T2*-weighted GRE scan)

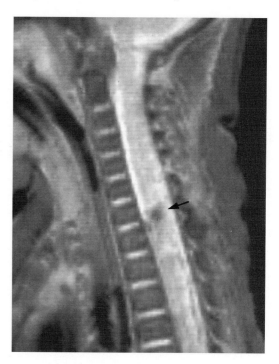

**Spinal Cord Contusion**

As illustrated on the preceding pages, MR scans can provide important soft tissue information in cases of spinal injury when osseous trauma is apparent on CT examinations or plain films. MR studies may also disclose neural injury when CT scans and routine radiographs are negative.

The pediatric spine is flexible and can undergo considerable subluxation without fracture. If such displacement is subsequently reduced, there may be no bony evidence of major spinal injury. The acronym "SCIWORA" (*S*pinal *C*ord *I*njury *W*ithout *R*adiographic *A*bnormality) has been used to describe this situation.

In Case 1177, vertebral alignment is normal. However, a zone of contusion with small areas of T1-shortening indicating subacute hemorrhage is seen within the spinal cord at the cervicothoracic junction *(arrow)*. The child remained paraplegic, and a follow-up scan showed localized atrophy at this site.

Case 1178 demonstrates a focal area of low signal intensity within the spinal cord at the C7-T1 level *(arrow)*. This zone represents susceptibility effect due to a small region of acute intramedullary hemorrhage. Gradient echo sequences are more sensitive than spin echo techniques for detecting susceptibility changes caused by small amounts of blood within the brain or spinal canal (see also Case 1189B).

The demonstration of hemorrhage within an injured spinal cord has been correlated with poor prognosis. Patients whose cords contain nonhemorrhagic edema at the level of trauma have a better chance of neurological recovery.

Frank transection of the spinal cord may occur in the pediatric population and is well demonstrated by sagittal MR scans. Perinatal transection can complicate difficult breech deliveries. The most common site of transection in older children is the cervicothoracic junction, comparable to the level of cord injury in the above cases.

## Case 1179

39-year-old man with quadriparesis since an
automobile accident two years earlier.
(sagittal, noncontrast T2-weighted FSE scan)

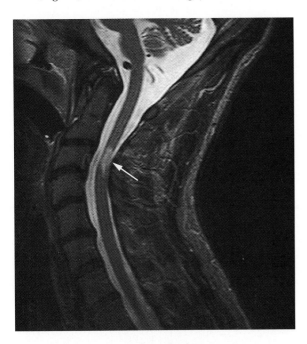

**Myelomacia**

## Case 1180

19-year-old woman, one year after
fracture/dislocation at C6-7.
(sagittal, noncontrast T1-weighted SE scan)

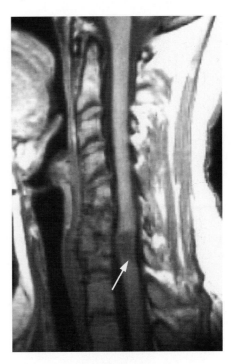

**Myelomalacia**

---

Focal injury to the spinal cord may lead to parenchymal loss and/or cyst formation. Localized myelomalacia frequently results from acute injuries like those on the preceding page. Chronic compressive or ischemic damage to the spinal cord (including cases of spinal stenosis) can also cause intramedullary necrosis and gliosis (see Cases 982 and 985).

In Case 1179, a well-defined intramedullary zone of prolonged T2 values is associated with focal volume loss at the C3 level *(arrow)*. The high signal intensity of the injured tissue implies increased water content, which may include microcystic and/or macrocystic components.

Case 1180 illustrates cystic myelomalacia at the site of old cord injury. Rather than being atrophic, as in Case 1179, the spinal cord is focally expanded by a small cyst that has developed in the damaged region. (Note that the cyst is confined to the level of prior injury, unlike the syrinxes in Cases 1183 and 1184.) A small cyst formed within a region of myelomalacia is usually not associated with further deterioration of function and rarely warrants evacuation.

However, an appearance similar to Case 1180 (i.e., localized cord "expansion") may alternatively indicate distortion of cord morphology by adhesions. Surgery to release tethering can lead to neurological improvement in such cases.

## Case 1181

21-year-old man with left arm weakness and sensory deficits two months after an automobile accident.
(axial, noncontrast T1-weighted SE scan; C7-T1 level)

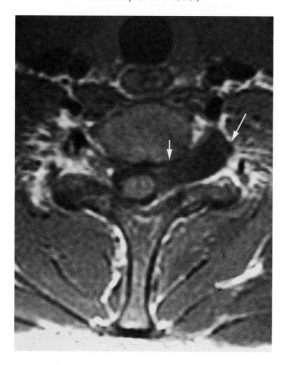

**Root Sleeve Injury with Pseudomeningocele**

## Case 1182

3-year-old girl with left arm weakness one year after an automobile accident.
(axial, noncontrast T2*-weighted GRE scan; C4 level)

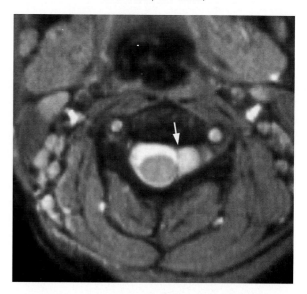

**Root Sleeve Injury with Pseudomeningocele**

---

When the head and neck of a patient are turned and pulled away from a restraining or distracting force on an arm, stretch injury may occur within the brachial plexus. In severe cases, cervical nerve roots are avulsed from the spinal cord. Scans performed acutely in this setting may demonstrate a column of hemorrhage along the lateral margin of the cord at the site of the avulsed fila radicularia.

Leakage of CSF (or intrathecal contrast) from a torn cervical root sleeve is presumptive evidence of severe injury to the contained nerve. Leaking spinal fluid may form a localized or extensive pseudomeningocele, often with persistent communication to the subarachnoid space at the level of injury.

In Case 1181, a pseudomeningocele occupied the left side of the spinal canal from C6 to T1. The intraspinal component of this fluid compartment *(short arrow)* causes mild compression of the thecal sac and displacement of the

spinal cord. A lateral extension of the pseudomeningocele *(long arrow)* traverses the nerve root canal to reach the paraspinal region. Note the lack of visualization of the presumably avulsed left C8 ventral and dorsal roots, compared to the normal appearance on the right side.

Case 1182 presents a T2-weighted scan of a similar posttraumatic pseudomeningocele in a pediatric patient. The dura is faintly seen as a thin membrane *(arrow)* separating the mildly deformed thecal sac from the epidural fluid pocket. The pseudomeningocele in this case extended over three vertebral levels and was associated with avulsion of the C4, C5, and C6 nerve roots.

Expansion of an intraspinal pseudomeningocele is a rare cause of delayed deterioration of neurological function after trauma. Posttraumatic syringomyelia (see Cases 1183 and 1184) and tethering adhesions are more common etiologies of worsening deficits.

### Case 1183

35-year-old man with a history of paraparesis,
now presenting with increasing
spasticity and arm weakness.
(sagittal, noncontrast T1-weighted SE scan)

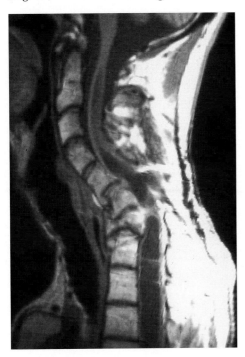

**Posttraumatic Syringomyelia**

### Case 1184

37-year-old man with a history of paraplegia due
to fracture/dislocation at C6-7, now complaining
of worsening arm numbness.
(coronal, noncontrast T1-weighted SE scan)

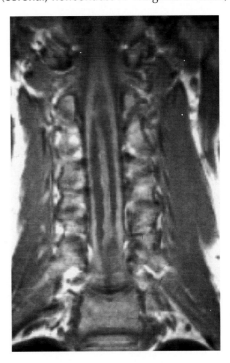

**Posttraumatic Syringomyelia**

Magnetic resonance imaging has demonstrated that syringomyelia is a common delayed consequence of spinal injury. This diagnosis should be suspected when neurological function deteriorates months or years after trauma. MR is the procedure of choice for evaluating such cases. The presence of orthopedic fixation hardware usually does not contraindicate an MR scan or prevent at least partial visualization of the spinal cord.

An old fracture deformity at C7 is apparent in Case 1183. A large intramedullary cyst is present above and below the level of trauma. (Compare to the localized cystic myelomalacia in Case 1180.) The rostral extension of this cyst into the cervical spinal cord is the basis for the patient's worsening condition. Decompression of a posttraumatic syrinx is warranted and often results in a return to baseline neurological function, as was true in this case.

Case 1184 presents an unusual double-barreled syrinx that has developed after trauma. This pattern, which has an "owl's eye" appearance on axial images, suggests symmetrical cord cavitation. In other cases, an eccentric posttraumatic syrinx is seen, resembling one of the two channels in Case 1184. Eccentric or twin-chambered morphology is rarely caused by congenital syringomyelia (see Cases 1228-1233).

Arachnoiditis occuring after spinal trauma may also be associated with the subsequent development of an intramedullary cyst, and release of adhesions may lead to resolution of syringomyelia. Tethering of neural elements by scar tissue is itself an important cause of late functional deterioration after spinal cord trauma, as discussed in Case 1180.

## Case 1185

26-year-old man with a three-day history
of increasing neck pain and leg weakness,
beginning after weight lifting.
(sagittal, noncontrast T1-weighted SE scan)

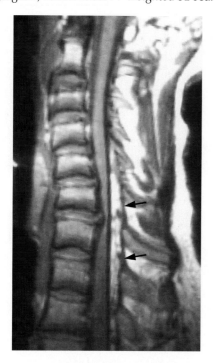

**Epidural Hematoma**
(subacute)

## Case 1186

62-year-old man presenting with recurrent
back pain one week after laminectomy.
(sagittal, noncontrast T1-weighted SE scan)

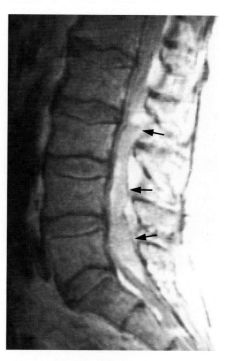

**Epidural Hematoma**
(subacute)

Epidural hemorrhage within the spinal canal may occur in association with disc herniation or vertebral fracture (see Case 1173). In other patients, spinal epidural hematomas develop spontaneously or as an isolated consequence of trauma.

Spinal epidural hematomas vary widely in size and morphology. Relatively thin layers of epidural blood may cause early symptoms within small canals, as in Case 1185. The dorsal hematoma in this patient *(arrows)* combines with a disc bulge at C6-7 to compress the spinal cord.

The postoperative epidural hematoma in Case 1186 is much thicker, occupying most of the lumbar canal. The dural sac is reduced to a thin layer compressed anteriorly against the vertebral bodies. (Compare the morphology of the hematoma in Case 1186 to the postoperative pseudomeningocele in Case 954.)

T1-shortening due to methemoglobin causes the subacute epidural hemorrhages in Cases 1185 and 1186 to be well defined. More acute epidural hematomas may be isointense on T1-weighted scans (see Case 1189), resembling other epidural pathologies. An isointense epidural (or subdural) hematoma (or empyema) is one cause of a featureless spinal canal lacking the normal definition of intrathecal nerve roots. (Imagine the appearance of Case 1186 if the hematoma did not demonstrate prominent T1-shortening.)

Both of the above hematomas extend over several vertebral levels, which is characteristic of epidural hemorrhage. Multilevel involvement is also typical of epidural abscesses and of some epidural tumors (e.g., lymphoma).

Subdural hemorrhages occur within the spinal canal and can be difficult to distinguish from epidural collections. Occasional spinal subdural hematomas develop as an extension of an intracranial hematoma or in association with spinal subarachnoid hemorrhage (see Case 1227).

### Case 1187

84-year-old woman presenting with paraplegia
one week after a minor fall.
(sagittal, noncontrast T1-weighted SE scan)

### Case 1188

53-year-old man presenting with
severe interscapular pain.
(sagittal, noncontrast T1-weighted SE scan)

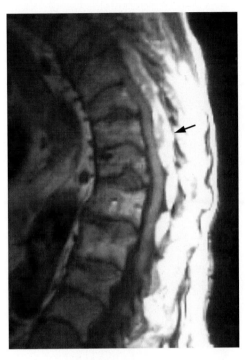

**Epidural Hematoma**
(subacute)

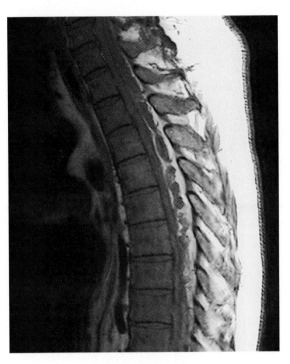

**Epidural Abscess**

Case 1187 illustrates that spinal epidural hemorrhage may be "spontaneous," occurring after trivial or unrecognized trauma. The morphology of this hematoma is distinctly lobulated, contrasting with the more linear collections on the preceding page. The superior pole of the hematoma contains central areas of isointensity. Cases 1185 to 1187 demonstrate the variable clinical context, morphology, and signal intensity of spinal epidural hemorrhage.

The dorsal epidural mass in Case 1188 is characterized by peripheral zones of high intensity surrounding central areas of longer T1 values. The loculations within this lesion represent fluid-filled abscess cavities, outlined by a perimeter of displaced epidural fat. Epidural abscesses, which can also be hemorrhagic, should be included in the differential diagnosis of thick epidural tissue containing short T1 values.

Lipomatosis is another potential cause of thickened epidural tissue with high signal intensity on T1-weighted scans (see Cases 1192 and 1193). Abnormal accumulation of epidural fat is most often seen in the thoracic canal of patients who are obese or are exposed to high levels of endogenous or exogenous corticosteroids. The condition may cause symptomatic cord compression.

Metastases containing paramagnetic substances or subacute hemorrhage (e.g., melanoma or leukemia) may cause epidural masses with short T1 components. Rare epidural angiolipomas and hemangiomas (see Case 996) can involve the dorsal thoracic region and resemble the more common pathologies discussed above.

The abscess in Case 1188 causes severe compression of the thecal sac. Prolonged T1 values throughout vertebral marrow in this case suggest a background of hematological abnormality or marrow infiltration (compare to Cases 1005 and 1006).

Cases 1123-1126 present a general discussion of spinal epidural abscesses. Compare the morphology of the abscess in Case 1188 to Case 1124.

# ACUTE SPINAL EPIDURAL HEMATOMAS

## Case 1189A

80-year-old woman with the sudden onset of neck
pain and right hemiparesis three days earlier.
(sagittal, noncontrast T1-weighted SE scan)

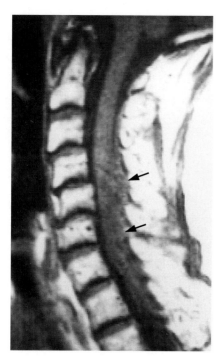

**Epidural Hematoma**
(acute)

## Case 1189B

Same patient.
(sagittal, noncontrast T2*-weighted GRE scan)

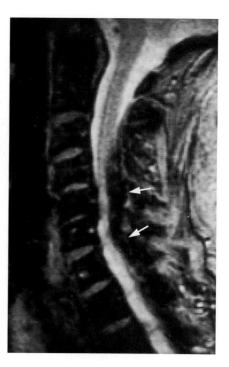

**Epidural Hematoma**
(acute)

The characteristic evolution of signal intensities described for intracerebral hematomas in Chapter 13 is less
rapid and less regular within extraparenchymal hemorrhages, either cranial or spinal. In particular, spinal
hematomas may appear isointense on T1-weighted scans for
many days after the onset of bleeding. This prolonged
"acute" phase may cause diagnostic confusion, mimicking
other epidural processes.

In Case 1189A, a dorsal epidural mass extends from C3
to C7 *(arrows).* The nonspecific mass is nearly isointense
to cord parenchyma. However, the gradient echo sequence
in Case 1189B demonstrates low signal intensity within the
same region. This evidence of local magnetic susceptibility
effect correctly suggests the presence of blood products
within the epidural tissue and identifies the lesion.

In some cases, low signal intensity on gradient echo
scans due to susceptibility effects is seen only at the margins of an epidural hematoma. The resulting dark rim
around the lesion resembles the morphology of the contrast enhancement in Case 1190.

The above scans demonstrate moderate compression of
the spinal cord at the C5 level due to the combination of
mild subluxation and the doral hematoma. Susceptibility
effects at interfaces on gradient echo images often exag-
gerate the degree of canal compromise associated with extradural deformities. The spinal canal in Case 1189B is
probably not as tight as it appears.

See Case 997 for another example of recent epidural
hemorrhage.

# DIFFERENTIAL DIAGNOSIS:
## EPIDURAL MASS WITH PERIPHERAL ENHANCEMENT

### Case 1190

80-year-old woman presenting with
neck pain and right hemiparesis.
(axial, postcontrast T1-weighted SE scan; C4-5 level)

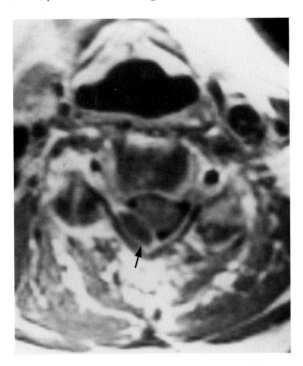

**Epidural Hematoma**
(same patient as Case 1189)

### Case 1191

69-year-old man presenting with
right-sided radicular back pain.
(axial, postcontrast T1-weighted SE scan; T8-9 level)

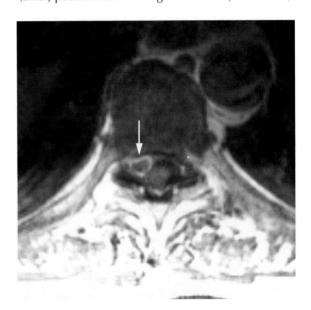

**Epidural Abscess**

---

A number of pathologies can cause peripherally enhancing epidural masses. The most common etiology, disc herniation surrounded by granulation tissue, is usually encountered in the lumbar region (see Case 945).

The posterolateral location of the cervical lesion in Case 1190 would be highly unusual for a herniated disc. A synovial cyst could be considered in the differential diagnosis (see Cases 969, 970, and 972), but these are rare in the cervical region. The dorsolateral position and the elliptical morphology of the mass are both common for spinal epidural hemorrhage, which was documented at surgery in this case.

Case 1191 illustrates a small epidural abscess with peripheral enhancement. The character of the lesion is indistinguishable from a localized epidural hematoma. These two pathologies must often be considered together in the differential diagnosis of an epidural mass.

A lateral thoracic disc herniation could also cause an appearance similar to Case 1191 on an axial scan but would probably be more limited in rostral/caudal extent than an epidural hematoma or abscess.

## Case 1192

27-year-old man, moderately obese but otherwise well, presenting with mild spasticity of the legs. (sagittal, noncontrast T1-weighted SE scan)

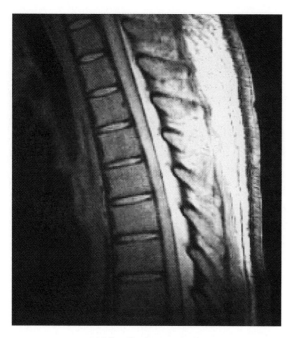

**Epidural Lipomatosis**

## Case 1193

82-year-old man presenting with back pain. (sagittal, noncontrast T1-weighted SE scan)

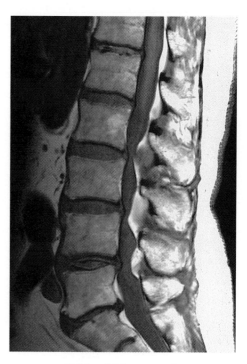

**Epidural Lipomatosis**

Abnormal accumulation of epidural fat may distort the thecal sac and compress the spinal cord or cauda equina. Epidural lipomatosis is most common in the thoracic canal of patients who are obese or are exposed to high levels of endogenous or exogenous corticosteroids.

Case 1192 is a typical example. Prominent thickening of epidural fat is present posterior to the thecal sac. The underlying subarachnoid space is partially effaced, and the spinal cord is mildly compressed. (Compare cord definition in the mid thoracic region to the appearance at the cervicothoracic junction.)

Epidural lipomatosis may present a more lobulated morphology, as in Case 1193. Thickening of dorsal epidural fat in this patient combines with disc bulges to cause central stenosis at multiple lumbar levels.

The above scans indicate that epidural lipomatosis can cause intraspinal masses demonstrating short T1 values and extending over long segments of the spinal canal with either linear or lobulated morphology. This appearance overlaps the spectrum of spinal epidural hematomas (compare to Cases 1185-1187), potentially causing diagnostic confusion.

Scans performed with fat-suppression techniques can distinguish between these two pathologies in ambiguous cases. The signal intensity of lipomatous tissue will be reduced by such sequences, whereas the T1-shortening of aqueous protons caused by the presence of paramagnetic methemoglobin within a hematoma will be unaltered.

### Case 1194A

35-year-old woman presenting with back pain.
(sagittal, noncontrast T2-weighted FSE scan)

### Case 1194B

Same patient.
(axial, noncontrast T1-weighted SE scan; T6 level)

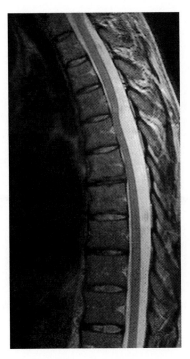

**Spinal Cord Herniation**

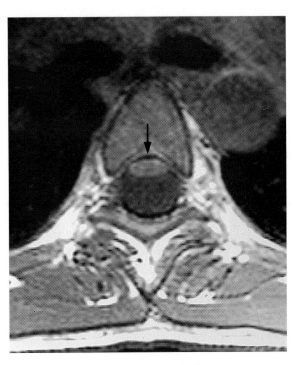

**Spinal Cord Herniation**

Spontaneous transdural herniation of the spinal cord is typically midthoracic in location and ventral in direction, as illustrated above. The age of reported patients ranges from the third to sixth decades; about two-thirds have been women.

The development of a spontaneous cord hernia presumably begins with a congenital or acquired defect in the ventral dura. The normal position of the thoracic spinal cord at the anterior margin of the subarachnoid space allows CSF pulsations to push it against and eventually into the dural defect. Over time, the bulging of the cord becomes more pronounced and less reducible, until incarceration and/or tethering adhesions cause permanent restriction and deformity.

Case 1194 demonstrates the typical imaging characteristics of this condition. The spinal cord in Case 1194A is focally deviated to abut the anterior margin of the thecal sac at the T6 level. The normally thin but patent ventral subarachnoid space is effaced, the cord diameter is mildly reduced, and the dorsal subarachnoid space is widened.

These features resemble the appearance of a dorsal intradural arachnoid cyst (compare to Case 1195). Diffusion-weighted studies or phase contrast sequences demonstrating CSF flow patterns may be useful to document or to exclude compartmentalization of the dorsal CSF space.

The axial scan in Case 1194B confirms the extreme anterior location of the mildly flattened spinal cord *(arrow)*, with a widely patent dorsal subarachnoid space. It is not possible to directly image extradural extension of cord parenchyma in most cases of spontaneous thoracic herniation; the diagnosis is instead suggested by the focal apposition of the cord to the anterior margin of the thecal sac.

Associated intramedullary signal abnormality is seen in a minority of cases of spinal cord herniation, implying edema, ischemia, and/or myelomalacia. Back pain and motor myelopathy are relieved in most cases by surgery to reduce the hernia and repair the dural defect; sensory deficits may persist.

Preoperative diagnosis of ventral cord herniation is important. Posterior exploration will encounter the widened dorsal subarachnoid space. This fluid "collection" can be misinterpreted as an arachnoid loculation causing cord displacement and dysfunction, with consequent failure to appreciate and address the ventral hernia.

### Case 1195

59-year-old woman presenting with back pain.
(sagittal, noncontrast T1-weighted SE scan)

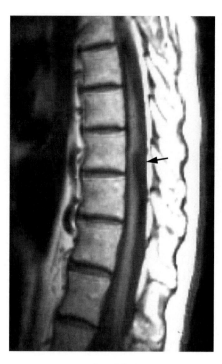

**Arachnoid Cyst**

### Case 1196

72-year-old woman presenting with
thoracic radiculopathy.
(axial, noncontrast T2-weighted FSE scan; T9 level)

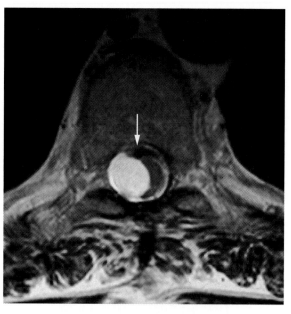

**Arachnoid Cyst**

Spinal arachnoid cysts most frequently occur within the thoracic canal, particularly dorsal to the spinal cord (as in the above cases). The formation of cysts in this region likely reflects loculation of the dorsal subarachnoid space, which is normally traversed by multiple arachnoid septations. Partial obstruction of CSF circulation within a subarachnoid compartment may lead to progressive enlargement and eventual cord compression. Arachnoiditis due to hemorrhage or meningitis may also cause subarachnoid loculation.

Like arachnoid cysts overlying the cerebral convexity (see Cases 808 and 809), spinal arachnoid cysts often demonstrate linear or angular margins. In Case 1195, the interface between the cyst and the spinal cord is quite straight. Cord compression is present.

The cyst in Case 1196 is more laterally based and rounder in morphology (compare to the intracranial cysts in Cases 810 and 811). The spinal cord is contralaterally displaced and compressed. A zone of low signal intensity at the anterior margin of the thecal sac *(arrow)* represents flow void from rapid and/or turbulent motion of CSF in the small residual channel of patent subarachnoid space.

The lesions in Cases 1195 and 1196 appear to be benign and extramedullary (but see Case 1200). A contrast-enhanced scan could be considered to exclude the rare possibility of an exophytic, cystic tumor (e.g., hemangioblastoma arising at the pial surface).

# EXTRADURAL ARACHNOID CYSTS ("MENINGEAL CYSTS")

## Case 1197

60-year-old woman presenting with back pain.
(sagittal, noncontrast T1-weighted SE scan)

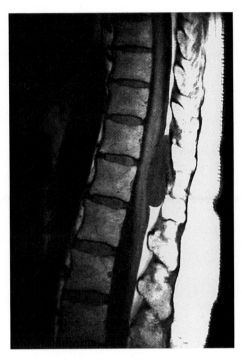

**Extradural Arachnoid Cyst**

## Case 1198

65-year-old woman presenting with back pain.
(axial, postcontrast T1-weighted SE scan; L1 level)

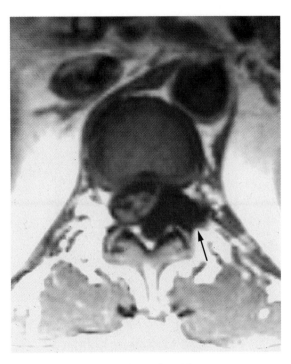

**Extradural Arachnoid Cyst**

Occasional arachnoid cysts are encountered in the epidural space, most commonly in the dorsal thoracic or lumbar region. This occurrence requires a congenital or acquired defect in the dura through which a loculation of the subarachnoid space can extend. Transmitted pulsation from the thecal sac and/or ball-valve restriction of bidirectional flow at the neck of the cyst may then lead to its enlargement. Some epidural "meningeal cysts" arise from a pedicle that originates where a dorsal nerve root penetrates the dura.

In contrast to the typically flat morphology of small intradural arachnoid cysts such as Case 1195, extradural cysts are often round and lobulated. The spherical margins of the lesion in Case 1197 are outlined by dorsal epidural fat. The underlying subarachnoid space is compressed.

In Case 1198, a left-sided dorsal meningeal cyst extends into the intervertebral foramen *(arrow)*. The intraspinal portion of the lesion causes mild displacement of the tip of the conus medullaris and proximal cauda equina. Together, the epidural and intraforaminal components of the cyst resemble a pseudomeningocele (compare to Cases 1181 and 1182), but the latter would be rare in the thoracolumbar region.

Compare the long-standing lobulated extradural cysts in the above cases to the chronic dural diverticula in Case 955 and to the acquired dorsal pseudomeningocele in Case 954. Also compare the morphology of the epidural cyst in Case 1197 to the schwannoma in Case 1055.

### Case 1199A

10-year-old boy presenting with
back pain and leg numbness.
(sagittal, noncontrast T2-weighted FSE scan)

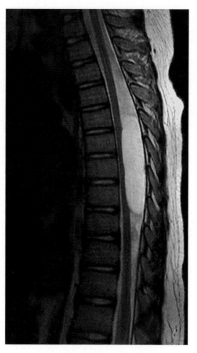

**Neuroepithelial Cyst**

### Case 1199B

Same patient.
(axial, noncontrast T2*-weighted GRE scan; T8 level)

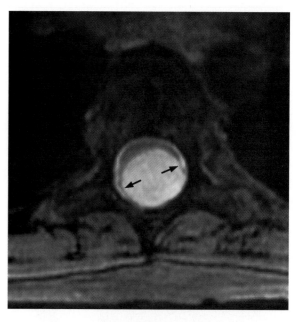

**Neuroepithelial Cyst**

Neuroepithelial (or "ependymal") cysts may arise from the spinal cord as well as within the intracranial compartment (see Cases 843 and 844). These benign masses are widely variable in size and morphology. They are often eccentric and exophytic, mimicking an intradural extramedullary process.

The large cyst in Case 1199A has expanded the spinal canal, indicating chronicity. The lesion is clearly intradural, with widening of the subarachnoid space at the rostral and caudal poles of the mass. Although the homogeneous T2 prolongation within this cyst suggests simple fluid, its thick, sausage-like morphology would be unusual for an arachnoid loculation (compare to Case 1195). More importantly, the axial scan in Case 1199B demonstrates a thin rim of cord parenchyma stretched around the lesion *(arrows)*, implying intramedullary origin.

There was no enhancement at the margins of the cyst on postcontrast scans. Surgery demonstrated a simple cyst filled with CSF and lined by neuroepithelium.

Compare the morphology of the intramedullary cyst causing circumferential thinning of the encircling cord in Case 1199B to the crescentic deformity of the cord compressed by an extramedullary arachnoid cyst in Case 1196.

# DIFFERENTIAL DIAGNOSIS:
## FOCAL CYST DEFORMING THE SPINAL CORD

### Case 1200

44-year-old man presenting with
progressive myelopathy.
(sagittal, noncontrast T1-weighted SE scan)

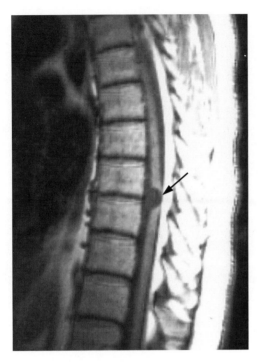

**Neuroepithelial Cyst**

### Case 1201

6-year-old girl presenting with spastic paraparesis.
(sagittal, noncontrast T2-weighted FSE scan)

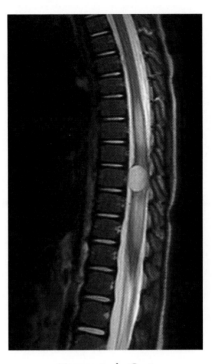

**Neurenteric Cyst**

---

The round, low intensity lesion in Case 1200 is much smaller than the neuroepithelial cyst in Case 1199 but is similarly eccentric and well defined. An axial image resembled the morphology of Case 1199B, except that the greatest thinning and distortion of cord parenchyma were ventral rather than dorsal. A postcontrast scan demonstrated no abnormal enhancement at the perimeter of the cyst or within the spinal cord.

Surgery in Case 1200 disclosed a benign neuroepithelial cyst arising exophytically from the spinal cord. Although this lesion is relatively rare, the characteristic appearance as demonstrated above has enabled preoperative diagnosis in a number of cases.

The mass in Case 1201 also appears simple and sharply defined as it deforms the ventral aspect of the spinal cord. Many spinal neurenteric cysts are more complex and/or are associated with adjacent vertebral anomalies (see Cases 1266 and 1267). The ventral location of the lesion in Case

1201 is typical for enterogenous cysts of the spinal canal, but comparison of Cases 1200 and 1201 indicates that this feature is nonspecific.

Spinal neurenteric cysts may be epidural, intradural but extramedullary, and/or intramedullary. Surgery in Case 1201 demonstrated a ventral endodermal cyst embedded within the spinal cord. The edema rostral and caudal to the cyst in the above scan resolved on postoperative studies.

The differential diagnosis in these cases includes an unusual invaginating arachnoid cyst, a parasitic cyst (e.g., cysticercosis), and an inclusion cyst (epidermoid or dermoid). An extramedullary tumor with long T1 and T2 values (e.g., schwannoma) or a cystic, exophytic primary tumor of the spinal cord (e.g., hemangioblastoma) could present a similar appearance on noncontrast scans but would be characterized by abnormal enhancement.

## Case 1202

61-year-old man presenting with back pain.
(sagittal, noncontrast T1-weighted SE scan)

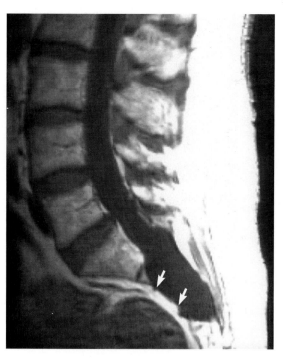

**Intrasacral Meningocele**

## Case 1203

18-year-old man presenting with
left S1 radiculopathy.
(axial, noncontrast scan; SE 2500/45; S1 level)

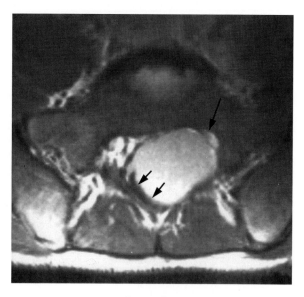

**Perineural Cyst**
("Tarlov" cyst)

---

CSF-containing masses are commonly found within the sacral canal. These may arise from the thecal sac or from sacral nerve roots. The benign and long-standing nature of the lesions is indicated by smooth erosion of adjacent bone, as seen in the above cases.

Among sacral cysts arising from the thecal sac are intrasacral or "occult" meningoceles, illustrated by Case 1202. Instead of tapering and terminating normally, the dural sac broadens within the sacral canal. Mass effect and CSF pulsation have caused erosion of the sacrum both anteriorly *(arrows)* and posteriorly. In some cases, an enlarged caudal sac balloons into the pelvis as an anterior sacral meningocele.

Another variety of sacral cyst is analogous to the extradural arachnoid cysts occasionally found at higher levels of the spinal canal (see Cases 1197 and 1198). A pedicle or neck communicates from the tip of the caudal sac to a sacral epidural cyst, which can fill and expand the sacral canal. Such lesions lack the broad communication with the dural sac seen in Case 1202. As a result, their signal intensity is usually higher than normal CSF due to elevated protein content and/or lack of pulsation-related signal loss.

"Tarlov" or perineural cysts arise from nerve root sleeves rather than from the dural sac. These cystic diverticula or ectasias may occur at any level (see Case 1059) but are particularly common in the sacral region. They are a frequent incidental finding but can enlarge to cause compressive radiculopathy.

In Case 1203, a large perineural cyst occupies much of the sacral canal. The left S1 nerve is displaced and compressed at the anterolateral margin of the cyst *(long arrow)*. The cyst displaces the dural sac and other roots posteriorly and to the right *(short arrows)*.

# DIFFERENTIAL DIAGNOSIS:
## MULTIPLE NERVE ROOT MASSES WITH LONG T2 VALUES

### Case 1204

58-year-old woman presenting with back pain.
(axial, noncontrast T2-weighted FSE scan; S2 level)

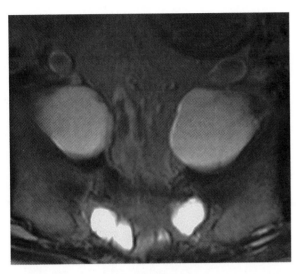

**Perineural Cysts**

### Case 1205

10-year-old boy presenting with back pain.
(axial, noncontrast T2-weighted FSE scan; S1 level)

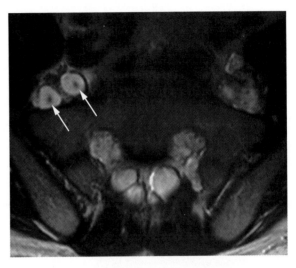

**Multiple Neurofibromas**

---

Perineural cysts are often multiple and bilateral, with variable symmetry. Case 1204 illustrates large cysts accompanying the S1 roots as they exit from their canals and enter the pelvis. Small intrasacral cysts are demonstrated involving the S2 roots bilaterally and the right S3 root. The homogeneous prolongation of T2 values throughout these masses is typical for simple CSF.

The masses within the sacral canal in Case 1205 also demonstrate high signal intensity on a T2-weighted scan. Close inspection suggests that these enlarged nerves are not as bright as the true cysts in Case 1204. More importantly, the enlarged presacral nerves of the lumbosacral plexus (and the smaller nerves within the S1 canals) demonstrate a central zone of low signal intensity *(arrows)*. This feature indicates that the expanded roots contain structured tissue rather than amorphous fluid. In particular, the target morphology of cross sections through these nerves is characteristic of neurofibromas, which typically have a dense fibrous core (see Case 1071).

The differential diagnosis in Case 1204 would include dural ectasia in a connective tissue disorder such as Marfan's syndrome.

The child in Case 1205 was known to have neurofibromatosis type 1. Both multiple and plexiform neurofibromas of the lumbar region and pelvis may be encountered in this disorder (see Cases 1069 and 1071).

An epidermoid cyst could also be considered among possible etiologies for a multilobulated intraspinal mass with long T1 and T2 values.

### Case 1206A

27-year-old woman who developed paraplegia
following surgery to remove a
herniated disc at T10-11.
(sagittal, noncontrast T2-weighted SE scan)

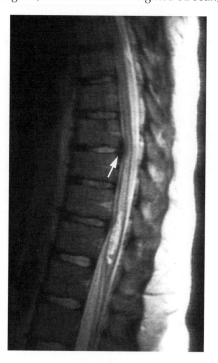

**Spinal Cord Infarct**

### Case 1206B

Same patient.
(sagittal, postcontrast T1-weighted SE scan)

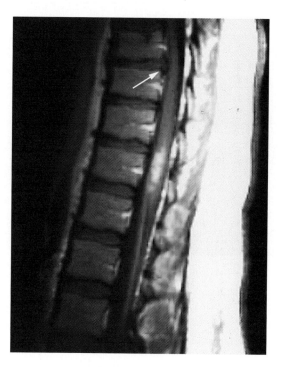

**Spinal Cord Infarct**

---

Infarction of the spinal cord may occur in a variety of clinical contexts. The most common association is an atherosclerotic aneurysm of the thoracolumbar aorta, either before or after surgery. Other possible etiologies include vasculitis (e.g., syphilis, collagen vascular disease), systemic embolization, trauma, and coagulopathy.

The thoracic spinal cord and conus medullaris are the regions most commonly affected by cord ischemia, although cervical cord infarcts also occur. Central gray matter of the cord is more severely damaged by ischemia than the peripheral white matter tracts (see Cases 1207 and 1208).

Case 1206 demonstrates typical findings in an atypical context. Abnormal high signal intensity involves central gray matter of the conus medullaris on a T2-weighted scan (Case 1206A). The center of the lesion is sharply defined, with an adjacent zone of less distinct signal abnormality extending rostrally into the thoracic region. Intense contrast enhancement is present within the infarct (Case 1206B).

The disc herniation at T10-11 *(arrows)* indents the ventral subarachnoid space and causes mild deformity of the spinal cord. It is conceivable that this epidural compression could lead to local compromise of the anterior spinal artery. A number of cases of spinal cord infarction secondary to disc herniation have been reported, including demonstration of embolic nuclear material within the anterior spinal artery. No other etiology for cord infarction was apparent in this young patient.

Equivocal swelling of the conus medullaris is seen in the above scans. Occasional cord infarcts demonstrate sufficient mass effect to resemble intramedullary tumors. In most cases the cord margins are not significantly expanded, and the differential diagnosis includes inflammatory or degenerative disorders (e.g., multiple sclerosis or amyotrophic lateral sclerosis).

Compare the enhancing lesion in Case 1206B to Cases 1140-1142, 1224, and 1225.

### Case 1207

68-year-old woman with a history of an aortic aneurysm, now presenting with abdominal pain, hypotension, and acute paraparesis. (axial, noncontrast T2-weighted SE scan; T10 level)

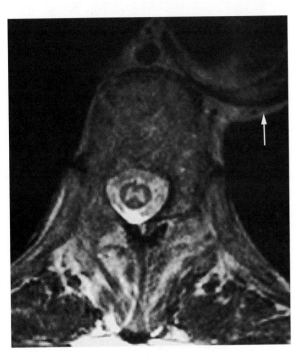

**Spinal Cord Infarct**

### Case 1208

67-year-old man with a history of diabetes mellitus who presented two weeks earlier with acute quadriparesis. (axial, noncontrast T2*-weighted GRE scan; C4-5 level)

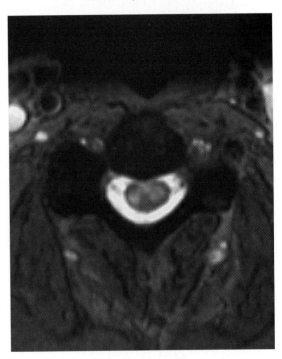

**Spinal Cord Infarct**

---

Acute or subacute infarction of the spinal cord can present variable patterns of intramedullary edema. Central gray matter is usually most severely affected, probably reflecting both the greater metabolic demand of cell bodies and the collateral blood supply at the perimeter of the cord.

In Case 1207, sharply defined regions of T2 prolongation conform to the anterior and posterior horns of intramedullary gray matter. Abnormal high signal intensity in Case 1208 is less distinctly marginated, but predominantly involves the anterior horns. Ischemic changes limited to the anterior horns may present an even more striking "snake eyes" or "owl's eyes" morphology in some cases.

Ventral or central edema symmetrically involving all or part of the distribution of gray matter within the cord should suggest the possibility of infarction. However, this pattern is not specific. Similar images may be obtained in patients with inflammatory or degenerative neuronal disorders (e.g., poliomyelitis). Intramedullary edema due to dural arteriovenous fistulae (see Cases 1209-1211) may also predominantly involve central gray matter.

The MR spectrum of spinal cord infarction includes diffuse edema in cases of severe ischemia affecting both the anterior and posterior spinal arteries. Unilateral ischemic changes may occur with occlusion of an individual, lateralized sulcoradicular branch of the anterior spinal artery.

Infarction of the spinal cord is most common near the thoracolumbar junction, with frequent involvement of the conus medullaris. Collateral supply to the anterior spinal artery is relatively sparse in this region, and occlusion of a single major radiculomedullary artery may cause symptomatic ischemia. Infarction of the cervical and superior thoracic segments of the spinal cord is infrequent due to redundancy of radicular supply to the anterior spinal artery at these levels.

Infarction should be included in the differential diagnosis of a conus lesion, particularly in patients with atherosclerotic disease. In Case 1207, thickening of the posterior margin of the descending aorta *(arrow)* suggests dissection, thrombus, and/or atherosclerotic plaque and supports the diagnosis of spinal cord infarction.

## Case 1209

81-year-old man presenting with
progressive myelopathy.
(sagittal, noncontrast T2-weighted FSE scan)

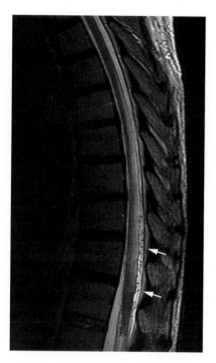

**Dural Arteriovenous Fistula**

## Case 1210

58-year-old man presenting with quadriparesis.
(sagittal, postcontrast T1-weighted SE scan)

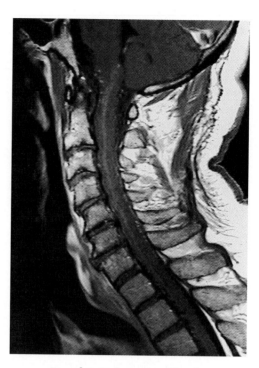

**Dural Arteriovenous Fistula**

Several types of arteriovenous malformations may be found within the spinal canal. The most common is the dural arteriovenous fistula or "radiculomedullary fistula." This lesion consists of an arteriovenous shunt occurring within the dura near the exit of spinal nerve root. Intradural venous drainage from the fistula floods the valveless coronal venous plexus on the surface of the spinal cord. The transmitted pressure and flow distend perimedullary veins for multiple levels rostral and/or caudal to the shunt. Venous hypertension impairs drainage of spinal cord parenchyma, causing intramedullary edema and occasional frank infarction.

A broad range of findings has been noted on MR scans of patients with spinal dural arteriovenous fistulae. In some cases, the MR scan is normal, with no evidence of a fistula that is subsequently proven angiographically and/or surgically.

Many patients demonstrate nonspecific cord edema and swelling, reflecting passive congestion due to venous hypertension. Dorsal intramedullary edema is present from T8 to T12 in Case 1209 (see also Case 1211).

Distended intradural veins may be visualized on MR scans with variable definition. In some cases, the presence of dilated pial vessels causes a subtle irregularity or fuzziness along the surface of the spinal cord. In other patients, tortuous flow voids can be specifically identified at the cord margin, as seen within the dorsal subarachnoid space in the inferior thoracic region in Case 1209 *(arrows)*.

Contrast enhancement may help to demonstrate abnormal vascular channels on the surface of the cord, as in Case 1210. The distended pial veins in this patient represented caudal drainage from a dural arteriovenous fistula of the posterior fossa (see Cases 744 and 745). The cervical spinal cord is expanded, effacing the ventral and dorsal subarachnoid spaces. A T2-weighted scan demonstrated extensive intramedullary edema.

The presence of dilated perimedullary vessels is not specific for spinal vascular malformations. Occasional tumors (especially ependymomas and hemangioblastomas) may cause a similar appearance (see Case 1094A). Postcontrast scans define the intramedullary masses in such cases.

Patchy intramedullary contrast enhancement may be noted in association with dural arteriovenous fistulae, probably reflecting venous congestion and correlating negatively with prognosis.

# DIFFERENTIAL DIAGNOSIS:
## MULTIPLE SUBARACHNOID FOCI OF LOW SIGNAL INTENSITY

### Case 1211

58-year-old man presenting with bilateral
leg pain and foot numbness.
(sagittal, noncontrast T2-weighted FSE scan)

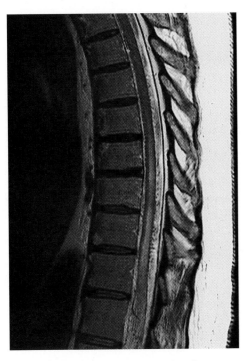

**Dural Arteriovenous Fistula**

### Case 1212

6-year-old boy presenting with back pain.
(sagittal, noncontrast T2-weighted FSE scan)

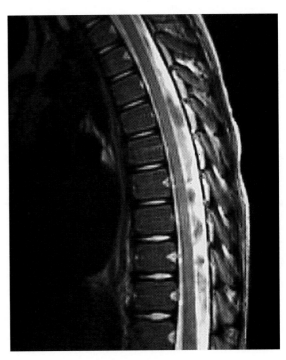

**Normal CSF Pulsation**

---

The dorsal subarachnoid space in the thoracic region is traversed by multiple arachnoid strands and septations. These bands produce a network of multiple partially divided chambers and channels. Localized turbulence of pulsatile CSF flow in this area normally causes multiple zones of low signal intensity, most apparent on T2-weighted scans such as Case 1212.

Flow-related areas of signal loss in the subarachnoid space may raise the question of enlarged intrathecal vessels. However, comparison of the CSF pulsation artifacts in Case 1212 with the enlarged intradural vessels in Case 1211 demonstrates their dissimilarity. Vascular channels, even when hypertrophied, are typically smaller and more sharply defined than zones of diminished signal due to disorganized CSF motion.

Central intramedullary edema in Case 1211 reflects congestion due to venous hypertension. This finding (and the associated myelopathy) often resolves when the responsible fistula is occluded.

The age and sex of the patient in Case 1211 are typical for spinal dural arteriovenous fistulae. These acquired lesions usually present between ages 50 and 70 years, with a male to female ratio of about 8 to 1. Many patients complain of pain prior to the onset of gradually progressive myelopathy.

Redundant nerve roots in cases of spinal stenosis can be serpentine intrathecal structures potentially resembling hypertrophied vessels (see Cases 957 and 1094A). Clinical context and the associated narrowing of the central canal establish the correct diagnosis in such cases.

### Case 1213

64-year-old man presenting with a two-year
history of worsening myelopathy.
(sagittal, noncontrast T1-weighted SE scan)

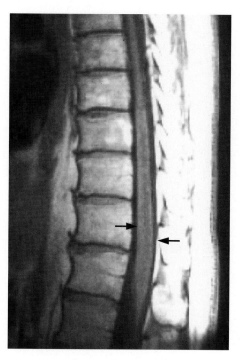

**Dural Arteriovenous Fistula**

### Case 1214

68-year-old woman presenting with
progressive conus dysfunction.
(sagittal, noncontrast T1-weighted SE scan)

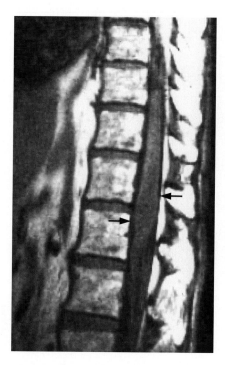

**Metastatic Carcinoma of the Breast**

The expansion and low signal intensity involving the thoracic cord and conus medullaris in Case 1213 were due to edema caused by a spinal dural arteriovenous fistula. Distended intradural vessels are only equivocally suggested on the MR scan but were demonstrated angiographically.

A history of long-standing progressive myelopathy is characteristic of patients with spinal dural AV fistulae. Such symptoms should suggest the diagnosis, particularly in middle-aged or elderly men. Intramedullary edema is a common finding in such cases and may be diffuse (as in Case 1213) or confined to central gray matter (resembling Case 1207).

Spinal dural arteriovenous fistulae can be successfully obliterated angiographically or sugically. They represent an important treatable cause of myelopathy. The prognosis is best when the diagnosis is made prior to the onset of extensive intramedullary edema.

Case 1214 is a reminder that metastatic disease should always be suspected when a lesion is found within the conus medullaris of an adult. An enhancing intramedullary nodule was demonstrated on a postcontrast scan.

Inflammatory and ischemic processes can also cause edema of the conus. (See Cases 1150 and 1206 for examples.)

### Case 1215A

48-year-old man presenting with leg
weakness and bladder dysfunction.
(sagittal, noncontrast T2-weighted FSE scan)

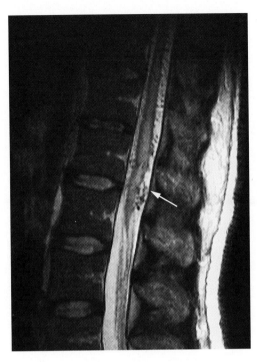

**Perimedullary Arteriovenous Fistula**

### Case 1215B

Same patient.
(sagittal, postcontrast T1-weighted SE scan)

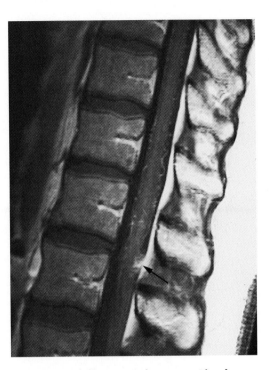

**Perimedullary Arteriovenous Fistula**

---

Dural arteriovenous fistulae ("radiculomedullary fistulae"), illustrated in Cases 1209-1211, are the most common vascular malformations of the spinal canal.

Arteriovenous fistulae may also occur at the pial surface of the spinal cord or conus medullaris, as in Case 1215. The average patient presenting with a perimedullary fistula is younger (age 15 to 50) than the usual patient presenting with a dural arteriovenous malformation (over age 50).

Angiography in Case 1215 demonstrated a direct arteriovenous connection at the site of the tissue nodule on the posterior surface of the conus medullaris (*arrows*). The findings above are otherwise similar to the appearance of the dural arteriovenous fistulae presented on the preceding pages. Enlarged veins are seen as channels of low signal intensity at the surface of the spinal cord and within the subarachnoid space in Case 1215A. These slowly flowing vessels are opacified with contrast material in Case 1215B.

Edema and faint, patchy enhancement within the conus medullaris are indistinguishable from the potential sequelae of a dural arteriovenous fistula.

Venous hypertension is the presumed cause of intramedullary edema and enhancement in both dural arteriovenous fistulae and perimedullary fistulae. However, the arterial supply to the lesion is distinctly different in these two malformations: dural supply from a radicular spinal artery in the former, and pial supply from the anterior and/or posterior spinal arteries in the latter.

True intramedullary arteriovenous malformations occur as a third major category of spinal vascular abnormality (see Cases 1218 and 1219). These lesions usually come to attention before age 40, often presenting with spinal subarachnoid hemorrhage. Mass effect of the malformation, arterial steal, and venous hypertension may all contribute to neurological deficits in these cases.

# DIFFERENTIAL DIAGNOSIS:
## NODULAR ENHANCEMENT WITHIN THE CAUDA EQUINA

### Case 1216

48-year-old man presenting with paraparesis.
(axial, postcontrast T1-weighted SE scan; L1-2 level)

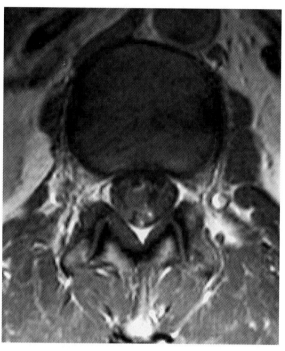

**Perimedullary Arteriovenous Fistula**
(same patient as Case 1215)

### Case 1217

64-year-old man presenting with
leg pain and weakness.
(axial, postcontrast T1-weighted SE scan; L1 level)

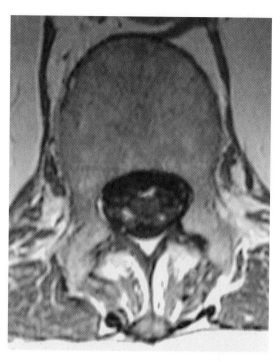

**Metastatic Carcinoma of the Lung**

Case 1216 is an axial scan of the patient presented in Case 1215. The nodular areas of enhancement among the roots of the cauda equina represent enlarged vessels. Accompanying sagittal views should minimize potential confusion with inflammatory or neoplastic pathologies in such cases, although the imaging features are occasionally ambiguous.

Intradural metastases from systemic or intracranial tumors have been discussed in Chapter 19. Case 1217 is a typical example of spinal leptomeningeal carcinomatosis, with multiple nodular metastases studding the surface of nerve roots.

Inflammatory disorders (e.g., sarcoidosis, tuberculosis, herpes zoster, and cytomegalovirus) should be considered among the potential etiologies for nodular enhancement in-volving intrathecal nerve roots. Polyradiculitis (e.g., Guillain-Barré syndrome; see Cases 1151-1153) usually involves nerves more uniformly and over longer segments than illustrated in the cases above.

Radicular enhancement may be noted for several centimeters proximal to a site of neural compression (see Cases 946 and 947). Such enhancement is more intense than the normal mildly increased signal of intrathecal roots on postcontrast scans.

Prominent, asymmetrical contrast enhancement of a single intrathecal nerve root is occasionally seen as a normal variant due to a large accompanying vein. (The largest vein of the cauda equina usually courses along the filum terminale before exiting with an inferior lumbar or sacral nerve root.)

# OCCULT INTRADURAL ARTERIOVENOUS MALFORMATIONS

## Case 1218

59-year-old woman presenting with paraparesis.
(sagittal, noncontrast T1-weighted SE scan)

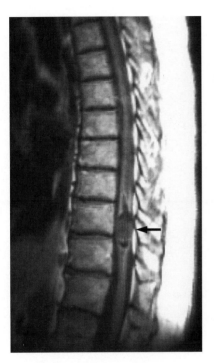

**Arteriovenous Malformation**

## Case 1219

45-year-old man presenting with back and leg pain.
(sagittal, noncontrast T2-weighted SE scan)

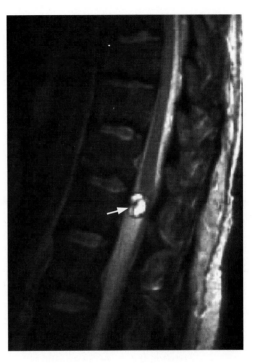

**Arteriovenous Malformation**

---

True arteriovenous malformations (AVMs) are much less common within the spinal canal than dural arteriovenous fistulae. Intradural AVMs may occur within the spinal cord (as in Case 1218) or in an extramedullary location (as in Case 1219) and demonstrate variable patency. The surgically proven AVMs in both of the above cases were thrombosed and angiographically "occult."

Low signal intensity capping the rostral and caudal portions of the lesion in Case 1218 may reflect calcification and/or hemosiderin from old hemorrhage. This appearance resembles the common finding of blood products at the margins of some intramedullary tumors (see Case

1223). The potential resemblance of intramedullary AVMs and primary neoplasms is compounded by the occasional presence of dilated superficial vessels adjacent to cord tumors (due to hyperemia and/or partial venous obstruction).

The extramedullary mass at the surface of the conus medullaris in Case 1219 is nonspecific. A thrombosed vascular malformation is a rare etiology for such a lesion. Differential diagnosis would include a necrotic or hemorrhagic schwannoma (see Case 1062) or an unusual ependymoma. The mass demonstrated intense enhancement on a postcontrast scan.

**Case 1220**

10-year-old boy presenting with
back pain and leg weakness.
(sagittal, noncontrast T1-weighted SE scan)

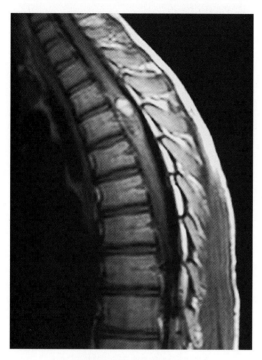

**Cavernous Angioma**

**Case 1221**

43-year-old man presenting with neck
pain and left arm numbness.
(axial, noncontrast T2*-weighted
GRE scan; C4 level)

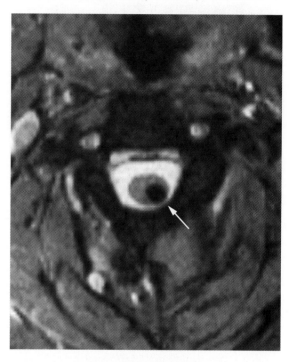

**Cavernous Angioma**
(presumed)

Cavernous angiomas are malformations consisting of thin-walled vascular spaces with no intervening neuroglial tissue. The sinusoidal channels of the hemangioma are often lined and surrounded by hemosiderin reflecting recurrent small hemorrhages. Occasional cavernous angiomas present with macroscopic hemorrhage, as illustrated intracranially in Cases 771 and 772.

MR imaging has demonstrated that cavernous angiomas occur at all levels of the spinal cord. They may be single or multiple, isolated or associated with intracranial lesions. Many intramedullary angiomas are incidental; the importance of recognizing these lesions is primarily to distinguish them from neoplasms. Occasional cavernous angiomas within the spinal cord cause myelopathy or radiculopathy, as in the above cases.

The MR features of intramedullary cavernous angiomas are comparable to the appearance of the intracranial lesions discussed in Chapter 14. A heterogeneous reticular architecture with short T1 components is characteristic. Short T2 values due to susceptibility effects are usually present with a peripheral and/or interstitial pattern.

The superior thoracic mass in Case 1220 is typical. At surgery, the superior pole of the lesion proved to be a subacute hematoma, whereas the inferior component was angiomatous tissue.

The lesion in Case 1221 has not been biopsied. The small area of signal loss within the left posterolateral aspect of the cervical spinal cord *(arrow)* suggests focal accumulation of hemosiderin, likely due to a small cavernous angioma. The differential diagnosis would include a site of old hemorrhage, but the mild mass effect (rather than tissue loss) and the absence of an acute event in the patient's history argue against this alternative.

# DIFFERENTIAL DIAGNOSIS:
## COMPLEX INTRAMEDULLARY MASS CONTAINING BLOOD PRODUCTS

### Case 1222

10-year-old boy presenting with
thoracic myelopathy.
(sagittal, noncontrast T2-weighted FSE scan)

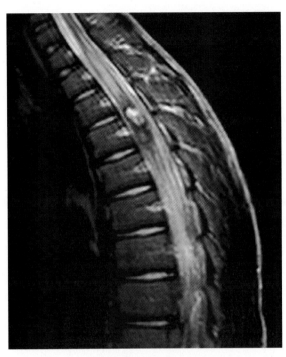

**Cavernous Angioma**
(same patient as Case 1220)

### Case 1223

48-year-old man presenting with
back pain and paraparesis.
(sagittal, noncontrast T2-weighted FSE scan)

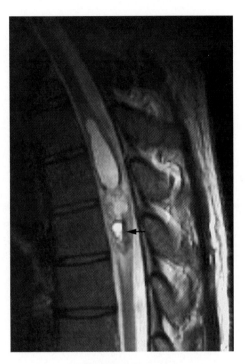

**Ependymoma**

---

Both vascular malformations and neoplasms can present as hemorrhagic intramedullary masses. Blood products may be seen within or capping the poles of either pathology.

Case 1222 is a T2-weighted scan of the patient presented in Case 1220. Signal loss due to blood products (mainly hemosiderin) is present at the margin of the intramedullary mass and surrounds the subacute hematoma at the superior pole. Edema is noted both rostral and caudal to the lesion.

The ependymoma in Case 1223 is comparably heterogeneous. Cysts of variable size are present, both within and adjacent to the central tissue nodule. Components of low signal intensity suggest blood products or calcification; a small sedimentation level of erythrocytes may be present

*(arrow).* This complex morphology including cysts and hemorrhage is typical for ependymomas of the spinal cord, as discussed in Cases 1080-1083.

A small amount of intramedullary edema is present inferior to the tumor in Case 1223. The rostral cyst in this case proved to be reactive rather than neoplastic (compare to Cases 1085 and 1100-1102). Cord expansion is more prominent in Case 1223 than in Case 1222.

Abnormal contrast enhancement can be seen in both cavernous angiomas and intramedullary tumors but is a more constant feature of the latter. That is, the absence of enhancement favors an occult vascular malformation as the etiology of a hemorrhagic intramedullary mass.

### Case 1224

41-year-old man presenting with
diminished position sense.
(axial, postcontrast T1-weighted SE scan; C3 level)

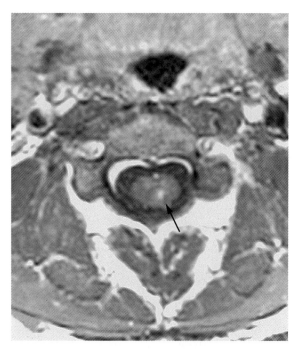

**Cavernous Angioma**

### Case 1225

54-year-old woman presenting with
gait abnormality.
(axial, postcontrast T1-weighted SE scan; C4 level)

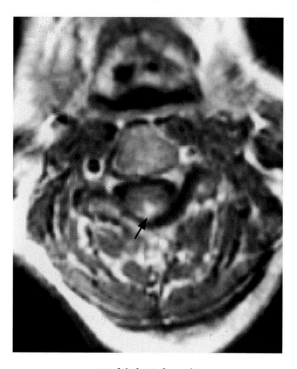

**Multiple Sclerosis**

---

Contrast enhancement within cavernous angiomas may be minimal or intense, diffuse or localized. The small focus of enhancement within the dorsal intramedullary lesion in Case 1224 *(arrow)* falls within the wide spectrum seen in cavernous malformations. A T2-weighted scan in this case resembled Case 1221. The position of the lesion within the posterior columns correlates with the patient's impaired sense of position.

As discussed in Chapter 20, multiple sclerosis is among the pathologies that may cause focal or multifocal enhancement within the spinal cord. The enhancing plaque in Case 1225 is nonspecific. However, the dorsal location is suggestive of demyelinating disease, which typically spares central gray matter.

Primary or metastatic tumors should be included in the differential diagnosis, as demonstrated in Cases 1099, 1101, 1106, and 1141. In particular, a pial-based hemangioblastoma or focal leptomeningeal carcinomatosis could resemble the appearance of Case 1225.

A number of additional inflammatory etiologies may present with focal intramedullary or pial-based enhancement. Examples include tuberculosis (see Case 478) and sarcoidosis (see Case 1142).

## Case 1226

58-year-old woman scanned three days after the acute onset of severe backache and headache. (sagittal, noncontrast T1-weighted SE scan)

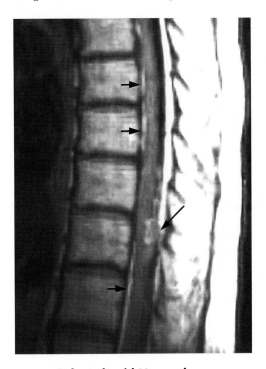

**Subarachnoid Hemorrhage**

## Case 1227

26-year-old man with back pain following suboccipital craniotomy for medulloblastoma. (sagittal, noncontrast T2-weighted FSE scan)

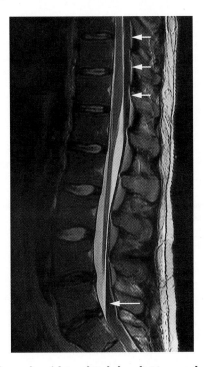

**Subarachnoid (and Subdural) Hemorrhage**

---

Linear and nodular areas of T1-shortening are present along the margins of the spinal cord in Case 1226. Axial images confirmed the intradural, extramedullary location of the high intensity zones, which are due to subarachnoid hemorrhage. Despite a thorough work-up including spinal angiography, the source of the bleeding was not determined.

In Case 1227, a sedimentation level of blood products is seen as a zone of low signal intensity within the dependent portion of the lumbar subarachnoid space *(long arrow)*. This clear separation of erythrocytes from more normal CSF requires an undisturbed period of gravitational settling. In ambulatory patients, spinal subarachnoid hemorrhage instead presents as homogeneously abnormal signal intensity throughout the thecal sac, often most easily appreciated as mildly shortened T1 values in the lumbosacral region. As in the intracranial compartment, FLAIR images increase the conspicuity of abnormal cellularity and/or protein within the spinal subarachnoid space.

Spinal subarachnoid hemorrhage may accumulate locally to form a focal hematoma. This sequestration of blood is common in the dorsal thoracic canal, where arachnoid septations are numerous. Such subarachnoid hematomas may mimic vascular intradural masses. The small dorsal accumulation of blood at the T10 level in Case 1226 *(long arrow)* resembles the perimedullary arteriovenous fistula in Case 1215.

A spinal source should be considered when no other etiology is found for intracranial subarachnoid hemorrhage. This is particularly true if (1) the hemorrhage is concentrated in the posterior fossa and/or (2) back pain is a prominent initial symptom.

Spinal origin of recurrent subarachnoid hemorrhage should also be suspected when superficial siderosis is discovered with no apparent intracranial etiology (see Cases 721 and 722). Ependymomas of the spinal canal are among the pathologies to be sought in this context.

The layer of blood products causing low signal intensity along the posterior margin of the thoracic and superior lumbar canal in Case 1227 *(short arrows)* was localized to the subdural space on axial images.

# REFERENCES

Amano Y, Machida T, Kumazaki T: Spinal cord infarcts with contrast enhancement of the cauda equina: two cases. *Neuroradiology* 40:669-672, 1998.

Avrahami E, Tadmor R, Ram Z, et al: MR demonstration of spontaneous acute epidural hematoma of the thoracic spine. *Neuroradiology* 31:89-92, 1989.

Baker LL, Goodman SB, Perkash I, et al: Benign versus pathologic compression fractures of vertebral bodies: assessment with conventional spin-echo, chemical-shift, and STIR MR imaging. *Radiology* 174:495-502, 1990.

Barkovich AJ, Sherman JL, Citrin CM, Wippold FJ II: MR of postoperative syringomyelia. *AJNR* 8:319-328, 1987.

Barnwell SL, Dowd CF, Davis RL, et al: Cryptic vascular malformations of the spinal cord: diagnosis by magnetic resonance imaging and outcome of surgery. *J Neurosurg* 72:403-407, 1990.

Barrena R, Guelbenzu S, Eiras J, et al: Cavernous angiomas of the spinal cord: clinical-radiologic factors predisposing to hemorrhage. *Int J Neurorad* 4:132-141, 1998.

Bauer A, Huber A, Ertl-Wagner B, et al: Diagnostic value of increased diffusion weighting of a steady-state free precession sequence for differentiating acute benign osteoporotic fractures from pathologic vertebral compression fractures. *AJNR* 22:366-372, 2001.

Baur A, Stabler A, Bruning R, et al: Diffusion-weighted MR imaging of bone marrow: differentiation of benign versus pathologic compression fractures. *Radiology* 207:349-356, 1998.

Beers GJ, Raque GH, Wagner GG: MR imaging in acute cervical spine trauma. *J Comput Assist Tomogr* 12:755-761, 1988.

Bhalla S, Reinus WR: The linear intravertebral vacuum: a sign of benign vertebral collapse. *Am J Roentgenol* 170:1563-1569, 1998.

Borges LF, Zervas NT, Lehrich JR: Idiopathic spinal cord herniation: a treatable cause of the Brown-Sequard syndrome—case report. *Neurosurgery* 36:1028-1032, 1995.

Boukobza M, Guichard J, Boissonet M, et al: Spinal epidural haematoma: report of 11 cases and review of the literature. *Neuroradiology* 36:456-459, 1994.

Bowen BC, Fraser K, Kochan JP, et al: Spinal dural arteriovenous fistulas: evaluation with MR angiography. *AJNR* 16:2029-2043, 1995.

Brugieres P, Malapert D, Adle-Biassette H, et al: Idiopathic spinal cord herniation: value of MR phase-contrast imaging. *AJNR* 20:935-940, 1999.

Brunereau L, Gobin YB, Meder J-F, et al: Intracranial dural arteriovenous fistulas with spinal venous drainage: relation between clinical presentation and angiographic findings. *AJNR* 17:1549-1554, 1996.

Bundschuh CV, Modic MT, Kearney F, et al: Rheumatoid arthritis of the cervical spine: Surface-coil MR imaging. *AJNR* 9:565-571, 1988.

Campi A, Filippi M, Comi G, Scotti G: Recurrent acute transverse myelopathy associated with anticardiolipin antibodies. *AJNR* 19:781-786, 1998.

Carvalho GA, Nikkhah G, Matthies C, et al: Diagnosis of root avulsions in traumatic brachial plexus injuries: value of computerized tomography myelography and magnetic resonance imaging. *J Neurosurg* 86:69-76, 1997.

Casselman JW, Jolie E, Dehaene I, Meeus L: Gadolinium-enhanced MR imaging of infarction of the anterior spinal cord. *AJNR* 12:561-562, 1991.

Chakeres DW, Flickinger F, Bresnahan JC, et al: MR imaging of acute spinal cord trauma. *AJNR* 8:5-10, 1987.

Chen CJ, Fang W, Chen CM, Wan YL: Spontaneous spinal epidural haematomas with repeated remission and relapse. *Neuroradiology* 39:739-740, 1997.

Chen CJ, Ro L-S: The MRI signs of spinal arachnoid diverticula. *Neuroradiology* 39: 446-449, 1997.

Choi BY, Chang K-H, Choe G, et al: Spinal intradural extramedullary capillary hemangioma: MR imaging findings. *AJNR* 22:799-802, 2001.

Coffe MJ, Hadley MN, Herrera GA, Morawetz RB: Dialysis-associated spondyloarthropathy. *J Neurosurg* 80:694-700, 1994.

Curati WL, Kingsley DPE, Kendall BE, Moseley IF: MRI in chronic spinal cord trauma. *Neuroradiology* 35:30-35, 1993.

Cuenod CA, Laredo J-D, Chevret S, et al: Acute vertebral collapse due to osteoporosis or malignancy: appearance on unenhanced and gadolinium-enhanced MR images. *Radiology* 199:541-550, 1996.

Davis PC, Reisner A, Hudgins PA, et al: Spinal injuries in children: role of MR. *AJNR* 14:607-617, 1993.

Davis SW, Levy LM, LeBihan DJ, et al: Sacral meningeal cysts: evaluation with MR imaging. *Radiology* 187:445-448, 1993.

Deutsch H, Jallo GI, Faktorovich A, Epstein F: Spinal intramedullary cavernoma: clinical presentation and surgical outcome. *J Neurosurg Spine* 93:65-70, 2000.

Dietemann JH, De la Palavesa MMF, Kastler B, et al: Thoracic intradural arachnoid cyst: possible pitfalls with myelo-CT and MR. *Neuroradiology* 33:90-91, 1991.

Dix JE, Griffitt W, Yates C, et al: Spontaneous thoracic spinal cord herniation through an anterior dural defect. *AJNR* 19:1345-1348, 1998.

Do HM, Jensen ME, Cloft HJ, et al: Dural arteriovenous fistula of the cervical spine presenting with subarachnoid hemorrhage. *AJNR* 20:348-351, 1999.

Doppman JL: Epidural lipomatosis. *Radiology* 171:581-1348, 1998.

Doppman JL, DiChiro G, Dwyer AJ, et al: Magnetic resonance imaging of spinal arteriovenous malformations. *J Neurosurg* 66:830-834, 1987.

Dormont D, Assouline E, Gelbert F, et al: MRI study of spinal arteriovenous malformations. *Neuroradiology* 14:351-364, 1987.

Dormont D, Gelbert F, Assouline E, et al: MR imaging of spinal cord artetiovenous malformations at 0.5T: study of 34 cases. *AJNR* 9:833-838, 1988.

Duke BJ, Levy AS, Lillehei KO: Cavernous angiomas of the cauda equina: case report and review of the literature. *Surg Neurol* 50:442-445, 1998.

Dupuy DE, Palmer WE, Rosenthal DI: Vertebral fluid collection associated with vertebral collapse. *Am J Roentgenol* 167:1535-1538, 1996.

El-Khoury GY, Whitten CG: Trauma to the upper thoracic spine: anatomy, biomechanics, and unique imaging features. *Am J Roentgenol* 160:95-102, 1993.

Elksnis SM, Hogg JP, Cunningham ME: MR imaging of spontaneous cord infarction. *J Comput Assist Tomogr* 15:228-232, 1991.

Enzmann DR, O'Donohue J, Rubin JB, et al: CSF pulsations within non-neoplastic spinal cord cysts. *Am J Roentgenol* 149:149-157, 1987.

Ernst RJ, Gaskill-Shipley M, Tomsick TA, et al: Cervical myelopathy associated with intracranial dural arteriovenous fistula: MR findings before and after treatment. *AJNR* 18:1330-1334, 1997.

Ewald C, Kuhne D, Hassler WE: Progressive spontaneous herniation of the thoracic spinal cord: case report. *Neurosurgery* 46:493-496, 2000.

Faig J, Busse O, Salbeck R: Vertebral body infarction as a confirmatory sign of spinal cord ischemic stroke: report of three cases and review of the literature. *Stroke* 29:239-243, 1998.

Falcone S, Quencer RM, Green BA, et al: Progressive posttraumatic myelomalacic myelopathy: imaging and clinical features. *AJNR* 15:747-754, 1994.

Fessler RG, Johnson DL, Brown FD, et al: Epiudural lipomatosis in steroid-treated patients. *Spine* 17:183-188, 1992.

Flanders AE, Spettell CM, Friedman DP, et al: The relationship between the functional abilities of patients with cervical spinal cord injury and the severity of damage revealed by MR imaging. *AJNR* 20:926-934, 1999.

Flanders AE, Spettell CM, Tartaglino LM, et al: Forecasting motor recovery after cervical spinal cord injury: value of MR imaging. *Radiology* 201:649-655, 1996.

Fontaine S, Melanson D, Cosgrove R, Bertrand G: Cavernous hemangiomas of the spinal cord: MR imaging. *Radiology* 166:839-842, 1988.

Friedberg SR, Fellows T, Thomas CB, et al: Experience with symptomatic spinal epidural cysts. *Neurosurgery* 34:989-993, 1994.

Friedman DP, Flanders AE: Enhancement of gray matter in anterior spinal infarction. *AJNR* 13:983-985, 1992.

Friedman DP, Flanders AE, Tartaglino LM: Vascular neoplasms and malformations, ischemia, and hemorrhage affecting the spinal cord: MR imaging findings. *Am J Roentgenol* 162:685-690, 1994.

Fukui MB, Swarnkar AS, Williams RL: Acute spontaneous spinal epidural hematomas. *AJNR* 20:1365-1372, 1999.

Gasparotti R, Ferraresi S, Pinelli L, et al: Three-dimensional MR myelography of traumatic injuries of the brachial plexus. *AJNR* 18:1733-1742, 1997.

Gebarski SS, Maynard FW, Gabrielson TO, et al: Posttraumatic progressive myelopathy: clinical and radiologic correlation employing MR imaging, delayed CT-metrizamide myelography, and intraoperative sonography. *Radiology* 157:379-386, 1985.

Gelbert F, Assouline E, Houdart E., et al: Classification and diagnosis of spinal vascular malformations. *Int J Neurorad* 5:205-211, 1999.

Georgy BA, Chong B, Chamberlain M, et al: MR of the spine in Guillain-Barré syndrome. *AJNR* 15:300-301, 1994.

Gilbertson JR, Miller GM, Goldman MS, et al: Spinal dural arteriovenous fistulas: MR and myelographic findings. *AJNR* 16:2049-2057, 1995.

Goldberg AL, Rothfus WE, Deeb ZL, et al: The impact of magnetic resonance on the diagnostic evaluation of acute cervicothoracic spinal trauma. *Skeletal Radiol* 17:89-94, 1988.

Goyal RN, Russell NA, Benoit BG, Belanger JMEG: Intraspinal cysts: a classification and literature review. *Spine* 12:209-213, 1987.

Grabb PA, Pang D: Magnetic resonance imaging in the evaluation of spinal cord injury without radiographic abnormality in children. *Neurosurgery* 35:406-414, 1994.

Greitz D, Ericson K, Flodmark O: Pathogenesis and mechanics of spinal cord cysts: a new hypothesis based on magnetic resonance studies of cerebrospinal fluid dynamics. *Int J Neurorad* 5:61-78, 1999.

Hackney DB, Asato R, Joseph PM, et al: Hemorrhage and edema in acute spinal cord compression: demonstration by MR imaging. *Radiology* 161:387-390, 1986.

Haddad MC, Aabed al-Thagafi MY, Djurberg H: MRI of spinal cord and vertebral body infarction in the anterior spinal artery syndrome. *Neuroradiology* 38:161-162, 1996.

Hader WJ, Fairholm D: Giant intraspinal pseudomeningoceles cause delayed neurological dysfunction after brachial plexus injury: report of three cases. *Neurosurgery* 46:1245-1249, 2000.

Hasuo K, Mizushima A, Mihara F, et al: Contrast-enhanced MRI in spinal arteriovenous malformations and fistulae before and after embolization therapy. *Neuroradiology* 38:609-615, 1996.

Hausmann ON, Moseley IF: Idiopathic dural herniation of the thoracic spinal cord. *Neuroradiology* 38:503-510, 1996.

Hayashi N, Yamamoto S, Okubo T, et al: Avulsion injury of cervical nerve roots: enhanced intradural nerve roots at MR imaging. *Radiology* 206:817-822, 1998.

Henderson FH, Crockard HA, Stevens JM: Spinal cord oedema due to venous stasis. *Neuroradiology* 35:312-315, 1993.

Hierholzer J, Beendorf G, Lehman T, et al: Epidural lipomatosis: case report and literature review. *Neuroradiology* 38:348-345, 1996.

Hirono H, Yamadori A, Komiyama M, et al: MRI of spontaneous spinal cord infarction: serial changes in gadolinium-DTPA enhancement. *Neuroradiology* 34:95-97, 1992.

Holtas S, Heiling M, Lonntoft M: Spontaneous spinal epidural hematoma: findings at MR imaging and clinical correlation. *Radiology* 199:409-414, 1996.

Hong SH, Chang KH, Han MH, et al: Cervical root avulsion: magnetic resonance imaging findings and comparison of diagnostic accuracy between magnetic resonance imaging and conventional myelography. *Int J Neurorad* 2:182-187, 1996.

Hurst RW, Grossman RI: Peripheral spinal cord hypointensity on T2-weighted MR images: a reliable imaging sign of venous hypertensive myelopathy. *AJNR* 21:781-786, 2000.

Isu T, Iwasaki Y, Akino M, et al: Magnetic resonance imaging in cases of spinal dural arteriovenous malformation. *Neurosurgery* 24:919-923, 1989.

Jinkins JR, Reddy S, Leite CC, et al: MR of parenchymal spinal cord signal change as a sign of active advancement in clinically progressive posttraumatic syringomyelia. *AJNR* 19:177-182, 1998.

Kalfas I, Wilberger J, Goldberg A, Prostko ER: Magnetic resonance imaging of acute spinal cord trauma. *Neurosurgery* 23: 295-299, 1988.

Kataoka H, Miyamoto S, Nagat I, et al: Venous congestion is a major cause of neurological deterioration in spinal arteriovenous malformations. *Neurosurgery* 48:1224-1230, 2001.

Kendall BE, Stevens JM, Crockard HA: The spine in rheumatoid arthritis. *Riv di Neuroradiol* (Suppl 2):23-28, 1992.

Kirsch EC, Khangure MS, Holthouse D, McAuliffe W: Acute spontaneous spinal subdural haematoma: MRI features. *Neuroradiology* 42:586-590, 2000.

Kochan JP, Quencer RM: Imaging of cystic and cavitary lesions of the spinal cord and canal: the value of MR and intraoperative sonography. *Radiol Clin North Am* 29:867-912, 1991.

Koyanagi I, Yoshinobu I, Hida K, et al: Acute cervical cord injury without fracture or dislocation of the spinal column. *J Neurosurg Spine* 93:15-20, 2000.

Kulkarni MV, Boundurant FJ, Rose SL, Narayama PA: 1.5T MR imaging of acutre spinal trauma. *Radiographics* 8:1059-1082, 1988.

Kulkarni MV, McArdle CB, Kopanicky D: Acute spinal cord injury: MR imaging at 1.5T. *Radiology* 164:837-843, 1987.

Kurata A, Miyasaka Y, Yoshida T, et al: Venous ischemia caused by dural arteriovenous malformation. Case report. *J Neurosurg* 80:552-555, 1994.

La Rosa G, D'Avella D, Conti A: et al: Magnetic resonance imaging-monitored conservative management of traumatic spinal epidural hematomas. Report of four cases. *J Neurosurg Spine* 91:128-132, 1999.

Larsson E-M, Desai P, Hardin CW, et al: Venous infarction of the spinal cord resulting from dural arteriovenous fistula: MR imaging findings. *AJNR* 12:739-743, 1991.

Larsson E-M, Holtas S, Zygmunt S: Pre- and postoperative MR imaging of the craniocervical junction in reheumatoid arthritis. *AJNR* 10:89-94, 1989.

Masaryk TJ, Ross JS, Modic MT, et al: Radiculomeningeal vascular malformations of the spine: MR imaging. *Radiology* 164:845-849, 1987.

Mascalchi M, Arnetoli G, Dal Pozzo G, et al: Spinal epidural angiolipoma: MR findings. *AJNR* 12:744-745, 1991.

Mascalchi M, Bianchi MC, Quilici N, et al: MR angiography of spinal vascular malformations. *AJNR* 16:289-298, 1995.

Mascalchi M, Cosottini M, Ferrito G, et al: Posterior spinal artery infarct. *AJNR* 19:361-363, 1998.

Mascalchi M, Ferrito G, Quilici N, et al: Spinal vascular malformations: MR angiography after treatment. *Radiology* 219:346-353, 2001.

Mascalchi M, Scazzeri F, Prosetti D, et al: Dural arteriovenous fistula at the craniocervical junction with perimedullary venous drainage. *AJNR* 17:1137-1142, 1996.

Mathis JM, Wilson JT, Barnard JW, Zelenik ME: MR imaging of spinal cord avulsion. *AJNR* 9:1232-1233, 1988.

Mawad ME, Rivera V, Crawford S: Spinal cord ischemia after resection of thoracoabdominal aortic aneurysms: MR findings in 24 patients. *AJNR* 11:987-991, 1990.

Mikulis DJ, Ogilvy CS, McKee A, et al: Spinal cord infarction and fibrocartilagenous emboli. *AJNR* 13:155-160, 1992.

Miller SF, Glasier CM, Griebal ML, Boop FA: Brachial plexopathy in infants after traumatic delivery: evaluation with MR imaging. *Radiology* 189:481-484, 1993.

Minami S, Sagoh T, Nishimura K, et al: Spinal arteriovenous malformations: MR imaging. *Radiology* 169:109-116, 1988.

Mirvis SE, Geisler FH, Jelinek JJ, et al: Acute cervical spine trauma: evaluation with 1.5T MR imaging. *Radiology* 166:807-816, 1988.

Mirvis SE, Wolf AL: MRI of acute cervical spine trauma. *Applied Radiology* 15-22, December 1992.

Miyake S, Tamaki N, Nugashima T, et al: Idiopathic spinal cord herniation. *J Neurosurg* 88:331-335, 1998.

Murphy MD, Batnitzky S, Bramble JM: Diagnostic imaging of spinal trauma. *Radiol Clin North Am* 27:855-872, 1989.

Nabors MW, Pait TG, Byrd EB, et al: Updated assessment and current classification of spinal meningeal cysts. *J Neurosurg* 68:366-377, 1988.

Ogilvy CS, Louis DN, Ojemann RG: Intramedullary cavernous angiomas of the spinal cord: clinical presentation, pathological features, and surgical management. *Neurosurgery* 31:219-230, 1992.

Paramore CG: Dorsal arachnoid web with spinal cord compression: variant of an arachnoid cyst? Report of two cases. *J Neurosurg Spine* 93:287-290, 2000.

Pathria MN, Petersilge CA: Spinal trauma. *Radiol Clin North Am* 29:847-866, 1991.

Paulsen RD, Call GA, Murtagh FR: Prevalence and percutaneous drainage of cysts of the sacral nerve root sheath (Tarlov cysts). *AJNR* 15:293-297, 1994.

Petersilge CA, Pathria MN, Emery SE, Masaryk TJ: Thoracolumbar burst fractures: evaluation with MR imaging. *Radiology* 194:49-54, 1995.

Petterson H, Larsson EM, Holtas S, et al: MR imaging of the cervical spine in rheumatiod arthritis. *AJNR* 9:573-577, 1988.

Popovich MJ, Taylor FC, Helmer E: MR imaging of birth-related brachial plexus avulsion. *AJNR* 10(Suppl):S98, 1989.

Post MJD, Becerra JL, Madsen PW, et al: Acute spinal subdural hematoma: MR and CT findings with pathologic correlates. *AJNR* 15:1895-1906, 1994.

Preul MC, Leblanc R, Tampieri D, et al: Spinal angiolipomas. Report of three cases. *J Neurosurg* 78:280-286, 1993.

Quencer RM: The injured spinal cord: evaluation with magnetic resonance and intraoperative sonography. *Radiol Clin North Am* 26:1025-1046, 1988.

Quencer RM, Nunez D, Green BA: Controversies in imaging acute cervical spine trauma. *AJNR* 18:1866-1868, 1997.

Quencer RM, Sheldon JJ, Post MJD, et al: Magnetic resonance imaging of the chronically injured cervical spinal cord. *AJNR* 7:457-464, 1986.

Quint DJ, Boulos RS, Sanders WP, et al: Epidural lipomatosis. *Radiology* 169:485-495, 1988.

Rabin BM, Roychowdhury S, Meyer JR, et al: Spontaneous intracranial hypotension: spinal MR findings. *AJNR* 19:1034-1039, 1998.

Ricolfi F, Gobin PY, Aymard A, et al: Giant perimedullary arteriovenous fistulas of the spine: clinical and radiologic features and endovascular treatment. *AJNR* 18:677-687, 1997.

Rimmelin A, Clouet PL, Salatino S, et al: Imaging of thoracic and lumbar spinal extradural arachnoid cysts: report of two cases. *Neuroradiology* 39:203-206, 1997.

Rohrer DC, Burshiel KJ, Gruber DP: Intraspinal extradural meningeal cysts demonstrating ball-valve mechanism of formation. *J Neurosurg* 78:122-125, 1993.

Roncaroli F, Scheithauer BW, Krauss WE: Capillary hemangioma of the spinal cord. Report of four cases. *J Neurosurg Spine* 93:148-151, 2000.

Rothfus WE, Chedid MK, Deeb ZL, et al: MR imaging of the diagnosis of spontaneous spinal epidural hematomas. *J Comput Assist Tomogr* 11:851-854, 1987.

Ryken TC, Menezes AH: Cervicomedullary compression in achondroplasia. *J Neurosurg* 81:43-48, 1994.

Schwartz ED, Falcone SF, Quencer RM, Green BA: Posttraumatic syringomyelia: pathogenesis, imaging, and treatment. *Am J Roentgenol* 173:487-492, 2000.

Shaw DWW, Weinberger E, Brewer DK, et al: Spinal subdural enhancement after suboccipital craniectomy. *AJNR* 17:1373-1378, 1996.

Shimada Y, Sato K, Abe E, et al: Spinal subdural hematoma. *Skeletal Radiol* 25:477-480, 1996.

Shin JH, Lee HK, Jeon SR, Park SH: Spinal intradural capillary hemangioma: MR findings. *AJNR* 21:954-956, 2000.

Silbergleit R, Brunberg JA, Patel SC, et al: Imaging of spinal intradural arachnoid cysts: MRI, myelography and CT. *Neuroradiology* 40:664-668, 1998.

Silberstein M, Tress BM, Hennessy O: Delayed neurologic deterioration in the patient with spinal trauma: role of MR imaging. *AJNR* 13:1373-1382, 1992.

Silberstein M, Tress BM, Hennessy O: Prediction of neurologic outcome in acute spinal cord injury: the role of CT and MR. *AJNR* 13:1597-1608, 1992.

Sklar E, Quencer RM, Green BA, et al: Acquired spinal subarachnoid cysts: evaluations with MR, CT myelography, and intraoperative sonography. *AJNR* 10:1097-1104, 1989.

Sklar EML, Post JMD, Falcone S: MRI of acute spinal epidural hematomas. *J Comput Assist Tomog* 23:238-243, 1999.

Stern Y, Spiegelmann SM: Spinal intradural arachnoid cysts. *Neurochirurgie* 34:127-130, 1991.

Stevens JM, Olney JS, Kendall BE: Posttraumatic cystic and noncystic myelopathy. *Neuroradiology* 27:48-56, 1985.

Suh DC, Kim SJ, Jung SM, et al: MRI in presumed cervical anterior spinal artery territory infarcts. *Neuroradiology* 38:56-58, 1996.

Takahashi S, Yamada T, Ishii K, et al: MRI of anterior spinal artery syndrome of the cervical spinal cord. *Neuroradiology* 33:25-29, 1992.

Tarr RW, Drolshagen LF Kerner TC, et al: MR imaging of recent spinal trauma. *J Comput Assist Tomogr* 11:412-417, 1987.

Tekkok IH: Spontaneous spinal cord herniation: case report and review of the literature. *Neurosurgery* 46:485-492, 2000.

Terk MR, Hume-Neal M, Fraipont M, et al: Injury to the posterior ligament complex in patients with acute spinal trauma: evaluation by MR imaging. *Am J Roentgenol* 168:1481-1485, 1997.

Terwey B, Becker H, Thron AK, Vahldiek G: Gadolinium-DTPA-enhanced MR imaging of spinal dural arteriovenous fistulas. *J Comput Assist Tomogr* 13:30-37, 1989.

Tomlinson FH, Rufenacht DA, Sundt TM Jr, et al: Arteriovenous fistulas of the brain and spinal cord. *J Neurosurg* 79:16-27, 1993.

Turjman F, Joly D. Monnet O, et al: MRI of intramedullary cavernous haemangiomas. *Neuroradiology* 37:297-306, 1995.

Verstraete KLA, Martens, F, Smeets P, et al: Traumatic lumbosacral nerve root meningoceles: the value of myelography, CT and MRI in the assessment of nerve root continuity. *Neuroradiology* 31:425-429, 1989.

Watters MR, Stears JC, Osborn AG, et al: Transdural spinal cord herniation: imaging and clinical spectra. *AJNR* 19:1337-1344, 1998.

Welsh CT, Palmer CA, Townsend JJ, Jacobs JM: Radiologic-pathologic correlation of spinal dural arteriovenous fistula (Foix-Alajouanine syndrome). *Int J Neurorad* 4:51-55, 1998.

Willinsky R, terBrugge K, Montanera W, et al: Posttreatment MR findings in spinal dural arteriovenous malformations. *AJNR* 16:2063-2071, 1995.

Yuh WTC, March EE, Wang AK, et al: MR imaging of spinal cord and vertebral body infarction. *AJNR* 13:145-154, 1992.

# CHAPTER 22

# Syringomyelia and Congenital Abnormalities of the Spinal Canal

### Case 1228

7-year-old girl presenting with back pain.
(sagittal, noncontrast T1-weighted SE scan)

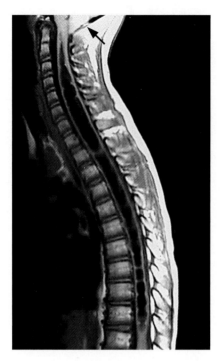

**Syringomyelia**

### Case 1229

15-year-old girl presenting with numbness
and weakness of the hands.
(axial, noncontrast T1-weighted SE scan; C7 level)

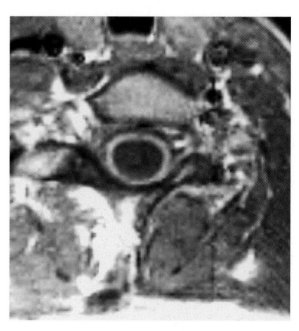

**Syringomyelia**

Purists describe dilatation of the ependymal-lined central canal of the spinal cord as "hydromyelia," reserving the term *syringomyelia* for acquired intramedullary cavities lined by glial reaction. In practice, the two terms are often interchanged, or combined as *syringohydromyelia.* In view of common application, this chapter will use "syringomyelia" to include true hydromyelia as well as other types of benign intramedullary cysts.

Abnormal hydrodynamics within the spinal canal probably play a major role in syrinx formation. The most common anatomical correlate is crowding of tissue within the foramen magnum in the Chiari I hindbrain malformation (see Cases 847-848). Acquired anatomical distortions at the foramen magnum may also lead to syringomyelia (see, for example, Case 824).

Although syringomyelia in association with Chiari hindbrain malformations may be considered to be of congenital origin, symptoms often do not occur until adolescence or adulthood. It is likely that the enlargement of the cyst over many years precedes the onset of myelopathy.

Intramedullary cysts are defined on T1-weighted scans as sharply marginated zones of low signal intensity. Intensity values within a syrinx may be slightly higher than those of subarachnoid CSF due to reduced signal loss from pulsation effects and/or mild elevation of protein. Cysts differing substantially in intensity from spinal fluid may be neoplastic and should be evaluated by contrast-enhanced studies.

The diameter of the cyst in Case 1228 varies from level to level, and the margins of the syrinx are mildly irregular. A septated, loculated, or "chain of lakes" morphology is common in syringomyelia. The compartments of the lesion usually communicate.

Case 1229 illustrates a large, smoothly marginated, central intramedullary cyst surrounded by a uniformly thin rim of compressed parenchyma.

A Chiari I hindbrain malformation is demonstrated in Case 1228 *(arrow)* and was also present in Case 1229 (see Case 1234).

## Case 1230

55-year-old woman with a history of decompressive cervical laminectomy for a presumed spinal cord tumor.
(sagittal, noncontrast T1-weighted SE scan)

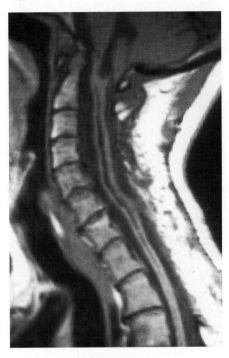

**Syringomyelia**

## Case 1231

37-year-old man presenting with cervical myelopathy.
(axial, noncontrast T1-weighted SE scan)

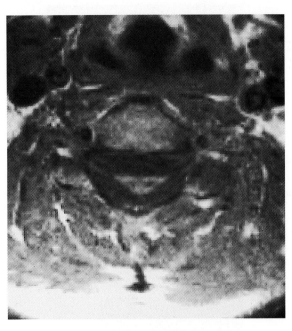

**Syringomyelia**

Some patients with syringomyelia present with collapsed cysts and atrophic spinal cords. Cord atrophy may be the result of prolonged compression from a previously distended syrinx or prior injury leading to both parenchymal damage and cavitation (see Cases 1183 and 1184).

In Case 1230, myelopathy with cord expansion had been thought to represent an intramedullary tumor when the patient was first evaluated as a young adult. Surgery at that time demonstrated benign syringomyelia. The follow-up scan above shows an abnormally thin cord with a collapsed central syrinx, associated with a Chiari hindbrain malformation.

Case 1231 illustrates an axial scan through an atrophic spinal cord containing small bilateral cysts (compare to

Case 1184). Anteroposterior narrowing of the cord is frequently seen in syringomyelia, whereas the transverse diameter is relatively preserved.

Compare the cross section of the spinal cord in Cases 1229 and 1231 to appreciate the potential variation in morphology of syringomyelia. Between these extremes are some cases with normal cord dimensions and contour.

Other causes of cord atrophy include trauma, multiple sclerosis, ischemia, arteriovenous malformation, and amyotrophic lateral sclerosis.

Cervical syringomyelia may extend superiorly into the dorsal medulla. The small cyst caudal to the fourth ventricle in Case 1230 probably represents such "syringobulbia."

## Case 1232

51-year-old woman presenting with
progressive quadriparesis.
(sagittal, noncontrast T1-weighted SE scan)

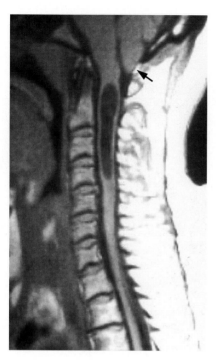

**Syringomyelia**

## Case 1233

3-year-old boy presenting with abnormal gait.
(sagittal, noncontrast T1-weighted SE scan)

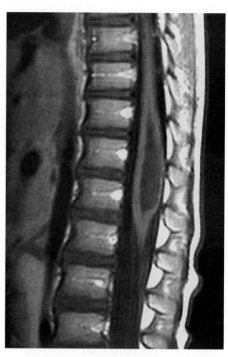

**Syringomyelia**
("terminal ventricle")

Syringomyelia often involves long segments of the spinal cord, as illustrated on the preceding pages. In other cases a benign, presumably congenital intramedullary cyst is quite localized.

Case 1232 demonstrates an expansile cyst involving the spinal cord from C2 to C4. The association of a Chiari I hindbrain malformation *(arrow)* suggests congenital origin of this localized syrinx. No enhancement was present on a postcontrast scan performed to exclude the alternative possibility of a cystic tumor. Subsequent drainage of this cyst (with simultaneous decompression of the foramen magnum) led to dramatic clinical improvement.

Localized dilatation of the caudal end of the central canal may be encountered with no evidence of syringomyelia in the cervical or thoracic region. These benign and probably congenital intramedullary cysts have been called *terminal ventricles.* Although they are often small and asympto-

matic, distal syrinxes may cause significant distortion of the conus medullaris with associated neurological deficits, as in Case 1233. Surgery in this patient demonstrated a benign cyst filled with clear CSF.

Congenital abnormalities of the spinal cord are often multiple. The presence of a terminal ventricle of any size should prompt a search for malformations at other levels. Gross expansion of a terminal syrinx may herniate through a defect in the posterior neural arch in patients with spinal dysraphism, forming a "myelocystocele."

Compare the central position and elongated morphology of the intramedullary cysts in the above cases to the neuroepithelial cyst in Case 1200 and the neurenteric cyst in Case 1201.

High signal intensity at the mid posterior aspect of vertebral bodies in Case 1233 probably represents fat surrounding the basivertebral vein at each level.

# DIFFERENTIAL DIAGNOSIS:
## EXTENSIVE INTRAMEDULLARY CYST

### Case 1234

15-year-old girl presenting with numbness
and weakness of the hands.
(sagittal, noncontrast T1-weighted SE scan)

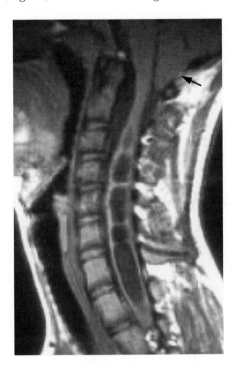

**Benign Syringomyelia**
(same patient as Case 1229)

### Case 1235

27-year-old woman presenting with
progressive quadriparesis.
(sagittal, noncontrast T1-weighted SE scan)

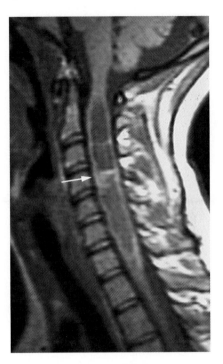

**Cystic Ependymoma**

---

The cysts expanding the cervical spinal cord in the above cases are similar in overall size and morphology. However, several clues argue against a diagnosis of benign syringomyelia in Case 1235, even on this noncontrast scan. Signal intensity within the lesion is mildly but definitely higher than that of normal CSF within the foramen magnum. A small zone of tissue near the center of the cyst *(arrow)* is more nodular than the usual band-like septations seen in benign syrinxes like Case 1234. Finally, there is no evidence of tissue crowding at the foramen magnum in Case 1235, arguing against abnormal CSF hydrodynamics as a mechanism for formation of an intramedullary cyst.

Postcontrast scans are important when atypical cysts are discovered within the spinal cord. In Case 1235, intense enhancement was present within the central tissue nodule. Other margins of the cyst were nonenhancing.

As discussed in Chapter 19, benign, reactive cysts are often found at the rostral and/or caudal poles of intramedullary neoplasms. Such cysts may contribute significantly to preoperative myelopathy but usually resolve following resection of the central tumor.

Intramedullary edema due to inflammatory or neoplastic lesions can cause large zones of homogeneously prolonged T2 values resembling the appearance of syringomyelia on long TR spin echo scans (see Case 1138). T1-weighted images are usually more helpful in distinguishing true intramedullary cysts from edematous parenchyma. If the margination of an abnormal region is not as sharply defined as in Case 1234, diagnoses other than syringomyelia should be suspected.

A Chiari I hindbrain malformation is demonstrated in Case 1234 *(arrow)*.

## Case 1236

6-year-old boy presenting with difficulty walking.
(sagittal, noncontrast T1-weighted SE scan)

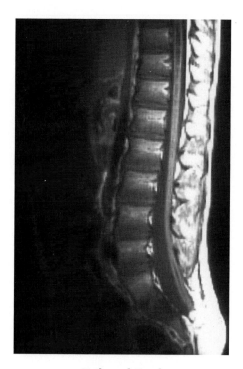

**Tethered Cord**

## Case 1237

62-year-old woman presenting with
leg weakness and bladder dysfunction.
(sagittal, noncontrast T2-weighted FSE scan)

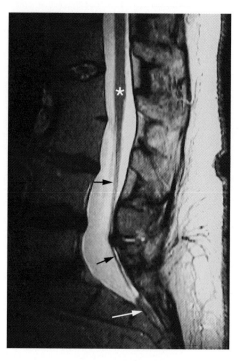

**Tethered Cord**

An abnormally low-lying spinal cord may be encountered as an isolated abnormality or in association with a malformation of the spinal canal. In the former circumstance, the cord may extend through the lumbar region to the termination of the thecal sac or be attached to a taut and/or thickened filum terminale at a mid lumbar level. In more complex malformations, the low-lying spinal cord may enter a lipomatous mass or a meningocele sac.

In Case 1236, the spinal cord extends inferiorly through the lumbar canal to terminate at the S2 level. Associated hypoplasia of the sacrum, sacral dysraphism, thoracic syringomyelia, and a small terminal ventricle are present.

On sagittal scans it may be difficult to distinguish between a stretched and thinned spinal cord and a thickened filum terminale within the lumbar spinal canal. Axial scans resolve this ambiguity by demonstrating nerve roots arising from spinal cord parenchyma (see Case 1240).

Case 1237 illustrates congenital abnormalities of the lumbar canal presenting in adulthood. The L2 and L3 vertebral bodies are fused. The conus medullaris *(asterisk)* is abnormally low-lying and stretched by a taut, thickened filum terminale *(black arrows)* that terminates in a small lipoma *(white arrow)*. (Compare the tight configuration of the conus medullaris and filum terminale in this case with the normally relaxed contour in Case 925.)

Tethering of the spinal cord may be discovered in the absence of related symptoms. Children with tethered cords frequently develop increasing dysfunction of the conus medullaris as somatic growth causes stretching of anchored neural tissue. The adult presentation of tethered cords presumably reflects traumatic or ischemic events superimposed on the developmental abnormality.

Cases 1246, 1247, and 1272 present T2-weighted sagittal scans of tethered cords in association with lipomas and sacral agenesis.

## Case 1238

4-year-old girl with a history of myelomeningocele repair at birth.
(sagittal, noncontrast T1-weighted SE scan)

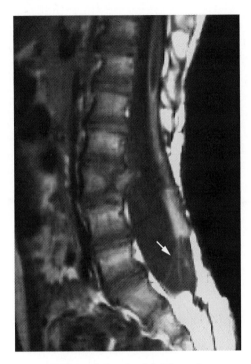

**Tethered Cord with Placode**

## Case 1239

1-week-old boy with a subcutaneous sacral mass.
(sagittal, noncontrast T1-weighted SE scan)

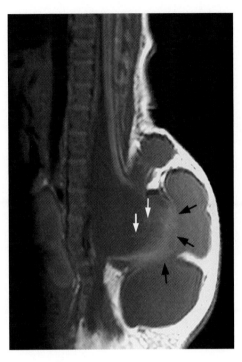

**Tethered Cord with Placode**
(and subcutaneous myelomeningocele)

---

Tethering of the spinal cord may be one component of a complex malformation. When dorsal dysraphism is present, the caudal termination of a tethered cord is often a plaque-like layer of neural tissue within or at the margin of the thecal sac. Such placodes represent neuroectoderm that failed to condense and organize normally as the inferior spinal cord and conus medullaris.

In Case 1238, a large dysraphic defect and repaired myelomeningocele are apparent at the posterior margin of the spinal canal. The caudal sac is ectatic. Osseous abnormality involving the L3 vertebral body includes a posterior spur that was shown on axial images to represent diastematomyelia. A localized syrinx occupies the cord at the T11-T12 level. A plate of neural tissue is present at the dorsal border of the ectatic sac, appearing to be tethered posteriorly at the site of myelomeningocele repair. Nerve

roots *(arrow)* extend caudally from this neural placode, identifying the more rostral tissue band as low-lying spinal cord rather than a thickened filum terminale.

Case 1239 demonstrates a large, lobulated subcutaneous myelomeningocele. The low-lying spinal cord deviates posteriorly to enter this sac, joining an obliquely oriented neural placode *(black arrows)*. The placode is established as neural tissue by the emergence of several roots from its ventral surface *(white arrows)*.

The presence of CSF posterior to the neural placode in Case 1239 is unusual, reflecting the occult nature of the myelomeningocele (and the absence of surgery). In patients with overt and repaired myelomeningoceles, placodes of malformed neural tissue are characteristically positioned at the dorsal margin of the thecal sac, as in Case 1238.

## Case 1240

8-year-old boy with a history of
repaired myelomeningocele.
(axial, noncontrast T1-weighted SE scan; L3-4 level)

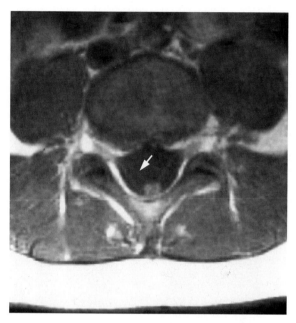

**Tethered Cord**

## Case 1241

5-year-old girl with a dorsal soft tissue
bulge at the lumbosacral junction.
(axial, noncontrast T1-weighted SE scan; S1-S2 level)

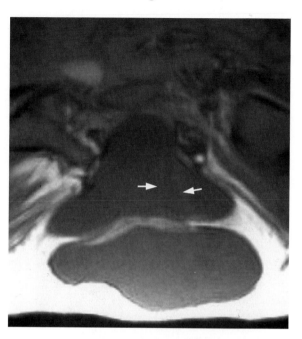

**Tethered Cord with Placode**

Axial scans confirm the nature of low-lying spinal cord parenchyma by demonstrating the presence of exiting nerve roots. By itself, the thick band of soft tissue within the dorsal subarachnoid space in Case 1240 is nonspecific; it could represent either a thick filum terminale or a thinned, low-lying spinal cord. (Clumping of intrathecal roots due to arachnoiditis may present a similar appearance; see Case 1159.) Visualization of emerging nerve roots *(arrow)* establishes the presence of spinal cord tissue at this level. Such documentation is important to identify the appropriate level for sectioning of the filum terminale to release a taut spinal cord.

Case 1241 is an axial view through the flat neural placode in a patient with a subcutaneous myelomeningocele (comparable to Case 1239). The plate of soft tissue traversing the meningocele sac represents the caudal portion of the spinal cord, which failed to close dorsally into a tube. Ventral and dorsal nerve roots *(arrows)* can be faintly seen extending anteriorly from the lateral margins of the placode. The dorsal nerve root usually arises at the edge of the unfolded neural plate, where it joins high intensity fat. This junction is therefore an important surgical landmark.

### Case 1242

2-year-old girl with a history of
repaired myelomeningocele.
(sagittal, noncontrast T1-weighted SE scan)

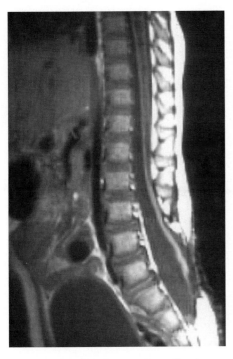

**Dorsal Cord Tethering by Adhesions**

### Case 1243

1-year-old boy with a history of myelomeningocele
repair at birth.
(sagittal, noncontrast T2-weighted FSE scan)

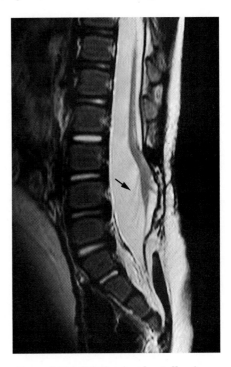

**Dorsal Cord Tethering by Adhesions**

---

Tethering of a low-lying spinal cord in the lumbar region may occur dorsally as well as caudally. Dorsal tethering may be primary, due to failed dysjunction of cutaneous and neuroectoderm (see Cases 1264 and 1265). Secondary or acquired dorsal tethering of neural elements may develop due to the formation of adhesions after surgery to repair a myelomeningocele or release a caudally tethered cord.

The usual dorsal position of neural tissue within a repaired myelomeningocele causes the spinal cord to drape across the last intact neural arch as it enters the meningocele sac. Such proximity does not by itself establish the presence of adhesions in this location. However, if the spinal cord appears tightly adherent to the dorsal dura, with abnormal angulation and/or absence of dorsal subarachnoid spaces, the possibility of acquired tethering should be considered.

In Case 1242, the low-lying cord deviates dorsally as it enters the area of dural ectasia and myelomeningocele repair. Dense adhesions were found at the previous operative site.

Case 1243 demonstrates focal dorsal angulation of the low-lying conus medullaris to abut the posterior margin of the thecal sac. This localized deformity and the obliteration of the dorsal subarachnoid space imply tethering of the cord to the dura. Dorsal adhesions frequently occur at the transition from the normal spinal canal to the dysraphic segment, as was true in this case.

Syringomyelia is present within the thoracic spinal cord in Case 1242. Nerve roots are demonstrated arising from the ventral aspect of the low-lying conus medullaris in Case 1243 *(arrow)*.

Infolding of cutaneous tissue may occur during closure of a myelomeningocele defect in the neonatal period. Subsequent intraspinal proliferation of squamous epithelium can produce an enlarging epidermoid mass. Like acquired adhesions, this possibility is among diagnostic considerations in children (or adults) whose neurological function deteriorates some time after initial surgery.

### Case 1244

4-year-old boy presenting with
bladder dysfunction.
(sagittal, noncontrast T1-weighted SE scan)

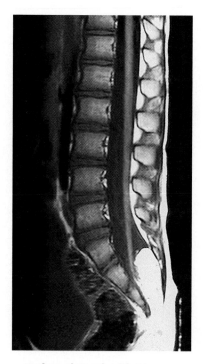

**Tethered Cord with Lipoma**

### Case 1245

8-year-old girl presenting with a
lipomatous lumbosacral mass.
(sagittal, noncontrast T1-weighted SE scan)

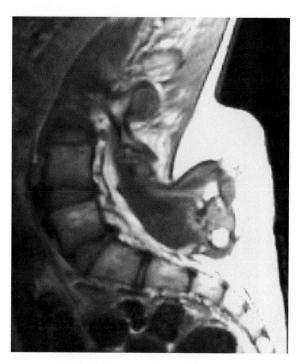

**Occult Lipomyelomeningocele**

---

Lipomas at the caudal end of the dural sac commonly accompany tethering of the spinal cord and spinal dysraphism. Abnormal fatty tissue within the lumbosacral canal may be intradural, extradural, or both. Intraspinal lipomas are often continuous with dorsal subcutaneous fat through dysraphic defects in the posterior neural arch. Lipomatous tissue may ascend along the dorsal surface of the cord, infiltrate the filum terminale, or surround and compress the spinal cord and cauda equina.

The characteristically short T1 of lipid protons readily identifies intraspinal fatty tissue on short TR spin echo images. In Case 1244, the high intensity of a lipoma surrounds the sacral termination of the tethered spinal cord. (See Case 1249 for an axial image of this lesion.) The intraspinal fat is most prominent along the dorsal surface of the low-lying cord, as is commonly the case. The lipoma extends inferiorly through a dysraphic defect to blend with subcutaneous fat. When a meningocele sac accompanies a lipoma through a spina bifida defect, the combined malformation is called a *lipomeningocele*.

Case 1245 illustrates an occult lipomyelomeningocele covered by a large mound of thickened subcutaneous fat. A complex mixture of lipomatous tissue and neural placode is present within the meningocele sac. The spinal cord enters the rostral pole of this heterogeneous mass. Associated scoliosis and exaggerated lumbosacral lordosis are present.

The taut configuration of the low-lying spinal cord in Case 1244 supports the diagnosis of symptomatic tethering (compare to Cases 1236 and 1237). The sacrum is mildly hypoplastic. (See the discussion of sacral agenesis in Cases 1271 and 1272.)

### Case 1246

7-year-old boy with a history of imperforate anus,
now presenting with urinary and fecal incontinence.
(sagittal, noncontrast T2-weighted SE scan)

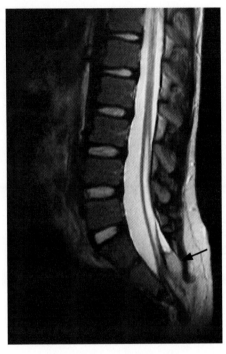

**Tethered Cord with Lipoma**

### Case 1247

69-year-old woman presenting with
progressive gait abnormality.
(sagittal, noncontrast T2-weighted SE scan)

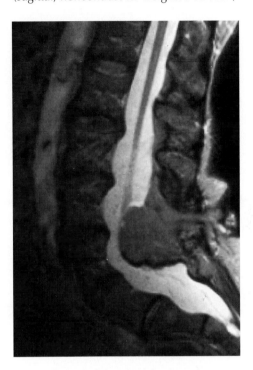

**Tethered Cord with Lipoma**

---

The signal intensity of spinal lipomas is characteristically low on conventional T2-weighted images. The above examples are typical. (Compare to the appearance of the intracranial lipomas in Case 862.)

In Case 1246, a small lipoma *(arrow)* occupies the caudal end of the spinal canal, blending inferiorly with subcutaneous fat and resembling Case 1244. The low-lying spinal cord extends through the lumbar region to terminate in the lipoma. A small syrinx cavity is present from L3 to S2.

Case 1247 illustrates the adult presentation of a congenital spinal lesion (see also Cases 1254 and 1255). A large, spherical, dorsally based lipoma occupies most of the ectatic spinal canal at the L4 level. Signal intensity within the mass is homogeneously low, and chemical shift artifact is present along its inferior and superior margins (see dis-

cussion of Cases 861 and 862). There appears to be communication between the intraspinal lipoma and dorsal subcutaneous tissues, suggesting dysraphism. The low-lying spinal cord is tightly stretched over the ventral margin of the intradural lipoma. Prominent scalloping of vertebral bodies indicates long-standing dural ectasia.

Lipid material may appear relatively higher in signal intensity on T2-weighted images produced by fast spin echo sequences than on conventional T2-weighted scans. This reduced signal loss is attributable to decreased spin–spin coupling. Phase modulation causing destructive interference on late echoes of a standard spin echo sequence is suppressed by the close echo spacing used in fast spin echo protocols.

**Case 1248**

2-year-old boy presenting with difficulty walking.
(axial, noncontrast T1-weighted SE scan; L5 level)

**Case 1249**

4-year-old boy presenting with bladder dysfunction.
(axial, noncontrast T1-weighted SE scan; S1 level)

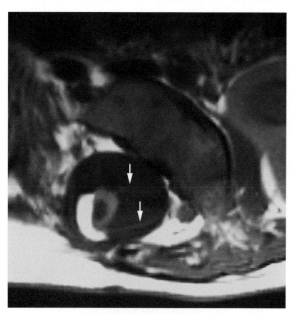

**Intraspinal Lipoma**
(with tethered cord and syringomyelia)

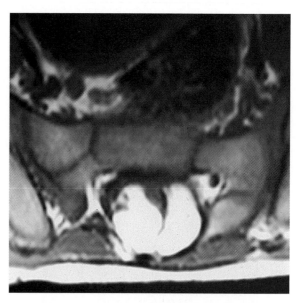

**Intraspinal Lipoma**
(with tethered cord; same patient as Case 1244)

Axial views demonstrate the variable relationship of spinal lipomas to low-lying spinal cords and/or neural placodes.

Lipomatous tissue is often applied to the dorsal aspect of the cord/placode. This characteristic appearance reflects premature dysjunction of neuroectoderm from cutaneous ectoderm, allowing mesenchymal cells to gain access to the posterior surface of the neural tube. In cases of spinal canal deformity with substantial rotation of the spinal cord, the location of lipomatous tissue may help to identify the originally dorsal surface of neural tissue.

Mild rotation of the cord is present in Case 1248. Nerve roots emerging on the left *(arrows)* indicate the anatomically ventral surface, whereas the lipoma on the right corresponds to the anatomically dorsal margin. A small intramedullary cyst represents a terminal ventricle (see Case 1233).

A larger lipoma surrounds the dorsal and lateral aspects of the tethered cord in Case 1249. (See Case 1244 for a sagittal scan of this patient.) The bulky lipoma occupies the majority of the spinal canal, which is mildly expanded.

The lipoma in Case 1248 is completely intradural. The lipomatous mass in Case 1249 is also largely intrathecal, although it was continuous inferiorly with subcutaneous fat. Other spinal lipomas may be partially or predominantly extradural (see, for example, Cases 1252 and 1253).

# LIPOMATOUS INFILTRATION OF THE FILUM TERMINALE

### Case 1250

4-month-old girl.
(axial, noncontrast T1-weighted SE scan; L4-5 level)

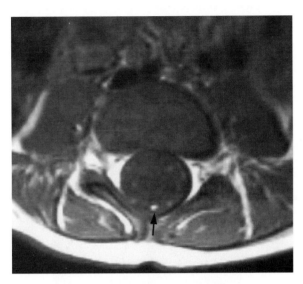

**Lipoma of the Filum Terminale**

### Case 1251

3-year-old girl presenting with back pain.
(axial, noncontrast T1-weighted SE scan; L3 level)

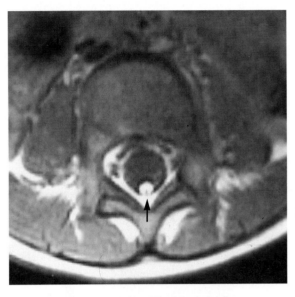

**Lipoma of the Filum Terminale**

---

Fatty infiltration of the filum terminale may be an incidental finding, alone or in combination with other congenital abnormalities. In other cases, a lipoma involving the filum terminale is associated with symptomatic tethering of the spinal cord. Evidence of cord traction (i.e., a tight or stretched configuration with a low-lying conus medullaris) and clinical correlation are important in assessing the significance of filum fat.

Prominent T1-shortening highlights lipomatous infiltration of the filum terminale in each of the above cases. The amount of thickening of the filum correlates with the likelihood of significant cord tethering. A filum diameter of more than two or three millimeters is frequently sympto-

matic. The child in Case 1251 had a normally positioned conus medullaris and no evidence of neurological dysfunction, but she will be carefully followed as somatic growth continues.

It is important to emphasize that fatty infiltration of the filum terminale is not synonymous with thickening of the filum or tethering of the spinal cord. Pathologically thickened fila often contain no fat. Conversely, fat may be present within a filum of normal dimensions and without associated traction on the spinal cord (as in Case 1250).

See Case 1271 for an additional example of lipomatous infiltration of the filum terminale.

### Case 1252

8-month-old boy presenting with a mound
of lipomatous tissue overlying
the thoracolumbar junction.
(sagittal, noncontrast T1-weighted SE scan)

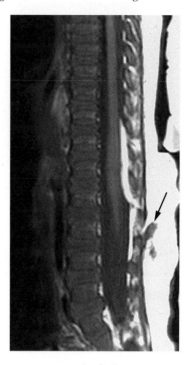

**Intraspinal Lipoma**

### Case 1253

4-month-old girl presenting with a mound
of lipomatous tissue overlying
the thoracolumbar junction.
(sagittal, noncontrast T1-weighted SE scan)

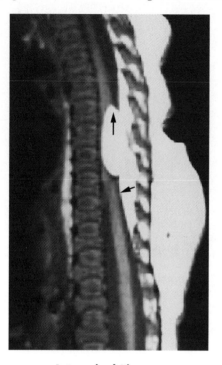

**Intraspinal Lipoma**

---

The intraspinal lipomas presented on preceding pages have involved the lumbosacral region and have been predominantly intradural. Lipomas are less commonly found in the cervical and thoracic canal, often demonstrating large dorsal epidural components associated with thickening of overlying subcutaneous fat.

Cases 1252 and 1253 illustrate this appearance. The dorsal band of intraspinal lipoma in Case 1252 seems to be anchored posteriorly at the L1-2 level, possibly merging with thickened subcutaneous fat. The close application of the lipomatous mass to the dorsal surface of the spinal cord suggests intradural extension. Axial images would help to confirm this impression.

The bulky lipoma in Case 1253 compresses the spinal cord. The subarachnoid space is narrowed along the inferior margin of the lesion *(short arrow)* but widened near the superior pole of the lobulation *(long arrow).* These features, together with the button-like shape of the mass, suggest that a globular intradural component of the lipoma extends ventrally from a dorsal epidural base. Subcutaneous fat of the back is markedly thickened in the region of the intraspinal lipoma.

The small zone of muscle-like signal intensity within the subcutaneous lipoma in Case 1252 *(arrow)* was associated with an accessory ossicle (or rudimentary appendage) on adjacent sections. (The material seen posterior to subcutaneous fat in the superior thoracic region of Case 1252 is a cushion.)

Compare the localized lipomas in the above scans to the more uniform appearance of epidural lipomatosis in Case 1192.

## Case 1254

70-year-old woman presenting with
back pain and paraparesis after a fall.
(sagittal, noncontrast T1-weighted SE scan)

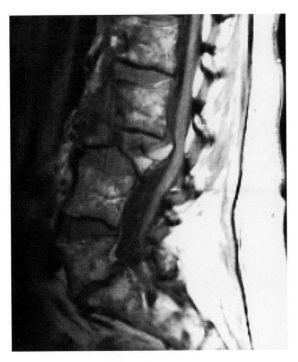

**Tethered Cord**
(and compression fracture)

## Case 1255

69-year-old woman presenting with
progressive gait abnormality.
(sagittal, noncontrast T1-weighted SE scan)

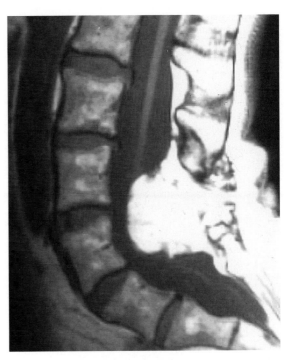

**Tethered Cord with Lipoma**
(same patient as Case 1247)

Spinal cord malformations usually become symptomatic during childhood or adolescence, as growth of the spine increases the tension on tethered neural structures. Occasionally, adults present with symptoms arising from congenital lesions. The adult onset of dysfunction in such cases may be due to superimposed acquired pathology or time-related worsening of congenital abnormalities.

Case 1254 illustrates the former mechanism. A tethered spinal cord is present, extending through the lumbar region. This congenital abnormality had not caused symptoms until the fracture of L3 resulted in cord compression. Conversely, the compression fracture might have displaced the cauda equina without neurologic impairment in the absence of cord tethering.

The scan in Case 1255 is a T1-weighted view of the lipoma presented in Case 1247. Stretching of the spinal cord over the long-standing lipoma in this case has proba-

bly worsened gradually over decades, finally causing increasing symptoms and leading to evaluation.

Serial MR studies of patients with intraspinal lipomas have demonstrated growth in occasional cases. Enlargement of a lipoma is a rare cause of new or recurrent symptoms in children after surgery for congenital cord lesions. More common etiologies include recurrence of syringomyelia, development of tethering adhesions, or increased tension on the spinal cord due to somatic growth.

Diastematomyelia (see Cases 1256-1261) is another congenital abnormality of the spine that may present in adulthood, typically with gait abnormality or bowel and/or bladder dysfunction.

The ectatic dural sac with scalloping of vertebral bodies in Case 1255 is a common finding in congenital malformations of the spinal canal. (Compare to the expansion of the lumbar canal due to mass lesions in Cases 1020 and 1094.)

# DIASTEMATOMYELIA WITH RIGID SEPTUM
## (SPLIT CORD MALFORMATION TYPE I)

### Case 1256

15-year-old girl being evaluated for scoliosis.
(axial, noncontrast T1-weighted SE scan; L3 level)

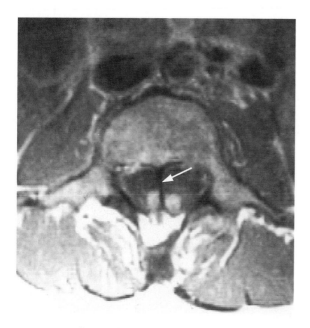

**Split Cord Malformation (Type I)**

### Case 1257

16-year-old girl presenting with
bowel and bladder dysfunction.
(axial, noncontrast T1-weighted SE scan; L4 level)

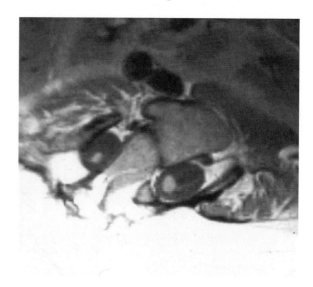

**Split Cord Malformation (Type I)**

Diastematomyelia is a congenital malformation characterized by division of the spinal cord. In at least 50% of such cases, the two hemicords are enclosed within a single arachnoidal and dural tube, with no apparent intervening septation. In the remaining cases, an osteocartilaginous septum divides the spinal canal. These two groups of congenital abnormalities have been categorized as split cord malformation (SCM) type I (separate dural tubes with an osteocartilaginous septation) and SCM type II (single dural tube with no rigid septation).

Axial views are the most reliable images for evaluating split cord malformations. Septa are well documented when present, and the size and morphology of the hemicords are clearly demonstrated.

Septations in diastematomyelia are variable in composition and morphology. Fibrous, cartilaginous, and osseous septa may occur. Bony partitions may be thin or thick, sagittal or oblique.

Case 1256 illustrates a thin plate of cortical bone in the midline *(arrow)*, bisecting the spinal canal. The low signal intensity of this structure is due to the low concentration of imageable hydrogen nuclei.

The septum in Case 1257 is a thick, obliquely oriented osseous structure containing cancellous bone. The two dural tubes are widely separated. Rotation of the hemicords within the dural sac(s), as seen in this case, is a common component of split cord malformations, with or without intervening septations.

The division of the dural sac and spinal cord in type I split cord malformations is approximately equal in about two thirds of cases.

# DIASTEMATOMYELIA WITHOUT RIGID SEPTUM
## (SPLIT CORD MALFORMATION TYPE II)

### Case 1258

4-year-old girl presenting with
leg weakness and numbness.
(axial, noncontrast T1-weighted SE scan; L2 level)

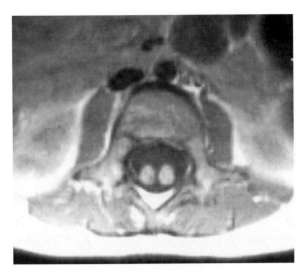

**Split Cord Malformation (Type II)**

### Case 1259

5-year-old girl presenting with
constipation and abnormal gait.
(axial, noncontrast T1-weighted SE scan; L2 level)

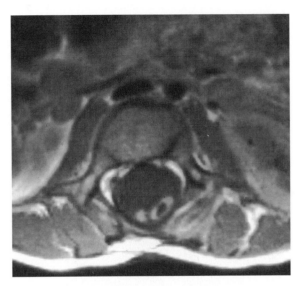

**Split Cord Malformation (Type II)**

The above cases illustrate type II split cord malformations. Although division of cord parenchyma is apparent, there is no evidence of an intervening osteocartilaginous septum or duplication of the dural tube.

As demonstrated here, the hemicords of diastematomyelia may be nearly equal in size or grossly asymmetrical. One or both hemicords may contain a syrinx (seen on the left in Case 1259) or be associated with a lipoma. The hemicords may be positioned side by side in the same coronal plane, as in Case 1258, or rotated with respect to each other, as in Case 1259.

In each of these cases the spinal cord extends abnormally far inferiorly within an ectatic dural sac. Diastematomyelia is usually associated with spinal cord tethering by adhesions even in the absence of mesodermal septations. Septae and adhesions associated with split cord malformations are often quite vascular and may be best seen on postcontrast scans.

Accompanying cutaneous stigmata (hypertrichosis, nevi, lipomas, and dimples) are present in about 50% of patients with split cord malformations.

## Case 1260

15-year-old girl scanned as a preoperative routine
prior to scheduled surgery for scoliosis.
(sagittal, noncontrast T1-weighted SE scan)

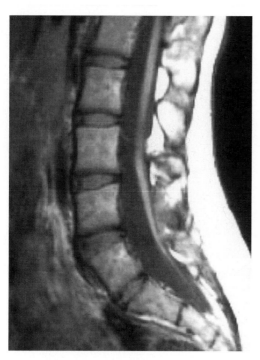

**Split Cord Malformation (Type I)**
(same patient as Case 1256)

## Case 1261

55-year-old woman with a history of
thoracolumbar myelomeningocele.
(sagittal, noncontrast T2-weighted FSE scan)

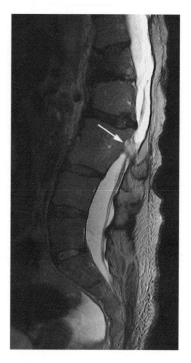

**Split Cord Malformation (Type I)**

---

Sagittal scans are the least reliable views for the diagnosis and assessment of split cord malformations. The division between the two hemicords is usually sagittally oriented. As a result, sagittal scans may only partially image the dividing plane, resulting in negative studies or the false suggestion of syringomyelia. Poorly defined low signal intensity within the low-lying spinal cord at the L3 level in Case 1260 represents the site of diastematomyelia, which was clearly demonstrated (with a thin bony partition) on axial and coronal views (see Case 1256).

A thick osseous septum crosses the anteroposterior diameter of the spinal canal in Case 1261 *(arrow)*. Bone spurs associated with diastematomyelia often arise from malformed vertebrae, illustrated by the fusion of the L2 and L3 vertebral bodies in this patient.

As seen in the above scans, diastematomyelia may be associated with abnormally low-lying spinal cords and the "tethered cord syndrome." Fibrous septation dividing the hemicords in type II SCM is often not apparent on preoperative imaging studies. However, such septa (and other fibroneurovascular bands) are usually present and can have the same tethering effect as the obvious bone spurs in type I SCM. Many surgeons now advocate exploration of SCMs of either type to release tethering.

Postoperative changes are present at the thoracolumbar junction in Case 1261. The abnormal appearance of the intradural compartment in this region suggests a combination of myelomalacia and arachnoiditis (see Cases 1155 and 1156).

# DIFFERENTIAL DIAGNOSIS:
## CSF-FILLED CLEFT WITHIN THE SPINAL CORD

### Case 1262

3-year-old girl presenting with scoliosis.
(coronal, noncontrast T1-weighted SE scan)

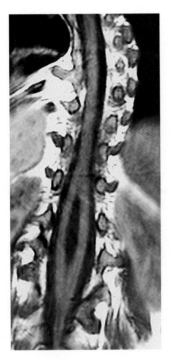

**Split Cord Malformation (Type II)**

### Case 1263

4-year-old girl presenting with mild gait abnormality.
(coronal, noncontrast T1-weighted SE scan)

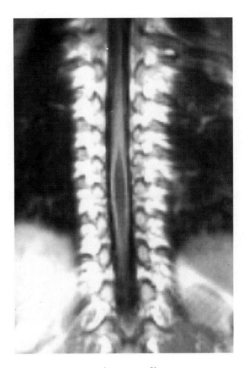

**Syringomyelia**

Coronal and axial scans are much more reliable than sagittal images for demonstration of split cord malformations. In Case 1262, the intramedullary cleft is clearly defined at the junction of the spinal cord and conus medullaris. No septation is apparent.

Localized syringomyelia (usually representing true hydromyelia) can present a similar appearance on coronal scans, as seen in Case 1263. Axial views are necessary to determine whether central CSF on coronal images represents a cleft traversing the anteroposterior diameter of the spinal cord or an intramedullary cavity enclosed by cord parenchyma.

Tethering of the spinal cord was demonstrated in the lumbar region in Case 1263. Both diastematomyelia and syringomyelia are commonly associated with other malformations of the spinal canal. The discovery of one congenital lesion should prompt a search for others.

About 90% of diastematomyelic hemicords reunite at a level below the split. A fibrous or osteocartilaginous septum passing between the hemicords represents an important potential cause of tethering in such cases.

Diastematomyelia, syringomyelia, and cord tethering are among the congenital abnormalities that can present with scoliosis in childhood, as in Cases 1260 and 1262. Intraspinal or paraspinal neoplasms form the other major category of pathology to be distinguished from idiopathic scoliosis (see Cases 1072 and 1268). MR surveys of the spinal canal are an important screening procedure prior to surgical correction of spinal curvatures.

Compare the above scans to the astrocytoma in Case 1073.

## Case 1264A

50-year-old man presenting with
back pain and leg weakness.
(sagittal, noncontrast T1-weighted SE scan)

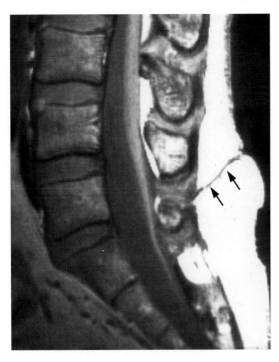

**Dorsal Dermal Sinus Syndrome**

## Case 1264B

Same patient.
(same image with different photography)

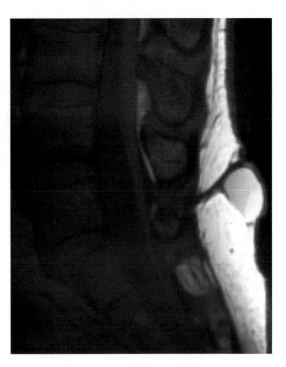

**Dorsal Dermal Sinus Syndrome**

---

The "dorsal dermal sinus syndrome" includes a group of disorders caused by failed dysjunction of neuroectoderm from cutaneous ectoderm. In most cases, the persistent connection of the neural tube to the skin surface leads to the invagination of a dermal sinus. This tract extends from the skin of the back through subcutaneous tissues and between spinous processes to terminate at the dura or within the thecal sac. Intradural dermal sinus tracts may ascend for several levels along the spinal canal. Associated intradural dermoid or epidermoid tumors are present in about 50% of cases and may be either intramedullary or extramedullary.

Dorsal dermal sinus tracts are variably patent. Fibrous obliteration of the lumen of the tract may still be associated with symptomatic cord tethering. Patent dermal sinus tracts are a potential source of intradural infection and may present with isolated or recurrent meningitis.

Case 1264 is unusual in that failure of dysjunction has lead to eversion of neuroectoderm rather than inversion of cutaneous ectoderm. The dorsal subcutaneous mass at the L5 level, best seen in Case 1264B, proved to be a meningocele linked to the dura and the dorsal surface of the tethered spinal cord by a fibrous stalk. The angled course of the tethering stalk in this case (*arrows,* Case 1264A) is typical of a lumbar dorsal dermal sinus: the tract angles inferiorly as it extends anteriorly from the skin surface, reaches the interspinous region, and then angles superiorly as it passes into the spinal canal. Both the cutaneous origin and the dural or intradural termination of a dorsal dermal sinus tract are usually superior to the level where it enters the spinal canal.

Spinal dermoid cysts often have predominantly long T1 and T2 values resembling simpler arachnoid or parasitic cysts. Heterogeneity (especially T1-shortening) within a small portion of the lesion and/or the presence of an associated dermal sinus tract (which is found in about 20% of cases) are clues to the correct diagnosis.

# CERVICAL DORSAL DERMIS SINUS SYNDROME

## Case 1265A

59-year-old man presenting with
mild cervical myelopathy.
(sagittal, noncontrast T1-weighted SE scan)

## Case 1265B

Same patient.
(axial, noncontrast T1-weighted SE scan; C4 level)

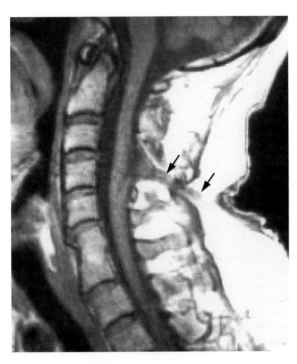

**Dorsal Dermal Sinus Syndrome**

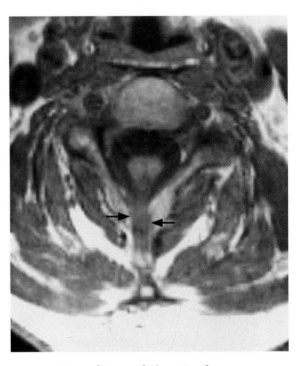

**Dorsal Dermal Sinus Syndrome**

---

Manifestations of the dorsal dermal sinus syndrome are rare in the cervical region. When present, the lesions may have any of the various morphologies discussed on the preceding page.

Case 1265A demonstrates a band of fibrous tissue *(arrows)* connecting the dorsal surface of the spinal cord with a thickened and invaginated area of skin on the back of the neck. This tract represents a site of failed separation of neuroectoderm and cutaneous ectoderm ("nondysjunction").

The lesion tethers the cervical spinal cord, as demonstrated in Case 1265B. The cord is pulled against the dorsal margin of the dural sac, and the posterior surface of the cord is tented.

Congenital fusion of the C6 and C7 vertebral bodies is present but unrelated to the dorsal dermal tract. (See Cases 1266 and 1267 for discussion of vertebral anomalies accompanying ventral adhesions of the neural tube.)

The differential diagnosis of an intraspinal mass associated with a dorsal dermal sinus includes abscesses as well as dermoid and epidermoid cysts.

## Case 1266

67-year-old man presenting with increasing difficulty walking and a fifty-year history of atrophic hands and arms.
(sagittal, noncontrast T1-weighted SE scan)

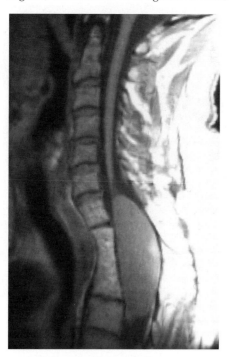

**Neurenteric Cyst**

## Case 1267

51-year-old man presenting with gradually worsening quadriparesis.
(sagittal, noncontrast T1-weighted SE scan)

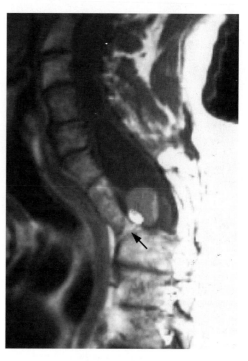

**Neurenteric Cyst**

Neurenteric cysts represent one form of the "split notochord syndrome." This group of congenital disorders arises from abnormally persistent connection between embryonic endoderm and neuroectoderm. The presence of such midline ventral adhesions prevents normal induction and formation of the notochord, which typically splits around the area of endodermal/neuroectodermal connection. Aberrant notochordal development leads to vertebral anomalies at the affected level.

Like the dorsal dermal sinuses discussed on the preceding pages, ventral tracts between the embryonic endoderm and the spinal canal (or extending further to the dorsal surface of the embryo) may be variably patent. Enteric fistulae may communicate from the foregut to the spinal canal or the dorsal skin surface. Alternatively, localized cysts may form at any point along this potential tract, with fibrous obliteration or involution of adjacent segments. When such cysts occur within the spinal canal, they are termed "neurenteric" cysts.

Neurenteric cysts are most commonly found near the cervicothoracic junction. Adjacent vertebral anomalies are usually present, as in the above cases. (Case 1201 presents a neurenteric cyst in the thoracic region with no associated spinal malformation.) The cysts are often intradural but extramedullary, although they may occur in epidural or intramedullary locations. They are frequently ventral and may become deeply embedded within the overlying spinal cord. Neurenteric cysts are typically unilocular, but irregular thickening of the wall is common. The signal intensity of the cyst content is variable.

The long-standing cyst in Case 1266 has caused expansion of the spinal canal and atrophy of the spinal cord. In Case 1267, a smaller cyst has become embedded in the ventral portion of the spinal cord, causing secondary syringomyelia superior to the lesion. A cleft in the spinal column is present at the anterior-inferior margin of the lesion *(arrow),* filled with high signal intensity that may reflect mucinous material of endodermal origin.

## Case 1268A

2-year-old girl with a history of surgery
for a spinal cord tumor.
(sagittal, noncontrast T1-weighted SE scan)

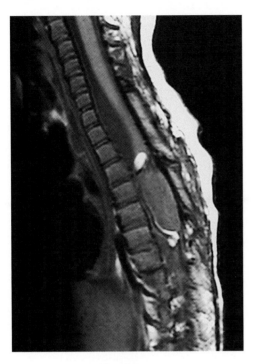

**Teratoma**

## Case 1268B

Same patient.
(sagittal, noncontrast T2-weighted FSE scan)

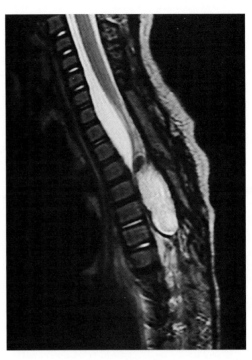

**Teratoma**

---

Teratomas of the spinal canal are rare lesions that can oc-cur at any level with a variety of appearances. These tu-mors may be predominantly solid, largely cystic, or both solid and cystic. Cysts can be solitary or multilocular, con-taining simple aqueous fluid or highly proteinaceous mate-rial. Bone, cartilage, and lipid material may be present. Hemorrhage and calcification can contribute to heterogeneity. (See the discussion of intracerebral teratomas in Case 309.) Some intraspinal teratomas are entirely in-tramedullary, whereas others are extramedullary masses but closely adherent to the spinal cord.

The location, cyst-like morphology, and mixed signal in-tensity of the mass in Case 1268 resemble the neurenteric cysts on the previous page. The lack of associated verte-bral anomalies argues weakly against a form of the split no-tochord syndrome but does not exclude this possibility (see Case 1201). The short T1 components of the lesion in Case 1268A become low in signal intensity on the fast spin echo image in Case 1268B. This pattern of signal change may represent blood products or thickly proteinaceous ma-terial rather than lipid tissue (see discussion of Case 923).

Expansion of the spinal canal and localized atrophy of the spinal cord at the cervicothoracic junction suggest that a previous component of the mass occupied this region and was resected at the time of the earlier surgery. Note the presence of scoliosis in association with this intraspinal tumor.

## Case 1269

6-year-old girl presenting with bilateral leg weakness and a neurogenic bladder. (sagittal, noncontrast T1-weighted SE scan)

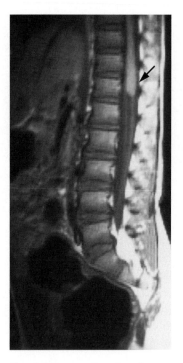

**Caudal Regression Syndrome**

## Case 1270

5-year-old girl presenting with vesicoureteral reflux. (sagittal, noncontrast T2-weighted FSE scan)

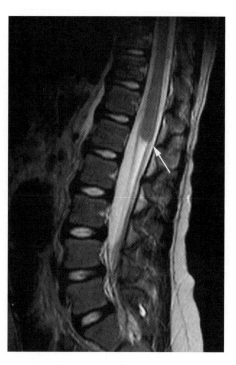

**Caudal Regression Syndrome**

---

The syndrome of "caudal regression" includes a complex group of congenital malformations potentially involving the legs, genitourinary tract, gastrointestinal tract, and caudal spinal canal. Spinal manifestations include aplasia or hypoplasia of vertebrae and the terminal portion of the spinal cord. This syndrome occurs in about 1% of infants born to diabetic mothers, but only 15% of all caudal regression cases have this association.

Vertebral hypoplasia or aplasia may be limited to the sacrum. Such sacral agenesis may be partial or complete, unilateral (including "scimitar sacrum") or bilateral. In Case 1269, the sacrum is hypoplastic and a lipoma is present within the sacral canal. Mild sacral hypoplasia is partially imaged in Case 1270. In more severe cases, multiple sacral, lumbar, and lower thoracic vertebrae may be absent.

A wedge-shaped or club-shaped deformity at the termination of an abnormally short spinal cord is characteristic of caudal regression syndrome. This morphology, illustrated in each of the above cases *(arrows)*, reflects greater hypoplasia of the ventral portion of the distal spinal cord than is present dorsally. There is often an associated clinical disparity in the level of residual neurological function, with sensation preserved to lower anatomical levels than motor abilities.

Although the cord hypoplasia in caudal regression syndrome is static, patients may experience progressive symptoms due to bony or fibrous compression of the dural sac, which commonly occurs near the level of vertebral aplasia/hypoplasia. Surgery is indicated to relieve cord distortion and stabilize residual neurological function in such cases.

## Case 1271

15-month-old boy with a history of imperforate
anus, now presenting with difficulty walking.
(sagittal, noncontrast T1-weighted SE scan)

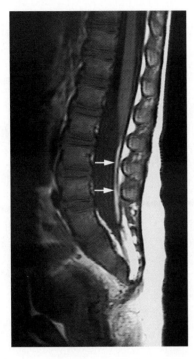

**Sacral Agenesis with Tethered Cord**

## Case 1272

13-year-old boy presenting with
urinary incontinence.
(sagittal, noncontrast T2-weighted SE scan)

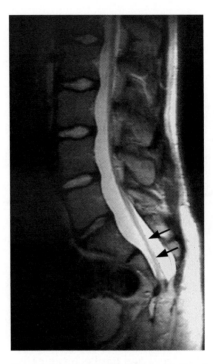

**Sacral Agenesis with Tethered Cord**

In cases of caudal regression syndrome, hypoplasia of the sacrum (and potentially of more rostral vertebrae) is associated with abnormally high position of the conus medullaris. The scans on the previous page are typical examples of this association.

Sacral agenesis may alternatively be associated with tethering of the spinal cord. The distal segments of the sacrum are absent in Cases 1271 and 1272. Instead of demonstrating truncation, the conus medullaris is clearly low-lying in Case 1271 and elongated in Case 1272.

The filum terminale in Case 1271 is short and thick *(arrows)*, with lipomatous infiltration (see Cases 1250 and 1251).

Cord tethering in Case 1272 is due to a thick, taut band of intradural tissue *(arrows)* extending to the termination of the moderately ectatic sacral sac. It is not possible to distinguish a low-lying spinal cord from a thickened filum terminale on this sagittal scan (see discussion of Case 1240).

## Case 1273

34-year-old man presenting with headaches.
(sagittal, noncontrast T1-weighted SE scan)

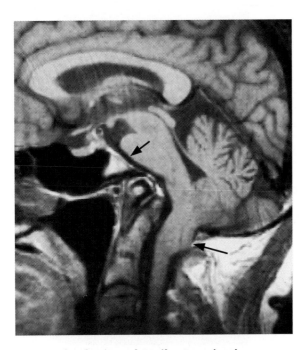

**Platybasia and Basilar Invagination**
(and Chiari I malformation)

## Case 1274

58-year-old woman presenting with occipital pain
and a history of posterior decompression
of the foramen magnum.
(sagittal, noncontrast T1-weighted SE scan)

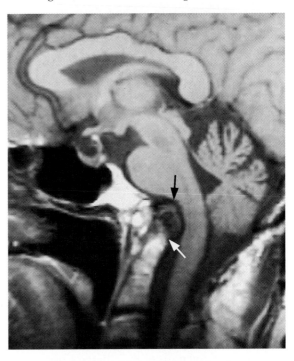

**Platybasia and Basilar Invagination**

---

As noted in Cases 1167 and 1168, both congenital deformity and acquired pathology can cause abnormal alignment (and instability) at the craniocervical junction. Superimposed degenerative changes often contribute to clinical consequences in either instance.

In Case 1273, the clivus is congenitally short and flat *(short arrow)*. The elongated odontoid process forms the anterior margin of the foramen magnum. The belly of the pons is flattened, and the medulla is kinked. Cerebellar tissue extends through the foramen magnum dorsal to the spinal cord *(long arrow)*, representing a Chiari I hindbrain deformity (see Cases 847 and 848). Basilar invagination is associated with parenchymal malformation in about 30% of cases.

The clivus in Case 1274 is also somewhat flat. The odontoid process projects above the plane of the atlas *(white arrow)*. A degenerative pseudomass consisting of calcified fibrous tissue has developed at the top of the odontoid process *(black arrow)*, deforming the ventral medulla.

Soft tissue thickening in the region of the odontoid process may reflect old trauma and/or ligamentous laxity, with excessive motion between C1 and C2. (See Case 1041 for another example.) Whatever the cause, the mound of degenerative change can act as an anterior epidural mass and cause myelopathy, requiring resection and/or decompression.

Acquired disorders such as Paget's disease and osteomalacia can soften the skull base and lead to basilar impression, resembling the anatomical distortion of the above cases.

# DOWN SYNDROME INVOLVING THE CRANIOCERVICAL JUNCTION

## Case 1275

31-year-old man with a six-month history
of abnormal gait due to increasing
leg spasticity and ataxia.
(sagittal, noncontrast T1-weighted SE scan)

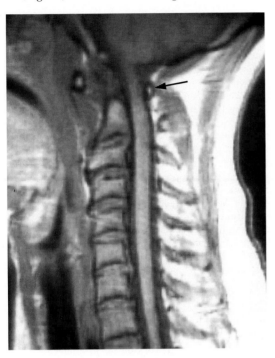

**Down Syndrome**

## Case 1276

2-year-old boy presenting with mild spasticity.
(sagittal, noncontrast T1-weighted SE scan)

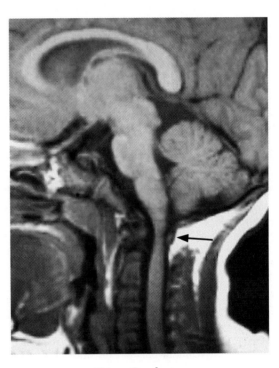

**Down Syndrome**

---

Subluxation at C1-2 due to ligamentous laxity is common in Down syndrome (trisomy 21). Case 1275 illustrates wide separation between the anterior arch of C1 and the hypoplastic odontoid process. The spinal canal is correspondingly narrowed, with reduced distance between the posterior arch of C1 *(arrow)* and the base of the dens. Compression of the spinal cord may be exacerbated by head movement or trauma in such cases.

Atlantoaxial subluxation is less prominent in Case 1276. However, constriction of the craniocervical junction is present, predominantly due to the abnormally short posterior arch of C1 *(arrow)*. This common malformation in patients with Down syndrome may be superimposed on C1-2 subluxation, resulting in severe cord compression.

In addition to causing neural compression, lesions crowding or narrowing the foramen magnum may predispose to the development of syringomyelia (see Cases 824 and 847).

Other congenital syndromes often associated with compromise of the foramen magnum are achondroplasia (see discussion of Case 960), osteopetrosis, and the mucopolysaccharidoses. The latter are characterized by ligamentous laxity at C1-2, a hypoplastic odontoid process, and intraspinal soft tissue masses due to the deposition of mucopolysaccharides.

Occipitoatlantal instability may accompany atlantoaxial subluxation in Down syndrome.

# REFERENCES

Altman NR, Altman DH: MR imaging of spinal dysraphism. *ANJR* 8:533-538, 1987.

Armonda RA, Citrin CM, Foley KT, et al: Quantitative cine-mode magnetic resonance imaging of Chiari I malformations: an analysis of cerebrospinal fluid dynamics. *Neurosurgery* 35:214-224, 1994.

Banna M: Syringomyelia in association with posterior fossa cysts. *AJNR* 9:867-873, 1988.

Barkovich AJ, Edwards MSB, Cogen PH: MR evaluation of spinal dermal sinus tracts in children. *AJNR* 12:123-129, 1991.

Barkovich AJ, Raghavan N, Chuang S, Peck WW: The wedge-shaped cord terminus: a radiographic sign of caudal regression. *AJNR* 10:1223-1231, 1989.

Barkovich AJ, Sherman JL, Citrin CM,et al: MR of postoperative syringomyelia. *AJNR* 8:319, 1987.

Barnes P: Imaging in spinal dysraphism. *Contemp Diagn Radiol* 12:1, 1990.

Barnes PD, Lester PD, Yamanashi WS, et al: Magnetic resonance imaging in infants and children with spinal dysraphism. *AJNR* 7:465-472, 1986.

Bassi P, Corona C, Contri P, et al: Congenital basilar impression: correlated neurological syndromes. *Eur Neurol* 32:238-243, 1992.

Bogdanov EI, Ibatullin MM, Mendelevich EG: Spontaneous drainage in syringomyelia: magnetic resonance imaging findings. *Neuroradiology* 42:676-678, 2000.

Brooks BS, Duvall ER, El Gammal T, et al: Neuroimaging features of neurenteric cysts: analysis of nine cases and review of the literature. *AJNR* 14:735-746, 1993.

Brophy JD, Sutton LN, Zimmerman RA, et al: Magnetic resonance imaging of lipomyelomeningocele and tethered cord. *Neurosurgery* 25:336-340, 1989.

Brugieres P, Idy-Peretti I, Iffenecker C, et al: CSF flow measurement in syringomyelia. *AJNR* 21:1785-1792, 2000.

Brunberg JA, Latchaw RE, Kanal E, et al: Magnetic resonance imaging of spinal dysraphism. *Radiol Clin North Am* 26:181-205, 1988.

Byrd SE, Darling CF, McLone DG: Development disorders of the pediatric spine. *Radiol Clin North Am* 29:711-752, 1991.

Caro PA, Marks HG, Keret D, et al: Intraspinal epidermoid tumors in children: problems in recognition and imaging techniques for diagnosis. *J Ped Orthopaed* 11:288-293, 1991.

Clifton AG, Stevens JM, Kendall BE: Idiopathic and Chiari-associated syringomyelia in adults: observation on cerebrospinal fluid pathway at the foramen magnum using static MRI. *Neuroradiology* 33(suppl):167-169, 1991.

Coleman LT, Zimmerman RA, Rorke LB: Ventriculus terminalis of the conus medullaris: MR findings in children. *AJNR* 16:1421-1426, 1995.

Davis PC, Hoffman JC Jr, Bell TI, et al: Spinal abnormalities in pediatric patients: MR imaging findings compared with clinical, myelographic, and surgical findings. *Radiology* 166:679-685, 1988.

Davis SW, Levy LM, LeBihan D, et al: Sacral meningeal cysts: evaluation with MR imaging. *Radiology* 187:445-448, 1993.

DePena CA, Lee Y-Y, Van Tassel P, et al: MR appearance of acquired spinal epidermoid tumors. *AJNR* 10:597, 1989.

Fischbein NJ, Dillon WP, Cobbs C, Weinstein PR: The "presyrinx" state: a reversible myelopathic condition that may precede syringomyelia. *AJNR* 20:7-20, 1999.

Gao P-Y, Osborn AG, Smirniotopoulos JG, et al: Neurenteric cysts: pathology, imaging spectrum, and differential diagnosis. *Int J Neurorad* 1:17-27, 1995.

Hoffman CH, Dietrich RB, Pais MJ, et al: The split notochord syndrome with dorsal enteric fistula. *AJNR* 14:622-628, 1993.

Hofmann E, Warmuth-Metz M, Bendszus M, Solymosi L: Phase-contrast MR imaging of the cervical CSF and spinal cord: volumetric motion analysis in patients with Chiari I malformation. *AJNR* 21:151-158, 2000.

Isu T, Iwasaki Y, Akino M, Abe H: Hydromyelia associated with a Chiari I malformation in children and adults. *Neurosurgery* 26:591-597, 1990.

Kaffenberger DA, Heinz, ER, Oakes JW, Boyko O: Meningocele Manque: Radiologic findings with clinical correlation. *AJNR* 13:1083-1088, 1992.

Kochan PJ, Quencer RM: Imaging of cystic and cavitary lesions of the spinal cord and canal. *Radiol Clin North Am* 29:867-880, 1991.

Kuharik MA, Edwards MK, Grossman CB: Magnetic resonance evaluation of pediatric spinal dysraphism. *Pediatr Neurosci* 12:213-218, 1985-1986.

Lee BCP, Zimmeraman RD, Manning JJ, Deck MDF: MR imaging of syringomyelia ad hydromyelia. *AJNR* 6:221-228, 1985.

Levy EI, Heiss JD, Kent MS, et al: Spinal cord swelling preceding syrinx development. *J Neurosurg Spine* 92:93-97, 2000.

Levy LM, Dechiro G, McCullough DC,e t al Fixed spinal cord: diagnosis with MR imaging. *Radiology* 169:773-778, 1988.

Lippman CR, Arginteanu M, Purohit D, et al: Intramedullary neurenteric cysts of the spine. Case report and review of the literature. *J Neurosurg Spine* 94:305-309, 2001.

Long FR, Hunter JV, Mahboubi S, et al: Tethered cord and associated vertebral anomalies in children and infants with imperforate anus: evaluation with MR imaging and plain radiography. *Radiology* 200:377-382, 1996.

Machado MADC Jr, deSouza PEM, Matos HDS, et al: Syringomyelia: imaging findings and review of the pathogenesis in 28 cases. *Int J Neurorad* 5:285-291, 1999.

Matsubayashi R, Uchino A, Kato A, et al: Cystic dilatation of ventriculus terminalis in adults. MRI. *Neuroradiology* 40:45-47, 1998.

Merx JL, Bakker-Niezen SH Thijssen HOM, Walder HAD: The tethered spinal cord syndrome: a correlation of radiological features and preoperative findings in 30 patients. *Neuroradiology* 31:63-70, 1989.

Milhorat TH, Capocelli ALJ, Anzil AP, et al: Pathological basis of spinal cord cavitation in syringomyelia: analysis of 105 autopsy cases. *J Neurosurg* 82:802-812, 1995.

Milhorat TH, Johnson WD, Miller JI, et al: Surgical treatment of syringomyelia based on magnetic resonance imaging criteria. *Neurosurgery* 31:231-245, 1992.

Milhorat TH, Miller JI, Johnson WD, et al: Anatomical basis of syringomyelia occurring with hindbrain lesions. *Neurosurgery* 32: 748-754, 1993.

Moufarrij NA, Palmer JM, Hahn JF, Weinstein MA: Correlation between magnetic resonance imaging and surgical findings in tethered spinal cord. *Neurosurgery* 25:341-346, 1989.

Munshi I, Frim D, Stine-Reyes R, et al: Effects of posterior fossa decompression with and without duraplasty on Chiari malformation-associated hydromyelia. *Neurosurgery* 46:1384-1390, 2000.

Muras I, Cioffi FA, Punzo A, Bernini FP: The occult intrasacral medningocele. *Neuroradiology* 33(suppl) 492-494, 1991.

Naidich TP, Harwood-Nash DC: Diastematomyelia. Part I. Hemicords and meningeal sheaths. Single and double arachnoid and dural tubes. *AJNR* 4:633-636, 1983.

Naidich TP, McLone DG, Mutleur A: A new understanding of dorsal dysraphism with lipoma (lipomyeloschisis: radiological evaluation and surgical correction. *AJNR* 4:103-116, 1983.

Nelson MD Jr, Bracchi M, Naidich TP, McLone DG: The natural history of repaired myelomeningocele. *Radiographics* 8:695-706, 1988.

Nievelstein RAJ, Valk J, Smit LME, et al: MR of the caudal regression syndrome: embryologic implications. *AJNR* 15:1021-1029, 1994.

O'Connor JF, Cranley WR, McCarten KM, Radkowski MA: Radiographic manifestations of congenital anomalies of the spine. *Radiol Clin North Am* 29:407-430, 1991.

Okumura R, Minami S, Asato R, Konishi J: Fatty filum terminale: assessment of MR imaging. *J Comput Assist Tomogr* 14:571-573, 1990.

Oldfield EH, Muraszko K, Shawker TH, Patronas NJ: Pathophysiology of syringomyelia associated wit Chiari I malformation of the cerebellar tonsils. Implications for diagnosis and treatment. *J Neurosurg* 80:3-15, 1994.

Pang D: Sacral agenesis and caudal spinal cord malformations. *Neurosurgery* 32:755-779, 1993.

Pang D: Split cord malformation: Part II: clinical syndrome. *Neurosurgery* 31:481-500, 1992.

Pang D, Dias MS, Ahab-Barmada M: Split cord malformation: Part I: a unified theory of embryogenesis for double spinal cord malformations. *Neurosurgery* 31:451-480, 1992.

Pena CA, Lee Y-Y, Van Tassel P, et al: MR appearance of acquired epidermoid tumor. *AJNR* 10:597, 1989.

Pojunas K, Williams AL, Daniels DL, Haughton VM: Syringomelia and hydromyelia: magnetic resonance evaluation. *Radiology* 153:679-683, 1984.

Raghavan N, Barkovich AJ, Edwards M, Norman D: MR imaging in the tethered spinal cord syndrome. *AJNR* 10:27-36, 1989.

Rindahl MA, Colletti PM, Zee CS, et al: Magnetic resonance imaging of pediatric spinal dysraphism. *Mag Reson Imaging* 7:217-224, 1989.

Rogg JM, Benzil DL, Haas RL, Knuckey NW: Intramedullary abscess, an unusual manifestation of a dermal sinus. *AJNR* 14:1393-1396, 1993.

Samuelsson L, Bergstrom K, Thuomas K-A, et al: MR imaging of syringohydromyelia and Chiari malformations in myelomeningocele patients with scoliosis. *AJNR* 8:539, 1987.

Scatliff JH, Kendall BE, Kingsley DPE, et al: Closed spinal dystraphism: analysis of clinical, radiological and surgical findings in 104 consecutive patients. *AJNR* 10:269-277, 1989.

Sherman JL, Barkovich AJ, Citrin CM: The MR appearance of syringomyelia: new observations. *AJNR* 7:985-995, 1986.

Sherman JL, Citrin CM, Barkovich AJ: MR imaging of syringobulbia. *J Comput Assist Tomogr* 11:407-411, 1987.

Sigal R, Denys A, Halimi P, et al: Ventriculus terminalis of the conus medullaris: MR imaging in four patients with congenital dilatation. *AJNR* 12:733-738, 1991.

Slasky BS, Bydder GM, Niendorf HP, Young JR: MR imaging with gadolinium-DTPA in the differentiation of tumor, syrinx, and cyst of the spinal cord. *J Comput Assist Tomogr* 11:845-850, 1987.

Smoker WRK: Craniovertebral junction: normal anatomy, craniometry, and congenital anomalies. *Radiographics* 14:255-277, 1994.

Stovner W, Rinck P: Syringomyelia in Chiari malformations: relation to extent of cerebellar tissue herniation. *Neurosurgery* 31:913-917, 1990.

Terae S, Miyasaka K, Abe S, et al: Increased pulsative movement of the hindbrain in syringomyelia associated with the Chiari malformation: cine-MRI with presaturation bolus tracking. *Neuroradiology* 36:125-129, 1994.

Tortori-Donati P, Cama A, Rosa ML, et al: Occult spinal dystraphism: neuroradiological study. *Neuroradiology* 31:512-522, 1990.

Tortori-Donati P, Rossi A, Cama A: Spinal dysraphism: a review of neuroradiological features with embryological correlations and proposal for a new classification. *Neuroradiology* 42:471-491, 2000.

Uchino A, Mori T, Ohno M: Thickened fatty filum terminale: MR imaging. *Neuroradiology* 33:331-333,1991.

Vaquero J, Martinez R, Arias A: Syringomyelia-Chiari complex: magnetic resonance imaging and clinical evaluation of surgical treatment. *J Neurosurg* 73:64-68, 1990.

Warder DE, Oakes WJ: Tethered cord syndrome: the low-lying and normally positioned conus. *Neurosurgery* 34:597-600, 1994.

White KS, Ball WS, Prenger ED, et al: Evaluation of the craniocervical junction in Down syndrome: correlation of measurements obtained with radiography and MR imaging. *Radiology* 186:377-382, 1993.

Wilberger JE Jr, Maroon J, Prostko R, et al: Magnetic resonance imaging and intraoperative neurosonography in syringomyelia. *Neurosurgery* 20:599-605, 1987.

Wilson DA, Prince JR: MR imaging determination of the location of the normal conus medullaris throughout childhood. *Am J Roentgenol* 152:1029, 1989.

Witkamp TD, Vandertop WP, Beek FJA, et al: Medullary cone movement in subjects with a normal spinal cord and in patients with a tethered spinal cord. *Radiology* 220:208-212, 2001.

Wolpert SM, Bhadelia RA, Bogdan AR, Cohen AR: Chiari I malformations: assessment with phase-contrast velocity MR. *AJNR* 15:1299-1308, 1994.

Zimmerman RA, Bilaniuk LT, Bury EA: Magnetic resonance of the pediatric spine. *Magn Reson Q* 5:169-204, 1989.

# Selected Pictorial Index

The following pages provide an abbreviated pictorial index to the cases in this book. Topics have been chosen to emphasize the various categories of pathology that may cause a particular appearance on MR images. An attempt has been made to minimize repetition of comparisons that are highlighted by "Differential Diagnoses" and/or chapter organization within the text.

The pictorial index is incomplete in several respects. To maintain reasonable image size, each topic is illustrated by a maximum of nine pathologies. Only one example of any specific diagnosis is included on each page. Most importantly, the index is limited to the preceding case collection, which is itself selective.

For these reasons, each page of the index should be viewed as a partial survey rather than as a comprehensive gamut. The cases listed will lead to adjacent cases, neighboring pages, and cross references that more fully discuss the general subject and the individual pathologies.

## CONTENTS

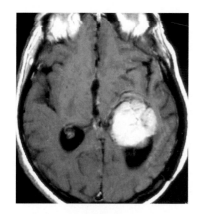

Meningioma
Case 68

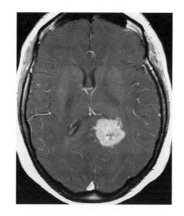

Metastasis
Case 70

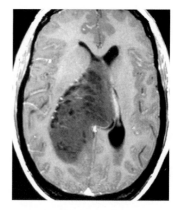

Astrocytoma
Case 109

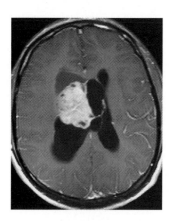

Ependymoma
Case 123

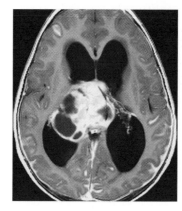

Pineoblastoma
Case 306

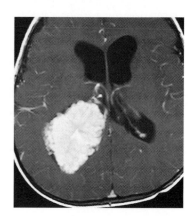

Choroid Plexus Papilloma
Case 330

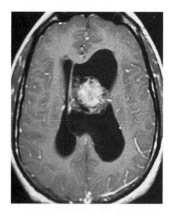

Central Neurocytoma
Case 343

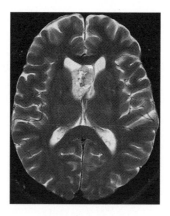

Subependymoma
Case 344

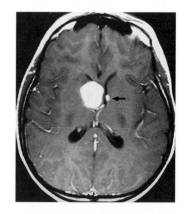

Giant Cell Astrocytoma
Case 897

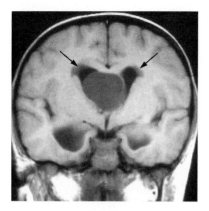

**Cystic Astrocytoma**
**Case 106**

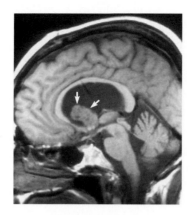

**Subependymoma**
**Case 129**

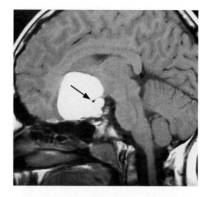

**Craniopharyngioma**
**Case 251**

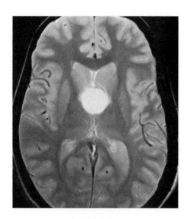

**Colloid Cyst**
**Case 285**

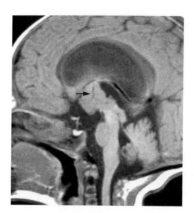

**Choroid Plexus Papilloma**
**Case 334**

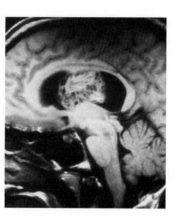

**Central Neurocytoma**
**Case 342**

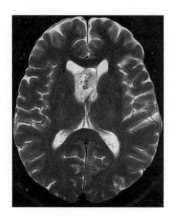

**Subependymoma**
**Case 344**

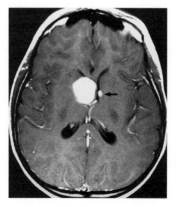

**Giant Cell Astrocytoma**
**Case 897**

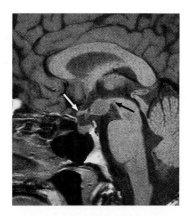

**Hypothalamic Hamartoma**
Case 274

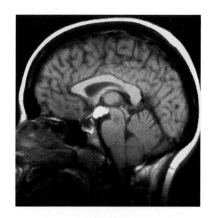

**Lipoma**
Case 276

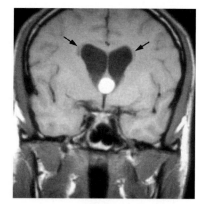

**Colloid Cyst**
Case 282

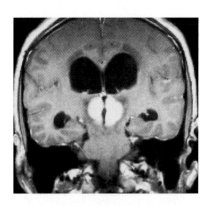

**Germinoma**
Case 301

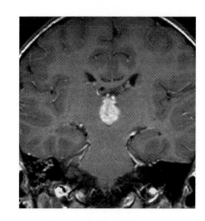

**Pineoblastoma**
Case 307

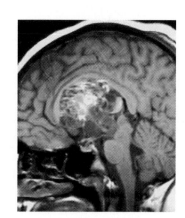

**Teratoma**
Case 309

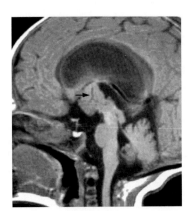

**Choroid Plexus Papilloma**
Case 334

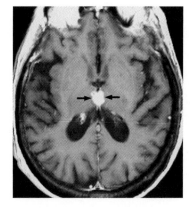

**Primary CNS Lymphoma**
Case 352

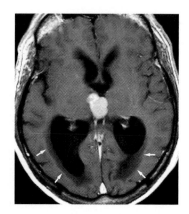

**Metastasis**
Case 353

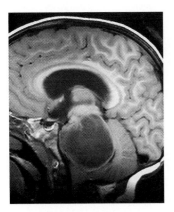

**Brainstem Glioma**
**Case 131**

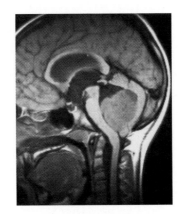

**Medulloblastoma**
**Case 150**

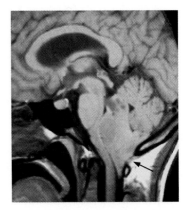

**Ependymoma**
**Case 157**

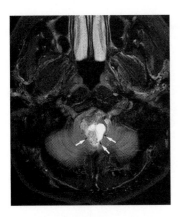

**Hemangioblastoma**
**Case 184**

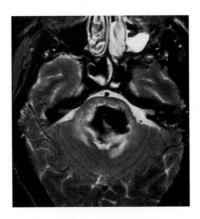

**Pontine Hemorrhage**
**Case 190**

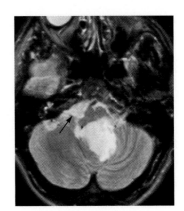

**Epidermoid Cyst**
**Case 327**

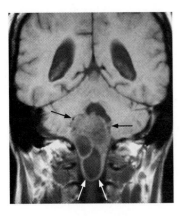

**Choroid Plexus Papilloma**
**Case 335**

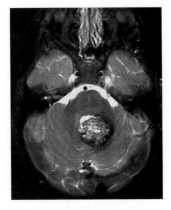

**Cavernous Angioma**
**Case 764**

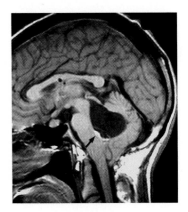

**Cysticercosis**
**Case 807**

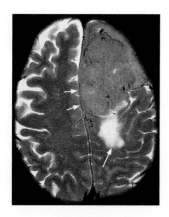

**Meningioma**
**Case 37**

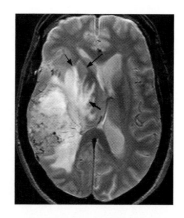

**Glioblastoma Multiforme**
**Case 92**

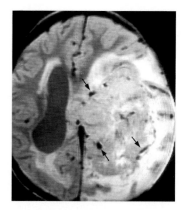

**Malignant Ependymoma**
**Case 124**

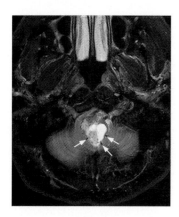

**Hemangioblastoma**
**Case 184**

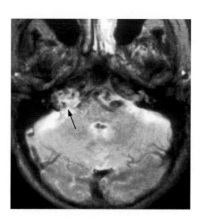

**Glomus Jugulare**
**Case 209**

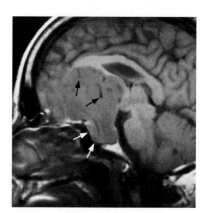

**Pituitary Adenoma**
**Case 235**

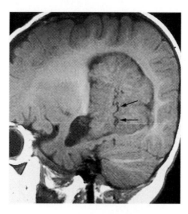

**Choroid Plexus Papilloma**
**Case 328**

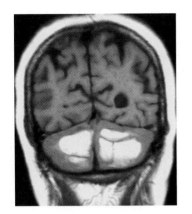

**Metastasis**
**Case 10**

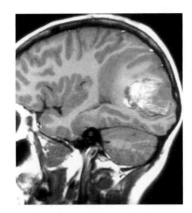

**Glioblastoma Multiforme**
**Case 96**

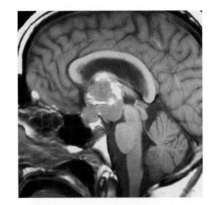

**Germinoma**
**Case 254**

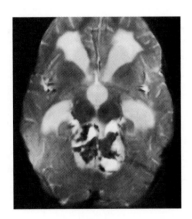

**Teratoma**
**Case 298**

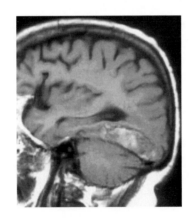

**Subacute Infarct**
**Case 573**

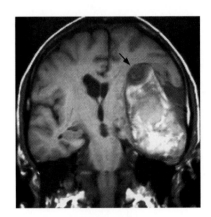

**Thrombosed Aneurysm**
**Case 733**

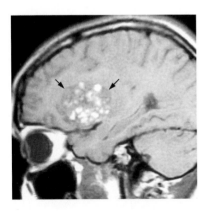

**Thrombosed AVM**
**Case 749**

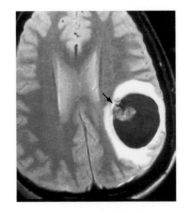

**Cavernous Angioma**
**Case 771**

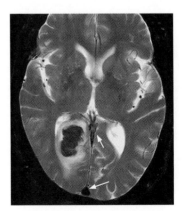

**Dural Sinus Thrombosis**
**Case 783**

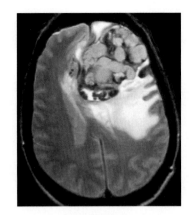

Metastasis
Case 12

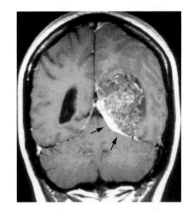

Meningioma
Case 53

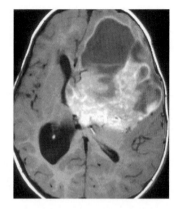

Grade III Astrocytoma
Case 99

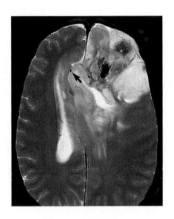

Oligodendroglioma
Case 115

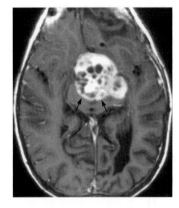

Hypothalamic Glioma
Case 268

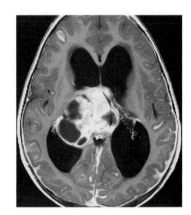

Pineoblastoma
Case 306

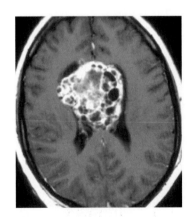

Teratoma
Case 309

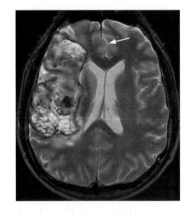

Hemorrhagic Infarct
Case 575

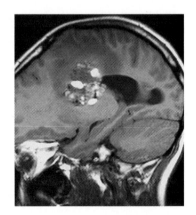

Cavernous Angioma
Case 762

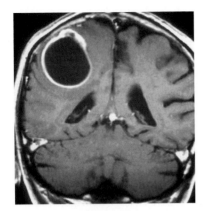

**Metastasis**
**Case 16**

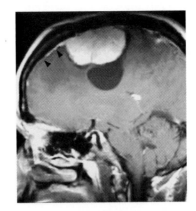

**Meningioma**
**Case 52**

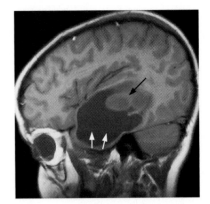

**Grade III Astrocytoma**
**Case 94**

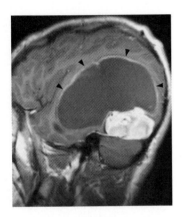

**Pleomorphic Xanthoastrocytoma**
**Case 121**

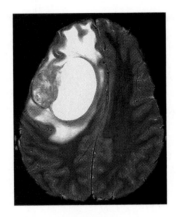

**Ependymoma**
**Case 126**

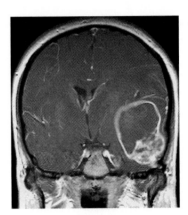

**Ganglioglioma**
**Case 128**

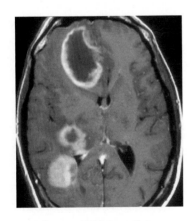

**Primary CNS Lymphoma**
**Case 357**

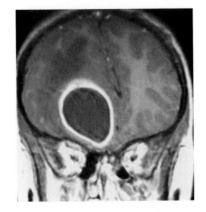

**Abscess**
**Case 465**

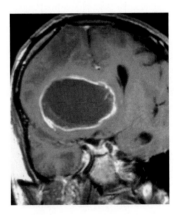

**Glioblastoma Multiforme**
**Case 466**

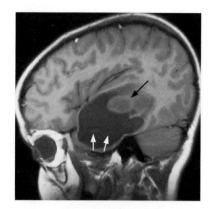

**Grade III Astrocytoma**
**Case 94**

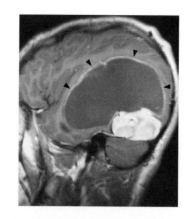

**Pleomorphic Xanthoastrocytoma**
**Case 121**

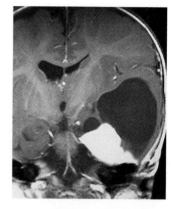

**Desmoplastic Ganglioglioma**
**Case 122**

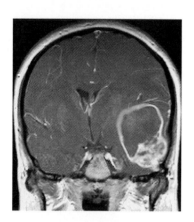

**Ganglioglioma**
**Case 128**

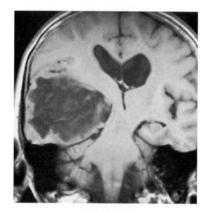

**Dermoid Cyst**
**Case 314**

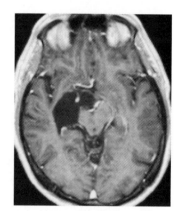

**Epidermoid Cyst**
**Case 321**

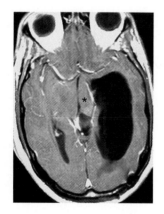

**Trapped Temporal Horn**
**Case 791**

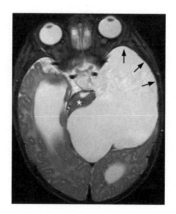

**Arachnoid Cyst**
**Case 814**

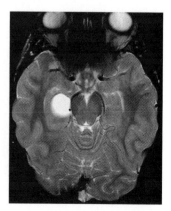

**Choroid Fissure Cyst**
**Case 840**

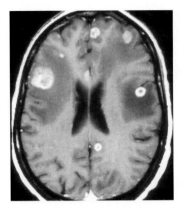

Metastases
Case 15

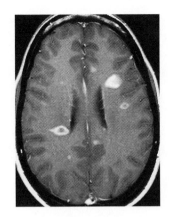

Multiple Sclerosis
Case 382

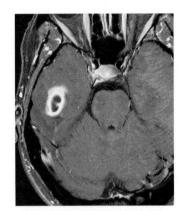

Abscess
Case 467

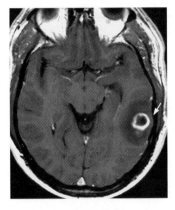

Glioblastoma Multiforme
Case 468

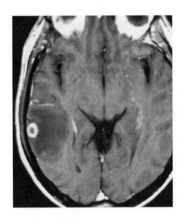

Cysticercosis
Case 469

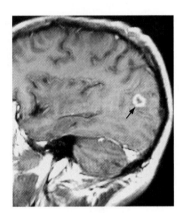

Toxoplasmosis
Case 477

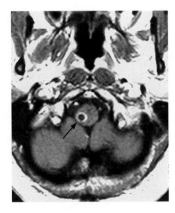

Tuberculosis
Case 478

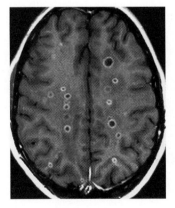

Histoplasmosis
Case 479

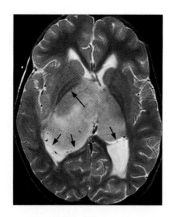

**Thalamic Astrocytoma**
**Case 80**

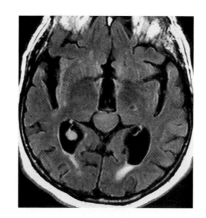

**Pineal Cyst**
**Case 291**

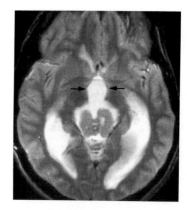

**Germinoma**
**Case 294**

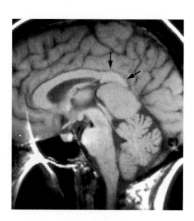

**Meningioma**
**Case 296**

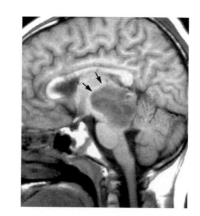

**Pineoblastoma**
**Case 305**

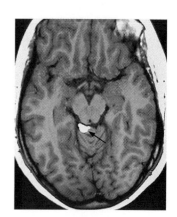

**Lipoma**
**Case 318**

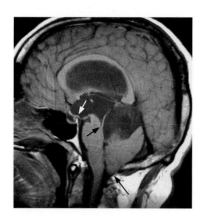

**Epidermoid Cyst**
**Case 326**

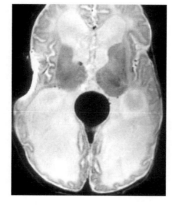

**Vein of Galen Aneurysm**
**Case 747**

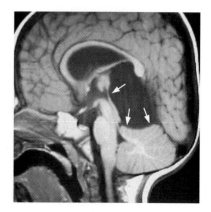

**Arachnoid Cyst**
**Case 818**

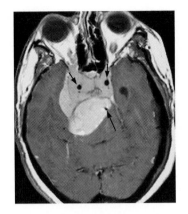

**Meningioma**
**Case 61**

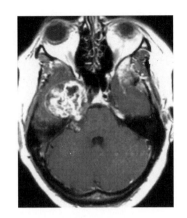

**Trigeminal Schwannoma**
**Case 203**

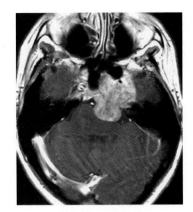

**Chondrosarcoma**
**Case 218**

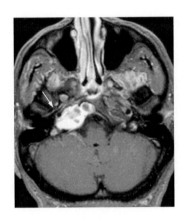

**Chordoma**
**Case 219**

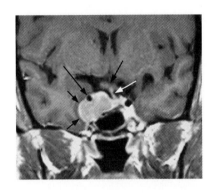

**Pituitary Adenoma**
**Case 233**

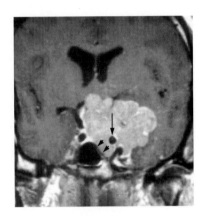

**Craniopharyngioma**
**Case 260**

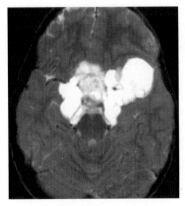

**Hypothalamic Glioma**
**Case 265**

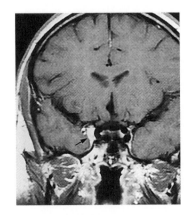

**Tolosa-Hunt Syndrome**
**Case 277**

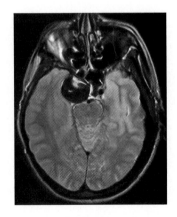

**Aneurysm**
**Case 280**

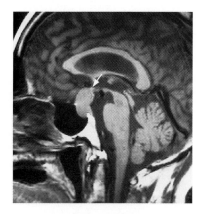

**Pituitary Adenoma**
**Case 224**

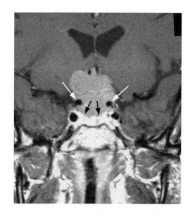

**Meningioma**
**Case 237**

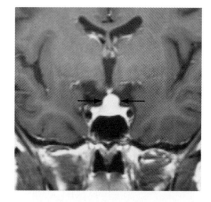

**Pituitary Hyperplasia**
**Case 243**

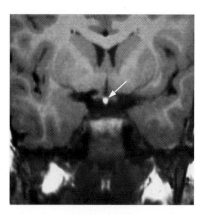

**Ectopic Neurohypophysis**
**Case 247**

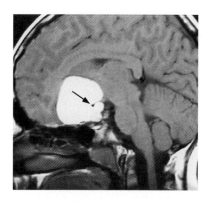

**Craniopharyngioma**
**Case 251**

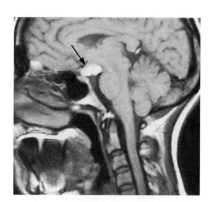

**Rathke's Cleft Cyst**
**Case 256**

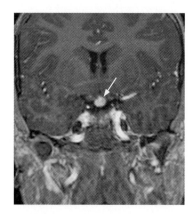

**Langerhans Cell Histiocytosis**
**Case 271**

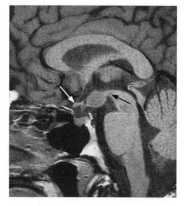

**Hypothalamic Hamartoma**
**Case 274**

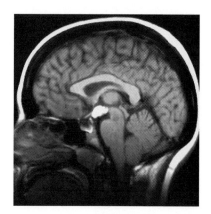

**Lipoma**
**Case 276**

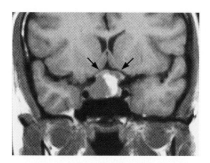

**Pituitary Adenoma**
**Case 228**

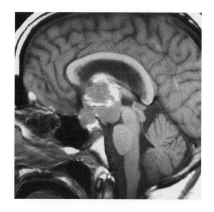

**Germinoma**
**Case 254**

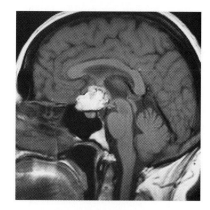

**Dermoid Cyst**
**Case 257**

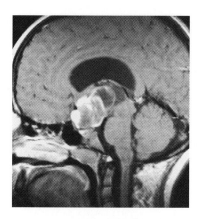

**Hypothalamic Glioma**
**Case 267**

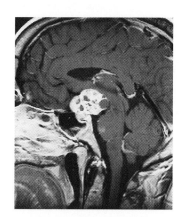

**Craniopharyngioma**
**Case 269**

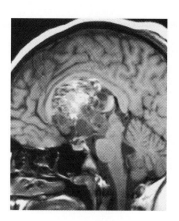

**Teratoma**
**Case 309**

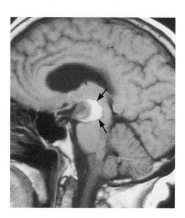

**Aneurysm**
**Case 732**

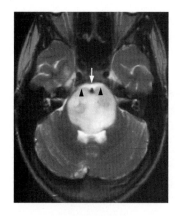

**Astrocytoma**
**Case 133**

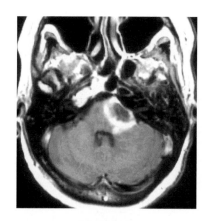

**Metastasis**
**Case 189**

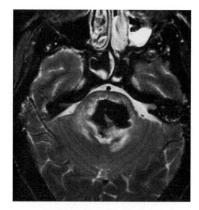

**Pontine Hemorrhage**
**Case 190**

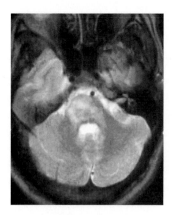

**Multiple Sclerosis**
**Case 379**

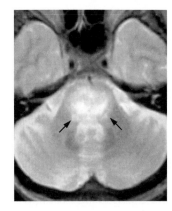

**Central Pontine Myelinolysis**
**Case 406**

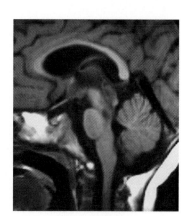

**Leigh Disease**
**Case 501**

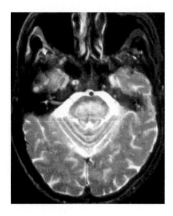

**Ischemic Changes**
**Case 612**

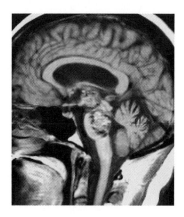

**Cavernous Angioma**
**Case 767**

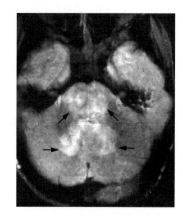

**Neurofibromatosis**
**Case 906**

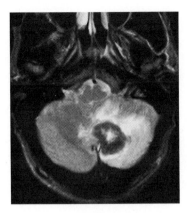

**Metastasis**
**Case 5**

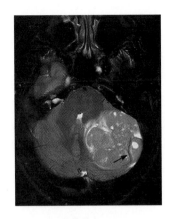

**Medulloblastoma**
**Case 177**

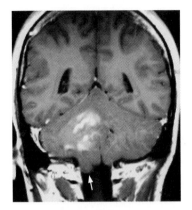

**Astrocytoma**
**Case 181**

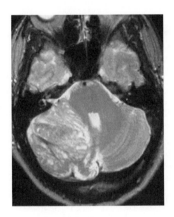

**Lhermitte-Duclos**
**Case 182**

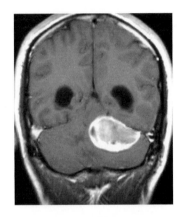

**Hemangioblastoma**
**Case 187**

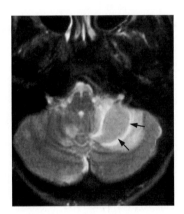

**Primary CNS Lymphoma**
**Case 348**

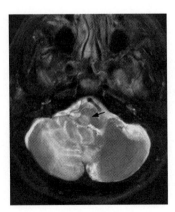

**PICA Infarct**
**Case 620**

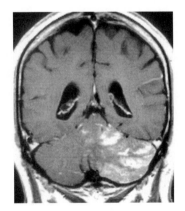

**Dural AVM**
**Case 745**

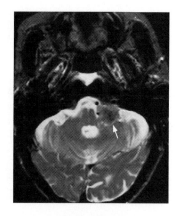

**Meningioma
Case 63**

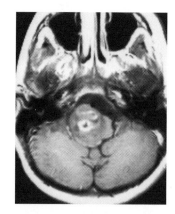

**Exophytic Brainstem Glioma
Case 141**

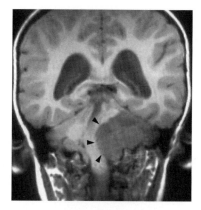

**Ependymoma
Case 162**

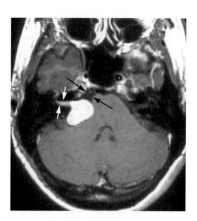

**Acoustic Schwannoma
Case 195**

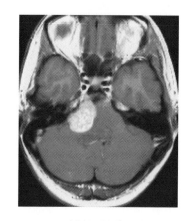

**Metastasis
Case 198**

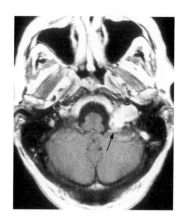

**Glomus Jugulare
Case 211**

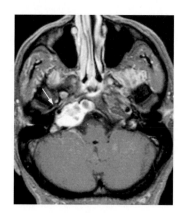

**Chordoma
Case 219**

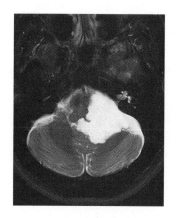

**Epidermoid Cyst
Case 323**

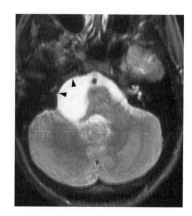

**Arachnoid Cyst
Case 829**

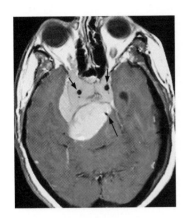

Meningioma
Case 61

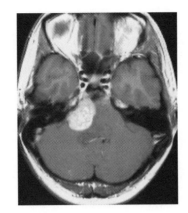

Metastasis
Case 198

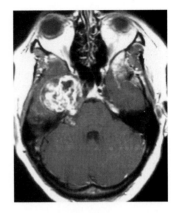

Trigeminal Schwannoma
Case 203

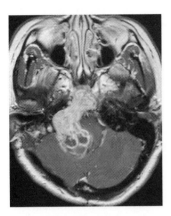

Hypoglossal Schwannoma
Case 204

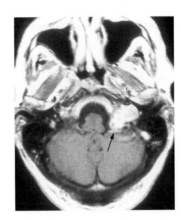

Glomus Jugulare
Case 211

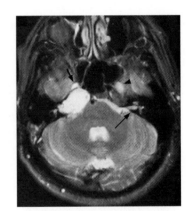

Epidermoid Cyst (Petrous)
Case 215

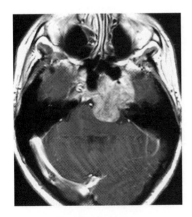

Chondrosarcoma
Case 218

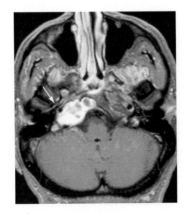

Chordoma
Case 219

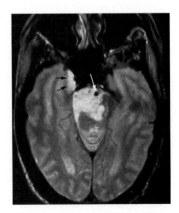

Epidermoid Cyst (Cisternal)
Case 322

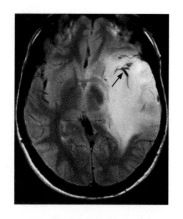

**Grade III Astrocytoma**
**Case 88**

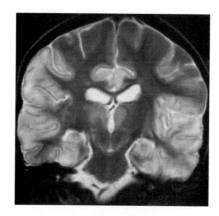

**Viral Meningitis**
**Case 427**

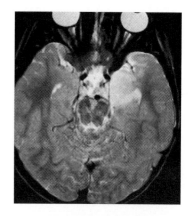

**Herpes Encephalitis**
**Case 445**

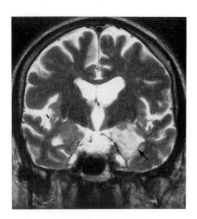

**Limbic Encephalitis**
**Case 446**

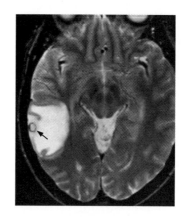

**Cysticercosis**
**Case 469**

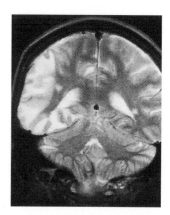

**Systemic Lupus Erythematosus**
**Case 483**

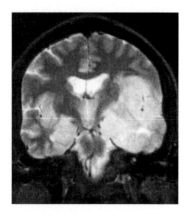

**Gliomatosis Cerebri**
**Case 484**

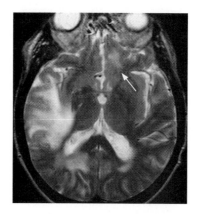

**Primary Angiitis of CNS**
**Case 641**

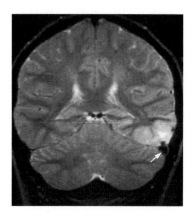

**Transverse Sinus Thrombosis**
**Case 659**

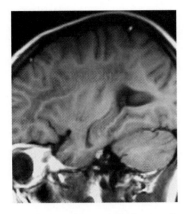

**Metachromatic Leukodystrophy**
**Case 408**

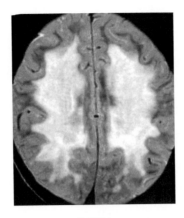

**ADEM**
**Case 409**

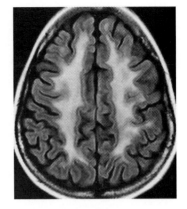

**Chemotherapy Toxicity**
**Case 410**

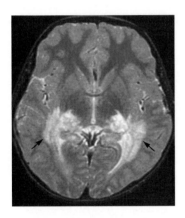

**Adrenoleukodystrophy**
**Case 411**

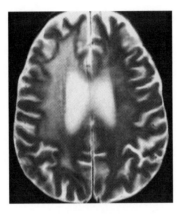

**HIV Encephalitis**
**Case 458**

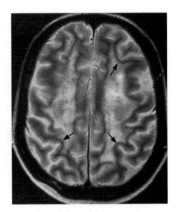

**Radiation Changes**
**Case 548**

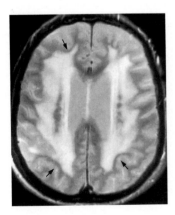

**Aging/Ischemic Changes**
**Case 609**

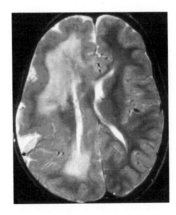

**Unilateral Megalencephaly**
**Case 881**

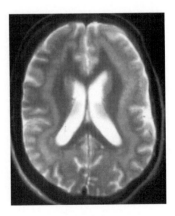

**Band Heterotopia**
**Case 883**

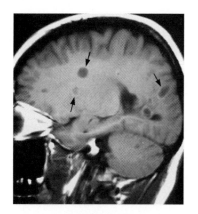

Metastases
Case 1

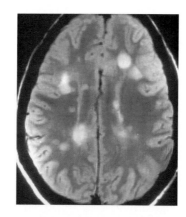

Multiple Sclerosis (Active)
Case 372

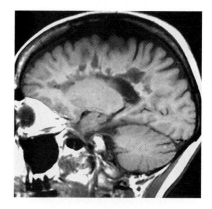

Multiple Sclerosis (Old)
Case 386

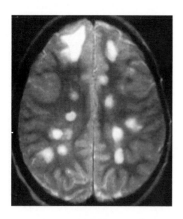

ADEM
Case 392

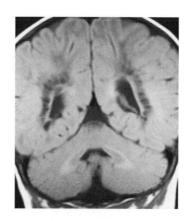

Canavan's Disease
Case 418

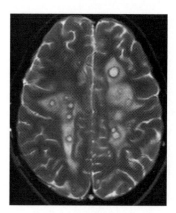

Histoplamosis
Case 470

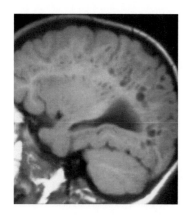

Hurler's Disease
Case 520

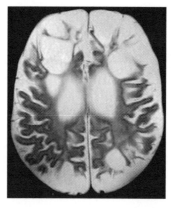

Cystic Encephalomalacia
Case 837

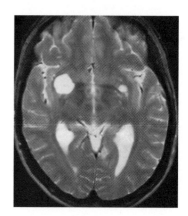

Sublenticular Cysts
Case 838

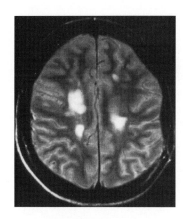

**Multiple Sclerosis**
**Case 371**

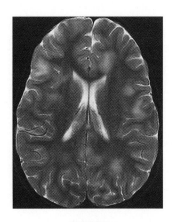

**ADEM**
**Case 391**

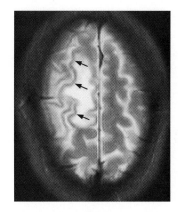

**PML**
**Case 401**

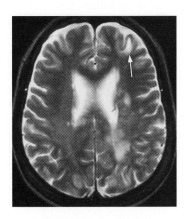

**Sjögren's Syndrome**
**Case 482**

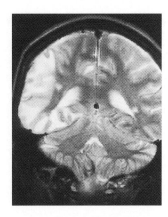

**Systemic Lupus Erythematosus**
**Case 483**

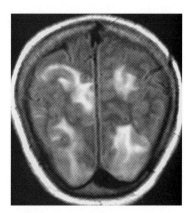

**Hypertensive Encephalopathy**
**Case 545**

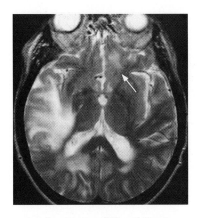

**Primary Angiitis of CNS**
**Case 641**

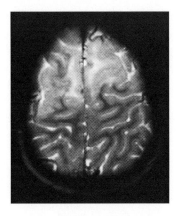

**Dural Sinus Thrombosis**
**Case 649**

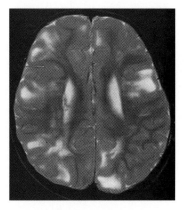

**Tuberous Sclerosis**
**Case 902**

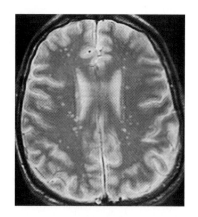

**Metastases**
**Case 19**

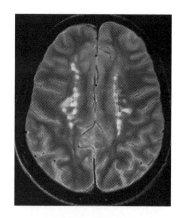

**Multiple Sclerosis**
**Case 360**

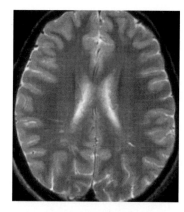

**Perivascular Spaces**
**Case 365**

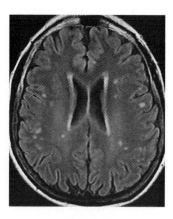

**Lyme Disease**
**Case 493**

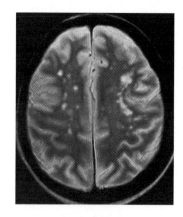

**Sarcoidosis**
**Case 496**

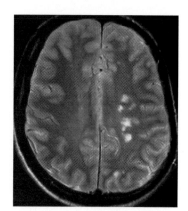

**Border Zone Infarcts**
**Case 591**

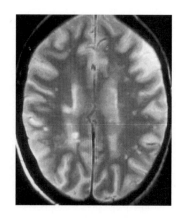

**Small Artery Infarcts**
**Case 606**

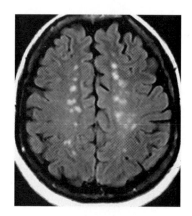

**Vasculitis**
**Case 645**

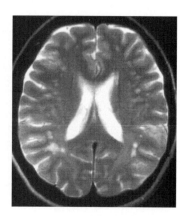

**Diffuse Axonal Injury**
**Case 695**

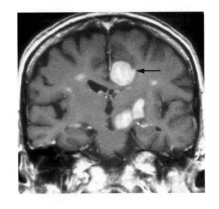

**Metastases**
**Case 15**

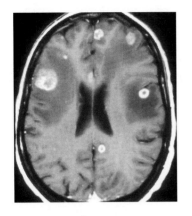


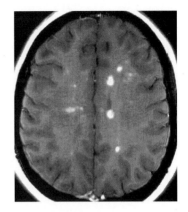

**Primary CNS Lymphoma**
**Case 351**

**Multiple Sclerosis**
**Case 384**

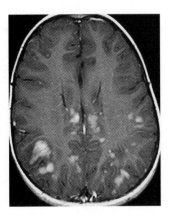

**ADEM**
**Case 397**

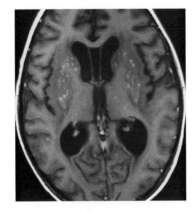

**Bacterial Encephalitis**
**Case 455**

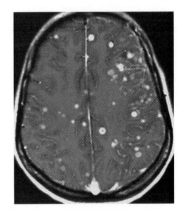

**Tuberculosis**
**Case 472**

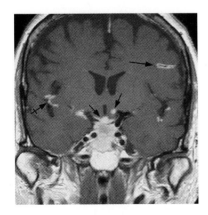

**Sarcoidosis**
**Case 487**

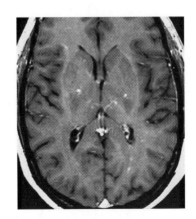

**Lyme Disease**
**Case 494**

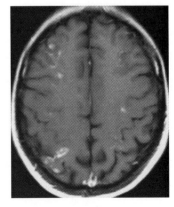

**Border Zone Infarcts**
**Case 587**

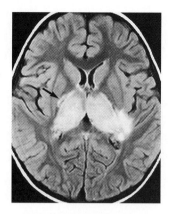

**Bithalamic Astrocytoma**
**Case 79**

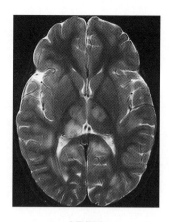

**ADEM**
**Case 394**

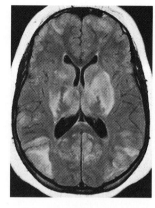

**Systemic Lupus Erythematosus**
**Case 481**

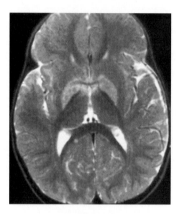

**Leigh Disease**
**Case 506**

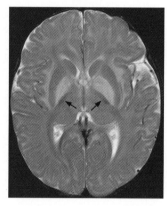

**Maple Syrup Urine Disease**
**Case 507**

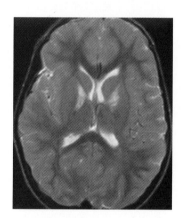

**Adrenoleukodystrophy**
**Case 508**

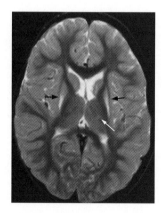

**Old Hypoxic/Ischemic Injury**
**Case 511**

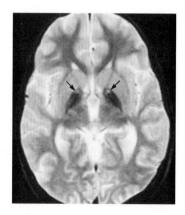

**Hallervorden-Spatz Disease**
**Case 514**

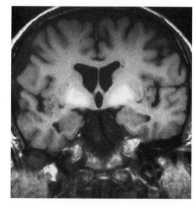

**Hepatocerebral Degeneration**
**Case 517**

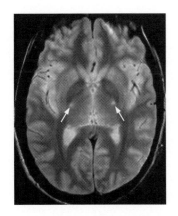

**Amyotrophic Lateral Sclerosis**
Case 528

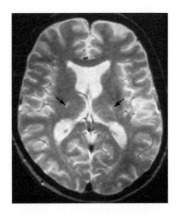

**Extrapontine Myelinolysis**
Case 530

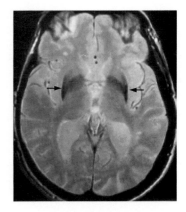

**Parkinson's Disease**
Case 531

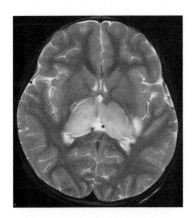

**Deep Venous Thrombosis**
Case 654

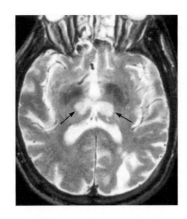

**Basilar Artery Ischemia**
Case 655

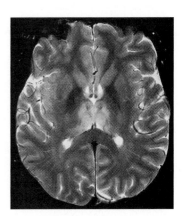

**Viral Encephalitis**
Case 656

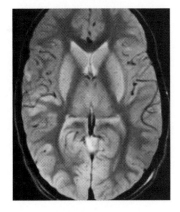

**Anoxia**
Case 665

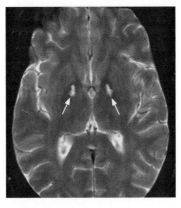

**Carbon Monoxide Poisoning**
Case 672

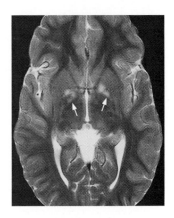

**Neurofibromatosis**
Case 904

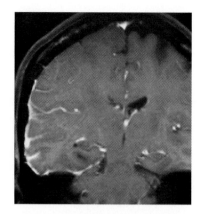

**Meningeal Carcinomatosis**
**Case 29**

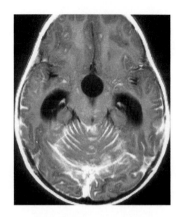

**CSF Tumor Seeding**
**Case 166**

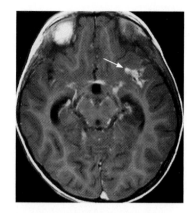

**Tuberculous Meningitis**
**Case 429**

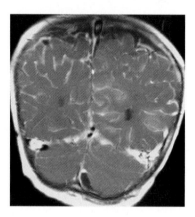

**Bacterial Meningitis**
**Case 430**

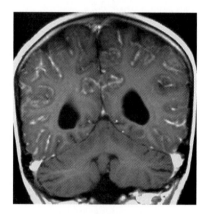

**Leukemia**
**Case 431**

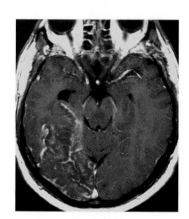

**Acute Infarct**
**Case 578**

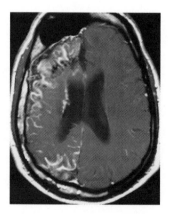

**Sturge-Weber Syndrome**
**Case 910**

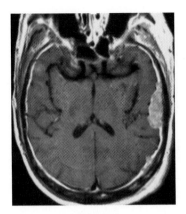

**Metastasis**
**Case 25**

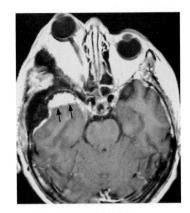

**Meningioma**
**Case 49**

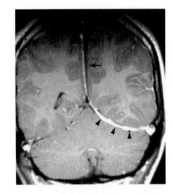

**Subdural Empyema**
**Case 439**

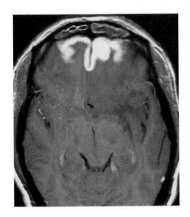

**Sarcoidosis**
**Case 488**

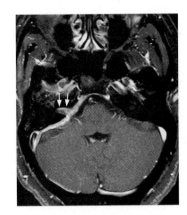

**Systemic Lymphoma**
**Case 492**

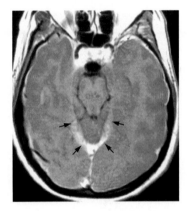

**Intracranial Hypotension**
**Case 540**

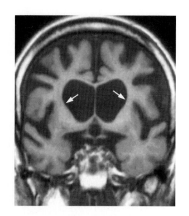

**Huntington's Disease**
Case 533

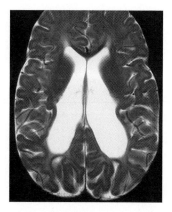

**Periventricular Leukomalacia**
Case 595

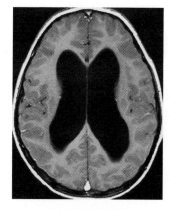

**Hydrocephalus**
Case 784

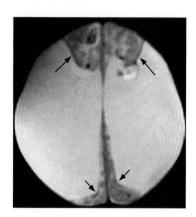

**Hydranencephaly**
Case 789

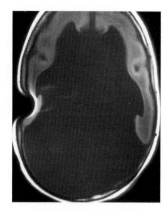

**Holoprosencephaly**
Case 790

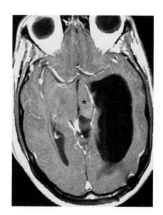

**Trapped Temporal Horn**
Case 791

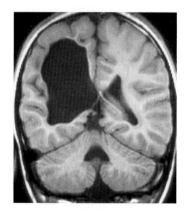

**Porencephaly**
Case 832

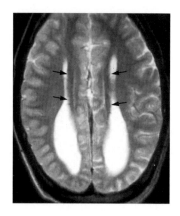

**Colpocephaly**
Case 857

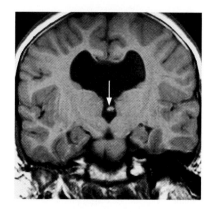

**Septo-Optic Dysplasia**
Case 864

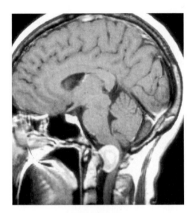

**Meningioma**
**Case 64**

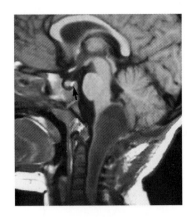

**Astrocytoma**
**Case 138**

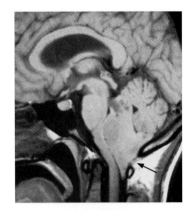

**Ependymoma**
**Case 157**

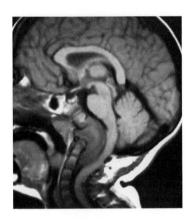

**Chordoma**
**Case 168**

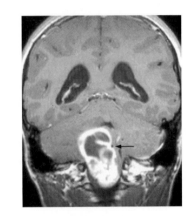

**Hemangioblastoma**
**Case 186**

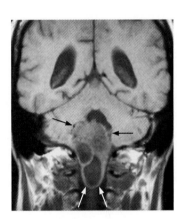

**Choroid Plexus Papilloma**
**Case 335**

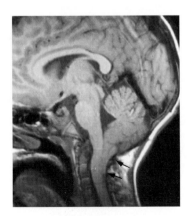

**Chiari Malformation**
**Case 848**

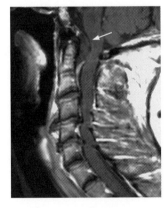

**Fibrous Pseudotumor**
**Case 1041**

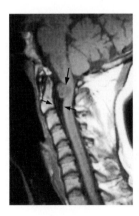

**Schwannoma**
**Case 1054**

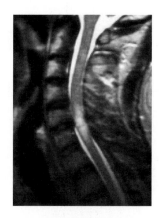

**Astrocytoma**
**Case 1075**

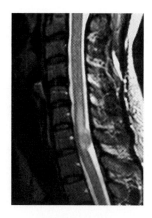

**Ependymoma**
**Case 1088**

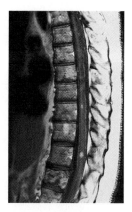

**Metastases**
**Case 1106**

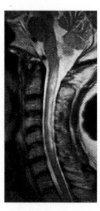

**Multiple Sclerosis**
**Case 1136**

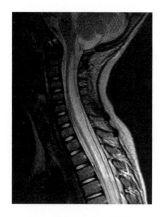

**Transverse Myelitis**
**Case 1138**

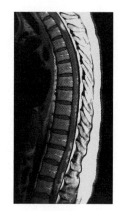

**Sarcoidosis**
**Case 1144**

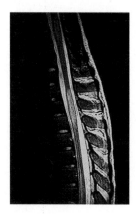

**Systemic Lupus Erythematosus**
**Case 1149**

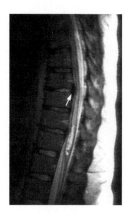

**Spinal Cord Infarct**
**Case 1206**

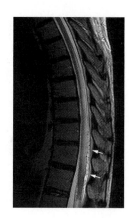

**Dural AV Fistula**
**Case 1209**

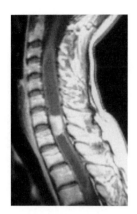

**Ependymoma**
**Case 1085**

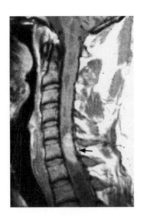

**Hemangioblastoma**
**Case 1100**

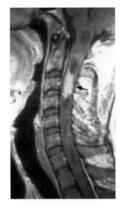

**Astrocytoma**
**Case 1102**

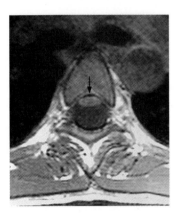

**Spinal Cord Herniation**
**Case 1194**

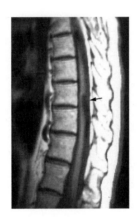

**Arachnoid Cyst**
**Case 1195**

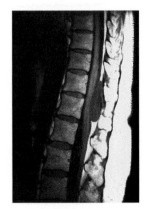

**Meningeal Cyst**
**Case 1197**

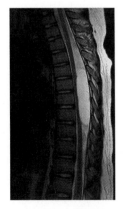

**Neuroepithelial Cyst**
**Case 1199**

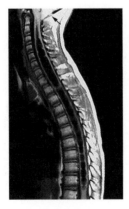

**Syringomyelia**
**Case 1228**

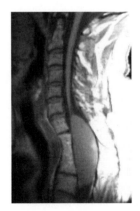

**Neurenteric Cyst**
**Case 1266**

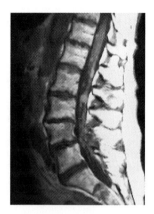

**Systemic Metastases**
**Case 1046**

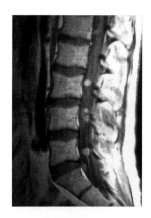

**Drop Metastases**
**Case 1047**

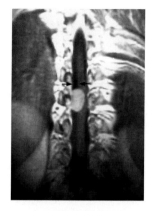

**Meningioma**
**Case 1052**

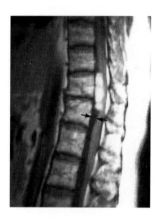

**Schwannoma**
**Case 1067**

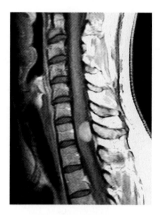

**Exophytic Ependymoma**
**Case 1090**

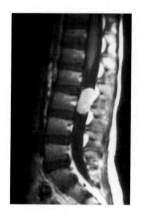

**Ependymoma of the Filum**
**Case 1095**

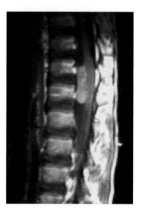

**PNET**
**Case 1098**

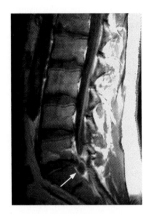

**Disc Compression**
**Case 946**

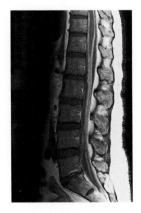

**Bacterial Meningitis**
**Case 1049**

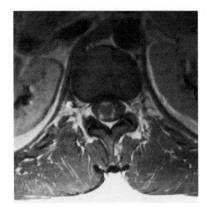

**CMV Radiculitis**
**Case 1148**

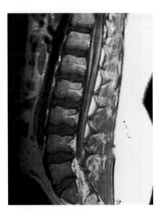

**Guillain-Barré Syndrome**
**Case 1151**

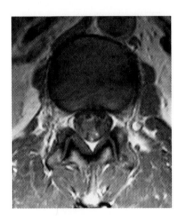

**AV Fistula**
**Case 1216**

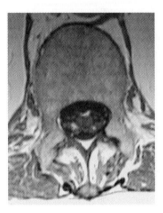

**Leptomeningeal Metastases**
**Case 1217**

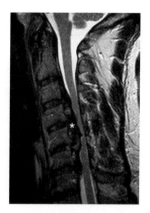

**OPLL**
**Case 989**

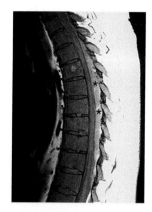

**Extramedullary Hematopoiesis**
**Case 1006**

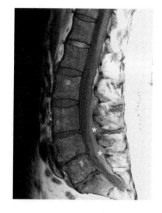

**Lymphoma**
**Case 1014**

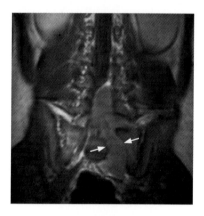

**Neuroblastoma**
**Case 1021**

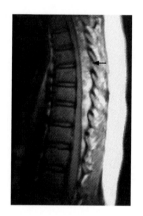

**Epidural Abscess**
**Case 1124**

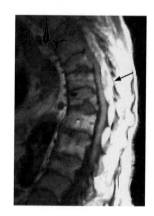

**Epidural Hematoma**
**Case 1187**

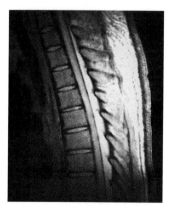

**Epidural Lipomatosis**
**Case 1192**

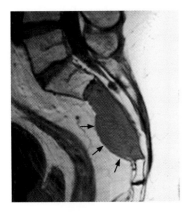

**Plasmacytoma**
**Case 1011**

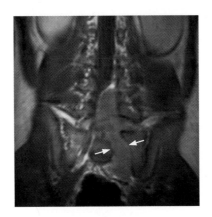

**Neuroblastoma**
**Case 1021**

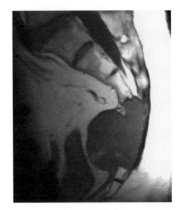

**Chordoma**
**Case 1028**

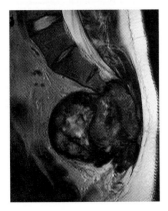

**Giant Cell Tumor**
**Case 1030**

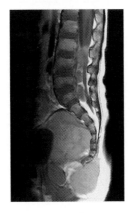

**Sacrococcygeal Teratoma**
**Case 1032**

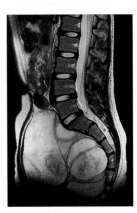

**Ganglioneuroma**
**Case 1034**

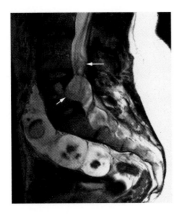

**Plexiform Neurofibroma**
**Case 1071**

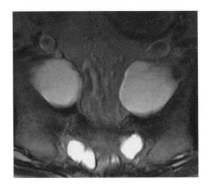

**Perineural Cysts**
**Case 1204**

Annulus fibrosus
  disruption of, 568-569
Anoxia
  cerebral, 406, 408-409
  cerebral atrophy from, 330
  hypoxic/ischemic injuries and, 318
  neonatal, 407
Anterior cerebral artery distribution infarction, 351, 360
Anterior clinoid process
  pneumatized, 447
Antiphospholipid antibody syndrome, 394
  versus cerebral vasculitis, 396
Antoni "B" zones, 651
Aortic aneurysms
  spinal cord infarction and, 738-739
Apical petrous air cell
  abscess within, 134
Aqueductal obstruction, hydrocephalus due to, 493
Aqueductal stenosis, 492
  benign, 85, 487
  congenital hydrocephalus from, 522
  hydrocephalus due to, 482
  third ventriculostomy and, 489
Arachnoid cyst(s)
  of cerebellopontine angle, 506-507
  complex, 499
  convexity of, 496
  epidermoid cysts versus, 501, 506-507
  extradural, 733
  invaginating, 497
  large cisterna magna versus, 503
  of middle cranial fossa, 498
  of posterior fossa
    mimicking Dandy-Walker malformations, 494
  of quadrigeminal cistern, 184-185, 501
  suprasellar, 487, 500
Arachnoiditis
  cauda equina syndrome and, 585
  clumping of intrathecal nerve roots from, 709
  due to subarachnoid hemorrhages, 732
  focal enhancement of nerve roots from, 579
  lymphomatous meningitis versus, 707
  thickened nerve roots from, 645
  T1-weighted images of, 706
  T2-weighted images of, 708
Artery(ies)
  basilar, 136
    aneurysm of, 450
    dolichoectasia of, 476
    emboli, occlusion of, 403
    exophytic tumor surrounding, 82
    stenosis of, 389
    thrombosis of, 388
  dissection, 390-391
  internal carotid, 389, 390, 391

Artery(ies)—cont'd
  posterior inferior cerebellar, 382, 383, 385
    abberrant, 475
  superior cerebellar, 386, 387
  tortuous, 474, 475
Arteriovenous malformation, 454-456
  dural, 457
  large vascular channels, 455
  occult intradural, 745
  radiculomedullary fistulae as, 740
    spinal cord atrophy and, 757
Arteriovenous shunts, 458
Arthritis, rheumatoid, 710-711
Aspergillosis, 26
Aspergillus, 290
Astrocytoma(s)
  associated with intramedullary cysts, 675
  with calcified cerebral mass, 70
  conus medullaris, 673
  cystic cerebellar, 88-90
  diffuse, 114
  exophytic, 82
  fibrillary, 82
  low grade, 46-50, 277, 349, 405
  mimicking colloid cysts, 182
  multiple sclerosis versus, 695
  pilocytic, 82
    enhancement characteristics of, 84
  sarcoidosis versus, 699
  spinal, 660-663
  subependymal giant cell, 77
Atlantoaxial subluxation
  in Down syndrome, 781
  in rheumatoid arthritis, 710-711
Atypical meningioma, 32
Atypical teratoid/rhabdoid tumor, 194
Atypical teratoma, 195
Auditory canal, internal; see Internal auditory canal
Axonal injury
  callosal lesions from, 424-425

**B**

Band heterotopia, 539
Basal arteries
  encasement of, 149
Basal ganglia
  gelatinous pseudocysts within, 511
  miliary enhancement in, 282
  primary CNS lymphoma and, 214
  signal abnormality
    with Leigh disease, 314
  symmetrical lesions
    in children, 315
Basilar arteries, 136
  bilateral anterior exophytic extension surrounding, 82
  stenosis of, 389

Craniopharyngioma(s)
contrast enhancement, 162
mimicking dermoid cyst, 196
near foramen of Monro, 183
of the skull base, 104
T1-weighted images of, 158
T2-weighted images of, 159
Cyst(s)
aneurysmal bone, 621, 637
arachnoid, 496, 706-709
in Canavan's disease, 256
care in labeling masses as, 58
cerebellar masses, 505
of choroid fissure, 512
in dysembryoplastic neuroepithelial tumors, 76, 211
convexity arachnoid, 509
of cysticercosis, 289, 495
dermoid, 161, 196-197, 559
in desmoplastic infantile gangliogliomas in, 73
dorsal interhemispheric, 525
with holoprosencephaly, 485
midline, 529
epidural dermoid, 558
extensive intramedullary, 758
focal deforming spinal cord, 735
of fourth ventricle, 207, 495
hematic, 419
in high and low grade glioma, 58
hypothalamic, 165
interhemispheric, 485, 525, 529
localized with syringomyelia, 758
midline developmental, 515
in mucopolysaccharidoses, 322
nasal dermal sinus and, 557
neurenteric, 676, 735, 776
neuroepithelial, 514, 734, 735
neurenteric and, 735
in oligodendroglioma, 68-69
pineal, 184-185
in pleomorphic xanthoastrocytomas, 72
porencephalic, 508
posterior fossa
Dandy-Walker malformations *versus,* 494
rapidly-growing brain, 514
Rathke's cleft, 161
of sacral canal, 627, 736
in schwannoma, 120-122
small developmental, 511
solitary multinodular, 777
spinal arachnoid, 732
spinal astrocytomas and, 662
spinal neuroepithelial, 734
sublenticular, 511
suprasellar dermoid, 171

Cyst(s)—cont'd
synovial, 594, 595, 654, 729
within teratomas, 194
typical for ependymomas, 747
of velum interpositum, 515
within white matter, 290
Cysticercosis, 289
near foramen of Monro, 183
cerebral, 290
intraventricular, 495
with multiple enhancing nodules, 237
racemose cysts of, 507
resembling epidermoid cyst, 203
within temporal horn, 325
tentorial thickening in, 274
Cytomegalovirus
focal enhancement of nerve roots from, 579
intrauterine encephalitis from, 270
myelitis, 702
with nodular enhancement
of intrathecal nerve roots, 744
ventriculitis, 720
Cytotoxic edema
with acute infarction, 385
with carbon monoxide poisoning, 411

**D**

Dandy-Walker malformation, 494, 504
Deep venous thrombosis, 402
Demyelinating disease; *see* Multiple sclerosis
Dermoid cyst(s), 196-197, 514, 559
epidural, 558
Rathke's cleft cysts *versus,* 161
resembling epidermoid cyst, 197
rupture of, 198
within sella turcia, 157
signal intensity of, 558
spinal, 774
suprasellar, 171
Desmoplastic infantile ganglioglioma, 73
Developmental abnormalities, 520-559
Diabetes insipidus
Langerhans cell histiocytosis and, 168-169
suprasellar germinomas and, 160, 195
Diabetes mellitus
scattered white matter infarcts with, 373
spinal cord infarction with, 739
Dialysis spondyloarthropathy, 684
Diastematomyelia, 770-773
with rigid septum, 770
without rigid septum, 771
Diastematomyelia hemicords, 773
Diencephalic gliomas, 187
Diffuse axonal injury, 424-426
Diffuse necrotizing leukoencephalopathy, 251, 258

## K

Kernicterus, 314, 408

Kyphosis, idiopathic, 605

## L

Lacunar infarcts, 227, 371

Laminar erosions in ankylosing spondylitis, 713

Laminar necrosis, 477

Langerhans cell histiocytosis, 105, 168, 169

  dural thickening and, 301

  vertebral, 636, 637

Lateral stenosis

  cervical, 603

  lumbar, 591

Leigh disease, 312

  brainstem lesions, 312-313

  deep nuclear lesions, 314

Lenticulostriate arteries, infarction involving, 370

Lentiform nuclei

  in Leigh disease, 314

  in Maple syrup urine disease, 315

  in Parkinson's disease, 328

Leptomeningeal carcinomatosis, 16, 17, 101, 645

Leptomeningeal enhancement, 17, 269, 553

Leptomeningeal involvement

  by CSF-borne tumor, 66, 100, 101

Leptomeningeal metastases, 11, 387, 644

  versus bacterial meningitis, 647

Leukemia

  abnormal vertebral signal intensity with, 619

    epidural disease with, 15, 626

    leptomeningeal infiltration by, 128

    skull base lesions, 105

    tentorial thickening with, 274

    vertebral body collapse with, 636

Leukodystrophy, metachromatic, 250

Leukoencephalopathy

  in carbon monoxide poisoning, 259

  ischemic, 374

  progressive multifocal, 244-246

  radiation, 338

  toxic, 259

Leukomalacia, periventricular, 366

Lhermitte-Duclos disease, 115

  mimicking hemispheric medulloblastoma, 95

Limbic encephalitis, 277

Lipoma(s)

  of corpus callosum, 526

  dorsal thoracic, 768

  intraspinal, 768-769

  suprasellar, 161

  with tethered cord, 760

  intracranial, 199

  spinal canal, 764-766

  with split cord malformations, 771

Lipomatosis, epidural, 727, 730

Lipomatous infiltration

  of filum terminale, 767

Lipomeningocele, 764

Lipomyelomeningocele, occult, 764

Lissencephaly, 532-533

Listeria rhombencephalitis, 119

Lumbar, lateral recess, stenosis of, 590

Lumbosacral neuroblastoma, 627

Lupus anticoagulant, 394

Lupus cerebritis; *see* Systemic lupus erythematosus

Lupus erythematosus, systemic; *see* Systemic lupus
  erythematosus

Lyme disease, 302

  cranial neuritis with, 304

  mimicking meningeal leukemia, 128

  mimicking multiple sclerosis, 397

  sarcoidosis *versus,* 303

  with thickening tentorial, 274

Lymphocytic (adeno)hypophysitis, 154, 168

Lymphoma, primary CNS; *see* Primary CNS lymphoma

Lymphoma, sytemic

  calvarial metastasis, 13

  causing dural thickening, 301

  epidural masses from, 15, 626

  causing meningeal carcinomatosis, 16

  causing parasellar mass, 173

  skull base lesions and, 105

  as small blue cell tumors, 628-629

  spinal, 624

  causing subependymal enhancement, 271

  tentorial thickening with, 274

Lymphomatous meningitis, 707

## M

Machiafava Bignami syndrome, 63

Malformations of cortical development; *see* Neuronal
  migration disorders

Malignant ependymoma, 74

Malignant gliomas; *see* Gliomas, Anaplastic astrocytomas,
  and Glioblastoma multiforme

Maple syrup urine disease, 315

Marfan's syndrome, 390, 453, 737

  dural diverticulae and, 585

Maroteaux-Lamy syndrome, 322

Marrow, vertebral

  changes with disc degeneration, 566

  edema from discitis, 682-684

  replacement by tumor, 616, 685

Medulla

  gliomas of, 86, 87, 99

  infarcts, 383

Medullary infarcts, 383

Medulloblastoma(s)

  contrast enhancement of, 94, 114

  CSF seeding in, 101

Middle cerebral artery
  aneurysm of, 446
  infarction in distribution of, 352
  thrombosed aneurysm of, 450
Middle cranial fossa
  arachnoid cysts of, 498
Migration lines of tuberous sclerosis, 547
Mitochondrial encephalomyopathy(ies), 317
Morquio's disease, 322
Moyamoya disease, 393
  collateral hypertrophy with, 393, 456
Mucocele, within apical petrous air cell, 134
Mucopolysaccharidoses, 322
  megalencephaly and, 491
Multicentric gliomas, 67
Multiple myeloma, 620, 621; *see also* Plasmacytoma
  extending between vertebral bodies, 685
Multiple sclerosis, 224-238
  *versus* astrocytoma, 695
  axonal injuries *versus,* 427
  brainstem involvement, 119, 234
  *versus* cavernous angiomas, 748
  chronic, 239
  contrast enhancement of, 236
  corpus callosum involvement in, 63, 228
  FLAIR images of, 226
  focally enhancing lesions, 473
  giant plaques as mass lesions, 233
  intramedullary enhancement, 699, 701
  large peripheral lesions, 230
  mimicking gliomas
    in young adults, 83
  *versus* multiple infarcts, 397
  myelitis from, 694, 697-699
    with multifocal lesions, 696
  nondeforming periventricular lesions, 229
  ring lesions, 232
  with ring-enhancing lesions, 295
  spinal cord atrophy, 757
  T1-weighted images of, 224
  T2-weighted images of, 225
Myelitis
  in AIDS, 702
  due to multiple sclerosis, 697-698
    focal lesions, 694
    multifocal lesions, 696
  due to sarcoidosis, 700
  transverse, 697
Myelocystocele, 758
Myelofibrosis
  abnormal vertebral signal intensity with, 619
  extramedullary hematopoiesis in, 619
Myelomalacia
  from acute spinal cord injuries, 723
  with spinal cord herniation, 731

Myeloma, multiple, 619, 620, 637
Myelomeningocele, 763
  with Chiari II malformations, 521-522
  dorsal tethering after repair, 763
  subcutaneous, 761
  with tethered spinal cord, 761-762
  thoracolumbar, 772
Myelopathy
  accompanying edema and swelling
    of conus medullaris, 742
  from adrenomyeloneuropathy, 255
  from arteriovenous malformations, 740
  progressive with transverse myelitis, 697
  from vertebral hemangiomas, 614
Myoblastoma (choristomas), 155
Myxopapillary ependymoma, 670-672

## N

Nasoethmoidal encephalocele, 556
Nasopharyngeal carcinoma, 139
Nerve root(s)
  adhesions, 706
  compression, due to spondylolisthesis, 593
  cysts of sleeve, 652
  dural diverticulae and, 585
  enhancement of, 579, 647, 705
  far lateral compression of, 576
  lumbar, compression of, 591
  redundant, 741
  thickened, 644, 645, 707
  tumors of, 657, 658
Neurenteric cyst, 507, 676, 776
Neuritis, cranial, 304
  differential diagnosis, 128
  due to herpes, 126
  due to Lyme disease, 304
Neuroblastoma
  epidural, 626
  lumbosacral, 627
  olfactory, 149, 209
Neurocytomas, central, 212
Neuroepithelial cyst, 514, 734, 735
Neurofibromas, 657-658
  extraspinal, 655
  plexiform, 658-659
  *versus* schwannoma, 657
  spinal, 657
Neurofibromatosis
  dural diverticulae and, 585
  ganglionic signal abnormality, 550
  posterior fossa, signal abnormalities, 551
  paraspinal masses with, 655
  type 1, 550, 551, 658
  type 2, 35, 39, 129
Neurohypophysis, 86; *see also* "Bright spot" pituitary

Wegener's granulomatosis
    dural thickening with, 14, 301
    inflamed cerebral vessels with, 396
    mimicking Tolosa-Hunt syndrome, 172
Wernicke's encephalopathy, 320
    producing bilateral thalamic lesions, 403
White matter
    aging, 374
    causes of symmetrical abnormalities, 258-259
    cysts within, 290
    diffusely abnormal in children, 251
    disorders of, 224-259
    "heart of the gyrus" edema, 245
    infarcts, 372, 373
    loss of with periventricular leukomalacia, 366

White matter—cont'd
    multifocal ischemia within, 372
    multiple round masses in, 231, 241
    multiple sclerosis and, 226, 230, 231
    PML effect on, 245
    primary CNS lymphoma and, 214
    radiation effects on, 338
    subcortical signal abnormality, 303
Wilson's disease
    with basal ganglia lesions, 321
    producing bilateral thalamic lesions, 403

## X

Xanthoastrocytoma, pleomorphic, 72